PHARMACOLOGY FOR HEALTH PROFESSIONALS

PHARMACOLOGY FOR HEALTH PROFESSIONALS

EVELYN SALERNO, RPh, BS, PharmD, FASCP

Courtesy Professor
School of Nursing
Florida International University
Clinical Assistant Professor
Nova-Southeastern College of Pharmacy
Miami, Florida

www.mosby.com

Mosby
An Imprint of Elsevier Science
St. Louis London Philadelphia Sydney Toronto

Mosby
An Imprint of Elsevier Science

Editor-in-Chief: Sally Schrefer
Acquisitions Editor: Jeanne Allison
Developmental Editor: Kristin Geen
Project Manager: Dana Peick
Senior Production Editor: Jeffrey Patterson
Manufacturing Manager: Karen Boehme
Designer: Pati Pye

A NOTE TO THE READER:
The author and publisher have made every attempt to check dosages and nursing content for accuracy. Because the science of pharmacology is continually advancing, our knowledge base continues to expand. Therefore we recommend that the reader always check product information for changes in dosage or administration before administering any medication. This is particularly important with new or rarely used drugs.

Printed in the United States of America
Composition by Clarinda
Printing by World Color

Mosby, Inc.
11830 Westline Industrial Drive
St. Louis, Missouri 63146

ISBN 0-8151-2711-1
31383

01 / 9 8 7 6 5 4 3 2

PREFACE

Pharmacology for Health Professionals by Evelyn Salerno, PharmD, is a unique textbook combining clearly-written, comprehensive pharmacology content with student-friendly pedagogy and features. The special features and consistent chapter pedagogy help the student focus on key content and therefore use the book more effectively as a learning tool.

This text will serve students not only throughout their pharmacology course but also as a valuable reference for their career as a health care provider. Following is a brief description of the text's organization, features, and ancillaries.

ORGANIZATION

Text Organization

Chapters 1 to 6 discuss pharmacology basics and issues important in today's health care settings, including legal foundations, over-the-counter and alternative medications, principles of drug action, life span aspects of drug therapy, and substance misuse and abuse. Chapters 7 to 65 discuss drugs classified by body system and drug function. The body system format facilitates easy access to this challenging content.

Chapter Format

- **Chapter Overviews, Objectives,** and **Key Terms** appear at the beginning of each chapter to help students focus and mentally organize content.
- **Chapter Summaries** and **Review Questions** appear at the end of each chapter to help students master material in manageable sections.
- **The Key Drug approach** helps students assimilate this challenging content. Key drugs are listed in chapter openers and highlighted with an icon ( ) throughout the chapter for quick reference.
- **Discussions of drug groups *and* individual drugs** provide students with the most thorough and comprehensive information available.
- **Drug reference tables** are utilized to make information more accessible and facilitate the text's utility as a reference.

FEATURES

This solid content is enhanced with the following special features:

- **Management of Drug Overdose boxes** alert the student to important information and guidelines regarding overdoses for specific medications.
- **Pregnancy Safety boxes** provide FDA pregnancy classifications.
- **Geriatric and Pediatric Implications boxes** stress important lifespan content.
- **Serious drug interactions are highlighted** to emphasize the interactions that the health care professional must take special care to prevent.
- **Over 100 illustrations** help explain how drugs work in the body and help define other pharmacologic principles.
- **Drug name pronunciations** precede the discussion of each drug.
- **Key Terms** are bold-faced and listed in chapter openers to emphasize essential terminology.
- **The Disorders index** features alphabetical reference to disorders, conditions, and diseases in the text for easier access.

ANCILLARIES

The ancillaries for *Pharmacology for Health Care Professionals* have been carefully prepared to aid the instructor as well as promote student learning.

Instructor's Resource Manual: This manual includes teaching objectives, chapter focus, key terms, case studies, lecture strategies, chapter outlines, and review questions for each chapter.

Mosby's Pharmacology Update: This e-mail newsletter written by Evelyn Salerno is provided 4 times each year.

Mosby's Electronic Image Collection for Pharmacology: This innovative CD-ROM product contains 150 full-color pharmacology images that can be imported into PowerPoint for use in lectures.

Mosby's PowerPoint Lecture Outlines: Available via the Mosby website, these presentations are organized by body system to cover principles of pharmacology and key drug information.

Quick Medication Administration Reference: This reference includes content on dosage calculations, the five rights of medication administration, life span considerations, client assessment, home health care, and medication administration techniques presented in an easy-to-access format in a portable booklet.

CONTENTS

UNIT VII

Drugs Affecting the Urinary System 415

UNIT VIII

Drugs Affecting the Respiratory System 445

UNIT IX

Drugs Affecting the Gastrointestinal System 481

UNIT X

Drugs Affecting the Visual and Auditory Systems 509

UNIT XI

Drugs Affecting the Endocrine System 529

UNIT XII

Drugs Affecting the Reproductive System 579

UNIT XIII

Drugs Used in Neoplastic Diseases 613

UNIT XIV

Drugs Used in Infectious Diseases and Inflammation 637

DETAILED CONTENTS

UNIT V

Drugs Affecting the Cardiovascular System 307

UNIT VI

Drugs Affecting the Blood..........379

UNIT VII

Drugs Affecting the Urinary System 415

UNIT XVI

UNIT XVII

UNIT XVIII

APPENDIXES

UNIT I

Principles of Pharmacology

CHAPTER 1

Introduction to Pharmacology

CHAPTER FOCUS

Proper selection and use of medication requires a thorough knowledge of pharmacologic principles. This chapter focuses on the origin and development of pharmacology, drug nomenclature, classification, sources and dosage measurements, and selected reference sources. An understanding of the key pharmacology terms and objectives is important in the development of a knowledge base for pharmacology.

OBJECTIVES

After reading and studying this chapter, the student should be able to do the following:

1. *Define and discuss the key terms.*
2. *Trace and describe the major significant historical events in the development of pharmacology.*
3. *Explain the difference between chemical, generic, and trade or brand drug names.*
4. *Briefly describe an alkaloid, glycoside, gum, resin, and oil.*
5. *Name the four primary sources of drug and biologic products.*
6. *Identify authoritative sources for drug information.*

KEY TERMS

adverse reaction, (p. 6)
chemical name, (p. 5)
drug, (p. 4)
generic name, (p. 5)
indication, (p. 6)
key, or prototype, drug, (p. 6)
nonprescription, or over-the-counter, drug, (p. 5)
pharmacodynamics, (p. 6)
pharmacokinetics, (p. 6)
pharmacology, (p. 4)
pharmacopeia, or compendium, (p. 4)
pregnancy safety, (p. 6)
prescription, or legend, drug, (p. 5)
side effect, (p. 6)
trade name, (p. 5)

Pharmacology is the study of drugs, including their actions and effects in a living system. It deals with all drugs used in society today—legal and illegal, prescription and over-the-counter (OTC) medications. The pharmacologic agents available today have controlled, prevented, cured, and in some instances eradicated disease. The result has been an improved quality of life and, perhaps, an extension of the life span.

However, medications also have the potential to cause harm, as indicated by the term *pharmaceutical,* which was actually derived from the Greek word for poison (Siler et al, 1982). Therefore, the healthcare professional should be thoroughly informed about each medication before administering it to a patient. To safely administer a medication, one must know the usual dose, route of administration, indications, significant side effects and adverse reactions, major drug interactions, contraindications, and appropriate monitoring techniques and interventions.

Key terms are listed at the beginning of each chapter along with the corresponding page on which the term is defined. Understanding key terms is essential in the development of a knowledge base in pharmacology.

HISTORICAL TRENDS

Since the beginning of time, people have searched for substances to treat illness and cure disease. The oldest prescriptions known were found on a clay tablet written by a Sumerian physician around 3000 B.C., nearly 5000 years ago.

Primitive people through the Egyptian period believed that disease was caused by evil spirits living in the body. Asclepias, who lived between 600 and 700 B.C., was considered to be the principal Greek god of healing. He combined religion and healing in a temple setting, and his large family represented health or medical ideology. For example, his wife Epione soothed pain; his daughter Hygeia, the goddess of health, represented the prevention of disease; and Panacea, another daughter, represented treatment. His large temple settings were used to treat both the rich and poor to cure their illnesses.

Hippocrates (fifth century B.C.) advanced the idea that disease results from natural causes and can only be understood through a study of natural laws. He believed that the body has recuperative powers and saw the healthcare provider's role as assisting the recuperative process. Called the "father of medicine," Hippocrates influenced the principles that control the practice of medicine today.

The fall of the Roman Empire marked the beginning of the medieval period (400 to 1580 AD). When the Germanic barbarians overran Western Europe, the practice of medicine reverted to folklore and tradition similar to that of the Greeks before Hippocrates. At the same time, Christian religious orders built monasteries that became sites for all learning, including pharmacy and medicine. They aided the sick and needy with food, rest, and medicinals from their monastery gardens. The Arabs' interest in medicine, pharmacy, and chemistry was reflected in the hospitals and schools they built, the many new drugs they contributed, and their formulation of the first set of drug standards.

In 1240 Emperor Frederick II declared pharmacy to be separate from medicine. However, pharmacy was not truly established separately until the sixteenth century, when Valerius Cordus wrote the first pharmacopeia as an authoritative standard. A **pharmacopeia,** or **compendium,** is a collected body of drug information in a country or a specified geographic area. This compendium usually contains all of the authorized drugs available within a country, including their descriptions, formulas, strengths, standards of purity, and dosage forms.

Paracelsus (1493 to 1541), a professor of physics and surgery at Basel, denounced "humoral pathology" and substi-

BOX 1-1 Summary of Major Drug Discoveries

Drug	*Time Period*	*Comments*
opium tincture, coca (cocaine), and ipecac	17th century	Important drugs, still used today
digitalis	1785	Cardiac medication, source of cardiac glycosides (digoxin, digitoxin)
smallpox vaccine	1796	Important vaccine in its time; now smallpox has been eradicated worldwide
morphine	1815	Most important analgesic derived from opium; used to treat severe pain
quinine, atropine, and codeine	19th century	Still available for use today
ether and chloroform	1840s	First general anesthetics; rare or obsolete today
insulin	1922	Most important discovery for treatment of diabetes mellitus
penicillin	mid-1940s	Revolutionized treatment of microbial infections; precursor of many other antibiotics
cortisone	1949	Important hormone from adrenal gland cortex; also synthetically prepared
polio vaccines	1955, 1961	Discovery of inactivated and live oral poliovirus vaccine were very significant in eliminating polio epidemics
oral contraceptives	late 1950s	Chemicals similar to natural estrogen or progesterone hormones that have been used by millions of women worldwide
antivirals	mid-1970s	Useful for the prophylaxis and treatment of viral diseases

tuted the idea that diseases are actual entities to be combated with specific remedies. He improved pharmacy and therapeutics for succeeding centuries, introducing new remedies and reducing the overdosing so prevalent in that period.

In the seventeenth and eighteenth centuries, great progress was made in pharmacy and chemistry. The first London pharmacopeia appeared in 1618 and many preparations introduced at that time are still in use today, including opium tincture, coca, and ipecac. The first important national pharmacopeia was the French Codex (1818), followed by the United States' Pharmacopeia in 1820, Great Britain's in 1864, and Germany's in 1872. See Box 1-1 for a summary of major drug discoveries.

The study of accurate dosages in the nineteenth century led to the establishment of large-scale manufacturing plants to produce drugs. Drug dosages and knowledge of their expected actions became more precise. Rational medicine had begun to replace empiricism. As the twenty-first century draws near, dramatic changes are occurring to reform the healthcare systems in the United States and Canada. The emphasis on providing quality healthcare in a more cost-effective manner is leading to a redefinition of professional roles and decision-making responsibilities among health professionals (Blumengold, 1995; McCombs et al, 1995). An integrated healthcare delivery team (i.e., an interdisciplinary team approach that centers on patient-focused care) is evolving. At a minimum, this approach includes assessment, planning, monitoring, counseling, accountability for therapeutic outcomes, and patient advocacy. Managed care and a health promotion focus will require changes in professional education. Because medications are the primary therapies used in treatment and rehabilitative care, the healthcare professional needs to have a solid foundation in pharmacology.

DRUG NOMENCLATURE

A **drug** is any substance used in the diagnosis, cure, treatment, or prevention of a disease or condition. As a drug passes through the investigational stages before it is approved and marketed, it collects three different types of names—the chemical name; the generic, or nonproprietary, name; and the trade, or brand or proprietary, name.

The **chemical name** is a precise description of the drug's chemical composition and molecular structure. It is particularly meaningful to the chemist. The generic name is a shorter name derived from the chemical name. For example, the chemical name of a popular analgesic is N-(4-hydroxyphenyl) acetamide. Its generic name is acetaminophen, and it is marketed under a number of brand or trade names—Tylenol, Tempra, and Datril among others.

The **generic name** is often assigned by the manufacturer with the approval of the United States Adopted Name Council (USAN). Since the generic name is simpler than the chemical name, it is the official name listed in official compendia, such as The United States Pharmacopeia. When drug companies market a particular drug product, they often select and copyright a **trade name** for their drug. This copyright restricts the use of the name to only the individual drug company. Since numerous brand names may exist for the same ingredient, such as for acetaminophen, prescribers are encouraged to use the generic name. The use of generic names is also widely advocated to avoid confusion between drugs with similar trade names.

With some exceptions the majority of generic drug products sold are considered therapeutically equivalent to the brand name product. In addition, such generic products are often much less expensive than the brand name drug.

To encourage physicians to prescribe and to promote sales of trade name drugs, extensive advertising is usually necessary. This expense is borne mainly by the consumer. However, much of the research in new drugs is done in laboratories of reputable drug firms. To realize a legitimate return for the cost of research, drug companies need to patent their products and have exclusive rights to their manufacture and sale for a specified period. The trade name of drugs discussed in this book appears in parentheses after the generic name.

A drug may be considered a **prescription,** or **legend, drug,** which means that it requires a legal prescription to be dispensed, or it may be a **nonprescription,** or **over-the-counter, drug,** which means that it may be purchased without a prescription. Some prescription drugs may be purchased OTC; they are usually lower drug dosages that are considered to be relatively safe for sale. An example is ibuprofen, which is sold as an OTC drug in a 200 mg strength as Advil or Motrin IB, but requires a prescription for the 300, 400, 600, or 800 mg tablet.

SOURCES OF DRUGS

Drugs and biologic products have been identified or derived from four main sources: (1) plants (e.g., digitalis, vincristine, and colchicine), (2) animals and humans (from which drugs such as epinephrine, insulin, and ACTH are obtained), (3) minerals or mineral products (e.g., iron, iodine, and Epsom salts), and (4) synthetic or chemical substances made in the laboratory. The drugs made of chemical substances are pure drugs, and some of them are simple substances, such as sodium bicarbonate and magnesium hydroxide. Others are products of complex synthesis, such as sulfonamides and adrenocorticosteroids.

Active Constituents of Plant Drugs

The leaves, roots, seeds, and other parts of plants may be dried or otherwise processed for use as a medicine and, as such, are known as *crude drugs.* Their therapeutic effect is produced by the chemical substances they contain. When the pharmacologically active constituents are separated from the crude preparation, the resulting substances are more potent and usually produce effects more reliably than the crude drug does. Some of the types of pharmacologically active compounds found in plants, grouped according to their physical and chemical properties, are alkaloids, glycosides, gums, and oils.

- *Alkaloids* are organic compounds that are alkaline in nature and are chemically combined with acids in the laboratory to form water-soluble salts, such as morphine sulfate and atropine sulfate. Synthetic alkaloids formulated in the laboratory have activity similar to that of plant alkaloids.
- *Glycosides* are active plant substances that, on hydrolysis, yield a sugar plus one or more additional active substances. The sugar is believed to increase the solubility, absorption, permeability, and cellular distribution of the glycoside. An important cardiac glycoside used in medicine is digoxin.
- *Gums* are plant exudates. When water is added, some of them will swell and form gelatinous masses. Others remain unchanged in the gastrointestinal tract, where they act as hydrophilic (water-attracting) colloids; they absorb water, form watery bulk, and exert a laxative effect. Agar and psyllium seeds are examples of natural laxative gums, whereas methylcellulose and sodium carboxymethylcellulose are synthetic colloids. Gums are also used to soothe irritated skin and mucous membranes.
- *Oils* are highly viscous liquids and are generally of two kinds, volatile or fixed. A volatile oil imparts an aroma to a plant; because of their pleasant odor and taste, these oils are frequently used as flavoring agents. Peppermint and clove oil are examples of volatile oils occasionally used in medicine. Fixed oils are generally greasy and, unlike volatile oils, do not evaporate easily. Olive oil is a fixed oil used in cooking, whereas castor oil is an example of a fixed oil used in medicine.

DRUG CLASSIFICATION

Drug classification can be approached from two perspectives—by clinical indication or by body system. This book uses both approaches where appropriate. Examples of drugs classified by clinical indication include "Chapter 32: Mucokinetic and Bronchodilator Drugs" and "Chapter 52: Antifungal and Antiviral Drugs." An example of drugs classified by body system is "Unit 3: Drugs Affecting the Central Nervous System."

Such drug classifications can help the healthcare professional understand and learn about the individual agents available for drug therapy. When a **key,** or **prototype, drug** representative of each drug class is reviewed, pharmacology is easier to understand. Then when a new drug becomes available, the practitioner will be able to associate it with its drug classification and make inferences about many of its basic qualities before reading about its specific properties. Focusing on qualities that are different from the prototype drug is important in the differentiation.

The basic information to be learned about each major drug includes generic name and primary trade name, category, indications, mechanisms of action, side and adverse effects, contraindications, precautions, significant drug interactions, and monitoring techniques. The pregnancy safety section in each monograph lists the Food and Drug Administration (FDA) pregnancy safety category that indicates the documented problems with the use of a drug during pregnancy. Pregnancy categories are discussed in Chapter 2. See Box 1-2 for definitions of pharmacology terms.

BOX 1-2 Pharmacology Terms

Adverse reaction An unintended and undesirable response to a drug.

Indication An illness or disorder for which a drug has a documented usefulness.

Pharmacokinetics How the body processes a specific drug, that is, how a drug is altered as it travels through the body (absorption, distribution, any special tissue binding or affinity, metabolism, and excretion).

Pharmacodynamics What drugs do to the body and how they do it. It refers to the interaction of drug molecules with their target cells; their biochemical and physiologic effects at the site(s).

Pregnancy safety A method of classifying drugs according to documented problems in pregnancy. The FDA issues a drug category scale that grades the risk to benefit with each drug.

Side effect A drug effect that is not necessarily the primary purpose for giving the drug. Side effects may be desirable or undesirable.

Sources of Drug Data

New information on old drugs and the release of new drugs is an ongoing event. News releases and numerous articles, journals, and books are written in an attempt to keep up with the new discoveries. It is unrealistic to assume that one can know everything about all medications on the market; therefore the practitioner must know how and where general and detailed drug information can be obtained. Many excellent drug references are available, each with its own focus or emphasis. Because no one reference is a complete source of drug data to meet the varied and specialized needs of clinical practice today, the student should be familiar with the primary drug reference sources available (Table 1-1).

Other Drug Information Sources

Drug information centers located throughout the United States disseminate information about drugs, treatment of drug overdoses, and other related information. The centers are usually located in large medical centers, and their advice is based on medical-scientific literature. They are excellent sources of information for difficult pharmacologic questions. In addition, drug manufacturers, package inserts, and pharmacists are usually available to provide drug information. With the proliferation of medical sites on the Internet, many search engines and directories are available to provide both general and specialized drug information for healthcare

TABLE 1-1 Drug Information Resources

Reference	***Comments***
American Hospital Formulary Service (AHFS) Drug Information (Bethesda, MD: American Society of Hospital Pharmacists, Inc.)	Objective overview in monograph form. Comprehensive source of comparative, unbiased information on nearly every drug available in the United States. Issues supplements; updated annually. Widely used drug information source for all healthcare professionals.
Drug Facts and Comparisons (St Louis, MO: Facts and Comparisons, Inc.)	Loose-leaf edition updated monthly. Comprehensive drug information arranged to facilitate comparisons and evaluations. Contains a variety of manufacturers' package sizes and strengths plus cost index information. Includes manufacturers' addresses and phone numbers. Contains section on orphan drugs, diagnostic aids, radiopaque agents, antidotes, and drugs in development (investigational). Widely used reference source, especially for pharmacists.
Handbook of Nonprescription Drug (Washington, DC: American Pharmaceutical Association)	Comprehensive over-the-counter (OTC) drug information. Each chapter reviews physiology, the primary minor illnesses, and the drugs used in treatment. Contains tables with specific OTC drug information.
Mosby's GenRx (St Louis, MO: Mosby)	Comprehensive drug information. Contains drug product identification charts. Includes product ratings (equivalent, not equivalent classifications) from FDA. Includes drug costs and comparisons. Published annually.
Physicians' Desk Reference (PDR) (Oradell, NJ: Medial Economics)	Widely used drug source for physicians. Pharmaceutical industry finances the book. Information same as drug package insert. Lacks comparative information on safety and efficacy. Contains drug product identification section and manufacturers' addresses and phone numbers.
United States Pharmacopeia, USP DI (Rockville, MD: U.S. Pharmacopeial Convention)	Available in several volumes; volume 1 is for healthcare professionals, and volume 2 offers advice for patients in lay language. Consists of extensive drug monographs with practical information. Highlights clinically significant information to reduce drug risks. Issues monthly updates; updated annually. Highly recommended drug reference for all healthcare professionals.

professionals and for the patient. It has been estimated that there are over 10,000 medical sites available on the Internet (Hutchinson, 1997). Many professional journals (medical, pharmacy, nursing) also provide current drug information, and some are also available on the Internet. The student is urged to carefully select the Internet site when seeking drug information because erroneous information may also be posted. There is no screening tool used to determine the accuracy of Internet information. Therefore the best approach may be to consider the reputation of the provider of the information (such as drug information from drug information centers, information posted by pharmacy, medical, or nursing schools; professional journals; American Cancer Society; Food and Drug Administration; National Institute of Health; and numerous other organizations).

At least three references (USP DI, Mosby's GenRx, and Physicians' Desk Reference, or PDR) provide actual photographs of drugs to assist the healthcare professional in identifying an unknown tablet or capsule. In addition, manufacturers often place numbers with letters on their solid dose medication that aids in identifying the individual dosage form.

An up-to-date pharmacology textbook is also a valuable source of drug information and highly recommended for inclusion in the healthcare professional's library. Many other sources of drug information are available, and the criteria for using any particular source should be based on the information desired and the currency and accuracy of the source. See Table 1-1 for selected drug information sources.

DOSAGE MEASUREMENTS

There are three systems of measurement in use for administering medications: the metric system (most widely used and the most convenient), the apothecary system (nearly phased out), and the household system (least accurate system; usually limited to the home setting).

Metric System

The metric system has three basic units of measure: the meter (m), liter (L), and gram (g). The meter is the unit for linear measurement, the liter is for volume or capacity, and the gram is for weight. A meter is a little longer than a yard, a liter is a little more than a quart, and a gram is a little more than the weight of a steel paper clip.

The metric system is a decimal system in which the basic units can be divided or multiplied by 10, 100, or 1000 to form a secondary unit. The names of the secondary units are formed by joining a Greek or Latin prefix to the name of the primary unit (Table 1-2). Subdivisions of the basic units are made by moving the decimal point to the left, whereas multiples of the basic units are indicated by moving the decimal point to the right. For example, the gram is the metric unit of weight used in weighing chemicals and various pharmaceutical preparations. As noted in Table 1-2, a decigram is 10 times greater than a centigram and 100 times greater than a milligram. To change a decigram to centigram, multiply by 10; to change decigram to milligram, multiply by 100. To change milligrams to centigrams, divide by 10; to change

TABLE 1-2 Metric Prefixes, Meanings, and Relationships

Prefix	*Meaning*
giga	Billions
kilo	Thousands
hecto	Hundreds
deka	Tens
Base Units of Water, Liter, Gram	***One Unit***
deci	Tenths
centi	Hundredths
milli	Thousandths
micro	Millionths
nano	Billionths

milligrams to decigrams, divide by 100; to change milligrams to grams, divide by 1000.

Centimeters and millimeters are the chief linear measures used in health care. Measurement of the size of body organs is made in centimeters and millimeters, and the sphygmomanometer used to measure blood pressure is calibrated in millimeters of mercury. Approximately 2.5 cm (25 mm) is equivalent to 1 inch.

The liter is a unit of volume, or capacity, and is equal to approximately 1000 cc, or 1000 ml. Fractional parts of a liter are usually expressed in milliliters or cubic centimeters. For example, 0.6 liter is written as 600 ml, or 600 cc. Multiples of a liter are similarly expressed; 1.4 liters is 1400 ml, or 1400 cc. According to the National Bureaus of Standards, the abbreviation cc is becoming obsolete; either ml or mL may be used.

The following is the recommended style of notation as proposed by the International System of Units from the National Bureau of Standards.

- Units are not capitalized (gram, not Gram)
- No period should be used with unit abbreviations (ml, not m.l. or ml.)
- Use only decimal notations, not fractions (0.25 kg, not ¼ kg)
- Quantities less than 1 should have a zero placed to the left of the decimal point (0.75 mg, not .75 mg)
- Abbreviations should not be pluralized (kg, not kgs)

Apothecary System

Only a few medications are now available in units of the apothecary system. This system is less convenient and less precise than the metric system. However the practitioner needs to be familiar with this system to avoid medication errors when such terms are used in ordering medications.

The basic unit of weight is the grain, which is today accepted as being approximately equivalent to 60 mg. Other units of weight commonly used are the fluid dram, the fluid ounce, and the pound.

The basic unit of fluid volume is the minim, approximately equal to the volume of water that would weigh a grain, a very small amount (about 0.05 or 0.06 ml). Other volume measures, also considered household measures, are the pint and quart.

In written apothecary prescriptions, the placement of abbreviations and the type of numerals follow a more complex arrangement. The abbreviation is placed before the numeral and whole numerical quantities are usually expressed in Roman numerals (e.g., gr X for 10 grains). Fractional quantities are usually expressed by Arabic numerals instead of decimals (e.g., gr ¼ not gr 0.25 for one-quarter grain).

Household System

Both household and apothecary measurements include the quart, pint, glass, cup, tablespoon, teaspoon, and drop. Because standardized measurements of household equipment usually do not exist in the home, more accurate measuring devices are necessary. For example, the average household teaspoon can hold 4, 5, or even more of a liquid medication rather than the standard 5 ml. A drop and a minim cannot be considered equivalent since drop size varies with the viscosity of the medication, even when measured by an approved dropper. Therefore any listing of household measurements on an equivalency table must be considered only an approximation. See Table 1-3 for the common approximate equivalents of weights and measures among the three systems.

DOSAGE CALCULATIONS

A thorough understanding of basic math (fractions and ratios) is necessary for safe drug administration in the healthcare setting. When in doubt, the student is advised to double check all calculations with another healthcare professional. The pharmacist is highly trained in medication calculations and, when available, is recommended for this check. The following problems are examples of the types of problems that may be encountered in the healthcare setting. For additional information and medication problems, the student is referred to the texts available to cover this topic, several of which are listed in the reference list at the end of this chapter.

Fraction Conversion

The prescriber ordered acetaminophen suppositories 600 mg rectally every 6 hours for a patient with a temperature over 102° F. The label on the package states acetaminophen gr X. How much do you administer to the patient?

Known:

$$1 \text{ gr} = 60 \text{ mg, or } \frac{1 \text{ gr}}{60 \text{ mg}}$$

Therefore:

$$\frac{1 \text{ gr}}{60 \text{ mg}} = \frac{10 \text{ gr}}{X \text{ mg}}$$

Note that the grain-to-mg ratio is set up the same on both sides. This is very important because the same measurements should be in the same position on both sides of the formula. Cross multiply:

$$X = 600 \text{ mg, so the dose is one suppository.}$$

TABLE 1-3 Common Approximate Equivalents of Weights and Measures

Metric	*Apothecary*	*Household*
Weight		
1 kg*	2.2 lb	
1000 mg = 1 g*	gr xv	
60 mg* (occasionally seen as 65 mg)	gr ī	
30 mg	gr ss (one half)	
1 μg (mcg) = 0.001 mg		
Volume		
	4 quarts	1 gal
1000 ml* = approx 1 L = 1000 cc	Approx 1 qt	1 qt
500 ml	Approx 1 pint (½ qt)	16 oz
240 or 250 ml	℥ viii (8 fluidounces)† = approx ½ pint	1 cup or 1 glass
30 ml* = approx 30 cc	℥ ī (1 fluidounce)	2 tbsp
Approx 16 ml = approx 16 cc	ʒ iv (4 fluidrams)	1 tbsp
Approx 8 ml	ʒ iī (2 fluidrams)	2 tsp
4 to 5 ml	ʒ ī (1 fluidram)	1 tsp
1 ml* = approx 1 cc	Minims xv or xvi	Minims cannot be compared with drops

*These equivalents may be committed to memory for ready application to dosage problems.
†Note the small difference in the symbols for fluidounce and fluidram.

The second way to solve this problem follows:

$$\frac{\text{dose ordered}}{\text{dose on hand}} \times \text{dose of one unit (suppository)}$$

$$\frac{10\ \text{gr}}{600\ \text{mg}} \times 600\ \text{mg} = 6000/600 = 10\ \text{gr, or one suppository}$$

Ratio Conversion

1. The prescriber ordered sulfamethoxazole (Gantanol) 2 g bid. Gantanol is available in 500 mg tablets. How many tablets do you administer? First convert to the same measurement:

$$1\ \text{g} : 1000\ \text{mg} :: 2\ \text{g} : X\ \text{mg}$$

Multiply the outer and inner portions of the ratio

$$X = 1000 \times 2, \text{ or } 2000\ \text{mg}$$

Set up the second ratio:

$$500\ \text{mg} : 1\ \text{tablet} :: 2000\ \text{mg} : X\ \text{tablets, or}$$

$$500X = 2000, \text{ then}$$

X = 2000/500 = 4 tablets. The dose is 4 tablets of the 500 mg strength.

2. The prescriber ordered gentamicin 1.7 mg per kg of body weight every 8 hours for 1 week. The patient weighs 158 lb. Calculate the dose of gentamicin.

$$1\ \text{kg} = 2.2\ \text{lb, therefore}$$
$$\frac{1\ \text{kg}}{2.2\ \text{lb}} = \frac{X\ \text{kg}}{158\ \text{lb}}$$
$$2.2\ X = 158\ \text{lb}$$
$$X = \frac{158}{2.2} = 71.8\ \text{kg}$$

Therefore, 1.7 mg per kg is 1.7 × 71.8 = 122 mg of gentamicin every 8 hours.

3. The patient has a prescription for Nitroglycerin SL tablets gr 1/200, but the bottles are the shelf are labeled 0.15 mg, 0.3 mg, and 0.4 mg sublingual tablets. Which is the correct equivalent for gr 1/200?

$$\frac{1\ \text{gr}}{60\ \text{mg}} = \frac{1/200}{X}$$

$$X = 60 \times 1/200, \text{ or } 60/200 = 0.3\ \text{mg}$$

GOALS OF THIS TEXT

The purpose of this text is to present a strong theoretical foundation and a practical approach to drug therapy. Chapters 1-6 provide the basic concepts and general principles about drugs and their administration. Chapters 7-65 discuss the clinical aspects, including specific drug information and application.

To find information about a particular drug in this book, do the following:

1. Look up the generic or brand name in the index.
2. When you find the drug monograph, it is recommended that you read the chapter or unit that precedes the specific discussion. This material will provide a more complete overview of the topic and will help place the drug in proper context within the chapter.

The key drugs are highlighted in this book by the key drug symbol ( ). Study these drugs as representative of the drug classification or category. Other drugs within the same drug classification or category can be identified by their differences from the key drug. An understanding of the drug's mechanism of action, indications, pharmacokinetics, major side and adverse reactions, contraindications, precautions, and significant drug interactions is necessary to safely prescribe and administer any medication.

Each generic name is followed by some of the common trade names by which the particular drug is known. Trade names of drugs available in Canada but not in the United States are followed by a maple leaf symbol (🍁).

SUMMARY

The history of pharmacology, or the study of drugs and their actions and effects in a living system, has intrigued and interested mankind throughout recorded history. Some drug preparations discovered in the seventeenth and eighteenth centuries have been refined or synthesized and are still in use today. Each drug is identified by three names: chemical, generic, and trade or brand name. With a few exceptions, many states permit or mandate that pharmacists dispense less expensive generic drugs for brand name products.

The four primary sources of drugs are plants, animals and humans, minerals, and chemical formulations. The pharmacologically active compounds that are derived from plants are alkaloids, glycosides, gums, resins, and oils. Drugs may be classified by clinical indication or by body system. Drug classifications help facilitate the student's understanding of pharmacology by comparing the common characteristics of a drug group or classification (key, or prototype, drug) with any new drugs released in the same classification or category.

Maintaining a current source of drug information is an absolute necessity in clinical practice today. For drug dosage calculations and administration of medications, the healthcare professional must have a working knowledge of the three systems of measurement and the methods of performing drug calculations.

REVIEW QUESTIONS

1. Name the three measuring systems used for administering medications. Which system is the recommended one that is most widely used and convenient?
2. The physician orders an investigational drug for a patient. Which drug reference would you select to find information on this drug? Which reference is only a compilation of package inserts?
3. What is the difference between an alkaloid, glycoside, gum, and oil? Name one medication from each category.
4. Supply the equivalents for the following dosages:

gr 2	=	______	mg
two tsp	=	______	ml
one tbsp	=	______	ml
250 lb	=	______	kg
90 kg	=	______	lb

REFERENCES

Blumengold JG: Strategic and financial considerations for integrated health care delivery, *Medical Interface* 8(5):77, 1995.

Hutchinson D: *A pocket guide to the medical Internet,* Sacramento, Calif, 1997, New Wind Publishing.

McCombs JS, Nichol MB, Johnson KA et al: Is pharmacy's vision of the future too narrow? *Am J Health-Syst Pharm* 52(11):1208, 1995.

Siler WA et al: *Death by prescription,* Tallahassee, Fla, 1982, Rose Publishing.

ADDITIONAL REFERENCES

Anderson KL et al, editors: *Mosby's medical, nursing, and allied health dictionary,* ed 5, St Louis, 1998, Mosby.

Brown M, Mulholland JL: *Drug calculations: process and problems for clinical practice,* ed 5, St Louis, 1996, Mosby.

Gray DC: *Calculate with confidence,* ed 2, St Louis, 1998, Mosby.

Leake CD: *An historical account of pharmacology to the twentieth century,* Springfield, Ill, 1975, Charles C Thomas.

Lyons AS, Petrucelli RJ II: *Medicine: an illustrated history.* New York, 1978, Harry N Abrams.

Mosby: *Mosby's GenRx,* St Louis, 1998, Mosby.

Ogden SJ: *Radcliff and Ogden's calculation of drug dosages,* ed 5, St Louis, 1995, Mosby.

Olin BR: *Facts and comparisons,* Philadelphia, 1998, Facts and Comparisons.

Roger FB: *A syllabus of medical history,* Boston, 1972, Little, Brown, & Co.

United States Pharmacopeial Convention: *USP DI: drug information for the health care professional,* ed 18, Rockville, Md, 1998, the Convention.

CHAPTER 2

Legal Foundations

CHAPTER FOCUS

Healthcare professionals who prescribe, dispense, or administer medications are legally accountable for their actions, especially as they relate to drug therapy. This chapter reviews the essential laws relating to prescription and nonprescription drugs, controlled substances, and investigational drugs in the United States and Canada. An understanding of the key terms and objectives is important for the development of a knowledge base in the legal aspects relating to medications.

OBJECTIVES

After reading and studying this chapter, the student should be able to do the following:

1. *Define and discuss the key terms.*
2. *Describe the impact of the Food, Drug, and Cosmetic Act and the Kefauver-Harris Amendment on public safety.*
3. *Explain the purpose of the Controlled Substances Act.*
4. *Discuss the three primary aspects of drug product liability.*
5. *Explain drug substitution and the purpose of a negative drug formulary.*
6. *List and describe the FDA pregnancy categories for drugs.*
7. *Identify and explain the three human study phases for investigational drugs.*

KEY TERMS

abbreviated new drug application (ANDA), (p. 20)
assay, (p. 18)
bioassay, (p. 18)
controlled substances, (p. 13)
Controlled Substances Act, (p. 13)
International Narcotics Control Board, (p. 19)
Investigational New Drug (IND), (p. 19)
LD_{50}, (p. 19)
MedWatch, (p. 20)
negative drug formulary, (p. 15)
new drug application (NDA), (p. 19)
product liability, (p. 15)
Pure Food and Drug Act, (p. 12)
therapeutic index, (p. 19)

Before the twentieth century, most medications lacked the detailed information available today, such as content analysis and strength, drug consistency from one bottle to another of the same preparation, and research studies proving the safety and effectiveness of the preparation. In the United States, the early 1900s marked the beginning of drug legislation.

UNITED STATES DRUG LEGISLATION

Before 1906, patent medicines and remedies were sold by medicine men in traveling wagon shows, in drugstores, by mail order, and by doctors (real or self-titled). Such products were not required to list ingredients on the label, and many contained potent and dangerous drugs such as opium, morphine, heroin, chloral hydrate, and alcohol. Many persons (especially infants) were reportedly injured, became addicted, or died as a result of the ingredients contained in these preparations.

In 1906 the **Pure Food and Drug Act** was the first U.S. law passed to protect the public from adulterated or mislabeled drugs. The law required drug companies to declare on the package label the presence of any of 11 identified dangerous and perhaps addictive drugs (including some on the list in the previous paragraph). This first law had loopholes that were used by the patent medicine dealers for their own gain:

1. False and misleading claims about the curative value of the product were not allowed on the package, which was described as a bottle, label, or wrapper that encircled the bottle. Claims made in advertisements, newspapers, or drug almanacs; by word of mouth; and on signs in store windows were not covered under the law. Unscrupulous nostrum dealers took full advantage of this oversight.
2. Serial numbers were required for products containing any of the 11 dangerous drugs, and each label was to bear the words "Guaranteed under the Food and Drugs Act." The dealer registered the product and was legally responsible for it if it was improperly sold under this act. However, many patent medicine dealers implied that this was the government seal of approval. In response to this abuse, this clause was abolished in 1919.
3. Only drugs sold in interstate commerce (made in one state and sold to persons living in other states) were covered. Drugs made and sold within the same state did not fall under the jurisdiction of this law.

The Food and Drug Act of 1906 designated the *United States Pharmacopeia* (*USP*) and the *National Formulary* as official standards and empowered the federal government to enforce them. It was required that drugs comply with the standards of strength and purity professed and that labels indicate the kind and amount of morphine or other narcotic ingredients present. In 1912, Congress passed the Sherley Amendment, prohibiting the use of fraudulent therapeutic claims.

A further update of the drug legislation occurred in 1938 with the passage of the Food, Drug, and Cosmetic Act. More than 100 deaths occurred in 1937 as a result of ingestion of a diethylene glycol solution of sulfanilamide. This preparation had been marketed as an "elixir of sulfanilamide" without investigation of its toxicity. Under the 1906 law the only charge that could be made against the drug company was mislabeling, since it was labeled an "elixir" and the drug failed to meet the definition of an elixir (an alcoholic solution). The 1938 act prevented the marketing of new drugs before they had been properly tested for safety.

BOX 2-1 Prescription (Legend) Drugs

Legend drugs must bear the legend "Caution: Federal law prohibits dispensing without prescription." These include all drugs given by injection as well as the following:

- Hypnotic, narcotic, or habit-forming drugs or derivatives thereof as specified in the law.
- Drugs that, because of their toxicity or method of use, are not safe unless they are administered under the supervision of a licensed practitioner (physician, dentist, or nurse practitioner).
- New drugs that are limited to investigational use or new drugs that are not considered safe for indiscriminate use by the public.

The Durham-Humphrey Amendment of 1952 further changed the 1938 drug act by specifying how prescription drugs and refills could be ordered and dispensed (Box 2-1). This amendment also recognized a second class of drugs, over-the-counter drugs (OTCs), for which prescriptions are not required.

In 1958 a U.S. Senate investigation into the drug industry began when it became known that drug companies were making huge profits and that some drug promotion was false or misleading. This investigation received little support until fueled by the thalidomide tragedy, although for the United States it was more a might-have-been catastrophe than a real one. Thalidomide, a hypnotic marketed in Europe, was found to be responsible for severe deformities in babies whose mothers had taken the drug during the early stages of pregnancy. These events led to passage of the Kefauver-Harris Amendment in 1962. Currently thalidomide has limited availability in the United States for the treatment of leprosy, bone marrow transplantation, acquired immunodeficiency syndrome (AIDS), and several other conditions. It was classified as an orphan drug (Olin, 1998). See explanation of orphan drugs on p. 21.

The Kefauver-Harris Amendment required proof of both safety and efficacy before a new drug could be approved for use. This meant that all drugs introduced under the safety-only criteria in effect from 1938 to 1962 had to be evaluated. To do this, the FDA signed a contract in 1966 with the National Academy of Sciences and the National Research Council (NAS/NRC) to study all supporting data for all therapeutic claims. This program of study was called the Drug Efficacy Study Implementation (DESI).

Under the DESI study, thousands of drugs and therapeutic claims have been evaluated and many ineffective drugs have been withdrawn from the market. Those rated as *possibly effective* or *probably effective* are being withdrawn or reformulated, although a drug may remain on the market while claims are being modified and scientific data are being collected to substantiate the claims. However, an approved drug can be prescribed for a disorder for which the drug has not been approved by the FDA. Informed consent for this nonresearch application of the drug is generally not required.

Over-the-Counter Drug Review

Of the estimated 400,000 drug products marketed in the United States, more than 300,000 are OTC drugs (Covington, 1996). The 300,000 individual drug products contain approximately 700 to 1000 active ingredients. In 1972 the FDA assembled an advisory review panel to perform an ingredient review, asking primarily the following questions: Are the ingredients safe and effective for consumers to self-medicate? Are the labeling, indications, dosage instructions, and warnings provided sufficient? If they were found lacking, appropriate recommendations had to be developed.

This study, completed in 1983, found that approximately one third of the ingredients reviewed were safe and effective for labeled indications. Ingredients found particularly or potentially dangerous were either transferred to prescription status only (such as hexachlorophene, an antibacterial topical with a potential for inducing neurologic toxicities) or removed entirely from the market (such as camphorated oil or camphor liniment). See Chapter 3 for a discussion of OTC medications.

Prescription Drugs Switched to OTC Drug Status

The OTC review panels are primarily responsible for switching a number of prescription drugs to nonprescription, or OTC, status. These drug products are considered to be safe for self-treatment by consumers without professional guidance. Cimetidine (Tagamet HB), famotidine (Pepcid AC), diphenhydramine (Benadryl), and topical hydrocortisone are examples of products switched from prescription to OTC status.

Control of Opioids (Narcotics) and Other Dangerous Drugs

Narcotic and Drug Abuse Laws

The Harrison Narcotic Act (1914) was the first federal law aimed at curbing drug addiction or dependence. This law not only established the word *narcotic* as a legal term but also regulated the importation, manufacture, sale, and use of opium and cocaine and all their compounds and derivatives. Marijuana and its derivatives were also included in this act, as were many synthetic analgesic drugs proved to produce or sustain either physical or psychologic dependence.

This act and other drug abuse amendments now have only historical importance, since they have been superseded by the Comprehensive Drug Abuse Prevention and Control Act of 1970, also called the **Controlled Substances Act** (CSA), which became effective May 1, 1971. This law was designed to provide increased research into, and prevention of, drug abuse and drug dependence; to provide for treatment and rehabilitation of drug abusers and drug dependent persons; and to improve the administration and regulation of the manufacture, distribution, and dispensing of controlled substances by legitimate handlers of these drugs to help reduce their widespread dispersion into illicit markets. Drugs covered by this act have a potential for causing drug dependence, abuse, or both and are classified according to their use and abuse potential.

The CSA classifies **controlled substances** into numbered levels, or schedules, from Schedule I to Schedule V (Table 2-1). Drugs with the highest abuse potential are placed in Schedule I; those with the lowest potential for abuse are in Schedule V. These classifications are flexible because drugs may occasionally be added or changed from one schedule to another without new legislation. It might be anticipated, for example, that marijuana will be changed to another schedule if and when it is accepted for use in treating nausea associated with cancer chemotherapy or for treatment of glaucoma. Some drugs with potential for dependence, such as ethanol and certain analgesics, are not listed as controlled substances. Anyone handling controlled substances must follow the more inclusive or stringent requirements of the laws, whether it be federal or state law.

In July 1973, the Drug Enforcement Administration (DEA) in the Department of Justice became the nation's sole legal drug-enforcement agency.

Possession of Controlled Substances

It is unlawful for any person to possess a controlled substance unless it has been obtained by a valid prescription or order or unless its possession is pursuant to actions in the course of professional practice. It is a federal offense to transfer a drug listed in Schedule II, III, or IV to any person other than the individual for whom the drug was ordered.

Drug suppliers and hospitals, as well as physicians, pharmacists, and nurses, are individually and collectively responsible for accounting for inventory and management of the flow and distribution of controlled substances. Institutional control of the flow of controlled substances is maintained by carefully recorded checks of the balance on hand, supplies added, and doses administered. Generally in a hospital setting, each dose is accounted for as it is administered, discarded, wasted, or withheld. Patient prescriptions or opioid drug supplies are stored in double-locked cabinets or other secure areas, with the keys assigned to a designated nurse or individual. Such protocols are necessary to safeguard the control of drug flow.

TABLE 2-1 Schedule of Controlled Substances

Schedule	Characteristics	Dispensing Restrictions	Examples
I	High abuse potential No accepted medical use—for research, analysis, or instruction only May lead to severe dependence	Approved protocol necessary	Opioids: heroin and many others Cannabis: hashish, marijuana Psychedelic: LSD, mescaline, PCP, psilocybin Other: methaqualone
II	High abuse potential Accepted medical uses May lead to severe physical or psychologic dependence	Written prescription necessary (signed by the practitioner)—emergency verbal prescriptions must be confirmed in writing within 72 hours No prescription refills allowed Container must have warning label*	Opioids: alfentanil, codeine, fentanyl, hydromorphone, levorphanol, meperidine, methadone, morphine, opium, oxycodone, oxymorphone, and others Barbiturates: amobarbital, pentobarbital, secobarbital Stimulants: amphetamine, cocaine, dextroamphetamine, methamphetamine, methylphenidate, and others Other: glutethimide
III	Less abuse potential than Schedules I and II Accepted medical uses May lead to moderate to low physical dependence or high psychologic dependence	Written or oral prescription required Prescription expires in 6 months No more than 5 prescription refills allowed within a 6-month period Container must have warning label*	Opioids: preparations that contain limited opioid quantity (hydrocodone liquids, paregoric) of opioid combined with one or more noncontrolled active ingredients (such as acetaminophen with codeine, aspirin with codeine, etc.) Barbiturates: aprobarbital, butabarbital, thiopental, and others. Steroids, anabolic: fluoxymesterone, dihydrotestosterone, methyltestosterone, nadrolone, stanozolol, testosterone, and others. Stimulants: benzphetamine, phendimetrazine
IV	Lower abuse potential than Schedule III Accepted medical uses May lead to limited physical or psychologic dependence	Written or oral prescription required Prescription expires in 6 months with no more than 5 prescription refills allowed Container must have warning label*	Opioids: d-proproxyphene, pentazocine Barbiturates: methohexital and others Benzodiazepines: alprazolam, chlordiazepoxide, clonazepam, clorazepate, diazepam, estazolam, flurazepam, lorazepam, midazolam, prazepam, temazepam, triazolam, and others. Stimulants: diethylpropion, fenfluramine, mazindol, pemoline, phentermine, and others Others: chloral hydrate, ethchlorvynol, meprobamate, paraldehyde, and others
V	Lower abuse potential than Schedule IV Accepted medical uses May lead to limited physical or psychologic dependence	May require written prescription or be sold without prescription (check state law)	Prescription: Opioids: buprenorphine, diphenooxylate with atropine Nonprescription: various cold or cough combinations with codeine

*Caution: Federal law prohibits the transfer of this drug to any person other than the patient for whom it was prescribed.
From *DEA pharmacist's manual—an informational outline of the Controlled Substance Act of 1970*, US Dept of Justice, Washington, DC, Red Book, 1996.

Additional Regulatory Bodies or Services

Food and Drug Administration

The Food and Drug Administration (FDA) is charged with the enforcement of the federal Food, Drug, and Cosmetic Act. Seizure of offending (improperly manufactured or packaged) goods and criminal prosecution of responsible persons or firms in federal courts are among the methods used to enforce the Act. In addition, pharmaceutical firms must report at regular intervals to the FDA all adverse effects associated with their new drugs.

The FDA also has an adverse-reaction reporting program. All healthcare professionals are encouraged to relate an unusual occurrence or unusually high number of occurrences associated with a drug, its formulation, or its packaging. Communication may be made directly to the FDA by telephone or by completing a Drug Experience Report form. A response from the FDA will follow. The purpose of this program is to detect reactions that have not been revealed by previous clinical or pharmaceutical studies. Changes in the drug package insert may result, or in some instances the drug may be withdrawn from the market.

Public Health Service

The Public Health Service is part of the U.S. Department of Health and Human Services. One of this agency's many functions is the regulation of biologic products. This refers to viral preparations, serums, antitoxins, or analogous products that are used for the prevention, treatment, or cure of diseases. The Public Health Service exercises control over these products by inspecting and licensing the establishments that manufacture them and by examining and licensing the products.

Product Liability

In most states, the rule of strict manufacturer's liability has been adopted. This doctrine holds manufacturers liable for injuries caused by defects in their products, drugs, or devices. **Product liability** exists if (1) a product is defective or not fit for its reasonably foreseeable uses, (2) the defect arose before the product left the control of the manufacturer, and (3) the defect caused some person harm. If these three criteria are met, the manufacturer must pay monetary damages for harm unless the liability can be shifted to some other party. Anyone harmed by a defective product has the right to sue the manufacturer for compensation.

Manufacturers are legally responsible for knowing the effects of their products. If an unknown risk could have been discovered through a reasonable amount of research, the manufacturer will be held liable for any resulting harm. Although many drug manufacturers have quality assurance programs, drug product errors in the manufacturing, packaging, and delivery processes may still occur. Detecting a chemical defect is difficult, but detecting a visual physical defect is common. Changes in color, a precipitate, or a foreign substance in a previously known clear solution are some warning signals to the professional. Such changes should be reported to the pharmacy department, drug manufacturer, or FDA for investigation. If a drug product is contaminated or defective, a drug recall is issued.

Drug Substitution

Nearly every state has a drug substitution law that either permits or mandates substitution on the part of the pharmacist, although the prescriber retains the prerogative to require the dispensing of a particular brand of drug. In permissive states, the prescriber must give express permission for substitution by either signing a special section on the prescription form or by checking the correct phrase on the prescription. If substitution is not wanted, the prescriber may note this by writing "dispense as written," "brand necessary," or "medically necessary."

In states with a mandatory law, the pharmacist is required to dispense approved, less-expensive, generic drugs to the patient. Several exceptions apply in such situations; for example, the consent of the patient may be required before substitution, or the prescriber may mark the individual prescription with a term that prohibits substitution, such as "medically necessary." Some states, such as Florida, have enacted a **negative drug formulary**, a list of drugs that have a proven potential for different bioavailabilities or therapeutic problems and that may not be substituted for trade name drugs (Box 2-2). If the prescriber orders a brand name for these products, then only that specific brand may be dispensed. If the prescriber orders any of these products by a generic name, then the pharmacist may select a generic drug product that is FDA approved (a drug with an approved new drug application [NDA] or abbreviated new drug application [ANDA]).

BOX 2-2 Florida Negative Drug Formulary List*

1. digoxin
2. digitoxin
3. quinidine gluconate
4. theophylline (controlled release)
5. warfarin
6. conjugated estrogens
7. chlorpromazine (solid oral dosage forms)
8. dicumarol
9. phenytoin
10. levothyroxine sodium
11. pancrelipase (oral dosage forms)

*This list may change in response to the publication of new information or evidence that can alter previous reviewed data (1997 data).

CANADIAN DRUG LEGISLATION

In Canada the Health Protection Branch (HPB) of the Department of National Health and Welfare is responsible for administration and enforcement of the Food and Drugs Act as well as the Proprietary or Patent Medicine Act and the Narcotic Control Act. These acts are designed to protect the consumer from health hazards and fraud or deception in the sale and use of foods, drugs, cosmetics, and medical devices. Canadian drug legislation began in 1875 when the Parliament of Canada passed an act to prevent the sale of adulterated food, drink, and drugs. Since that time foods and drugs have been controlled on a national basis.

Canadian Food and Drugs Act

In 1953 the present Canadian Food and Drugs Act was passed by the Senate and House of Commons of Canada. Since that time, the law has been amended often. The Act stipulates that no food, drug, cosmetic, or device is to be advertised or sold to the general public as a treatment, preventive, or cure for certain diseases listed in Schedule A of the Act. Among the diseases included in the list are alcoholism, arteriosclerosis, and cancer. When it is necessary to provide adequate directions for the safe use of a drug used to treat or prevent diseases mentioned in Schedule A, that disease or disorder may be mentioned on the labels and inserts accompanying the drug. In addition, the Act prohibits the sale of drugs that are contaminated, adulterated, or unsafe for use and those whose labels are false, misleading, or deceptive. According to the Act, drugs must comply with prescribed standards as stated in recognized pharmacopeias and formularies listed in Schedule B of the Act or with the professed standards under which the drug is sold. Recognized pharmacopeias and formularies include the following:

- Pharmacopoeia Internationalis
- The *British Pharmacopoeia* (*BP*)
- The *USP*
- Pharmacopée Française
- The Canadian Formulary
- British Pharmaceutical Codex

The legend "Canadian standard drug" or the abbreviation CSD must appear on the inner and outer labels of a drug to signify that it meets the standards prescribed for it.

Sale of certain drugs is prohibited unless the premises where the drug was manufactured and the process and conditions of manufacture have been approved by the Minister of National Health and Welfare. These drugs are listed in Schedules C and D and include injectable liver extracts, all insulin preparations, anterior pituitary extracts, radioactive isotopes, antibiotics for parenteral use, serums, drugs other than antibiotics prepared from microorganisms or viruses, and live vaccines. Distribution of samples of drugs is also prohibited except for distribution to duly licensed individuals such as physicians, dentists, or pharmacists. Schedule F of the Act contains a list of drugs that can be sold and refilled only by prescription. Refills may be permitted at specified intervals but cannot exceed 6 months. Drugs listed in Schedule F include antibiotics, hormones, and tranquilizers. They must always be properly and clearly labeled and include directions for use. Labels on containers of Schedule F drugs must be marked with the symbol uPr (prescription required). These drugs cannot be advertised to the general public other than giving the name, price, and quantity of the drug. See Table 2-2 for a summary of Canadian prescription (Schedules F and G) and restricted (Schedule H) drugs.

Controlled drugs are those listed in Schedule G of the Act and include amphetamines, barbituric acid and its derivatives (barbiturates), and phenmetrazine. Controlled drugs must be marked with the symbol eC in a clear and conspicuous color and size on the upper left quarter of the label. The proper name of the drug must appear on the labels, either immediately before or after the trade name. Controlled drugs can be dispensed only by prescription.

TABLE 2-2 Canadian Prescription and Restricted Drugs

Category	*Description*
Prescription Drugs	
Schedule F	May be used only after professional consultation; includes over 200 drugs, identified by uPr on the label
Schedule G (also called *controlled drugs*)	Affect the central nervous system (stimulants, sedatives); identified by eC on the label
Restricted Drugs	
Schedule H	Available only to institutions for research; present dangerous physiologic and psychologic side effects and have no recognized medical use

*For more specific information, see Health Protection and Drug Laws from Supply and Services Canada, Canadian Government Publishing Centre, Ottawa, Canada, KIA 059.

When a controlled drug is dispensed by prescription, the labels must carry the following:

- Name and address of the pharmacy or pharmacist
- Date and number of the prescription
- Name of the person for whom the controlled drug is dispensed
- Name of the practitioner
- Directions for use
- Any other information that the prescription requires be shown on the label

Prescriptions for controlled drugs cannot be refilled unless at the time the prescription was issued the practitioner so directed in writing and specified the number of times it could be refilled and the dates for or intervals between refilling. All information on the labels must be clearly and prominently displayed and readily discernible. Controlled drugs cannot be advertised to the general public.

Designated drugs are the following controlled drugs: (1) amphetamines, (2) methamphetamines, (3) phenmetrazine, and (4) phendimetrazine. Physicians may prescribe a designated drug for the following conditions: (1) narcolepsy, (2) hyperkinetic disorders in children, (3) mental retardation (minimal brain dysfunction), (4) epilepsy, (5) parkinsonism, and (6) hypotensive states associated with anesthesia. Permission can be obtained to prescribe amphetamines for patients with diagnoses other than those listed.

Restricted drugs are those listed in Schedule H of the Act and include the hallucinogenic drugs lysergic acid diethylamide (LSD), diethyltryptamine (DET), dimethyltryptamine (DMT), and dimethoxyamphetamine (STP, DOM). Sale of these drugs is prohibited. These drugs may be obtained for research by a qualified investigator if authorized by the Minister of National Health and Welfare. Precautions must be taken to ensure against loss or theft of a restricted drug.

Following are some of the additional requirements found in the Canadian food and Drugs Act:

1. Labels of drugs must show the following:
   a. Proper name of the drug immediately before or after the trade name
   b. Name and address of the manufacturer or distributor
   c. Lot number of the drug
   d. Adequate directions for use
   e. Quantitative list of medicinal ingredients and their proper or common names
   f. Net amount of drug
   g. Common or proper name and proportion of any preservatives used in parenteral drugs
   h. Expiration date if the drug does not maintain its potency, purity, and physical characteristics for at least 3 years from the date of manufacture
   i. Recommended single and daily adult dose; if the drug is for children, the label must state "Children: As directed by physician" or the following:

Age (yr)	Proportion of Adult Dose
10-14	One-half
5-9	One-fourth
2-4	One-sixth
Under 2	As directed by physician

   j. A warning that the drug be kept out of the reach of children and any precautions to be taken (e.g., "Caution: May be injurious if taken in large doses for a long time. Do not exceed the recommended dose without consulting a physician." Warning is to be preceded by a symbol—octagonal in shape, red in color, and on a white background)
   k. Contraindications and side effects if it is a nonprescription drug
   l. On and after July 1, 1974, the drug identification number assigned to the drug, preceded by the words "Drug Identification Number" or the abbreviation "D.I.N.", to be shown on the main labels of a drug sold in dosage form (i.e., one ready for use by the consumer)
2. Other specific regulations include the following:
   a. Manufacturers must be able to demonstrate that a drug in oral dosage form represented as releasing the drug at time intervals actually is released and available as represented.
   b. Oral tablets must disintegrate within 45 minutes. Enteric-coated tablets must not disintegrate for 60 minutes when exposed to gastric juice but must disintegrate within an additional 60 minutes when exposed to intestinal juices.
   c. Drugs containing boric acid or sodium borate as a medicinal ingredient must carry a statement that the drug should not be administered to infants or children under 3 years of age.
   d. Safety factors such as sterility and absence of pyrogens must be ensured in parenteral drugs.

The regulations allow the government to withdraw from the market drugs found to be unduly toxic. New drugs introduced to the market must have shown effectiveness and safety in human clinical studies to the satisfaction of the manufacturer and the government.

Canadian Narcotic Control Act

The regulations of the Canadian Narcotic Control Act govern the possession, sale, manufacture, production, and distribution of narcotics. The Canadian Narcotic Control Act was passed in 1961 and revoked the Canadian Opium and Narcotic Act of 1952. The 1961 Act has been amended several times.

Only authorized persons can be in possession of a narcotic. Authorized persons include a licensed dealer, pharmacist, practitioner, person in charge of a hospital, or a person acting as an agent for a practitioner. A licensed dealer is one who has been given permission to manufacture, produce, import, export, or distribute a narcotic. Practitioners include persons registered under the laws of a province to practice the profession of medicine, dentistry, or veterinary medicine. However, persons other than these may be licensed by the Minister of National Health and Welfare to cultivate and produce opium poppy or marijuana or to purchase and possess a narcotic for scientific purposes. Members of the Royal Canadian Mounted Police and members of technical or scientific departments of the government of Canada or of a province or university may possess narcotics in connection with their employment. A person who is undergoing treatment by a medical practitioner and who requires a narcotic may possess a narcotic obtained by prescription. This person may not knowingly obtain a narcotic from any other medical practitioner without notifying that practitioner that he or she is already undergoing treatment and obtaining a narcotic by prescription.

All persons authorized to be in possession of narcotics must keep a record of the name and quantity of all narcotics received, from whom narcotics were obtained, and to whom narcotics were supplied (including quantity, form, and dates of all transactions). In addition, they must ensure the safekeeping of all narcotics, keep full and complete records on all narcotics for at least 2 years, and report any loss or theft within 10 days of discovery.

The schedule of the Act lists those drugs, as well as their preparations, derivatives, alkaloids, and salts, that are subject to the Canadian Narcotic Control Act. Included in the schedule are opium, coca, and marijuana. Before a pharmacist may legally dispense a drug included in the schedule or a medication containing such a drug, he or she must receive a prescription from a physician. A signed and dated prescription issued by a duly authorized physician is essential in the case of any narcotic medication prescribed as such or any preparation containing a narcotic in a form intended for parenteral administration. Medications containing a narcotic and two or more nonnarcotic ingredients may be dispensed by a pharmacist on the strength of a verbal prescription received from a physician who is known to the pharmacist or whose identity is established. Prescriptions of any narcotic drug may not be refilled.

There is one exception to the prescription requirement. Certain codeine compounds with a small codeine content may be sold to the public by a pharmacist without a prescription. In such instances the narcotic content cannot exceed 8 mg per tablet or 20 mg/28 ml. In products of this kind, codeine must be in combination with two or more nonnarcotic substances and in recognized therapeutic doses.

Additionally, items of this nature are required to be labeled in such a fashion as to show the true formula of the medicinal ingredients and a caution to the following effect: "This preparation contains codeine and should not be administered to children except on the advice of a physician." These preparations cannot be advertised or displayed in a pharmacy. It is also unlawful to publish any narcotic advertisement for the general public.

Labels on containers of narcotics must legibly and conspicuously bear the trade name and generic names of the narcotic, the names of the manufacturer and distributor, the symbol "N" in the upper left-hand quarter, and the net contents of the container and of each tablet, capsule, or ampule.

Although the administration of the Canadian Narcotic Control Act is legally the responsibility of the Department of National Health and Welfare, the enforcement of the law has been made largely the responsibility of the Royal Canadian Mounted Police. Prosecution of offenses under the Act is handled through the Department of National Health and Welfare by legal agents specially appointed by the Department of Justice.

The Narcotic Control Act defines a narcotic addict as "a person who through the use of narcotics has developed a desire or need to continue to take a narcotic, or has developed a psychological or physical dependence upon the effect of a narcotic." A person brought into court for a narcotic offense may be placed in custody by the court for observation and examination. If the person is convicted of the offense and found to be a narcotic addict, the court can sentence him or her to custody for treatment for an indefinite period.

Amendments to this Act place special restrictions on methadone. No practitioner can administer, prescribe, give, sell, or furnish methadone to any person unless the practitioner has been issued an authorization by the Minister of National Health and Welfare.

STANDARDIZATION OF DRUGS

Drugs may vary considerably in strength and activity. Drugs obtained from plants such as opium and digitalis may fluctuate in strength from plant to plant depending on where the plants are grown, the age at which they are harvested, and how they are preserved. Since accurate dosage and reliability of a drug's effect depend on uniformity of strength and purity, standardization is necessary.

The technique, either chemical or biologic, by which the strength and purity of a drug are measured is known as **assay.** Chemical assay is a chemical analysis to determine the ingredients present and their amounts. For example, opium is known to contain certain alkaloids, and these may vary greatly in different preparations. The United States' official standard demands that opium must contain no less than 9.5% and no more than 10.5% of anhydrous morphine. Opium of a higher morphine content may be reduced to the official standard by admixture with opium of a lower percentage or with certain other pharmacologically inactive diluents such as sucrose, lactose, glycyrrhiza, or magnesium carbonate.

In the case of some drugs, either the active ingredients are not known or there are no available methods of analyzing and standardizing them. These drugs may be standardized by biologic methods, or **bioassay.** Bioassay is performed by determining the amount of a preparation required to produce a defined effect on a suitable laboratory animal under certain standard conditions. For example, the potency of a certain sample of insulin is measured by its ability to lower the blood glucose level of rabbits.

Drug Standards in the United States

Since 1980 the only official book of drug standards in the United States has been the *USP.* Any drug included in this book has met high standards of quality, purity, and strength. Drugs meeting these criteria can be identified by the letters U.S.P. after the official name.

Although numerous additional reference books and guides are available on the market, two very valuable resources for drug information in a clinical setting are *USP DI: Volume 1, Drug Information for the Health Care Professional* and the *AHFS Drug Information.* The *USP DI* contains information for both the healthcare provider and the patient. Drug information resources are reviewed in Chapter 1.

Drug Standards in Great Britain and Canada

The *BP* is similar to the *USP* in scope and purpose. Drugs listed in the *BP* are considered official and subject to legal control in the United Kingdom and those parts of the British Commonwealth in which the *BP* has statutory force. The *USP* is used a great deal in Canada, and some preparations used in Canada conform to the *USP* instead of the *BP* because many of the drugs used in Canada are manufactured in the United States.

The *British Pharmaceutical Codex* is published by the Pharmaceutical Society of Great Britain. In general, it resembles the *National Formulary.* The Canadian formulary contains formulas for preparations used extensively in Canada. It also contains standards for new drugs prescribed in Canada but not included in the *BP.* The Canadian formulary has been given official status by the Canadian Food and Drugs Act.

The Physician's Formulary contains formulas for preparations that are representative of the needs of medical practice in Canada. It is published by the Canadian Medical Association.

INTERNATIONAL DRUG CONTROL

International control of drugs legally began in 1912 when the first "Opium Conference" was held at The Hague. International treaties were drawn up legally obligating governments to (1) limit to medical and scientific needs the manufacturing of and trade in medicinal opium, (2) control the production and distribution of raw opium, and (3) establish a system of governmental licensing to control the manufacture of and trade in drugs covered by the convention.

In 1961, government representatives formulated the "Single Convention on Narcotic Drugs," which became effective in 1964. This act consolidated all existing treaties into one document for the control of all narcotic substances by doing the following:

- Outlawing the production, manufacture, trade, and use of narcotic substances for nonmedicinal purposes.
- Limiting possession of all narcotic substances to authorized persons for medical and scientific purposes.
- Providing for international control of all opium transactions by the national monopolies (countries designated to produce opium, such as Turkey) and authorizing production only by licensed farmers in areas and on plots designated by these monopolies.
- Requiring import certificates and export authorizations.

An **International Narcotics Control Board** was established to enforce this law. This Board is an international organization of governmental representatives established to enforce the "Single Convention on Narcotic Drugs." Since enforcement is an immense task, it is impossible to prevent illicit trafficking in drugs. For example, during a 1-year period it was estimated that 1200 tons of opium were circulated in the illicit market when 800 tons were considered sufficient for world medical needs. Laws need to be frequently updated and strictly enforced, but the unfortunate fact is that financial support for regulation and enforcement is sometimes not equal to the task.

INVESTIGATIONAL DRUGS

The multibillion dollar pharmaceutical industry is constantly screening substances with potential to market as new drugs. Prospective drugs may take years and large amounts of capital to progress through the following FDA-required testing sequence:

1. Animal studies, to ascertain the following:
   a. Toxicity
      (1) Acute toxicity. As represented by the **LD_{50}** (the median lethal dose; the dose that is lethal to 50% of the laboratory animals tested).
      (2) Subacute toxicity
      (3) Chronic toxicity
   b. **Therapeutic index.** A quantitative measure of the relative safety of a drug; the ratio of the LD_{50} to the median effective dose
   c. Modes of absorption, distribution, metabolism (biotransformation), and excretion (pharmacokinetics)
2. Human studies
   a. *Phase I.* Initial pharmacologic evaluation
   b. *Phase II.* Limited controlled evaluation
   c. *Phase III.* Extended clinical evaluation

A noteworthy lack of correlation exists between levels of toxicity in animals and adverse effects in humans. In addition, many symptoms of adverse effects in humans simply cannot be determined in animals. A partial list of common human symptoms that are not measurably distinguishable in animals includes dizziness, nausea, drowsiness, nervousness, indigestion, headache, and weakness.

FDA Approval Process

The FDA approval process and specifications are as follows:

1. **Investigational New Drug (IND).** If a pharmaceutical company or individual desires to investigate a new drug substance or an old drug for a new indication or at a different unapproved dosage in humans, an IND application must be completed and submitted to the FDA. The IND will include evidence of drug safety by providing animal or clinical information, proof of the investigator's qualifications to perform this research, and evidence of the drug product's proven quality and strength. The investigation covered under the IND is divided into three phases:
   a. *Phase I: Initial pharmacologic evaluation.* A small number of normal individuals (usually volunteers) take the drug so that the investigators can determine the pharmacokinetics of the agent (absorption, distribution, metabolism, routes of elimination or excretion). Blood tests, urine analysis, vital signs, and specific monitoring tests are performed during this phase.
   b. *Phase II: Limited controlled evaluation.* The drug is administered at gradually increasing dosages to selected individuals with the targeted disease. For example, if the product is believed to have antihypertensive properties, individuals with documented hypertension would be chosen for this phase. During this phase, the individual is closely monitored for drug effectiveness and for side effects. If no serious side or adverse effects occur, the study progresses to phase III.
   c. *Phase III: Extended clinical evaluation.* The drug is now ready for testing in various centers in the United States in larger numbers of individuals. Standards (protocols) have been developed and are to be followed at all investigative sites. The three objectives for this phase are (1) determination of clinical effectiveness, (2) drug safety determination, and (3) establishment of tolerated dosage or dosage range.

   Several other factors are involved with this program. First, the investigator reports to the FDA after completion of each phase and needs FDA approval before progressing to the next phase. Second, a double-blind study may be instituted, usually in phase II or phase III. A double-blind study involves the administration of the research drug or a placebo (such as lactose) or a marketed drug with the same pharmacologic effects as the drug being studied. All of the products are formulated to look the same and then packaged, usually by code numbers. Generally no one involved with the study knows whether the patient is taking the study (active) drug or the placebo. By this method, bias is eliminated and the evaluation is done accurately on the basis of therapeutic response.
2. **New Drug Application (NDA).** After the completion of phase II of the IND and assuming that the data collected indicate that the new drug is very promising, investigators submit all the collected data to the FDA. After careful review of the information, the FDA may approve or reject the NDA. If the NDA is approved, the drug product can be marketed for the selected indication in the dosing schedules as studied. If the NDA is rejected, the FDA may require additional studies or information before reconsideration.

3. **Abbreviated New Drug Application** (ANDA) (for generic drug approval). Generic formulations of currently marketed medications are not usually required to repeat all the previous steps before marketing. A company is required to prove that its product can produce the same therapeutic effects as the already marketed drug. Although nearly all generic drugs require the ANDA, the FDA may require different methods to prove generic equivalency, depending on the drug. For example, chlordiazepoxide (Librium) and amitriptyline (Elavil) require in vivo studies; that is, the generic drug must be given to humans, and data from blood and urine studies should be equivalent to data obtained when the name brand product is given, according to statistical analysis. Other drug products, such as chlorpheniramine (Chlor-Trimeton) and dexamethasone (Decadron), only need to prove that the manufacturing process is in compliance with Good Manufacturing Practice guidelines and that their quality control standards are equivalent. Thus the FDA establishes the criteria according to the drug product, the possibility of bioequivalency problems, or the lack of such problems. Drugs marketed before 1938, such as chloral hydrate and phenobarbital, do not require an approved ANDA before marketing.

The professional should be aware of several limitations in the testing and marketing process. The number of persons studied and the time allotted for the study are limited. Also, certain types of individuals are excluded from the study, such as children, pregnant women, persons with multiple disease states, and the elderly. If a drug is considered safe and effective during the time of study, with the previously mentioned limitations, it is marketed. Once marketed, the drug is used in much greater numbers of patients, probably for longer periods; thus it is inevitable that the drug will be reported to produce additional effects (possibly therapeutic but often adverse) that were not noted during the trial studies.

Therefore a phase IV, or postmarketing surveillance period, has been advocated to monitor and tabulate information about new drugs to disseminate it to healthcare professionals and consumers. This is a more difficult phase to supervise since it depends on the voluntary reports of persons in the medical field. The importance of this phase should not be underestimated because it will affect many more people than the previous three phases combined. See Box 2-3 on classifications for newly approved drugs.

In 1993 the FDA initiated **MedWatch,** a voluntary program to enhance the reporting by healthcare professionals of adverse effects they suspect are related to medications and medical devices. The verification of an adverse effect is not necessary. It is important to inform the agency of medication or medical device related events that are suspected to have resulted in death or the risk of death, hospitalization, persistent or permanent disability, birth defect, or the need for medical intervention to prevent permanent impairment. The FDA is requesting information about products even if patients are not involved in the incident, such as possible contaminated products or a product labeling that might be confusing. Confidentiality is maintained in the reporting. The paperwork is a one-page form that can be obtained from the hospital's pharmacy or risk manager.

BOX 2-3 FDA Classifications for Newly Approved Drugs

To assist the professional in immediately classifying new drug entities, the FDA has developed the following method of drug classification. A number and a letter are assigned to each new drug at the IND phase or at the NDA review by the FDA. The manufacturer has a right to contest this classification and have it changed before the final classification is established.

Numerical Classification (Chemical)

1. A new molecular drug
2. A new salt of a marketed drug
3. A new formulation or dosage form not previously marketed
4. A new combination not previously marketed
5. A drug that is already on the market, a generic duplication
6. A product already marketed by the same company (this designation is used for new indications for a marketed drug)
7. A drug product on the market without an approval NDA (drug was marketed prior to 1938)

Letter Classification (Treatment or Therapeutic Potential)

P Drug offers an important therapeutic gain (P-priority)
S Drug that is similar to drugs already on the market (S-standard)

Other Classifications

AA Drugs indicated for AIDS or HIV-related disease
E Drug developed to treat life-threatening or severely debilitating illnesses
V An orphan drug

The above classification is available by request from the Freedom of Information Staff at the Bureau of Drugs (Food and Drug Administration, 5600 Fishers Lane, Rockville, MD, 20857).

Informed Consent

Any participant in an investigational drug study should be an informed volunteer. The informed consent form should contain detailed information about the study, potential benefits, and side and adverse effects. This information should be discussed with the individual by a designated member of the research team before obtaining a signed approval. All guidelines (federal, state, and institutional) are closely adhered to in this process.

Pregnancy Safety Categories

The FDA has assigned pregnancy safety categories for drugs studied in humans and animals, based on documentation. The categories are as follows:

Category A Adequate and well-controlled studies indicate no risk to the fetus in the first trimester of pregnancy (and there is no evidence of risk in later trimesters).

Category B Animal reproduction studies indicate no risk to the fetus, and there are no well-controlled studies in pregnant women.

Category C	Animal reproduction studies have reported adverse effects on the fetus; and there are no well-controlled studies in humans, but potential benefits may indicate use of the drug in pregnant women despite potential risks.
Category D	Positive human fetal risk has been reported in data from investigational or marketing experience, or human studies. Considering potential benefit versus risk may, in selected cases, warrant the use of these drugs in pregnant women.
Category X	Fetal abnormalities reported and positive evidence of fetal risk in humans is available from animal or human studies. The risks involved clearly outweigh the potential benefits. These drugs should not be used in pregnant women.

Orphan Drugs

In 1983 the FDA established an Orphan Drug Act that provided grants that encourage research to find drugs for treatment of rare chronic diseases. Because such research was unprofitable, it was very limited before this act. Among the disorders that benefit from this research are cystic fibrosis, Von Willebrand's disease, leprosy (Hansen's disease), AIDS, and rare cancers. Nearly 500 drugs were discovered under this Act (Olin, 1998).

SUMMARY

The road to market of a new drug product requires an initial drug discovery, drug standardization, animal and human testing, FDA approval, and marketing requirements before a new drug reaches the consumer. Each step along the way, the various laws and legal requirements previously reviewed were established to remove or eliminate unsafe or ineffective drugs from reaching the marketplace. The ultimate purpose of this lengthy process was to protect the consumer by approving only medications that were proved to be safe and effective.

Because the investigational studies before FDA approval are limited, postmarketing surveillance (MedWatch) is very important in identifying adverse reactions or serious problems not previously identified. The success of this voluntary program requires the cooperation of healthcare professionals.

The distinction between prescription and over-the-counter (OTC) drugs and the regulations that govern controlled substance use and limit potential abuse directly impact the individual in clinical practice.

Canadian legislation also regulates to protect its citizens. The Canadian Food and Drugs Act establishes drug standards and the Narcotic Control Act governs narcotic manufacture, production, and distribution. The only official book of drug standards in the United States is the *United States Pharmacopeia* (*USP*), whereas Canada uses the *USP*, the *Canadian Formulary*, and the *British Pharmacopoeia* (*BP*).

The healthcare professional must have a thorough working knowledge of the federal drug acts and individual state laws and practice acts to safely practice in the healthcare profession today.

REVIEW QUESTIONS

1. Discuss the importance of the Durham-Humphrey Amendment to the professional and consumer today.
2. Describe the five schedules under the Controlled Substances Act. Name two drugs that fall under each schedule.
3. How does the Controlled Substances Act affect you as a health professional?
4. Describe the advantages and disadvantages of investigational animal and human studies. Trace the three phases of human studies.
5. Discuss the pregnancy safety categories. Which category of drugs should definitely be avoided for use in the pregnant woman?

REFERENCES

Covington TR, editor: *Handbook of nonprescription drugs,* ed 10, Washington, DC, 1996, American Pharmaceutical Association.

Drug Enforcement Administration: *Pharmacist's manual: an informational outline of the Controlled Substance Act of 1970,* Washington, DC, 1996, US Department of Justice.

Olin BR: *Facts and comparisons,* Philadelphia, 1998, Facts and Comparisons.

ADDITIONAL REFERENCES

Anderson KN et al, editor: *Mosby's medical, nursing, & allied health dictionary,* ed 5, St Louis, 1998, Mosby.

Blake JB, editor: *Safeguarding the public: historical aspects of medicinal drug control.* Baltimore, Md, 1968, The Johns Hopkins University Press.

Couig MP, Merkatz RB: MedWatch: the new medical products reporting program, *Am J Nurs* 93(8):66, 1993.

Cowen DL, Helfand WH: *Pharmacy: an illustrated history.* New York, 1990, Harry N Abrams.

Dippel JVH: Legally speaking: reporting to the FDA, *RN* 56(12):61, 1993.

Farley D: How FDA approves new drugs, *FDA Consum* 21(10):6, 1988.

Florida negative drug formulary, *Florida Pharmacy Law & Information Manual,* Board of Pharmacy: Rule 59X-27.500, 100-Pharmacy, 1997, p. 40.

Mosby: *Mosby's GenRx,* St Louis, 1998, Mosby.

New FDA classification system, *Am Pharm* NS32(4):11, 1992.

Shapiro RS: Legal bases for the control of analgesic drugs, *J Pain Sympt Manag* 9(3):153, 1994.

United States Pharmacopeial Convention: *USP DI: drug information for the health care professional,* ed 18, Rockville, Md, 1998, the Convention.

CHAPTER 3

Over-the-Counter and Alternative Medications

KEY DRUGS

acetaminophen (p. 25)
aspirin (p. 28)

CHAPTER FOCUS

With proper use, over-the-counter (OTC), or nonprescription, drugs are considered safe for the treatment of minor illnesses without the supervision of a licensed healthcare professional. Problems relating to the use of these products can occur, such as side effects, drug-drug interactions, drug toxicity, and drug misuse or abuse. Alternative medicines such as herbal therapies are commonly employed today. Because the Food and Drug Administration (FDA) does not review these agents for safety and effectiveness, healthcare professionals need to be informed about the use of and potential problems associated with such products.

OBJECTIVES

After reading and studying this chapter, the student should be able to do the following:

1. *Define and discuss the key drugs and key terms.*
2. *Discuss the effect of product ingredients in treating a minor illness and their effects on patient drug allergies, special diets, and underlying medical conditions.*
3. *Describe the recommended procedure for taking solid dosage form medications.*
4. *Explain the basic information necessary for proper selection of an OTC product in the following categories: analgesics, antacids, laxatives, cough-cold preparations, and antidiarrheal agents.*
5. *Discuss the difference between Eastern and Western approaches to illness; the laws governing herbals in the United States; and the healthcare professional's role regarding safe OTC drug and herbal consumption.*

KEY TERMS

analgesic, (p. 25)
antacids, (p. 30)
antihistamines, (p. 41)
antitussive, (p. 41)
chronic diarrhea, (p. 38)
constipation, (p. 32)
decongestants, (p. 42)
diarrhea, (p. 35)
expectorants, (p. 42)
Food and Drug Administration (FDA), (p. 23)
laxatives, (p. 32)

OTC medications are used by the general public to self-treat minor illnesses. Such preparations are readily available in pharmacies, supermarkets, and other nonpharmacy outlets for selection by individuals who want to avoid the time and expense involved with going to a prescriber. The Nonprescription Drug Manufacturers' Association reports that Americans visit their physicians for only 10% of their illnesses and injuries, and the Health Care Financing Administration (HCFA) states that 6 out of every 10 medications purchased are OTC medications. OTC drugs are a tremendous market; it has been estimated that there are over 300,000 OTC products available in the United States. These products contain from 700 to 1000 active ingredients (Burns, 1991; Zimmerman, 1993). When used wisely, they result in time and money savings for the individual and ultimately a reduction in overall healthcare costs. A good example of these cost savings is hydrocortisone cream, a product commonly used to treat rash and pruritus. When the cream became available as an OTC preparation, it was estimated to have saved Americans more than $1 billion over a 3-year period as compared with the medical model of physician visits, prescriptions, and other related costs (Burns, 1991).

Although OTC medications are generally considered to be safe and effective for consumer use, it is apparent that problems can result from their usage. For example, self-medication requires self-diagnosis of the signs and symptoms of a clinical condition. Generally, the public may consider most illnesses to be minor. However, if a potentially serious condition is self-treated with OTC medications, the condition may be masked, and the seeking of professional help for appropriate treatment may be delayed (Covington, 1996). Also, OTC drugs may contain potent chemicals, many of which were previously prescription drugs. The biggest trend in the 1990s is to transfer more prescription medications to OTC status. Thus the healthcare professional should be aware that many OTC products (new and old) are capable of producing both desired and undesirable effects, drug interactions, and drug toxicity. This potential problem has been recognized by a current pharmacy law (Omnibus Budget Reconciliation Act, or OBRA), which mandates that OTC drugs be considered an important part of the individual's medical record (Fitzgerald, 1994).

Although the **Food and Drug Administration (FDA)** issued regulations that require OTC package labeling be stated in terms that are likely to be read and understood by the average consumer, many consumers believe that the labels are confusing and that often the print is too small to read. Approximately 35% of Americans read at a sixth to tenth grade level, and an estimated 20% are considered functionally illiterate (that is, they have a reading level below the fifth grade level) (Covington, 1996). Therefore OTC labeling that is difficult to understand and apply may result in unsafe and possibly improper use of the medication.

This chapter reviews the regulatory difference between a prescription and OTC drug and discusses the process of a drug being changed from prescription to OTC status, general considerations on drug marketing, consumer education for safe administration of OTC drugs, and selected major OTC drug categories.

DIFFERENCE BETWEEN A PRESCRIPTION AND OVER-THE-COUNTER DRUG

The FDA regulates and makes decisions about the safety and effectiveness of drugs, the classification of a product as a prescription or OTC drug, and the information printed on the drug labels. Thus drug substances are subjected to regulation, review, and various study requirements before being released and to a limited extent may be monitored afterward. Medications not considered safe enough for use by the general public without medical supervision are restricted to prescription status only. OTC drugs are defined as safe and effective drugs for self-treatment by the public, assuming good manufacturing practices are followed by the manufacturer and the label directions are followed by the consumer.

Because many drugs were marketed without the more current standards of proof of documented safety and effectiveness, in 1972 the FDA established a number of OTC expert advisory panels to review drug categories and make recommendations to the FDA. As a result of this review, many ingredients used in such products were removed from the market, mainly because they lacked proof of effectiveness for their claims. Examples include aphrodisiacs, hair growers, and hexachlorophene products. These drugs were found to be either ineffective, dangerous, or both. In 1991 the FDA established an OTC Drugs Advisory Committee to assist in the review and evaluation and to advise the FDA Commissioner on its findings and recommendations. The Committee may also suggest prescription drugs to change to OTC status based on expert findings that the medication is safe and effective for use by the general public. The definitions for OTC drug safety and effectiveness include the following:

- *Safety:* The drug product has a low incidence of severe side effects and a low potential for harm assuming that proper instructions and adequate warnings are given on the label.
- *Effectiveness:* The drug ingredient when properly used will provide relief of the minor symptom or illness in a significant portion of the population.

CHANGE OF A DRUG FROM PRESCRIPTION TO OTC STATUS

In the past few years the FDA has approved a number of ingredients in prescription drugs to be sold as OTC medications, including 17 new products in 1995 (Newton, Pray, Popovich, 1996). With some products a lower strength of the active ingredient in the OTC product was required, whereas with others the same prescription strength was released OTC. For example, ibuprofen (Motrin) was released in a 200 mg strength as an OTC drug, whereas the higher dose tablet strengths, 400 or 800 mg, still require a prescrip-

TABLE 3-1 Prescription Drugs Changed to OTC Status

Ingredient Prescription Name	OTC Name	Principal Use
brompheniramine (Dimetane, etc.)	Dimetane, Bromphen, etc.	antihistamine
clemastine (Tavist)	Tavist, etc.	antihistamine
chlorpheniramine (Chlor-Trimeton, etc.)	Chlor-Trimeton, Aller-chlor, etc.	antihistamine
cimetidine (Tagamet)	Tagamet HB	heartburn, acid indigestion
clotrimazole (Lotrimin, etc.)	Lotrimin AF, Zeasorb-AF, etc.	antifungal
diphenhydramine (Benadryl)	Benylin Cough, Diphen Cough, etc.	cough
diphenhydramine (Benadryl)	Nytol, Sominex, etc.	sleeping aid
famotidine (Pepcid)	Pepcid AC	heartburn, acid indigestion
hydrocortisone (Cort Dome, etc.)	Cortizone, Dermolate, etc.	topical for itching and rash
ibuprofen (Motrin)	Advil, Nuprin, etc.	analgesic
ketoconazole	Nizoral	dandruff shampoo
loperamide (Imodium, etc.)	Imodium A-D, Kaopectate II, etc.	antidiarrheal
miconazole (Monistat)	Micatin, etc.	antifungal
nicotine polacrilex	Nicorette	smoking cessation
nicotine transdermal	Nicotrol, Nicoderm CQ	smoking cessation
nizatidine (Axid)	Axid AR	heartburn, acid
pyrantel (Antiminth)	Reese's Pinworm, etc.	pinworm remedy
sodium fluoride	Fluorigard, ACT, etc.	dental rinse
tioconazole	Vagistat-1	anticandidal
triprolidine (Myidyl, etc.)	Actidil, etc.	antihistamine

tion. The lower strength of ibuprofen is considered to be safe and effective for self-treatment of a minor illness, if the label instructions are followed. Use of higher strength ibuprofen requires medical supervision and a prescription because it has the potential of causing serious side or adverse effects. See Table 3-1 for examples of prescription drugs that have been changed to OTC drugs.

Drug Marketing

In contrast to prescription drugs, OTC medications may be marketed without FDA approval. Monographs of information developed by the OTC drug review identified specific drugs "generally recognized as safe and effective" (GRASE). Therefore any drug manufacturer may produce such products for market without government approval. The manufacturer, however, has flexibility in package labeling. Although it is required to use certain approved terminology (e.g., heartburn, acid indigestion, and sour stomach for antacids), other terms may also be used that have not been approved as long as they are not false or misleading.

In contrast to prescription medications, no regulations require the reporting of OTC adverse reactions. Also the manufacturer may substitute a GRASE ingredient in an OTC preparation for another GRASE ingredient without changing the name of the OTC drug and without indicating the change to the public by placing a warning on the package or label. The only method of determining a product's ingredients is to check the label for the listing of ingredients before each purchase (Covington, 1996).

Another important concept to understand is the difference between drug potency and drug effectiveness. Drug potency is the amount of drug required to produce a desired effect. When drug manufacturers claim that their product is more potent than another product, this usually means that less of the drug is necessary to produce the same effect as the comparison drug. This does not mean that the more potent drug is also the more effective drug (unless greater effectiveness has been proven and clearly stated); it only refers to the amount of drug necessary to produce a desired effect. This terminology is often used and may be misleading if the difference between potency and effectiveness is not understood by healthcare providers or consumers.

OTC analgesics have many extra strength dosage forms that imply greater potency than the regular strength of the same brand or the competitor's usual adult strength product (usually 500 mg compared with 325 mg of analgesic). However, if a more potent drug does not have documented proof of greater effectiveness when compared with an equivalent dose of the second drug, then there is no advantage to a "more potent" medication. When the only difference is drug strength, the therapeutic effect expected with either drug is the same, and the potential disadvantages in using a more potent drug may increase costs and side effects and have unknown long-term effects.

CONSUMER EDUCATION FOR OVER-THE-COUNTER DRUGS

OTC drugs are misconceived as being very safe and thus not requiring the special precautions necessary to take a prescription drug safely. These products also have the potential for being misused, abused, and inducing side and adverse effects. They also may be very dangerous if taken in certain concurrent disease states or if taken concurrently with other drugs, food, or alcohol. The healthcare professional needs to be aware of this information before administering or advising about an OTC preparation.

Product ingredients have either proven or questionable effectiveness; therefore a careful check of ingredients is necessary to select the appropriate product in a specific drug category. Teach the consumer to select the proper ingredient for treatment of the specific symptom the consumer is experiencing. Combination products may contain substances that are not necessary for the person's symptoms. If the individual has an adverse reaction to the combination drug, it would be difficult to determine the responsible ingredient.

In addition, many different products may also have the same active ingredients that may or may not differ in strength, dosage forms (liquid, tablet, capsule), or with other ingredients in combination. If the ingredients are not carefully checked, accidental overdosing is possible by taking the same ingredient in many different products. Another aspect of having the same ingredients is that it may allow for product substitution. For example, thousands of antacid products are available throughout the United States that primarily contain only four or five recognized active ingredients. Thus many OTC antacids are duplicate preparations. The generic product is often as effective as the advertised product; therefore there is usually little, if any, advantage in purchasing the more expensive item.

Consumers should check the selected product for tampering. Most products are now packaged in tamper-resistant packaging or tampering-evident packaging, which allows the consumer to detect signs of tampering. If the package is suspect, it should be taken to the pharmacist or store manager. The expiration date should also be checked to ensure that it has not passed.

Consumers should read labels very carefully if they have ever had an allergic or unusual response to any medication, food, or other substance, such as yellow dye or sulfites, to ensure that such an ingredient is not included. Caution should be used if the individual is on a special diet, such as low-sugar or low-sodium, because many OTC drugs contain more than their active ingredients, and the liquid preparations may contain sugar or alcohol. Women who are pregnant or breastfeeding should not take OTC medications without first consulting the healthcare provider. Individuals with underlying medical conditions, such as hypertension or diabetes, should read labels carefully to assess whether the medication may be contraindicated with their condition.

OTC medications are just that—medications. They should be reported to any healthcare provider when a drug history is being taken. Instructions and warnings on the label are to be followed carefully. If the instructions seem unclear, ask the pharmacist for clarification. If the symptoms for which the OTC drug is being taken are not relieved in an appropriate time as indicated on the label, a healthcare provider should be consulted.

Unless instructed otherwise, store both prescription and OTC medications in closed containers in a cool, dry place, out of the reach of children. Do not store in the bathroom, near sinks, or in damp places because heat, moisture, and strong light may cause deterioration or loss of medication potency.

All solid-dose medications (tablets and capsules) should be taken with a full glass of water (8 oz). The individual should be advised to sit up for approximately 15 to 30 minutes after taking the solid-dose medication to help reduce the potential for esophageal irritation or injury. If the person has a problem with dry mouth or minor problems in swallowing, taking a small amount of water before taking a tablet or capsule is very helpful. If the drug is a long-acting medication, it should be swallowed whole. If the medication is in a liquid form, the specially marked measuring spoon or other device provided by the manufacturer should be used to measure each dose accurately.

SELECTED OTC DRUG CATEGORIES

The following is a review of the most commonly purchased OTC drug categories: analgesics, antacids, laxatives, antidiarrheals, and cold-cough preparations. The information includes a review of the ingredients in each category, mechanisms of action, indications, pharmacokinetics, warnings, drug interactions, and specific tips on the proper and safe use of the individual product. This information should assist the healthcare professional in identifying and evaluating the multitude of OTC medications on the market. By understanding the basic information presented in this chapter and checking package ingredients, a safer and more logical approach to product selection can be made.

ANALGESICS

Pain is one of the most common and feared symptoms. For minor pain such as headache, toothache, muscle and joint aches, swelling (inflammation), and fever, many people can obtain relief inexpensively with an OTC medication. **Analgesic** is the term used to describe a drug that relieves pain.

Since OTC analgesics have different therapeutic effects, side effects, drug interactions, and other characteristics, they are divided into the three major categories available OTC: acetaminophen, aspirin, and nonsteroidal antiinflammatory drugs (NSAIDs).

acetaminophen [a seat a min′ oh fen]

Many brand name products of acetaminophen are available, including Tylenol, Anacin-3, Feverall Sprinkle, Liquiprin, Panadol, and Tempra. The mechanism of action for acetaminophen is primarily inhibition of prostaglandin synthesis in the central nervous system (CNS) and to a lesser degree blocking of the generation of peripheral pain impulses. Acetaminophen is equivalent to aspirin as an analgesic and antipyretic agent, but it does not have antiinflammatory effects. Acetaminophen has been used to treat mild forms of arthritis (osteoarthritis), but aspirin or NSAIDs are preferred in moderate to severe arthritis, especially rheumatoid arthritis (Box 3-1).

BOX 3-1 **Common Types of Arthritis**

Osteoarthritis, or degenerative joint disease, affects 85% of persons over 70 years of age, although symptoms may start in the fifth or sixth decade of life. This common form of arthritis is the result of deformation or dismatched joint surfaces rather than an inflammatory disease as in rheumatoid arthritis. Symptoms include joint stiffness that usually lasts only a few minutes after initiating joint movement and perhaps an aching pain in weight-bearing joints. Early disease stages may respond to local heat and OTC analgesics. Later stages may require orthopedic or other interventions.

Rheumatoid arthritis usually occurs between 30 to 70 years of age, more often in women than in men. Early symptoms may include feelings of fatigue and weakness, joint pain and stiffness and several weeks later, joint swelling. Joints are inflamed (warm, red, swollen) and often are limited in range of motion. This is a progressive disease that leads to joint deformity. Aspirin and aspirin type products (NSAIDs) are usually necessary to reduce the inflammation around the joints. Heat therapy, weight control, and exercise may also be helpful.

Acetaminophen offers several advantages over aspirin, including the following:

- May be used by people allergic to aspirin
- Rarely causes abdominal upset, tinnitus, or gastric bleeding (inhibition of platelet aggregation) as reported more often with aspirin
- May be used by patients taking anticoagulant medications
- May be used by children with colds and flu symptoms because it has not been associated with Reye's syndrome as reported with aspirin (Box 3-2)

Pharmacokinetically, acetaminophen taken orally is rapidly absorbed, reaching peak serum levels in ½ to 1 hour and its half-life in 2 to 3 hours. It is metabolized in the liver and excreted by the kidneys. Side or adverse effects are rare with acetaminophen, although in some instances nausea and rash have occurred. However, the drug should be discontinued and a healthcare provider should be contacted immediately if an allergic type of reaction (hives, pruritus, respiratory difficulties), blood in the urine or stool, severe pain in the side or lower back, or unusual bleeding, bruising, weakness or tiredness occurs.

Acetaminophen overdose can cause serious damage to the liver and kidneys. (See Chapter 8 for management of an acetaminophen overdose.) The maximum acetaminophen dose per day for adults is 4 g/day; for children the single dose is 40 to 480 mg depending on age and weight but no more than five doses should be given in 24 hours (Insel, 1996).

Prescription and OTC drug interactions with acetaminophen include the following:

Drug	Possible effect and management
Alcohol	Increased possibility of hepatotoxicity, especially in persons who regularly drink large amounts of alcoholic beverages, if more acetaminophen is taken than recommended on the label, or if acetaminophen is taken over a long period. Avoid alcoholic beverages when taking acetaminophen.
Anticoagulants such as warfarin (Coumadin) and heparin	High doses and frequent use of acetaminophen may increase anticoagulant action of these drugs, increasing the risk of bleeding. Occasional use of acetaminophen in persons taking anticoagulants is usually not a problem.
Prescription drugs containing acetaminophen, such as Tylenol with codeine, Darvocet, Percocet, and others	Combined use may result in an acetaminophen overdose. See Chapter 8 for symptoms and treatment of an acetaminophen overdose.
Other OTC drugs that contain acetaminophen	Use of two or more OTC products containing acetaminophen may result in acetaminophen overdose.

Box 3-2 describes acetaminophen and aspirin OTC warnings.

OTC acetaminophen is available in powder, tablet, chewable tablet, liquid, drops, and suppository dosage forms. The usual adult dose is 325 to 650 mg every 4 hours, 325 to 500 mg every 3 hours, or 650 to 1000 mg every 6 hours as needed. The usual pediatric dose is 10 to 15 mg/kg every 4 to 6 hours as needed.

acetaminophen combinations

Analgesic combinations of acetaminophen with other ingredients are also available OTC. At one time, combination products were thought to be stronger because of the extra ingredients and also to have fewer side effects because the dose of each ingredient was usually less than the full dose of a single ingredient alone. This reasoning is outdated and highly questionable today. Most combination products offer little advantage over acetaminophen or aspirin alone.

The more common combinations include acetaminophen with salicylates (aspirin, salicylamide), with a salicylate and caffeine, or with an antacid (sodium bicarbonate, calcium carbonate, or "buffered"). Box 3-3 lists acetaminophen and aspirin formulations.

Salicylates, salicylamide, and aspirin are from the salicylate drug family; thus they have analgesic, antipyretic, and

BOX 3-2 Acetaminophen and Aspirin OTC Warnings

General Precautions for Both Analgesics

One should consult with prescriber before taking any analgesic if he or she is allergic to an analgesic or has had a severe allergic analgesic reaction such as asthma, swelling, hives, rash, or other symptoms.

One should avoid taking analgesics if he or she has kidney disease, liver damage, is pregnant or breastfeeding, has taken the analgesics for more than 10 days (adult) or 5 days (child) for pain or 3 days for fever, if pain increases or painful site is inflamed, if new symptoms develop, or if sore throat is very painful or lasts more than 2 days.

If stomach distress occurs, one should take analgesic after meals or with food.

Aspirin

Special Dosing Information

- Children and teenagers (under 17 years of age) should avoid aspirin use for fever or symptoms of a viral infection, especially flu or chickenpox, without prescriber approval. The use of aspirin in viral illnesses may cause a very serious condition known as Reye's syndrome in children. Symptoms include severe vomiting, weakness, stupor that may progress into coma, convulsions, and even death.
- Aspirin use should be stopped at least 5 to 7 days before a scheduled surgery.
- Aspirin products should never be placed directly on a tooth or gum surface because they can burn the tissues and cause injury.
- Aspirin that has a strong, vinegar-like odor should not be used because the odor indicates that the aspirin is deteriorating.

The prescriber should be informed about an individual who has aspirin or salicylate allergy, asthma, nasal polyps, anemia, gout, ulcers or ulcer symptoms, or hemophilia or other bleeding problems.

BOX 3-3 Acetaminophen and Aspirin Formulations*

- Acetaminophen with salicylates
  - acetaminophen with salicylates (Gemnisyn)
  - acetaminophen and salicylamide (Duoprin)
- Acetaminophen with aspirin/salicylate and caffeine
  - acetaminophen, aspirin, salicylamide, and caffeine (Saleto; Tri-pain)
  - acetaminophen, aspirin, and caffeine (Goody's Extra Strength Tablets; Duradyne; Excedrin Extra-strength)
  - acetaminophen, salicylamide, and caffeine (Rid-A-Pain Compound; S-A-C)
- Aspirin/salicylates combined with caffeine
  - aspirin and caffeine (Anacin, Instantine, Nervine, 217 Strong, McNess Pain Tablets)
- Acetaminophen combinations with antacid
  - buffered acetaminophen, aspirin, and caffeine (Gelprin; Supac; Buffets; Vanquish)
  - buffered acetaminophen, aspirin, and salicylamide (Presalin)
  - acetaminophen, sodium bicarbonate, and citric acid (Bromo-Seltzer)
  - acetaminophen with calcium carbonate (Extra Strength Tylenol)
- Aspirin-salicylates with antacid (buffering agents)
  - aspirin, sodium bicarbonate, citric acid (Alka-Seltzer Original, Alka-Seltzer Flavored, Alka-Seltzer Extra Strength†)
  - aspirin, aluminum hydroxide, magnesium hydroxide (Arthritis Pain Formula, Magnaprin, Maprin)
  - aspirin, calcium carbonate, magnesium carbonate, magnesium oxide (Bayer Plus Buffered Aspirin and Bayer Plus, Extra Strength Buffered Aspirin)
  - aspirin, magnesium oxide (Buffaprin, Buffaprin Extra, Buffasal, Buffasal Max, Buffinol)
  - aspirin, calcium carbonate, magnesium oxide, magnesium carbonate (Bufferin Tri-Buffered, Bufferin Arthritis Extra Strength, Tri-Buffered)
- Enteric-coated or delayed-release aspirin (Ecotrin, Bayer 8-hour, Extra Strength Bayer Caplets, etc.)

*Extra strength usually refers to 500 mg analgesic as compared with 325 mg in regular strength products.

†Primary difference between the Alka-Seltzer products is taste and 500 mg aspirin in the extra strength product compared with 325 mg in the other two products.

antiinflammatory effects. The antiinflammatory effect depends on the amount of salicylates in the product, but because the combination dosages of aspirin are usually low, they are not recommended for treatment of severe inflammation or severe arthritic pain.

Salicylamide is also considered to be much less effective than either acetaminophen or aspirin. In addition, the FDA has stated that salicylamide lacks documented proof of being effective as an analgesic or antipyretic.

Caffeine and analgesic combinations may enhance or produce a better pain relief effect than the individual analgesic alone. Although some studies report that the caffeine-analgesic combination may provide better pain-relieving effects, the FDA indicates that sufficient proof is lacking for this effect (USP DI, 1998).

The addition of an antacid buffer to acetaminophen or aspirin is also of questionable benefit. If acetaminophen causes little if any stomach upset, then the addition of an antacid is unnecessary. If the purpose is to avoid gastric distress caused by the other ingredients (aspirin or salicylates), this is also questionable, because studies have indicated that there is no difference between buffered and unbuffered tablets in the production of gastric damage. It appears that the amount of antacid or buffering agent added in the tablets may not be in a sufficient quantity to produce this effect.

If the buffer hastens drug dissolution, then a more rapid absorption of the analgesic may occur, which is why the effervescent antacid preparations (Alka Seltzer, Bromo Seltzer, and others) are more rapidly absorbed. In general, liquid dosage forms of medication are faster and better absorbed. Evidence is lacking, however, that such products produce a more rapid or more effective analgesia than the tablet dosage form, especially when the tablets or capsules are taken with a full glass of water (8 oz). The professional should also be aware that effervescent medications usually contain a large amount of sodium, which must be avoided in persons with cardiac problems or renal failure (Lipman, 1996).

In summary, combination analgesic products are no more effective and are often more expensive than taking either acetaminophen or aspirin alone. The healthcare provider should also be aware that acetaminophen is often included in numerous products that contain more than one ingredient, such as cold, cough, allergy, menstrual or premenstrual, and sleeping aid products.

aspirin [as′ pir in]

Aspirin available OTC includes acetylsalicylic acid (ASA), Bayer, Ecotrin, Norwich, St. Joseph, and many other commercial products. The mechanism of action for aspirin and the NSAIDs is inhibition of prostaglandin synthesis in both the CNS and periphery. See Chapter 8 for more information on analgesics and NSAIDs.

Aspirin has analgesic, antipyretic, antiplatelet, and antiinflammatory effects. It is indicated for the treatment of pain, fever, rheumatic fever, rheumatoid arthritis, and osteoarthritis and for the prevention of myocardial infarction (MI) or reinfarction and prevention of platelet aggregation in ischemia and thromboembolism. The advantages of aspirin over acetaminophen include its antiinflammatory effects and its effectiveness in preventing MI and thrombi.

Pharmacokinetically, aspirin in tablets for oral administration is rapidly absorbed, reaching peak serum level within 1 to 2 hours or more rapidly with liquid preparations; the peak antirheumatic effect occurs in 2 to 3 weeks. Tissue and blood esterases hydrolyze aspirin to acetic acid and salicylate; salicylates are then metabolized in the liver and excreted primarily by the kidneys.

Common side and adverse effects include stomach irritation, cramps or discomfort, heartburn or indigestion, and nausea or vomiting. Taking aspirin with a full glass of water helps reduce these effects. Less common or rare adverse effects include severe abdominal pain, blood in stools, tinnitus, hematemesis, allergic reaction, confusion, weakness, flushing, visual disturbances, severe nausea or vomiting, and gastric ulcers. See the box on p. 144 in Chapter 8 for clinical management of aspirin overdose.

Prescription and OTC drug interactions with aspirin include the following:

Drug	Possible effect and management
alcohol, NSAIDs, and corticosteroids	Increased risk of GI side effects such as irritation, bleeding, and ulceration. Avoid taking aspirin concurrently with these substances.
Anticoagulants (such as warfarin [Coumadin], heparin); thrombolytic agents; antibiotics; carbenicillin (Geopen), cefamandole (Mandol), cefoperazone (Cefobid), cefotetan (Cefotan), plicamycin (Mithracin), ticarcillin (Ticar), and anticonvulsants, such as divalproex (Depakote), valproic acid (Depakene)	Can increase anticoagulant effects, resulting in increased risk of bleeding and hemorrhage. Avoid taking aspirin concurrently with these drugs.
Antidiabetic drugs, oral	May increase therapeutic and side effects of the antidiabetic agents, especially when large doses of aspirin or salicylates are taken. Avoid taking aspirin or salicylates concurrently.
furosemide (Lasix)	Increased risk for hearing loss, especially if high doses of aspirin or salicylates are consumed routinely. Limited intermittent use may not be problematic.
methotrexate (Mexate)	May increase methotrexate plasma levels, leading to severe systemic toxic effects. Avoid taking salicylates while taking this drug.
probenecid (Benemid), sulfinpyrazone (Anturan)	Concurrent administration decreases the effect of antigout medications. Avoid use of aspirin or salicylates if taking these medications.
vancomycin (Vancocin)	Increased potential for hearing loss, which can progress to deafness. Avoid taking aspirin or salicylates concurrently with vancomycin.

Color type indicates an unsafe drug combination.

Antacid analgesic combinations: The same drug interactions as listed above. In addition, the following may occur:

Drug	Possible effect and management
bismuth subsalicylate (Pepto-Bismol)	Taking large repeated dosages of this product with frequent use of aspirin products increases the risk of toxicity (overdose). If taking this product for traveler's diarrhea or chronic diarrhea, be careful or avoid taking additional aspirin-containing products.
Bulk-forming laxatives (Metamucil, Perdiem, and others)	If taken with aspirin or salicylate products, they may reduce the absorption and effect of aspirin or salicylates. Take these products 2 hours apart.
ketoconazole (Nizoral)	Antacids or buffering agents may increase stomach acidity, which reduces the absorption and effectiveness of ketoconazole. Buffered aspirin products should be taken at least 3 hours before or after ketoconazole.
oral tetracycline (Achromycin V)	Antacids and the magnesium in some salicylate medications can interfere with absorption of the tetracyclines. To reduce this effect, take the aspirin or salicylate preparation 3 to 4 hours apart from the tetracycline.

Enteric-coated aspirin products, in addition to the interactions noted above, may also interact with the following:

Drug	Possible effect and management
Antacids or H_2-blocking such as cimetidine (Tagamet), ranitidine (Zantac), nizatidine (Axid), and famotidine (Pepcid)	The increase in gastric pH produced by these drugs agents may cause enteric-coated tablets to dissolve early, thus losing the benefit of the enteric coating in the stomach.

Caffeine in analgesic medications, in addition to the interactions noted above, may also cause the following to occur:

Drug	Possible effect and management
Other caffeine products, appetite suppressants, theophylline, pemoline (Cylert), selegiline (Eldepryl), tranylcypromine (Parnate), fluoxetine (Prozac), methylphenidate (Ritalin), sertraline (Zoloft), and sympathomimetics in oral, inhaler, and injectable dosage forms	An increase in CNS-stimulating effects occurs, such as nervousness, tremors, increased irritability, insomnia, and possibly cardiac dysrhythmias. Reducing or avoiding caffeine-containing products can reduce this effect.
lithium	Caffeine may increase lithium excretion from the body, which results in a reduction of lithium effects. Reduce or avoid use of caffeine-containing products.
monoamine oxidase (MAO) inhibitors such as tranylcypromine (Parnate), procarbazine (Matulane), and possibly selegiline (Eldepryl)	May result in an increase in CNS-stimulating effects (see above), hypertension, and dangerous cardiac dysrhythmias. Avoid use of large amounts of caffeine-containing products.

Color type indicates an unsafe drug combination.

Aspirin products are available in tablet, chewable tablet, chewing gum tablet, extended-release tablet, and suppository dosage forms. The usual adult dose is one to two regular strength tablets (325 to 650 mg) every 4 hours or 500 to 1000 mg (extra strength) every 6 hours as needed. The adult maximum OTC aspirin dose per day is 4 g/day. The pediatric dose is 1.5 g/m^2 daily, in four to six divided doses. Check package labels for further dosing information.

aspirin combinations

Pain-relieving combinations of aspirin with other ingredients are available without a prescription. Aspirin and salicylates have been combined with acetaminophen, caffeine, and antacids (buffering agents) like acetaminophen; therefore the same comments from acetaminophen apply to aspirin. For examples of acetaminophen and aspirin formulations, see Box 3-3.

nonsteroidal antiinflammatory drugs

NSAIDs and aspirin have analgesic, antipyretic, and antiinflammatory effects. Unlike aspirin, NSAIDs were all prescription drugs before approval by the FDA for the change to OTC status. Currently, ibuprofen (Advil, Motrin lB, and others), naproxen (Aleve), and ketoprofen (Actron, Orudis

KT) are available OTC, with manufacturers of other NSAIDs expected to seek OTC approval in the near future.

The difference between the prescription and OTC NSAID is the strength of the product. For example, prescription strengths for ibuprofen are 300 mg, 600 mg, and 800 mg tablets, whereas the OTC product is 200 mg. Naproxen prescription strengths are 250 mg, 375 mg, and 500 mg tablets, whereas the OTC product is 200 mg. Ketoprofen prescription strengths are 25 mg, 50 mg, 75 mg, and a 200 mg extended-release dosage form, whereas the OTC product is 12.5 mg. As mentioned previously, OTC strengths are considered to be safe and effective for consumer use without professional supervision, assuming the label instructions and warnings are closely followed. The higher-strength products are prescription medications in the United States because of their potential side and adverse effects.

The mechanism of action for NSAIDs is inhibition of cyclooxygenase, which results in a decrease synthesis of prostaglandins. The decrease in prostaglandins may be responsible for both therapeutic and adverse effects associated with this drug category. (See Chapter 8 for additional information.)

Pharmacokinetics

Ibuprofen, naproxen, and ketoprofen are well absorbed orally, although concurrent food and antacids may decrease absorption. The onset of action is ½ hour for ibuprofen, 1 hour for naproxen, and unknown for ketoprofen. The peak effect for ibuprofen is 1 to 2 hours; ketoprofen, ½ to 2 hours; and naproxen, 2 to 4 hours. The duration of action is 6 hours for ibuprofen, up to 7 hours for naproxen, and not available for ketoprofen (Olin, 1998; USP DI, 1998). Metabolism of NSAIDs is primarily hepatic with excretion by the kidneys.

Side effects and adverse effects

Side effects and adverse effects of NSAIDs are primarily GI distress (nausea, vomiting, diarrhea, cramps, gas), gastric ulcers, and bleeding. (See Chapter 8 for additional side effects and adverse effects and drug interactions.) Box 3-4 describes OTC NSAID warnings.

The usual adult ibuprofen dose is one (200 mg) tablet every 4 to 6 hours when necessary. If the pain or fever does not respond to one tablet, two may be taken, but the maximum is six tablets in 24 hours without prescriber approval.

The usual adult ketoprofen dose is one (12.5 mg) tablet every 4 to 6 hours. If pain or fever is not improved within an hour, a second dose may be taken. Do not take more than two tablets in any 4-to 6-hour period nor more than six doses in 24 hours. Do not administer to children under 16 years of age.

The usual adult naproxen dose is one (200 mg) tablet every 8 to 12 hours when necessary. Some persons may need two tablets initially and then one 12 hours later. Do not take more than three tablets in 24 hours. The elderly should not take more than two tablets in 12 hours and children under 12 years of age should not take this product.

BOX 3-4 Nonsteroidal Antiinflammatory OTC Drug Warnings

General Precautions

With NSAIDs, contact the prescriber if the person reports that they had a severe allergic reaction to any analgesic, such as asthma, swelling, hives, rash, or any other reaction, because the NSAIDs are capable of causing similar reactions.

- Avoid taking NSAIDs with any other OTC analgesics (acetaminophen, aspirin, or other NSAIDs).
- Avoid taking these products for more than 10 days for pain, 3 days for fever, if painful area is inflamed, if pregnant or breastfeeding, if new symptoms occur or current symptoms worsen, or if abdominal pain occurs. Contact prescriber for advice.
- Do not use NSAIDs during the last 3 months of pregnancy because it may adversely affect the fetus or result in complications during the delivery.
- Alcohol (especially 3 or more drinks daily) and many other medications may result in adverse drug interactions. Review all medications with the prescriber or pharmacist before taking an NSAID.

ANTACIDS

Various medical conditions, overeating, or eating certain foods may result in stomach upset, gas, heartburn, and indigestion. **Antacids**—drugs that buffer, neutralize, or absorb hydrochloric acid in the stomach—are commonly used for these conditions. Americans have been estimated to spend $1 billion annually on antacids (Cornacchia, Barrett, 1993). (See Chapter 41 for additional information on antacids.) Antacids buffer or neutralize hydrochloric acid in the stomach, increasing gastric pH. The major ingredients in antacids include aluminum salts, calcium carbonate, magnesium salts, magaldrate (aluminum-magnesium combination), and sodium bicarbonate. Simethicone may be added to these preparations as a defoaming or antigas agent.

Antacids generally have a rapid onset of action. A small amount of absorbable antacid is absorbed systemically (15% to 30%), but the remainder is broken down via the digestive process and excreted in the feces. Table 3-2 lists side effects and adverse effects related to antacids. Long-term use of antacids or their use in the presence of impaired renal function may result in increased adverse effects from metal ion absorption, especially of calcium carbonate or magnesium hydroxide.

Dosage and administration

The amount of antacid necessary to neutralize hydrochloric acid depends on the individual, the condition being

TABLE 3-2 Antacid Side Effects and Adverse Reactions

Name	***Side Effects and Adverse Reactions****
Aluminum aluminum carbonate (Basaljel) aluminum hydroxide (Alterna-GEL, Alu-Cap, Amphojel) aluminum-magnesium compounds (Aludrox, Gaviscon, Maalox, Mylanta)	Constipation (combination products with magnesium reduce this) Phosphate depletion via feces (including weakness, apnea, hemolytic anemia, tetany) Delay in gastric emptying Concretions (intestinal and renal) Encephalopathy from aluminum intoxication Bone demineralization (osteomalacia, osteoporosis)
Bicarbonate sodium bicarbonate (Alka-Seltzer, Instant Metamucil)	Systemic alkalosis or sodium overload (elevated plasma pH and carbon dioxide, anorexia, mental confusion) Gastric acid hypersecretion ("acid rebound") Enhanced effects of amphetamines, quinidine, quinine
Calcium calcium carbonate (Tums)	Milk-alkali syndrome (including metabolic alkalosis, anorexia, nausea, vomiting, confusion, hypercalcemia, possibly renal impairment) Increased potential for calcium stone formation Nephrocalcinosis Gastric acid hypersecretion ("acid rebound") Antagonism of digitalis preparations Elevated serum and urine calcium levels Kidney failure Constipation Decreased phosphate levels (if dietary phosphate intake is low)
Magnesium magnesium hydroxide (Milk of Magnesia) magnesium trisilicate	Diarrhea (combination products with aluminum reduce this) Decreased potassium levels (hypokalemia) Increased magnesum levels (hypermagnesemia) in clients with renal failure or severe kidney impairment (causing low blood pressure, nausea, vomiting, respiratory depression, CNS depression, coma)
Sodium sodium bicarbonate	Sodium overload or systemic alkalosis Salt and water retention (causing edema, ascites, effusion, hypertension) Metabolic alkalosis Milk-alkali syndrome (see under calcium) Gastric acid hypersecretion ("acid rebound")

*Chronic, high-dose usage.

treated, and the buffering capability of the preparation used. The acid-neutralizing property of antacids varies for the individual patient. Antacids taken before meals have a duration of action of approximately 30 minutes. If the antacid is taken after meals, the duration may be up to 3 hours. Duodenal ulcer, Zollinger-Ellison syndrome, and other hypersecretory conditions may require 80 to 160 mEq of acid-neutralizing effect per dose (USP DI, 1998); for pain relief, the dose of antacids should provide 40 to 80 mEq neutralizing effect (Table 3-3) (Pinson, Weart, 1996). Antacids are not very effective for the treatment of gastric ulcers (Brunton, 1996).

Liquid and powder dosage forms have been found to be more effective antacids than the tablet dosage formulations. Most tablets require chewing before swallowing to be effective. The majority of antacids contain 10 mg or less of sodium per recommended adult dose. Patients on sodium-restricted diets should read ingredient listings carefully. Examples of antacids containing more than 10 mg per recommended adult dose (Pinson, Weart, 1996) include the following:

Alka-Seltzer Extra Strength	588 mg sodium/tablet
Alka-Seltzer Original	567 mg sodium/tablet
Bell/ans	144 mg/tablet

The maximum dosages listed on antacid packages should be followed. Many individuals exceed the FDA recommendations, thus increasing the potential for producing many of the potential side effects or adverse reactions.

Pregnancy safety

Antacids are generally considered safe for use in pregnancy if prolonged or high doses are avoided.

Antacid Combinations

Although there are numerous antacid preparations on the market, the magnesium-aluminum combinations (e.g., Gelusil, Maalox, and Mylanta) are the most common antacids selected by individuals and healthcare professionals alike. Antacid recommendation should be based on its ingredients relative to the patient's health status. Combination antacids have been formulated to reduce the risk of diarrhea or con-

TABLE 3-3 Antacids: Acid-Neutralizing Capacity

Antacid	Primary Ingredients	Acid-Neutralizing Capacity	Dose to Neutralize 80 mEq HCl
Liquid Preparations		**mEq/5 ml**	**ml Needed**
Gelusil	aluminum hydroxide, magnesium hydroxide, simethicone	12	33
Maalox	aluminum hydroxide, magnesium hydroxide	13.3	30
Maalox Plus Extra Strength	aluminum hydroxide, magnesium hydroxide, simethicone	29	14
Mylanta	aluminum hydroxide, magnesium hydroxide, simethicone	12.7	31
Mylanta Double Strength	aluminum hydroxide, magnesium hydroxide, simethicone	25.4	16
Riopan Plus Susp	magaldrate, simethicone	15	27
Tablet Preparations		**mEq/Tablet**	**Tablets Approx. Needed**
Gelusil	aluminum hydroxide, magnesium hydroxide, simethicone	11	7
Maalox	aluminum hydroxide, magnesium hydroxide	8.5	9
Maalox Plus	same as Maalox plus simethicone	10.6	7
Mylanta	aluminum hydroxide, magnesium hydroxide, simethicone	11.5	7
Mylanta Gelcaps	same as above, double strength	23	3.5
Riopan Plus	magaldrate, simethicone	13.5	6
Rolaids	calcium carbonate, magnesium hydroxide	7.5	10.5
Tums	calcium carbonate	10	8

From *USP DI*, 1998.

stipation as a side effect. However, the antacid combination Gaviscon deserves particular attention because of its uniqueness and widespread use.

antacid combination plus alginic acid
(Gaviscon)

Gaviscon forms a viscous cohesive foam that floats on the surface of the stomach contents, neutralizing stomach acid. This helps to protect the sensitive mucosa from irritation because the foam precedes the stomach contents into the lower esophagus when reflux occurs. The foam is caused by the alginic acid contained in the product; the other ingredients are aluminum hydroxide, magnesium trisilicate, and sodium bicarbonate.

Antiflatulents

simethicone [si meth′ i kone] (Mylicon, Phazyme)

Simethicone, a defoaming agent, relieves flatulence by dispersing and preventing the formation of mucus-surrounded gas pockets in the gastrointestinal (GI) tract. Gas retention is a problem in conditions such as air swallowing, diverticulitis, functional dyspepsia, peptic ulcer, postoperative gaseous distention, and spastic or irritable colon.

The tablets are taken four times daily and chewed thoroughly after meals, at bedtime, and as needed for flatulence. Antacid liquid combination products also often contain simethicone.

LAXATIVES

Laxatives, drugs given to induce defecation, may be classified according to their source, site of action, degree of action, or mechanism of action. Fig. 3-1 and Table 3-4 summarize the traditional laxatives that can be bought without a prescription.

One of the major indications for the use of laxatives is constipation. **Constipation** is difficult fecal evacuation as a result of hard stool and perhaps infrequent movements. The primary causes of constipation are reviewed in Chapter 35. Failure to respond to the normal defecation impulse, insufficient time to permit the bowel to produce an evacuation, inadequate fluid and dietary fiber intake, sedentary habits, and insufficient exercise may be factors. Constipation is also a side effect of many medications, such as antacids, diuretics, morphine, tricyclic antidepressants, codeine, aluminum hydroxide, and anticholinergics.

In addition to constipation, laxatives may be administered within a healthcare agency setting for a variety of purposes, such as preparation for surgery, in cases of food and drug poisoning, and to promote the elimination of an offending substance from the GI tract. Saline cathartics are considered useful for this purpose.

Laxatives are also used to keep the stool soft when it is essential to avoid the irritation or straining that accompanies the passage of a hardened stool. This indication might include rectal disorders, irritated polyps in the bowel, hem-

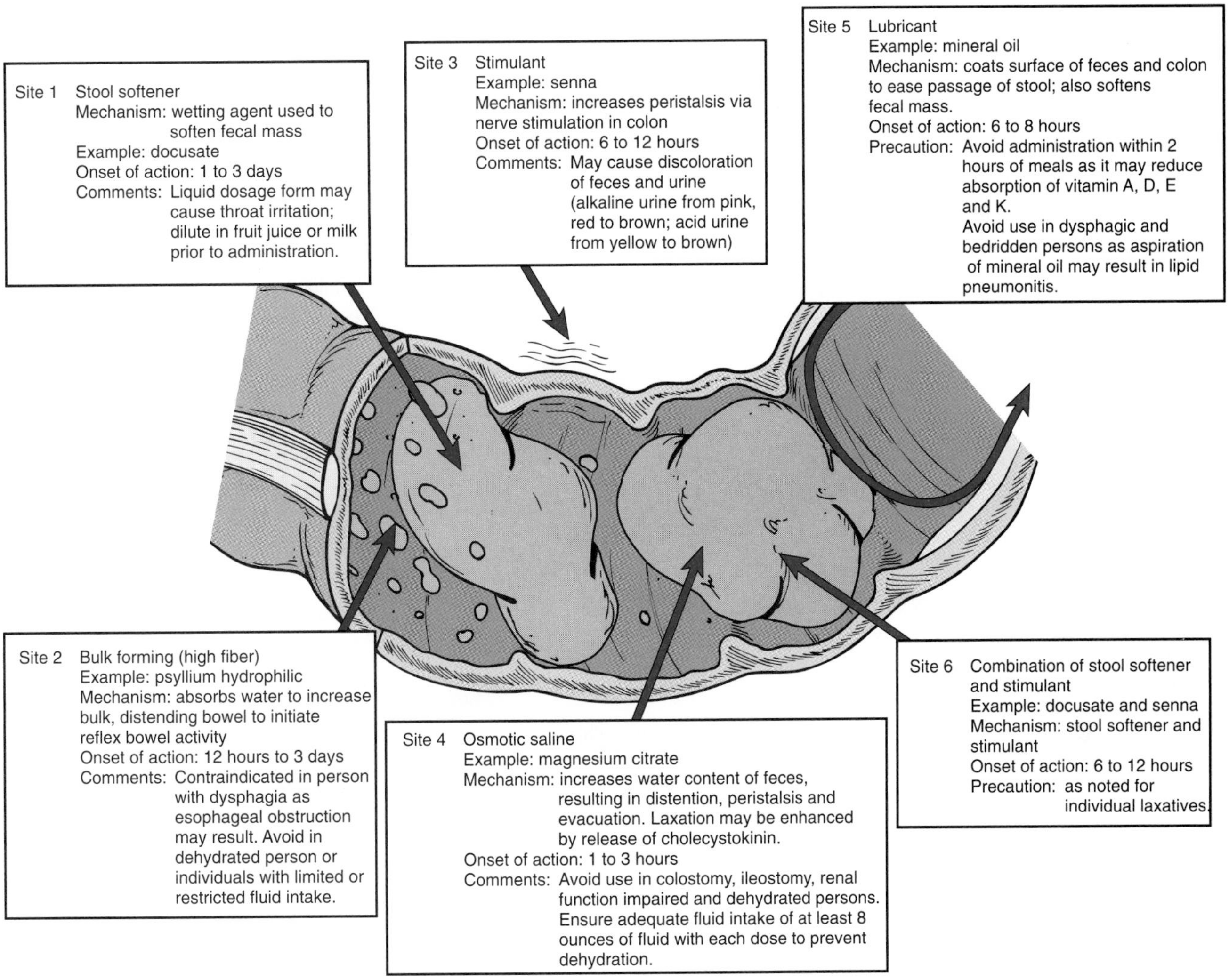

FIGURE 3-1
Classification of laxatives according to site of action.

orrhoidectomy, and perianal abscess, or the recovery phase of an MI, cerebrovascular accident, or the repair of a hernia. Saline laxatives are routinely used to expel parasites and toxic anthelmintics and to secure a stool specimen to be examined for parasites.

Laxatives should not be taken if the individual is experiencing undiagnosed abdominal pain because this may be due to an inflammatory disorder of the alimentary tract, such as appendicitis, typhoid fever, or chronic ulcerative colitis. If the pain is caused by an inflamed appendix, a laxative may bring about a rupture of the appendix by increasing intestinal peristalsis. Laxatives should be taken with caution after some operations, such as repair of the perineum or rectum (at least for a time); during pregnancy and breastfeeding; by patients with severe anemia, and by debilitated patients. Other conditions in which caution is needed include chronic and spastic constipation.

Because constipation is common in children, parents need to be informed about problems associated with indiscriminate use of laxatives. The following factors may contribute to or cause constipation in children: emotions, environmental changes (new home, new school, new friends), dietary changes, and febrile illnesses. Adding or increasing fluids, vegetables, fruits, and bran products may be very helpful. A malt soup extract is often suggested for infants up to 2 months of age, but for older children, glycerin suppositories or docusate sodium may be appropriate.

The elderly may have an increased incidence of constipation because of multiple illnesses that require a variety of medications, the aging process with its associated decline in physiologic functions, plus a progressive decrease in physical activity (see Geriatric Implications box). An increase in fluid intake, a moderate exercise program if permitted, and an increase in intake of bran products, vegetables, and fruit will help to correct this problem. Laxative abuse or the chronic or excessive use of laxatives is often reported with this age group. While this syndrome may take several years to develop, it is frequently not diagnosed. Interventions are

TABLE 3-4 Laxatives: Over-the-Counter Varieties

	Stimulant (Contact)	*Osmotic Saline*	*Stool Softener Surfactant or Wetting Agent*	*High-Fiber and Bulk-Forming*	*Lubricant*
Disadvantages with repeated frequent (long-term) administration	Watery stools, gripping	Watery stools, cramps	Unreliable results, may contribute to liver toxicity	Obstruction of narrowed lumen, some difficulty in chewing and swallowing	Anal leakage, lipid pneumonia
Increases rate of transit in small bowel	Yes	Yes	Yes	Yes	Unknown
Causes net secretion of water and electrolytes in small bowel	Yes	Yes	Yes	Yes	No
Inhibits absorption in small bowel	Yes	Yes	Yes	Yes	Yes
Increases mucosal permeability in small bowel	Yes	Not studied	Yes	Not reported	Not reported
Causes mucosal damage in small bowel	Yes	Not studied	Yes	Not reported	Not reported
Acts only in colon (not small bowel)	No	No	No	No	Yes
Indicated for long-term treatment	No	No	No	Probably	No
Examples of type	anthraquinone, bisacodyl, phenolphthalein, castor oil, danthron	magnesium salts, MOM, sodium salts, glycerin	DSS, DCS Polomaxer 188	methylcellulose, karaya gum, sodium CMC, malt soup extract, psyllium seed, agar, plantago bran (unprocessed), polycarbophil	mineral oil
Physical or chemical property responsible for action	Mucosal surface irritation to stimulate or increase intestinal motor function or activity	Hyperosmolar ingredients trap water in intestinal lumen; hypertonicity of colon increases liquid in colon; hyperosmotic or saline	Changes surface tension of fecal mass, provides increased penetration of colonic water; penetrates and softens fecal mass by wetting agents	Absorbs water on surface, increases soft fecal mass, adds bulk and moisture to feces causing distention and elimination	Coats over fecal mass, passes with ease, lubricates gastrointestinal tract and softens feces

MOM, milk of magnesia; *DSS*, dioctyl sodium sulfosuccinate; *DCS*, docusate sodium; *CMC*, carboxymethylcellulose.

necessary for patients who chronically abuse laxatives or permanent bowel damage may occur. Because there may be many factors contributing to constipation, a complete and thorough history by the healthcare professional is always necessary.

Constipation is commonly reported during pregnancy. It is usually caused by colon compression as a result of the increase in the size of the uterus or a decrease in muscle tone and peristalsis. Vitamins containing iron and calcium are often prescribed for pregnant women, and such products also tend to be constipating. Laxatives used in pregnancy should be limited to emollients or bulk-forming laxatives. Most of the other laxatives have the potential for undesirable effects (e.g., castor oil may induce premature labor, mineral oil may decrease absorption of fat-soluble vitamins, and osmotic agents may induce dangerous electrolyte alterations). The childbearing woman should be advised about proper diet, adequate fluid intake, appropriate exercise programs, and the importance of discussing the problem with her prescriber.

Saline Laxatives

Saline laxatives are soluble salts that are only slightly absorbed from the alimentary canal. Because of their osmotic

GERIATRIC IMPLICATIONS

Nonpharmacologic Laxative Therapy

The elderly often use or abuse laxatives because they believe that regularity implies a daily bowel movement (Ahronheim, 1992).

To reduce the potential for chronic laxative use or dependency, the client should be taught nonpharmacologic measures, such as encouraging an increase in fluid intake to 6 to 8 glasses of water/day if permitted and tolerated. Also recommended is a regular exercise routine, such as a daily walk or active and passive exercise for bedridden clients.

The healthcare professional should obtain a dietary and laxative history from the patient. Advise individuals who regularly consume a low-fiber diet or foods that tend to harden stools (such as cheese, hard-boiled eggs, liver, cottage cheese, foods high in sugar content, and rice) that such foods are associated with constipation.

A high-fiber diet with adequate fluid intake helps to reduce constipation by exerting a mild laxative effect. High-fiber foods include orange juice with pulp or fresh citrus fruits, bran or whole grain cereals and breads, and leafy vegetables. Other fruits high in dietary fiber are prunes, bananas, figs, and dates. Prunes contain a laxative substance in addition to being high in dietary fiber. Therefore daily consumption of prunes or a small glass of prune juice is often recommended for constipation.

Avoid fiber supplements in nonambulatory patients or those who are on restricted or limited fluid intake. Bulk or fiber laxatives are also contraindicated in cases of fecal impaction.

effect of drawing water in the small intestine, they retain and increase the water content of feces. The water in the intestinal lumen produces fluid accumulation and distention, leading to peristalsis and eventual evacuation of bowel contents. The result is a fecal mass of liquid or semiliquid stools. The laxative effect may be enhanced by the intestinal release of cholecystokinin (CCK). **Diarrhea** is created in the small intestine to overcome constipation in the colon. Laxation may result in 30 minutes to 3 hours.

Saline laxatives are the laxative of choice for securing a stool specimen for examination, for fecal impaction, for use with certain anthelmintics, and in some cases of food and drug poisoning.

Phosphate enemas are useful as preparations for a barium enema. When the object is merely to empty the intestine, magnesium sulfate, sodium phosphate, or magnesium hydroxide (milk of magnesia [MOM]) is effective. MOM is the mildest of the salines and is often the cathartic of choice for children. Sodium salts are contraindicated for those on a sodium restricted diet. Magnesium and potassium salts are contraindicated in individuals with renal disease.

The intestinal membrane is not entirely impermeable to the passage of saline laxatives. Electrolyte disturbances have been reported with their long-term daily use. Some saline laxatives find their way into the general circulation only to be excreted by the kidney, in which case they act as saline diuretics. Hypertonic saline solutions in the bowel may result in so much fluid loss that little or no diuretic effect will be possible. Some saline laxatives contain up to 1 g or more of sodium per dose. Some ions may have a toxic effect in impaired renal function if they accumulate in the blood in sufficient quantity. This may occur with magnesium ions if a solution is retained in the intestine for a long time or if the patient suffers from renal impairment. Magnesium acts as a depressant of the CNS and neuromuscular activity.

Dosage and administration

The following salts, when taken for their laxative effect, are usually taken orally. Some of them may be given rectally as an enema. The salts tend to have a rapid action, especially if ingested before breakfast. They may be taken at bedtime with food for early morning evacuation (food delays the effect). Patients sometimes complain of gaseous distention after taking saline laxatives. All preparations should be dissolved and accompanied by a liberal (8 oz) intake of water, since the salts do not readily leave the stomach and may cause vomiting if not well diluted.

When a salt such as magnesium sulfate is taken, it should not only be dissolved in an adequate amount of water and taken on an empty stomach but it should also be disguised in fruit juice, plain water (chilled), citrus-flavored carbonate beverage, or chipped ice to increase palatability.

magnesium sulfate [mag nee′ zhum] (Epsom salt)

Magnesium sulfate occurs as a crystal or white powder that is readily soluble in water. It has a bitter saline taste. The usual dose for laxative effect is 15 g in 8 oz of water. Children over 6 are given 5 to 10 g in 4 oz of water.

magnesium hydroxide (milk of magnesia [MOM])

Magnesium hydroxide is also used as an antacid. In the stomach the magnesium hydroxide reacts with hydrochloric acid to form magnesium chloride, which is responsible for the laxative effect. The usual dose for adults is 30 to 60 ml with additional liquids, and the usual dose for children 1 to 12 years of age is 7.5 to 30 ml.

magnesium citrate solution

Magnesium citrate solution is not very soluble, hence the need for a relatively large dose. It is not unpleasant to take because it is carbonated and flavored. The usual adult dose is 240 ml, and the usual dose for children 6 to 12 years of age is 50 to 100 ml.

TABLE 3-5 Stimulant Laxatives

Name	Therapeutic Effect (hr)	Stool Consistency	Remarks
bisacodyl (Dulcolax)	6-10	Soft	Not to be taken with or within 1 hr after ingestion of milk or antacids to prevent premature dissolving of enteric coating and gastrointestinal irritation
castor oil (Neoloid emulsion, Castor Oil)	2-6	Watery	Chilling, mixing with fruit juice or carbonated drinks increases palatability
cascara sagrada	6-10	Soft, formed	Gives a yellowish brown color to acid urine; reddish color to alkaline urine
phenolphthalein (Ex-Lax, Feen-A-Mint, Phenolax, Doxidan)	6-10	Semifluid	Gives pink color to alkaline urine or feces; action may persist for 3-4 days; may cause skin eruptions as dermatitis
senna (X-prep, Senokot)	6-12	Soft	Crude senna may cause urine discoloration like cascara sagrada

effervescent sodium phosphate

Sodium phosphate is made effervescent by the addition of sodium bicarbonate, citric acid, and tartaric acid. The usual dose is 10 g. A concentrated aqueous solution of sodium biphosphate and sodium phosphate is available under the name Fleet Phospho-Soda as a laxative. The usual oral adult dose is 20 to 45 ml mixed with ½ glass of cold water. Children 6 to 9 years of age are given 5 ml, whereas children over 10 years of age receive 10 ml, diluted in 4 oz of water. It is also marketed in a disposable enema unit for rectal administration.

Stimulant (Contact) Laxatives

With the exception of bisacodyl, the principal stimulant laxatives (cascara, senna, rhubarb, and aloe) are botanical glycoside drugs obtained from the bark, seed pods, leaves, and roots of many plants. These laxatives are absorbed and later secreted to produce stimulation and peristalsis in the intestines. Their exact mechanism of action is unknown. The stimulant laxatives usually act in 6 to 8 hours. Their primary effect is on the small and large intestines, which explains their tendency to produce cramping. Aloe and rhubarb are almost obsolete because of their irritating properties.

Stimulant laxatives are used in preparation for barium enemas, in some cases of acute constipation, and before a proctologic examination.

Side effects of stimulant laxatives include abdominal cramping, nausea, diarrhea, and flatulence. Adverse reactions that should be reported to a healthcare provider if they occur include allergic reactions, esophageal or intestinal obstruction, change in heart rate, disorientation, cramping of muscles, increased weakness, and skin rash. Senna, cascara sagrada, and aloe are passed through the breast milk, initiating laxation in the nursing infant. Their occasional use should be restricted to 1 week because long-term abuse may lead to a poorly functioning large intestine. Contact stimulant laxatives may also lead to mucus secretion and fluid evacuation. Table 3-5 compares the stimulant laxatives in use today. Laxatives are habit forming and should be used judiciously.

bisacodyl [bis a koe′ dill] (Dulcolax)

Bisacodyl is a relatively nontoxic laxative agent that reflexively stimulates peristalsis on contact with the mucosa of the colon. Bisacodyl has been successful in the treatment of various types of constipation. In larger doses, it is also widely used for cleansing the bowel before some surgeries and before proctoscopic and roentgenographic examinations.

Bisacodyl has an insoluble coating that was formulated to dissolve in intestinal fluids and, when released, produces its stimulating effects on the colon. It should not be chewed, crushed, or taken with milk or antacids because it can have an irritating effect on the stomach that might manifest as severe abdominal cramps. If antacids are to be taken, they should be taken at least several hours apart from the bisacodyl.

Oral adult dosage is two to three tablets (10 to 15 mg). The tablets produce evacuation of the bowel in 6 to 8 hours, and suppositories and enemas act within 15 to 60 minutes. The suppositories may cause a burning sensation and proctitis.

cascara sagrada [kas′ kar a / sa grah′ da]

Cascara sagrada was one of the most extensively used laxatives in the past. It is considered to be the mildest laxative belonging to this group. Its action is mainly on the small and large bowel. The active ingredients reach the large bowel by way of the bloodstream, as well as by passage along the alimentary tract. Bowel evacuation occurs in about 8 hours. Cascara sagrada may discolor urine to pink, red, violet, or brown depending on the urinary pH. The patient should be alerted to this possibility.

Aromatic cascara sagrada fluid extract contains 18% to 20% alcohol. Each milliliter represents 1 g cascara sagrada.

The usual dose is 5 ml (range 5 to 15 ml). For infants up to 2 years of age the dose is 1 to 3 ml. Cascara sagrada is also available in tablets.

senna [sen′ a] (Senexon, Senokot)

Senna is obtained from the dried leaves of the *Cassia* plant. It produces a thorough bowel evacuation in 6 to 12 hours, which may be accompanied by abdominal pain or gripping. Senna resembles cascara sagrada but is more powerful. It is also found in proprietary remedies, such as Fletcher's Castoria and Black Draught. Senna tea is an infusion of senna leaves made from adding a teaspoonful of leaves to a cup of hot water.

A powdered concentrate of senna (X Prep Liquid) is said to contain the desirable laxative components but to be free of the impurities that cause cramping. This compound is sold under the name Senokot (tablets, syrup, granules, and suppositories). The usual adult dose of Senokot is two tablets, 10 to 15 ml of the syrup, or 1 teaspoon of the granules twice daily. For children over 6 years of age, the dose is one tablet twice daily.

castor oil [kas′ tor]

Castor oil is obtained from the seeds of the castor bean. It is a bland, colorless, emollient glyceride that passes through the stomach unchanged. However, like other fatty substances, it retards the emptying of the stomach. For this reason it is usually given when the stomach is empty. In the small intestine the oil is hydrolyzed by pancreatic lipase to glycerol and a hydroxy fatty acid, ricinoleic acid. Ricinoleic acid is responsible for irritation of the bowel, especially the small intestine. Its irritating effect causes a rapid propulsion of contents from the small intestine, including any of the oil that may have escaped hydrolysis.

A therapeutic dose produces several copious semiliquid stools in 2 to 6 hours, so it should not be taken at bedtime. The fluid nature of the stool is caused by the rapid passage of the fecal content rather than by a diffusion of fluid into the bowel. The drug is excreted into the milk of nursing mothers.

Castor oil is used much less often today, although it may be used in the preparation of certain patients scheduled for a roentgenographic examination of abdominal viscera. The usual adult dose of castor oil is 15 to 60 ml orally. The dose for children 2 years of age and older is 5 to 15 ml.

phenolphthalein [fee nole thay′ leen] (Ex-Lax, Phenolax)

Phenolphthalein is a synthetic stimulant laxative that has been available for many years. It was banned by the FDA (1997), and the OTC products that contained this ingredient have been reformulated with a safer ingredient. Check ingredients and avoid purchasing any product that may still contain phenolphthalein.

Bulk-Forming Laxatives

The laxatives constituting this group are polycarbophil (Mitrolan) and other natural or semisynthetic cellulose derivatives such as psyllium and methylcellulose. Hydrophilic colloids stimulate peristalsis by swelling, increasing bulk and modifying the consistency of the stool. This mechanism of laxative action is a normal stimulus and is one of the least harmful. These drugs do not interfere with absorption of food, but if not administered with sufficient fluids (8 oz of water or juice), they can cause esophageal obstruction or fecal impaction or obstruction.

The effect of these laxatives may not be apparent for 12 to 24 hours, and their full effect may not be achieved until the second or third day after administration. Some prescribers maintain that bran and dried fruits (e.g., prunes, prune juice, and figs) exert the same effect, and they prefer to suggest these foods rather than the bulk-forming laxatives. Bulk-forming laxatives are used in irritable bowel syndrome, diverticular disease, and postpartum constipation. Because of the altered bulk consistency, they have also been found to be useful in the treatment of diarrhea. Side effects are minimal, the most commonly reported being flatulence and bulky stools.

polycarbophil calcium [pol i kar′ boe fil] (Mitrolan)

Polycarbophil is used to normalize stools both in diarrhea and in constipation by restoring the normal moisture level and providing bulk in the intestinal tract. In diarrheal conditions the intestinal mucosa is unable to absorb the excess fecal water. This agent absorbs water (up to 60 times its weight) by forming a gel in the intestinal lumen, thus creating formed stools. In constipation the agent retains water in the lumen.

Polycarbophil has a low sodium content; each tablet contains 150 mg of calcium. The maximum dosage of calcium recommended by the FDA is much higher than the 1800 mg a patient would receive by taking the maximum dosage of 12 tablets per day. Nevertheless, patients with hypercalcemia or those susceptible to hypercalcemia should not take this product without prior consultation with their prescriber (Curry, Jr, Tatum-Butler, 1996).

psyllium [sill′ i yum] (Metamucil, Konsyl)

Psyllium hydrophilic mucilloid is a powder that contains about 50% powdered mucilaginous portion (outer epidermis) of psyllium seeds and about 50% dextrose or sucrose. This mixture is used to treat constipation because it promotes the formation of a soft, water-retaining, gelatinous residue in the lower bowel within 12 to 72 hours. In addition, it has a demulcent effect on inflamed mucosa. The dosage is 4 to 7 g, administered one to three times daily.

Sugar-free Metamucil contains aspartame (Nutra-Sweet). Products containing aspartame should not be taken by patients on a phenylalanine-restricted diet.

Lubricant Laxatives

mineral oil

Mineral oil (liquid petrolatum; MO), a mixture of liquid hydrocarbons obtained from petroleum, is not digested, and absorption is minimal. Mineral oil penetrates and coats the fecal mass and also prevents excessive absorption of water.

Mineral oil is especially useful when it is desirable to keep feces soft and when straining at stool must be reduced, as after abdominal surgery, rectal operations, repair of hernias, eye surgery, aneurysm, or MI, or for prevention of hemorrhoidal tearing. It is also indicated for patients who have chronic constipation because of prolonged inactivity, as in the case of patients with orthopedic conditions.

Some healthcare providers object to the use of mineral oil on the basis that it impairs the absorption of fat-soluble vitamins A, D, E, and K. If mineral oil is taken with meals, gastric emptying time is delayed. Another objection to its use is that in large doses it tends to leak or seep from the rectum, which may cause anal pruritus and interfere with healing of postoperative wounds in the region of the anus and perineum. This leakage is often an embarrassment to the patient.

Although absorption of mineral oil is limited, after prolonged use it may cause a chronic inflammatory reaction in tissues where it is found. Indiscriminate use by elderly or weak individuals should be discouraged because of the increased potential for aspiration leading to lipid pneumonia.

Concurrent use with fecal moistening agents should be avoided because they increase absorption of mineral oil. The adult dose ranges from 15 to 45 ml. For children over 6 years of age, doses range from 5 to 15 ml.

Emollient, or Fecal Moistening, Agents

Emollient, or fecal moistening, agents include stool softeners and surfactants. They decrease the consistency of stools by reducing surface tension, allowing water to penetrate the feces. They are commonly used for the treatment of hard or dry stools.

docusate or dioctyl sodium sulfosuccinate

[dok′ yoo sate] (Colace, Doxinate)

Docusate acts like a detergent, permitting water and fatty substances to penetrate and be well mixed with the fecal material. It may also inhibit water absorption from the bowel and stimulate water secretion into the GI tract. Thus this agent promotes the formation of soft-formed stool and is useful in the treatment of constipation. Formed stools are usually excreted in 1 to 3 days. Docusate is available in three different salt formulations: calcium (Surfak), potassium (Dialose, Diocto-K), and sodium (Colace, Regulex, DSS, Modane Soft).

These agents are indicated for patients with rectal impaction, hemorrhoids, chronic constipation, postpartum constipation, painful conditions of the rectum and anus, and for persons who should avoid straining (e.g., after rectal surgery or MI) at time of defecation. Docusate may be useful for immobile patients, especially children. It is said to have a wide margin of safety and few potential adverse reactions. The following dosages should be given with a full glass of water:

- *sodium docusate:* Adults and children over 12 years of age: 50 to 500 mg daily orally; children 6 to 12 years of age: 40 to 120 mg daily
- *calcium docusate* (Surfak): Adults: one capsule daily, 50 to 240 mg daily orally
- *docusate potassium* (Dialose): Adults, 100 to 300 mg daily; children over 6 years of age: 100 mg at bedtime

hyperosmotic suppository

Glycerin suppositories are available in adult, child, and infant sizes. The suppositories are osmotic agents that absorb water, lubricate, and increase stool bulk. They may also promote peristalsis through local irritation of the mucous membrane of the rectum. Evacuation occurs 15 to 60 minutes after insertion. The adult dose is 3 g, and the dose for children under 6 years of age is 1 to 1.5 g held high in the rectum for 15 minutes. Effects are achieved in 15 minutes to 1 hour.

ANTIDIARRHEAL AGENTS

The term **diarrhea** describes the abnormal passage of stools with increased frequency, increased fluidity, or increased weight and an increase in stool water excretion. Diarrhea is acute when it is of sudden onset in a previously healthy individual, lasts about 3 days to 1 to 2 weeks, is self-limiting, and resolves without sequelae. Morbid and mortal consequences are seen in malnourished populations, the elderly, infants, and debilitated persons.

Chronic diarrhea lasts for more than 3 to 4 weeks, with the recurring passage of diarrheal stools, fever, anorexia, nausea, vomiting, weight reduction, and chronic weakness. It is the result of multiple causative factors, as listed in Box 3-5. Chronic diarrhea necessitates definitive treatment directed to the organic cause or causes. The causes vary from psychogenic to neoplastic origins.

This section focuses on the OTC drugs with a direct pharmacologic effect on the GI tract. The drugs providing symptomatic therapy do not alter the pathophysiology of diarrhea and do not prevent electrolyte and fluid loss. Antidiarrheal agents diminish stool water by inhibiting intestinal fluid secretion or by increasing intestinal fluid absorption. Although these drugs decrease the number, consistency, and fluidity of the stool, there is no absolute clinical evidence that an effective antidiarrheal therapeutic benefit accrues to the patient. However, there is a relief of the bothersome symptoms that interrupt daily routines.

Adsorbents

Adsorbents act by coating the walls of the GI tract, absorbing the bacteria or toxins causing the diarrhea, and passing them out with the stools. Examples of OTC drugs in this

BOX 3-5 Causes of Acute and Chronic Diarrhea

Causes of Acute Diarrhea

Bacterial

1. Invasive organisms
   a. *Campylobacter fetus* (jejuni)
   b. *Clostridium difficile*
   c. *Escherichia coli* (enteropathogenic)
   d. *Salmonella*
   e. *Shigella dysenteriae*
   f. Staphylococci
2. Noninvasive toxigenic organisms
   a. Cholera *(Vibrio cholerae)* enterotoxin
   b. *Escherichia coli* (enterotoxigenic) toxin
3. Food poisoning as toxin mediated
   a. *Bacillus cereus*
   b. *Clostridium perfringens*
   c. *Salmonella*
   d. *Staphylococcus aureus*

Viral

1. Adenoviruses
2. Coxsackievirus
3. Coronaviruses
4. Eshoviruses
5. Norwalk agent
6. Rotavirus

Protozoal

1. Amebic dysentery *(Entomoeba histolytica)*, amebiasis
2. Giardiasis *(Giardia lamblia)*

Nutritional

1. Allergy
2. Ingestion without discretion (spices, fats, roughage, seeds, preformed toxin)
3. Enteral nutrition

Other

1. Bile acids
2. Carcinoma
3. Diverticulitis
4. Fatty acids
5. Neurogenic
6. Psychogenic
7. Radiation therapy
8. Regional and ulcerative colitis
9. Stress

Causes of Chronic Diarrhea

1. Addison's disease
2. Diabetic enteropathy or neuropathy
3. Iatrogenic
   a. Bacterial overgrowth
   b. Postsurgical
4. Inflammatory bowel disease
   a. Chronic ulcerative and granulomatous colitis
   b. Crohn's enteritis
5. Irritable bowel syndrome
6. Malabsorption syndrome
7. Pancreatic adenoma—nongastrin secreting, such as syndrome of watery diarrhea-hypokalemia-achlorhydria (WDHA)
8. Pancreatic insufficiency
9. Thyroid—hyperthyroidism
10. Tumors
    a. Carcinoma of colon and rectum
    b. Intestinal
    c. Lymphoma
    d. Polyposis
    e. Villous adenoma
11. Other
    a. Blind loops, ileostomy, colostomy
    b. Carcinoid syndrome
    c. Enteritis
    d. Gardner's syndrome
    e. Gastrointestinal hormones
    f. Gluten enteropathy
    g. Zollinger-Ellison syndrome
    h. Many other conditions

class are activated charcoal, aluminum hydroxide, bismuth salts, attapulgite, kaolin, and pectin. Attapulgite, activated charcoal, polycarbophil, and bismuth salts are the GI adsorbents in clinical use today. Bismuth salts are used for adsorption, astringency, and protection.

The adsorbent preparations are usually taken after each loose bowel movement until the diarrhea has been controlled. Constipation may develop because of the large amounts of the adsorbent products that must be used. A caution with all adsorbents is that they may interfere with the absorption of medications given concurrently (e.g., digoxin and clindamycin).

The drugs and nutrients adsorbed include a wide range of ingested substances. These may be decreased by administering the adsorbent 2 hours or more before or after a drug (except when used to inactivate a drug or for a specific poison in overdose situations).

bismuth subsalicylate [bis′ meth] (Pepto-Bismol)

Bismuth subsalicylate is an antidiarrheal, antacid (weak), and antiulcer medication. It has several actions, including (1) inhibition of GI secretions (i.e., it stimulates absorption of fluid and electrolytes in the intestine), (2) inhibition of synthesis of prostaglandins that produce intestinal inflammation and hypermotility, and (3) suppression of the growth of *Helicobacter pylori.* It is the only bismuth preparation available in the United States (Pinson, Weart, 1996; USP DI, 1998).

Administered orally, more than 90% of the dose is absorbed; it is bound to plasma proteins and excreted by the kidneys. Because bismuth subsalicylate is a salicylate and may be taken in large amounts to control diarrhea, it will enhance the effects of oral anticoagulants (i.e., increased bleeding time, bruising). Methotrexate may be displaced from its protein binding sites causing toxicity. Probenecid, an antigout agent, promotes the renal excretion of uric acid. When combined with bismuth subsalicylate, the uricosuric effects of probenecid can be inhibited by the salicylate.

Bismuth salicylate may antagonize the effects of hypoglycemic agents and could require a change in the dosage of the hypoglycemic agent. Be aware of possible salicylate toxicity when the drug is taken in large doses by persons taking large amounts of aspirin daily. Bismuth salicylate also has the potential for drug interactions if taken with oral anticoagulants, methotrexate, or any other drug that interacts with aspirin. The suspension of bismuth salicylate contains 130 mg of salicylate in 15 ml; the original tablet contains 102 mg, whereas the caplets and cherry flavored tablets contain 99 mg of salicylate (Longe, 1996).

The usual adult dose of bismuth subsalicylate is 30 ml or two tablets chewed or dissolved every 30 to 60 minutes (up to eight doses in 24 hours).

activated charcoal (Charcocaps, Charcodoteo, charcoal)

Activated charcoal is used for the relief of intestinal gas, diarrhea, and for GI distress associated with indigestion. It acts as an adsorbent, adsorbing toxic substances, irritants, and gas. It may also adsorb medication, nutrients, and enzymes.

The activated charcoal is administered as two capsules repeated every 30 to 60 minutes as needed up to eight doses (16 Charcocaps) for treatment of diarrhea symptoms. Tablets may be chewed or dissolved in the mouth and followed by water.

attapulgite (Kaopectate)

Attapulgite, a hydrated magnesium aluminum silicate, is a GI adsorbent and protective agent that has replaced the kaolin and pectin in Kaopectate. Kaolin and pectin are being reviewed by the FDA, and currently the evidence for kaolin is better that the combination of kaolin and pectin for treatment of acute, nonspecific diarrhea (Longe, 1996). Attapulgite is also being reviewed for both safety and efficacy. Therefore the healthcare professional should carefully watch for labeling changes on these products in the future.

Synthetic Opioids

loperamide [loe per′ a mide] (Imodium)

Loperamide is a synthetic OTC opioid that decreases GI motility by inhibiting propulsive movements in the gut. It produces a direct musculotropic effect that decreases hyperperistalsis, slows passage of intestinal contents, and allows reabsorption of water and electrolytes, resulting in a reduction in stool frequency.

Loperamide is indicated for the treatment of acute nonspecific and chronic diarrhea. Peak plasma levels after administration is 5 hours with the capsule dosage form or 2.5 hours for the oral liquid; the half-life ranges from 9 to 14 hours with a duration of action up to 24 hours. Loperamide is metabolized in the liver and excreted both fecally and by the kidneys.

Side effects are usually minimal, including dizziness, dry mouth, and skin rash. Drug-induced GI side effects are difficult to separate from those of diarrhea itself (epigastric pain, abdominal cramps, nausea, vomiting, and anorexia).

The usual adult OTC dose is 4 mg (two tablets) initially, followed by 2 mg after each loose stool, not exceeding 8 mg/day for more than 2 days.

COUGH-COLD PREPARATIONS

In 1990, it was estimated that more than $10 billion was spent on OTC medications; nearly $3 billion of this amount was used to buy cough, cold, and influenza (flu) preparations (Popovich, Newton, Pray, 1992). Box 3-6 describes the major differences between cold, allergic rhinitis, and influenza. This section is devoted to a description of the symptoms of these conditions and the medications used to treat coughs and colds, such as antitussives, antihistamines, expectorants, and decongestants. Many cough-cold products contain a combination of ingredients, some of which are

BOX 3-6 Colds, Allergic Rhinitis, and Influenza: Signs or Symptoms

Signs or Symptoms	*Common Cold*	*Allergic Rhinitis*	*Influenza*
Fever	Rare	Absent	Common–sudden onset, may range 102-104° F
Aches and pains	Slight	Absent	May be severe
Sneezing	Usual	Common	Infrequent
Pruritus	Absent or rare	Common	Absent
Cough	Mild-moderate	Uncommon	Common
Headaches	Rare	Can occur	Prominent
Causative	Usually viruses	Usually allergens	Usually viruses
Occurrence	Anytime	Usually seasonal	Anytime
Complications	Sinus congestion, earache	Uncommon	Bronchitis, pneumonia

subtherapeutic dose combinations or are unnecessary for the particular symptoms for which they are purported to treat. Such preparations are not considered rational and may not be safe and effective.

Although some combination products are very useful, they should be carefully selected according to the presenting symptoms. Generally, cough-cold preparations that contain analgesic and antipyretic agents should be avoided. Routine use of such products may mask a fever secondary to a bacterial infection, and if side effects or adverse effects occur, it would be difficult to determine the causative ingredient. In fact, the American Academy of Pediatrics Committee on Drugs has recommended against the use of combination cough-cold preparations (Tietze, 1996).

Products that do not provide full information on the label, such as the strength or amount of each ingredient, should also be avoided. It is difficult to evaluate such products when essential information is missing. How to select a combination product is discussed later in this chapter.

Cough

Coughing is defined as protective reflex for clearing the respiratory tract of environmental irritants, foreign bodies, or accumulated secretions and thus should not be depressed indiscriminately. The afferent impulses that arise from irritated pharyngeal and laryngeal tissues initiate the central cough reflex. A productive cough occurs when irritants or secretions are removed from the respiratory tract and generally should not be suppressed because it is helping to clear the airways. If a nonproductive cough is dry, irritating, frequent, and prolonged, it should be treated, since it can be exhausting, painful, and taxing to the circulatory system and the elastic tissue of the respiratory system, particularly in the elderly and young children.

Treatment of the cough is secondary to treatment of the underlying disorder. An **antitussive,** or cough suppressant, may act in the central or peripheral nervous system to suppress the cough reflex. Antitussives should not be taken in situations in which retention of respiratory secretions or exudates may be harmful. The therapeutic objective is to decrease the intensity and frequency of the cough yet permit adequate elimination of tracheobronchial secretions and exudates.

Drugs act either by suppressing the cough center in the medulla or by lessening irritation of the respiratory tract peripherally. Intake of fluids and inhalation of fully water-saturated vapors (steam) should be stressed as one of the most important means of producing increased amounts of mucus and thinning such secretions.

Antitussives

The primary OTC cough suppressant agents that affect the cough center centrally are codeine and dextromethorphan. Diphenhydramine (Benadryl), an antihistamine, and benzonatate (Tessalon) also have antitussive effects. Benzonatate is a prescription drug in the United States, so it is reviewed in Chapter 33, and diphenhydramine is reviewed in the antihistamine section of this chapter.

Codeine is included in selected combination products, and dextromethorphan is the preferred antitussive agent in OTC preparations. Codeine is an effective antitussive, but as an opioid, many laws govern its use as an OTC drug. The amount of codeine permitted in OTC products is also limited because codeine has a higher potential for misuse and abuse than other products. Dextromethorphan has no addictive properties and works centrally to raise the coughing threshold. It also has fewer side effects (drowsiness and gastric distress) than codeine. As an antitussive, 8 to 15 mg of codeine is considered equivalent to 15 to 30 mg of dextromethorphan (Olin, 1998).

dextromethorphan [dex troe meth or′ fan] (Sucrets Cough Control and others)
dextromethorphan combinations (Pertussin ES, Benylin DM, and others)

Dextromethorphan is well absorbed orally with an onset of action between 15 and 30 minutes and a duration of activity up to 6 hours. In usually recommended doses, side effects are minimal. Nausea, mild dizziness, and drowsiness have been reported.

Significant drug interactions have been reported with CNS depressant and MAO inhibitor medications. The former may result in enhanced CNS depressant effects, whereas concurrent use with MAO inhibitors may result in increased excitability, tremors, sedation, severe hypertension, intracranial bleeding, hyperpyrexia, or psychosis. Dextromethorphan should not be taken by persons taking an MAO inhibitor.

The dosage of adults and children 12 years of age and older is 10 to 20 mg orally every 4 hours or 30 mg every 6 to 8 hours, up to a maximum of 120 mg/day. For children 6 to 12 years of age, the recommended dosage is 5 to 10 mg every 4 hours up to a maximum of 60 mg/day; for children 2 to 6 years of age, 2.5 to 5 mg every 4 hours to a maximum of 30 mg/day. Dextromethorphan is not recommended for use in children under 2 years of age. Pregnancy safety is not established.

Many other products have been used as antitussive agents in various preparations, but the FDA advisory review panel on OTC cold, cough, allergy, bronchodilator, and antiasthmatic products has indicated that more evidence is needed to prove their effectiveness. Some of the products in this category include noscapine, beechwood creosote, elm bark, cod liver oil, and horehound.

Antihistamines

Antihistamines are drugs that compete with histamine for its receptor sites. With the discovery of two histamine receptors, H_1 and H_2, the antihistamines related to cold and allergy symptoms, such as diphenhydramine (Benadryl), chlorpheniramine (Chlor-Trimeton), and others, are H_1 receptor antagonists. The H_2 receptor antagonists related to the symptoms of gastric hyperacidity, such as cimetidine (Tagamet) and ranitidine (Zantac), are discussed in Chapter 35.

Receptor Antagonists

Antihistamines block histamine (H_1) receptors to reduce the histamine physiologic and pharmacologic effects such as sneezing, increased nasal secretions, and itching and watering eyes. These antihistamines have the greatest therapeutic effect on nasal allergies, particularly on seasonal hay fever and colds with histamine-like symptoms. In allergies, they relieve symptoms better at the beginning of the hay fever season than during its height but fail to relieve asthma that may frequently accompany hay fever. Antihistamines are palliative agents. Their action is comparatively short-lived and provides only symptomatic relief.

Many OTC preparations contain antihistamines, and some contain two or more different ones. Antihistamines may be used in a variety of OTC medications including antitussives, cough-cold products, sleep-inducing products, oral analgesic products, menstrual formulations, and many others. For example, diphenhydramine depresses the cough center in the medulla of the brain (antitussive effect), has antihistamine effects (blocks H_1 receptors), central antimuscarinic effects (antiparkinson action), sedative-hypnotic effects, and is used to prevent or treat nausea and vomiting associated with motion sickness. The consumer should check ingredients of all medications that they buy, consume, or administer. Often individuals have unwanted side effects or are accidentally overdosed by the same product available in several different medications that they are consuming, which unfortunately is often overlooked in a community setting. The antihistamines currently available OTC include the following:

- *brompheniramine* [brome fen air′ uh meen] (Dimetane, generics)
- *chlorpheniramine* [klor fen air′ uh meen] (Allerchlor, Chlor-Trimeton, and others)
- *diphenhydramine hydrochloride* [dye fen hye′ dra meen] (AllerMac, Benadryl 25, and others]
- *phenindamine* [fen in′ da meen] (Nolahist)
- *pyrilamine* [peer il′ uh meen] (generics available)

The primary difference between OTC and prescription antihistamines is the strength of the product. For example, OTC chlorpheniramine is 4 mg, whereas prescription products are 8 mg, 12 mg time-release, and injectable dosage forms.

Absorption of oral doses of antihistamines is good, with onset of action within 15 to 60 minutes. The time to peak effect can vary with each individual preparation. For example, brompheniramine has a peak effect in 3 to 9 hours, chlorpheniramine in 6 hours, and diphenhydramine in 1 to 4 hours. Duration of action is also variable with that of brompheniramine being 4 to 8 hours, chlorpheniramine 4 to 8 hours, diphenhydramine 6 to 8 hours, and pyrilamine 8 hours. These agents are primarily metabolized in the liver and excreted in the kidneys.

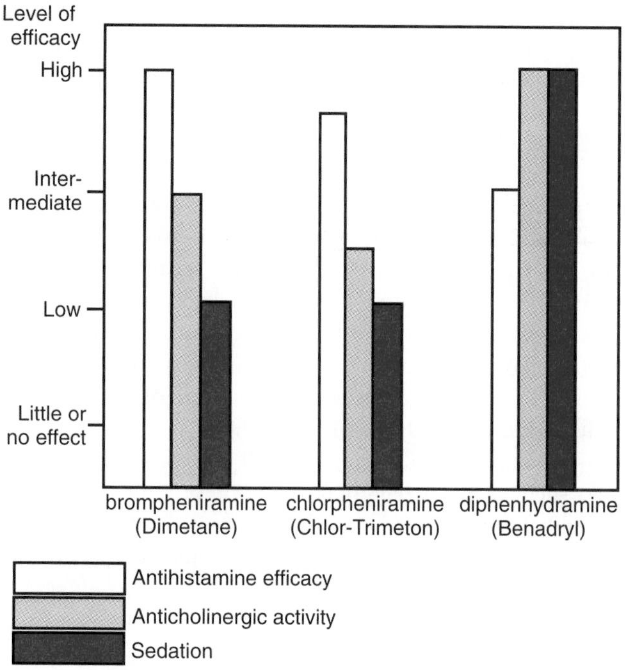

FIGURE 3-2
Comparison of efficacy and side effects of selected antihistamines

The most frequently reported OTC antihistamine side effects include constipation; decrease in sweating; difficulty in initiating urinary stream in elderly males; sedation; visual disturbances; photosensitivity; nausea or vomiting; and dry mouth, nose, or throat. Less often reported effects are orthostatic hypotension, headaches, anxiety, weak hands or feet, sore mouth and tongue, abdominal pain or increased excitability, and muscle cramps. Rarely reported adverse effects include glaucoma or eye pain in susceptible persons (individuals with predisposition to angle-closure glaucoma), skin rash, and confusion, especially in elderly persons having taken high doses. Fig. 3-2 shows a comparison of selected antihistamines, efficacy, and side effects.

Expectorants

Expectorants are substances that reduce the viscosity of secretions, thus promoting the ejection of mucus or other exudates from the lungs, bronchi, and trachea. In OTC preparations the only expectorant with evidence of safety and effectiveness is guaifenesin. Many other expectorants, such as ammonium chloride, iodides, and terpin hydrate, are listed as Category III (i.e., safe but not proven to be effective) (Tietze, 1996).

Decongestants

Decongestants are vasoconstricting agents used to shrink engorged nasal mucous membranes in mild upper respiratory tract infections. In OTC products, they are available in oral and nasal preparations.

TABLE 3-6 Topical and Oral Nasal Decongestants: Dosage

Drug/Strength	*Adults*	*Children (6 to 12 Years of Age)*
ephedrine, 0.5% (in Va-Tro-Nol and others)	2-3 drops q4h	1-2 drops q4h
naphazoline (Privine and others)		
0.05%	1-2 drops/spray, q6h	Not recommended
0.025%	—	1-2 drops q6h
oxymetazoline (Afrin, Allerest, Dristan Long-Lasting and others)		
0.05%	2-3 drops twice daily	Same as for adults
phenylephrine (Neo-Synephrine and others)		
1%	1-2 drops/spray q4h	Not recommended
0.25%	Same as for 1%	1-2 drops q4h
xylometazoline (Otrivin)		
0.1%	2-3 drops/spray q8-10h	Not recommended
0.05%	Same as for 0.1%	2-3 drops/spray q8-10h
Oral Nasal Decongestants (Usually Combined with Other Drug Products)		
phenylephrine	10 mg q4h	5 mg q4h
phenylpropanolamine	25 mg q4h	12.5 mg q4h
pseudoephedrine	60 mg q6h	30 mg q6h

The oral agents are sympathomimetic amines, and their vasoconstricting properties are not limited to the nasal mucosa. They can also elevate blood pressure in individuals with hypertension, induce cardiac stimulation and dysrhythmias in some people, and depending on the sympathomimetic, may increase blood glucose in those with diabetes. For this reason, warnings on the labels instruct the consumer with hypertension, hyperthyroidism, diabetes mellitus, or ischemic heart disease to contact their prescriber before using the product. Reported side effects and adverse effects include CNS stimulation or nervousness, insomnia, restlessness, dizziness, headaches, and increased irritability.

Three agents (phenylephrine, phenylpropanolamine, and pseudoephedrine) have been classified as Category I (safe and effective if label instructions are followed). These ingredients are often incorporated into combination products for their decongestant effects.

Many drugs are used exclusively as nasal vasoconstrictors or topical decongestants. Because of their popular use and lack of serious hazard (when used topically), many preparations have been provided by the pharmaceutical industry for direct sale to the public.

The FDA advisory review panel has recommended the following products as safe and effective topical nasal decongestants: ephedrine 0.5%; naphazoline (Privine) 0.05%, 0.025%; oxymetazoline (Afrin, Dristan) 0.05%, 0.025%; phenylephrine (Neo-Synephrine) 0.125%, 0.25%, 1%; and xylometazoline (Otrivin) 0.1%, 0.05%. Table 3-6 lists recommended dosages for topical nasal decongestant products and oral decongestant products. These drugs are adrenergic agents that act on alpha receptors of blood vessels in the nasal mucosa to produce vasoconstriction and so a decrease in mucosal swelling. Some nasal decongestant products (those containing ephedrine, epinephrine, metaproterenol, and others) also possess beta-stimulating effects, which may cause the CNS stimulation and perhaps the adverse effect of vasodilation after vasoconstriction.

Nasal decongestant drugs are used to shrink engorged mucous membranes of the nose and to relieve nasal stuffiness. However, there is a tendency on the part of the public to misuse them by using them excessively or too frequently. Excessive use may result in "rebound" engorgement, or swelling of the mucous membranes and a paradoxical bronchospasm. If an infection is present, there is always the possibility of spreading the infection deeper into the sinuses or to the middle ear with the use of nasal sprays or drops. Additives such as preservatives, antihistamines, and detergents are sometimes included in a decongestant preparation. In some cases, reactions may be caused by the additive rather than by the decongestant. Sprays and nose drops are beneficial when used judiciously. Table 3-6 lists topical and oral dosages of nasal decongestants.

Selection of Combination Cough-Cold Preparations

Combination OTC products require careful selection because some of these multidrug formulations contain unnecessary drugs for the individual. As previously mentioned, combinations that contain an analgesic or antipyretic agent should be avoided for several reasons:

1. There is the risk of masking a bacterial infection.
2. A fixed amount of analgesic or antipyretic is taken with other ingredients on a regular basis, whether needed or not.
3. If a side effect or adverse effect occurs, it would be difficult to identify the offending agent. If an analgesic or antipyretic is necessary, the proper dose should be selected and administered separately.

BOX 3-7 Selected Cough-Cold Combinations

Brand Name	Ingredients	Pharmacologic Effect
Robitussin	guaifenesin	Expectorant
Robitussin A-C	guaifenesin, codeine	Expectorant, cough suppressant
Robitussin-CF	guaifenesin, phenylpropanolamine, dextromethorphan	Expectorant, decongestant, cough suppressant
Robitussin-DM	guaifenesin, dextromethorphan	Expectorant, cough suppressant
Robitussin-PE	guaifenesin, pseudoephedrine	Expectorant, decongestant
Robitussin Night Relief	pyrilamine, pseudoephedrine, dextromethorphan, acetaminophen	Antihistamine, decongestant, cough suppressant, analgesic, alcohol-free solution
Robitussin Night-Time Cold Formula	doxylamine, pseudoephedrine, dextromethorphan, acetaminophen	Antihistamine, decongestant, cough suppressant, analgesic
Benylin Expectorant	guaifenesin, dextromethorphan	Expectorant, cough suppressant, alcohol free and sugar free
Cheracol Syrup	guaifenesin, codeine	Expectorant, cough suppressant, contains alcohol (4.75%)
Cheracol D Cough Solution	guaifenesin, dextromethorphan	Expectorant, cough suppressant, contains alcohol (4.75%)
Cheracol Plus Syrup	chlorpheniramine, phenylpropanolamine, dextromethorphan	Antihistamine, decongestant, cough suppressant, contains alcohol (8%)

From *USP DI*, 1998.

When only one drug effect is necessary, such as a nasal decongestant, expectorant, or an antihistamine effect, a therapeutic dose of that single drug entity should be taken. If the individual has several symptoms that need to be addressed, selection of a combination product should be limited to addressing just those symptoms with few if any additional substances. For example, for a cough suppressant and expectorant, an OTC product that contains guiafenesin and dextromethorphan (Robitussin DM and many others) may be selected. To treat allergy, nasal congestion, sneezing, and rhinorrhea, an antihistamine and decongestant combination is used, such as triprolidine and pseudoephedrine (Actifed) or chlorpheniramine and phenylpropanolamine (Allerest, etc.) or many others. With nasal or sinus congestion alone, an oral or a nasal decongestant may be selected (pseudoephedrine [Sudafed] or oxymetazoline [Afrin, Allerest]). See Box 3-7 for examples of cough-cold combinations.

ALTERNATIVE MEDICATIONS

In the past 20 years there has been a vast increase in the interest and use of alternative medical approaches reported in the United States. According to Eisenberg et al (1993), the number of visits to unconventional medicine practitioners in 1990 exceeded the number of visits to primary care physicians, with the cost of alternative therapies estimated at $14 billion dollars annually. Alternative medicine is also prevalent worldwide with an estimated 48% of the Australian population and 20% to 50% of Europeans reported as utilizing such therapies (MacLennan et al, 1996). Unfortunately, scientific evidence concerning the safety and efficacy of alternative medicine is often lacking. The U.S. National Institute of Health, which includes the Office of Alternative Medicine, is devoting millions of dollars annually to alternative and complementary medical research. Although the terms alternative and complementary have been used interchangeably, there is believed to be a distinction between them. *Alternative medicine* generally refers to practices that are either scientifically unfounded or lacking in support data, whereas *complementary* indicates that some scientific documentation exists, the practice is accepted, and it may be integrated in mainstream medical practice (Child Health 2000, 1998). Usually, complementary medical therapies include diet, exercise, counseling, biofeedback, massage therapy, relaxation, and hypnosis or imagery. Most other therapies such as homeopathy, herbals, macrobiotics, and many others are often classified under the alternative label.

The primary pharmacologic alternative therapy is herbals or natural products. Use of such products dates back to the earliest records of mankind when it was believed that an herbal tea, home remedy, or folk medicine could treat or cure many illnesses. Table 3-7 lists common home or folk remedies.

This interest in what is commonly referred to as the "back to nature movement" may have evolved from the numerous warnings that were issued on food additives, preservatives, and synthetic products that were said to be cancer-producing substances. In addition, dissatisfaction with an expensive, hard-to-access, and technologically oriented medical system may also have contributed to this movement. Whatever the reason, the general public appears to be more interested than ever in taking personal responsibility for their health and well being and for trying alternative methods to self-treat their health problems. The result is a vast proliferation of alternative healers, health food stores, natural products, organic fruits and vegetables, and the use of herbal remedies. This movement has evolved into a mul-

TABLE 3-7 Common Home or Folk Remedies

Remedy	Potential Uses or Illnesses	Comments
Garlic (Allium sativum)	Antiseptic, antibiotic, antiplatelet, coronary artery disease, lowers high blood cholesterol, hypertension, antitumor	Garlic contains alliin, which is converted to allicin and is responsible for both the garlic odor and the potential antibacterial effects. Other ingredients such as ajoene are considered to be at least as potent as aspirin and may be responsible for its antithrombotic and antiplatelet effects. Published studies and other trials are underway (Tyler, 1993; Tyler, 1994; Weiner, Weiner, 1994).
Onion (Allium cepa)	Stomach and intestinal distress, coronary heart disease, blood-clotting disorders	Onion is from the same family as garlic. It has been used for many purposes as noted, and in addition, some cultures use the following home remedies: • To reduce fever, place raw onion slices on feet and cover • To treat a cold, place a slice of cut onion in a glass of hot water, then remove after a few second. Allow the water to cool, and sip fluid throughout the day. May also inhale onion vapors to help breathing. • For headaches, apply raw onion poutice to back of neck, calves of legs, and soles of the feet. Numerous other home remedies are available (Tyler, 1993; Vogel, 1991).
Lemon in water	Colds, congestion	Hot lemon is mixed with water and honey; garlic or onion may be added. Drink.
Potato juice	Arthritis	The potato is grated, and juice is squeezed out and mixed in warm water or soup. Take daily before breakfast (Vogel, 1991).

timillion dollar enterprise that is not limited to any specific cultural or ethnic groups but rather is widespread.

Eastern versus Western Medicine

There is a major difference between the Eastern (Asian) and Western philosophical approaches to healthcare. In Eastern practice, such as Traditional Chinese Medicine (TCM), maintaining an energy balance in the body is most important; a balance between yin (negative) and yang (positive) forces is necessary to maintain good health. Thus the Chinese physician may prescribe a variety of interventions such as herbal therapy, acupuncture, diet changes, exercise, meditation, or the services of a spiritual healer. In this culture, herbals have been studied for thousands of years, so this knowledge is used with other therapies to achieve a balance within the body to help regain and maintain good health.

In Chinese herbal medicine, herbs are either taken orally or applied externally to correct the physical disorder. It is believed that herbals are much more effective when used in a balanced formula. For example, ginseng may energize the body (especially lungs, spleen, and pancreas), but it can also cause strong side effects if used alone. The ginsenosides in ginseng can constrict arteries. However, if ginseng is combined with other herbs such as kudzu or astragalus, the side effects are believed to be balanced. Another example is the combination of bitter orange, ginseng, and ginger; the bitter orange stimulates the bodies vital energy (Qi), ginseng energizes the body, and ginger is included as an assisting herbal (i.e., it helps to relax muscle tissue). Therefore this combination was chosen for their individual effects and their effects in combination together. In this formula the key herbal may be the bitter orange for the person who needs to strengthen his or her body Qi energy (cold). The balancing herbal is ginseng because it energizes the body by providing a warmer energy, and ginger serves as an assistant herbal. This combination may be used to treat muscle aches (muscle relaxant) and digestive tract problems and in persons who need to strengthen their Qi energy (Zhou, 1998).

Eastern or Asian interest is in health promotion or stabilization, as opposed to the American concept of illness intervention and treatment. In the West the concentration is on treating symptoms or treating the area where the symptoms originated with pharmacologic and nonpharmacologic treatments. For example, bronchitis symptoms may include excessive mucus secretion in the bronchi, cough, frequent chest infections, and cyanosis. Treatment may include a systemic antibiotic for the infection, an expectorant and postural drainage for the mucus, and advising the patient not to smoke. If necessary, a bronchodilator and oxygen may be ordered. As previously mentioned, the Western focus is on the symptoms and the organ affected. Eastern treatment might use some of these therapies but would also include approaches to help the individual regain energy balance to hopefully reduce further episodes. Depending on the practitioner, the approaches can vary considerably.

Herbal Products in the United States

Herbals are marketed as food supplements in the United States; therefore it is not necessary to prove safety nor effectiveness, before packaging them for resale. When the FDA suggested stricter regulation, thousands of letters from the general public were sent to Congress to block such regulations. Instead, the Dietary Supplement and Health Education Act of 1994 was created to separate supplements from food and drug. This act made these products independent of the previous FDA rules that governed questionable prod-

TABLE 3-8 Selected Herbals Used in the United States

Herbal (Scientific Name)	***Part Used***	***Uses***	***Comments***
Alfalfa *(Medicago sativa)*	Leaves, sprouted seed	Appetite stimulant, antiarthritic, diuretic, and many others	1. Studies on effectiveness for these claims is lacking. 2. Consuming large quantities of alfalfa tablets has been reported to activate inactive and dormant SLE (Tyler, 1993).
Aloe *(Aloe vera)*	Leaves	Orally, for constipation; topical, heals external wounds and burns; also promoted as a cleanser, antipyretic, anesthetic, antiinflammatory, and dozens of others.	1. Use of aloe to treat burns dates back to ancient Egypt (Cleopatra). 2. Fresh aloe is effective for burns (sunburn, radiation burns) and wound healing. 3. Oral aloe is a potent laxative that should be used to treat chronic constipation only, because its effect is mainly in the colon where it can cause pain resulting from bowel muscle spasms (Weiner, Weiner, 1994).
Damiana *(Turnera aphrodisiaca)*	Leaves	Aphrodisiac	1. There is no evidence to support this claim (Tyler, 1993; Weiner, Weiner, 1994).
Dandelion *(Taraxacum officinale)*	Leaves, root	Tonic, GI distress, mild diuretic, mild laxative	1. Old Indian remedy and food. 2. Good source of vitamin A. 3. Used to make wine and coffee substitute (roasted roots) (Tyler, 1993; Weiner, Weiner, 1994).
Ginseng, American *(Panax quinquefolius)*	Root, leaf	Aphrodisiac, tonic, panacea for many illnesses	1. This species is similar in effect to the Asian variety. A remedy used by many Indian tribes in the United States. 2. Most research on ginseng was done in Asia, and until recently, nearly 95% of all American ginseng was exported from there. 3. All ginsengs are adaptogens, that is they help the person to adapt to physical and mental stress, fatigue, and cold (i.e., help to normalize an abnormal condition in the body) (Chevallier, 1996, Weiner, Weiner, 1994). 4. The root of red American ginseng does not have any ginseng properties and when ingested produces a laxative effect (Weiner, Weiner, 1994). 5. Panex ginseng is often referred to as Chinese or Korean ginseng, and *Eleutherococcus senticosus* is Siberian ginseng. The latter has been researched in Russia, and extracts of it appear to stimulate cellular immunity (Weiner, Weiner, 1994). 6. Some products that claim to be Siberian ginseng have been analyzed and found to contain no *Eleutherococcus senticosus* root (Weiner, Weiner, 1994). 7. Chevallier (1996) claims that ginseng is abused in the West where it is taken as a tonic instead of a medicine, (i.e., it should not be taken for more than 6 weeks).
Hawthorn *(Crataegus oxycantha)*	Flowers, leaves, and berries	Heart remedy, diuretic, nerve tonic, hypertension	1. Prescribed in Europe as a substitute for digitalis (Weiner, Weiner, 1994). 2. Hawthorn has flavonoids with cardiotonic effects. It is used to treat mild congestive heart failure, irregular heartbeats, angina, and coronary artery disease but may take months to produce effects (Chevallier, 1996). 3. Further research with Hawthorn is necessary because self-treatment for cardiac problems is not recommended (Tyler, 1993).
Juniper *(Juniperus communis)*	Ripe berries	Diuretic, for indigestion	1. Some oils it contains can cause kidney damage. 2. In very small amounts it is used to flavor gin. This use is not considered harmful (Tyler, 1994).
Slippery Elm *(Ulmus fulva)*	Bark	GI distress, cough, sore throat, and topically as a lubricant and poultice for boils and splinters.	1. Has demulcent properties, therefore it soothes irritating surfaces such as GI tract and throat. 2. Used in many ways by Americans Indians (Chevallier, 1996; Weiner, Weiner, 1994).

ucts (Herbal Supplements, 1998). The Act created a new category for herbs, vitamins, minerals, and nearly anything else that was sold as a dietary supplement before October 15, 1994. It was estimated that there are approximately 20,000 such products covered by this act.

Previously, a supplement manufacturer had to prove that its product was safe if challenged by the FDA; now the FDA has to prove the product is unsafe. Such information, in many instances, would come after the marketing of the product or after a problem is reported. Therefore the healthcare professional and consumer should be aware that "natural" does not always mean safe. Some natural products can cause harm, depending on the herbal itself, the quantity consumed, whether the proper plant or part of the plant is present in the package, the presence of contaminants in the supplement, and other factors. Although one does not hear of many herbal toxicities in consumer literature, some very serious problems have been reported in medical literature. For example, chaparral was promoted as a blood purifier and cancer cure (not on the label, which would then involve the FDA as this is a medicinal use promotion), but its usage has caused serious liver damage in some patients. In at least one case, the need for a liver transplant was reported after 10 months of chaparral usage (Stashower et al, 1995).

The mushroom Kombucha has also been associated with illnesses and death. Liquid from Kombucha is said to be a tonic, but several people were hospitalized and one woman died after taking this product (Herbs, 1998). The cause could not directly be attributed to the Kombucha, but several theories were offered: (1) the tea may have reacted with other medications that the woman was taking, or (2) bacteria may have grown in the Kombucha liquid, and in patients with suppressed immunity, it might prove to be fatal.

The latter reasoning indicates potential problems that may not have been considered before taking the product; that is, what effect would the active ingredients in the herbal have on other medications that the individual may be consuming? Many active medications in current use were originally discovered from plants, such as digitalis glycosides from foxglove, vinca alkaloids from periwinkle, or ephedra (ephedrine) from MaHuang, which was promoted as Herbal Fen-Phen (Weiner, Weiner, 1994; FDA talk paper, 1998). Therefore various natural or herbals may contain active ingredients that have or have not been identified, and which, in combination with other medications, may cause serious drug interactions.

Since many herbal remedies may be harmful to some individuals, healthcare professionals taking a medication his-

TABLE 3-9 Herbals with a Potential for Toxicity

Botanical Name	Common Names	Comments
Arnica montana	Arnica flowers, Wolfsbane, mountain tobacco, *Flores Arnicae*	Substances extracted affect the heart and vascular systems. Arnica is extremely irritating and can induce a toxic gastroenteritis, nervous system disturbances, extreme muscle weakness, collapse, and perhaps, death
Artemisia absinthium	Wormwood, absinthe, madderwort, absinthium, Mugwort	Contains a narcotic poison (oil of wormwood); can cause nervous system damage and mental impairment
Atropa belladonna	Belladonna, deadly nightshade	Considered a poisonous plant that contains the toxic alkaloids of atropine, hyoscyamine, and hyoscine. Anticholinergic symptoms range from blurred vision, dry mouth, and inability to urinate to unusual behaviors and hallucinations
Aesculus hippocasteranum	Buckeyes, horse chestnut, aesculus	Contains coumarin glycoside, aesculin; may interfere with normal blood clotting; a toxic plant
Conium maculatum	Hemlock, conium, spotted hemlock, spotted parsley, St. Bennet's herb, spotted cowbane, fool's parsley	Contains toxic alkaloid coniine and perhaps, four other related alkaloids
Lobelia inflata	Lobelia, Indian tobacco, wild tobacco, asthma weed, emetic weed	Toxic plant that contains lobeline plus other alkaloids; excessive use of plant or its leaves or fruit extracts can result in severe vomiting, pain, sweating, paralysis, decreased temperature, collapse, coma, and death
Ma-Huang	Ephedra	Herb contains ephedrine (30% to 90% depending on species); pseudoephedrine also discovered in some species. Both substances are sympathomimetics, producing effects similar to epinephrine. Therefore it can increase systolic and diastolic blood pressure, heart rate, and many side effects associated with sympathomimetics (Tyler, 1993; Weiner, Weiner, 1994). This herbal has been used to make methamphetamine (speed) and is used as an alternative drug in ecstasy, also an illegal street drug. Herbal Fen-Phen's main ingredient is ephedra. (There are over 800 adverse reports with its use that range from headaches, heart attacks, and death. The FDA has issued warnings, and some states have restrictions that regulate the sale of this herbal (FDA Update, 1998; HHS News, 1996; Tyler, 1993)
Vinca major *Vinca minor*	Periwinkle, vinca, greater or lesser periwinkle	Contain toxic alkaloids (vinblastine, vincristine) that are cytotoxic and may cause liver, kidney, and neurologic damage

From Tyler, 1993.

tory should inquire about the use of OTC, health food store, and herbal products. Such products are often not considered to be drugs or medications by the consumer, and therefore are not generally reported. See Table 3-8 for selected herbals used in the United States and Table 3-9 for herbals with a potential for toxicity.

Since the safety and efficacy of herbals are not monitored by the FDA, the consumer should seek as much information as possible on these products before consumption. Checking reliable herbal references or contacting a knowledgeable healthcare professional or prescriber is highly recommended.

SUMMARY

With proper use, over-the-counter (OTC) drugs are considered safe for use in the treatment of minor illnesses without the supervision of a healthcare professional. Because of the widespread use of these drugs, problems relating to these products can occur, such as prescription drug-OTC drug interactions and drug misuse or abuse. This chapter reviews pharmacologic information about the most commonly used OTCs, including analgesics, antacids, laxatives, cough-cold preparations, and antidiarrheals.

Consumers should be informed on how to review the label on OTC medications before purchase (e.g., ingredients, precautions, and contraindications as related to their documented health problems). Wise selection and use of OTC drug products can be very cost effective.

With the increased interest and use of herbal, home, and natural remedies today, the healthcare professional needs to be informed on such products. A thorough medication history and close patient monitoring is recommended. The consumer or the healthcare professional is primarily responsible for detecting any unusual or adverse reactions with these products because the FDA, by law, does not approve herbals for safety or effectiveness before marketing.

REVIEW QUESTIONS

1. Name the laxative category that is contraindicated for use in patients who are on restricted or limited fluid intake or who have a fecal impaction. Name one laxative from this category. Explain why it is contraindicated.
2. A patient is administered 2 tablets of bisacodyl (Dulcolax) and 30 ml of an antacid at 9 pm, as ordered by the physician. Within 1 hour, the patient is complaining of severe stomach cramps and pain. The healthcare provider informed the patient that this was a normal indication that the laxative is working. Is this a correct response? Discuss the cause of this problem and a method for prevention.
3. Name three serious drug-drug interactions with the use of bismuth subsalicylate (Pepto-Bismol). How can the healthcare provider help to prevent these interactions?

REFERENCES

Ahronheim JC: *Handbook of prescribing medications for geriatric patients,* Boston, 1992, Little, Brown, & Co.

Brunton LL: Agents for control of gastric acidity and treatment of peptic ulcers. In Hardman JF, Limbird LE, editors: *Goodman & Gilman's the pharmacological basis of therapeutics,* ed 9, New York, 1996, McGraw-Hill.

Burns J, editor: *OTC drugs can be a low-cost alternative: the value of pharmaceuticals, Business & Health Special Report,* Montvale, NJ, 1991, Medical Economics Publishing.

Chevallier A: *The encyclopedia of medicinal plants,* New York, 1996, DK Publishing.

Child health 2000: the meaning of alternative and complementary medicine: information superhighway and telemedicine, http://edie.cprost.sfu.ca/gcnet/iss4-45a.html (Feb 3, 1998).

Cornacchia HJ, Barrett S: *Consumer health: a guide to intelligent decisions.* St Louis, 1993, Mosby.

Covington TR: Self-care and nonprescription pharmacotherapy. In Covington TR, editor: *Handbook of nonprescription drugs,* ed 11, Washington, DC, 1996, American Pharmaceutical Association.

Curry CE, Jr, Tatum-Butler D: Laxative products. In Covington TR, editor: *Handbook of nonprescription drugs,* ed 11, Washington, DC, 1996, American Pharmaceutical Association.

Eisenberg DM, Kessler RC et al: Unconventional medicine in the United States: prevalence, costs, and patterns of use. *N Engl J Med* 328:246, 1993.

FDA talk paper, http://vm.cfsan.fda.gov/~ lrd/tpfenphn.html (Feb 4, 1998).

FDA update: warning about herbal Fen-Phen, http://www.fda.gov/fdac/departs/1998/198_upd.html (February 7, 1998).

Fitzgerald WL: Legal control of pharmacy services. In OBRA '90: *A practical guide to effecting pharmaceutical care,* Washington, DC, 1994, American Pharmaceutical Association.

Herbal supplements: promises and pitfalls, http://www.vitawise.com/danger.htm. (Feb. 4, 1998).

Herbs: does natural = safe? http://www.vitawise.com/safsup.htm (Feb. 4, 1998).

HHS news: search '97 information server document news release, http://www.fda.gov/medwatch/safety/1997/ephedr.htm. (Feb. 2, 1998).

Insel PA: Analgesic-antipyretic and antiinflammatory agents and drugs employed in the treatment of gout. In Hardman JG, Limbird LE, editors: *Goodman & Gilman's the pharmacological basis of therapeutics,* ed 9, New York, 1996, McGraw-Hill.

Lipman AG: Internal analgesic and antipyretic products. In Covington TR, editor: *Handbook of nonprescription drugs,* ed 11, Washington, DC, 1996, American Pharmaceutical Association.

Longe RL: Antidiarrheal products. In Covington TR, editor: *Handbook of nonprescription drugs,* ed 11, Washington, DC, 1996, American Pharmaceutical Association.

MacLennan AH, Wilson DH, Taylor AW: Prevalence and cost of alternative medicine in Australia, *Lancet* 347:569, 1996.

Newton GD, Pray WS, Popovich NG: New OTC drugs and devices: a selected review, *J Am Pharmaceut Assoc* S36(2):108, 1996.

Olin BR: *Facts and comparisons.* Philadelphia, 1998, Lippincott.

Pinson JB, Weart CW: Acid-peptic products. In Covington TR, editor: *Handbook of nonprescription drugs,* ed 11, Washington, DC, 1996, American Pharmaceutical Association.

Popovich MG, Newton GD, Pray WS: New OTC drugs: a selected review, *Am Pharm* NS32(2):26, 1992.

Stashower ME, Torres H et al: Letters: chaparral and liver toxicity, *JAMA* 273:489, 1995.

Tietze KJ: Cold, cough, and allergy products. In Covington TR, editor: *Handbook of nonprescription drugs,* ed 11, Washington, DC, 1996, American Pharmaceutical Association.

Tyler VE: *The honest herbal,* ed 3, New York, 1993, Pharmaceutical Products Press.

Tyler VE: *Herbs of choice: the therapeutic use of phytomedicinals,* New York, 1994, Pharmaceutical Products Press.

United States Pharmacopeial Convention: *USP DI: drug information for the health care professional,* vol I. *Advice for the patient,* vol II, ed 18, Rockville, Md, 1998, the Convention.

Vogel HCA: *The nature doctor.* New Canaan, Conn, 1991, Keats Publishing.

Weiner MA, Weiner JA: *Herbs that heal,* Mill Valley, Calif, 1994, Quantum Books.

Zhou J: *Chinese herbal medicine: Dr. James Zhou explains traditional Chinese herbs,* http://www.arxc.com/herbaswy/zhoucol.htm. (Feb. 2, 1998).

Zimmerman DR: *Complete guide to nonprescription drugs,* ed 2, Detroit, 1993, Gale Research.

ADDITIONAL REFERENCES

Anderson KN et al, editors: *Mosby's medical, nursing, and allied health dictionary,* ed 5, St Louis, 1998, Mosby.

Mosby: *Mosby's GenRx,* St Louis, 1998, Mosby.

UNIT II

Physiologic Aspects of Pharmacology

CHAPTER 4

Principles of Drug Action

CHAPTER FOCUS

To meet the knowledge challenge of the numerous drugs on the market today combined with the many new drugs released annually, the healthcare professional must develop a basic theoretical framework based on the principles of drug action. This chapter reviews the general properties of drugs, mechanisms of action, pharmacokinetics, pharmacodynamics, and other factors that influence drug therapies.

OBJECTIVES

After reading and studying this chapter, the student should be able to do the following:

1. *Define and discuss the key terms.*
2. *Explain the three general properties of drugs.*
3. *Describe the mechanisms of drug action including the pharmaceutical, pharmacokinetic, and pharmacodynamic phases.*
4. *Cite six examples of variables that affect drug absorption.*
5. *Discuss the major theories of drug action.*
6. *Explain the relationship between drug dose and patient response, including plasma level, biologic half-life, and therapeutic index.*
7. *Discuss the differences between side and adverse effects and predictable and unpredictable adverse responses.*

KEY TERMS

absorption, (p. 56)
active or carrier transport, (p. 55)
bioavailability, (p. 65)
biotransformation, (p. 61)
dissolution, (p. 54)
distribution, (p. 59)
excretion, (p. 62)
half-life, (p. 64)
iatrogenic, (p. 70)
ionized, (p. 55)
loading doses, (p. 57)
maintenance doses, (p. 57)
nonionized, (p. 55)
passive transport, (p. 55)
receptor, (p. 63)

The number of drugs used in medical treatment today has increased dramatically and continues to grow annually. To meet this challenge, healthcare professionals need to develop a fundamental approach and framework within which to study and apply an understanding of drug therapy. This chapter reviews the general properties of drugs, mechanisms of action, pharmacokinetics, pharmacodynamics, dosage formulations, side effects and adverse drug reactions, and other related topics on principles of drug action.

GENERAL PROPERTIES OF DRUGS

As stated previously, a drug is a chemical that interacts with a living organism to produce a biologic response. This section addresses drug dosages that are administered to obtain therapeutic, prophylactic, or diagnostic effects. These effects are achieved by some underlying biochemical or physiologic interaction between the drug and a functionally important tissue component (usually a receptor) in the body. Thus it is important to recognize the following general properties of drugs:

1. Drugs do not confer any new functions on a tissue or organ in the body; they only modify existing functions. Therefore the effects of drugs can be recognized only by alterations of a known physiologic function or process such as replacing, interrupting, or potentiating a physiologic process in specialized tissues. An example is ferrous sulfate, which is used to treat anemia by replacing iron to restore the adequate production of red blood cells. Atropine, on the other hand, reduces the rate of salivation in preoperative patients, which is an essentially abnormal state but a necessary one to decrease the surgical risk of aspiration. Finally, the administration of a potent laxative can potentiate the rate of evacuation of the large intestine.
2. Drugs in general exert multiple actions rather than a single effect. Consequently, drugs may in varying degrees produce undesirable responses because of their potential to modify more than one function of the body. These unwanted effects may be avoided somewhat by administering more specific or more selective drugs. For example, metaproterenol is a selective beta$_2$-adrenergic agent used to produce bronchodilation. Yet a common side effect is beta$_2$-mediated muscle tremors.
3. Drug action results from a physicochemical interaction between the drug and a functionally important molecule in the body. Some drugs act by combining with a small molecule (e.g., antacids neutralize gastric acid) or producing an alteration of cell membrane activity (e.g., local anesthetics). However, the major mechanism by which drugs interact is by combining with macromolecular components of tissues, such as receptors.

MECHANISMS OF DRUG ACTION

To produce its optimal effect, a drug must reach appropriate concentrations at its site of action. This means that the molecules of the chemical compound must proceed from their point of entry into the body to the tissues with which they react. In addition, the magnitude of the response depends on the dosage and the frequency of doses of the drug in the body. Therefore the concentration of the drug at its site of action is influenced by various processes, which may be divided into three phases of drug activity: pharmaceutical, pharmacokinetic, and pharmacodynamic. The sequential order of these phases is depicted in Fig. 4-1.

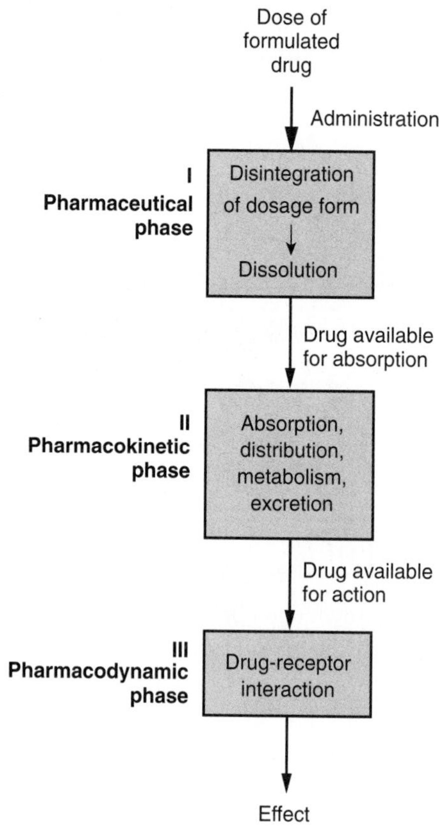

FIGURE 4-1
Phases affecting drug activity.

Pharmaceutical Phase

Pharmaceuticsis the study of the ways in which various drug forms influence pharmacokinetic and pharmacodynamic activities. An oral drug may appear in solid form (tablet, capsule, or powder) or in liquid form (solution or suspension).

Disintegration of solid dosage forms must occur before **dissolution,** a process by which a drug goes into solution and becomes available for absorption. The drug dosage form is important because the more rapid the rate of dissolution, the more readily the compound crosses the cell membrane to achieve absorption. Therefore oral drugs in liquid form are more rapidly available for gastrointestinal absorption than those in solid form (Fig. 4-2 and Box 4-1).

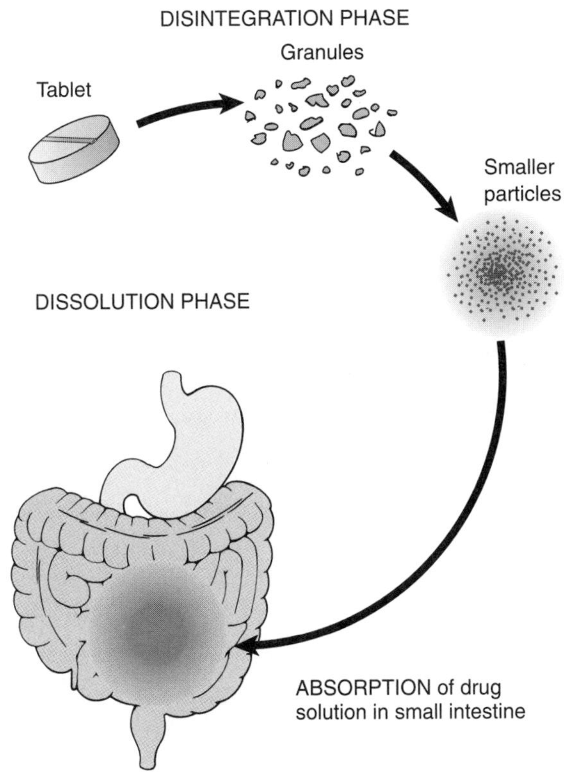

FIGURE 4-2
Pharmaceutical phase.

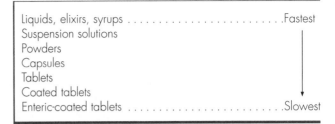

Pharmacokinetic Phase

Pharmacokinetics is the study of the concentration of a drug during the processes of absorption, distribution, biotransformation, and excretion. The concentration that a drug attains at its site of action is influenced by four primary factors: the rate and extent to which a drug is (1) absorbed into body fluids, (2) distributed to sites of action or storage areas, (3) biotransformed or metabolized to breakdown or active metabolites, and (4) excreted from the body by various routes (Fig. 4-3).

Factors Influencing Pharmacokinetic Activity

Physiochemical properties of drugs

In general, drugs exist as weak acids or weak bases, and in body fluids they appear in either ionized or nonionized (un-ionized) forms. The **ionized** (polar) form is usually water soluble (lipid insoluble) and does not diffuse readily through the cell membranes of the body. By contrast, the **nonionized** (nonpolar) form is more lipid soluble (less water soluble) and is more apt to cross the cell membranes. The influence of pH on these compounds is discussed under Absorption in this chapter.

Physiochemical properties of cell membranes

The extent to which a drug attains pharmacokinetic activity depends on the rate at which it crosses the cell membrane. The membrane consists of a bimolecular layer of lipids that contain protein molecules, which are irregularly dispersed throughout the lipid bilayer. The protein molecule itself may act as a carrier, an enzyme, a receptor, or an antigenic site. The drugs that are lipid (fat) soluble can easily pass through the lipid membrane, while ionized or water-soluble drugs have difficulty crossing cell membranes. The membrane, which appears to contain pores, permits the passage of small water-soluble substances such as urea, alcohol, electrolytes, and water itself.

Drug molecules, when free to move to sites of action, are transported from one body compartment to another by way of the plasma. However, free movement can be somewhat limited because these various sites are enclosed by membranes. Barriers to drug transport may consist of a single layer of cells, such as the villus in intestinal epithelium, or several layers of cells, such as skin. Nevertheless in order for a drug to gain access to the interior of a cell or a body compartment, it has to penetrate cell membranes. All the physiologic processes mediating drug action—absorption, distribution, metabolism, and excretion—are predicated on three drug transport systems: membrane openings or pores, passive transport, and active or carrier transport.

Membrane openings or pores. These openings or pores are very small so only a few of the smallest drugs can be transported by this method.

Passive transport. **Passive transport** is the transfer of drug substance from a region of higher concentration to a region of lower concentration until an equilibrium is established at the membrane. No energy is required for this process. The vast majority of drugs are transported by this system. This transport mechanism also forms the basis for many of the extended-release tablet formulations and the rectal drug dosage form (Sjoqvist et al, 1997).

Active or carrier transport. **Active or carrier transport** is necessary for the transport of amino acids, glucose, and a few drugs such as methyldopa and levodopa. These moderate-sized ions and water-soluble drugs are transported by carriers that form complexes with drug molecules on the membrane surface to carry them through the membrane and then dissociate from them. The dynamics of active transport require an energy source. Active transport involves the movement of drug molecules against the concentration gradient (from areas of low concentration to

BOX 4-1 Absorption of Preparations

Liquids, elixirs, syrups	Fastest
Suspension solutions	↓
Powders	
Capsules	
Tablets	
Coated tablets	
Enteric-coated tablets	Slowest

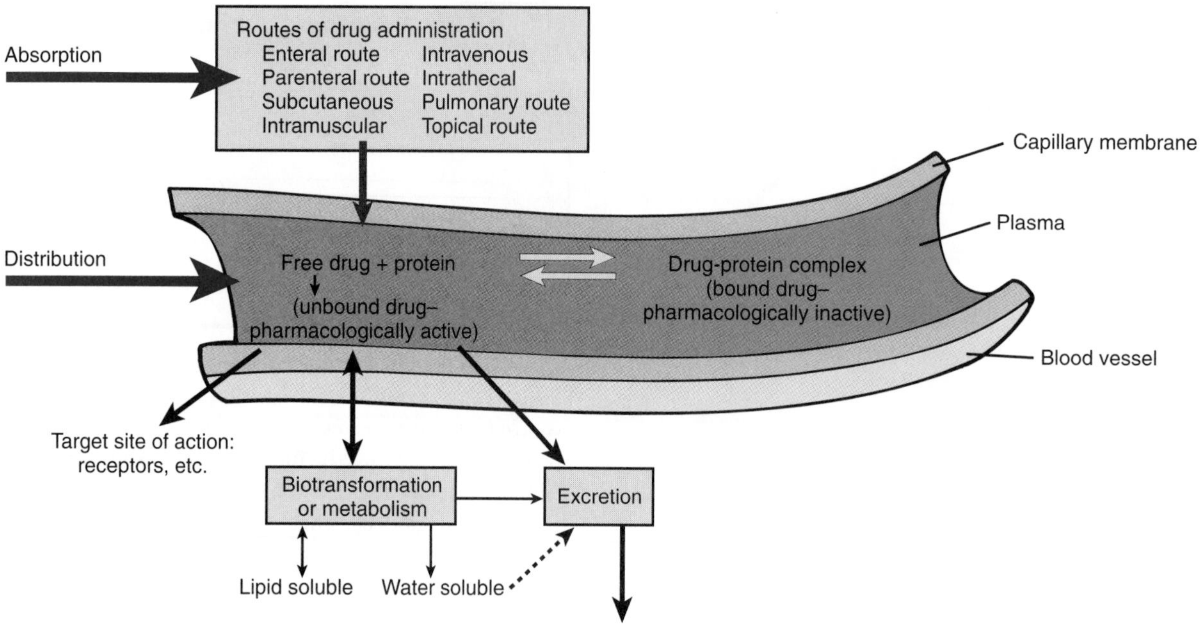

FIGURE 4-3
Schema of pharmacokinetic phase of drug action, showing absorption, distribution, biotransformation, and excretion of drugs. Note that only free drug is capable of movement for absorption, distribution to the target site of action, biotransformation, and excretion; the drug-protein complex represents bound drugs; and because the molecule is large, it is trapped in the blood vessel and serves as a storage site for the drug.

areas of high concentration) or, in the case of ions, against the electrochemical potential gradient such as that occurring with the "sodium pump." Active transport is usually more rapid than passive diffusion.

Pharmacokinetic Activity

Absorption

Absorption is a process involving the movement of drug molecules from the site of entry into the body to the circulating fluids. Absorption begins at the site of administration and is essential to the three subsequent processes—distribution, metabolism, and excretion. The rate of drug absorption is significant because it determines when a drug becomes pharmacologically available to exert its action. Of importance is that both the duration and the intensity of drug action are greatly influenced by the rate of this process. Accordingly, this type of response depends on the selection of the route of administration, the dose of the drug, and the dosage form (tablet, capsule, or liquid) of the agent administered.

Variables that affect drug absorption. The rate and extent to which a drug is absorbed are influenced by the following variables.

1. *Nature of the absorbing surface (cell membrane) through which the drug must traverse.* The drug molecule may pass through a single layer of cells (intestinal epithelium), in which case transport is faster than when it traverses several layers of cells (skin). In addition, the size of the surface area of the absorbing site is an important determinant of drug absorption. Generally, the more extensive the absorbing surface, the greater the drug absorption and the more rapid its effects. Anesthetics are absorbed immediately from the pulmonary epithelium because of the vast surface area. Absorption from the small intestine, which offers a massive absorbing area, is more rapid than from a smaller absorbing surface, such as the stomach.
2. *Blood flow to the site of administration.* Circulation to the site of administration is a significant factor in the absorption of drugs. A rich blood supply (sublingual route) enhances absorption, whereas a poor vascular site (subcutaneous route) delays it. An individual in shock, for example, may not respond to intramuscularly administered drugs because of poor peripheral circulation. Drugs injected intravenously, on the other hand, are placed directly into the circulatory system and are totally available. Intravenous administration is desirable when speedy drug effects are necessary, but it carries the potential danger of achieving temporarily toxic responses in vital organs such as the heart or the brain. Therefore to prevent deleterious effects, some drugs must be injected slowly. In addition, the decreased peripheral blood flow in patients with congestive heart failure or circulatory shock may cause a significant reduction in the rate of transport of injected drugs to the target tissues, thereby considerably altering their efficacy.
3. *Solubility of the drug.* To be absorbed, a drug must be in solution; the more soluble the drug, the more rapidly it will be absorbed. Because cell membranes contain a fatty

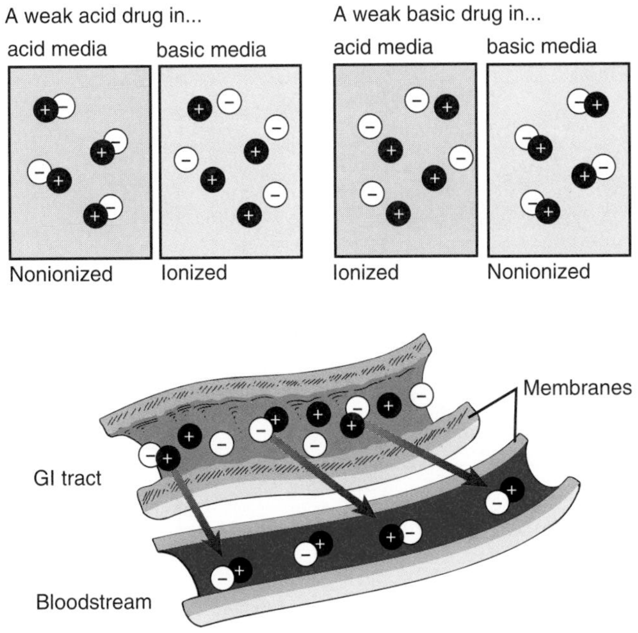

FIGURE 4-4
Effect of pH on drug ionization and transport. **A,** Effects of pH on drug molecules. **B,** Effects of pH on the transport of drug molecules through membranes.

acid layer, lipid solubility is a valuable attribute of drugs to be absorbed from certain areas, for example, the alimentary tract and the placental barrier. Chemicals and minerals that form insoluble precipitates in the gastrointestinal tract, such as barium salts, or drugs that are not soluble in water or lipids cannot be absorbed. Parenterally administered drugs prepared in oily vehicles, such as streptomycin, will be absorbed more slowly than drugs dissolved in water or isotonic sodium chloride.

4. *pH.* When in solution, drugs are a mixture of ionized and nonionized forms. The nonionized drug is lipid soluble and readily diffuses across the cell membrane; the ionized drug is lipid insoluble and nondiffusible. An acidic drug (e.g., aspirin) becomes relatively undissociated in an acid environment such as the stomach and therefore can readily diffuse across the membranes into the circulation. In contrast, a basic drug tends to ionize in the same acid environment and is not absorbed through the gastric membrane. Absorption is enhanced in the less acidic or more basic sites, such as the small intestine. The reverse occurs when a drug is in an alkaline medium (Fig. 4-4).
5. *Drug concentration.* Drugs administered in high concentrations tend to be more rapidly absorbed than drugs administered in low concentrations. In certain situations, a drug may be initially administered in large or **loading doses** that temporarily exceed the body's capacity for excretion of the drug. In this way, active drug levels are rapidly reached at the receptor site. Once an active drug level is established, smaller daily doses of the drug can be administered to replace only the amount of the drug excreted since the previous dose. The initial large drug dose is used to rapidly reach a therapeutic drug response, while the smaller daily doses are **maintenance doses** used to maintain a therapeutic drug response (Fig. 4-5). Such manipulation of drug dosage is frequently used, for example, with digitalis and steroid preparations in acute situations.
6. *Dosage form.* Drug concentration can be manipulated by pharmaceutical processing. It is possible to combine an active drug with a resin or another substance from which it is slowly released or to prepare a drug in a vehicle that offers relative resistance to the digestive action of stomach contents (enteric coating). Enteric coatings on drugs are used (1) to prevent decomposition of chemically sensitive drugs by gastric secretions (e.g., penicillin G and erythromycin are unstable in an acid pH), (2) to prevent dilution of the drug before it reaches the intestine, (3) to prevent nausea and vomiting induced by the drug's effect in the stomach, or (4) to provide delayed action of the drug.

Routes of drug administration. The mode of drug administration affects both the rate at which onset of action occurs and the magnitude of the therapeutic response that results. Therefore the choice of the route of administration is crucial in determining the suitability of a drug for an individual patient. For example, a patient who is vomiting will have little or no appreciable gastrointestinal absorption of an oral drug. Obviously rectal or parenteral administration would be more beneficial to obtain a therapeutic drug response.

Drugs are given for either local or systemic effects. The local effect of a drug usually occurs at the immediate site of application, in which case absorption is a disadvantage. When a drug is given for a systemic effect, absorption is an essential first step before the agent appears in the circulation and is distributed to a location distant from the site of administration.

A drug may enter the circulation either by being injected there directly (intravenously) or by absorption from depots in which it has been placed. The routes of drug administration can be classified into the following categories: (1) enteral or drugs administered along any portion of the gastrointestinal tract; (2) parenteral—subcutaneous, intramuscular, intravenous, intrathecal, or epidermal; (3) pulmonary; and (4) topical (see Fig. 4-3).

Enteral route. Oral or enteral ingestion is usually the most commonly used method of giving medications. It is also the safest (because drug may be retrieved), most convenient, and most economical route of administration. However, the frequent changes in the gastrointestinal environment produced by food, emotion, physical activity, and other medications may make it unreliable and the slowest of the commonly used routes. Drugs may be absorbed from several sites along the gastrointestinal tract.

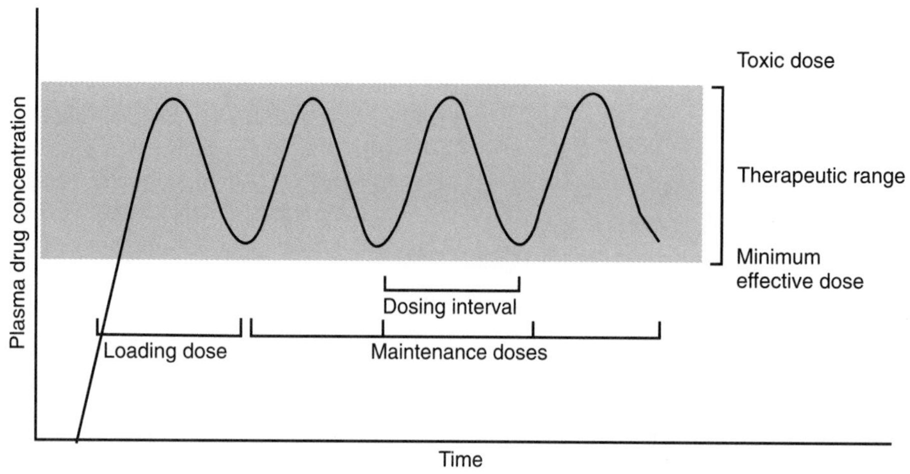

FIGURE 4-5

A loading dose is administered to reach a therapeutic response level rapidly. Maintenance doses are administered at prescribed intervals to maintain a therapeutic drug response.

ORAL ABSORPTION. Although the oral cavity possesses a thin lining, a rich blood supply, and a slightly acidic pH, little absorption occurs in the mouth. Despite its small surface area, the oral mucosa is capable of absorbing certain drugs as long as they dissolve rapidly in the salivary secretions (i.e., drugs given by the sublingual and buccal routes). In sublingual administration the drug is placed under the tongue to permit tablet dissolution in salivary secretions. Nitroglycerin is administered in this manner, and the patient is advised to refrain as long as possible from swallowing the saliva containing the tablet form of the drug. Because nitroglycerin is nonionic with a high lipid solubility, the drug readily diffuses through the lipid mucosal membranes. After absorption, it enters the systemic circulation without preliminary passage through the liver. Accordingly, absorption is rapid, and the effects of the drug may become apparent within 2 minutes. In buccal administration the drug (tablet) is placed between the teeth and the mucous membrane of the cheek. Some hormones and enzyme preparations are administered by this route and are rapidly absorbed. Both sublingual and buccal routes avoid drug destruction by gastrointestinal fluids and the first-pass effect of the liver by avoiding the portal circulation.

GASTRIC ABSORPTION. Although the stomach has a rich blood supply and a large surface area, which provide excellent potential for drug absorption, it is not an important absorption site. The length of time a substance remains in the stomach is a significant variable in determining the extent of gastric absorption. This is governed by the pH of the drug and gastric motility.

In the stomach the pH is low (about 1.4), and drugs such as the barbiturates, which are slightly acidic, tend to remain nonionized and thus are readily absorbed into the circulation. Morphine and quinine are slightly basic; they ionize in the stomach and thus are poorly absorbed. As the majority of drugs are weak bases on entry into the small intestine, they are absorbed because of the alkaline pH of the environment.

Generally, slowing the gastric emptying rate decreases drug absorption and vice versa. This is the reason so many drugs are administered on an empty stomach with sufficient water (8 ounces) to ensure dissolution, rapid passage into the small intestine, and drug absorption in the larger surface area. Since some drugs cause gastric irritation, they are usually given with food. In addition, after solid-dose drug administration, the patient should be encouraged to sit upright for at least 30 minutes to hasten gastric emptying time (the time required for the drug to reach the small intestine) and also to reduce the potential for tablets or capsules to lodge in the esophageal area. Prolongation of emptying time increases the risk of destruction of unstable drugs (e.g., acetaminophen [Tylenol]) by gastric juices.

SMALL INTESTINE ABSORPTION. The small intestine is highly vascularized and with its many villi has a larger absorption area than the stomach. Drugs that are poorly soluble in the stomach pass into this region and are absorbed primarily in the upper part of the small intestine. The pH of the intestinal fluid is alkaline (7 to 8), which strongly influences the rate of absorption of the nonionized basic drugs. Increased intestinal motility caused, for example, by diarrhea or cathartics may decrease exposure to the intestinal membrane and thereby diminish absorption. Prolonged exposure, on the other hand, allows more time for absorption.

RECTAL ABSORPTION. The surface area of the rectum is not very large, but drug absorption does occur because of extensive vascularity. Rectal suppositories are used for both local and systemic effects. Disadvantages to rectal drug administration include erratic absorption because of rectal contents, local drug irritation with some medications, and uncertainty of drug retention.

Parenteral route. The parenteral route refers to the administration of drugs by injection. It is the most rapid form of systemic therapy.

SUBCUTANEOUS. A subcutaneous injection of a drug is given beneath the skin into the connective tissue or fat im-

BOX 4-2 **Other Parenteral Routes**

Drugs may be injected into other cavities of the body:
- Intraarticular—drug delivery into the synovial cavity of a joint to relieve joint pain and reduce inflammation
- Intraosseous—drug delivery into the bone marrow
- Intraperitoneal—drug administration into the peritoneal cavity
- Intrapleural—drug administration to pleura

mediately underlying the dermis. This site can be used only for drugs that are not irritating to the tissue; otherwise severe pain, necrosis, and sloughing of tissue may occur. The rate of absorption is slow and can provide a sustained effect.

INTRAMUSCULAR. Intramuscular administration means a drug is injected into skeletal muscle. Absorption occurs more rapidly than with subcutaneous injection because of greater tissue blood flow.

INTRAVENOUS. The intravenous route produces an immediate pharmacologic response because the desired concentration of drug is injected directly into the bloodstream, thereby circumventing the absorption process. Intravenous drugs should generally be administered slowly to prevent adverse effects.

INTRATHECAL. Intrathecal drug administration means the drug is injected directly into the spinal subarachnoid space, bypassing the blood-brain barrier. Many compounds cannot enter the cerebrospinal fluid or are absorbed in this region very slowly. When rapid effects of drugs are desired, as with spinal anesthesia or in treatment of acute infection of the central nervous system, this route may be used.

EPIDURAL. Epidural drug administration refers to the injection of a drug within the spinal canal on or outside the dura mater that surrounds the spinal column. This is sometimes called extradural or peridural. For other parenteral routes, see Box 4-2.

Pulmonary route. To ensure that normal gas exchange of oxygen and carbon dioxide is continuous in the lungs, drugs must be in the form of gases or fine mists (aerosols) when they are administered by inhalation. The lungs provide a large surface area for absorption, and the rich capillary network adjacent to the alveolar membrane tends to promote ready entry of medication into the bloodstream. Drugs such as bronchodilators and antibiotics are administered by various inhalation devices (nebulizers, pressure tanks) that propel the agents into the alveolar sacs and produce primarily local effects and at times unwanted systemic effects.

Topical route. Absorption of drugs applied topically to the skin and mucous membranes of various structures in the body is generally rapid.

SKIN. Drugs applied to the skin are used to produce a local or systemic effect through ointments or transdermal patches. Only lipid-soluble compounds are absorbed through the skin, which acts as a lipid barrier. To prevent adverse effects from systemic absorption of toxic chemicals, only an intact skin surface should be used. Massaging the skin enhances absorption of the drug because capillaries become dilated and local blood flow is increased as a result of the warmth created by the friction of rubbing.

Transdermal administration is usually done with a patch that may contain a 1-, 3- or 7-day supply of medication, depending on the drug product. Examples of drugs that are applied transdermally are estrogen, nitroglycerin and scopolamine.

EYES. Ophthalmic administration of drugs in the eye produces a local effect on the conjunctiva or anterior chamber. Eyeball movements promote the distribution of drug over the surface of the eye.

EARS. Otic administration of drops into the auditory canal may be chosen to treat local infection or inflammatory conditions or to help remove wax in the external ear.

NOSE. Nasal drops or sprays containing medications may be applied or sprayed directly to the intranasal mucosa.

Distribution

Distribution is defined as the transport of a drug in body fluids from the bloodstream to various tissues of the body and ultimately to its site of action (see Fig. 4-3). The rate at which a drug enters the different areas of the body depends on the permeability of capillaries for the drug's molecules. As already discussed, lipid-soluble drugs can readily cross capillary membranes to enter most tissues and fluid compartments, whereas lipid-insoluble drugs require more time to arrive at their point of action. However, cardiovascular functions also affect the rate and extent of distribution of a drug; specifically, cardiac output (the amount of blood pumped by the heart each minute) and regional blood flow (the amount of blood supplied to a specific organ or tissue) determine how much time is required. Most of the drug is first distributed to organs that have a rich blood supply: heart, liver, kidney, and brain. Afterward, the drug enters organs with a poor blood supply, which include muscles and fat.

Drug reservoirs. Storage reservoirs allow a drug to accumulate by binding to specific tissues in the body. This sustains the pharmacologic effect of a drug at its point of action. The body's storage reservoirs involve two general types of drug pooling: plasma protein binding and tissue binding.

Plasma protein binding. On entry into the circulatory system, drugs may become attached to proteins, mainly albumin contained in the blood. Thus as free drug enters the plasma, it binds to the protein to form a drug-protein complex. This combination can also be reversed:

$$\text{Free drug} + \text{protein} \leftrightarrow \text{drug-protein complex}$$

The formula indicates that equilibrium is established between the amount of free drug and the amount of drug that is bound to protein (drug-protein complex). Protein binding decreases the concentration of free drug in the circulation; therefore it limits the amount that travels to the site of action. The drug-albumin molecule is too large to diffuse through the membrane of the blood vessel, so the bound molecule is trapped in the bloodstream and is pharmacologically inactive. It becomes a circulating drug reservoir or storage depot (see Fig. 4-3).

The equilibrium process is dynamic. As free drug is eliminated from the body, the drug-protein complex dissociates so that more free drug is released to replace what is lost. As a result, the fact that the body temporarily stores the drug molecules in the drug-protein complex allows the drug to be available for a longer period of time. For example, a sulfonamide is highly bound to protein; and because free drug molecules are released slowly from the bound form, the antiinfective action of the antibiotic is long-lasting.

DEGREE OF DRUG BINDING. Plasma protein binding is expressed as a percentage, which represents the percentage of total drug bound. Among the highly protein-bound drugs are warfarin (Coumadin), which is 99% protein bound, and propranolol, which is 93% protein bound. Accordingly, a ratio exists between free and bound drug. In the case of propranolol this means that in a given period of time, 93% is bound to plasma proteins and only 7% of free drug is available for therapeutic use, eventual biotransformation, and excretion. Therefore if more than 7% of the drug is free to act within this same period of time, toxicity may occur. The USP DI (1998) defines protein binding in general terms with ranges as follows:

- Very high: >90%
- High: 65% to 90%
- Moderate: 35% to 64%
- Low: 10% to 34%
- Very low: <10%

COMPETITION FOR BINDING SITES. Since albumin and other plasma proteins provide a number of binding sites, two drugs can compete with one another for the same site and displace each other. This competition may have dangerous consequences if particular combinations of drugs are administered. For example, serious problems can arise when a patient who is stabilized on a maintenance dose of warfarin, an anticoagulant, is simultaneously given aspirin, an analgesic. The aspirin may displace some of the protein-bound warfarin, increasing the free drug level that induces severe bleeding. Because warfarin is normally highly protein bound, its continued administration may raise the concentration of free drug with the potential of causing further severe adverse reactions. The healthcare professional must be alert to the potential danger of drug interactions occurring when certain agents are prescribed concurrently.

HYPOALBUMINEMIA. Hypoalbuminemia, or low levels of albumin in the blood, may be cause by hepatic damage, such as cirrhosis of the liver, by some type of body cavity drainage, or by failure of the liver to synthesize enough plasma proteins. The decrease in albumin levels results in more free drug available for distribution to tissue sites. Therefore when a patient is given the usual dosage of a drug that normally is plasma protein bound, more of the free form of drug is allowed into the circulation, resulting in possible overdosage and toxicity. The drug dosage should be adjusted (reduced) until the normal level of plasma protein is reported.

Tissue binding.

FAT TISSUE. Lipid-soluble drugs have a high affinity for adipose tissue, which is where these drugs are stored. Moreover, the relatively low blood flow in fat tissue makes it a stable reservoir for drugs. As an example, a lipid-soluble drug such as the barbiturate anesthetic thiopental may accumulate in fatty tissues at levels 6 to 12 times those in the plasma. Continued administration of thiopental that does not allow time for the drug to metabolize will lead to drug accumulation and toxicity.

BONE. Some drugs have an unusual affinity for bone; for example, the antibiotic tetracycline accumulates in bone after being absorbed onto the bone-crystal surface. This site serves as a storage site for tetracycline, which later can interfere with bone growth when it accumulates in skeletal tissues of the fetus (by crossing the placenta from the mother) or young children. Distribution of tetracycline to the teeth in a fetus or young child results in discoloration. Brownish pigmentation of permanent teeth also may result if this drug is given during the prenatal period or early childhood.

Barriers to drug distribution. Specialized structures made up of biologic membranes can serve as barriers to the passage of drugs at certain sites in the body, such as the blood-brain barrier and the placental barrier.

Blood-brain barrier. The blood-brain barrier allows distribution of only lipid-soluble drugs (e.g., general anesthetics, barbiturates) into the brain and cerebrospinal fluid. The barrier is made up of a row of capillary endothelial cells covered by a fatty sheath of glial cells joined by continuous tight intercellular junctions; therefore drugs that are strongly ionized and poorly soluble in fat cannot enter the brain. An antibiotic that has difficulty crossing the blood-brain barrier should not be used to treat infections of the central nervous system. However, if a drug is instilled intrathecally, it bypasses the blood-brain barrier and can directly treat the bacterial infection.

Placental barrier. The membrane layers that separate the blood vessels of the mother and the fetus constitute the placental barrier. In addition, tissue enzymes in the placenta can metabolize some agents (e.g., catecholamines) by inactivating them as they travel from the maternal circulation to the embryo. Despite the thickness of the structure, it does not afford complete protection to the fetus. Unlike the blood-brain barrier, the nonselective passage of drugs across the placenta to the fetus is a well-established fact. Although lipid-soluble substances preferentially diffuse across the placenta, the barrier is also permeable to a great number of lipid-insoluble drugs. Consequently, many agents intended to produce a therapeutic response in the mother also may cross the placental barrier and exert harmful effects on the developing embryo. Among the drugs easily transported across the placenta are steroids, narcotics, anesthetics, and some antibiotics.

Metabolism or biotransformation

Drug metabolism, or **biotransformation**, is the process of chemical inactivation of a drug by conversion into a more water-soluble compound or metabolite, which can then be excreted from the body (see Fig. 4-3). The liver is the primary site of drug metabolism, but with certain drugs, other tissues also may be involved in this process (plasma, kidneys, lungs, and intestinal mucosa).

Hepatic metabolism. The vast majority of drugs are metabolized in the liver by the hepatic microsomal enzyme system. A key element of the enzyme system is the cytochrome P-450 system. The microsomal enzymes usually affect biotransformation of lipid-soluble, nonpolar drugs. To increase polarity or water solubility, they undergo one or both of two general types of chemical reactions. One type of transformation consists of oxidation, hydrolysis, or reduction. These chemical reactions increase the water solubility of drug molecules. The second type, called conjugation, involves the union of the polar group of a drug with another substance in the body (glucuronide, glycine, methyl, or other alkyl groups). The conjugated molecule also becomes more polar or more water soluble, and therefore the result is an acceleration in renal excretion. Generally these responses convert an active drug to an inactive substance (decrease or loss of pharmacologic activity) and to a substance that is more easily excreted in the urine.

Secondly, many drugs can affect the hepatic enzymes by either inducing or increasing hepatic enzymes that will increase selected drug metabolism or by inhibiting the cytochrome P-450 system. This would decrease drug metabolism and possibly increase the potential for drug interactions and toxicity. An example is cimetidine (Tagamet); it inhibits the P-450 system, which then can affect the metabolism of warfarin (Coumadin), phenytoin (Dilantin), and other drugs.

A third example of hepatic metabolism is the chemical or enzymatic alterations needed to activate a prodrug. A prodrug is an inactive substance that must be converted to an active substance, in the liver. Some examples of prodrugs include losartan (Cozaar), benazepril (Lotensin), and sulindac (Clinoril).

The fourth example of hepatic metabolism is the conversion of an active drug to other active metabolites with similar therapeutic effects. Examples include the conversion of codeine in part to morphine, which increases the analgesic effect of codeine. Another is the conversion of the antidepressant amitriptyline (Elavil) to the active metabolite nortriptyline, which was later marketed individually as Aventyl and Pamelor.

Other considerations. The rates at which drugs are metabolized can vary considerably in individuals. For example, starvation and obstructive jaundice affects hepatic function, resulting in depression of the microsomal enzyme system. Other physical problems, such as liver disease or severe cardiac or renal impairment, may also affect drug metabolism. Infants with immature metabolizing enzyme systems and the aged with degenerative enzyme function are major groups that experience depressed biotransformation. Genetically determined differences may affect metabolism. Some drugs (e.g., procainamide, hydralazine, and isoniazid) are metabolized by the acetyltransferase system. This system divides the population into "rapid acetylators" and "slow acetylators." The rapid acetylators metabolize a greater proportion of a drug dose than do the slow acetylators. The rapid acetylators may develop reactions caused by the drug metabolic products, whereas the slow acetylators may appear more sensitive to drugs that produce severe toxic or adverse effects. For example, an individual who is a slow acetylator and is receiving procainamide (Pronestyl) may develop a lupus-like syndrome, which is a serious adverse response. If drug metabolism is delayed, cumulative drug effects may be expected and may be manifested as excessive or prolonged responses to ordinary doses of drugs.

A variety of chemicals can cause an increase in hepatic microsomal enzyme activity, such as central nervous system (CNS) depressants, xanthine derivatives, dyes, pesticides, and food preservatives. Chronic administration of some drugs may stimulate the formation of new microsomal enzymes, which may be the case with some hypnotic drugs, whose effect diminishes with prolonged administration. Stimulated drug metabolism may produce a state of drug tolerance.

Hepatic first-pass effect. Orally administered drugs absorbed normally travel first to the portal system and the liver before entering the general circulation. Some drugs though may first be taken up by the hepatic microsomal enzyme system, so that a significant drug dosage is metabolized before the drug ever reaches the systemic circulation. Consequently, only a small fraction of the dose is available for distribution to produce a pharmacologic effect. For such medications, the oral drug dose was calculated to compensate for this effect. For example, propranolol (Inderal) has a very significant hepatic first-pass effect, that is, the oral dose may range from 10 to 80 mg while the parenteral usual dose is usually 1 to 3 mg. This hepatic first-pass effect described here helps to explain why an intravenous dose of some drugs is so much smaller than an equally potent oral dose.

Some drugs may have a hepatic first-pass effect that totally eliminates pharmacologic activity. Such medications (such as lidocaine) require a different route of drug administration, such as parenteral, which bypasses the first pass through the liver.

Excretion

A drug continues to act in the body until it is biotransformed and/or excreted. Drug molecules (intact, changed, or inactivated) ultimately must be removed from their sites of action by physiologic channels involving mechanisms of excretion. **Excretion** is a process whereby drugs and pharmacologically active or inactive metabolites are eliminated from the body, primarily through the kidneys.

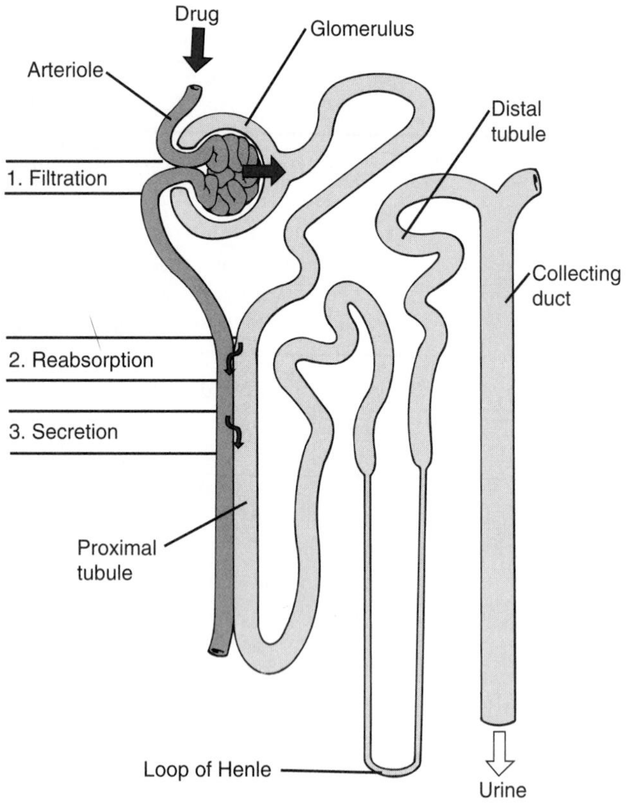

FIGURE 4-6
The drug excretion process.

Organs of excretion: kidneys. Drug excretion via the kidneys is the most important route for elimination; some drugs are excreted unchanged in the urine, while other drugs are so extensively metabolized that only a small fraction of the original chemical substance is excreted unchanged.

The process of excretion is accomplished primarily through passive glomerular filtration, active tubular secretion, and partial reabsorption (Fig. 4-6). For example, the availability of a drug for glomerular filtration depends on its concentration in unbound form in plasma that is, free, unbound drugs and water-soluble metabolites are filtered by the glomeruli, whereas protein-bound substances do not pass through this structure. After filtration, lipid-soluble compounds are not excreted; instead, they are reabsorbed by the tubular nephron and reenter the systemic circulation. The water-soluble compounds, on the other hand, fail to be reabsorbed and therefore are eliminated from the body.

Urinary pH varies between 4.6 and 8.2 and affects the amount of drug reabsorbed in the renal tubule by passive diffusion. Weak acids are excreted more readily in alkaline urine and more slowly in acidic urine; the reverse is true for weak bases. In cases of poisoning by weak organic acids such as aspirin or phenobarbital, alkalinizing the urine can result in increased urinary drug excretion. Raising the pH of the urine causes weak acids to become ionized, and subsequently these agents are excreted.

Urine may be alkalinized by administering sodium bicarbonate or tromethamine (Tham-E). By contrast, high doses of vitamin C or ammonium chloride acidify the urine and promote the excretion of basic drugs such as quindine and amphetamines. By altering the pH of urine, increased elimination of certain drugs can be facilitated, thus preventing prolonged action or overdosage of a toxic compound.

Another technique to alter the rate of excretion of a drug is to produce a competitively blocking effect. For example, probenecid may be used to block the renal excretion of penicillin. This prolongs the effect of the antibiotic by maintaining a higher therapeutic plasma level.

Additional excretion sites.

- Some drugs may be excreted by *biliary excretion.* After metabolism by the liver, the metabolite is secreted into the bile, passed into the duodenum, and eliminated with feces.
- Other drugs, such as fat-soluble agents, may be reabsorbed by the bloodstream and returned to the liver. This is the *enterohepatic cycle.* These compounds are later excreted by the kidney.
- Gases and volatile liquids (general anesthetics) are administered and excreted via the *pulmonary route,* generally in intact form. On inspiration, these agents enter the bloodstream and after crossing the alveolar membrane are distributed by the general circulation. The rate of gas loss depends on the rate of respiration. Therefore exercise or deep breathing, which causes a rise in cardiac output and a subsequent increase in pulmonary blood flow, promotes excretion. By contrast, decreased cardiac output, such as that occurring in shock, prolongs the period of time for drug elimination. Other volatile substances, such as ethyl alcohol and paraldehyde, are highly soluble in blood and are excreted in limited amounts by the lungs. These compounds can be easily detected because the individual expires the gases into the atmosphere.
- Drug excretion through *sweat* and *saliva* is relatively unimportant because this process depends on diffusion of lipid-soluble drugs through the epithelial cells of the glands. The elimination of drugs and metabolites in sweat may be responsible for side effects such as dermatitis and several other skin reactions.
- Many drugs or their metabolites cross the epithelium of the *mammary glands* and are excreted in breast milk. Breast milk is acidic (pH 6.5), and therefore basic compounds such as narcotics (e.g., morphine and codeine) achieve high concentrations in this fluid. A major concern arises over the transfer of drugs from mothers to their breastfed babies, which can result in an accumulative drug effect because of the infant's undeveloped metabolizing system. The nursing mother should be warned against taking any medications without physician approval.

Pharmacodynamic Phase

Pharmacodynamics is the study of the mechanism of drug action on living tissue, that is, the response of tissues to specific chemical agents at various sites in the body. The effects of drugs can be recognized only by alterations of a known physiologic function as drugs modify physiologic activity but do not confer any new function on a tissue or organ in the body. They may increase, decrease, or replace enzymes, hormones, or body metabolic functions. Some drugs inhibit or destroy foreign organisms or malignant cells in the body, while other drug substances may protect cells from foreign agents. The goal of drug therapy is to attain a therapeutic effect in an individual. Therefore, drugs may be used to treat symptoms, cure a disease, or diagnose and prevent disease.

Essentially, pharmacokinetics refers to the way the body processes or handles the drug while pharmacodynamics is the effect the drug has on the body (Katzung, 1992).

Theories of Drug Action

The term "mechanism of action" refers to a drug's effect at the sites of action. The mechanism of action of most compounds is believed to involve a chemical interaction between the drug and a functionally important component of the living system. Most drugs produce their effects by one of the following ways: a drug-receptor interaction, a drug-enzyme interaction, or a nonspecific drug interaction.

Drug-receptor interaction

Structural specificity is an essential postulate of the receptor theory of drug action. This theory hypothesizes that drugs are selectively active substances that have a high affinity for a specific chemical group or a particular constituent of a cell. In essence, the drug-receptor interaction theory states that a certain portion (active site) of the drug molecule selectively combines or interacts with some molecular structure (a reactive site on the cell surface or within the cell) to produce a biologic effect. Thus a **receptor** is a reactive cellular site with which a drug interacts to produce a pharmacologic response. The relationship of a drug to its receptor has often been likened to that of the fit of a key in a lock. The drug represents the key that fits into the lock, or receptor. Thus some sort of reciprocal or complementary relationship exists between a certain portion of the drug molecule and the receptor site of the cell.

It has been postulated that the drug molecule with the best fit to the receptor will produce the greatest response from the cell. It has also been suggested that there must be some force that attracts a receptor and holds it in combination with a specific drug long enough to produce a pharmacologic response. After absorption, a drug gains access to the receptor after it leaves the bloodstream and is distributed to tissues that contain receptor sites. Box 4-3 lists terms used in this theory of drug action.

BOX 4-3 Drug-Receptor Interaction Terms

affinity the propensity of a drug to bind or attach itself to a given receptor site.

efficacy (intrinsic activity) the drug's ability to initiate biologic activity as a result of such binding.

agonist a drug that combines with receptors and initiates a sequence of biochemical and physiologic changes; possesses both affinity and efficacy.

antagonist an agent designed to inhibit or counteract effects produced by other drugs or undesired effects caused by cellular components during illness.

competitive antagonist an agent with an affinity for the same receptor site as an agonist; the competition with the agonist for the site inhibits the action of the agonist; increasing the concentration of the agonist tends to overcome the inhibition. Competitive inhibition responses are usually reversible.

noncompetitive antagonist an agent that combines with different parts of the receptor mechanism and inactivates the receptor so that the agonist cannot be effective regardless of its concentration. Noncompetitive antagonist effects are considered to be irreversible or nearly so.

partial agonist an agent that has affinity and some efficacy but that may antagonize the action of other drugs that have greater efficacy. Not infrequently, antagonists share some structural similarities with their agonists.

Drug-enzyme interaction

The second method of a drug producing an effect is the interaction between the drug and a cellular enzyme. Enzymes are indispensable biologic catalysts that control all biochemical reactions of the cell. Drugs can inhibit the action of a specific enzyme and alter a physiologic response, such as neostigmine (Prostigmin), an agent that combines with acetylcholinesterase to prevent the breakdown of acetylcholine at the neuromuscular junction. This drug is used to manage the muscle weakness caused by myasthenia gravis.

Drugs that combine with enzymes are thought to do so by virtue of their structural resemblance to an enzyme's substrate molecule (the substance acted on by an enzyme). A drug may resemble an enzyme's substrate so closely that it can combine with the enzyme instead of with the normal substrate. Drugs resembling enzyme substrates are termed "antimetabolites" and can either block normal enzymatic action or result in the production of other substances with unique biochemical properties. The antimetabolites then become the receptors for the drug. However, although enzymes may be receptors, not all receptors are enzymes. An example of an antimetabolite is the anticancer drug methotrexate.

Nonspecific drug interaction

Some drugs demonstrate no structural specificity and presumably act by more general effects on cell membranes and cellular processes. These drugs may penetrate into cells

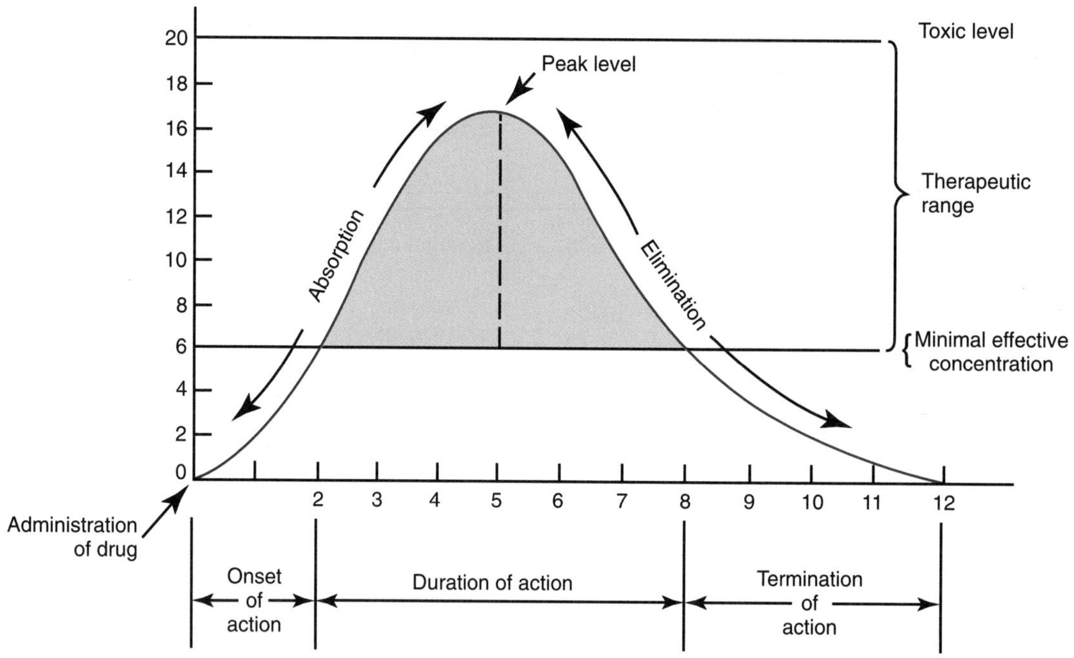

FIGURE 4-7
Plasma level profile of a drug.

or accumulate in cellular membranes, where they interfere by physical or chemical means with some cell function or some fundamental metabolic processes.

Cell membranes are complex lipoprotein structures that regulate the flow of ions and metabolites in a highly selective manner, thereby maintaining an electrochemical gradient between the interior and exterior surfaces of the cell. Examples of structurally nonspecific drugs are the general anesthetics, which are lipid-soluble compounds of unrelated chemical structure but with similar properties. It is believed that general anesthetics alter the properties of lipids in cell membranes of nerves rather than act on specific receptors.

Other structurally nonspecific drugs may act by biophysical means that do not affect cellular or enzymatic functions. Drugs may produce an effect as a result of their obvious physical properties, such as ointments and emollients. Hydrophilic indigestible substances exert a cathartic effect because of their physical action on the bowel. Examples of true chemical reactions that produce biologic effects are the interaction of a molecule such as lead with an antidote and the neutralization effect of antacid drugs on hydrochloric acid present in gastric juice. Neither is considered a receptor interaction because no macromolecular tissue elements are involved. Detergents, alcohol, hydrogen peroxide, and phenol derivatives such as Lysol are also structurally nonspecific and act by irreversibly destroying the functional integrity of the living cell.

Drug-Response Relationship

After administration each drug has its own characteristic pharmacokinetic effects that can be analyzed by performing a plasma level profile. The prescriber uses this information to alter the dose, drug scheduling, or route of drug administration for an individual patient. Plasma drug levels may also provide information about the drug reaching therapeutic, subtherapeutic, or toxic dose range. Such data are instrumental in helping to diagnose and prevent serious adverse reactions.

Plasma level profile of a drug

The plasma or serum level profile graphically demonstrates the relationship between the plasma drug concentration and the level of therapeutic effectiveness over a course of time. After the administration of a single dose, the time course of the amount of drug in the body depends on the rates of absorption, distribution, metabolism, and elimination. For example, the drug in Fig. 4-7 has an onset of action of approximately 2 hours, a peak level at 5 hours, and a 6-hour duration of action (length of time in the therapeutic range) or effect. By monitoring the plasma level of a compound, the efficacy and safety of drug therapy can be more closely controlled. See Box 4-4 for key terms used in plasma level profiles.

Biologic half-life

The rate of biotransformation and excretion of a drug determines its biologic **half-life** ($t_{1/2}$), which is the time required to reduce by one half the amount of unchanged drug that is in the body at the time equilibrium is established. Moreover, the duration of a dose can be demonstrated by the biologic half-life. The half-life of each drug may be different; for example, a drug with a short $t_{1/2}$, such as 2 or 3

BOX 4-4 **Plasma Level Profile Terms**

onset of action or latent period interval between the time a drug is administered and the first sign of its effect
termination of action point at which a drug effect is no longer seen
duration of action period from onset of drug action to the time when response is no longer perceptible
minimal effective concentration lowest plasma concentration that produces the desired drug effect
peak plasma level highest plasma concentration attained from a dose
toxic level plasma concentration at which a drug produces serious adverse effects
therapeutic range range of plasma concentrations that produce the desired drug effect without toxicity (the range between minimal effective concentration and toxic level)

hours, will need to be administered more often than one with a long $t_{1/2}$, such as 6 hours.

The half-life does not change with the drug dose; it always takes the same amount of time to eliminate one half of the drug present in the body. If, for example, 10,000 units of a drug are administered and that drug has a half-life of 4 hours, then 5000 units of the drug will be excreted in 4 hours. In the next 4 hours, 2500 units will be excreted, with 1250 units more being excreted in the third 4-hour period. The drug's elimination can be altered in patients with hepatic dysfunction or renal disorders. Then drug elimination may be prolonged and drug half-life is lengthened, which usually necessitates a reduction of drug dosage.

Therapeutic index

The therapeutic index (TI) provides a quantitative measure of the relative safety of a drug. It represents a ratio between two factors: (1) lethal dose (LD_{50}), which is the dose of a drug that is lethal in 50% of laboratory animals tested, and (2) effective dose (ED_{50}), which is the dose required to produce a therapeutic effect in 50% of a similar population. The therapeutic index is calculated as follows:

$$TI = \frac{LD_{50}}{ED_{50}}$$

The closer the ratio is to 1, the greater the danger involved in administration of that drug to human beings. Obviously, in humans, the dose that promotes a side effect or the first sign of a toxic response is of greater importance than the therapeutic index of the drug, since the prescriber's major concern is avoiding even an isolated fatality caused by drug toxicity.

Drug bioavailability

Drug **bioavailability** refers to the percentage of active drug substances absorbed and available to reach the target tissues after drug administration. Drugs are considered to be biologically equivalent if they attain similar concentrations in blood and tissues at similar times; they are therapeutically equivalent if they provide equal therapeutic effectiveness in clinical trials. Of importance is the similarity of the absorption and therapeutic performances of drugs, which can be altered markedly by the ingredients and method of drug manufacture. Furthermore, different brands of the same drug can vary, and even different lots from a single manufacturer may show different levels of effectiveness. Thus the Food and Drug Administration (FDA) is paying more attention to drug preparation and trying to ensure that the bioavailability of a drug conforms to uniform standards. Both the proportion of active drug and the percentage of its absorption are essential to attain therapeutic equivalence among all chemically similar drugs.

SIDE EFFECTS AND ADVERSE REACTIONS

Although drugs have the potential of producing the desired therapeutic effect, they may also induce an undesirable response such as a side effect or adverse reaction. Side effects are usually predictable, and in many instances, this secondary (usually undesirable) effect(s) is produced at therapeutic drug dosages. For example, a drug such as an opioid analgesic often causes the side effects of drowsiness and constipation. These effects occur at the usual prescribed dose, but drowsiness may occur soon after drug administration while constipation is often a delayed side effect that occurs later in therapy. The intensity of the side effects, however, is often dose dependent.

The most commonly reported side effects are nausea, vomiting, dizziness, drowsiness, dry mouth, abdominal gas or distress, constipation, and diarrhea. For some side effects, healthcare providers may provide nonpharmacologic advice such as telling the individual to use caution when getting up suddenly from a lying or sitting position (to reduce the potential for dizziness or hypotension); to use sugarless gum or candy or ice chips for relief of dry mouth; or to not drive or use dangerous machinery until the individual's response to the medication can be assessed. Persistent or troublesome side effects though may require pharmacologic interventions such as laxatives, antiemetics, and antidiarrheals for constipation, vomiting, and diarrhea. In most instances, side effects are manageable, and in some instances tolerance may develop to the side effect. Patients should be informed about the most common side effects reported with a particular medication and also how to avoid or manage the effect, when possible.

An adverse drug effect or reaction is unintended, undesirable, and often unpredictable. Every medication has a potential for causing harm, and sometimes these effects are immediate while at other times they may take weeks or months to develop. Because only several thousand persons are exposed to each drug before release, all potential adverse effects may not be detected before the drug is marketed. Therefore, the healthcare provider should be monitoring each patient for any unusual individual response to a medication. As the least information is available for newly released medications, these agents should be very closely monitored.

Adverse reactions can range from mild to fatal, but with the increasing numbers of drugs being used, the incidence of adverse reactions has increased and is presently a significant problem in clinical practice (Nies, Spielberg, 1996).

Predictable Adverse Responses

Some factors such as age, body mass, sex, environment, time of administration, pathologic state, genetic factors, and psychologic characteristics can alter the response to drug therapy. Therefore the healthcare professional should be aware of characteristics that modify cell conditions and, possibly, drug activity.

Age

Young children and the elderly are usually highly responsive to medications. Infants often have immature hepatic and renal systems and therefore incomplete metabolic and excretory mechanisms. Elderly persons may demonstrate different responses to drug therapy because of a decline in hepatic and renal function, which is often accompanied by a concurrent disease process.

Body Mass

The relationship between body mass and amount of drug administered influences the distribution and concentration of a drug. To maintain a desired drug level in individuals of various sizes, the drug dose may need to be adjusted in proportion to body mass. For a given dose of drug, the greater the volume of distribution, the lower the concentration of drug reached in various body compartments. Because the volume of interstitial and intracellular water is related to body mass, weight has a marked influence on the quantitative effects produced by drugs. The average adult drug dose is calculated on the basis of the drug quantity that will produce a particular effect in 50% of persons who are between the ages of 18 and 65 and weigh about 150 lb (70 kg). Therefore, particularly for children and for very lean and very obese individuals, drug dosage is frequently determined on the basis of amount of drug per kilogram of body weight or body surface area.

Sex

Differences in drug effects related to the variable of sex result, in part, from size differences between men and women. Women are usually smaller than men, which will lead to high drug concentrations if dosage is prescribed indifferently. Demonstrable differences also exist in relative proportions of fat and water in the bodies of men and women, and some drugs may be more soluble in one or the other. It is best to avoid drugs during pregnancy unless an absolute necessity exists.

Environmental Milieu

Drugs affecting mood and behavior are particularly susceptible to the influence of the individual's environment. With such drugs, one has to consider effects of (1) the drug itself, (2) the personality of the user, (3) the environment of the user, and (4) the interaction of these three components. Sensory deprivation and sensory overload may also affect responses to drugs. Physical environment can also modify drug effects; for example, temperature affects drug activity: heat relaxes peripheral vessels and thus intensifies the actions of vasodilators, while cold has the opposite effect. The relative oxygen deprivation at high altitudes may also increase sensitivity to some drugs.

Time of Administration

It is well known that drugs are absorbed more rapidly if the gastrointestinal tract is free of food and that irritating drugs are more readily tolerated if administered with food. Research has indicated that the time of drug administration in relation to human biologic rhythms can significantly affect the response to certain medications. It seems quite plausible that in humans the sleep-wake rhythm, drug-metabolizing enzyme rhythms, and circadian (24-hour) variations contribute to the effective, ineffective, adverse, or toxic response to particular drugs. For example, cyclophosphamide, an antineoplastic agent, should be administered in the morning to reduce the risk of hemorrhagic cystitis (blood in the urine) (USP DI, 1998). Chronopharmacology and chronotoxicology are new areas that healthcare professionals are monitoring with great interest.

Pathologic State

The presence of a pathologic condition and the severity of symptoms may call for careful consideration of the type and dose of drug administered. For example, the presence of severe pain tends to increase a patient's requirement for an analgesic, and an extremely anxious individual can prove resistant to very large doses of tranquilizing and sedating drugs. Aspirin administered to a patient with a fever will produce a decrease in temperature, whereas a patient taking the drug for its analgesic effects will show no temperature change at all. Also, the presence of cardiovascular, hepatic, or renal dysfunctions will interfere with the physiologic processes of drug action.

Genetic Factors

Genetic differences may arise from genetic deficiencies in drug metabolism or in receptor sensitivity. These pharmacogenetic abnormalities often manifest themselves as "idiosyncrasies" and may be mistakenly diagnosed as drug allergies. For example, some individuals may lack pseudocholinesterase activity in their plasma. If they receive an injection of succinylcholine, which is normally hydrolyzed by plasma cholinesterase, they may become paralyzed and remain that way for a long time. Malignant hyperpyrexia with general anesthesia is another example of a genetic based difference (Edwards, 1997). The field of pharmacogenetics is of great interest, since it may provide a rational explanation for many so-called drug idiosyncrasies.

Psychologic Factors

The patient's symbolic investment in drugs and faith in their effects strongly influence and usually potentiate drug effects. The placebo effect is an outstanding example of how strong motivation can influence the emergence of desired drug effects, whereas hostility and mistrust of medicine and health personnel can diminish drug effects. Healthcare professionals should realize that their attitudes and the impressions created at the time of drug discussion or administration may influence the therapeutic result.

Unpredictable Adverse Responses

The most common and best-defined, unpredictable adverse drug reactions include the following:

Allergic Drug Reactions

A drug allergy is an altered state of reaction to a drug, resulting from previous sensitizing exposure and the development of an immunologic mechanism. Substances foreign to the body act as antigens to stimulate the production of antibodies or immunoglobulins (IgE, IgG, IgM). Later, when a previously sensitized individual is again exposed to the foreign substance, the antigen reacts with the antibodies to release substances such as histamine, which then provoke allergic symptoms. "Hypersensitivity," "drug allergy," and "chemical allergy" are all terms used to describe an allergic drug reaction (Klaassen, 1996). There are four different types of allergic drug reactions.

- Type I (anaphylactic) reaction is an immediate reaction that occurs within minutes of exposure to the chemical in a previously sensitized person. This reaction is mediated by IgE antibodies located on the surface of mast cells and basophils. An immediate, severe reaction results, which may be fatal if not recognized and treated quickly. The most dramatic form of anaphylaxis is sudden, severe bronchospasm, vasospasm, severe hypotension, and rapid death. Signs and symptoms are largely caused by contraction of smooth muscles and may begin with irritability, extreme weakness, nausea, and vomiting and then proceed to dyspnea, cyanosis, convulsions, and cardiac arrest. Drugs associated with this type of reaction include penicillins and cephalosporins. Antihistamines, epinephrine, and bronchodilators are indispensable in the treatment of anaphylactic shock.
- Type II (cytotoxic) reaction involves a drug and IgG or IgM; it has sometimes been called an autoimmune response. This reaction may manifest as hemolytic anemia (methyldopa or penicillin induced), thrombocytopenia (quinidine induced), or systemic lupus erythematosus (procainamide induced). Removal of the medication usually results in improvement, although it may take several months for the reaction to subside.
- Type III (or Arthus, an immune complex) reaction is sometimes called "serum sickness." With this reaction, the drug forms a complex with IgG antibodies in the blood vessel, resulting in angioedema, arthralgia, fever, swollen lymph nodes (lymphadenopathy), and splenomegaly in approximately 1 to 3 weeks after drug exposure. Penicillins, sulfonamides, and phenytoin can cause this type of delayed reaction.
- Type IV is a cell-mediated or delayed hypersensitivity reaction. For example, direct skin contact between the drug and sensitized cells results in an inflammatory reaction, such as contact dermatitis from poison ivy. This type of reaction involves sensitized T lymphocytes and macrophages (Klaassen, 1996).

Drug-Induced Reactions

An individual who has had a mild allergic response to a particular drug should avoid overexposure to that drug and, optimally, should have skin tests performed to more definitively diagnose the response. Mild allergic reactions may be characterized by the development of a rash, angioedema, rhinitis, fever, asthma, and pruritus. Reinstitution of the

BOX 4-5 Drug-Drug Effects

Drug interaction occurs when the effects of one drug are modified by the prior or concurrent administration of another drug, thereby increasing the pharmacologic action of one drug. Drug interactions may be either beneficial (e.g., probenecid prolongs the action of penicillins) or detrimental (e.g., aspirin increases the action of anticoagulants, causing hemorrhage).

Drug antagonism occurs when the combined effect of two drugs is less than the sum of the drugs acting separately.

Summation (additive effect) occurs when the combined effect of two drugs produces a result that equals the sum of each individual drug's effects. The mathematical equivalent is $1 + 1 = 2$. For example, codeine and aspirin both act as analgesics and when given together they provide an additive or greater pain relief than when either one is used alone. The combination allows the administration of a lower dosage of each drug, with a resultant decrease in side effects or adverse reactions.

Synergism describes a drug interaction in which the combined drug effect is greater than the sum of each agent acting independently. Mathematically the response can be written as $1 + 1 = 3$ or more. For example, a combination of antihypertensive agents may produce a greater decrease in blood pressure than either drug given alone, primarily because the drugs lower blood pressure via a different mechanism of action.

BOX 4-6 Various Forms of Drug Preparations

Preparations for Oral Use

Liquids

Aqueous solutions (substances dissolved in water and syrups)
Aqueous suspensions (solid particles suspended in liquid)
Emulsions (fats or oils suspended in liquid with an emulsifier
Spirits (alcohol solution)
Elixirs (aromatic, sweetened alcohol and water solution)
Tinctures (alcohol extract of plant or vegetable substance)
Fluid extracts (concentrated, alcoholic liquid extract of plant or vegetables)
Extracts (syrup or dried form of pharmacologically active drug, usually prepared by evaporating solution)

Solid

Capsules (soluble case [usually gelatin] that contains liquid, dry, or beaded drug particles)
Tablets (compressed, powdered drug(s) in a small disk)
Troches/lozenges (medicated tablets that dissolve slowly in mouth)
Powders/granules (loose or molded drug substance for drug administration, with or without liquids)

Preparations for Parenteral Use

Ampules (sealed glass container for liquid injectable medication)
Vials (glass container with rubber stopper for liquid or powdered medication)
Cartridge/Tubex (single-dose unit of parenteral medication to be used with a specific injecting device)

Intravenous Infusions (Suspended on Hanger at Bedside)

Glass bottles, flexible collapsible plastic bags, and semirigid plastic containers in sizes from 150 to 1000 ml used for continuous infusion of fluid replacement with or without medications
Intermittent intravenous infusions—usually a secondary IV setup of a small plastic or glass bottle (volume between 50 to 250 ml) to which medication is added. It runs as a "piggyback," hung separately from the primary IV infusion via a secondary administration tubing set usually for a period of 20 to 120 minutes. The primary IV solution is run during the time between medication doses.
Heparin lock or angiocath—a port site for direct administration or intermittent IV medications without the need for a primary IV solution

Preparations for Topical Use

Liniments (liquid suspensions for lubrication that are applied by rubbing)
Lotions (liquid suspensions that can be protective, emollient, cooling, astringent, antipruritic, cleansing, etc.)
Ointment (semisolid medicine in a base for local protective, soothing, astringent, or transdermal application for systemic effects [such as nitroglycerin, scopolamine, estrogen])
Paste (thick ointment primarily used for skin protection)
Plasters (solid preparations that are adhesive, protective, or soothing)
Creams (emulsions that contain an aqueous and an oily base)
Aerosols (fine powders or solutions in volatile liquids that contain a propellant)
Transdermal patches (patches containing medication that is absorbed continuously through the skin and acts systemically)

Preparations for Use on Mucous Membranes

Drops are aqueous solutions with or without gelling agent to increase retention time in the eye, used for eyes, ears, or nose.
Aqueous solutions of medications are usually for topical action but occasionally used for systemic effects, including enemas, douches, mouthwashes, throat sprays, and gargles.
Aerosol sprays, nebulizers, and inhalers deliver aqueous solutions of medication in droplet form to the target membrane, such as bronchial tree (e.g., bronchodilators).
Foams are powders or solutions of medication in volatile liquids with a propellant, such as vaginal foams for contraception.
Suppositories usually contain medicinal substances mixed in a firm but malleable base (cocoa butter) to facilitate insertion into a body cavity (e.g., rectal or vaginal).

Miscellaneous Drug Delivery Systems

Intradermal implants are pellets containing a small deposit of medication that are inserted in a dermal pocket and are designed to allow medication to leach slowly into tissue. Usually used to administer hormones such as testosterone or estradiol.
Micropump system is a small, external pump attached by belt or implanted that delivers medication via a needle in a continuous steady dose. Insulin, anticancer chemotherapy, and opioids are examples
Membrane delivery systems are drug-laden membranes that are instilled in the eye to deliver a steady flow of medications, such as pilocarpine or corticosteroids.

same drug therapy in a patient who manifests allergic reactions is always dangerous, since an anaphylactic reaction may occur. The following are brief descriptions of important drug-induced reactions.

Tolerance is the decreased physiologic or therapeutic response to a drug after repeated drug administration. It is a reaction that necessitates an increase in drug dosage to maintain a given therapeutic effect. When tolerance develops, a cross-tolerance to pharmacologically similar drugs may also develop. That is, drugs that act at the same receptor sites may also need increased dosage to maintain an effect.

TABLE 4-1 Common Abbreviations and Symbols*

Abbreviation	*Unabbreviated Form*	*Meaning*
ac	ante cibum	before meals
ad lib	ad libitum	freely
AM	ante meridiem	morning
bid	bis in die	twice each day
c̄	cum	with
caps	capsule	capsule
cc, cm^3	cubic centimeter	cubic centimeter (mL)
D/C or DC	discontinue	terminate
elix	elixir	elixir
g, gm	gram	1000 milligrams
gr	grain	60 milligrams
gtt	gutta	drop
h, hr	hora	hour
hs	hora somni	at bedtime
IM	intramuscular	into a muscle
IV	intravenous	into a vein
IVPB	IV piggyback	secondary IV line
kg	kilogram	2.2 lb
KVO	keep vein open	very slow infusion rate
L	liter	liter
µg, mcg	microgram	one millionth of a gram
mg	milligram	one thousandth of a gram
mEq	milliequivalent	the number of grams of solute dissolved in one milliliter of a *normal* solution
min or mn	minim	minim (1/15 or 1/16 mL)
ml, mL	milliliter	one thousandth of a liter
ng	nanogram	one billionth of a gram
OD	oculus dexter	right eye
OS	oculus sinister	left eye
os	os	mouth
OTC	over-the-counter	nonprescription drug
OU	oculus uterque	each eye
pc	post cibum	after meals
PM	post meridiem	after noon
PO	per os	by mouth, orally
prn	pro re nata	according to necessity
q	quaque	every
qd	quaque die	every day
qh	quaque hora	every hour
q4h	every 4 hours	every 4 hours
qid	quater in die	four times each day
qod	quaque aliem die	every other day
qs	quantum satis	sufficient quantity
℞	receipt	take
s̄	sine	without
SL	sub linguam	under the tongue
ss	semis	a half
stat	statim	at once
SC, SQ	subcutaneous	into subcutaneous tissue
tbsp	tablespoon	tablespoon (15 mL)
tid	ter in die	three times a day
TO	telephone order	order received over the telephone
tsp	teaspoon	teaspoon (4 or 5 mL)
U	unit	a dosage measure for insulin, penicillin, heparin
VO	verbal order	order received verbally
ʒ	dram	4 or 5 mL
℥	ounce or fluid-ounce	ounce (30 ml)
×	times	as in two times a week
>	greater than	greater than
<	less than	less than
=	equal to	equal to
↑, ↗	increase or increasing	increase or increasing
↓, ↙	decrease or decreasing	decrease or decreasing

*It is recommended that certain abbreviations be abandoned if they are found to be confusing.

While the actual mechanism of tolerance is unknown, multiple mechanisms have been proposed, such as an increase in hepatic drug-metabolizing enzymes and pharmacodynamic tolerance. *Pharmacodynamic tolerance* refers to chronic or long-term drug use in an individual that then requires larger drug dosages to produce the same effect as before. Drugs well known for their propensity to produce tolerance are opium alkaloids, nitrites, and ethyl alcohol. While the exact reason for this is unknown, it is believed that receptor or cellular adaptation may have occurred (Nies, Spielberg, 1996).

Tachyphylaxis refers to a quickly developing tolerance after repeated administration of a drug over a short time period. It is rapid in onset and the patient's initial response to the drug cannot be reproduced, even with larger doses of the drug. Nitroglycerin administered transdermally is an example that requires an intermittent dosing schedule (12 on, 12 hours off) to maintain its effect. A cumulative effect occurs when the body cannot metabolize one dose of a drug before another dose is administered. In other words, when drugs are excreted more slowly than they are absorbed, each new dose adds more to the total quantity in the blood and organs than is lost in the same amount of time by excretion. Unless drug administration is adjusted, high concentrations can be reached, producing toxic effects. Cumulative toxicity can occur rapidly, as dramatically illustrated in ethyl alcohol intoxication, or it can occur insidiously, as is the case in poisoning with heavy metals such as lead. Lead is stored in many body tissues and deposited in bones, therefore having prolonged effects on the body while accumulation continues. The terms "drug dependence" and "addiction" will be discussed in Chapter 6. See Box 4-5 for additional drug-drug effects.

Iatrogenic Response

An **iatrogenic** drug response is an unintentional drug effect or disease induced by a physician's prescribed therapy. The five major syndromes commonly reported with iatrogenic response include blood dyscrasias, hepatotoxicity, nephrotoxicity, teratogenicity, and dermatologic effects. With careful prescribing and monitoring, iatrogenic conditions may be reduced or avoided. An example of iatrogenic disease is Cushing's disease induced when a patient takes corticosteroids for an extended time period.

PRESCRIPTION ORDERS

A prescription order written by a licensed prescriber (physician, dentist, and others) may present in two formats: a prescription blank or an institutional order sheet. Such orders are filled by a registered pharmacist. A prescription order has eight elements that can be correlated with the five nursing rights of medication administration: the patient's name (Right Patient), date written, drug name (Right Drug), drug strength, dosage (Right Dose), route of administration (Right Route), dosage instructions or frequency (Right Time), and signature of the prescriber. All the elements should be clearly written to avoid any chance for error. If any doubt exists, the prescriber is contacted for clarification.

Pharmaceutical Preparations

Various formulations of drug preparations are available for use on the market. This variety assists the prescriber in choosing a formulation that is best suited for the individual patient. See Box 4-6 for a listing of various forms of drug preparations.

Abbreviations and Drug Orders

A clearly written drug order specifies the conditions for drug administration. For example, a routine order means the drug is administered until discontinued by the prescriber; a prn order is only administered when needed by the patient while a stat order is for immediate administration of one dose of medication. Many abbreviations and symbols are used in drug ordering. See Table 4-1 for a list of common abbreviations and symbols. Abbreviations for specific drugs are also used by some prescribers. This method of drug ordering should be discouraged as the abbreviation may be misinterpreted, thus endangering the patient. Healthcare professionals should closely follow the approved abbreviation lists as published by their facility. See Table 4-2 for a drug abbreviation list.

TABLE 4-2 Drug Abbreviations

Abbreviation	Definition
ACTH	adrenocorticotropic hormone
ASA	acetylsalicylic acid (aspirin)
DES	diethylstilbestrol
DM	dextromethorphan
D_5W	5% dextrose in water
D_5S	5% dextrose in normal saline
DSS or DOSS	dioctyl sodium sulfosuccinate
DW	distilled water
EC	enteric coated
ETH & C	elixer terpin hydrate with codeine
Fe	iron
5-FU	5-fluorouracil
FUD	floxuridine
HC	hydrocortisone
HCTZ	hydrochlorothiazide
INH	isoniazid
K	potassium
KCl	potassium chloride
LOC	laxative of choice
MOM	milk of magnesia
6-MP	6-mercaptopurine
MS	morphine sulfate
Na	sodium
NS	normal saline
NSAID	nonsteroidal antinflammatory drug
NTG	nitroglycerin
PAS	*para*-aminosalicyclic acid
PB	phenobarbital
PCN	penicillin

SUMMARY

A drug is a chemical that interacts within a living organism to produce a biologic response. This chapter reviews the three major properties of drugs, that is (1) drugs modify existing functions in the body but can not create new ones; (2) drugs produce multiple effects, desirable and undesirable, and (3) the actual drug action depends on an interaction between the drug and a functionally important molecule in the body.

The mechanisms of drug action depend on three major phases of drug activity: the factors that affect pharmaceutical, pharmacokinetic, and pharmacodynamic phases. The theories of drug action involve a chemical interaction between the drug and a functionally important component of the living system; a receptor, an enzyme or a nonspecific, cell membrane interaction.

The drug-response relationship is very important as this information is used to adjust the drug dose, drug schedule, or route of drug administration. In addition to producing a desired therapeutic effect, drugs may also induce an undesirable side effect or adverse reaction. An adverse drug effect is more problematic as this effect is unintended, undesirable, and often unpredictable.

A clear understanding of the principles of drug action is vital for the understanding of various drugs and drug therapies.

REVIEW QUESTIONS

1. Name and explain the six variables that affect drug absorption.
2. Select two of the four examples involving the hepatic liver enzymes and drug metabolism and explain the importance of each of them in clinical practice.
3. Explain why a parenteral dose of propranolol is not equivalent to the oral drug dose.
4. A patient with a history of amphetamine drug abuse is admitted to your facility and immediately requests large dosages of sodium bicarbonate for a "stomach ache."

How would this product alter the urine pH? What effect would it have on amphetamine serum levels?

REFERENCES

Edwards IR: Pharmacological basis of adverse drug reactions. In Speight TM, Holford NHG, editors: *Avery's drug treatment,* ed 4, Auckland, NZ, 1997, Adis International Limited.

Katzung BG: *Basic and clinical pharmacology,* ed 5, Norwalk, Conn, 1992, Appleton & Lange.

Klaassen CD: Principles of toxicology and treatment of poisoning. In Hardman JG, Limbird LE, editors: *Goodman & Gilman's the pharmacological basis of therapeutics,* ed 9, New York, 1996, McGraw-Hill.

Nies AS, Spielberg SP: Principles of therapeutics. In Hardman JG, Limbird LE, editors: *Goodman & Gilman's the pharmacological basis of therapeutics,* ed 9, New York, 1996, McGraw-Hill.

Sjoqvist F, Borga O et al: Fundamentals of clinical pharmacology. In Speight TM, Holford NHG, editors: *Avery's drug treatment,* ed 4, Auckland, NZ, 1997, Adis International Limited.

United States Pharmacopeial Convention: *USP DI: drug information for the health care professional,* ed 18, Rockville, Md, 1998, the Convention.

ADDITIONAL REFERENCES

Miller SW, Strom JG Jr: Drug-product selection: implications for the geriatric patient, *Consult Pharmacist* 5(1):30, 1990.

Young LY, Koda-Kimble MA, editors: *Applied therapeutics: the clinical use of drugs,* ed 6, Vancouver, Wash, 1997, Applied Therapeutics.

CHAPTER 5

Life Span Aspects of Drug Therapy

CHAPTER FOCUS

The administration of drugs across the life span may result in a wide variety of drug responses, from undertreatment and therapeutic dose to overdosing. Such variations may be individual and are altered by both physiologic and pathophysiologic factors present in patients of different ages. If the healthcare professional understands the rationales behind these effects, he or she may maximize drug benefits while reducing the potential for adverse effects and toxicity.

OBJECTIVES

After reading and studying this chapter, the student should be able to do the following:

1. *Define and discuss the key terms.*
2. *Name and describe the physiologic changes that occur during pregnancy and their affect on drug pharmacokinetics (i.e., absorption, distribution, metabolism, and excretion).*
3. *List the three most important variables to review when considering the administration of drugs during pregnancy.*
4. *Describe pharmacokinetic alterations related to breastfeeding.*
5. *Discuss the factors that influence an increase in drug use and misuse in the elderly.*
6. *Review the physiologic effects in aging that may affect drug pharmacokinetics and pharmacodynamics. List an example for each effect.*

KEY TERMS

carcinogenic, (p. 74)
fetal alcohol syndrome, (p. 76)
mutagenic, (p. 74)
phocomelia, (p. 75)
polypharmacy, (p. 82)
teratogenic, (p. 74)

The effects of drug therapy in the pregnant woman, infant, child, and elderly patient differ from those in the rest of the adult population. For example, drugs taken by the pregnant woman may reach the fetus via maternal circulation and cause birth defects. Furthermore drugs consumed by a breastfeeding woman may be excreted in milk; if the drug levels are high enough, this can be problematic or toxic to the nursing infant. In addition, pediatric and geriatric patients are often more sensitive to medications, primarily because infants have an immature organ system, whereas in the elderly, organ function may be compromised or impaired. Therefore management of drug therapy must be based on the physiologic and pathophysiologic factors present in the individual.

PREGNANCY AND BREASTFEEDING

During pregnancy, any chemical or drug substance that is consumed and absorbed may reach the fetus by way of maternal circulation or be transferred to the neonate via breast milk. The drug concentration in the maternal circulation depends on individual drug factors such as dose, route of administration, and the drug's pharmacokinetics in the mother and infant.

PREGNANCY

Even though many drugs cross the placenta, the potential for inducing adverse fetal effects depends on the drug type, drug concentration, and fetal age. The Food and Drug Administration (FDA) established five pregnancy categories (A, B, C, D, and X) to indicate the risk level of drugs to the fetus (see Chapter 2 for more information on pregnancy safety). Although this schedule is useful clinically, unfortunately a number of drugs in use today have not been rated, and most of the studies were performed in animals. In this scheme, category A is considered the least dangerous, while drugs in categories B, C, and D are progressively more dangerous. Drugs in category X are considered the most dangerous and should be avoided during pregnancy.

Evaluation of drug therapy in a pregnant woman should consider the risk to benefit ratio. This ratio is evaluated based on the mother's condition and the potential effect of the drug(s) on the mother and the developing fetus. It is important to understand that no drug can really be labeled as totally safe. For example, the use of the estrogen diethylstilbestrol (DES) during pregnancy initially did not cause any problems. However, years later, it was linked to an increased risk of vaginal and cervical cancer in female offspring and genital abnormalities in both male and female offspring. It has been theorized that the DES consumed during the first trimester of pregnancy accumulated in the fetus unable to metabolize it, thus resulting in problems later in life. The incidence was low (0.01% to 0.1%) according to the FDA (Williams, Stancel, 1996), but the origin of the problem, a drug taken during developmental stages in pregnancy that has the potential of causing problems later in offspring, is a concern.

The first trimester is when the developing embryo is most vulnerable to the teratogenic (causing fetal defects or abnormalities) effects of various medications and chemicals. The healthcare professional should keep in mind that drugs in this context includes prescription and over-the-counter (OTC) drugs, alcohol, drugs of abuse, and any other chemical substance consumed by the mother during this time period.

Drug Transfer to the Fetus

Pharmacokinetics

Many physiologic changes that occur during pregnancy may affect drug pharmacokinetics. Although pregnancy does not directly affect drug absorption from the gastrointestinal tract, it does delay gastric emptying and decreases motility, which can increase or decrease drug absorption. For example, drugs that require an acidic environment for absorption may have a delayed absorption pattern due to the previous changes and because of the typical decrease in production of hydrochloric acid in the stomach during pregnancy.

However drug absorption from other sites may be increased. For example, an increase in pulmonary drug absorption and an increase in cutaneous or topical drug absorption may be seen secondary to a greater minute ventilation pattern and a larger surface area and blood flow during pregnancy (Wingard et al, 1991).

Changes in the woman's body mass and fluid distribution may also change the volume of drug distribution. During pregnancy there is an increase in fatty tissue (especially during the 10th to 30th week of pregnancy), which decreases the ratio of albumin to water and alters or reduces drug protein binding. Maternal renal blood flow and glomerular filtration rate increase during the first 8 months of pregnancy, while the hepatic enzyme activity appears to decline or decrease during pregnancy.

The results of these changes on drug therapies are difficult to predict as the alterations can vary among individual patients. Even though drug biotransformation in the liver may be delayed, the increase in renal excretion may offset this alteration. Nevertheless, if drugs are absolutely necessary during pregnancy, they should be carefully selected and titrated to the desired clinical response.

Many drugs ingested during pregnancy can cross the placenta and reach the fetus. The transfer of drugs across the placenta depends on the chemical properties of the drug, protein binding, and lipid solubility. The transport mechanisms primarily involve simple diffusion, although other transport processes may also be involved to a much lesser degree. Early in pregnancy, low-molecular-weight drugs freely cross the placenta by various transport mechanisms. In late gestation, the enhanced uteroplacental blood flow and thinner membranes that separate maternal blood flow and placental capillaries result in an increased placental transfer of un-ionized, lipophilic (lipid-soluble) drugs in their free or unbound state. Disease states such as

BOX 5-1 Drugs and Potential Teratogenic Effects

Drug	Critical Time Period	Potential Defect
angiotensin-converting enzyme (ACE) inhibitors	2nd-3rd trimester	renal dysgenesis, defects in skull ossification
alcohol, chronic use	<12 weeks	heart defects, central nervous system (CNS) abnormalities
	>24 weeks	delay in development, low birth weight
aminopterin	<14 weeks	spontaneous abortion
	1st trimester	limb, craniofacial, and neural tube defects
androgens	>10 weeks	external female genitalia masculinization
carbamazepine	<30 days after conception	spina bifida
cigarette smoking	<20 weeks	miscarriage
	>20 weeks	low birth weight and perhaps delay in development
cocaine	2nd-3rd trimester	abruptio placentae
	3rd trimester	premature labor and delivery; intracranial bleeding
diethylstilbestrol (DES)	<12 weeks	vaginal adenosis, vaginal carcinoma, uterine abnormalities, male infertility
isotretinoin (Accutane)	>15 days after conception	hydrocephalus, CNS abnormalities, fetal death
lithium	<2 months	Ebstein's anomaly
methotrexate	6-9 weeks after conception	skull ossification defect, limb and craniofacial defects
phenytoin (Dilantin)	1st trimester	craniofacial defects, phalanges/nails underdevelopment
tetracycline	>20 weeks	stained teeth, bone growth defect
valproic acid	<1 month after conception	spina bifida
	1st trimester	craniofacial defects
vaccines (measles, mumps, rubella)	1st trimester	spontaneous abortions, premature births, possibly congenital defects
vitamin A (high doses and parenteral)	—	fetal abnormalities including urinary tract malformations, growth retardation

Modified from Jennings, 1996.

pregnancy-induced hypertension or diabetes mellitus can also affect drug transfer.

The majority of drugs cross the placenta by simple diffusion; therefore fetal serum levels may equal maternal levels. In some instances, the fetal drug serum level may range from 50% to over 100% of the maternal level (McCombs, 1993). Certain drugs are contraindicated during pregnancy or are used only when the risk-benefit situation has been carefully reviewed and discussed with the patient. Some of the drugs considered to be potential teratogens, along with the critical time periods and potential defects, are noted in Box 5-1.

Fetal Drug Effects

Drug effects in the fetus can be more significant and prolonged than in the mother because the fetus usually has an immature liver enzyme metabolizing system and a slower excretion rate. Fetal excretion occurs by the kidneys into amniotic fluid, which then is reabsorbed by the mother. An immature or underdeveloped physiologic mechanism in the fetus may result in an altered drug responses or toxicity.

Several chronic medical disorders in the mother often need to be treated during pregnancy. For example, pregnancy in the patient with diabetes, hypertension, epilepsy, or asthma requires close monitoring and carefully selected therapies to minimize or reduce fetal abnormalities and disease complications.

The use of alcohol and abuse drugs, however, should be avoided as they can be extremely harmful to the fetus and newborn. Drugs given before delivery, such as alcohol, barbiturates, or opioid analgesics, may result in withdrawal symptoms in the neonate. These symptoms include hyperactivity, increased irritability, persistent crying, convulsions, and, perhaps, sudden death. Table 5-1 lists drugs that are associated with neonatal withdrawal symptoms.

Various medications can be toxic or **teratogenic, mutagenic** (causing genetic mutation), or **carcinogenic** (causing or accelerating the development of cancer). An example of the latter is DES, a drug associated with precancerous or cancer cell changes that occurred in offspring of mothers who took DES during pregnancy as previously discussed in this chapter.

Embryo Development

Each embryo undergoes a series of precisely programmed steps from cell proliferation, to differentiation, to organogenesis. The critical periods for drug effects on the fetus are the first 2 weeks of rapid cell proliferation, when exposure

TABLE 5-1 Drugs Associated with Neonatal Withdrawal Symptoms*

	Symptoms	
	General	***CNS***
Alcohol	Irritability, poor sleep pattern, diaphoresis	Crying, hyperactivity, increased sensitivity to sound, hypertonicity, tremor, seizures
Cocaine	Tremulousness, poor sleep pattern	Hypotonia, hyperreflexia
Antihistamines		
diphenhydramine (Benadryl)	Tremulousness	
hydroxyzine (Atarax, Vistaril)	Irritability	Hyperactivity, tremor, jitteriness, shrill cry, hypotonia, seizures
Barbiturates		
amobarbital (Amytal) ethchlorvynol (Placidyl) phenobarbital, secobarbital (Seconal)	Irritability, poor sleep pattern, diaphoresis, skin abrasions	Excessive crying, hyperreflexia, increased sensitivity to sound, hypertonicity, tremor, seizures
Benzodiazepines		
chlordiazepoxide (Librium)	Irritability	Tremors
diazepam (Valium)	Hypothermia	Hyperactivity, hypotonia, hypertonia, apnea/tremor, hyperreflexia
Opiates		
codeine heroin meperidine (Demerol) methadone morphine pentazocine (Talwin)	Irritability, wakefulness, yawning, tearing, fever, diaphoresis Skin excoriations, voracious sucking Poor sleep pattern Hypothermia Respiratory (stuffy, runny nose, sneezing, tachypnea, respiratory alkalosis) Gastrointestinal (hiccups, salivation, vomiting, diarrhea, failure to thrive)	Coarse tremors, seizures, twitching Hyperactivity (high-pitched cry), hypertonicity Hyperreflexia, increased sensitivity to sound, photophobia, apneic spells
propoxyphene (Darvon)	Irritability, fever	Hyperactivity, tremor, high-pitched cry

*Modified from Levy, Spino, 1993.

to drugs can be lethal to the embryo, and weeks 3 to 12 of pregnancy, the period of organogenesis. This is when the extremities (arms, fingers, legs, and toes), central nervous system (CNS), muscles, and organs are developing most rapidly (Wingard et al, 1991).

Thalidomide is an unfortunate example of a drug that caused teratogenic effects during organogenesis. It was used as a sedative-hypnotic drug from the 1950s to early 1960s, mostly in Europe. Its wide use resulted in abnormal limb development (**phocomelia**), a rare birth defect that is characterized by the absence or malformation of arms or legs in many children whose mothers received this drug during pregnancy. When administered after the 10th to 12th week of pregnancy, physiologic or behavioral alterations and growth delays were more likely. Thalidomide is currently available in the United States as an orphan drug or an investigational drug for use in bone marrow transplantation, in treatment of leprosy, and in human immunodeficiency virus (HIV)-associated wasting syndrome (Olin, 1998). However, the history of this product should not be overlooked; every precaution needs to be instituted if it is prescribed for women of childbearing age.

The abuse of cocaine during pregnancy has resulted in spontaneous abortions, fetal hypoxia, premature delivery and congenital abnormalities (skull defects, cardiac abnormality), and cerebral infarction or stroke. At birth the newborn may exhibit symptoms of cocaine drug withdrawal: irritability, increased respiratory and heart rates, diarrhea, irregular sleeping patterns, and poor appetite. It has been reported that long-term behavioral patterns of infants born to cocaine-abusing women may also occur, such as poor attention spans and a decrease in organizational skills (Hall et al, 1990). Cocaine abuse is discussed further in Chapter 6.

Drug Use During Pregnancy

Drug use during pregnancy should be avoided or limited to only those women who absolutely require treatment. Some drugs considered relatively safe during pregnancy are listed in Table 5-2.

TABLE 5-2 Some Drugs Considered Relatively Safe for Use in Pregnancy

Agent	Recommendations and Cautions*
Analgesics	
acetaminophen	Considered safest analgesic during pregnancy
Antiasthmatics	
cromolyn sodium	Relatively safe
metaproterenol (aerosol)	Relatively safe for mild, intermittent episodes: avoid oral form
theophylline	Relatively safe if blood levels are closely monitored
Anticoagulants	
heparin	For use during first trimester; use caution if given during last trimester
Anticonvulsants	
phenobarbital	Can cause malformations: for use only if necessary to maintain seizure control; if given during pregnancy, monitor neonate during first 24 hours for neonatal coagulation defect (bleeding)
Antidiabetics	
insulin	Relatively safe; drug of choice
Antiemetics	
pyridoxine	Relatively safe for morning sickness
doxylamine	For use as necessary for severe nausea or vomiting
prochlorperazine	
trimethobenzamide	
cyclizine	
meclizine	
Antihypertensives	
methyldopa	Safest of antihypertensives during pregnancy (especially as substitute for diuretics in pregnancy for diastolic blood pressure > 110 mm Hg in the third trimester)
hydralazine	Safest for hypertensive crises in pregnancy
Antiinfectives	
cephalosporins	Safe during pregnancy
erythromycin	For use as substitute for penicillin hypersensitivity
metronidazole	Not to be used during the first trimester
miconazole	Relatively safe
penicillin and derivatives	Relatively safe
Antituberculosis Drugs	
rifampin	Relatively safe
ethambutol	
Cardiac Glycosides	
digoxin	Relatively safe; maternal plasma levels should be closely monitored

*Recommendations are likely to change; therefore manufacturers' package inserts should always be consulted. No drugs are known to be *absolutely* safe during pregnancy. The use of many substances, including most drugs not on this list, should be carefully considered by the obstetrician as to risks and benefits. See drug monographs for specific drug information; see also bibliography. Consult references for sources of information about drugs in this table.

If it is necessary to administer drug therapy, the most important variables to be considered include the following:

1. Fetal gestational age at time of exposure
2. Duration of therapy planned
3. Any other drugs administered concurrently

The drug dose, dosing intervals, and duration of treatment should be adjusted carefully to avoid harmful effects.

Excessive maternal intake of alcohol, especially at or near time of conception, is associated with **fetal alcohol syndrome,** which produces congenital anomalies and both growth and mental retardation (Box 5-2). Other common substances that are potentially dangerous during pregnancy include extended-release aspirin (pregnancy category D), parenteral vitamin A (category X), and nicotine chewing gum and nicotine transdermal systems (category X and category D, respectively) (USP DI, 1998).

A major problem with drug use is that the effects on the embryo may occur before a woman is aware that she is pregnant. Women of childbearing age who are not using contraceptives and who are sexually active should be prescribed drugs carefully and should be instructed to use over-the-counter medications cautiously. Education and prevention are considered the best therapy.

PEDIATRICS

Neonates

Newborns require special consideration because they lack many of the protective mechanisms of older children and adults. Their skin is thin and permeable, their stomachs lack acid, and their lungs lack much of the mucous barrier. Neonates regulate body temperature poorly and become dehydrated easily. Their liver and kidneys are immature and cannot manage foreign substances as well as older children and adults. Specific pharmacokinetic factors affecting medication use in neonates are reviewed in Table 5-3.

Breastfed Infants

Almost all forms of drugs in maternal circulation can be readily transferred to the colostrum and breast milk. Because drugs or their biotransformed products are handled

BOX 5-2 Alcohol and the Childbearing Patient: Fetal Alcohol Syndrome

Alcohol consumption during pregnancy can cause tragic effects on the fetus. As many people do not consider alcohol a drug; its danger during pregnancy may be overlooked. Alcohol easily crosses the placenta to enter the fetal bloodstream, which can result in fetal alcohol syndrome (FAS), a series of congenital abnormalities.

The symptoms of FAS include small head (microcephaly), a low birth weight, mental and growth retardation, impaired coordination, irritability in infancy, hyperactivity in childhood, cardiac murmurs, cleft lip or palate, hernias, and many other organic and structural abnormalities (see figure below).

As even limited amounts of alcohol during pregnancy may have tragic effects on a developing fetus, the only safe approach is total abstinence.

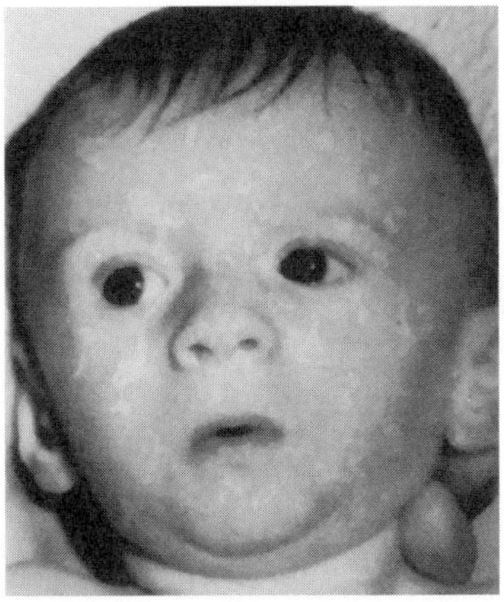

From Baldwin, Cook, 1995. Photo courtesy Dr. Charles Linder, Medical College of Georgia. From Goodman RM, Gorlin RJ: *Atlas of the face in genetic disorders*, ed 2, St Louis, 1977, Mosby.

by different pathways in the infant and the fetus, the impact of maternal medications on the infant probably differs (is probably less) than that on the fetus. This difference can guide in prescribing medications for the breastfeeding woman. Typical nontherapeutic or unexpected outcomes in the breastfed infant may be signs of the drug's usual side or toxic effects.

Adverse effects may also occur, such as allergic sensitization to penicillin, or gray-brown stains of the later-erupting teeth as a result of tetracycline therapy of more than 10 days duration. Most drug products that reach the neonate via breast milk have undergone maternal biotransformation and are probably less than the original dose. However, immaturity of the neonate's hepatic and renal systems may limit the infant's capacity for further metabolism and excretion.

Data about an infant's capabilities for drug absorption, digestion, distribution, metabolism, and excretion are scant and conflicting. In general, the proven benefits of continuing breastfeeding must be weighed on an individual basis against the risks of maternal medication to the infant. Although the mammary glands are a relatively insignificant route for maternal drug excretion and the drug level in breast milk is usually less than the actual maternal dose, the infant's actual dose depends largely on the volume of milk consumed. Thus a single measurement of a drug in human milk will not accurately reflect the total dose the infant receives.

The drug concentration in maternal circulation depends on the relationship of several factors: dosing and route of administration, the drug's distribution, its protein binding, and maternal metabolism and excretion. The mammary alveolar epithelium consists of a lipid barrier with water-filled pores; thus it is more permeable to drugs during the colostrum stage of milk production (first week of life). Drug factors that enhance drug excretion into milk are nonionization, low molecular weight, fat solubility, and concentration. Transfer of an active or passive form of a drug's metabolite into maternal plasma and then to milk depends mainly on passive diffusion.

It is believed that absorptive processes in the infant's gastrointestinal tract and drug distribution are similar to those in the adult and that lipid-soluble drugs are well absorbed. The infant's age (thus the amount of drug-containing milk consumed) and the relative immaturity of the infant's important organs bear greatly on the outcome. The following factors are also relevant: (1) if the drug is fat soluble, it may be more highly concentrated in breast milk at the end of feedings and at midday; (2) because the infant's total serum protein is lower in comparison to the adult's, more free drug may be available to the circulation; (3) metabolic reactions in the infant's liver are slower than in the older child's and consequently drug biotransformation may likewise be delayed; and (4) drug excretion is delayed in the neonate because it is largely via the kidneys, where immature glomerular filtration rates and tubular functioning are maintained for months. The extreme variability among drug effects and infants' capabilities makes it difficult to decide whether the mother should take a drug and whether or not she should breastfeed.

If human milk contains small, fixed amounts of substances absorbed by the mother, it is usually recommended that breastfeeding be temporarily interrupted (usually for 24 to 72 hours) and the breasts pumped to remove drug-containing milk. Less often, it is advisable to cease breastfeeding altogether. Dosages and routes may also be changed. It is recommended that certain drugs be avoided while breastfeeding (Box 5-3).

Drug effects may be minimized by substituting formula for the midday breastfeeding, since that is the feeding highest in fat content and thus more likely to contain higher amounts of fat-soluble drug products. In addition, breastfeeding mothers who must take medications can take the medication immediately after breastfeeding so as much time as possible elapses and the drug can reach a relatively low concentration before the next feeding (Table 5-4).

If diagnostic radioisotope testing is to be done, breastfeeding is interrupted until all radiation is absent from milk

TABLE 5-3 Pharmacokinetics that Influence Drug Dosing in Neonates

Physiologic Process	Neonate	Type of Drugs Affected
Absorption		
Gastric pH	Increased to 6 to 8 for first 24 hours; then usually a 10- to 15-day achlorhydria	Acid-labile drugs, such as oral penicillin, better absorbed Oral forms of phenobarbital or phenytoin: reduced bioavailability
Gastric emptying time	Prolonged, usually 6 to 8 hours	Oral absorption of penicillin increased; phenytoin, phenobarbital decreased
Distribution		
Total body water (TBW) content	75% to 79%	Average adults have about 60% TBW and 25% to 45% fat
Adipose (fat) content	5% to 12%	Vast differences in drug distribution across the age span Water-soluble drugs have a larger volume of distribution in newborns; fat-soluble drugs have considerably less Drug dosage adjustments largely based on this factor
Protein binding	Decreased	Highly protein-bound drugs require dose adjustment to avoid toxicity
Metabolism		
Liver metabolism	Decreased	Potent or potentially toxic drugs requiring liver metabolism are slowly metabolized; lower doses are necessary for such drugs (especially chloramphenicol and theophylline, among others)
Microsomal enzymes	Low	
Excretion		
Glomerular filtration	Decreased	Drugs excreted by filtration or secretion will accumulate in the neonate; dose adjustments necessary (especially aminoglycosides and digoxin)
Tubular secretion	Decreased	

BOX 5-3 Drugs Contraindicated During Breastfeeding

The American Academy of Pediatrics Committee on Drugs has suggested the following drugs be avoided by the woman who is breastfeeding:

amphetamines	gold salts
bromocriptine	heroin
cocaine	lithium
cyclophosphamide	marijuana
cyclosporine	methotrexate
doxorubicin	nicotine (smoking)
ergotamine	phenindione

samples. Breastfeeding will probably be terminated at any time when the drug is so potent that minute amounts may profoundly affect the infant when the drug has high allergenic potential, when the mother's renal function decreases (which augments drug excretion into breast milk), or when serious pathologic conditions require prolonged administration of high doses of the drug.

Changes in the activity levels of the fetus or nursing infant signal dangerous effects resulting from drug administration. Parents should be taught how to assess and report unusual fetal inactivity or infant apathy.

Nonbreastfed Infants

Infant formula feeding is used when the mother:

- Chooses not to breastfeed
- Is advised not to breastfeed because of illness or disease
- Has an infant with special formulation needs

Commercially available preparations prepared from nonfat cow's milk are available and are generally divided into two categories: general purpose and special purpose infant formulas (see Box 5-4 for selected formulas from each category).

Infant formulas contain essential and minor trace elements as found in human breast milk, plus the three sources of calories (protein, carbohydrate, and lipids) in a balanced proportion to promote growth. Many of the formulas contain vitamins and minerals and usually the vitamin K in these formulas is more than is contained in breast milk. Vitamin K is included because it reduces the risk of hemorrhagic disease in the infant.

Cow's milk differs from human milk in protein content. The protein (80%) in cow's milk is casein, whereas human milk contains whey protein (70%). Human milk protein (whey) is richer in immunoglobulins, albumin, lysozyme, amylase, transaminase, protease, and lipases. Casein provides lesser amounts of these ingredients. Although the protein in many of the formulations is of a higher quality than in cow's milk, some infant formulas may contain bovine whey, a protein that contains beta-lactoglobulin.

TABLE 5-4 Some Drugs Considered Relatively Safe during Breastfeeding

Agent	*Recommendations and Precautions**
Analgesics	
acetaminophen	Relatively safe
butorphanol	With usual dosages, drug levels in breast milk are usually low
codeine	
meperidine	
morphine	
propoxyphene	
Antiinfectives	
cefadroxil	Low concentrations distributed into breast milk, no problems reported
cefazolin	
cefoxitin	Relatively safe
ceftriaxone	No problems reported
isoniazid	
ethambutol	
Cardiovascular Drugs	
digoxin	Safe if maternal serum levels are closely monitored
guanethidine	Safe in recommended dosages
methyldopa	Distributed in breast milk, no documented problems in humans
propranolol	Relatively safe at lower maternal dosages (higher drug levels in breast milk than in maternal bloodstream because of high lipid solubility of drug)
Diuretics	
spironolactone	Safe
thiazides	May suppress lactation; avoid in first month of lactation
Bronchodilators	
cromolyn sodium	
theophylline	Observe for infant irritability or insomnia
Antidiabetics	
insulin	Safe; not distributed in breast milk
Thyroid Drugs	
thyroid hormones	Relatively safe if monitored for thyroid function and response
Gastrointestinal Drugs	
antacids	Relatively safe
cisapride	
laxatives (except cascara and danthron)	
Air Pollutants	Have not been found in human milk
Vaccines	
RhoGAM	Considered safe

*Over time recommendations may change; therefore manufacturers' package inserts should always be consulted by pediatricians and nurses. Most substances should be avoided during the period of breastfeeding. (Details about specific drugs are located under relevant chapter headings in this text.) Consult references for sources of information.

This substance contributes to the development of cow's milk allergies.

Infants can absorb 20% to 50% of the iron they need from breast milk, whereas iron from infant formulations is only minimally absorbed (4% to 7%). The reason for this difference in absorption is unknown. The Committee on Nutrition of the American Academy of Pediatrics checked the iron content in formulas and found that as many as 20% of infants receive a formula with a low-iron content (1.5 mg/L). The possible reason for the use of these products is prescribers believing that iron is responsible for colic, constipation, diarrhea, and regurgitation and thus recommending the lower iron formulations. Research indicates this belief is unfounded; thus the Committee has recommended that these formulations be removed from the market and iron-fortified formulas be used exclusively (Pray, 1993).

PEDIATRIC DRUG ADMINISTRATION

Drug administration to pediatric patients requires special knowledge and approaches. Pharmacokinetically hepatic drug metabolism in neonates is slow due to immaturity. For example, phenobarbital plasma half-life is 70 to 500 hours in a neonate (<7 days), 20 to 70 hours in infants (>1 month), 20 to 80 hours in children 1 to 15 years of age, and 60 to 180 hours in young adults (Walson, 1997).

When the infant is 1 year old, most pharmacokinetic patterns (other than hepatic) are similar to those in an adult. The liver metabolizing enzymes are increased; therefore children metabolize drugs at a faster rate than adults as illustrated by the phenobarbital example above. This alteration is primarily due to the liver being larger in proportion to body weight compared with an adult (Walson, 1997). The child reaches adult parameters at puberty. Therefore drugs primarily eliminated by hepatic metabolism may require dosage or frequency adjustments due to a shorter half-life. Such variations though must be individually determined and carefully monitored.

Renal excretion is decreased in neonates and reaches adult parameters for glomerular filtration rate between 3 to 6 months while tubular function does not mature until the infant is approximately 12 months old. Therefore for drugs excreted primarily by the kidneys, the serum half-life will be prolonged during the first week of life (the lower the renal drug clearance, the longer the drug half-life in the body). Then the elimination rate increases rapidly over the next few weeks. Later in childhood, renal function may exceed adult parameters and if not detected result in drug underdosing (Walson, 1997).

A standard medication dosage is nearly nonexistent in pediatrics; therefore medications are usually ordered according to the weight or body surface area of the child. The use of calculation formulas based on the child's weight, etc., are inaccurate and should not be used. Children are not small adults, and their physiologic differences will definitely affect the amount of drug needed to produce a therapeutic effect.

BOX 5-4 Selected Examples of Infant Formulations

Product Name/Manufacturer	Indications/Special Features
General Purpose	
Enfamil (Mead Johnson)	Supplement to breastfeeding
Good-Start (Carnation)	
PediaSure (Ross)	
Special Purpose	
Alimentum Liquid (Ross)	Severe food allergies, protein sensitivity or maldigestion, or fat malabsorption; corn and lactose free
Isomil Liquid & Powder (Ross)	Infants and children allergic to cow's milk, lactose deficient, or galactosemic; lactose free
Phenex-1 Powder (Ross)	Infants with phenylketonuria (PKU)
Pregestrimil Powder (Mead Johnson)	Severe malabsorption disorders
ProSobee (Mead Johnson)	Infants with family history of allergies; lactose, milk, and sucrose free
Infant Formulas with Iron	
Enfamil with Iron (Mean Johnson)	
Similac w/Iron (Ross)	
SMA Iron Fortified (Mead Johnson)	
Lofenalac Powder (Mead Johnson)	Low phenylalanine plus iron

For example, an infant's body composition is approximately 75% water (adults have 50% to 60%), and an infant has less fat content than the adult. Therefore, water-soluble drugs are generally administered in larger doses to infants and children in proportion to body weight than to adults. A good example of this is the water-soluble drug gentamicin, an intravenous antibiotic. Recommended dosages from USP DI (1998) are as follows: older neonates and infants, 2.5 mg/kg every 8 to 16 hours; children, 2 to 2.5 mg/kg every 8 hours; and adults weighing less than 60 kg, 1.5 mg/kg every 12 hours.

Although pharmaceutical companies are increasing their marketing of pediatric drug products, many medications are still only available in the standard adult dosage strength; therefore the healthcare professional must be able to calculate and formulate such products into the correct pediatric dosage.

Body Surface Area as a Basis

It was suggested years ago that drug dosages be calculated on size or the proportional amount of body surface area (BSA) to weight. Some prescribers continue to use weight as the basis for calculating drug dosages and BSA for calculating fluid requirements. However, most clinicians advocate using BSA for determining drug dosage for adults as well as children. Prescribers usually carry a simple slide rule or nomogram (Fig. 5-1) to make rapid BSA conversions from weight and height. It is believed that the larger amount of total body water (TBW) in children, as well as the percentage of water in body weight and the part of that percentage formed by extracellular water, accounts for the fact that children tolerate or require larger doses of some drugs on a mg/m^2 basis.

The surface area rule for pediatric drug calculations is the most accurate. As a relationship between height and weight, it can provide a more precise guide to the maturity of the child's organs and metabolic rate of functioning for effective pharmacokinetics. The dosage should be tailored to the individual child according to the amount of medication per square meter of body surface area. The BSA rule for pediatric dosages follows:

Approximate pediatric dose =
Child's BSA in square meters (from nomogram) ×
Adult dose/1.73

For example, using Fig. 5-1, a child with a height of 34 inches weighing 10 kg would be considered to have a BSA (m^2) of 0.5. The dosage calculation then would be:

Child's approximate dose = 0.5 × Adult dose/1.73

If the student is uncertain about dosage, the following sources are recommended: the drug monograph in a package insert, *USP DI* (1998), *AHFS* (1998), pediatric drug handbooks (such as the John Hopkins Hospital *Harriet Lane Handbook* and others), or consultation with a pharmacist.

Although these rules have been devised for converting adult dosage schedules to infants and children, it must be emphasized that no rules or charts are adequate to guarantee safety of dosage at any age, particularly in the neonate. No method takes into account all variables, particularly individual tolerance differences. Close observation of how the individual child reacts to medications is very useful in help-

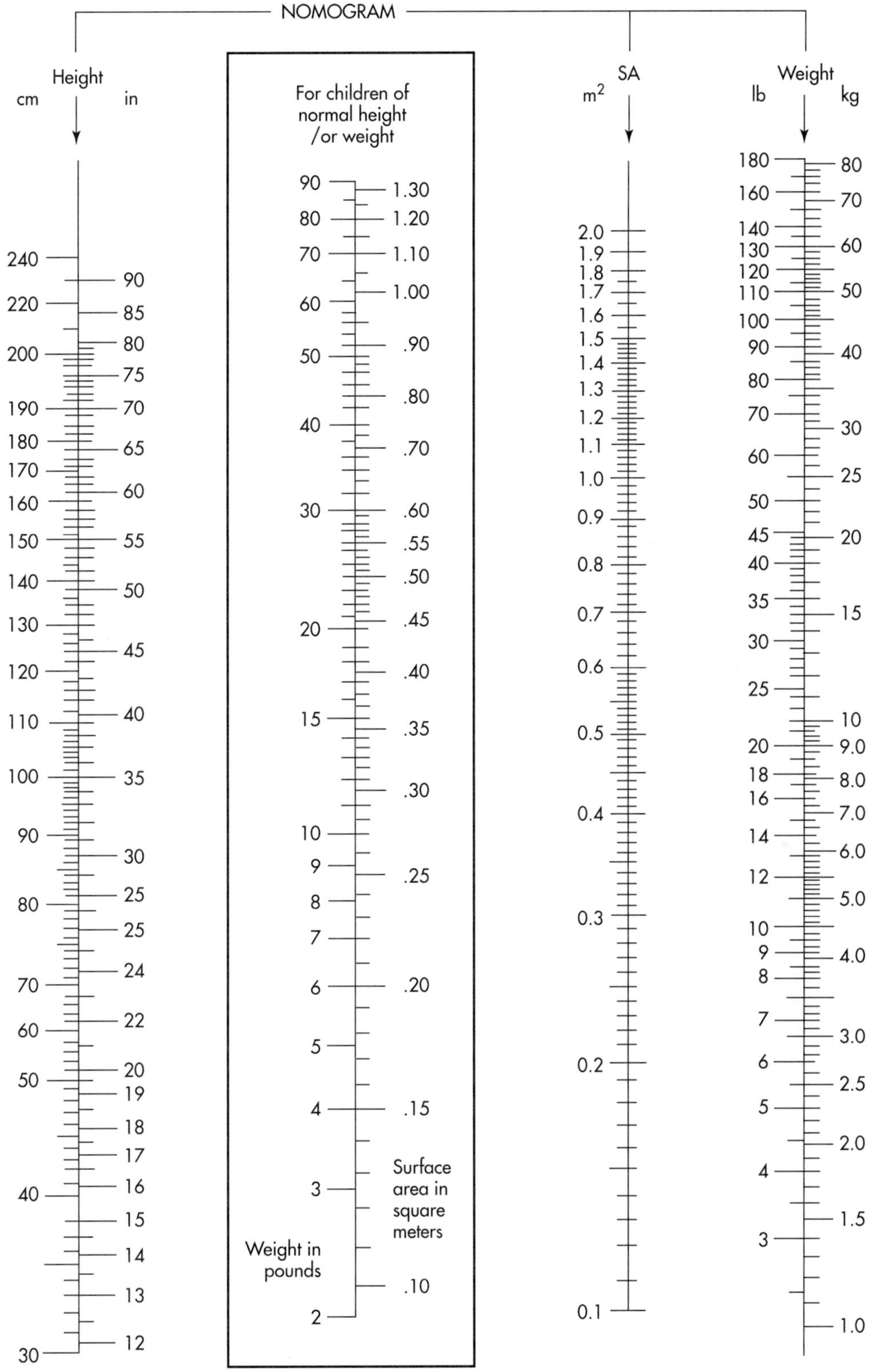

FIGURE 5-1
BSA is indicated where straight line that connects height (on the left) and weight (on the right) levels intersects BSA column or, if patient is above average size, from weight alone (enclosed area). From Barone MA: *The Harriet Lane handbook*, ed 14, St Louis, 1996, Mosby.

ing to determine the proper drug, dose, and dosing intervals that are necessary for the patient.

Topical Medications

Children have a large skin surface area in proportion to total body weight. Their skin, especially neonates' skin, is particularly thin and permeable and has limited protective oil. Although adults absorb much more medication through intact skin than was previously believed, the child is even more at risk than the adult for systemic absorption of topical medication. The discovery that hexachlorophene can cause encephalopathy in newborns and that topically applied boric acid can cause systemic poisoning testifies to the hazard of applying drugs to children's skin, especially for prolonged contact or over broken skin areas. Plain soap and water, not medicated dressings, may be the preferred treatment for abrasions or open lesions.

Other Factors Influencing Drug Dosages

Again, the dosage of most agents is related to the child's age, weight, and height. A child's body systems grow and develop at varying rates, which makes for unpredictable primary and secondary effects in pediatric medication administration. One example of secondary effects specific to children is discoloration of teeth and depression of enamel growth with administration of tetracycline liquid medications in children younger than 8 years of age. (This adverse reaction is well-documented, but the drug is still being prescribed for this age group, according to the FDA.) The skeletal growth of children receiving long-term adrenocortical steroids is also impaired.

Individual variations are noted in children's responses to digitalis, insulin, and opioids; doses require careful titration. Paradoxical responses are noted with a few drugs; responses may be directly opposite to those expected in the adult. Excessive reactivity to atropine by infants may be related to immaturity of the central nervous system. In addition, many drugs that are safe and effective for adults may not have been tested for use with children, nor have doses been established because of the complex medicolegal issues involved in experimentation on children.

ELDERLY

Although the geriatric population represents approximately 12% of the population in the United States and Canada today, it has been reported that they do the following:

- Consume 30% of all prescribed drugs and 50% of all OTC medications in the United States
- Are admitted to hospitals for adverse drug reactions (ADRs) three times more frequently than younger adults
- Represent 51% of the deaths and 39% of hospitalizations from ADRs (persons older than 60 years of age)
- Experience more drug-related incidents than other aged populations (25% of all admissions from a nursing home setting to a hospital are drug-related) (Trends & Analysis, 1995)

It has been projected that by the year 2030, more than 20% of the population will be 65 years of age or older (Trends & Analysis, 1995). Because the elderly are the most rapidly increasing segment of the U.S. population, an understanding of age-related alterations in pharmacokinetics and pharmacodynamics is necessary. Furthermore, the increased incidence of chronic diseases in the elderly often results in an increase in the number of prescriptions, OTC medications, and home remedies prescribed or self-selected. The age of specialization has in some ways added to this problem, because multiple physicians usually prescribe a variety of medications often without discontinuing the drugs the patient is currently taking. This practice is often referred to as **polypharmacy,** the indiscriminate use of numerous medications concurrently.

Polypharmacy can be a dangerous practice that may increase the risk of drug interactions and adverse reactions and the need for or prolonging of hospitalization. Jinks and Fuerst (1995) report that adverse drug reactions in the elderly in 1985 resulted in 243,000 hospitalizations, 32,000 hip fractures, and 163,000 cases of drug-induced mental alterations or impairments. Although the magnitude of problems caused by polypharmacy is enormous, it is frequently overlooked as being the causative factor. It is important that healthcare providers realize that the vast majority of undesirable drug effects resulting from polypharmacy are preventable.

To minimize the risks associated with use of multiple medications and adverse drug reactions in this population, the healthcare provider needs to provide continuous monitoring of the drug regimen, with a primary goal of reducing or eliminating inappropriate medications and improving the patient's quality of life.

Physiologic Changes of Aging

Aging persons undergo a variety of physiologic changes that may increase their sensitivity to drugs and drug-induced disease (Fig. 5-2). The loss in body weight in many elderly patients may require initiation of therapy at a lower adult dose or reevaluation of dosages of medications already in use. The criterion for dosage should be shifted from age to weight. Some older patients weigh no more than the average large child and some weigh a lot less, yet they are prescribed the larger "adult" doses.

Pharmacokinetics (Box 5-5) are altered in the aging patient because of reduced gastric acid and slowed gastric motility, resulting in unpredictable rates of dissolution and absorption of drugs. Changes in absorption may occur when acid production decreases, altering the absorption of weakly acidic drugs such as barbiturates. However, few studies of drug absorption have shown clinically significant changes occurring with advanced age.

Changes in body composition, such as increased proportion of body fat and decreased total body water, plasma volume, and extracellular fluid, have been noted in the elderly. The increased proportion of body fat increases the body's

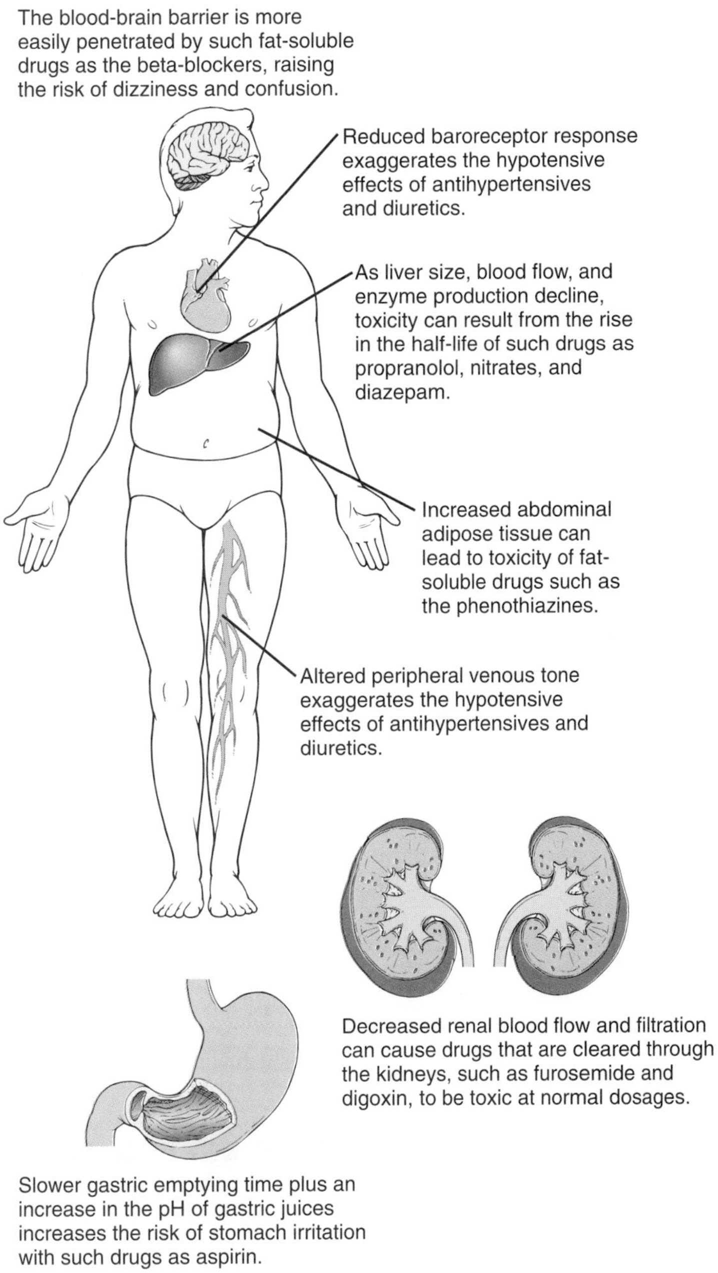
The blood-brain barrier is more easily penetrated by such fat-soluble drugs as the beta-blockers, raising the risk of dizziness and confusion.
Reduced baroreceptor response exaggerates the hypotensive effects of antihypertensives and diuretics.
As liver size, blood flow, and enzyme production decline, toxicity can result from the rise in the half-life of such drugs as propranolol, nitrates, and diazepam.
Increased abdominal adipose tissue can lead to toxicity of fat-soluble drugs such as the phenothiazines.
Altered peripheral venous tone exaggerates the hypotensive effects of antihypertensives and diuretics.
Decreased renal blood flow and filtration can cause drugs that are cleared through the kidneys, such as furosemide and digoxin, to be toxic at normal dosages.
Slower gastric emptying time plus an increase in the pH of gastric juices increases the risk of stomach irritation with such drugs as aspirin.

FIGURE 5-2

How pharmacokinetics change with age. *(Courtesy Dr. Charles Linder, Medical College of Georgia. From Goodman RM, Gorlin RJ:* Atlas of the face in genetic disorders, *ed 2, St Louis, 1977, Mosby.)*

ability to store fat-soluble compounds such as phenothiazines and barbiturates and thus increases the accumulation of those drugs. The reduced lean body mass affects drug distribution by decreasing the volume in which the drug circulates, thereby causing higher peak levels. The risk of toxicity with hydrophilic or water-soluble drugs increases as total body water decreases. Digoxin, theophylline, and the aminoglycosides are examples of hydrophilic drugs that may accumulate and result in an adverse reaction or toxicity.

Decreased serum albumin for highly protein-bound drugs may lead to increased amounts of free drug in the circulation. Warfarin (Coumadin), phenytoin (Dilantin), and diazepam (Valium) are a few examples of highly bound drugs.

Liver drug metabolism is also affected by aging. Medications that undergo phase I metabolism (reduction, oxidation, hydroxylation, or demethylation) may have a decreased metabolism while phase II metabolism (glucu-

BOX 5-5 Potential Altered Pharmacokinetics in the Elderly

Absorption
Increase in gastric pH
Altered gastric emptying and intestinal blood flow
Decrease in first-pass metabolism in the liver

Distribution
Altered body composition (decrease in lean body mass, increase in adipose [fat] stores)
Decrease in total body water
Decrease in serum albumin
Decrease in blood flow and cardiac output

Metabolism
Phase I metabolic reactions decrease with age
Decrease in enzymatic activity with age (P-450 system)
Decrease in hepatic blood flow and drug metabolism

Excretion
Decrease in renal function; most persons lose 10% renal function per decade after age 50

Modified from Trends & Analysis, 1995.

ronidation, acetylation, conjugation, etc.) is not affected by aging. Thus drugs that may have decreased hepatic metabolism in the elderly are the nitrates, barbiturates, propranolol (Inderal), and lidocaine (Jinks, Fuerst, 1995).

Disorders common to the aging person, such as congestive heart failure (CHF), may impair liver function and influence biotransformation by decreasing the metabolism of drugs and increasing the risk of drug accumulation and toxicity. Renal function may be impaired because of loss of nephrons, decreased blood flow, and decreased glomerular filtration rate. A reduction in renal function is also secondary to CHF. Decreased renal clearance may cause increased plasma drug concentrations and longer half-lives of drugs and active metabolites that the kidney usually excretes. Drugs that are highly dependent on the kidneys for excretion include the aminoglycosides, ciprofloxin (Cipro), digoxin (Lanoxin), lithium (Eskalith), and numerous other drugs (Jinks, Fuerst, 1995).

Alterations in Pharmacokinetics

It has been estimated that 70% to 80% of all adverse drug reactions in the elderly are dose related. The physiologic changes previously discussed may result in a decrease in drug metabolism, distribution in the body, and renal excretion. Therefore, higher blood and tissue levels of potent medications may result in an increased incidence of adverse drug reactions. Diazepam's (Valium's) half-life increases from 20 hours in a 20-year-old to 90 hours in individuals in their 80s because of the increase in volume of drug in the body of the elderly person. Although reduced or impaired renal function of drugs primarily excreted by the kidneys may result in drug accumulation and perhaps toxicity, up to one third of the elderly have little or no "age-related renal insufficiency" (McCue et al, 1993). Thus the previously described aging process does not necessarily affect all elderly people.

Alterations in Pharmacodynamics

Changes in target organ or receptor sensitivity in the elderly may result in a greater or lesser drug effect at these sites. The reason for this alteration is unknown, but it may be due to a decrease in the number of receptors at the site or an altered receptor response to the medication. The elderly often exhibit a decreased response to beta agonists and antagonists, but they have a greater response (CNS depression) with diazepam (Valium) (Erwin, 1993). It has also been reported that the muscarinic receptors in the cortex tend to decrease with aging so the elderly are often very sensitive to anticholinergic medications. Side effects of anticholinergic drugs including confusion, dry mouth, blurred vision, constipation, and urinary retention are frequently noted (Lucas et al, 1995). See Chapter 15 for additional information on anticholinergic drugs.

There is also believed to be a loss in responsiveness or an age-related decline in beta-adrenergic receptors and dopamine receptors in the elderly. The number of receptors may vary or the alteration may be in different areas of the aging body, which may result in altered drug responses or an increased risk for drug-induced Parkinson's disease (Lucas et al, 1995).

In summary, the elderly are perceived to have a greater sensitivity to drugs, especially to CNS-acting medications. If monitoring and dosage adjustments are not instituted, the elderly may encounter more adverse reactions than younger persons.

Medications in the Elderly

Potent medications available to treat the elderly often have a narrow index between effectiveness and toxicity. A study of more than 6000 persons 65 years or older living in the community indicated that physicians prescribe inappropriate medications for at least 25% of that elderly population (Willcox et al, 1994). Box 5-6 lists inappropriate drugs for the elderly. This list of potentially inappropriate medications was derived from a previously published list (Beers et al, 1991) and was limited to drugs that should be avoided entirely in the geriatric patient. For example, the three long-acting benzodiazepines (diazepam [Valium], chlordiazepoxide [Librium], and flurazepam [Dalmane]) have been associated with daytime sedation and an increased risk of falls while the antidepressant amitriptyline (Elavil), has been reported to cause the most anticholinergic and orthostatic hypotension side effects compared with other drugs in this category. Therefore, the prescribing of such medications in the aged patient increases the risk of inducing side effects, adverse drug reactions, and perhaps injury.

BOX 5-6 Inappropriate Drugs for the Elderly

Category	*Drug Examples*
analgesics	propoxyphene (Darvon) pentazocine (Talwin)
antidiabetic	chlorpropamide (Diabinese)
antidepressant	amitriptyline (Elavil)
antiemetic	trimethobenzamide (Tigan)
antihypertensives	propranolol (Inderal) methyldopa (Aldomet) reserpine (Serpasil)
hypnotic/sedative	diazepam (Valium) chlordiazepoxide (Librium) flurazepam (Dalmane) meprobamate (Miltown) pentobarbital (Nembutal) secobarbital (Seconal)
muscle relaxants	cyclobenzaprine (Flexeril) methocarbamol (Robaxin) carisoprodol (Soma) orphenadrine (Norflex)
nonsteroidal antiinflammatory agents (NSAIDs)	indomethacin (Indocin) phenylbutazone (Butazolidin)
platelet inhibitor	dipyridamole (Persantine)
peripheral vasodilators (dementia therapy)	cyclandelate (Cyclospasmol) isoxsuprine (Vasodilan)

Table 5-5 is a list of commonly prescribed medications for the elderly with the most common side or adverse effects reported. "Although all systems are altered by the aging process, the central nervous system and the cardiovascular system appear to be the most affected" according to Lucas et al (1995). To reduce the potential for adverse effects, it has been recommended that CNS-acting medications be reduced to approximately 50% of the usual adult recommended dose (Lucas et al, 1995). If the prescriber titrates slowly to the therapeutic effect, the potential of drug-induced adverse effects declines.

Avorn and Gurwitz (1995) report that nursing home residents receive more medications than noninstitutionalized elderly persons. Jinks and Fuerst (1995) report the elderly receive an average of 17 to 20 drugs annually while older patients in nursing homes consume an average of 6 to 8 different drugs a day. The use of inappropriate prescribed medications (see Box 5-6) was also documented in this setting. In addition, the prolonged use of oral antibiotics, short-acting benzodiazepines, and histamine-2 antagonists and high drug dosages of iron products, histamine-2 antagonists, and the antipsychotic medications were also reported. Inappropriate prescribing of psychotropic medications in long-term facilities has resulted in federal legislation (Omnibus Budget Reconciliation Act [OBRA]) that established guidelines for the proper use of such medications in the elderly. See Chapter 13 for additional information.

TABLE 5-5 Commonly Prescribed Medications in the Elderly

Medication	*Common Side/Adverse Effects*
aminoglycoside antibiotics (gentamycin, etc.)	Ototoxicity (hearing impairment or loss), renal impairment, or failure
analgesics, opioid	Confusion, constipation, urinary retention (morphine and others), nausea, vomiting, respiratory depression
anticholinergics, antispasmodics, especially antihistamines, anti-Parkinson's drugs, atropine, etc.	Blurred vision, dry mouth, constipation, confusion, urinary retention, nausea, delirium
anticoagulants (heparin, warfarin)	Bleeding episodes, hemorrhage, increase in drug-interaction potential
antihypertensive medications	Sedation, orthostatic hypotension, sexual dysfunction, CNS alterations, nausea
aspirin, aspirin-containing products	Tinnitus, gastric distress, ulcers, gastrointestinal (GI) bleeding
digoxin, digitalis preparations, especially at higher dosages	Nausea, vomiting, cardiac dysrhythmias, visual disorders, mental status changes, hallucinations
diuretics (thiazides, furosemide, etc.)	Electrolyte disorders, rash, fatigue, leg cramps, dehydration
hypnotics/sedatives (flurazepam, triazolam, etc.)	Confusion, daytime sedation, gait disturbances, lethargy, increased forgetfulness, depression, delirium
H_2 receptor antagonists (cimetidine, ranitidine, etc.)	Confusion, depression, mental status alterations
nonsteroidal antiinflammatory agents (NSAIDs)	Gastric distress, GI bleeding, ulceration
psychotropics (neuroleptic agents)	Sedation, confusion, hypotension, drug-induced parkinsonian effects, tardive dyskinesia
tricyclic antidepressants (amitriptyline, doxepin, and others)	Confusion, cardiac dysrhythmias, seizures, agitation, anticholinergic effects, tachycardia, etc.

SUMMARY

This chapter reviews drug therapy effects on the fetus, neonate, infant, child, and elderly, based on drug pharmacokinetics and the physiologic factors present across the life span. The inherent dangers and critical time period associated with drug transfer across the placenta and in breast feeding were also discussed. Fetal drug effects (teratogenic, mutagenic, and carcinogenic) are important considerations whenever drug therapy is contemplated for use during pregnancy.

The increase in the geriatric population and the age-related alterations in drug pharmacokinetic and pharmacodynamic parameters has resulted in an increase in drug use, polypharmacy, drug interactions, and adverse reactions. An understanding of the physiologic changes in aging along with careful drug selection, drug dose, and close monitoring will help to improve drug therapy in this population.

REVIEW QUESTIONS

1. Describe factors one must consider when evaluating the risk-to-benefit ratio of prescribing a drug for a pregnant woman.
2. Discuss the physiologic changes during pregnancy that affect drug transfer to the fetus.
3. Explain why the body surface area nomogram is preferred over using an infant's body weight formula for calculating drug dosage.
4. Review the issues that resulted in the elderly consuming 30% of all prescribed drugs in the United States even though they are only approximately 12% of the total population. What adverse outcomes have been reported from such usage?
5. As a healthcare professional working with a geriatric population, discuss the alterations in health status of concern with drug therapies. Name three or more interventions that could be used to prevent complications and improve drug therapy in this population.

REFERENCES

American Hospital Formulary Service: *AHFS drug information '98.* Bethesda, Md, 1998, American Society of Hospital Pharmacists.

Avorn J, Gurwitz JH: Drug use in the nursing home, *Ann Intern Med* 123(3):195, 1995.

Baldwin JN, Cook MD: Issues: psychoactive substance use disorders. In Young LY, Koda-Kimble MA, editors: *Applied therapeutics: the clinical use of drugs,* ed 6, Vancouver, Wash, 1995, Applied Therapeutics, Inc.

Beers MH, Ouslander JG, Rollingher I et al. Explicit criteria for determining inappropriate medication use in nursing homes, *Arch Intern Med* 151:1825, 1991.

Erwin WG: Geriatrics. In DiPiro JT et al., editors: *Pharmacotherapy,* ed 2, Norwalk, Conn, 1993, Appleton & Lange.

Hall WC et al.: Cocaine abuse and its treatment, *Pharmacotherapy* 10(1):47, 1990.

Jennings JC: Guide to medication use in pregnant and breastfeeding women, *Pharm Pract News* 23(4):10, 1996.

Jinks MJ, Fuerst RH: Geriatric drug use and rehabilitation. In Young LY, Koda-Kimble MA, editors: *Applied therapeutics,* ed 6, Vancouver, Wash, 1995, Applied Therapeutics, Inc.

Levy M, Spino M: Neonatal withdrawal syndrome: associated drugs and pharmacologic management, *Pharmacotherapy* 13(3):202, 1993.

Lucas DS, Noyes MA, Stratton MA: Principles of geriatric pharmacotherapy, *Clin Consult* 14(5):1, 1995.

McCombs J: Therapeutic considerations during pregnancy and lactation. In DiPiro JT, Talbert RL et al., editors: *Pharmacotherapy,* ed 2, Norwalk, Conn, 1993, Appleton & Lange.

McCue JD et al.: *Geriatric drug handbook for long term care.* Baltimore, 1993, Williams & Wilkins.

Olin BR: *Facts and comparisons.* Philadelphia, 1998, Lippincott.

Pray WS: Infant formulas and nutrition, *US Pharmacist* 18(3):29, 1993.

Trends & Analysis: Long-term care of elderly patients: chronic disease comorbidity and other considerations, *Consult Pharm* 10(6):583, 1995.

United States Pharmacopeial Convention: *USP DI: drug information for the health care professional,* ed 18, Rockville, Md, 1998, the Convention.

Walson PD: Paediatric clinical pharmacology and therapeutics. In Speight TM, Holford NHG, editors: *Avery's drug treatment,* ed 4, Auckland, NZ, 1997, Adis International Limited.

Willcox SM, Himmelstein DU, Woolhandler S: Inappropriate drug prescribing for the community-dwelling elderly, *JAMA* 272 (4):292, 1994.

Williams CL, Stancel GM: Estrogens and progestins. In Hardman JG, Limbird LE. editors: *Goodman & Gilman's the pharmacological basis of therapeutics,* ed 9, New York, 1996, McGraw-Hill.

Wingard LB, Brody TR et al: *Human pharmacology, molecular-to-clinical,* St Louis, 1991, Mosby.

ADDITIONAL REFERENCES

Anderson KN et al, editors: *Mosby's medical, nursing, and allied health dictionary,* ed 5, St Louis, 1998, Mosby.

Keene EF: Another way to administer antiepileptic medications in infants and children, *MCN* 18(6):270, 1993.

Mosby: *Mosby's GenRx,* St Louis, 1998, Mosby.

Wong DL et al: *Whaley & Wong's essentials of pediatric nursing,* ed 6, St Louis, 1999, Mosby.

CHAPTER 6

Substance Misuse and Abuse

CHAPTER FOCUS

Substance and drug misuse and abuse is widespread, despite legislation, enforcement, and educational efforts to curb drug use. Healthcare professionals must be able to recognize the signs and symptoms of various drugs of abuse. They must also be informed about the proper interventions (pharmacologic and nonpharmacologic) used for treatment in clinical practice.

OBJECTIVES

After reading and studying this chapter, the student should be able to do the following:

1. *Define and discuss the key terms.*
2. *Describe the difference between drug misuse and drug abuse.*
3. *Discuss the scope and impact of substance and drug abuse in the United States.*
4. *Identify the pharmacologic basis of physical drug dependence and tolerance.*
5. *Explain the different formulations of cocaine and its usage and impact in society today.*
6. *Describe the pathophysiologic changes resulting from chronic drug abuse.*
7. *Identify the signs, symptoms, and treatment for amphetamine, opioid, and PCP overdose.*

KEY TERMS

abstinence or withdrawal syndrome, (p. 94)
Drug Abuse Warning Network (DAWN), (p. 89)
designer drugs, (p. 90)
drug abuse, (p. 88)
drug misuse, (p. 88)
euphoria, (p. 104)
flashback phenomena, (p. 107)
hallucinogen, (p. 107)
intrapsychic, (p. 89)
physical dependence, (p. 90)
pK_a, (p. 104)
psychologic dependence or addiction, (p. 88)
tolerance, (p. 90)

All drugs prescribed or self-administered have the potential to be misused or abused. The prescribing of drugs without adequate exploration of the patient's presenting complaint, for example, represents drug misuse by a prescriber. Prolonged and unsupervised administration of drugs for symptomatic relief is another example. In general, **drug misuse** refers to nonspecific or indiscriminate use of drugs, including alcohol. **Drug abuse** refers to self-medication or self-administration of a drug in chronically excessive quantities, resulting in physical and psychologic dependence, functional impairment, and deviation from approved social norms.

Psychologic dependence or addiction is a behavioral pattern characterized by drug craving, out-of-control drug usage, overwhelming concern with obtaining a drug supply, drug use causing personal and legal problems, denial, and continuing to use the drug despite personal and legal difficulties. Most importantly, the use of the drug does not improve the person's quality of life (Sees, Clark, 1993).

Drug abuse is neither a new nor a recent phenomenon. It has been known throughout history as one expression of an individual's search for relief of physical, psychologic, social, and economic problems. Contemporary drug abuse has attained prominence as an issue with moral, legal, religious, social, psychologic, and medical implications. Drug abuse is not a problem confined to any particular socioeconomic, cultural, or ethnic group.

Drug and alcohol abuse in the workplace has been estimated to cost businesses up to $100 billion per year in the United States (Malatestinic, Jorgenson, 1991). The impact on society of alcohol and drug abuse is tremendous. For example, alcohol played a role in the following societal problems:

- 40% of assaults reported and at least one third of all rape and child abuse cases are alcohol related.
- Nearly 50% of prisoners state they were under the influence of alcohol when they committed their crimes.
- One half of all U.S. traffic accidents and nearly 80% of accident fatalities that occur between 8 pm and 4 am involve alcohol-impaired drivers.
- In one rural state, alcohol was present in 35% of suicides, 63% of homicide victims, and 49% of unintentional injury fatalities (Baldwin, Cook, 1995).

Substance abuse is a major medical, social, economic, and interpersonal problem affecting individuals from all economic backgrounds and across the life span.

SUBSTANCE ABUSE

Professional Problems

In 1984, Bissell and Haberman studied alcoholism and the use of other drugs with alcohol in professionals, including doctors, nurses, dentists, attorneys, social workers, and college women. After following a group of approximately 400 professionals for 5 to 7 years, they found that alcoholism or alcohol abuse with other drugs was usually identified as a problem during the first 15 years of professional practice. The combination of alcohol and other drugs was quite prevalent, especially with physicians and nurses. This group reported the greatest addiction to hard narcotics. Their narcotic of choice was meperidine (Demerol) because it was readily available in their settings and also because it produced less pupillary constriction than the other opioids. Most physicians and nurses stated that they obtained their drugs through professional channels. Many started with a painful condition, such as back pain, or stress for which legitimate drugs were prescribed. One study of nearly 2000 chemically dependent healthcare professionals found that those who abused medications generally used more than four substances (Gallegos et al, 1988).

Although healthcare professionals most commonly abuse prescription drugs (opioids and benzodiazepines), alcohol, and tobacco, the choice of drug and route of administration may vary by profession. Nurses and physicians are more apt to abuse injectable drugs, pharmacists often use multiple oral drugs, dentists have a problem with nitrous oxide addiction, and anesthesiologists and nurse anesthetists commonly abuse fentanyl (Sublimaze) or similar products (Baldwin, Cook, 1995).

Career pressures and easy accessibility to drugs place healthcare professionals at greater risk for drug abuse. Unfortunately, impaired health professionals constitute a hazard to their patients' well-being and to themselves, so they cannot be ignored, overlooked, or left unreported. It is vital that health agencies be alert to suspected drug abusers on their staffs. Many agencies and most states have mandatory reporting of and active rehabilitation programs for impaired healthcare professionals.

Substance abuse (alcohol and drugs) is considered a "handicap," and such employees may be protected by state and federal employment discrimination laws. The Rehabilitation Act (29 USC, Section 706[7][B]) states that employers are required to employ these individuals if they can properly perform their job functions and are not a threat to safety or property (Malatestinic, Jorgenson, 1991). Many healthcare facilities and other businesses have established employee assistance programs to help impaired employees with rehabilitation.

Drug Testing

In an effort to identify persons with alcohol- and drug-related problems, many businesses, government agencies, and healthcare-related facilities are performing drug analysis or urine drug tests under specified conditions on their employees. Drug screens may also be part of a preemployment physical examination. Although a number of testing procedures are available, it is important to know the analytic techniques used and the purpose and limitations of any tests performed. Also, initial positive tests should be confirmed with more specific and accurate tests because false-positive and false-negative results may occur.

BOX 6-1 Time Versus Drug Detection in Urine

Drug	Detection in Urine*
alcohol	less than 1 day
amphetamines	up to 1 day
barbiturates	up to 1 day
benzodiazepines	up to 2 days
cocaine	up to 2 days
methadone	up to 3 days
marijuana	
single use	up to 6 days
chronic use	up to 29 days
opioids	
short acting	up to 1 day
phencyclidine	up to 6 days
phenobarbital	up to 6 days

*Chronic high doses may extend the time intervals.
From Baldwin, Cook, 1995.

BOX 6-2 Drug Abuse Characteristics

The four characteristics of drug abuse are:
1. Altered state of consciousness
2. Development of tolerance
3. Rapid onset of action of desired effects
4. Possibly abstinence syndrome if drug is discontinued abruptly after extended period of use

To ensure accuracy, a second test specific for the agent reported in the screening test is necessary. Healthcare providers interpreting the tests should be familiar with drugs known to cross-react or give a false-positive result with the test in use.

Urine testing for specific drugs may detect substances used days or even a week before the test (Box 6-1). Such tests only give evidence of use or prior exposure to a drug and are not indicative of the individual's pattern of drug abuse or degree of drug dependency.

It is beyond the scope of this chapter to explore all aspects of drug abuse in depth; instead, this chapter focuses on drug actions and the treatment of drug abuse.

Etiologic Factors

A characteristic common to most drugs that cause dependence is that they are initially taken because the individual believes that a desirable pharmacologic effect will result. The person who is dependent on a drug has found something that provides relief from personal problems, and the drug generally is used as a maladjustive coping mechanism. Since very few drugs or substances without central nervous system (CNS) effects are abused, one of the predominant factors contributing to drug abuse appears to be **intrapsychic**—a desire to alter one's state of mind.

This desire may arise from a number of factors, such as curiosity, boredom, peer pressure, alienation, hedonism (pleasure-seeking behavior), affluence, and the widely publicized attention to drug abuse in the mass media. All or any combination may lead to misuse of drugs and substances. Individual reasons for abusing drugs might include feelings of inadequacy or failure, personal conflicts, feeling of shame, and perhaps, a predisposition to depression, which may result in emotional and behavioral problems. The characteristics of drug abuse are listed in Box 6-2.

More specifically, some psychologic hypotheses have been proposed that persons use drugs as an escape mechanism. Individuals who have a predisposition for drug dependency may be described as having a strong psychologic dependence, a low threshold of frustration, fear, and feelings of failure and inadequacy. Other authorities dispute the "addiction-prone" personality theory, maintaining that everyone has the potential to become dependent on something. "In 1990 alcoholism and other chemical dependencies were described by the American Society of Addiction Medicine (ASAM) as primary, chronic, relapsing diseases with genetic, psychosocial, and environmental factors influencing their development and manifestations" as stated by Baldwin and Cook (1995, p. 81-1). Thus, treatment centers have evolved to address the biopsychosocial factors associated with substance abuse.

TYPES OF DRUGS AND SUBSTANCES ABUSED

Although all drugs have some abuse potential, the more frequently abused chemically active substances are the xanthines and caffeine, found in coffee, tea, chocolate, and colas (see Chapter 12). Although these substances rarely are perceived as drugs by the lay public, they produce mild stimulant and euphoric effects, and their use may lead to physical dependence. Nicotine and ethyl alcohol (ethanol) are the most frequently misused and abused drugs, with consequent physical and psychologic dependence. Other CNS drugs such as anticholinergics, steroids, amphetamines, pentazocine, and L-dopa are examples of agents that may induce altered states of perception, thought, and feelings and drug-induced psychoses as a result of prolonged and concentrated therapeutic use or abuse. Few drugs without CNS effects are misused or abused.

This chapter reviews the drugs most commonly reported to the **Drug Abuse Warning Network (DAWN)** as being involved in drug abuse-related emergency room episodes. DAWN is a federal agency that monitors data on medical and psychologic problems associated with drug use and changing patterns of drug abuse. Box 6-3 lists the top 15 drugs misused or abused in 1993. See Table 6-1 for selected drugs commonly abused and symptoms of abuse.

TABLE 6-1 Selected Drugs Commonly Abused and Symptoms of Abuse

Drug Category	*Street Names*	*Methods of Use*	*Symptoms of Use*	*Hazards of Use*
Marijuana/Hashish	Pot, grass, reefer, weed, Columbian, hash, hash oil, sinsemilla, joint	Most often smoked; can also be swallowed in solid form	Sweet, burnt odor Neglect of appearance Loss of interest, motivation Possible weight loss	Impaired memory, perception Interference with psychologic maturation Possible damage to lungs, heart, and reproduction and immune systems Psychologic dependence
Alcohol	Booze, hooch, juice, brew	Swallowed in liquid form	Impaired muscle coordination, judgment	Heart and liver damage Death from overdose Death from car accidents Addiction
Stimulants				
Amphetamines* Amphetamine Dextroamphetamine Methamphetamine	Speed, uppers, pep pills Bennies Dexies Moth, crystal Black beauties	Swallowed in pill or capsule form, or injected into veins	Excess activity Irritability; nervousness Mood swings Needle marks	Loss of appetite Hallucinations; paranoia Convulsions; coma Brain damage Death from overdose
Cocaine	Coke, snow, toot, white lady, crack, readyrock	Most often inhaled (snorted); also injected or swallowed in powder form, smoked	Restlessness, anxiety Intense, short-term high followed by dysphoria	Intense psychologic dependence Sleeplessness; anxiety Nasal passage damage Lung damage Death from overdose
Nicotine	Coffin nail, butt, smoke	Smoked in cigarettes, cigars and pipes, snuff, chewing tobacco	Smell of tobacco High carbon monoxide blood levels Stained teeth	Cancers of the lung, throat, mouth, and esophagus Heart disease; emphysema

Depressants				
Barbiturates Pentobarbital Secobarbital Amobarbital	Barbs, downers Yellow jackets Red devils Blue devils	Swallowed in pill form or injected into veins	Drowsiness Confusion Impaired judgment Slurred speech Needle marks	Infection after parenteral use Addiction with severe life-threatening withdrawal symptoms Loss of appetite Death from overdose
Opioids Dilaudid, Percodan Demerol, Methadone		Swallowed in pill or liquid form, injected	Constricted pupils Drowsiness Lethargy	Nausea Addiction with severe withdrawal symptoms Loss of appetite Death form overdose
Morphine Heroin	Dreamer, junk Smack, horse	Injected into veins, smoked	Needle marks	
Codeine	School boy	Swallowed in pill or liquid form		
Hallucinogens				
PCP (phencyclidine)	Angel dust, killer weed, supergrass, hog, PeaCe pill	Most often smoked; can also be inhaled (snorted); injected or swallowed in tablets	Slurred speech; blurred vision, uncoordination Confusion, agitation Aggression	Anxiety, depression Impaired memory, perception Death from accidents Death from overdose
LSD	Acid, cubes, purple haze	Injected or swallowed in tablets		
Mescaline	Mesc, cactus	Usually ingested in their natural form	Dilated pupils Delusions; hallucinations	Breaks from reality Emotional breakdown
Psilocybin	Magic mushrooms		Mood swings	Flashback
Inhalants Gasoline Airplane glue Pain thinner		Inhaled or sniffed, often with use of paper or plastic bag or rag	Poor motor coordination Impaired vision, memory and thought processes Abusive, violent behavior	High risk of sudden death Drastic weight loss Brain, liver, and bone marrow damage
Nitrites Amyl Butyl	Poppers, locker room, rush, snappers	Inhaled or sniffed from gauze or ampules	Slowed thought Headache	Anemia, death by anoxia

*Includes lookalike drugs resembling amphetamines that contain caffeine, phenylpropanolamine (PPA), and ephedrine.
From Blue Cross & Blue Shield Association, Chicago, Ill.

BOX 6-3 Leading Drugs Resulting in Emergency Department Visits in the United States*

Males	*Females*
1. alcohol in combination	1. alcohol in combination
2. cocaine	2. cocaine
3. heroin/morphine	3. acetaminophen
4. marijuana/hashish	4. heroin/morphine
5. acetaminophen (Tylenol)	5. aspirin
6. methamphetamine/speed	6. alprazolam (Xanax)
7. aspirin	7. ibuprofen (Motrin)
8. ibuprofen (Motrin)	8. marijuana/hashish
9. diazepam (Valium)	9. diazepam (Valium)
10. PCP/PCP combinations	10. lorazepam (Ativan)
11. benzodiazepine (unspecified)	11. clonazepam (Klonopin)
12. alprazolam (Xanax)	12. amitriptyline (Elavil)
13. clonazepam (Klonopin)	13. D-propoxyphene (Darvon products)
14. amitriptyline (Elavil)	14. acetaminophen with codeine
15. amphetamine	15. diphenhydramine (Benadryl)

*Trade names are in parentheses; many of these products are also available under other trade or generic names. Statistics are based on drug episodes caused by an illegal drug or nonmedical use of a legal drug resulting in emergency department visits.
From 1993 Emergency Department Data (DAWN, 1996).

Drug abuse may take several forms:

1. Experimental abuse occurs when individuals use drugs in an exploratory way and after which they accept or reject continuing use of the drugs.
2. Social-recreational drug abuse may occur only in social contexts; drugs that are frequently abused in social situations are alcohol, marijuana, cocaine, nicotine, and caffeine.
3. Episodic drug abuse refers to the periodic abuse of a drug.
4. Compulsive drug abuse is characterized by irrational, irresistible, or compelling abuse of a drug.
5. Ritualistic drug abuse may be related to religious practices. Polydrug or multiple drug abuse is common. Marijuana, alcohol, and other depressants frequently are used together and in conjunction with CNS stimulants. Heroin may be used with cocaine, and pentazocine (Talwin) with tripelennamine (PBZ), alcohol, or other depressants.

In the 1980s cocaine (especially crack cocaine) became popular, and its abuse was seen fairly often but initially was somewhat curtailed by its high cost. In the 1990s, cocaine usage increased as reported in emergency department statistics; its use was reported in 37% of emergency room episodes that involved men and in 18% of drug episodes involving women.

The 1980s also documented the development of synthetic **"designer drugs"** produced by illegal laboratories or chemists. The molecular structure of a controlled substance is modified to produce a new variant that mimics the effects of the original drug. The types of drugs most commonly modified and sold are analogs of meperidine (Demerol), fentanyl (Sublimaze), and 3,4-methylenedioxymethamphetamine (MDMA) from the illicit psychedelic agent methylenedioxyphenylethylamine (MDA). When designer drugs are identified, the Drug Enforcement Agency (DEA) enacts regulations to ban them. Until it is banned, such a substance is legal to make, sell, or use. Once outlawed, though, the underground chemists often make a new, legal variation of the product, and it will be sold until a ban against it is established. Thus designer drugs are constantly changing and should be considered potentially dangerous substances. Contaminants have been identified in these products, and overdoses and deaths have been reported with their use.

PHARMACOLOGIC BASIS OF DEPENDENCE AND TOLERANCE

Psychologic and physical dependence on a drug can exist independently or simultaneously. In contrast to psychologic dependence (defined above), **physical dependence** is an adaptive state, occurring after prolonged use of a drug, in which discontinuation of the drug causes physical symptoms that are relieved by readministering the same drug or a pharmacologically related drug. Both types of dependence can potentially lead to compulsive patterns of drug use in which the user's lifestyle is focused on procurement and administration of the drug. Several hypotheses attempt to explain the pharmacologic basis of the physiologic adaptation that occurs in tolerance and physical drug dependence.

Tolerance is the tendency to increase drug doses to maintain the same effect that was formerly produced by a lower dose. Tolerance may exist with either psychologic or physical dependence and may be viewed in two ways.

Receptor site (tissue) tolerance is a form of adaptation in which the effect produced depends both on the concentration of the drug and on the duration of the exposure. In this type of tolerance the clinical effect of the drug is reduced as the duration of exposure continues.

The second type of tolerance is metabolic (pharmacologic) tolerance, which refers to an aspect of drug disposition. Prolonged exposure to a drug can change the body's metabolic response to the drug, increasing drug clearance with repeated ingestion. For example, with prolonged exposure to barbiturates, the steady-state blood concentrations will fall progressively with continued administration of the same dose. This may be attributed to barbiturates' inducing effect on hepatic microsomal enzymes, which increases barbiturate metabolism.

Pathophysiologic Changes

Physical and psychologic dependence on drugs is frequently associated with debilitated physical states caused by the user's extensive abuse of the drug, which often results in malnutrition, dehydration, and hypovitaminosis. Respiratory complications such as pneumonia, pulmonary emboli, and abscesses frequently are associated with neglect, debilitation, and the respiratory depression produced by CNS depressants. The intravenous administration of illicit drugs often leads to a high incidence of sepsis, hepatitis, infective endocarditis, and acquired immunodeficiency syndrome (AIDS) as a result of the use of contaminated equipment. In addition, cellulitis, sclerosis of the veins, phlebitis, and skin abscesses may occur. Death from accidental overdose is common.

Overdosage is a particularly significant potential danger because illegal drugs are notoriously unreliable in regard to the potency of their active ingredient. The drugs are frequently adulterated (mixed) with various substances such as active (amphetamines, benzodiazepines, hallucinogens, etc.) and inactive substances (lactose, sugars) by the time they reach the user. If an individual who has been using such drugs unknowingly receives pure or stronger drugs, the risk of toxicity and death exists. Overdosage also may occur when an individual who has been withdrawn from drugs for some time (thereby having lost accumulated tolerance) injects the previous usual dose, which now is in excess of the tolerance level.

As a consequence of all these factors, the life expectancy of persons who are psychologically dependent on drugs is generally lower than the life expectancy of nondependent individuals. Table 6-2 presents common drug groups that are abused, along with signs and symptoms of acute intoxication.

Cultural Aspects of Drug Abuse

Different societies use and accept certain drugs as legal, while they may restrict or ban the use of other drugs. In the United States and some parts of Western Europe, the most commonly used substances include alcohol, caffeine, and nicotine. In Japan amphetamines are the major abuse drug probably because of the desired work ethic that requires increases in personal productivity and achievement. In the Middle East cannabis is considered a legal drug, but alcohol is usually a forbidden substance. In America some Native American tribes use peyote, a hallucinogen (a drug that causes auditory or visual hallucinations), for religious purposes, but such hallucinogens usually have no accepted therapeutic usage in the general population in the United States. In high-altitude regions such as the South American Andes and Peru, coca leaves (source of cocaine) are brewed as a tea or chewed to decrease hunger sensations, increase work performance, and increase a feeling of well-being. Therefore drug substances are used and accepted or rejected based on the individual group or society. In areas where particular drugs are illegal and are in short supply, the non-law-abiding persons in society are motivated to obtain and sell the banned substances. The selling of illicit drugs is usually a very profitable venture.

TYPES OF DRUGS MOST COMMONLY ABUSED

OPIOIDS (HEROIN, MORPHINE, AND OTHER AGONIST OPIOIDS)

One of the most abused drug categories is the opioids, often listed in the top five for drug-related emergency room episodes. The pharmacologic types of drugs from natural sources (opiate) include the opium alkaloids (heroin, morphine), the semisynthetic group (hydromorphone [Dilaudid], oxymorphone [Numorphan]), and the synthetic group (meperidine [Demerol], levorphanol [Levo-Dromoran], methadone [Dolophine]). Heroin, D-propoxyphene (Darvon), oxycodone combinations (Percodan, Percocet), and morphine are the most often abused. The term "opioid" is preferred because it refers to both natural and synthetic products that have morphine-like effects.

Mode of Administration

The opium derivatives generally can be administered percutaneously (absorbed through the mucous membranes) by sniffing (snorting), by subcutaneous injection (skin popping), or by direct IV injection (mainlining). The rate of absorption is correspondingly increased, with mainlining producing almost immediate drug effects.

Mechanism of Action and Effects

Opium derivatives are CNS depressants that probably act on the sensory cortex or higher centers and thalami. Because they can relieve pain, change or elevate mood, relieve tension, fear, and anxiety, and produce feelings of peace, euphoria, and tranquility, they are particularly likely to lead to physical and psychologic dependence. Rapid intravenous injection of these drugs produces warm, flushing sensations described as being similar to sexual orgasm followed by a soothing state that seems to be best characterized as a state of complete drive satiation. The individual "high" on opioids feels no need to satisfy drives for basic biologic needs and is often described as being "on the nod"—drowsy, content, and euphoric. The drugs do not produce hallucinogenic or psychotomimetic effects.

Acute Overdosage

Acute overdosage of opioid substances may result in severe pulmonary edema and respiratory depression. These outcomes are dose dependent and are related to the degree of individual tolerance. What constitutes a lethal dose depends on the individual's tolerance for the drug. Symptoms occur rapidly in most patients. See Table 6-2 for signs and symptoms of acute drug intoxication.

Opioid toxicity is manifested in various ways, such as slow, shallow breathing; cold, clammy skin; miosis (pinpoint pupils, common with most opioids; however, mydriasis may occur in meperidine overdose); severe hypoxia (AHFS, 1998); mixed overdose conditions; or severe acidosis. Bra-

TABLE 6-2 Signs and Symptoms of Acute Drug Intoxication

Drug(s) Abused	Signs and Symptoms
cannabis drugs	Tachycardia and postural hypotension, conjunctival vascular congestion, distortions of perception, dryness of mouth and throat, possible panic
cocaine	Increased stimulation, euphoria, increased blood pressure and heart rate, anorexia, insomnia, agitation; in overdose, increased body temperature, hallucinations, seizures, death
opiates	Depressed blood pressure and respiration; fixed, pinpoint pupils; depressed sensorium; coma; pulmonary edema
barbiturates and other general CNS depressants	Depressed blood pressure and respirations; ataxia, slurred speech, confusion, depressed tendon reflexes, coma, shock
amphetamines	Elevated blood pressure, tachycardia, other cardiac dysrhythmias, hyperactive tendon reflexes, pupils dilated and reactive to light, hyperpyrexia, perspiration, shallow respirations, circulatory collapse, clear or confused sensorium, possible hallucinations, paranoid feelings
hallucinogenic agents	Elevated blood pressure, hyperactive tendon reflexes, piloerection, perspiration, pupils dilated and reactive to light, anxiety, distortion of body image and perception, delusions, hallucinations

dycardia, hypotension, muscle spasm, lethargy, respiratory depression, and urinary retention may also occur, although meperidine's toxic effects may be more excitatory, causing significant tachycardia (Sinatra, Savarese, 1992). The presence of thrombophlebitis, scarred veins, and puckered scars from subcutaneous injections may help identify the patient with opioid toxicity.

Opioids tend to delay motility and gastric emptying time, so that the revival of the patient may increase peristalsis and thus further increase absorption of the drug, producing a coma cycle. Chronic abuse may result in abscesses, cellulitis, endocarditis, glomerulonephritis, encephalopathy, tetanus, and thrombophlebitis. These are caused by a spectrum of factors ranging from injection technique to adulterants in the substance of abuse.

The treatment of choice for acute overdosage is administration of an antagonist (e.g., naloxone) and respiratory support. The box on p. 95 describes management of an opioid overdose.

Physical Dependence and Acute Abstinence Syndrome

In a patient who is physically dependent on opioids, an abrupt and complete reversal of narcotic effects with naloxone may precipitate an acute **abstinence or withdrawal syndrome.** These symptoms are usually experienced by a chemically dependent person who is suddenly deprived of his or her intake of the substance of abuse. Although opioid abstinence syndrome may be reversed by administration of an opioid, to do so in a drug-dependent patient is prohibited by law unless the individual is an inpatient who was admitted for an emergency procedure or is being detoxified or maintained in an approved federal drug-treatment program. Methadone usually is considered the drug of choice in the treatment of this clinical condition.

Physical dependence on opioids is usually described in relation to heroin or morphine, but the other drug derivatives manifest similar symptoms. Physical dependence is evident in the withdrawal syndrome that develops if the drug is withheld and in the marked tolerance that develops with continued use of the drug.

Also, because persons dependent on heroin or morphine so frequently feel satiated, physical, emotional, and social deterioration often occurs. The individual may not feel hungry and thus may become grossly malnourished and weak. Preoccupation with obtaining the drug is the primary focus in life; therefore participation in the usual social and vocational aspects of life are reduced or eliminated. As the drug craving increases, tolerance develops, and eventually the individual needs more and more drug to maintain the original drug effect. Now the person may be more focused on avoidance of withdrawal symptoms and less focused on the achievement of euphoria.

Withdrawal Symptoms

The initial withdrawal symptoms are related to the half-life of the opioid being used. Symptoms of withdrawal from heroin are autonomic in origin and appear within 8 hours after the last dose in physically dependent individuals. These symptoms are less life-threatening than with other substances of abuse and manifest as restlessness, chills and hot flashes, restless sleep, piloerection on the skin (which gives rise to the term "cold turkey"), rhinorrhea, drowsiness, lacrimation, and mydriasis during the first 24 hours. As withdrawal progresses, these symptoms are more severe and additional symptoms may include sneezing, yawning, generalized anxiety, abdominal cramps, lower back pain, lower extremity cramps, vomiting and diarrhea, anorexia, diaphoresis, muscular twitching, insomnia, elevated pulse rate, blood pressure, and temperature, and a craving for the drug. Depending on the drug used, abstinence syndrome develops within 2 to 48 hours and peaks at 72 hours.

MANAGEMENT OF DRUG OVERDOSE

Opioids

GENERAL APPROACH

Provide symptomatic and basic supportive care of airway, breathing, and circulation (the "ABCs"). Maintain cardiac output, blood pressure, urinary output, and peripheral perfusion.

If oral opioids were consumed and client is not lethargic or unresponsive, empty stomach by emesis or gastric lavage.

SPECIFIC APPROACH

If apnea is present, maintain a patient airway, using assisted or controlled respiration and oxygen as necessary.

When the triad of miotic pupils, coma or stupor, and bradypnea (respirations slowed to a rate of four to six per minute) appears, the administration of naloxone (Narcan) is indicated and will help to differentiate narcotic poisoning from other conditions.

Naloxone, a pure narcotic antagonist, reverses opioid toxicity. The usual adult dose is 0.4 to 2 mg given intravenously, which may be repeated at 2- to 3-minute intervals if necessary. Larger doses may be required to treat acute overdoses of butorphanol (Stadol), nalbuphine (Nubain), propoxyphene (Darvon and Darvocet products), and pentazocine (Talwin). Failure to respond to high doses of a narcotic antagonism may indicate a mixed substance overdose or involvement of a nonopiate substance.

Support blood pressure and maintain respiration after response to naloxone (Narcan). Blood and urine samples should be examined with a multiple drug screen to aid in diagnosis. A positive response to naloxone is characterized by dilation of the pupils (if previously miotic) and an increase in respiratory function, blood pressure, and cardiac rate.

Children with a known or suspected narcotic overdose may receive 0.01 mg/kg of naloxone (Narcan) as the first dose. (Dilute naloxone with sterile water for injection.) If the child does not respond to the first dose, additional intravenous doses at 2- to 3-minute intervals may be administered.

Naloxone reverses apnea and coma within minutes and should be titrated to the client's arousal with a respiratory rate in a range of 10 to 20 breaths per minute. Continued patient monitoring is necessary because additional naloxone (IV bolus or by IV infusion) is often necessary to prevent the reemergence of opioid toxicity.

Occasionally withdrawal symptoms are severe enough to result in cardiovascular collapse. If withdrawal is untreated, it may continue for up to 7 to 10 days, after which the physical dependence of the body on the presence of opioids is eventually lost. Psychological dependence continues for a longer period with some authorities claiming it continues forever.

Treatment of Opioid Dependence

Withdrawal Programs

Generally, opioid withdrawal is difficult, and repeated relapses may be expected. Abrupt and complete withdrawal (cold turkey) can be accomplished, but should generally be avoided because this procedure is a dangerous (especially in patients with a coexisting medical illness) and inhumane approach. Therapeutic withdrawal from an opioid may be somewhat more comfortably achieved by successively tapering the drug's dosage over a period of several days.

The choice of withdrawal program is partly influenced by the following factors: the patient's physical condition, the duration of drug dependence, the type and amount of drug being taken, motivations for drug abuse and withdrawal, and whether the individual is also dependent on other drugs, such as alcohol. In some instances, depending on these factors, opioid withdrawal may need to be accomplished in a hospital with close medical supervision.

In identifying criteria for evaluating opioid withdrawal, one should note that recovery from morphine-type dependence is not equated with cure. Regardless of repeated relapses to drug abuse, the individual should continue in therapeutic programs. Progress in withdrawal is often measured by progressively longer periods of abstinence from opioids without resort to the use of other drugs or alcohol and by the patient's growing confidence in the ability to function effectively without drugs.

Therapeutic Community Programs

The ultimate goal of using any medication to treat dependency is to relieve the compulsive craving for the abuse drug. Rehabilitation, however, requires more than another drug. The individual also needs to receive and develop dignity, self-respect, compassion, and hope, along with positive reinforcement. To be an independent, self-sustaining, productive member in society, the abuser must be provided with medical, emotional, and social support. Unfortunately, these human resources have not been effectively addressed by many treatment programs, and failures have resulted.

Often persons withdrawing from drugs cannot easily make the transition necessary to be drug free; therefore groups of persons with a similar problem meet or live together in an attempt to support and guide one another. Therapeutic community programs such as Phoenix House and halfway houses have been established, which include group psychotherapy and support and self-help approaches. The ultimate goal for an individual is that he or she emerges from such a program with sufficient personal growth and appropriate support systems to be able to manage life satisfactorily without a return to drug abuse.

Methadone Detoxification and Withdrawal

A currently preferred method of withdrawal is substitution of methadone. Methadone is a synthetic opioid analgesic that, by virtue of cross-tolerance, permits effective substitution of methadone dependence for heroin dependence. Its effectiveness against heroin dependence results from its ability to forestall the euphoriant effects of heroin and the craving for the drug without producing heroin's deleterious physical and mental effects. When properly administered, methadone allows the individual to function adequately, without intellectual or emotional impairment.

For adults in detoxification, methadone is taken orally in 15 to 40 mg doses per day, titrated according to patient response, until withdrawal symptoms are controlled. Methadone therapy is initiated empirically based on the individual's symptoms. As a general guide, 1 mg of methadone is substituted for 20 mg of meperidine, 4 mg of morphine, or 2 mg of heroin (Baldwin, Benson, 1995). For a review of recommended dosages and dosage adjustments, refer to current drug abuse references or references cited in this section.

Regular administration results in the development of tolerance to methadone and a cross-tolerance to heroin. The patient will not experience the opioid-induced "rush" and euphoria unless higher doses than a tolerance dose are administered. Because of this, professionals should be aware that some patients might exaggerate their withdrawal symptoms to obtain more methadone. When the abuser is being treated with methadone, supportive psychologic or psychiatric counseling may help to relieve some of the problems that led to drug dependence. During this phase the methadone may be gradually withdrawn, usually at a rate of 20% reduction or 5 mg in daily dosage. However, methadone maintenance programs are controversial and are not always successful. Previous opioid abusers who are unable to negotiate life in a drug-free state may revert to their former dependence or alternative substance abuse or may return to the methadone therapy detoxification.

Methadone Maintenance

In the United States, maintenance methadone treatment programs require both Food and Drug Administration (FDA) and state licensing and approval. The ultimate goal of these programs is complete withdrawal from drug dependency for the participant, although some patients continue methadone therapy for an extended time. Methadone programs can include psychologic, vocational, and rehabilitation services in addition to medical support. Approved methadone programs are required to comply with all the requirements in the Federal Methadone Regulations.

Admittance to a methadone maintenance program usually requires evidence of current dependence on morphine-type drugs and at least a 1-year history of opioid dependence. Nurses should be aware that addicts hospitalized with medical conditions other than addiction may require pharmacologic support with methadone or opioids during their stay. Be aware also that a cross-tolerance to opioids is common, and thus these patients usually require higher analgesic doses to control pain. Usually verification of enrollment in an approved methadone maintenance program is required to continue methadone therapy during the hospital stay. The hospital pharmacist should be consulted on the regulations and for assistance in such matters.

The healthcare professional should also be aware that treatment centers vary in their methods and drugs used for opioid withdrawal. Some treatment centers report having accomplished withdrawal from methadone through the use of clonidine, whereas others maintain that methadone is the drug of choice.

Methadone dependence does occur, but withdrawal symptoms are less severe although they last for a longer time period. Methadone withdrawal programs generally include supplemental rehabilitation techniques such as vocational and social rehabilitation. After individuals have functioned free from heroin for a sufficient period, secured steady employment, and readjusted their lifestyle, theoretically they can be withdrawn from methadone maintenance.

Additional Agonist Analgesics

A second drug used in approved opioid treatment centers is levomethadyl (Orlaam). Similar to methadone but with a longer duration of action, it is given three times a week, usually Monday, Wednesday, and Friday (or Tuesday, Thursday, and Saturday). This product can only be dispensed through approved opioid addiction treatment programs, and it should never be given daily. Federal regulations do not allow take-home dosages of levomethadyl (Orlaam), so patients who are ill or require hospitalization usually are given methadone on a temporary basis (Baldwin, Benson, 1995; USP DI, 1998).

Heroin Maintenance

Diacetylmorphine (heroin), a Schedule I drug (see Chapter 2), is a substance with no accepted medical use in the United States. It was banned because of its high potential for abuse and the increasing number of heroin addicts. Today it is still one of the top drugs abused illegally in the United States and often is used in combination with cocaine.

While most countries have banned heroin use, it is a legal drug in Belgium, Canada, and England, although it is rarely used in Belgium and Canada. Physicians are permitted to prescribe heroin and other opioids for persons who have a history of intractable dependence, thereby maintaining them and preventing withdrawal symptoms. Prescriptions are issued through designated hospitals or clinics.

The approval of heroin as an analgesic for intractable pain has been proposed and denied numerous times in the United States. Pharmacologically, heroin is a prodrug—when it is administered it is converted in the liver to morphine—and thus opponents of heroin legislation state that legalized heroin is unnecessary because morphine and other opioids are available in the United States (Lipman, 1993).

Clonidine Treatment

Clonidine (Catapres), a sympatholytic antihypertensive, stimulates $alpha_2$ receptors in the brain, which decreases sympathetic outflow from the CNS. This effect produces a decrease in peripheral resistance, heart rate, and blood pressure. It is also under investigation for relieving the symptoms of acute drug withdrawal (e.g., opioids, nicotine, alcohol) and aid in the detoxification process. Withdrawal symptoms may be caused by the hyperactivity of the locus ceruleus, a major noradrenergic nucleus of the brain. When clonidine transdermal patches are used, the nurse should be aware that it takes 2 to 3 days to reach a peak effect, which is often too late to treat the worst effects seen with opioid withdrawal. The tablet dosage form offers a quicker and a more easily titratable method of preventing or reducing unwanted effects.

A clonidine dosage of 5 μg/kg/day, increasing to 17 μg/kg/day in divided doses, has been used to prevent withdrawal syndrome. The dose is individualized according to the patient's tolerance and quantity and type of opioid agonist used. The daily dosage is administered in equally divided doses over a 24-hour period for approximately 10 days. Then the dosage is reduced by 50% on days 11, 12, and 13 and discontinued on day 14 (USP DI, 1998).

The clinical usefulness of clonidine is limited by the drug's sedative and hypotensive effects. Close supervision of the patient is necessary to monitor side effects, adverse effects, and any manipulation of the dose by the patient.

OTHER ANALGESICS

pentazocine [pen taz′ oh seen] (Talwin)

Pentazocine (Talwin) 60 mg IM is considered approximately equivalent as an analgesic to 10 mg IM of morphine. Sharp increases in the incidence of pentazocine drug abuse led the Drug Enforcement Administration to place this drug in Class IV under the Controlled Substances Act. Pentazocine's potential for producing psychologic and physical dependence is significant even in low doses, and infants born to pentazocine-dependent women experience withdrawal immediately postpartum. Pentazocine can also cause psychotomimetic reactions such as visual hallucinations, feelings of depersonalization, and nightmares.

The CNS effects of pentazocine are similar to those of the opioids, including analgesia, sedation, and respiratory depression (reversed by naloxone [Narcan]). In high doses pentazocine causes increases in blood pressure and heart rate. Lung problems have been reported when tablets are crushed, dissolved, and administered intravenously. This may be due to the talc binders and other particulate matter in tablet dosage forms. The use and reuse of cotton as a filter may result in "cotton fevers," a type of allergic reaction caused by tiny cotton fibers. This syndrome occurs within 30 minutes of the injection, and the person experiences increased heart rate, hypotension, increased sweating, shaking chills, and fever. Often these symptoms resolve in approximately 4 to 24 hours without treatment although the healthcare provider should be aware that sepsis, embolism, and other complications are also possible. Other potential effects include seizures and ulceration and severe sclerosis of the skin and subcutaneous tissue and muscles, caused by subcutaneous or intramuscular injections. The combination of pentazocine with other CNS depressants such as barbiturates and alcohol may be lethal.

Pentazocine (Talwin) and tripelennamine (PBZ) abuse first appeared in the late 1960s to early 1970s as a result of shortages or the high cost of heroin in large metropolitan areas. This combination is known as Ts and blues (T for Talwin and blue for the color of the generic tablet of tripelennamine). Ts and blues are oral tablets crushed together, dissolved, and injected either through a cotton filter intravenously, like heroin, or subcutaneously. Abscesses and necrotic tissue have resulted, which require hospitalization and grafting. Drug abusers report that tripelennamine is used to increase the onset of action and prolong the duration of euphoria produced by pentazocine.

To discourage abuse, oral pentazocine now contains naloxone (Talwin-Nx). The addition of naloxone has no effect on the analgesic properties of oral pentazocine, but if this combination is administered intravenously, the naloxone will nullify or cancel the rush effect of the injected Ts and blues combination.

The treatment of pentazocine dependence is gradual reduction of the drug itself in a controlled environment. The psychotomimetic effects should be observed closely in a controlled environment because they may persist for 5 to 7 days.

propoxyphene [pro pox′ i feen] (Darvon)

Use of propoxyphene products in excessive doses, either alone or in combination with other CNS depressants including alcohol, is a significant cause of drug-related deaths. Because an overdose of propoxyphene may result in death, intensive supportive and symptomatic therapy must be instituted immediately.

Propoxyphene should not be taken in doses higher than those recommended by the manufacturer and patients should be so warned. The judicious prescribing of propoxyphene is essential for safe use of this drug. With patients who are depressed or suicidal, consideration should be given to the use of nonnarcotic analgesics.

Because of its depressant effects, propoxyphene should be prescribed with caution for individuals whose medical condition requires the concomitant administration of sedatives, tranquilizers, muscle relaxants, antidepressants, or other CNS depressant drugs. Patients should be cautioned against the concomitant use of propoxyphene products and alcohol because of potentially serious CNS additive effects of these agents. Some deaths have occurred as a consequence of the accidental ingestion of excessive quantities of propoxyphene alone or in combination with other drugs. Propoxyphene-related deaths have occurred in individuals with previous histories of emotional disturbances or of misuse of tranquilizers, alcohol, and other CNS-depressant drugs.

The clinical effects of an acute propoxyphene overdose are similar to those of acute opioid toxicity: coma, respiratory arrest, pulmonary edema, circulatory collapse, and death. Grand mal seizures have also been reported. Propoxyphene is metabolized in the liver to norpropoxyphene, which may be responsible for some of its toxicity. Toxic propoxyphene serum levels are between 0.6 and 10 μg/ml; lethal levels reportedly are more than 10 μg/ml (AHFS, 1998).

Norpropoxyphene has a lesser CNS-depressant effect than propoxyphene, but it has a greater anesthetic effect on the myocardium, similar to that of amitriptyline and antidysrhythmic drugs such as lidocaine and quinidine. Electrocardiographic monitoring is essential in management of overdose. The manufacturer recommends that in all suspected overdose cases, a poison control center should be contacted for the most current treatment of the overdose.

This drug has also been abused by parenteral administration of the oral dosage form. Propoxyphene napsylate (Darvon-N, Darvocet-N) is considered a less toxic propoxyphene formulation because of its delayed absorption orally and its relative insolubility in water. Thus the napsylate dosage form has less abuse potential than propoxyphene hydrochloride.

Propoxyphene is pharmacologically related to the opioids, so naloxone, may reverse the signs of toxicity. Overdose may be accompanied by seizures requiring anticonvulsants, and emergence from a coma may require restraints before administration of naloxone because of the patient's disorientation, agitation, and confusion. Patients need psychologic and emotional support during this time. A quiet, calm environment with reduced sensory stimulation may reduce the incidence of disorientation and agitation. The healthcare professional should use a simple, direct approach and communicate with reality orientation and reassurance.

ALCOHOL

Although there are many different kinds of alcohol, the term "alcohol" usually refers to ethyl alcohol. Methyl, propyl, butyl, and amyl alcohols are examples of other alcohols that are very toxic when taken orally.

ethyl alcohol (ethanol)

Ethyl alcohol is the only alcohol used extensively in medicine and in alcoholic beverages. Many over the counter (OTC) "nighttime" cough and cold remedies may be abused due to their considerable sedative potential because they contain alcohol (up to 25%, or 50-proof) with antihistamines. Table 6-3 lists the ethyl alcohol content of various OTC preparations. Ethyl alcohol is a colorless liquid that mixes readily with water and because it lowers surface tension, it is a good solvent for a number of substances. Ethyl alcohol, also referred to as grain alcohol, is the product of the fermentation of a sugar by yeast.

Therapeutically, ethyl alcohol has been used as a cardiac disease preventative, as an appetite stimulant for patients with poor appetite during periods of convalescence and debility, and as a hypnotic for older persons who do not tolerate other hypnotics.

Mechanism of action

Ethyl alcohol may have either a local or a systemic action.

Local effect. Ethyl alcohol denatures proteins by precipitation and dehydration, which may be the basis for its germicidal, irritant, and astringent effects. It irritates denuded skin, mucous membranes, and subcutaneous tissue. Subcutaneous injection of alcohol may cause considerable pain and sloughing of the tissues. When it is injected into or near a nerve, alcohol may cause nerve degeneration and anesthesia.

Systemic effect. Contrary to popular belief, alcohol is not a stimulant but a CNS depressant. What sometimes appears to be stimulation results from the depression of the higher faculties of the brain and represents the loss of inhibitions acquired by socialization.

Alcohol is thought to interfere with the transmission of nerve impulses at synaptic connections, but how this is accomplished is not known. It causes progressive and continuous depression of the CNS, the sequence being cerebrum, cerebellum, spinal cord, and medulla. Its action is comparable to that of the general anesthetics. The excitement stage, however, is longer, and when the anesthetic stage is reached, definite toxic symptoms are present. The margin between the anesthetic stage and the fatal dose is a narrow one.

The action of alcohol varies with the individual's tolerance, the presence or absence of extraneous stimuli, the rate of ingestion, and gastric contents. Small or moderate quantities produce a feeling of well-being, talkativeness, greater vivacity, and increased confidence in one's mental and physical power. There is a general loss of inhibitions. The finer powers of discrimination, insight, concentration, judgment, and memory are gradually dulled and lost. Large quantities may cause excitement, impulsive speech and behavior, laughter, hilarity, and in some persons, pugnaciousness, while others may become melancholy or unduly sentimental. Table 6-4 lists the content of ethyl alcohol in various beverages.

The effects of large quantities of alcohol may become apparent when the individual attempts to operate machinery such as an automobile. Visual acuity (especially peripheral vision) is diminished, reaction time is slowed, and judgment and self-control are impaired, and individuals tend to be complacent and pleased with themselves. Many drivers will take chances when under the influence of alcohol that they would never take ordinarily. This leads to disaster, as accident statistics reveal.

The intoxicated individual usually becomes ataxic, mutters incoherently, has disturbance of the special senses, is often nauseated, may vomit, and eventually may lapse into stupor or coma. The respiratory neurons are usually not depressed except by large doses of alcohol.

Cardiovascular. Alcohol depresses the vasomotor neurons in the medulla and causes dilation of the peripheral blood vessels, especially those of the skin. This causes a feeling of warmth. Heat is also lost from the interior, which ac-

TABLE 6-3 Content of Ethyl Alcohol in OTC Products

Medicinals	*Alcohol Content (%)*	*Alcohol Proof*
Cough-Cold Preparations		
Ambenyl-D	9.5	19
Comtrex Maximum	10	20
Vicks 44	10	20
Vicks NyQuil	10	20
Benadryl	0	0
Benylin Expectorant	0	0
Naldecon DX and EX	0	0
Triaminic	0	0
Mouthwash Preparations		
Cepacol	14.5	29
Listerine	26.9	53.8

Modified from APA, 1997.

TABLE 6-4 Content of Ethyl Alcohol in Various Beverages

Beverages	*Alcohol Content (%)*	*Alcohol Proof*
Beer	4	8
Wine (red/white)	12	24
Brandy	30-45	60-90
Whiskey, vodka	45	90
Martini, Manhattan	30	60
Daiquiri, Alexander	15	30

From Hinds, 1985.

counts for the fact that an intoxicated person may freeze to death more quickly than a nonintoxicated person. Alcohol also depresses the heat-regulating mechanism.

Small doses (10 to 25 ml) produce an insignificant increase in the pulse rate, caused mainly by the excitement and the reflex effect on the gastrointestinal tract. Larger doses (more than 25 ml) produce the same effect but may be followed by lowered blood pressure caused by the effect on the vasoconstrictor neurons. Chronic alcoholism may result in cardiomyopathy, hypertension, and a variety of cardiac dysrhythmias, especially atrial fibrillation and flutter. Epidemiology studies, though, report light to moderate consumption of alcohol (up to two drinks per day) reduces the risk for myocardial infarction and cardiac death (Jungnickel, Hunnicutt, 1995).

Gastrointestinal. The effect of alcohol on the function of the digestive organs depends on the presence or absence of gastrointestinal disease, the degree of alcohol tolerance, the concentration of the alcohol, and the type and amount of food present. Small doses of alcohol will stimulate the secretion of gastric juice rich in acid. Salivary secretion is also reflexively stimulated. Large and concentrated doses of alcohol tend to inhibit secretion and enzyme activity in the stomach, although the effect in the intestine seems to be negligible. Chronic alcohol ingestion causes pancreatitis and hepatic cellular damage, which results in fibrosis and scarring, cirrhosis, and hepatitis. In addition, when large quantities of alcohol are taken over a prolonged period, gastritis, nutritional deficiencies, and other untoward results have been observed.

Pharmacokinetics

Alcohol does not require digestion before absorption. A small amount is absorbed in the stomach while most is absorbed in the small intestine. Approximately 90% of the alcohol is metabolized in the liver. The liver enzyme, alcohol dehydrogenase, oxidizes alcohol (ethanol) to acetaldehyde; acetaldehyde oxidizes to acetic acid, which is buffered to an acetate that eventually oxidizes to carbon dioxide and water. Approximately 90% to 98% of ethanol is metabolized (oxidized) in the liver with the remainder primarily excreted by way of the lungs and kidneys. As plasma ethanol levels increase, though, the hepatic alcohol dehydrogenase pathway becomes saturated, resulting in an increase in the unmetabolized alcohol ratio. Chronic alcohol use may result in hyperlipidemia, fatty deposits in the liver, and ultimately alcoholic cirrhosis.

Alcohol produces an increased flow of urine because of the increase in fluid intake. Alcohol also acts as a diuretic through CNS depression and inhibition of antidiuretic hormone (ADH) release. If the individual has preexisting renal disease, the kidney may be further damaged. Large and concentrated doses of alcohol are thought to injure the renal epithelium.

After absorption, alcohol is distributed in every tissue of the body in approximately the same ratio as its water content. Therefore a rough estimate of the quantity consumed may be obtained from an analysis of the blood (Table 6-5).

Healthcare professionals should be aware of the approximate total amount of alcohol in different beverages: 12 oz of beer = 4 oz of wine = 1 oz of whiskey. Therefore, alcohol abuse can occur with any of the beverages, depending on the quantity consumed.

Drug interactions

The most commonly used and abused drug in North America is alcohol. It interacts with many prescription and OTC drugs, resulting in serious adverse effects that lead to emergency room admission or even death. The magnitude of this potential interaction is enormous. Most people, professionals and lay persons alike, may not be fully cognizant of some of the most significant alcohol-drug interactions (Table 6-6).

Alcohol Abuse

Signs of alcohol abuse typically include the following:

- Changes in drinking patterns, such as early morning drinking, drinking alone, hiding partial or full liquor bottles, or having the need for a drink before performing

TABLE 6-5 Concentration of Alcohol in Blood and Related Clinical Observations

Stage	Blood Alcohol mg/dl	Clinical Observations
Subclinical	30-100	Slight evidence of performance deterioration possible, such as motor function, coordination, personality, or mood and mental acuity
Emotional instability	100-200	Decreased inhibitions; emotional instability; slight muscular incoordination; slowing of responses to stimuli
Confusion	200-300	Disturbance of sensation; decreased pain sense; staggering gait; slurred speech
Stupor	300-400	Marked decrease in response to stimuli; muscular incoordination approaching paralysis
Coma, death	400	Complete unconsciousness; depressed reflexes; subnormal temperature; anesthesia; impairment of circulation; possible death

TABLE 6-6 Selected Significant Alcohol-Drug Interactions

Substances Interacting with Alcohol	Mechanism	Possible Effect(s)
I. antihistamines antidepressants opioid analgesics sedative-hypnotics antianxiety agents antipsychotic drugs	Additive	Enhanced CNS depressant effects
II. disulfiram (Antabuse) cefamandole and some other second and third generation cephalosporins chlorpropamide (Diabinese) other oral antidiabetic agents to varying degrees griseofulvin (Fulvicin) metronidazole (Flagyl) procarbazine (Matulane)	Inhibition of aldehyde dehydrogenase in metabolism of alcohol, leading to acetaldehyde accumulation (disulfiram or a "disulfiram-type reaction")	Most severe effects seen with disulfiram and alcohol: flushing, stomach pain, head throbbing, increased heart rate, hypotension, sweating, nausea, and vomiting With antidiabetic agents: mild to severe hypoglycemia
III. phenytoin (Dilantin)	Increase or decrease in liver metabolism	In chronic alcohol abuse: possible decrease in anticonvulsant effect caused by increased metabolism In acute alcohol use: a possible decrease in metabolism, causing increased serum level of phenytoin and toxicity
IV. salicylates	Additive	Increased gastrointestinal irritability and bleeding
V. nitrates nitroglycerin	Additive	Vasodilation leading to hypotension, syncope

a potentially stressful event (e.g., job interview, keeping an appointment); personality changes
- Family discord
- Job absenteeism
- Neglect of personal appearance
- Poor eating habits
- Memory lapses
- Blackouts

Sudden abstinence from alcohol in a heavy drinker can be very dangerous because alcoholic withdrawal syndrome may occur (Box 6-4).

The major objectives for treatment of ethyl alcohol withdrawal include a quiet environment, monitoring of health status, symptom relief, prevention or treatment of complications, and the development of long-term rehabilitation plans. Supportive care includes fluid and electrolyte replacement, adequate nutrition, thiamine to prevent development of Wernicke encephalopathy, and anticonvulsant medications if necessary. A sedative drug such as a long-acting benzodiazepine may be necessary for severe withdrawal reactions; its dosage can then be tapered and discontinued. In selected persons, beta-adrenergic blocking agents or clonidine may be used to reduce the sympathetic manifestations of alcohol withdrawal, such as increased anxiety, tachycardia, hypertension, and tremors.

Toxic Alcohols

Isopropyl alcohol and methyl or wood alcohol are toxic when taken internally. When some alcoholic individuals are unable to purchase ethanol (ethyl alcohol), they substitute agents such as isopropyl (rubbing) alcohol, methyl alcohol (antifreeze), or any available substance that might prevent alcohol withdrawal. This is a dangerous practice that can cause severe poisoning and death.

isopropyl alcohol

A clear, colorless liquid with a characteristic odor, isopropyl alcohol compares favorably with ethyl alcohol in its antiseptic action. It has been recommended for skin disinfection and for rubbing compounds and lotions used on the skin. Its bactericidal effects are said to increase as its concentration approaches 100%.

methyl alcohol (wood alcohol, methanol)

Methyl alcohol, if taken orally, is a central nervous system toxin. However, intoxication does not occur as readily as with ethyl alcohol unless large amounts are consumed. Methyl alcohol is oxidized in the tissues to formic acid, which is poorly metabolized, the basis for the development of a severe acidosis.

Symptoms of poisoning include nausea and vomiting, abdominal pain, headache, dyspnea, blurred vision, and cold, clammy skin. Symptoms may progress to delirium, convulsions, coma, and death. In nonfatal cases the individual may become blind or suffer from impaired vision. Treatment is focused on the relief of acidosis since this seems to be related to the severity of the visual symptoms. Large amounts of sodium bicarbonate may be needed to treat acidosis successfully. One dose of 60 ml of methyl alcohol has been known to cause permanent blindness. Fluids containing methyl alcohol usually bear a "Poison" label.

Drugs Used in Treatment of Chronic Alcoholism

disulfiram [dye sul' fi ram] (Antabuse)

Disulfiram is used to sensitize an individual to alcohol by inducing an unpleasant alcohol-disulfiram reaction. This disulfiram reaction begins with flushing of the face and develops into intense vasodilation of the face, neck, and upper part of the body. Hyperventilation and increased pulse rate may occur. Nausea occurs in 30 to 60 minutes along with facial pallor, hypotension, and copious vomiting. There is usually an intense feeling of discomfort, pulsating headache, palpitations, dyspnea, syncope, and a constrictive feeling in the neck. The reaction lasts from 30 minutes to several hours, as long as alcohol is being metabolized; it is then followed by drowsiness and sleep. Other drugs have been reported to cause a disulfiram-type reaction when taken with alcohol (Table 6-6 lists these drugs).

Mechanism of action

Disulfiram inhibits the enzyme aldehyde dehydrogenase, which converts acetaldehyde to acetate. This permits acetaldehyde to accumulate and cause the unpleasant toxic effects. Disulfiram has few effects unless the person ingests alcohol.

Pharmacokinetics

Metabolism is hepatic and the initial effect may be delayed from 3 to 12 hours because of drug storage in adipose tissue. Studies indicate that up to 20% of a dose remains in the body for up to 6 days. Elimination occurs via the kidneys with smaller amounts excreted in feces and lungs. Because of slow and incomplete absorption and elimination, effects persist for up to 2 weeks after therapy is discontinued. Patients should be instructed not to ingest any alcohol-containing substance during this time.

Drug interactions

The following effects may occur when disulfiram is given with the drugs listed below:

Drug	Possible effect and management
Alcohol	Will result in a disulfiram-alcohol reaction if alcohol or alcohol containing products such as cough syrups, tonics, sauces, aftershave lotions, etc. are consumed during or within 2 weeks of disulfiram therapy. See "Side effects and adverse reactions" section.
alfentanil (Alfenta)	May prolong the action of alfentanil.
Anticoagulants	Increased anticoagulant effects; dosage adjustments may be necessary; monitor closely for bleeding.
Anticonvulsants, especially phenytoin (Dilantin), hydantoins	Increased serum levels of hydantoins; monitor serum levels before and during concurrent drug therapy because dosage adjustments may be necessary.
isoniazid (INH)	May increase incidence of CNS side effects such as ataxia, insomnia, dizziness, and irritability. Monitor closely as disulfiram dosage may need to be reduced or stopped.
metronidazole (Flagyl)	Confusion and psychotic episodes reported with this combination. Metronidazole should not be administered concurrently or during the 2 weeks after disulfiram therapy.
paraldehyde	Inhibition of acetaldehyde dehydrogenase may occur, resulting in increased blood levels of paraldehyde and acetaldehyde. Do not administer concurrently.

Color type indicates an unsafe drug combination.

Side effects and adverse reactions

The disulfiram-alcohol reaction may range from facial flushing, severe throbbing headache, nausea, severe vomit-

BOX 6-4 Clinical Stages of Alcohol Withdrawal

Stage	Description	Time From Last Dose
Minimal	Mild expressed anxiety, fidgets, mentally clear, pulse and temperature normal	12 hr
Mild	Clear hyperactivity, appears anxious, sweaty, pulse rate up, mentally alert, restless	12-24 hr
Moderate	Momentary mental lapses, marked agitation, sweaty, rapid pulse, fearful, severely restless, fairly cooperative	24-48 hr
Severe	Hallucinations, mental lapses markedly interfering with communication, severe agitation, sweaty, tachycardia, unable to cooperate, may have convulsion	24-48 hr

*Remember that these symptoms may be delayed until the third or fourth day in trauma clients or those operated on in an emergency situation who have subsequently received analgesia.
From Iber, 1991.

ing, dyspnea, blurred vision, confusion, dizziness, tachycardia, diaphoresis, and weakness to the rarer, more severe adverse reactions of dysrhythmias, seizures, myocardial infarction, and death. Therefore patients should be advised to avoid drinking alcohol or using any alcohol-containing product while taking this medication and also for 2 weeks after this drug is discontinued.

The common side effects of disulfiram include drowsiness or sedation. Less frequently reported side effects are headache, impotency, rash, weakness, and a metallic or garlic-like taste in the mouth. An infrequent adverse effect reported is neurotoxicity, such as optic neuritis or peripheral neuropathy.

Warnings

Disulfiram should never be administered to an alcohol-intoxicated person nor should it be given without the patient's knowledge and approval. The intensity of the disulfiram-alcohol reaction is proportional to the amount of alcohol and disulfiram consumed although in some persons, it can be severe even with small amounts of alcohol. Use disulfiram with caution in patients with cerebral impairment, diabetes mellitus, epilepsy, hypothyroidism, liver or renal impairment, and severe pulmonary dysfunction.

Contraindications

Avoid use in patients with severe cardiac disease or psychoses and in those sensitive to disulfiram, rubber, and pesticides.

Dosage and administration

Initially, the patient is given up to 500 mg orally daily for 7 to 14 days; the maintenance dose is 250 mg orally daily.

CNS STIMULANTS

The primary CNS stimulants abused in the United States include cocaine and amphetamine products, especially methamphetamine.

cocaine

Cocaine, while classified as a controlled substance, is an alkaloid related to the belladonna alkaloids. Topically it has local anesthetic and vasoconstriction therapeutic effects; thus it has a limited use in a few selected surgical procedures, such as nasal surgery. Cocaine abuse has reached epidemic levels. In the United States it is one of the most frequently mentioned drugs resulting in emergency room visits, second only to alcohol in combination with other substances (DAWN, 1996).

It has been estimated that 3 million Americans are regular users of cocaine (Scott, Gabel, 1995). Cocaine is a very potent CNS stimulant that is highly addicting and is also a potentially lethal drug. As a social-recreational drug of abuse, it is popular for its euphoric effects. It also produces increased energy like the amphetamines and may lead to a similar psychotic state with strong elements of paranoia.

The purity of the illicitly produced drug varies greatly because this short-lived CNS stimulant is often diluted or cut with agents such as amphetamines, boric acid, quinine, mannitol, procaine, and lidocaine. The vasoconstricting effect of cocaine may be responsible for limiting its own absorption. Multiple drugs are often taken with or after cocaine, such as alcohol (84% of users), marijuana (98% of cocaine addicts), heroin, barbiturates, benzodiazepines, and phencyclidine (PCP) (Scott, Gabel, 1995). Cocaine is a very dangerous substance with high financial, psychologic, and physical control over the user.

Routes of administration

Cocaine may be taken by sniffing (snorting) the white, fluffy, crystalline powder (which resembles snow, hence its street name), by direct IV injection, or by smoking (transalveolar route) the converted base form, "freebase" or crack. In the United States, cocaine is usually found as the hydrochloride (HCl) salt or in the base form. Cocaine HCl is water soluble, and thus it can be snorted or injected intravenously. Freebase and crack cocaine (minus the HCl salt) are essentially the same free alkaloidal base; the difference between them is that different solvents are used in the manufacturing process (Scott, Gabel, 1995). Freebase is dangerous to make (ether and ammonia are involved) and dangerous to use. The freebase form is heat resistant, lending itself to smoking in any form including "coke pipes." Smoking freebase cocaine produces a more intense effect and is dangerous because of the possibility of an excessive dose being administered. The freebase solvents are flammable and may explode during the process, causing further harm to the user.

Freebase cocaine has largely been replaced by "crack" or "rock" cocaine. Crack cocaine is also a freebase, but it is made without any volatile chemicals. It became popular because of its availability in smaller amounts at a much lower cost than freebase cocaine and because its use does not require any elaborate paraphernalia. The cocaine market has thus become affordable to all economic groups. Freebase cocaine when dried looks like rocks and when smoked makes a cracking sound. Therefore the street names of freebase cocaine include "rock," "crack," "gravel," and "readyrock." Crack cocaine also produces a fast and very intense effect.

Cocaine HCl may be inhaled (snorted) from a small spoon, rolled dollar bills, a lengthened fingernail, or various other inhalation devices. Sniffing causes vasoconstriction, which limits the amount of cocaine absorbed from the nasal mucosa into systemic circulation; thus more intense effects are derived from freebase or crack cocaine.

Pharmacokinetics

Cocaine is rapidly metabolized in the liver, and the cocaine abuser may need to use the drug every half hour or less to maintain the high. Cocaine serum levels are not proportional to toxicity, and the elimination half-lives by oral, intranasal, and intravenous routes are similar (50, 80, and 60 minutes, respectively). Cocaine stimulation of the CNS initially affects the intellect (cognition) and behavior (affective domain).

At this time there is no absolute level known to be lethal. The rapidity of the increase in blood level may be as important in determining fatal reactions as the peak blood concentration. Factors other than blood concentration of cocaine must be examined. These factors include tolerance, reverse tolerance, previous history of cocaine abuse, individual susceptibility, the presence of other drugs, and the medical problems associated with cocaine abuse.

Initial symptoms of cocaine use are restlessness, mydriasis, hyperreflexia, vasoconstriction, tachycardia, hypertension, hallucinations, nausea, vomiting, and muscle spasms, which may be followed by respiratory failure, convulsions, coma, and circulatory collapse. In chronic abusers, a toxic cocaine psychosis (similar to paranoid schizophrenia) is often found, characterized by hallucinations and paranoid delusions. Skin eruptions (with itching and compulsive scratching) caused by self-inflicted skin irritation are also frequently observed. The energetic person may be prone to outbursts of violent behavior. Blood in the nose and a perforated nasal septum are frequently seen in those who chronically snort cocaine.

Medical complications associated with cocaine abuse may affect many body systems, including cardiovascular (hypertension, tachycardia, myocardial infarction, dysrhythmias, thrombosis, and sudden death), respiratory (pulmonary abscesses, lung infections, pulmonary edema and hemorrhage, and pneumonitis), renal (rhabdomyolysis [the release of skeletal muscle contents into the plasma], which results in generalized muscle aches and pains and, in one third of the reports, acute renal failure), and neurologic (seizures, stroke, and intracranial hemorrhage); psychiatric disorders (psychosis, suicide, delirium, and clinical depression) are also seen. Miscellaneous other conditions may also occur, including septicemia, hepatitis, and human immunodeficiency virus (HIV) infection. The medical complications are numerous and vary with the type cocaine used and the route of administration.

Cocaine is particularly dangerous in pregnant women. It has been associated with an increased risk of stillbirth and preterm labor and neonatal complications such as congenital malformations, cerebral infarction and hemorrhage, and sudden infant death syndrome. Other neonatal complications include acute withdrawal symptoms (increased irritability, tremors, abnormal reflexes, tachypnea, and poor eating and sleeping patterns) and neurobehavioral delays during the first year of life. Neonates may also be susceptible to cocaine-induced seizures and a variety of other complications (Young et al, 1992). Such effects have resulted in child-abuse convictions for mothers who used cocaine while pregnant (Schydlower, 1990).

See the box below for management of a cocaine overdose.

MANAGEMENT OF DRUG OVERDOSE

Cocaine

GENERAL APPROACH

Provide symptomatic and basic supportive care of airway, breathing, and circulation

Establish an intravenous line using an isotonic or hypotonic solution for administration of medications necessary to treat the adverse effects induced by cocaine.

Continuously monitor patient's vital signs and core body temperature.

Avoid or reduce sensory stimulation as it may provoke or worsen agitation and paranoid behavior.

SPECIFIC APPROACH

Treat medical complications as necessary, for example, for:

- metabolic acidosis, administer sodium bicarbonate
- hyperthermia, utilize external cooling measures such as sponging with cold water or use a cooling blanket.
- seizure, intravenously administer diazepam (Valium), lorazepam (Ativan), phenobarbital (Luminal), phenytoin (Dilantin), or thiopental (Pentothal) as necessary.
- cardiac arrhythmias, administer propranolol (Inderal), labetalol (Normodyne), phentolamine (Regitine), or lidocaine as necessary.
- hypertension, administer phentolamine (Regitine), labetalol (Normodyne), verapamil (Isoptin), or nitroprusside as indicated

Monitor and treat other side/adverse effects as necessary.

amphetamine products

Amphetamine abuse has been reported for more than 50 years and although it declined for a while, its use now has increased, as noted in Box 6-3. It was estimated that 3 million Americans used these drugs for nonmedical purposes in 1992 (Scott, Gabel, 1995). See Table 6-1 for street names and additional information.

Chemically, amphetamines are similar to the natural catecholamines, epinephrine, norepinephrine, and dopamine. They can activate catecholamine receptor sites to increase stimulation; therefore they have been classified as sympathomimetic agents. In addition, they also increase release of natural catecholamines and block their reuptake into the neurons, which results in the induction of an artificial "fight or flight" response (Scott, Gabel, 1995).

Oral amphetamine is absorbed from the gastrointestinal (GI) tract and concentrates in the brain, kidneys, and lungs. It is metabolized in the liver and excreted via the kidneys. Amphetamine is a basic drug with a **pK_a** (the point at which half the drug amount in the body is ionized and half nonionized) of 9.9; therefore a urine pH of 7 or more extends the half-life of amphetamine to approximately 20 hours. A pH of 5, however, reduces the half-life to 5 to 6 hours. Persons that abuse this drug are usually aware of the prolonged effect they can achieve by alkalizing their urine. Prescribers are also aware that acidifying the urine to a pH of 4.5 to 5.5 will enhance amphetamine excretion.

Effects

The amphetamines are usually abused because they produce mood elevation, reduction of fatigue, and a sense of increased alertness. They do not create extra physical or mental energy; instead they promote expenditure of present resources, often to the point of hazardous fatigue. Intravenous amphetamine injection results in marked **euphoria,** an orgasmic feeling knows as a "rush" that is accompanied by a sense of great physical strength and clear thinking. The person feels little or no need for rest, sleep, or food and may continually engage in vigorous activity that may be perceived as exhilarating and creative. To an observer, however, they are inefficient and performing repetitious type behaviors, which is common during an amphetamine high.

Termination of the drug's effect may result from exhaustion, fright, or inability to obtain more drug. Drug withdrawal is followed by long periods of sleep, and on awakening the individual often feels hungry, extremely lethargic, and profoundly depressed, a phenomenon known as "crashing." Suicide risk is quite possible during this period.

The stimulant properties of amphetamines can cause dramatic cardiorespiratory effects such as tachycardia, dyspnea, chest pain, and hypertension. The person may panic because these signs and symptoms are those of a myocardial infarction. To deal with these disturbing symptoms, amphetamine users often use depressants or "downers" such as large amounts of alcohol, marijuana, benzodiazepines, barbiturates, or heroin (Scott, Gabel, 1995) to offset the overstimulation effect.

Acute toxic amphetamine effects can be very serious and, in addition to the signs and symptoms mentioned previously, seizures and circulatory collapse have been reported. "Fatal intoxication usually is preceded by hyperpyrexia, convulsion, and shock" as reported by Scott and Gabel (1995). Detoxification and use of conventional therapies for medical complications are necessary in the treatment of the acute toxicity.

Amphetamines are also said to be psychotomimetic, although there is conflicting evidence as to the cause of amphetamine psychosis. The questions asked include: Is the psychosis caused by heavy use of amphetamines or is the user perhaps also mentally ill? Or are some of the symptoms (paranoia, aggression, delusions of persecution, and hallucinations) secondary to the insomnia (sleep deprivation) induced by prolonged amphetamine abuse?

The healthcare professional should be aware that amphetamine (especially methamphetamine) usage is on the increase, with much of it being made by illicit laboratories in the United States. Crystal methamphetamine (known as "ice" or "crystal meth") is gaining popularity because a high results in usually less than a minute when these crystals are heated and the vapor is inhaled (Scott, Gabel, 1995). In some instances, oral amphetamine users are also smoking methamphetamine concurrently to vastly increase the intensity of effect. Methamphetamine serum levels after smoking produce elevated plasma levels and a high that can persist for 12 hours (with a half-life of approximately 12 hours), whereas serum levels after smoking of freebase cocaine rapidly peak and decline because it has a half-life of about an hour. The toxicity resulting from the combination of smoking and oral administration of the drug produces an enhanced and potentially dangerous effect.

Preparations

Chemically there are three types of amphetamines—salts of racemic amphetamines, dextroamphetamines, and methamphetamines—all of which vary in degree of potency and peripheral effects. Dextroamphetamine is said to have fewest peripheral effects, such as hypertension and tachycardia.

See the box on p. 105 for management of an amphetamine overdose.

CANNABIS DRUGS (MARIJUANA/ HASHISH)

The cannabis drugs are derived from the leaves, stems, fruiting tops, and resin of both female and male hemp plants (*Cannabis sativa*). The potency of the active ingredient, tetrahydrocannabinol (THC), is greatest in the flowering tops of the plant and seems to vary according to the climatic conditions under which the plant is grown. In the United States the plants grow wild or are illegally cultivated and thus potency varies. The only legal cultivation is that by the federal government for research purposes.

MANAGEMENT OF DRUG OVERDOSE

Amphetamines

GENERAL APPROACH

No specific antidote is available to treat amphetamine overdose.

Psychotic symptoms usually occur within 36 to 48 hours after a single large overdose and disappear in approximately 1 week.

Treatment is mainly supportive and symptomatic.

SPECIFIC APPROACH

If a large overdose is discovered within an hour in a conscious, nonconvulsant patient, vomiting or gastric lavage may be used, followed by a saline cathartic.

The person should be closely monitored because of the potential for hypertension, hyperpyrexia, and seizures.

To increase renal excretion of amphetamines, an osmotic diuretic such as mannitol with a urinary acidifier (ammonium chloride) may be necessary.

After the acute episode, the amphetamine abuser will need intensive counseling, and perhaps desensitization techniques, on a long-term basis to overcome the craving and relapses common with abuse of this stimulant drug.

Both the availability of more potent species and varieties of marijuana and the increase in use among young teenagers (12 to 14 years of age) require a new attitude of concern toward the substance. The potency of THC in marijuana varies, with the typical leaf containing 3%. Imported marijuana, when carefully cultivated, may contain 6% to 10% THC (Jungnickel, 1995). Marijuana grown under scientifically controlled conditions is often much more potent than the domestic variety smoked in the past.

Preparations

Marijuana and hashish are the most common forms of cannabis in use. Hashish refers to the powdered form of the plant's resin, which contains 7% to 12% THC (Jungnickel, 1995). Other forms of cannabis, used in such countries as Jamaica, Mexico, Africa, India, and the Middle East, include banji, ganga, and charas, which correspond, respectively, to American marijuana, hashish, and unadulterated resin. In Morocco kif is used, whereas in South America a cannabis drug called dagga is often used.

Mode of administration

Cannabis drugs may be absorbed when administered by oral, subcutaneous, or pulmonary routes, but they are most potent when inhaled. Either the pure resin or the dried leaves of the cannabis plant may be smoked in pipes or cigarettes. Because the smoke is acrid and irritating, some users prefer to smoke marijuana through a water pipe. The smoke is inhaled deeply and retained in the lungs as long as possible to achieve maximal saturation of the absorbing surface. Powdered hashish and marijuana may also be mixed with foods, a mode of administration that delays the drug's absorption. The effects sought by users are mental relaxation and euphoria. The sedative-hypnotic effects of smoking are rapid and generally last 2 to 3 hours, while the effects of the orally ingested drugs may not begin for several hours. Hashish oil injected intravenously has a high incidence of mortality.

Marijuana plants contain hundreds of different chemicals. Approximately 100 chemicals have been isolated and are generally termed "cannabinoids." Of these, only THC (delta-9-tetrahydrocannabinol) and CBD (cannabidiol) have been studied in humans to identify their pharmacologic effects. While many questions are still unanswered, it is believed the major psychoactive ingredient in cannabis is THC.

Dronabinol (Marinol or THC) and nabilone (Cesamet) are synthetic cannabinoids available for the treatment of nausea and vomiting induced by cancer chemotherapy that are not responsive to standard therapies. Both products have a high potential for abuse, so they are closely regulated under the Federal Control Substances Act (Schedule II).

Mechanism of action

All the cannabis drugs seem to act as CNS depressants. They depress higher brain centers and consequently release lower centers from inhibitory influences. Although some controversy exists regarding their classification, the cannabis drugs are not narcotic derivatives but are legally classified as controlled substances. They are more frequently classified as sedative-hypnotic-anesthetics or psychedelic (capable of altering perception, thought, and feeling) drugs. Like the sedative-hypnotics, they appear to depress the ascending reticular activating system. As dosage increases, their effects proceed from relief of anxiety, disinhibition, and excitement to anesthesia. If dosage is high enough, respiratory and vasomotor depression and collapse may occur.

Pharmacokinetics

The peak plasma level of THC after smoking one marijuana cigarette is reported to occur within minutes. It is metabolized in the liver and the major route of elimination of THC is bile and feces. Only trace amounts of the unmetabolized THC are detected in the urine.

Marijuana may affect the metabolism of other drugs in the liver or compete with other drugs for protein-binding sites in the plasma; ethyl alcohol, barbiturates, amphetamines, cocaine, opiates, and atropine are some of the reportedly affected drugs.

Effects

Marijuana cigarettes ("joints") are illicitly used in the United States. Although potency varies with plant strain and cultivation, the cigarettes usually produce moderate to intense psychopharmacologic effects that reach a peak in 15 minutes and last 1 to 4 hours. The drug has intoxicating, mind-altering properties. It induces an anxiety-free state characterized by a feeling of well-being. Perceptions of time and space are distorted. Ideas flow freely and disconnectedly; interruptions in thought that are blanks or gaps similar to epileptic absence may occur. The individual may experience palpitations, loss of concentration, lightheadedness, and floating sensations followed by weakness, tremors, postural hypotension, incoordination, and ataxia. Hallucination can occur with high doses of the drug.

Dissociative phenomena are also reported; research suggests that impaired decision making and psychometric performance are related to the use of marijuana. The drug experience is highly subjective; the presence of an altered state of consciousness may be perceived by the novice until sensitized to it by colleagues. Some factors that influence the psychologic and behavioral effects of marijuana are drug dose, the user's personality, the user's expectations of the effects of the drug, environment, social influences, and life experiences.

Side effects include immediate tachycardia and delayed bradycardia, delayed hypotension, conjunctival vascular congestion (red eyes), dry mouth and throat, delayed gastrointestinal disturbances, possible vasovagal syncope, and enhanced appetite and flavor appreciation. More serious side effects are psychologic and include fear, panic (especially among first-time or naive users), paranoia, disorientation, memory loss, confusion, and a variety of perceptual alterations. Marijuana has been known to precipitate acute psychotic reactions and toxic psychoses in poorly organized personalities. The incidence of adverse effects appears to be highest in novice users of the drugs.

Withdrawal symptoms

Physiologic withdrawal symptoms have been reported on discontinuance of marijuana. Minor discomfort may pass in several days, but insomnia, anxiety, irritability, and restlessness may persist for weeks. Craving for the drug can recur intermittently for months after the drug is stopped. Generally, nonpharmacologic interventions and an exercise program are preferred over substitution of another drug product.

CNS DEPRESSANTS

Barbiturates and Nonbarbiturates

Barbiturate and nonbarbiturate sedative-hypnotic usage and abuse reports have declined greatly in recent years, probably as a result of newer agents available with greater safety and effectiveness profiles. It has been suggested that treatment of abuse and addiction to these agents should be familiar to the interventions reviewed for alcohol and benzodiazepine abuse (O'Brien, 1996). See Table 6-1 for barbiturate information.

Benzodiazepines (diazepam, alprazolam, lorazepam)

Benzodiazepines are commonly prescribed medications for anxiety or insomnia. Although they are not considered street or illegal drugs, misuse, abuse, and drug dependency have been reported, especially with diazepam (Valium), alprazolam (Xanax), and lorazepam (Ativan).

Benzodiazepine withdrawal syndrome is more likely to occur if the drug was taken regularly for more than 3 months, if the drug dose consumed was higher than recommended, if patients have a history of substance abuse or passive and dependent personality traits, or if the drug is discontinued abruptly. Withdrawal symptoms from short-acting benzodiazepines occur within 1 to 2 days and from long-acting benzodiazepines in 5 to 7 days. Symptoms include increased anxiety and irritability, twitching, aching, muscle weakness, tremors, headache, nausea, anorexia, depression, lethargy, blurred vision, sleep disturbance, hypersensitivity to stimuli (light, touch, sound), and hyperreflexia. Delirium, psychosis, and convulsions are rare but have been reported.

Management of benzodiazepine dependence should include gradual drug withdrawal. If the individual is dependent on a short-acting benzodiazepine, switching to a long-acting benzodiazepine is recommended for the withdrawal process. The symptoms occur more frequently and are more severe in individuals who suddenly withdraw from the short-acting benzodiazepines, while use of a long-acting benzodiazepine is associated with less prominent withdrawal symptoms (Box 6-5). Generally a 10% to 25% reduction in benzodiazepine dose every 1 to 2 weeks is recommended. While titration schedules and dose reduction

BOX 6-5 Benzodiazepine Classifications

Short-Acting (Half-Life Less than 24 Hours)
alprazolam (Xanax)
bromazepam (Lectopam)
clonazepam (Klonopin)
lorazepam (Ativan, Apo-Lorazepam)
nitrazepam (Mogadon)
oxazepam (Serax, Ox-Pam)
temazepam (Restoril)
triazolam (Halcion)

Long-Acting (Half-Life Longer than 24 Hours)
chloriazepoxide (Librium, Apo-Chlorax)
chlorazepate (Tranxene)
diazepam (Valium, Apo-Diazepam)
flurazepam (Dalmane, Novoflupam)
halazepam (Paxipam)
ketazolam (Loftran)
prazepam (Centrax)
quazepam (Doral)

may vary, the time frame is usually within 1 to 4 months. In very difficult withdrawals, the addition of carbamazepine (Tegretol), an anticonvulsant, or propranolol (Inderal), a beta-adrenergic blocker, may help reduce withdrawal symptoms (Grimsley, 1995).

Flumazepil (Romazicon) is a benzodiazepine receptor antagonist that is administered intravenously for the treatment of benzodiazepine toxicity. Although it appears to have no pharmacologic effects of its own, it has been reported to be associated with seizures, cardiac dysrhythmias, and other serious adverse effects in patients receiving benzodiazepines, or those with mixed drug overdoses (particularly with tricyclic antidepressants). Therefore, in high-risk patients the smallest effective dose should be used with close monitoring (Olin, 1998).

See Chapter 10 for benzodiazepine pharmacokinetics, additional pharmacologic information, and treatment of benzodiazepine overdose.

NONOPIOID ANALGESICS (ACETAMINOPHEN, ASPIRIN, IBUPROFEN)

Acetaminophen (Tylenol), aspirin, and ibuprofen (Motrin) are OTC drugs readily available in many outlets in the United States and Canada. These same ingredients may also be contained in additional combination formulations and sold with or without a prescription. Thus the potential for intentional and nonintentional drug overdose exists with this category of drugs.

Overdoses from nonopioid analgesics are commonly seen in emergency departments. Covington (1996) reports that 66% of OTC analgesic overdose reports in the United States are associated with acetaminophen, while ibuprofen and aspirin account for 19% and 15% respectively. Also approximately 58% of the overdoses occur in children younger that 6 years of age.

See Chapter 3 for additional information on this drug category.

HALLUCINOGENS

A **hallucinogen** is a drug that produces auditory and visual hallucinations. The most common hallucinogenic agents include lysergic acid diethylamide or lysergide (LSD) and its variants, mescaline, psilocybin, and phencyclidine (PCP). "Entactogen" is a term used today that refers to substances that have mind-altering effects (Jungnickel, 1995). A number of psychoactive hallucinogenic drugs have been used as adjuncts to religious services or were used experimentally on college campuses in the 1960s and are now experiencing a resurgence in popularity. LSD, dimethyltryptamine (DMT), PCP, mescaline, psilocybin, and 5-methoxy-3,4-methylenedioxyamphetamine (MDMA), known as "ecstasy" (Box 6-6) are examples of drugs that can produce distortions in perception or thinking at very low doses.

BOX 6-6 Other Hallucinogens

MDA an amphetamine type drug, similar in structure to MDMA. It destroys serotonin-producing neurons in the brain.

MDMA (ecstasy, Adam, XTC) a stimulant-hallucinogenic used largely by college students. Evidence indicates that it can destroy brain dopamine neurons. High dose or chronic use may lead to Parkinson's symptoms and eventually paralysis.

MPPP (meperidine analog) synthesis usually produces a toxic byproduct, MPTP, which has caused permanent, irreversible Parkinson's disease in users (Hall, 1989)

The use of most of these drugs declined in the 1970s to 1980s, with the exception of PCP, but use is increasing again in the 1990s (Kaufman, McNaul, 1992).

LSD (lysergide)

LSD is a very potent hallucinogenic drug that illicitly is usually available in doses of approximately 200 μg. After oral administration it will cause a central sympathomimetic effect within 20 minutes: hypertension, dilated pupils, hyperthermia, tachycardia, and enhanced alertness. The psychoactive effects occur in about 1 to 2 hours and have been described as heightened perceptions, distortions of the body, and visual hallucinations. The effect on mood is unpredictable, ranging from euphoria to severe depression and panic.

Unpleasant experiences with LSD are rather frequent. Clinically, evidence of impaired judgment in the toxic state is frequent and examples of such behavior are well known, as demonstrated, for example, by LSD users attempting to stop traffic with their bodies. Altered states of consciousness may cause psychosis to develop or trigger a latent psychosis into activity. Feelings of acute panic and paranoia during a toxic LSD psychosis can result in homicidal thoughts and actions. Toxic delirium, with altering and alternating levels of consciousness, follows toxic psychosis, and the experience generally resolves in a stage of exhaustion in which the user feels "empty," unable to coordinate thoughts, and depressed. During this time suicide is a definite risk.

Significant unfavorable reactions induced by LSD include prolonged, delayed, and recurrent reactions such as depression and long-term schizophrenic or psychotic reactions. The recurrent reactions have been described as **flashback phenomena,** referring to the transient, spontaneous repetition of a previous LSD-induced experience that is unrelated to renewed administration of the drug. Flashbacks occur in 15% to 77% of LSD users. Moreover a bad trip (anxiety or panic reaction) on LSD is likely to be a paranoid experience, and tendencies toward violence can be characteristic of LSD intoxication.

Treatment for bad trips has not changed over the years. A "talk-down" approach in a quiet, relaxed environment is often used. This helps to reassure individuals that they are safe and that the drug effects will dissipate in a few hours. If the panic cannot be helped by talking down, then drug therapy with an oral benzodiazepine such as diazepam (Valium) might be considered. Avoid the use of phenothiazines, especially chlorpromazine (Thorazine), as such agents can potentiate the panic reaction, induce postural hypotension, and perhaps induce anticholinergic toxicity. In any case, the administration of medication is recommended only as an adjunct to crisis intervention psychotherapy, which consists of directing the person's attention away from perceptions that produce panic and providing reassurance that the experience will dissipate and that no permanent harm has been done. Flashbacks are treated as acute drug-induced episodes (Jungnickel, 1995).

The practice of administering massive doses of tranquilizers, applying restraints, and isolating such individuals should be avoided. The person's dramatically heightened awareness of the environment and distorted perceptions may render these measures traumatic rather than therapeutic.

Pregnant women should be especially cautioned against taking LSD. Because lysergic acid is the base of all ergot alkaloids, it has uterine stimulant properties that can adversely affect a pregnancy.

mescaline

Mescaline is the chief alkaloid extracted from mescal buttons (flowering heads) of the peyote cactus, and it produces subjective hallucinogenic effects similar to those produced by LSD. It is usually ingested in the form of a soluble crystalline powder that is either dissolved into teas or capsulated. The usual dose of mescaline is 300 to 500 mg.

The effects of mescaline doses up to 500 mg are characterized by prodromal abdominal pain, nausea, vomiting, and diarrhea, which are followed by vivid and colorful visual hallucinations. After oral ingestion, a syndrome of sympathomimetic effects including anxiety, hyperreflexia, static tremors, and psychic disturbances with vivid visual hallucinations is encountered. The half-life of mescaline is about 6 hours, and it is excreted in the urine.

psilocybin

Psilocybin is a drug derived from Mexican mushrooms, and it produces subjective hallucinogenic effects similar to those produced by mescaline but of shorter duration. Within ½ to 1 hour after ingestion of 5 to 15 mg of psilocybin, a hallucinogenic dysphoric state begins. A dose of 20 to 60 mg may produce effects lasting 5 or 6 hours. The mood is pleasant to some users and others experience apprehension. The user has poor critical judgment capacities and impaired performance ability. Also seen are hyperkinetic compulsive movements, laughter, mydriasis, vertigo, ataxia, paresthesia, muscle weakness, drowsiness, and sleep.

PCP (phencyclidine)

PCP is a hallucinogen with a history of the most serious adverse outcomes; many suicides, assaults, and murders appear to result from its usage. It was developed in the late 1950s as an anesthetic for dissociative anesthesia, a cataleptic state in which the person appears to be awake but is detached from the surroundings and unresponsive to pain. As hallucinogenic effects were noted in patients emerging from this anesthetic, the drug was withdrawn from human use. It is, however, used in veterinary practice, and this use is the origin of one of its street names, "hog" (Katzung, 1992).

Pharmacokinetics

PCP is rapidly metabolized in the liver to inactive metabolites, and ingestion of large amounts results in high concentrations of the unmetabolized drug in urine. PCP is lipophilic and has a half-life of ½ to 1 hour in small doses and from 1 to 4 days in larger doses. The pK_a of the drug is 8.5. The "ion trapping" of the drug into extravascular areas, which are more acidic than the serum, is thought to be a major cause of prolonged toxicity. The recirculation of the drug, secretion into the acidic gastric fluid, and reabsorption in the small intestine may also account for the prolonged toxicity and offer a key to the management of the toxicity of overdosage. These observations have led to treatment using urine acidification with diuresis and continuous gastric drainage in severe intoxication to enhance elimination. Urinary excretion is enhanced when the urine is acidified to 5.5 pH or less with ascorbic acid. The fact that PCP may be found in adipose tissue may indicate that the long-term effects are related to its lipophilic nature. Possibly during a nutritional fast PCP is released, and resulting symptoms are interpreted as a flashback.

Effects

In humans, common peripheral signs include flushing, profuse sweating, nystagmus, diplopia, ptosis, analgesia, and sedation. Other effects of PCP are as follows:

- A state similar to alcohol intoxication with ataxia and generalized numbness of extremities
- Psychologic effects that usually proceed in three stages:
  1. Change in body image and feelings of depersonalization
  2. Perceptual distortions (visual or auditory)
  3. Discomforting feelings of apathy, estrangement, or alienation
- Disorganization of thought and derealization that is greater than with LSD
- Impairment of attention span, motor skills, and sense of body boundaries, movement, and position
- Hallucinations that can recur unpredictably for days, weeks, or months

PCP is similar to ketamine in producing stages of anesthesia. In addition, excitation, paranoid behavior, self-destructive acts (because sensation or feeling of pain is ab-

MANAGEMENT OF DRUG OVERDOSE

PCP

GENERAL APPROACH

The clinical symptoms and signs of PCP intoxication are dose related. The waxing and waning of the intoxicative signs may be related to the pharmacokinetics of enteric reabsorption for the alkalized (nonionized) PCP with the recirculation and redistribution of the agent, as described earlier.

The healthcare professional should be aware of these signs, as this time period will constitute the greatest threat for both the patient and healthcare provider.

The person often has alternating periods of paranoia, assaultiveness, terror, and hyperactivity followed by a calm demeanor, blank stare, or withdrawn period.

During the first 10 days after ingestion, the healthcare professional should never assume that the calm states are permanent. During an acute intoxication phase the patient is unable to process incoming sensory stimuli.

SPECIFIC APPROACH

Treatment is primarily symptomatic.

Keep patient in a dark room with minimal sensory stimulation and protected from self-inflicted injury. Do not attempt to talk down the PCP-anxious individual because it may provoke more serious anxiety or agitation.

Diazepam (Valium) and haloperidol (Haldol) have been used for their antianxiety and antipsychotic effects, respectively.

Urine acidification will enhance the excretion rate of PCP. Cranberry juice is frequently used to acidify the urine for this purpose.

The use of PCP causes a wide range of subjective effects requiring careful monitoring of the patient. Be aware that prolonged and severe behavioral disturbances may progress to respiratory and cardiovascular emergencies as serum levels of the drug change.

sent), horizontal and vertical nystagmus, tachycardia, hypertension, seizures, increased reflexes, muscle rigidity, respiratory depression, and coma with open eyes may ensue. PCP is a strong sympathomimetic and hallucinogenic dissociative anesthetic agent. Because the drug is now classified as a controlled substance, penalties for illegal manufacture have been enacted and enforced.

Effects of PCP are claimed by some investigators to mimic schizophrenia more accurately than those of other psychotomimetics or hallucinogenics. Like the symptoms of schizophrenia, the effects of PCP are reduced by sensory deprivation. Currently no chemical antidote exists for inhibiting the effects of PCP. Keeping the user quiet and away from sensory stimuli may decrease the intensity of some of the effects.

Toxic effects

The pressor effects of PCP may cause hypertensive crisis, intracerebral hemorrhage, convulsions, coma, and death. See the box at left for management of a PCP overdose.

INHALANTS

Volatile hydrocarbons and aerosols are other substances of abuse. Representatives of this group are toluene, xylene, benzene, gasoline, paint thinner, typewriter correction fluid, lighter fluid, airplane glue, and nitrous oxide.

Volatile hydrocarbons are often used as propellants in aerosol products. When sniffed (inhaled), these agents may produce a rapid general CNS depression with marked inebriation, dizziness, floating sensations, exhilaration, and intense feelings of well-being that are at times exhibited as reckless abandonment, disinhibition, and feelings of increased power and aggressiveness similar to those seen with alcohol intoxication. Inhalation may result in bronchial and laryngeal irritation, transient euphoria, headache, giddiness, vertigo, ataxia, and renal tubular acidosis, especially with glue sniffing. At high doses, confusion and coma occur as well as blood dyscrasia. Depression may follow these early excitatory effects.

Chronic toluene abuse will lead to hepatic and renal toxicity, and death from cardiac dysrhythmia and respiratory failure has been reported. Recovery from lower doses may be seen in 15 minutes to a few hours. Inhalants are used mainly by young children and preteens (6 to 15 years of age).

Butyl nitrite is a clear, yellow liquid sold as a room deodorizer under trade names such as Rush, Bolt, and Bullet. The substance is sold in drug paraphernalia shops and adult bookstores and by mail order. The opened container is placed under the nose; and the individual inhales deeply and becomes dizzy, feels faint, and possibly loses consciousness. This rush lasts less than 1 minute and may include a headache, perspiration, and flushing, all caused by rapid vasodilation. It strongly resembles the effects achieved from amyl nitrite (a prescription smooth muscle relaxant and vasodilator).

Amyl nitrite is sometimes abused to heighten a sexual orgasm in both partners. Both butyl nitrite and amyl nitrite lower blood pressure and reduce the heart's oxygen consumption. They diminish sexual inhibition and, by their physiologic action, may prolong sexual intercourse (Katzung, 1992).

Inhaled nitrite abuse has been implicated as being associated with or as being a contributory factor in the development of opportunistic infections and Kaposi's sarcoma in immunosuppressed homosexuals. Nitrites themselves are not considered a major risk factor, but as amyl nitrite (and other nitrite products) users tend to have more sexual partners, they could be at a higher risk of developing such infections (AHFS, 1998).

The development of tolerance also occurs with inhalants. For example, persons starting with one tube of sniffing glue per day may eventually increase to three, four, or more tubes per day to maintain the effect. In economically depressed populations inhalants are often the first drug of abuse used.

ANABOLIC (ANDROGENIC) STEROIDS

Anabolic-androgenic steroids are synthetic formulations produced from testosterone, the male hormone. Young people are taking these agents to increase strength and body weight, to look good, and to improve their chances of winning in sports (Box 6-7). The Council on Scientific Affairs (1990) reported that anabolic steroids are used by men and women of all ages who are involved in athletic activity. Use is estimated to be up to 80% in weight lifters and body builders while its use overall in competitors is approximately 50%. The abuse of these drugs is widespread and has been documented in young school-aged students and in older persons and in both males and females.

Since 1984, many organizations have publicly denounced or banned the use of anabolic steroids, including the American College of Sports Medicine, the American Medical Association, the National Collegiate Athletic Association, the International Olympic Committee, and the U.S. Powerlifting Federation. Many states have also passed laws to ban or limit the selling of such products (Council on Scientific Affairs, 1990).

Nevertheless the debate continues over the use of steroids. Anabolic steroids have been prescribed, especially for underweight persons and for athletes seeking an edge in the competitive field. Many steroidal preparations are available and are used orally and parenterally. Athletes often use the drugs in amounts far in excess of the recommended dosages. This misuse led to the withdrawal of anabolic steroid products from the market in 1982. "Stacking" of drugs or taking multiple anabolic steroids at one time is a practice used by a number of athletes. This usually includes taking very large dosages of the steroids on an 8-week cycle schedule while following a regular strenuous exercise program (perhaps on isolated muscle groups) and consuming a high-protein diet. The long-term effects of such a schedule have not been studied, but documented short-term effects include increased aggressive behavior and some masculinization in females.

The disqualification of Olympic athletes for using steroids, along with the many undesirable and harmful effects reported from their usage, has led to an increase in regulation of this category of drugs. In 1991 all anabolic steroids were placed in the Schedule III controlled substances category. Some states have or are considering placing these substances in the Schedule II category to further restrict the availability of these drugs for nontherapeutic usage (Surface, 1991). The general public should be informed of the serious health problems associated with short-term and long-term consumption of anabolic steroids (Box 6-8).

BOX 6-7 Major Effects Associated with Anabolic Steroids

Androgen-Type Effects

Increased growth and development of the seminal vesicles and prostate gland
Increased body and facial hair
Increased production of oil from the sebaceous glands
Deepening of the voice
Increased sexual interest and desire
Enhancement of abstract and spatial dimension thinking ability
Increased aggression

Anabolic-Type Effects

Increased organ and skeletal muscle mass
Increased calcium in bones
Increased retention of total body nitrogen
Increased hemoglobin concentration
Increased protein synthesis

Data from Council on Scientific Affairs, 1990.

BOX 6-8 Major Adverse Effects of Anabolic Steroids

Females

Oily skin; acne
Decrease in breast size, ovulation, lactation, or menstruation
Hoarse and deep voice tone (usually irreversible)
Clitoral enlargement
Unusual hair growth and/or male type baldness (usually irreversible)

Males

Prepuberty

Increased size of penis, number of erections, and secondary male characteristics

Postpuberty

Priapism (continuing erections), difficult/increased urination
Increase in breast size (gynecomastia)
Testicular atrophy, oligospermia, impotence

Both Sexes

Hypercalcemia
Edema of feet or legs
Jaundice, liver impairment
Liver carcinoma (rare)
Urinary calculi
Hypersensitivity
Insomnia
Iron deficiency anemia
Nausea, vomiting, anorexia, stomach pains

SUMMARY

Substance abuse and misuse is one of the top public health issues in society today. This chapter addresses drug misuse and abuse by identifying the problem and its effects on the individual and society, the issues that affect drug abuse in professionals, problems in drug testing, and the etiologic factors and pharmacologic basis of dependence and tolerance. The drugs most commonly abused are identified and discussed, especially opioids, alcohol, CNS stimulants and depressants, inhalants, anabolic steroids, and hallucinogens. As everyone is affected by drug abuse, professionals must strive to be informed on the current drug abuse issues, the reported signs and symptoms of drug abuse with each agent, and the recommended interventions and treatment approaches.

REVIEW QUESTIONS

1. Explain why an opioid drug such as methadone was selected as a substitute drug for heroin drug detoxification and withdrawal. Name the advantages and disadvantages of methadone use.
2. Why is clonidine, an antihypertensive drug, used to treat acute opioid, nicotine, and alcohol withdrawal and detoxification? Explain the pharmacologic effects and the primary side effects associated with its use.
3. Explain how the formulations of Talwin-Nx and Darvocet-N resulted in a reduction in intravenous drug abuse reports for these agents.
4. Ethyl alcohol abuse is a common problem in society today. Review its pharmacologic effects systemically on the cardiovascular system and the gastrointestinal organs in short-term use and in chronic alcohol consumption. Can alcohol abuse occur with any alcoholic beverage, such as beer and wine? Name at least three major drug interactions with alcohol and other drugs.
5. What is the difference between cocaine HCl, free base cocaine, and crack or rock cocaine? What are cocaine's effects on the body initially and with chronic use? What are some medical complications associated with cocaine abuse? Why is cocaine use particularly dangerous in pregnant women?
6. Discuss the use and abuse of anabolic steroids in society today.

REFERENCES

American Hospital Formulary Service: *AHFS drug information '98,* Bethesda, Md, American Society of Hospital Pharmacists, 1998.

American Pharmaceutical Association: *Nonprescription products: formulations and features '97-'98,* Washington, DC, 1997, the Association.

Baldwin JN, Benson B: Depressant and inhalant use. In Young LY, Koda-Kimble MA, editors: *Applied therapeutics: the clinical use of drugs,* ed 6, Vancouver, Wash, 1995, Applied Therapeutics, Inc.

Baldwin JN, Cook MD: Issues: psychoactive substance use disorders. In Young LY, Koda-Kimble MA, editors: *Applied therapeutics: the clinical use of drugs,* ed 6, Vancouver, Wash, 1995, Applied Therapeutics, Inc.

Bissell C, Haberman PW: *Alcoholism in the professions,.* Oxford, Oxford University Press, 1984.

Council on Scientific Affairs: Medical and nonmedical uses of anabolic-androgenic steroids, *JAMA* 264(22):2923, 1990.

Covington TR, editor: *Handbook of nonprescription drugs,* ed 11, Washington, DC, 1996, American Pharmaceutical Association.

DAWN: *Data from Drug Abuse Warning Network: statistical series: annual emergency department data for 1993,* Rockville, Md, 1996, US Department of Health and Human Services.

Gallegos K et al: Substance abuse among health professionals, *Md Med J* 37(3):191, 1988.

Grimsley SR: Anxiety disorders. In Young LY, Koda-Kimble MA, editors: *Applied therapeutics: the clinical use of drugs,* ed 6, Vancouver, Wash, 1995, Applied Therapeutics, Inc.

Hinds M, editor: How much blood alcohol content per drink? *Informed Families Dade County* 2(6):1, 1985.

Iber FL, editor: *Alcohol and drug abuse as encountered in office practice,* Boca Raton, Fla, 1991, CRC Press.

Jungnickel PW: Entactogen and phencyclidine abuse. In Young LY, Koda-Kimble MA, editors: *Applied therapeutics: the clinical use of drugs,* ed 6, Vancouver, Wash, 1995, Applied Therapeutics, Inc.

Jungnickel PW, Hunnicutt DM: Alcohol abuse. In Young LY, Koda-Kimble MA, editors: *Applied therapeutics: the clinical use of drugs,* ed 6, Vancouver, Wash, 1995, Applied Therapeutics, Inc.

Katzung BG: *Basic and clinical pharmacology,* ed 5, Norwalk, Conn, 1992, Appleton & Lange.

Kaufman E, McNaul JP: Recent developments in understanding and treating drug abuse and dependence, *Hosp Commun Psychiatry* 43(3):223, 1992.

Lipman AG: The argument against therapeutic use of heroin in pain management, *Am J Hosp Pharm* 50(5):996, 1993.

Malatestinic WN, Jorgenson JA: Dealing with substance abuse in the workplace, *Hosp Pharm* 26(1):102, 1991.

O'Brien CP: Drug addiction and drug abuse. In Hardman JG, Limbird LE, editors: *Goodman & Gilman's the pharmacological basis of therapeutics,* ed 9, New York, 1996, McGraw-Hill.

Olin BR: *Facts and comparisons.* Philadelphia, 1998, JB Lippincott.

Schydlower M: Current issues affecting drug-exposed infants and their mothers, *Healthcare Executive Currents,* 34(special issue):2, 1990.

Scott DM, Gabel TL: Central nervous system (CNS) stimulant abuse. In Young LY, Koda-Kimble MA, editors: *Applied therapeutics: the clinical use of drugs,* ed 6, Vancouver, Wash, 1995, Applied Therapeutics, Inc.

Sees KL, Clark HW: Opioid use in the treatment of chronic pain: assessment of addiction, *J Pain Sympt Manag* 8(5):257, 1993.

Sinatra RS, Savarese A: Parenteral analgesic therapy and patient-controlled analgesia for pediatric pain management. In Sinatra RS et al, editors: *Acute pain: mechanism and management,* St Louis, 1992, Mosby.

Surface, RE, editor: Drug information: anabolic steroids now, schedule 111, *The White Sheet* 25(3):3, 1991.

United States Pharmacopeial Convention: *USP DI: Drug information for the health care professional,* ed 18, Rockville, Md, 1998, the Convention.

Young SL, Vosper HJ, Phillips SA: Cocaine: its effects on maternal and child health, *Pharmacotherapy* 12(1):2, 1992.

ADDITIONAL REFERENCES

Anderson KN et al, editors: *Mosby's medical, nursing, and allied health dictionary,* ed 5, St Louis, 1998, Mosby.

Balkon J, Balkon N: Drug testing in the workplace, *US Pharm* 15(6):44, 1990.

Bennett EG, Woolf DS: *Substance abuse: pharmacologic, developmental and clinical perspectives,* ed 2, Albany, NY, 1991, Delmar Publishers.

Group for the Advancement of Psychiatry Committee on Alcohol and the Addictions: Substance abuse disorders: a psychiatric priority, *Am J Psychiatry* 148(10):1291, 1991.

Hall IN: US illicit drug production booming, *Street Pharmacol* 12 (Spring):4, 1989.

Henderson GL et al: Street and designer drugs, *Patient Care* 26(18):118, 129 135, 143, 146, 148,153, 157, 1992.

Milzman DP, Soderstrom CA: Substance use disorders in trauma patients: diagnosis, treatment, and outcome, *Crit Care Clin* 10(3):595, 1993.

Mosby: *Mosby's GenRx,* St Louis, 1998, Mosby.

Thomas DJ: Organ transplantation in people with unhealthy lifestyles, *AACN Clin Issues* 4(4):665, 1993.

UNIT III

Drugs Affecting the Central Nervous System

CHAPTER 7

Overview of the Central Nervous System

CHAPTER FOCUS

The central nervous system (CNS) is a complex system that regulates all body functions; therefore its activities allow the person to adapt to both the internal and external environment. An understanding of the anatomy and physiology of the CNS system is necessary for the comprehension of the various pharmacologic agents used to treat diseases and illnesses that affect or originate with this system.

OBJECTIVES

After reading and studying this chapter, the student should be able to do the following:

1. *Present an overview of the nervous system that includes both the central nervous system and peripheral nervous system.*
2. *Identify the major components of the brain, including site or location and function.*
3. *Describe the blood-brain barrier.*
4. *Name and describe three major functional systems of the CNS.*
5. *Describe synaptic transmission and the function of the common neurotransmitter substances in the CNS.*

KEY TERMS

acetylcholine, (p. 122)
blood-brain barrier, (p. 119)
brainstem, (p. 117)
catecholamines, (p. 122)
cerebellum, (p. 117)
cerebrum, (p. 116)
endorphins, (p. 122)
extrapyramidal system, (p. 121)
hypothalamus, (p. 117)
limbic system, (p. 121)
midbrain, (p. 117)
neurotransmitters, (p. 122)
pons, (p. 117)
reticular activating system (RAS), (p. 119)
synapse, (p. 121)
thalamus, (p. 117)

The nervous system consists of the central nervous system (CNS) and the peripheral nervous system (PNS) (Fig. 7-1). The PNS is discussed in Chapter 14. This chapter reviews the primary areas of the CNS, focusing on the specific areas affected by drug therapy.

The CNS, composed of the brain and spinal cord, essentially controls all functions in the body. The PNS is the network that transmits information to and from the CNS, thus alerting the CNS to internal and external changes, such as muscle tension, blood vessel alterations, pain, fever, sound, smell, taste, touch, and sight. This information is integrated, and instructions are then relayed to appropriate cells or tissues to produce the necessary actions and environmental adjustments. Information concerning these actions and adjustments is again fed back into the CNS. The constant feeding of information into the CNS permits continuous adjustments to be made in the instructions sent to various tissues to ensure effective control of body functions.

BRAIN

The brain can be physically divided in various ways. A simplified approach is to divide it into major components: cerebrum, parietal lobe, frontal lobe, thalamus, occipital lobe, temporal lobe, cerebellum, midbrain, pons, and medulla oblongata (Fig. 7-2). The following are the major areas of the brain affected by specific drug therapies.

Cerebrum

The **cerebrum,** the largest and uppermost section of the brain, is the highest functional area of the brain, where memory storage and sensory, integrative, emotional, language, and motor functions are controlled. The cerebrum consists of two hemispheres (right and left) connected by fibrous tracts. The outer surface of the cerebrum is called the cerebral cortex or gray matter of the brain, and it covers the four lobes into which each hemisphere is divided. These lobes are named for the bones of the skull under which they lie: frontal, parietal, occipital, and temporal. The frontal lobe contains the motor and speech areas. The sensory cortex is located in the parietal lobe, the visual cortex in the occipital lobe, and the auditory cortex in the temporal lobe. Association areas lie near these lobes and act in conjunction with them. In addition, large parts of the cortex are concerned with higher mental activity—reasoning, creative thought, judgment, and memory—those attributes that are unique to humans and separate them from other animals.

Drugs that depress cortical activity may decrease acuity of sensation and perception, inhibit motor activity, decrease alertness and concentration, and even promote drowsiness and sleep. Drugs that stimulate the cortical areas may cause more vivid impulses to be received and greater awareness of the surrounding environment. In addition, increased muscle activity and restlessness may occur. The specific re-

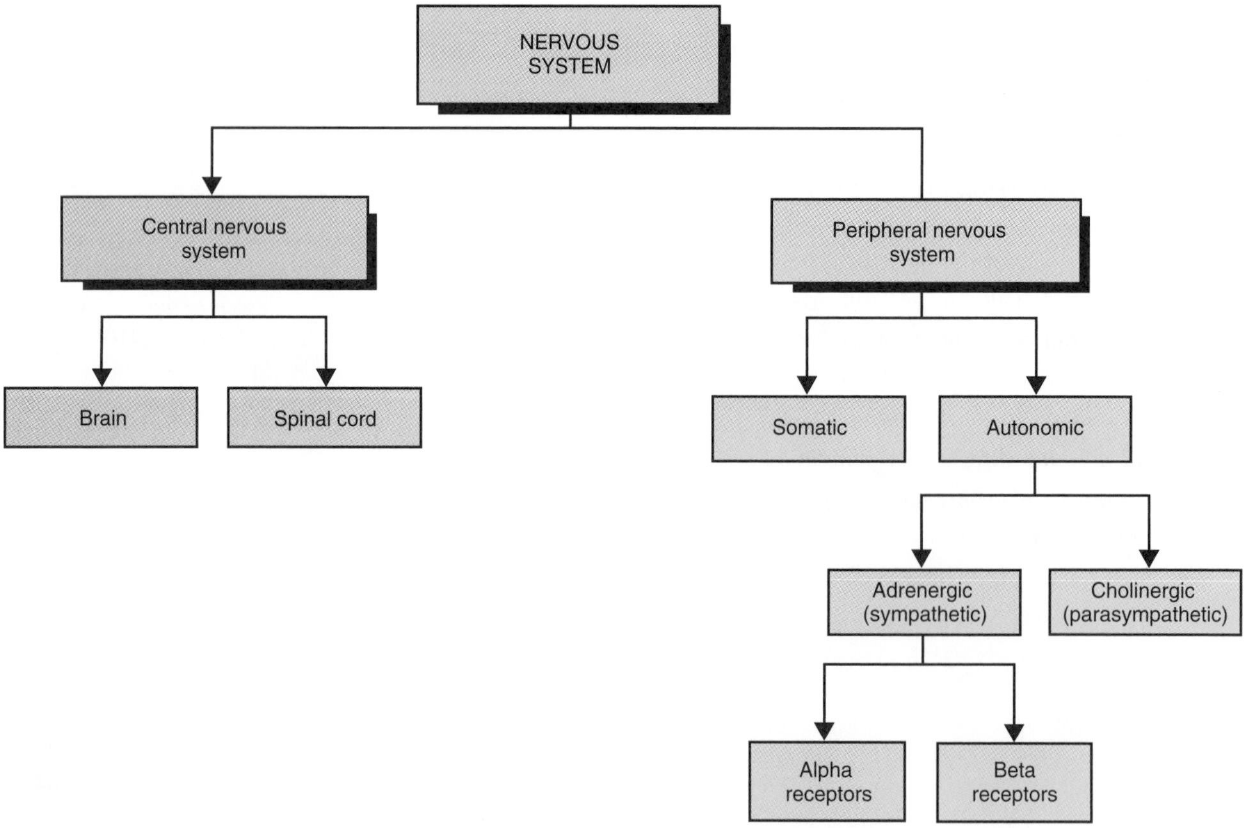

FIGURE 7-1
Overview of the nervous system.

sponse brought forth by a drug depends to a large extent on the personality of the individual, the emotional and physiologic state, the specific attributes of the drug, and a host of other factors.

Thalamus

The **thalamus** is composed of sensory nuclei and serves as the major relay center for impulses to and from the cerebral cortex. It also registers sensations such as pain, temperature, touch, and other sensory impulses and relays this information to the cerebrum.

The thalamus enables the individual to have impressions of pleasantness or unpleasantness, and it also appears to play a part (with the reticular activating system) in arousal or alerting signals. (See Reticular Activating System later in this chapter for a further description.) Drugs that depress cells in the various portions of the thalamus may interrupt the free flow of impulses to the cerebral cortex. This is one way in which pain may be relieved.

Hypothalamus

The **hypothalamus** lies below the thalamus and is vital for maintaining many body functions and for the well-being of the individual. It is a major link between the mind and the body, and it also regulates the release of anterior pituitary gland hormones. Functions of the hypothalamus include regulation of body temperature, carbohydrate and fat metabolism, and water balance; the appetite center and pleasure or reward centers are also believed to be located here. There is evidence that a center for sleep and wakefulness also exists within the hypothalamus. Some of the sleep-producing drugs are thought to depress hypothalamic centers.

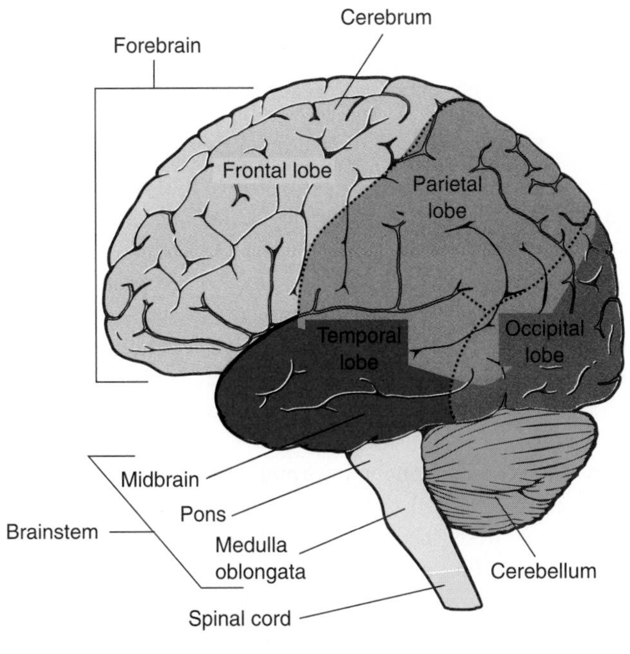

FIGURE 7-2
The human brain.

As part of its integrative role in neurohormonal regulation, neurons in the hypothalamus release hormones that affect the anterior pituitary gland. Growth hormone, hormones that affect sexual glands or functions, and thyroid and the adrenal cortex hormones are under the control of the hypothalamus.

The hypothalamus, along with other specific areas of the brain, is also involved with the control of emotions. These functions of the hypothalamus may be affected by drugs. An example is the use of antidepressants to treat the symptoms of depression. The action of tricyclic antidepressants on the hypothalamus often reverses the symptoms of weight loss, anorexia, decreased libido, and insomnia associated with depression. Other psychotherapeutic agents may cause a number of hypothalamic side effects, including breast engorgement, lactation, amenorrhea, appetite stimulation, and alterations in temperature regulation.

Brainstem

The **brainstem** is composed of the midbrain, pons, and medulla oblongata and is the source of 10 of the 12 cranial nerves (Table 7-1); the exceptions are the olfactory and optic nerves. The **midbrain** contains nerve tracts to and from the cerebrum. It is the source of the third (oculomotor) and fourth (trochlear) cranial nerves; some optic fibers are also located here. The midbrain serves as a relay station from higher areas of the brain to lower centers. The source of the fifth, sixth, seventh, and eighth cranial nerves is the **pons.** It also contains a center that controls involuntary respiratory regulation. The midbrain and pons are affected by drugs as they stimulate or depress the reticular activating system. The medulla oblongata contains the vital centers: the respiratory, vasomotor, and cardiac centers. Such centers are referred to as vital because they are necessary for survival. Other essential functions also originate here, such as vomiting, hiccuping, sneezing, coughing, and swallowing reflexes.

If the respiratory center is stimulated by drugs, it will discharge an increased number of nerve impulses over nerve pathways to the muscles of respiration. If it is depressed, it will discharge fewer impulses, and respiration will be correspondingly affected. Other centers in the medulla that respond to certain drugs are the cough center and the vomiting center. The medulla, pons, and midbrain contain many important correlation centers (gray matter), as well as ascending and descending pathways (white matter).

Cerebellum

The **cerebellum,** located in the posterior cranial fossa behind the brainstem, contains centers for muscle coordination, equilibrium, and muscle tone. It receives afferent impulses from the vestibular nuclei, as well as the cerebrum, and plays an important role in the maintenance of posture and voluntary muscular activity. Drugs that disturb the cerebellum or vestibular branch of the eighth cranial nerve cause dizziness and loss of equilibrium.

TABLE 7-1 Cranial Nerves

Cranial Nerve	*Type of Nerve*	*Function*
I Olfactory	Sensory	Smell
II Optic	Sensory	Sight
III Oculomotor	Motor	Movement of eye and eyelid muscles, pupillary constriction
IV Trochlear	Motor	Eye muscle for downward and inward motion of eye
V Trigeminal	Motor	Chewing, lateral jaw movement
	Sensory	Sensations of the face, scalp, oral cavity, teeth, and tongue
VI Abducens	Motor	Eye movements
VII Facial	Motor	Facial expressions
	Sensory	Taste
VIII Acoustic	Sensory	Hearing, equilibrium
IX Glossopharyngeal	Motor	Swallowing, salivation
	Sensory	Taste, throat sensations
X Vagus	Motor	Voice production, decrease in heartbeat, swallowing, increased peristalsis
	Sensory	Gag reflex; sensations of throat, larynx, and abdominal viscera
XI Spinal accessory	Motor	Head and shoulder movements
XII Hypoglossal	Motor	Tongue movements

Drug effects, toxicity, or both have been reported to affect various cranial nerve functions. For example, ototoxicity, or eighth cranial nerve damage, has been reported with aminoglycoside antibiotics. Vincristine, an antineoplastic agent, may produce ptosis (cranial nerve III), trigeminal neuralgia (cranial nerve VII), facial palsy (cranial nerve V), and jaw pain. Since various medications have the potential for affecting the cranial nerves adversely, the student should be familiar with the functions of the cranial nerves.

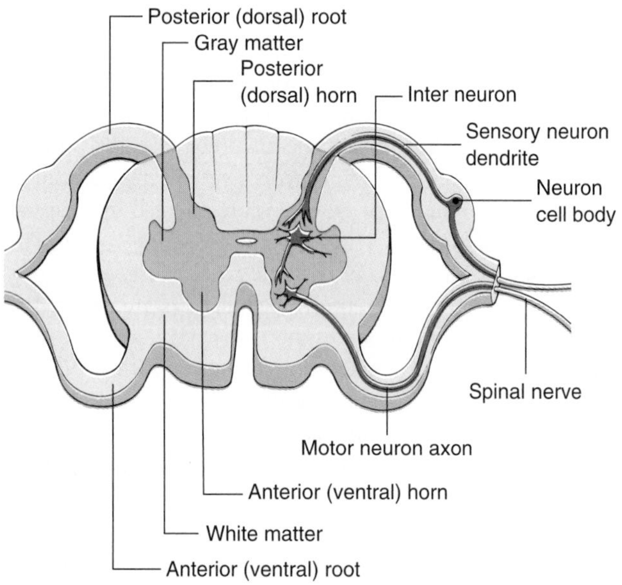

FIGURE 7-3
Cross-section of the spinal cord.

SPINAL CORD

The spinal cord, a center for reflex activity, also functions in the transmission of impulses to and from the higher centers in the brain and may be affected by the action of drugs. Ascending sensory tracts conduct impulses up from peripheral nerves to the brain, and descending motor tracts conduct impulses down from the brain to peripheral nerves.

A cross-section of the spinal cord reveals an internal mass of gray matter enclosed by white matter (Fig. 7-3). The butterfly-shaped gray matter is divided into horns; the afferent (sensory) nerve fibers are located in the dorsal or posterior section, whereas the efferent (motor) nerve fibers exit from the ventral or anterior horns. For example, when a pain impulse reaches the dorsal horn, the impulse will be transmitted along special tracts (lateral spinothalamic tract) to the thalamus, which then distributes the message to other areas of the brain. The brain responds by means of the descending efferent fiber pathways to inhibit or modify other incoming pain stimuli. (See the discussion of the gate theory of pain in Chapter 8.) Small doses of spinal stimulants may increase reflex excitability; larger doses may cause convulsions.

When a drug is described as having a central action, it means that it has an action on the brain or the spinal cord.

CELL TYPES

The two major cell types in the CNS are glial cells and neurons. The functions of the glial cells are not fully understood, although recent studies indicate that they are composed of many types of neurotransmitter receptors and ion channels. It is possible that this type of network might serve to support and assist neurons in the transfer and integration of information in the CNS (Wingard et al, 1991).

Neurons have four basic parts: dendrites, cell body, axon, and axon or nerve terminals (Fig. 7-4). The cell body contains the nucleus (genetic information) and the ribosomes, Nissl substance, and endoplasmic reticulum necessary for protein synthesis. The Golgi complex stores, processes, and concentrates the protein while the mitochondria in the cell body and dendrites provide the production of energy necessary for protein synthesis and lipid metabolism.

Dendrites also contain some neurotransmitter vesicles; thus incoming messages from other neurons are received in

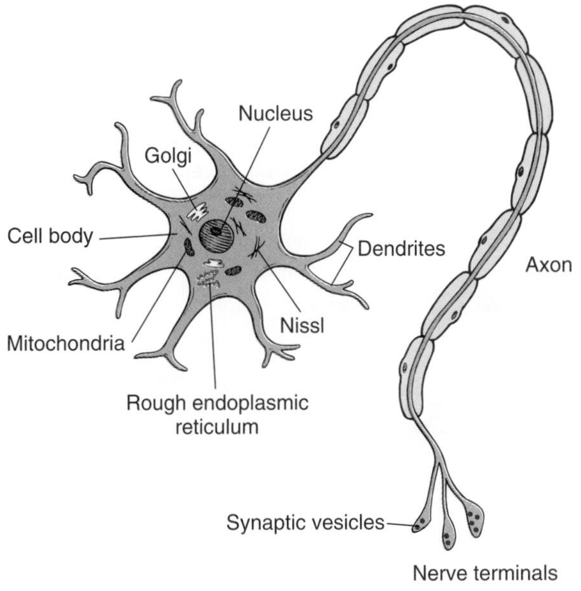

FIGURE 7-4
Structural components of nerve cells.

the dendrites, processed in the cell body, transported in the axon, and exit via the axon terminal. This process of conveying messages from one cell body to another usually involves electrical or chemical transport of the message across a synapse. Most information transmitted in the central nervous system is due to alterations in electrical currents; the following is a brief summary of this process. For more detailed information refer to a current anatomy and physiology textbook.

The electrical properties of nerve cells are generated by various ions, pumps and channels located in the cell membrane. A nerve cell in the resting state is illustrated in Fig. 7-5. A membrane difference or potential is caused by changes in the ion concentration of sodium, potassium, and chloride. Pumps are capable of actively moving charged ions from one side of the membrane to the other side, and channels are membrane pores that allow the movement of specific ions to pass.

In the resting state, sodium and chloride are found in large amounts outside the cell while potassium is in high concentration in the cell. The concentration gradients are stabilized by the sodium-potassium adenosine triphosphatase (ATPase) pump, which trades three sodium ions from the intracellular fluid for two potassium ions from the extracellular fluid. This helps to maintain the resting membrane potential. The movement and concentration of these ions in and around the cell are the primary determinants affecting the membrane potential of the nerve cells.

During rest or after an electrical potential, potassium ions selectively flow to outside the nerve cell, which allows sodium (positive ions) to enter the nerve cell. This action alters or reduces the membrane potential, and as the sodium influx increases, the cell depolarizes. Depolarization will result in the opening of more sodium channels, thus allowing more sodium to flow into the cell, which causes further depolarization of the nerve cell. This reduction in membrane potential generates an action potential as a result of the changes illustrated in Fig. 7-6.

Drugs can act directly on the ion channel or via receptors that affect ion channels. For example, general anesthetics and ethanol bind to specific receptors, which effectively reduces sodium influx, preventing regeneration of the action potentials and conduction of nerve impulses. The action of the sodium-potassium pump on cardiac cells will be discussed in the cardiac glycoside section in Chapter 19.

BLOOD-BRAIN BARRIER

The **blood-brain barrier** is actually a covering of nerve cells (astrocytes) that encircle the brain's capillary walls. This covering prevents the passage of many drugs or large molecules into the brain, but it will allow small molecules (such as water, alcohol, oxygen, and carbon dioxide), glucose, gases, and lipid-soluble substances to penetrate. Such selective processing allows the brain a degree of security against the toxic effects of some drugs on the CNS. However, in large doses or in instances of meningeal inflammation the permeation of such substances across the blood-brain barrier will increase. A focus of current research is studying methods to increase the permeability of the blood-brain barrier to specific therapeutic agents, such as antibiotics or antineoplastic agents, needed to treat a localized brain infection or brain tumors.

CNS FUNCTIONAL SYSTEMS

The three major CNS functional systems affected by selected drug or chemical administration include (1) the reticular activating system, (2) the limbic system, and (3) the extrapyramidal system.

Reticular Activating System

The **reticular activating system (RAS)** is a diffuse system of nuclei in the brainstem that permits a two-way communication among the spinal cord, thalamus, and the cerebral cortex. The primary functions of the RAS are as follows:

1. Consciousness and arousal effect
2. An alerting mechanism
3. A filter process that allows for concentration

When stimulated, the gray matter of the pons and the midbrain transmits impulses to the thalamus, which further transmits the impulse to various areas of the cerebral cortex. This results in consciousness or awakening and possibly an arousal effect. Arousal reactions require an external signal, such as a pain stimulus, an alarm clock, or bright lights. The cerebral cortex may signal the RAS or vice versa, but the end result is activation of both areas that may lead to additional transmission of impulses throughout the body (e.g., skeletal muscle activation). Inactivation of the RAS results in sleep, whereas injury or disease may produce a lack of consciousness or a comatose state.

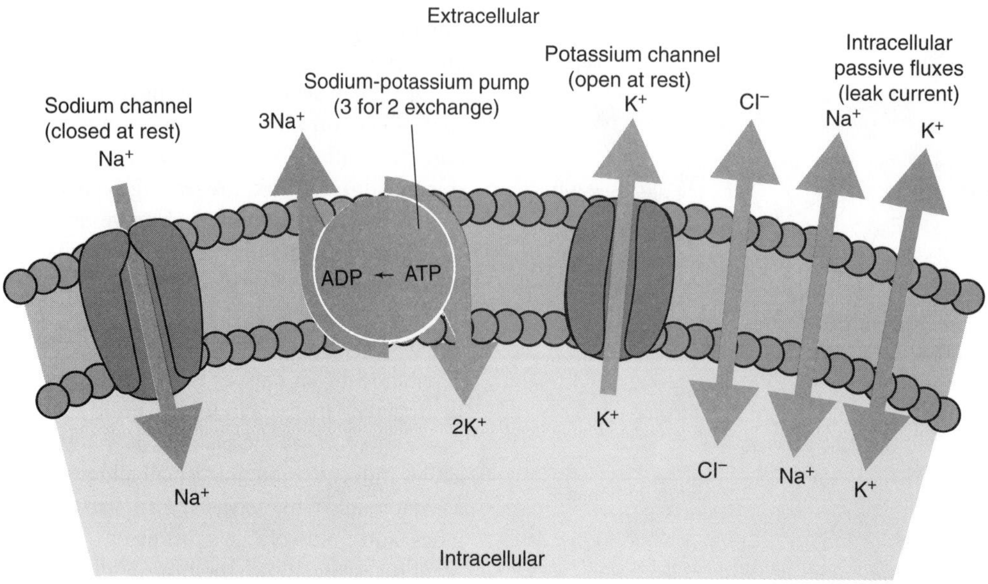

FIGURE 7-5

Primary determinants of resting membrane potential in nerve cells.

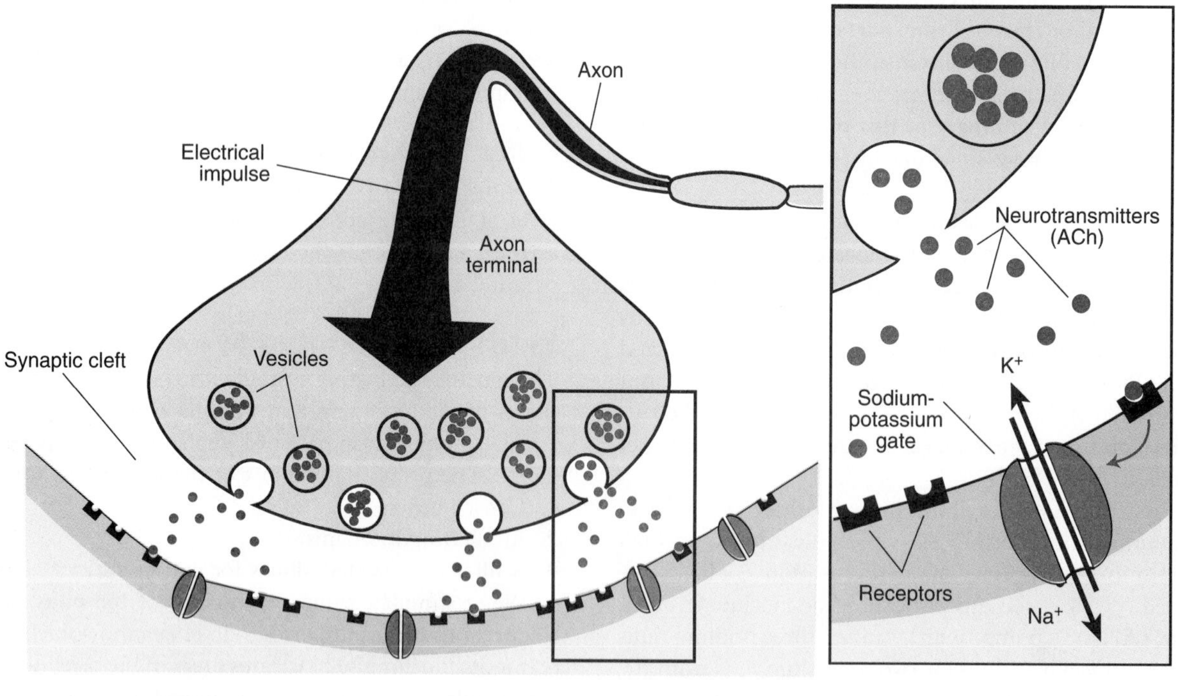

FIGURE 7-6

Nerve cell depolarization. Intracellular sodium is lower than extracellular sodium concentration in the resting state, which is regulated by the sodium-potassium ATPase pump. Electrical impulses release neurotransmitters that alter the membrane potential of the nerve cell. The sodium-potassium gate opens during cell depolarization, resulting in an increased Na^+ influx into the cell. Then the sodium channels are inactivated (gate closes) to start the beginning of the repolarization phase. See text for further information.

The alerting mechanism's primary function is self-preservation, for example, waking up at night because of a chilly sensation. Once awakened, the individual can assess the situation and discover the reason for awakening, such as the blanket on the bed having fallen to the floor. The sensation of feeling chilly activated the RAS and caused the awakening, but the situation had to be assessed to determine why the chilliness occurred.

The filter mechanism allows the individual to decrease the perception of monotonous stimuli that usually surround us. It permits us to concentrate on a specific stimulus at a given time. For example, imagine attending a large party where nearly everyone is talking at the same time. A functioning RAS will allow us to focus on the single conversation or person we are interested in by filtering out all the other conversations. In other words, it permits us to have selective concentration.

Many drugs act on the RAS. Anesthetics dampen its activity and induce sleep, whereas amphetamines stimulate or activate the system. Lysergic acid diethylamide (LSD) and some of the other hallucinogenic agents may act on the RAS by interfering with its ability to filter out stimuli; therefore the person taking this substance is bombarded by all kinds of wanted and sometimes unwanted stimuli. In contrast, it is a proposed theory that chlorpromazine stimulates the activity of the RAS and reinstates the activity of the filtering process, thus making it useful in reducing hallucinations in the psychotic patient and in individuals experiencing an untoward reaction to LSD, a hallucinogenic drug.

Limbic System

The **limbic system** is a border of subcortical structures that surround the corpus callosum (Fig. 7-7). This system forms a ring around the top of the brainstem that consists of the portions of the brain remaining after the cerebral hemispheres and cerebellum have been removed.

The emotions of anger, fear, anxiety, sexual feelings, pleasure, and sorrow are related to this system. Learning and memory have been associated with the hippocampus, a component of the limbic system.

The limbic system is extremely complex in its functioning. It may work with or inhibit other parts of the brain such as the cerebral cortex, brainstem, or hypothalamus to normalize expressions of emotions, influence their ultimate expression to other than normal, or affect the biologic rhythms, sexual behavior, and motivation of an individual.

Drugs that affect the limbic system are the benzodiazepines, meprobamate, and morphine. The benzodiazepines and meprobamate are believed to suppress the limbic system, preventing it from activating the reticular formation and thus resulting in drowsiness and sleep, especially in patients with anxiety. Morphine is thought to alter the subjective reactions of the individual to pain in addition to abolishing pain stimuli received by special areas within the limbic system.

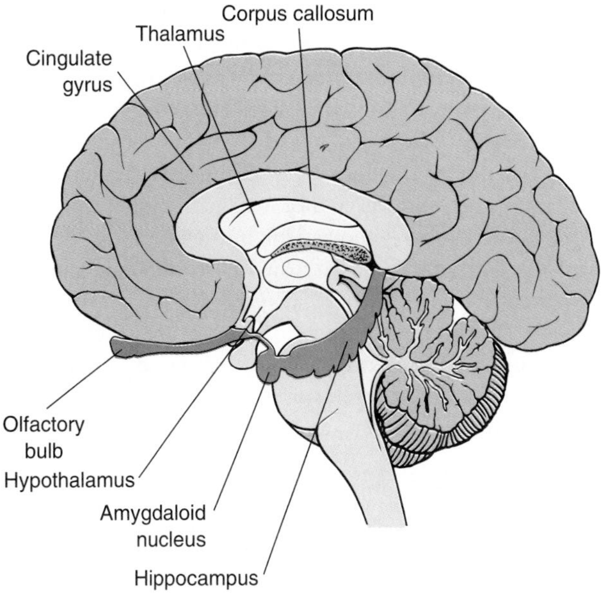

FIGURE 7-7
The limbic system.

Extrapyramidal System

The **extrapyramidal system** is a somatic motor pathway located in the CNS that affects skeletal muscles. This system is associated with coordination of muscle group movements and posture. Antipsychotic agents that block dopamine receptors may produce side effects or adverse effects related to this system. For further discussion of these effects, see Chapter 13.

SYNAPTIC TRANSMISSION IN THE CNS

The **synapse** is the junction point between two neurons or between a neuron and an effector organ. There is evidence that transmission of impulses at synapses in the CNS is humoral, through a neurotransmitter secretion. When the neurotransmitter is released, it either stimulates or inhibits the activity of the postsynaptic neurons.

Inhibition of motor neuron activity may be presynaptic or postsynaptic. Studies indicate that presynaptic inhibition occurs in the brain and is widespread at the spinal level, affecting transmission in afferent fibers from skin and muscle. The function of presynaptic inhibition is probably to suppress weak inputs that would otherwise cause unnecessary responses. This modulation of nerve impulses results in less transmitter substance being liberated. The net effect is a limiting or "inhibiting" of impulses to postsynaptic nerve fibers. Inhibition is important for orderly function.

Postsynaptic inhibition may be the result of changes in the membrane permeability of the postsynaptic cells caused by release of chemical transmitters from presynaptic nerve endings. Upper motor neurons are scattered throughout the cerebral cortex; a number of them are located in the motor cortex. About three fourths of the nerve fibers from these motor neurons cross to the opposite side at the level of the medulla, descend to the spinal cord, and synapse with interneurons, which in turn synapse with the lower motor neurons. Almost all motor neurons of one side are controlled by the motor cortex of the other side. Therefore injury to the motor cortex of the right side of the brain causes paralysis on the left side of the body (left hemiplegia). Systems other than the upper and lower motor neuron systems are concerned with voluntary movement, but lower motor neurons form the common final pathway for stimuli for voluntary movement.

Some of the **neurotransmitters** that are discussed are acetylcholine, the **catecholamines** (dopamine, norepinephrine, and epinephrine), serotonin, and neuroactive peptides (enkephalins, endorphins, and dynorphins).

Acetylcholine

Acetylcholine is the best known chemical transmitter of nerve impulses. Not all parts of the CNS contain acetylcholine. Those areas that have high concentrations are the motor cortex, thalamus, hypothalamus, and anterior spinal roots; very low concentrations are found in the cerebellum, optic nerves, and dorsal roots of the spine. Acetylcholine can cause cardiac inhibition, vasodilation, gastrointestinal peristalsis, and other parasympathetic effects.

Lower motor neurons release acetylcholine at the neuromuscular junction, causing contraction in striated (voluntary) muscle. The concentration of acetylcholine must be high, since a large number of muscle fibers must respond synchronously for striated muscle contraction to occur and also because acetylcholine is very rapidly destroyed by the enzyme cholinesterase.

Catecholamines and Related Substances

Dopamine, norepinephrine, and epinephrine, a group of sympathetic compounds, and the amine serotonin (5-hydroxytryptamine) are synthesized, stored, and metabolized in the brain. They act directly on sympathetic effector cells by binding to receptors. These substances do not easily penetrate the blood-brain barrier, but their precursors do. The effect of injected catecholamines on the CNS is slight in comparison with the effect on the autonomic nervous system. However, an increase in catecholamines and serotonin causes cerebral stimulation. Drugs such as reserpine that release catecholamines and reduce amine concentration in the brain have a depressing or sedative action. Methyldopa lowers the serotonin and norepinephrine levels and this, too, has a cerebral depressing effect.

Special staining techniques indicate that there are adrenergic (sympathomimetic) and serotoninergic tracts within the CNS. Dopamine, a catecholamine, is especially concentrated in the basal ganglia. The low level of dopamine at this site in individuals suffering from Parkinson's disease led to the therapeutic approach of using its precursor, L-dopa, with good results in many patients.

Neuroactive Peptides

Neuroactive peptides may be considered neuromodulators, neurohormones, or neurotransmitters. Studies indicate that a peptide may affect neuronal activity by increasing or decreasing the synthesis, release, or breakdown of neurotransmitters, neurohormones, or neuromodulators. The parenteral or intracerebral injection of these components causes potent behavioral effects. A number of these peptides exist in tissues other than the CNS, primarily in the gastrointestinal tract cells.

Enkephalins, endorphins, and dynorphins are three major polypeptides found in the brain that have opioid activity. Enkephalins may block opiate receptors in the dorsal horn of the spinal cord by blocking the release of substance P. Substance P, a transmitter of pain impulses in the nerve fibers, has been proposed to be a transmitter for the primary afferent sensory fibers. Enkephalins behave as inhibitory neurotransmitters, decreasing the perception and emotional aspect of pain. Studies indicated that enkephalins may bind to the same neuroreceptor membranes as morphine, and the concept of internal opiates or natural pain killers developed. The enkephalins allow modification and control of the perception of pain.

Endorphins (from "endogenous morphine") is a general term that includes many peptides in the brain that suppress pain. These peptides are also found in the pituitary gland, intermediate lobe, and the corticotrophin cells of the adenohypophysis. Subgroups of endorphins have been isolated and identified, including beta-endorphin, an analgesic substance that is much more potent than enkephalin.

Technology has shown that the brain, pituitary gland, and gastrointestinal tract each have enkephalins and beta-endorphins. These peptides are not found in the same cells. Further, the brain cells containing beta-endorphin are different from those that contain enkephalins.

Dynorphin is an endorphin found in the pituitary gland, hypothalamus, and spinal cord. This is the most potent pain-relieving substance discovered; dynorphin is 50 times more potent than beta-endorphin and 200 times more potent than morphine.

Naloxone, a potent opioid antagonist, reverses the analgesic effect of narcotics. Animal studies demonstrate that if naloxone is administered after enkephalins or endorphins are given, it will reverse the analgesic effect produced by the polypeptides.

Endorphin release in the body is higher after acupuncture and transcutaneous electrical nerve stimulation, and both effects may be reversed by the use of naloxone. It has been proposed that the analgesic response associated with the use of a placebo may result from an increased release of endorphins in the body. From peptide research may come pain relievers with fewer side effects and minimal to no addiction potential. We may also gain an increased understanding of mental disorders and addiction mechanisms from this research.

SUMMARY

The central nervous system (CNS) is a complex system that regulates all body functions; therefore its activities aid the individual in adapting to both internal and external changes in the environment. It is composed of the brain and the spinal cord. Essentially, the CNS integrates information it receives from the peripheral nervous system and then sends messages to the body to produce the necessary adjustments to maintain homeostasis.

The largest and highest functional section of the brain is the cerebrum, the storage site for memory; there many other functions are controlled. The outer surface of the cerebrum is the cerebral cortex, and drugs may affect it by decreasing mental activity, consciousness, and motor function. The thalamus serves as a relay station to the cerebral cortex in addition to being the site that registers pain, temperature, touch, and other sensory impulses. The hypothalamus is the major connection between the mind and body or the nervous and the endocrine systems, while the brainstem is the origin of 10 of the 12 cranial nerves and the involuntary respiratory center. This center is very sensitive to drugs as it also contains the respiratory center, as well as the centers for coughing and vomiting. Drugs that disturb the cerebellum cause dizziness and loss of balance.

The three major CNS functional systems include the reticular activating system, limbic system, and extrapyramidal system. These are responsible for the following: consciousness, filtering, and alerting to stimuli; the emotions of anger, fear, anxiety, pleasure, and sorrow and learning and memory; and muscle coordination, respectively. All systems may be affected by medications.

The neurotransmitters in the postsynaptic neurons serve to increase or decrease their activity. The most important of these are acetylcholine, the catecholamines (dopamine, norepinephrine, and epinephrine) serotonin, and the neuroactive peptides. Most of these transmitters are involved with drug therapies that will be discussed in future chapters.

REVIEW QUESTIONS

1. Name the site and component of the brain that performs the following functions:
   a. Registers pain sensations, temperature touch, and other sensory impulses and relays this information on to the cerebrum
   b. Maintains many of the body functions and the well-being of the individual
   c. Is the source of most of the cranial nerves with the exception of the olfactory and optic nerves

2. Describe the function of the blood-brain barrier and its effect on medications.

3. Describe the reticular activating system and give two examples of how it works to protect the individual.

4. Describe the location and functions of the limbic system. Name and describe the actions of two drugs on this system.

REFERENCES

Wingard LB et al: *Human pharmacology,* St Louis, 1991, Mosby.

ADDITIONAL REFERENCES

Anderson KN et al., editors: *Mosby's medical, nursing, and allied health dictionary,* ed 5, St Louis, 1998, Mosby.

Barker E: *Neuroscience nursing,* St Louis, 1994, Mosby.

Katzung BG: *Basic and clinical pharmacology,* ed 5. Norwalk, Conn, 1992, Appleton & Lange.

Martini F et al: *Fundamentals of anatomy and physiology,* ed 2, Englewood Cliffs, NJ, 1992, Prentice-Hall.

Melmon KL et al, editors: *Melmon and Morrelli's clinical pharmacology: basic principles in therapeutics,* ed 3, New York, 1992, McGraw-Hill.

Seeley RR, Stephens TD, Tate P: *Anatomy & physiology,* ed 3, New York, 1995, McGraw-Hill.

Thibodeau GA, Patton KT: *Anatomy and physiology,* ed 4, St Louis, 1999, Mosby.

Van Wynsberghe D, Noback CR, Carola R: *Human anatomy and physiology,* ed 3, New York, 1995, McGraw-Hill.

CHAPTER 8

Analgesics

KEY DRUGS

morphine (p. 134)
naloxone (p. 143)
pentazocine (p. 144)

KEY TERMS

acute pain, (p. 127)
agonist, (p. 134)
agonist-antagonist drug, (p. 134)
analgesics, (p. 125)
chronic pain, (p. 127)
equianalgesic, (p. 141)
gate control theory, (p. 128)
neuropathic (deafferentation) pain, (p. 128)
opioids, (p. 132)
prostaglandins, (p. 127)
pseudoaddiction, (p. 125)
selective tolerance, (p. 125)
somatic (nociceptive) pain, (p. 127)
visceral pain, (p. 127)

CHAPTER FOCUS

Pain is a universal symptom experienced by nearly everyone at some point in life. Each person's experience is individual, unique, and subjective. Only the person who is in pain can truly describe and rate the degree of his or her pain. As pain is the most commonly feared symptom for patients, the healthcare professional needs to be knowledgeable about types of pain and interventions that are useful in controlling or preventing pain.

OBJECTIVES

After reading and studying this chapter, the student should be able to do the following:

1. *Define and discuss the key drugs and key terms.*
2. *Discuss at least two factors (pro and con) associated with legislative approval of heroin for intractable pain in the United States.*
3. *Name and describe the two components of pain.*
4. *Define acute and chronic pain and give two examples of each.*
5. *Name the four primary opioid receptors in the CNS and their primary effects.*
6. *Discuss the special concerns and uses of analgesics in pediatric and geriatric patients.*
7. *Describe the actions of opioid agonist analgesics, antagonists, and agonist-antagonist agents and name one drug in each category.*
8. *Discuss the relationship between prostaglandin tissue effects and NSAID drugs in inflammation.*

Pain is one of the most common problems affecting the human race. It is more distressing and disabling than nearly any other patient symptom (Salerno, 1996). This is unfortunate, because the potent **analgesics** (pain-relieving drugs) currently available are safe and effective when properly selected and applied based on the drug pharmacokinetics and the individual patient's response. This chapter reviews the primary fears or myths that interfere with pain management; pain components, concepts, and classifications; pain assessment and responses in various populations; and the pharmacology of analgesics.

FEARS OR MYTHS THAT INTERFERE WITH PAIN MANAGEMENT

Addiction or Tolerance

The greatest abuse with opioid analgesics is not inducing addiction but the *fear* of inducing addiction. This **"pseudoaddiction"** (Weissman, Haddox, 1989) refers to patients who are inadequately treated for pain and, as a result, develop a pattern of drug-seeking behaviors to achieve pain control. This pattern is often mistaken for opioid addiction (Jacox et al, 1994).

Healthcare providers and the general public are overly concerned about the potential of inducing addiction with the use of opioid analgesics for the treatment of pain. This is unfortunate because addiction is very rare in clinical practice, and the fear of inducing addiction or even respiratory depression in a patient with severe pain is not an acceptable reason for undertreatment of pain (Salerno, 1996).

Studies have reported that the risk of addiction in hospitalized persons receiving opioids at regular intervals is minimal. Porter and Jick (1980) reviewed approximately 40,000 hospital charts and reported that nearly 12,000 patients had received opioid analgesics. Of this group, only four cases of addiction were documented in patients with no previous history of drug abuse. Another study of more than 10,000 hospitalized burn patients reported no cases of opioid or iatrogenic-induced addiction (Watt-Watson, Donovan, 1992). Thus, psychologic dependence (addiction) is a rare complication of opioid therapy.

Tolerance, or the need to increase the dose of an analgesic to maintain the desired effect, is another concern in practice. Tolerance is not usually seen in opioid-naive patients with severe acute or chronic pain for which there is a physical cause such as trauma, tumor growth, and surgery. Usually an increase in pain in such individuals is due to disease progression or complications. Persons in pain respond differently to an analgesic than drug-seeking individuals who crave opioids for a euphoric effect. One should not confuse physical or psychologic dependence with tolerance (Jacox et al, 1994). Physical dependence is an altered physiologic condition in a long-term drug user who requires consistent use of the drug to avoid withdrawal symptoms.

Opioids may be titrated to large amounts in persons with cancer to control pain without producing the adverse effects of respiratory depression or excessive sedation. Pain specialists believe this is the result of **selective tolerance,** tolerance to some of the effects of the drug without interference with the drug's analgesic effect (Jacox et al, 1994; Foley, 1991).

BOX 8-1 Time Required to Produce Maximal Respiratory Depression Effects with Opioid Analgesics

Route of Administration	Approximate Times
IV	Within 7 minutes
IM	Within 30 minutes
SC	Within 90 minutes

Fear of Inducing Respiratory Depression

An additional fear of healthcare professionals is the risk of inducing respiratory depression with the use of opioids. With careful assessment, prescribing, and monitoring, the potential for this adverse effect is low. See Box 8-1 for times required to produce maximal respiratory depression effects with the opioids. In patients with advanced cancer or terminally ill patients, very large amounts of opioids are often necessary to control pain. In such instances, tolerance develops to the respiratory depression effect but not to the analgesia. Therefore the patient in true pain may have opioid doses increased until pain control is achieved (Gossel, Wuest, 1993). Significant respiratory depression is rarely seen in this population because the dose of medication has been titrated to meet an individual's requirement.

Healthcare Professionals' Biases

Another area of concern is the influence of personal biases on the administration of pain medications. Cohen (1980) and McCaffery and Ferrell (1992) have raised the question of gender effect and bias in pain management. It was reported that nurses generally believe that there is a difference between male and female pain sensitivity, pain tolerance, and distress. This belief influences the nurse's assessment of the patient's pain and the amount of drug used in treatment. As a result, women were usually undertreated for pain.

Cleeland et al (1994) studied pain treatment in approximately 1300 outpatients with metastatic cancer from 54 cancer treatment centers ranging from university cancer centers to community-based hospitals and oncology programs. The study outcome indicated undertreatment with medication for pain: (1) women were at a greater risk for being undermedicated for pain, especially those younger than 50 years of age; (2) the elderly older than 70 years of age (both sexes) often received less potent pain medication, even with reports of significant pain; (3) clinics serving predominantly minority populations were nearly three times more likely to undertreat pain compared with nonminority centers; (4) there was a vast discrepancy between the physician's and the individual cancer patient's estimate of pain severity; and (5) over one half of the patients in this study had pain, with 62% reporting that pain interfered with their daily functioning.

Studies and research have identified the problems associated with inadequate cancer pain management and the Agency for Healthcare Policy and Research (AHCPR) issued *Clinical Practice Guidelines for Acute Pain Management and Cancer Pain Management* (Carr et al, 1992; Jacox et al, 1994) to help correct this problem.* However, additional studies are needed in the area of sex, age, and ethnic and cultural biases in pain management.

Fear of Legal Regulation of Opioids

Opioids have the potential for abuse and illegal diversion; therefore federal and state laws strictly monitor and regulate the availability, prescription, and use of these medications. The intent of federal law is not to interfere with a healthcare provider's appropriate prescribing of these substances. However, many states have enacted laws or regulations that limit, restrict, or so closely monitor opioid prescribing that healthcare providers are reluctant to prescribe opioids for fear of prosecution and suspension or loss of their professional licenses. Such regulations have resulted in undertreatment of pain, even in patients with severe pain from cancer (Jacox et al, 1994).

Need for More Potent Analgesics

During the past decade or two, congressional legislation for the approval of heroin (diacetylmorphine) for intractable pain has been proposed and denied. The proponents for this bill have used the argument that heroin is an alternate therapy comparable to other opioids and that it might be useful for persons in intolerable pain because of its analgesic and euphoric effects. Some advocates believe it is more potent, is faster acting, and produces a more prolonged analgesic and euphoric effect than other analgesics (McCarthy, Montagne, 1993).

The opponents of heroin in the United States contend that heroin is unnecessary because the opioids available, if properly prescribed, are sufficient for the treatment of intractable pain. Pharmacologically, heroin is a prodrug; that is, when it is administered orally or intravenously, it is converted in the liver to morphine and morphine metabolites. Although heroin given as a rapid IV injection crosses the blood-brain barrier faster than morphine to cause the euphoric or "high" effect, a potentially clouded sensorium is generally undesirable clinically. Most seriously ill persons want pain relief and also want to be able to communicate with their healthcare providers, friends, and family.

Although heroin is legitimately available in Belgium, Canada, and England, it is rarely used in Belgium and Canada. Heroin is a popular illegal drug of abuse, so an additional fear associated with legalizing it is that there may be an increased risk for drug diversion, pharmacy burglaries, and crime. If heroin offers few (if any) advantages over the already marketed opioids, then, as Lipman (1993, p. 998) has succinctly stated, ". . . legalization of heroin is not in the public interest."

*AHCPR Publications Clearinghouse, P.O. Box 8547, Silver Spring, MD 20907 (available in professional and consumer versions in English and Spanish).

PAIN COMPONENTS AND CONCEPTS

Because of its highly subjective nature, pain is difficult to define. Pain can be viewed as having two components: the physical component or the sensation of pain, which involves the nerve pathways and the brain; and the psychologic component or the emotional response to pain, which is the product of factors such as the individual's anxiety level, previous pain experience, age, sex, and culture.

Individuals have a relatively constant pain threshold under normal circumstances. For example, heat applied to the skin at an intensity of 45 to 48 °C will initiate the sensation of pain in almost all individuals. However, pain tolerance—the point beyond which pain becomes unbearable—varies widely among individuals and in a single individual under different circumstances. Fig. 8-1 shows factors affecting the pain threshold.

Welk (1991) described an educational model that illustrates pain and suffering and the various issues that influence suffering in a terminally ill patient (Fig. 8-2). As noted from this model, physical pain is only part of the suffering model and is not interchangeable with suffering. A person may be suffering without physical pain or may have physical pain without suffering. Suffering then is described as multiple issues that prevent a person from living without fear such as physical pain, emotional fear (fear of the unknown, fear of dying, fear of dying alone, etc.), social conflict (resolution of conflicts with family and friends, etc.), and spiri-

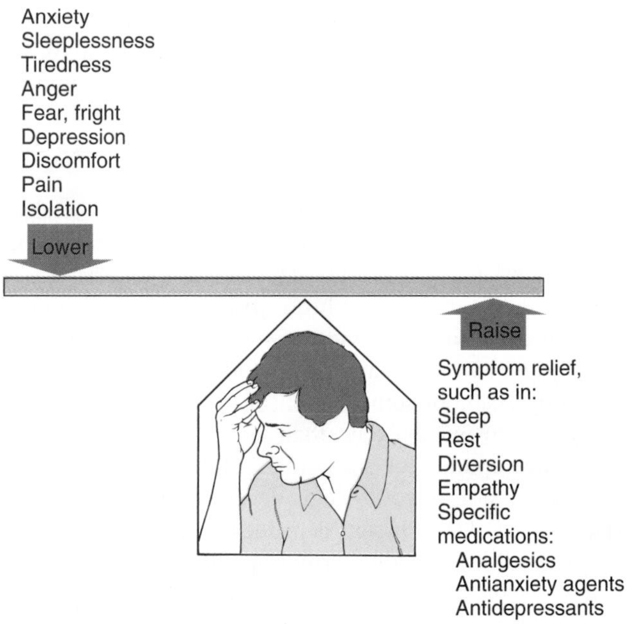

FIGURE 8-1
Factors affecting the pain threshold.

tual despair (not necessarily religious, but a spiritual dimension to meet an individual patient's need). Other persons with persistent, chronic pain may also have factors other than physical pain involved. Such concerns are often addressed by interdisciplinary teams in hospices and pain management programs.

Pain Classification

Pain can be classified in various ways; for instance it may be acute or chronic. **Acute pain,** a state in which an individual experiences the presence of severe discomfort or an uncomfortable sensation, has a sudden onset that usually subsides with treatment. Examples of acute pain include the pain of myocardial infarction, appendicitis, and kidney stones. **Chronic pain,** such as that accompanying cancer and rheumatoid arthritis, is a persistent or recurring pain that continues for more than 6 months and may be difficult to treat effectively (Table 8-1).

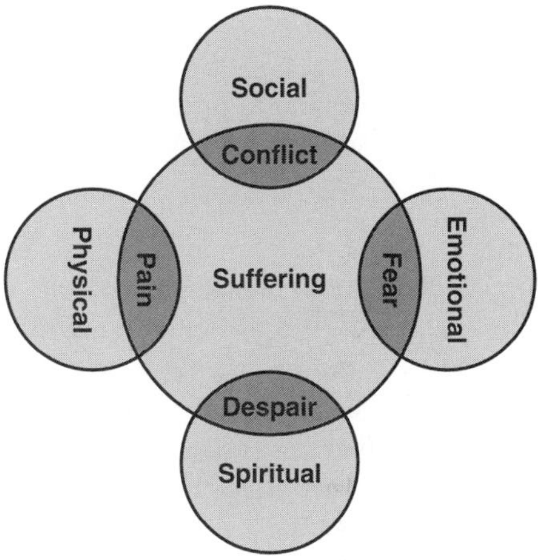

FIGURE 8-2
Education mode illustrating pain and suffering.

Pain may also be classified as visceral, somatic (nociceptive), or neuropathic (deafferentation). **Visceral pain** has its origin in smooth musculature or sympathetically innervated organ systems. This pain is often difficult to localize since it is dull and aching and may also be referred, that is, felt at a site distant from its origin (such as the pain of a myocardial infarction that is felt initially in the arm). **Somatic (nociceptive) pain** arises from activation of nociceptors in the skeletal muscles, fascia, ligaments, vessels, or joints. This pain is usually localized, constant, and may be described as aching or throbbing (Patt, 1993).

Direct cancerous infiltration of the bone causes a somatic pain mediated by prostaglandins. **Prostaglandins** are hormone-like unsaturated fatty acids that act on local target organs to affect vasomotor tone, capillary permeability, smooth muscle tone, platelet aggregation, endocrine and exocrine functions, and the autonomic and central nervous systems. They have been referred to as tissue hormones because they are secreted in many different tissues and only perform their activity within a short distance, usually to other cells within the same tissue. (They are rapidly metabolized in the bloodstream, so circulating prostaglandin levels are low.) At least 16 prostaglandins have been identified that produce a variety of diverse effects. For example prostaglandin F is involved in the reproductive system, causing uterine muscle contractions so it has been used to induce labor.

Prostaglandins and leukotrienes (found in the lungs, mast cells, leukocytes, and platelets) also are mediators of allergic and inflammatory reactions, that is, redness and heat in an inflamed area, swelling, and pain. Therefore, the cancer-induced somatic bone pain that is mediated by prostaglandins may present as a persistent ache that diffuses widely over the affected areas, usually unrelated to position or activity. In some persons it may appear as an intermittent piercing pain localized to a small area, which may be related to position, weight bearing, and activity (Kinzbrunner, Salerno, 1994). Somatic pain responds best to the nonsteroidal

TABLE 8-1 Pain: Acute versus Chronic

	Acute Pain	*Chronic Pain*
Onset	Usually sudden	Longer duration
Characteristics	Generally sharp, localized, may radiate	Dull, aching, persistent, diffuse
Signs and symptoms		
Physiologic response	Increased blood pressure and heart rate, sweating, pallor	Often absent
Emotional response	Increased anxiety and restlessness	Client may be depressed, withdrawn, expressionless, and exhausted
Therapeutic goals	Relief of pain Sedation often desirable	Prevention of pain Sedation not usually wanted
Drug administration		
Timing	As needed or upon request often adequate	Regular preventative schedule
Dose	Standard dosages are often adequate	Individualize according to client response
Route	Parenteral	Oral

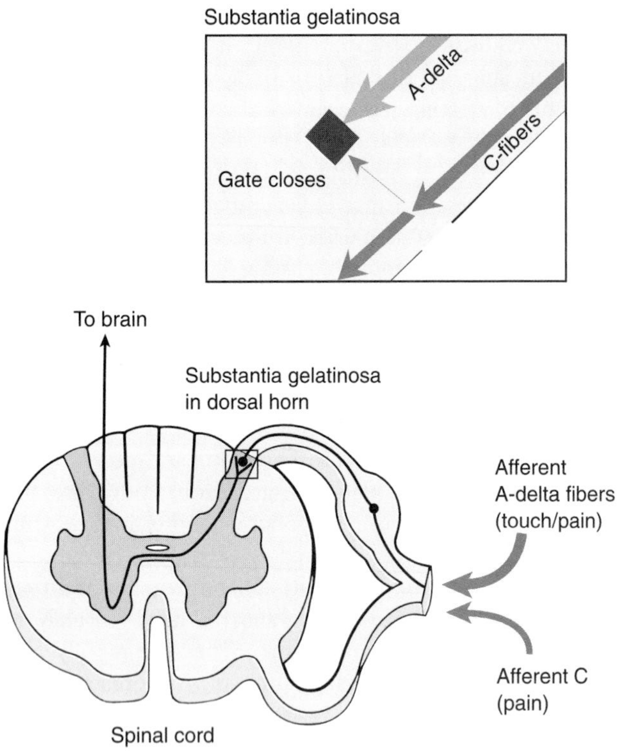

FIGURE 8-3
Gate control theory. Activity from A-delta (large afferent) fibers excites activity in the substantia gelatinosa, thus closing the gate to C, the pain-stimulating carrying fibers.

antiinflammatory agents, whereas visceral pain usually responds well to opioid analgesics.

Whereas nociceptive, or somatic, pain is usually the result of direct stimulation of intact afferent nerve endings, **neuropathic (deafferentation) pain** is caused by peripheral nerve injury and not stimulation. This pain has been described as burning, shooting, and/or tingling, and it is often associated with paresthesia or dysesthesia. This type of pain, caused by cancer tumor invasion or treatment-induced nerve damage, may be accompanied by sympathetic nervous system dysfunction. Neuropathic pain responds less well to opioid analgesics and often requires the addition of adjunct medication (e.g., anticonvulsant or tricyclic antidepressant.) to the patient's drug regimen.

Pain may also have psychogenic origins. Psychiatric illness or psychosocial issues, including anxiety, depression, and fear of dying have been known to cause severe somatic pain. In such patients, drug therapy alone does not usually bring relief; psychotherapy is indicated.

The great variation in the pain experience has prompted research and led to the proposal of several theories of pain transmission and pain relief. The **gate control theory,** proposed by Melzack and Wall in 1965, attempts to explain the modulations in the pain experience (Fig. 8-3). This theory proposes that a mechanism in the dorsal horn of the spinal cord (the "spinal gate") can alter the transmission of painful sensations from the peripheral nerve fibers to the thalamus and cortex of the brain, where the sensations are recognized as pain. The spinal gate is closed by large-diameter, low-threshold afferent fibers (the fast-acting A-delta fibers) and opened by small-diameter, high-threshold afferent fibers (the slower-acting C fibers). The gate is further influenced by descending control inhibition from the brain. Thus stimulation of large-diameter fibers will "close the gate" to stop perception of slower-acting painful stimuli (Warfield, 1993). This theory is the basis or foundation for many non-drug regimens, transcutaneous electrical nerve stimulation (TENS) units, and the Lamaze theory for pain relief.

Pain Management

Even though proper pain management techniques are available, the wide institution or application of such approaches has been slow. The foreword of the U.S. Department of Health and Human Services publication on acute pain management (Carr et al, 1992) states the following:

> Unfortunately, clinical surveys continue to indicate that routine orders for intramuscular injections of opioid "as needed"—the standard practice in many clinical settings—fail to relieve pain in about half of postoperative patients. Postoperative pain contributes to patient discomfort, longer recovery periods, and greater use of scarce healthcare resources and may compromise patient outcomes.

In the United States, cancer is diagnosed in over a million persons annually and is the reason for 20% of all reported deaths (Jacox et al, 1994). Pain is a common symptom identified in persons with cancer, with 20% to 50% reporting pain at the time of diagnosis and approximately 33% reporting pain during therapy (Hammack, Loprinzi, 1994). Gu and Belgrade (1993) reported that in the general population, nearly 35% of hospitalized medical inpatients identified pain as their major complaint. The undertreatment with analgesics of patients in pain is well documented in the literature (Cleeland et al, 1994; Zhukovsky et al, 1995).

Although several major reasons for such undertreatment were reviewed earlier in this chapter, the healthcare professional should be aware that a major difference exists between the expression of pain in patients with acute pain compared with the person with chronic, severe pain. The latter person experiences an adaptation process; thus there may be a decrease or absence of the observable signs and symptoms even in patients with very severe pain. McCaffery and Beebe (1989) have described the differences in both behavioral and physiologic responses (Fig. 8-4).

The undertreatment of pain has resulted in a court awarding a multimillion dollar settlement to the family of a nursing home resident because his pain was mismanaged by the nurses, and he died an unnecessarily painful death (Cushing, 1992). Despite healthcare providers being legally as well as morally responsible for pain relief, undertreatment or improper use of analgesics continues to be a major problem in both acute and chronic pain settings. Extensive

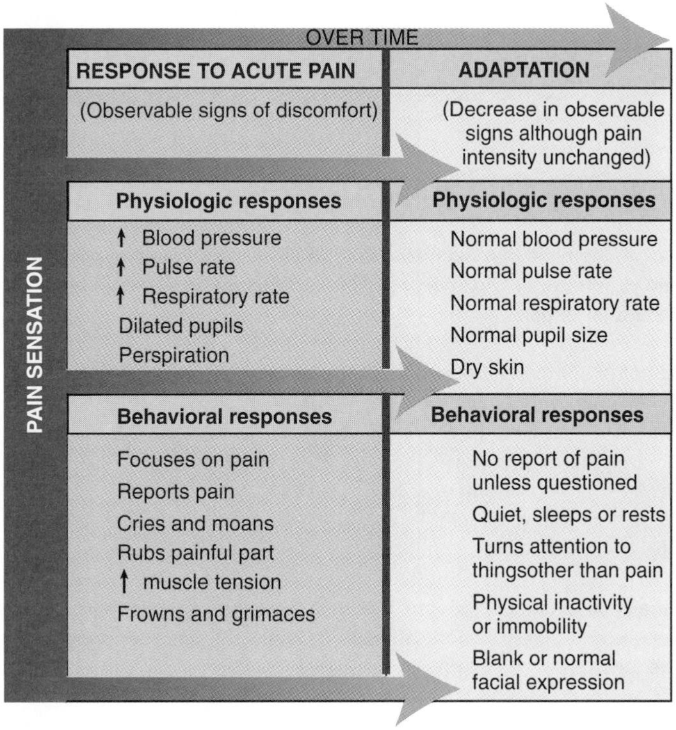

FIGURE 8-4
Acute pain mode versus adaption. *(Modified from McCaffery, Pasero, 1999.)*

information about the proper treatment of pain is available and should be used in practice today (Salerno, Wiens, 1996).

Opioid Use in Pregnancy, Labor, and Delivery

Most women experience pain during labor, and ideally the analgesic used should provide pain relief without any interference with labor and also without increasing the risk or danger to the mother or fetus. Currently there is no ideal analgesic available for use during pregnancy; therefore the prescriber should carefully choose the analgesic based on the individual and the prevailing conditions.

Opioid drugs may increase or decrease the time of labor, but the primary concern with their use is neonatal respiratory depression. These agents cross the placenta to enter fetal circulation; thus the dose administered to the mother should be sufficient to reduce the pain and discomfort to a level that can be tolerated by the woman but not large enough to cause respiratory depression in either the mother or fetus. Intravenously is the preferred method of drug administration, and meperidine is the most commonly used drug. In a primigravid women, the analgesic medication is usually not administered until contractions are occurring about every 2 to 3 minutes and the cervix is dilated (3 to 4 cm), while the multiparous women might receive the analgesic slightly earlier (McCombs, 1993).

Morphine is a potent analgesic, but it has been associated with more neonatal respiratory depression than meperidine and also has a slower onset of action (Eisenach, 1992; McCombs, 1993). Other opioids have also been used, but none appears to offer an advantage over meperidine (McCombs, 1993).

A second concern with the use of opioids during pregnancy (particularly in an addicted woman) is that these agents may lead to physical drug dependence in the fetus, causing severe withdrawal reactions in the neonate after birth. Pregnant women enrolled in methadone maintenance programs may present with fetal distress syndrome in utero and often they deliver an underweight baby at birth.

Naloxone (Narcan) should always be available to treat the mother or neonate if excessive central nervous system (CNS) depression occurs. If an opioid analgesic is administered to a woman who is breastfeeding her baby, the next scheduled feeding should be 4 to 6 hours after the drug to decrease the quantity of drug that is passed on to the infant.

Opioid Use in Children

Children are often untreated or inadequately treated for pain. It is unfortunate that they have suffered needlessly because of the many myths and misconceptions about pain and pain management in their population. Pain assessment in young children, though, is more difficult than in an older child or adult. At a minimum, it should be based on a knowledge of the procedure or event that caused the pain, as well as the child's nonverbal behavior. Be aware, however, that even when children can verbalize their feelings, they may be somewhat reluctant to report pain, often fearing that the results (diagnostic test, examination, or injection)

0	1	2	3	4	5
"no hurt"	"hurts little bit"	"hurts little more"	"hurts even more"	"hurts whole lot"	"hurts worst"

1. Explain to the child that each face is for a person who feels happy because he has no pain (hurt, or whatever word the child uses) or feels sad because he has some or a lot of pain.

2. Point to the appropriate face and state, "This face is ..."
   FACE 0 — "no hurt"
   FACE 1 — "hurts little bit"
   FACE 2 — "hurts little more"
   FACE 3 — "hurts even more"
   FACE 4 — "hurts whole lot"
   FACE 5 — "hurts worst"

3. Ask the child to choose the face that best describes how he feels. Be specific about which pain (e.g., "shot" or incision) and what time (e.g., now? earlier? before lunch?).

FIGURE 8-5
Scale for rating the intensity of pain with pediatric patients. *(Modified from Wong et al, 1999.)*

may be more painful than the pain they currently are experiencing. Some young children may not be able to make the distinction or connection between the pain from the injection and the pain relief they experience later.

The healthcare provider should consider giving medication to the pediatric patient for pain in the same circumstances as an adult would receive medication. Medicating a child younger than 2 years of age who cannot verbally report pain is justified if the child displays increased irritability, restlessness, crying, anorexia, and decreased activity. The approach to a child should be individualized based on the child's age and stage of development and the various assessment tools available, such as figure drawings to identify the area that hurts and scales that rate pain intensity (Fig. 8-5).

As with adults, it is best to medicate a child early for pain rather than waiting until the pain is severe. Children may deny pain to avoid receiving an injection; therefore the healthcare professional should be aware of alternate analgesic dosage forms, that is, suppositories and liquid preparations. Table 8-2 lists dosing data for opioid analgesics for infants, children, and adults.

Opioid Use in the Elderly

Analgesic dosing in the elderly usually requires dosage and dosing interval adjustments according to the person's therapeutic response and development of undesirable side effects (increased pain, confusion, excessive untoward CNS effects, or respiratory depression). The elderly reportedly have enhanced medication responses and may not tolerate side or adverse drug effects as well as younger patients. Elderly persons usually have multiple medical problems and often have additional medications prescribed for them (polypharmacy). Thus it is important to carefully assess, evaluate, and closely monitor the geriatric patient to reduce the potential for undertreatment or overtreatment and adverse effects. Height, weight, and body surface area are not accurate measurements for dosing analgesics in the elderly.

The elderly often report pain differently than younger persons, frequently because of physiologic, psychologic, and cultural differences (Carr et al, 1992). Cognitive impairment, dementia, and confusion may add to the barriers for pain assessment in this population. As traditional approaches are limited, pain assessment and management in this population require close supervision and monitoring of daily functioning and quality of life as outcomes. In the past, lower dosages of analgesics were often recommended for the aged, but this approach should not be the rule. Age is not a significant factor in determining analgesic dosage, but it is important in establishing the frequency of drug dosing. Because liver or kidney impairment may reduce drug clearance, less frequent drug dosing may be necessary. Both dosage and drug frequency should be carefully titrated to the individual's response to the analgesic medication. The presence of adverse effects would influence drug dosage and drug frequency.

Specific analgesics that may be considered inappropriate for use in the elderly include propoxyphene (Darvon products), pentazocine (Talwin) (Beers et al, 1992; Wallace, 1994; Willcox et al, 1994), and meperidine (Demerol)

TABLE 8-2 Dosing Data for Opioid Analgesics for Infants, Children, and Adults

Drug	Approximate Equianalgesic Oral Dose	Approximate Equianalgesic Parenteral Dose	Recommended Starting Dose (Adults More than 50 kg Body Weight)		Recommended Starting Dose (Children and Adults Less than 50 kg Body Weight)*	
			Oral	Parenteral	Oral	Parenteral
Opioid Agonist						
morphine†	30 mg q3-4h (around-the-clock dosing) 60 mg q3-4h (single dose or intermittent dosing)	10 mg q3-4h	30 mg q3-4h	10 mg q3-4h	0.3 mg/kg q3-4h	0.1 mg/kg q3-4h
codeine‡	130 mg q3-4h	75 mg q3-4h	60 mg q3-4h	60 mg q2h (intramuscular/ subcutaneous)	1 mg/kg q3-4h§	Not recommended
hydromophone† (Dilaudid)	7.5 mg q3-4h	1.5 mg q3-4h	6 mg q3-4h	1.5 mg q3-4h	0.06 mg/kg q3-4h	0.015 mg/kg q3-4h
hydrocodone (in Lorcet, Lortab, Vicodin, others)	30 mg q3-4h	Not available	10 mg q3-4h	Not available	0.2 mg/kg q3-4h§	Not available
levorphanol (Levo-Dromoran)	4 mg q6-8h	2 mg q6-8h	4 mg q6-8h	2 mg q6-8h	0.04 mg/kg q6-8h	0.02 mg/kg q6-8h
meperidine (Demerol)	300 mg q2-3h	100 mg q3h	Not recommended	100 mg q3h	Not recommended	0.75 mg/kg q2-3h
methadone (Dolophine, others)	20 mg q6-8h	10 mg q6-8h	20 mg q6-8h	10 mg q6-8h	0.2 mg/kg q6-8h	0.1 mg/kg q6-8h
oxycodone (Roxicodone, also in Percocet, Percodan, Tylox, others)	30 mg q3-4h	Not available	10 mg q3-4h	Not available	0.2 mg/kg q3-4h§	Not available
oxymorphone† (Numorphan)	Not available	1 mg q3-4h	Not available	1 mg q3-4h	Not recommended	Not recommended
Opioid Agonist-Antagonist and Partial Agonist						
buprenorphine (Buprenex)	Not available	0.3-0.4 mg q6-8h	Not available	0.4 mg q6-8h	Not available	0.004 mg/kg q6-8h
butorphanol (Stadol)	Not available	2 mg q3-4h	Not available	2 mg q3-4h	Not available	Not recommended
nalbuphine (Nubain)	Not available	10 mg q3-4h	Not available	10 mg q3-4h	Not available	0.1 mg/kg q3-4h
pentazocine (Talwin, others)	150 mg q3-4h	60 mg q3-4h	50 mg q4-6h	Not recommended	Not recommended	Not recommended

From Acute Pain Management Guideline Panel, 1992.

Note: Published tables vary in the suggested doses that are equianalgesic to morphine. Clinical response is the criterion that must be applied for each patient; titration to clinical response is necessary. Because there is not complete cross-tolerance among these drugs, it is usually necessary to use a lower than equianalgesic dose when changing drugs and to retitrate to response.

Caution: Recommended doses do not apply to patients with renal or hepatic insufficiency or other conditions affecting drug metabolism and kinetics.

***Caution:** Doses listed for patients with body weight less than 50 kg cannot be used as initial starting doses in babies less than 6 months of age. Consult the *Clinical Practice Guideline for Acute Pain Management: Operative or Medical Procedures and Trauma* section on management of pain in neonates for recommendations.

†For morphine, hydromorphone, and oxymorphone, rectal administration is an alternate route for patients unable to take oral medications, but equianalgesic doses may differ from oral and parenteral doses because of pharmacokinetic differences.

‡Caution: Codeine doses above 65 mg often are not appropriate due to diminishing incremental analgesia with increasing doses but continually increasing constipation and other side effects.

§Caution: Doses of aspirin and acetaminophen in combination opioid/NSAID preparations must also be adjusted to the patient's body weight.

Date ____________

Client's Name ____________ Age ______ Room ______

Diagnosis ____________ Physician ____________

Nurse ____________

I. Location: Client or nurse mark drawing

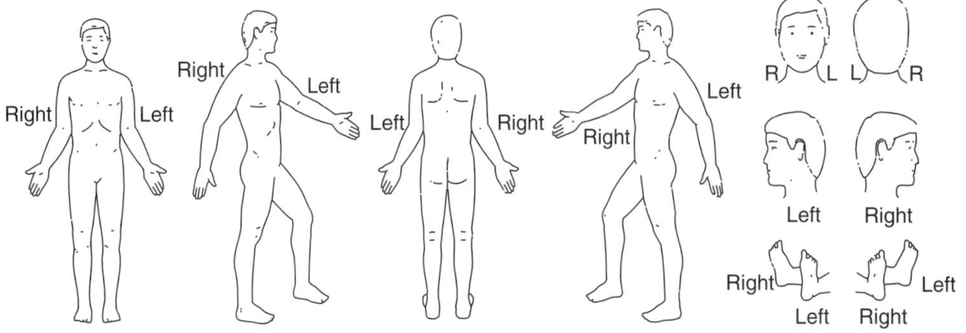

II. Intensity: Client rates the pain. Scale used ____________

Present: ____________

Worst pain gets: ____________

Best pain gets: ____________

Acceptable level of pain: ____________

III. Quality: (Use client's own words, e.g., prick, ache, burn, throb, pull, sharp) ____________

IV. Onset, duration variations, rhythms: ____________

V. Manner of expressing pain: ____________

VI. What relieves the pain? ____________

VII. What causes or increases the pain? ____________

VIII. Effects of pain: (Note decreased function, decreased quality of life.

Accompanying symptoms (e.g., nausea) ____________

Sleep ____________

Appetite ____________

Physical activity ____________

Relationship with others (e.g., irriability) ____________

Emotions (e.g., anger, suicidal, crying) ____________

Concentration ____________

Other ____________

IX. Other comments: ____________

X. Plan: ____________

FIGURE 8-6

Pain assessment tool developed by McCaffery and Pasero (1999).

(Wallace, 1994). It is generally believed that these agents are more toxic in the elderly and that much safer analgesics are available.

The intramuscular and subcutaneous routes of analgesic administration may also be influenced by the aging process. The elderly may have a diminished circulatory process, which results in slower absorption of drugs administered by these parenteral routes. Administering additional dosages in such a situation may result in unpredictable or increased drug absorption, which increases the potential for adverse effects.

Some elderly patients are less likely to ask for pain medication because of the belief that pain is a part of old age, because they do not want to be a bother to the healthcare professional, or because they deny their discomfort as a cultural and ethnic issue. In such instances, nonverbal communication should be carefully assessed, such as increased irritability, loss of appetite, decrease in activity, whining or crying easily, or tightly gripping an object. Decreased activity in the elderly because of pain may result in an increased risk of the complications of immobility.

Fig. 8-6 shows an example of a pain assessment tool developed by McCaffery and Pasero (1999) that is very useful for the assessment of pain. Crucial information in the assessment process includes the location of the patient's pain(s), the pain intensity, and a description of the pain. This information is then used to select the proper medication for the individual. Many facilities also use a pain scale

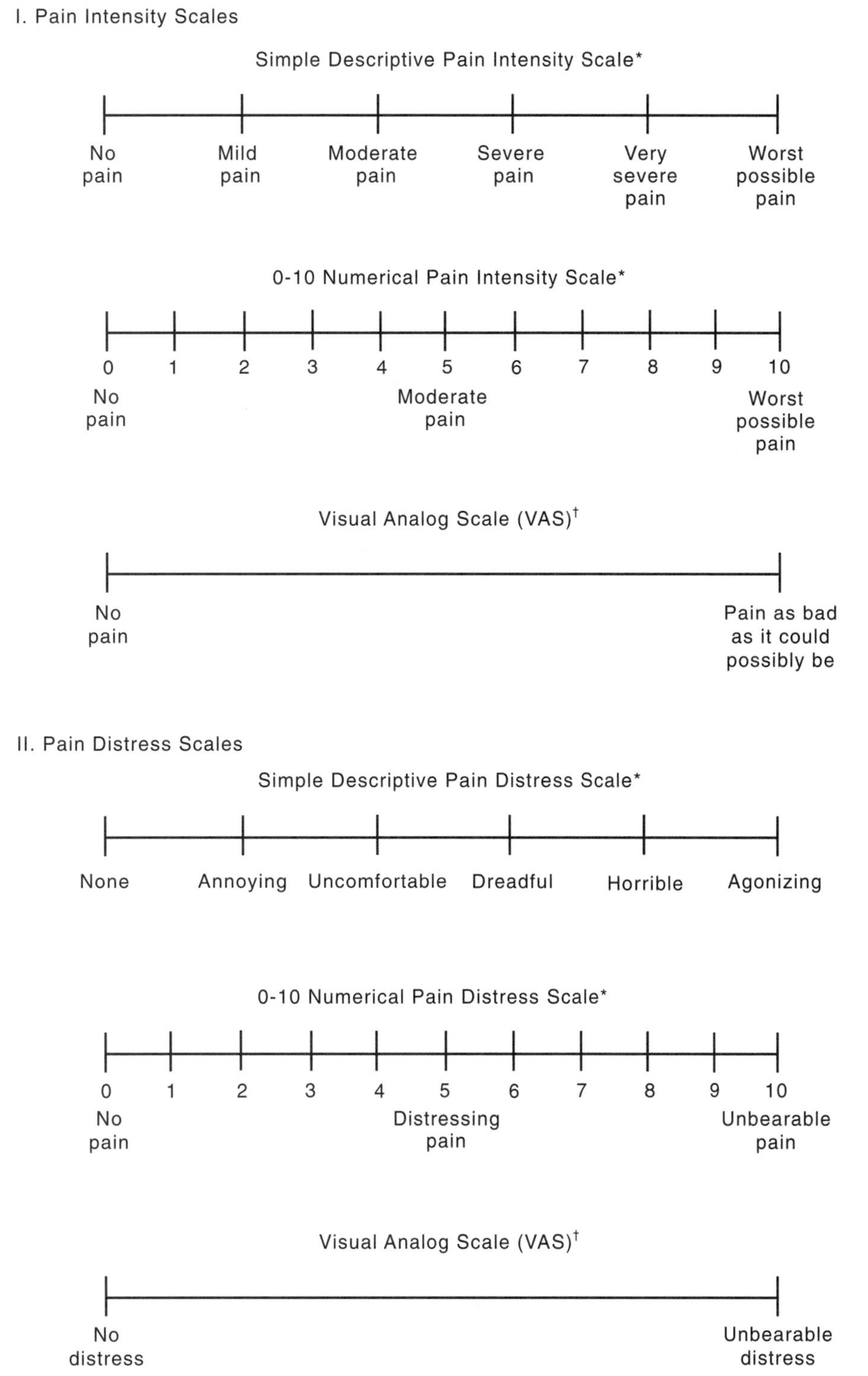

FIGURE 8-7
Scales for rating the intensity and distress of pain. *If used as a graphic rating scale, a 10-cm baseline is recommended. †A 10-cm baseline is recommended for visual analog scales. *(From Carr et al, 1992.)*

to determine pain intensity. See Fig. 8-7 for illustrations of some of the scales available.

OPIOID (AGONIST) ANALGESICS

Receptor Classification

The term "agonist" means "to do or to activate," and the term "antagonist" means "to block." **Opioids,** natural or synthetic agents that have a morphine-like effect, have been classified as agonist, partial agonist, or mixed agonist-antagonist medications. An **agonist** drug binds with the receptor(s) to activate and produce the maximum response of the individual receptor, whereas a partial agonist produces a partial response. A mixed opioid **agonist-antagonist drug** will produce mixed effects; it is a drug that acts as an agonist at one type of receptor and as a competitive antagonist at another receptor (Fig. 8-8). A review of selected examples of opioid receptor responses are listed in Table 8-3.

The mechanism of action for opioids is related to their binding to specific opioid receptors in and outside of the CNS (Jacox et al, 1994). The primary opioid receptors concentrated in the CNS are mu (μ), kappa (κ), delta (δ), and sigma (σ) receptors. Analgesia has been associated with the first three receptors, with limited research on the delta receptor. Therefore the primary analgesic receptors at this time are the mu and kappa receptors. The sigma receptors are primarily associated with psychotomimetic or unwanted effects, such as dysphoria, hallucinations, and confusion.

The agonist analgesics (e.g., morphine or hydromorphone) activate both the mu and kappa receptors while the agonist-antagonist agents (butorphanol, nalbuphine, and pentazocine) activate kappa receptors (agonist) and block or have minimal effects on the mu receptors (antagonist). The agonist-antagonist drugs (especially pentazocine) may induce the undesirable effects associated with sigma receptor activity.

In addition to analgesia, opioids are capable of altering perception and emotional responses to pain because the receptors are widely distributed in the CNS, especially in the

TABLE 8-3 Selected Opioid Receptor Responses

Receptor	*Medication Examples*	*Response*
mu	Strong agonist: morphine, hydromorphone Partial agonist: buprenorphine Weak agonist: meperidine	Supraspinal analgesia, euphoria, respiratory depression, sedation, constipation, urinary retention, drug dependence
	Antagonist: naloxone, opioid agonist-antagonist	Reverses opioid effects, induces acute withdrawal in opioid dependency
kappa	Agonist: pentazocine, morphine, nalbuphine, butorphanol Little or no activity: levorphanol, methadone, meperidine	Spinal analgesia, sedation
	Antagonist: naloxone, buprenorphine	Reverses opioid effects, induces acute withdrawal in opioid dependency

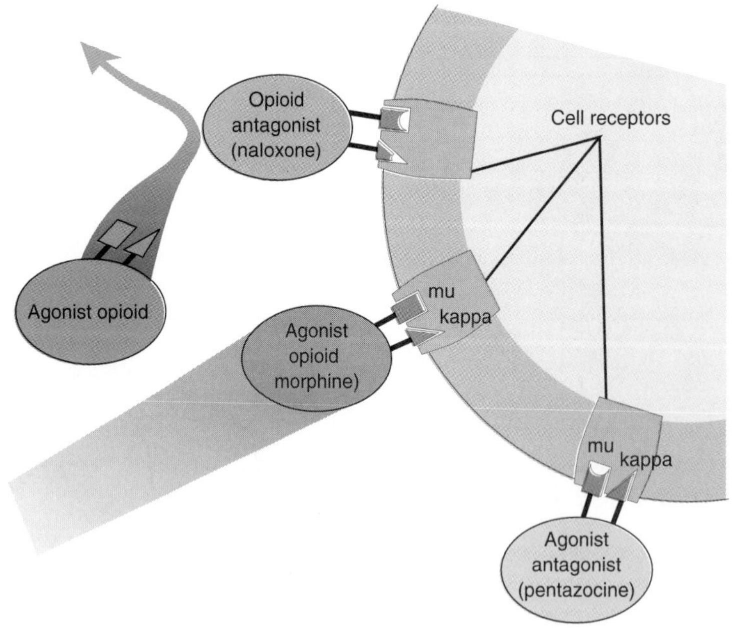

FIGURE 8-8
Receptor interactions of opioids.

spinal and medullary dorsal horn, limbic system, thalamus, hypothalamus, and midbrain. When these areas are stimulated, pain perception is inhibited (Willens, 1996), which enhances the analgesic effect of morphine.

Agonist Opioids

morphine (mor' feen)

Morphine is the prototype agonist opioid. It is still obtained from opium poppy because of the difficulty encountered in synthesizing morphine in the laboratory. Many analgesics are available now, but none has been proved to be clinically superior to morphine. In fact, all new analgesics are compared with morphine, which is the standard for potency and for side effects or adverse reactions. The World Health Organization (WHO) in 1990 recommended a three-step approach to the management of cancer pain, using nonopioid analgesics initially and progressing to stronger analgesics in the second and third steps. Morphine and other agonist opioids are used to treat step three, the treatment of severe pain. See Fig. 8-9 for a pharmacologic flow chart for the management of pain.

Mechanism of action

As mentioned previously, morphine produces its potent analgesic effects by combining with receptor sites in the brain called opioid receptors (see previous discussion of opioid receptors).

Although morphine is considered the drug of choice for cancer pain (Jacox et al, 1994), it has additional pharmacologic effects that are useful in treating symptoms other than pain. For example, morphine may be given to patients with lung cancer to treat pain aggravated by coughing or to suppress an unproductive nagging cough. Small doses of morphine may depress the cough center; this secondary effect is useful in selected situations. For persons with a cough caused by a cold, less potent and potentially safer medications should be used (such as the nonopioid antitussive dextromethorphan).

Another indication for morphine therapy is in the treatment of acute pulmonary edema secondary to left ventricular heart failure. Morphine's peripheral vasodilation effect on veins and arteries can be very useful in decreasing heart workload, resulting in enhanced cardiac function and a reduction of lung fluid. Morphine's effectiveness in treating myocardial infarction is a result of the fact that it does not significantly alter heart rate and blood pressure at usual doses, as well as its calming effect along with the peripheral vasodilation effect, which may result in a decrease in cardiac workload (Salerno, Willens, 1996).

Opioid drugs also act centrally and locally to alter intestinal motility (antidiarrheal effect). Morphine's gastrointestinal (GI) effects include decreases in peristalsis and glandular secretions, which usually result in the side effect of constipation.

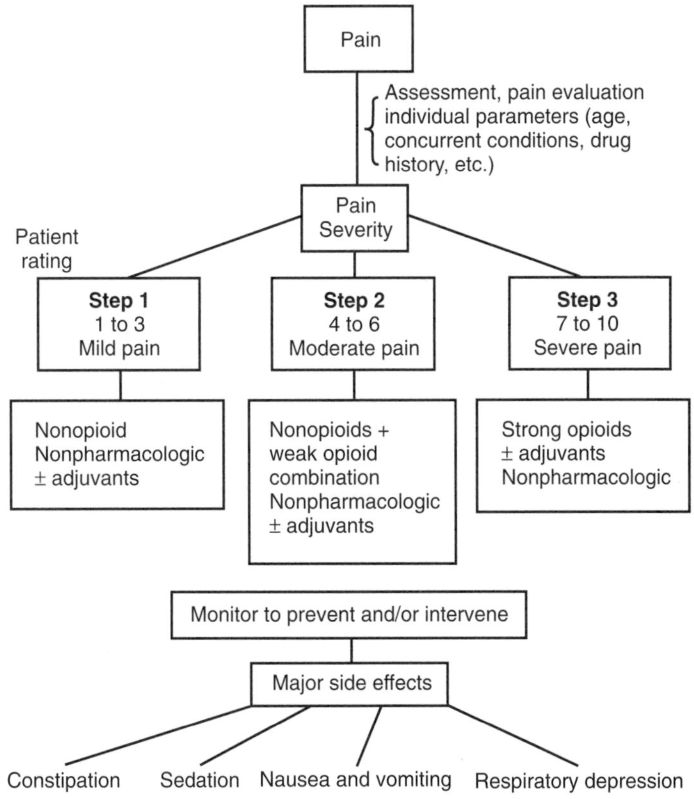

FIGURE 8-9
Pharmacologic flow chart for the management of pain. *(From Salerno, Willens, 1996.)*

TABLE 8-4 Selected Opioid Dosage Forms: Pharmacokinetic Overview

Drug/dosage Form	Onset of Action (min)	Peak Effect (min)	Duration of Action (hr)
codeine			
Oral	30-45	60-120	4
IM	10-30	30-60	4
SC	10-30		4
hydrocodone (Hycodan)			
Oral	10-30	30-60	4-6
hydromorphone (Dilaudid)			
Oral	30	90-120	4
IM	15	30-60	4-5
IV	10-15	15-30	2-3
SC	15	30-90	4
Rectal	Not available	Not available	6-8
Levorphanol (Levo-Dromoran)			
Oral	10-60	90-120	6-8
IM	Not available	60	6-8
IV	Not available	Within 20	6-8
SC	Not available	60-90	6-8
meperidine (Demerol)			
Oral	15	60-90	2-4 (usually 3)
IM	10-15	30-50	2-4 (usually 3)
IV	1	5-7	2-4 (usually 3)
SC	10-15	30-50	2-4 (usually 3)
methadone			
Oral	30-60	90-120	4-6*
IM	10-20	60-120	4-5*
IV		15-30	3-4
morphine			
Oral			
Solution,† syrup,‡ tablets	10-30	60-120	4-5
Extended-released tablets§	—	—	8-12
IM	10-30	30-60	4-5
IV		20	4-5
SC	10-30	50-90	4-5
Epidural‖	15-60	—	Up to 24
Intrathecal‖	15-60	—	Up to 24
Rectal**	20-60	—	4-5
oxycodone			
Oral	Not available	60	3-4
Controlled release	Not available	3-4	12
oxymorphone (Numorphan)			
IM	10-15	30-90	3-6
IV	5-10	15-30	3-4
SC	10-20	Not available	3-6
Rectal	15-30	120	3-6
propoxyphene (Darvon)			
Oral	15-60	120	4-6

*With active metabolites and continuous dosing, half-life and duration of action may increase to 22 to 48 hours.
†Roxanol, M.O.S., MSIR.
‡Morphite, Morphitex-1, Morphitec-5 (not commercially available in the United States).
§MS Contin, Roxanol SR.
‖Duramorph (prservative-free).
**RMS suppositories.

Indications

The analgesic effect of morphine is indicated for the treatment of severe pain.

Pharmacokinetics

Morphine may be administered orally, intramuscularly, intravenously, subcutaneously, epidurally, intrathecally, and rectally. Table 8-4 describes various opioid pharmacokinetics, and Table 8-5 lists the various routes of administration and dosages of morphine. Morphine is distributed widely in body tissues. It is metabolized in the liver primarily to morphine 3-glucuronide (M3G) and morphine 6-glucuronide (M6G), an active metabolite, and is excreted primarily via the kidneys.

Drug interactions

The following effects may occur when morphine or opioids are given with the drugs listed below:

Drug	Possible Effect and Management
Alcohol or other CNS depressants	May result in enhanced CNS depression, respiratory depression, and hypotension. Reduce dosage of one or both drugs and monitor closely for decreased respiration and blood pressure, slowed reflexes, and drowsiness.
buprenorphine (Buprenex)	May result in additive effect of respiratory depression if given concurrently with low doses of mu-receptor agonists or with a kappa-receptor agonist. Avoid concurrent usage. Buprenorphine has partial agonist effects on the mu receptor. If given before or after an opioid agonist, it may reduce the analgesic effects of the opioid.
carbamazepine (Tegretol)	Concurrent use with propoxyphene may result in decreased metabolism and increased carbamazepine serum concentration, thus increasing the potential for toxicity. Avoid concurrent drug administration.
Monoamine oxidase (MAO) inhibitors (furazolidone [Furoxone], procarbazine [Matulane], phenelzine[Nardil], tranylcypromine [Parnate])	Test dose with one fourth of the dose of morphine (or any prescribed opioid analgesics) to ascertain compatibility of the medications. The possibility exists for inducing excitability, hypertension, or hypotension; increased sweating; convulsions; respiratory depression; fever; and cardiac dysfunctions. Therefore, it is usually recommended that caution be taken and reduced dosages of opioids be prescribed for patients receiving MAO inhibitors. Concurrent administration with meperidine has resulted in very severe, and at times, fatal reactions. The effects include sudden excitation, increased sweating, rigidity, very severe hypertension (or hypotension in some persons), coma, seizures, hyperpyrexia, and collapse. The use of meperidine is contraindicated in any patients receiving or having received a MAO inhibitor within 2 to 3 weeks (USP DI, 1998).
naltrexone (ReVia)	Will produce withdrawal symptoms in patients dependent on opioid medications. Avoid concurrent administration in patients receiving opioids therapeutically.
rifampin (Rifadin)	May increase methadone metabolism, and so may precipitate withdrawal symptoms in patients being treated for opioid dependence. Methadone dosage adjustment may be required.
zidovudine(AZT)	Morphine may decrease clearance of zidovudine. Concurrent use should be avoided as toxicity of one or both drugs may occur.

Color type indicates an unsafe drug combination.

Side effects and adverse reactions

The most frequently reported side effects of morphine and the other opioids include vertigo, faintness, and lightheadedness, which occur most often in ambulatory patients. Fatigue, sleepiness, nausea and vomiting, increased sweating, constipation, and hypotension may also occur. Less frequent side effects include dry mouth, headache, anorexia, abdominal cramping, nervousness, increased anxiety, mental confusion, urinary retention or painful urination, visual disturbances, and nightmares.

Among the more serious adverse reactions reported are seizures (particularly with meperidine and propoxyphene), tinnitus, jaundice (hepatic toxicity), pruritus, skin rash or facial edema (allergic reaction), breathing difficulties, respiratory depression, excitability (paradoxical reaction seen mainly in children), confusion, and tachycardia (USP DI, 1998).

Warnings

Use opioids with caution in patients with acute asthma, a history of drug abuse, chronic obstructive pulmonary disease (COPD), any respiratory impairment, or any condition of preexisting respiratory depression or hypoxia. Also use with extreme caution in patients with increased intracranial

TABLE 8-5 Morphine Analgesic Dosage and Administration

Route	*Adult Dosage*
IV	4-10 mg diluted in 4-5 ml sterile water administered slowly
IM	5-20 mg q4h
SC	5-20 mg q4h
Epidural	1-5 mg initially; assess in 1 hr; if inadequate for pain relief, 1-2 mg increments may be administered; 10 mg in 24 hr maximum
Intrathecal	0.2-1 mg as single dose only; repeated dosage by this route not recommended
Oral (individualized)	Initially 10-30 mg q4h for morphine sulfate syrup, oral solution, and tablets; may be increased according to pain severity and client's response
Rectal suppositories	20-30 mg rectally q4-6h

MANAGEMENT OF DRUG OVERDOSE

Opioids

- If an oral opioid overdose occurs, emesis or gastric lavage is used to empty the stomach. If respiratory depression or any other life-threatening adverse effect is present, the treatment for these effects would take precedence.
- For respiratory depression establish a patent airway and controlled respiration. Administer naloxone (Narcan) to reverse the opioid-induced respiratory depression and sedation by displacing the opioids at the receptor site. In opioid-dependent individuals, it can also induce acute drug withdrawal. The intravenous route of administration is the preferred method of administering naloxone. Its effects are seen within 2 minutes. Naloxone can also be given intramuscularly or subcutaneously, but the onset of action is then seen within 2 to 5 minutes. Naloxone is shorter acting than most opioids; therefore to prevent the recurrence of respiratory depression, it must be administered by a continuous infusion or by repeated injections (intramuscularly or subcutaneously). See the drug monograph on naloxone, p. 143, for additional information.

PREGNANCY SAFETY

Category	Drug
B	diclofenac, flurbiprofen, ketoprofen, nalmefene, naloxone, naproxen
C	auranofin, aurothioglucose, buprenorphine, codeine, dezocine, diflunisal, etodolac, fentanyl, hydrocodone, hydromorphone, ketorolac, morphine, nabumetone, naltrexone, opium, oxaprozin, pentazocine, tolmetin, mefenemac acid
Unclassified	butorphanol, fenoprofen, indomethacin, levorphanol, meclofenamate, meperidine, methadone, nalbuphine, oxycodone, oxymorphone, penicillamine, piroxicam, propoxyphene, sulindac, tiaprofenic acid

pressure (may increase) or severe inflammatory bowel disease (risk of toxic megacolon). See the box for management of opioid overdose and the box for Food and Drug Administration (FDA) pregnancy safety classifications.

Contraindications

Avoid the use of opioids in patients with known opioid drug hypersensitivity, acute respiratory depression, or drug-induced diarrhea, that is, pseudomembranous colitis, which is caused by cephalosporins, lincomycins, and penicillins. In epidural or intrathecal drug administration, the contraindications include coagulation defects that may be caused by anticoagulant therapy or a hematologic disorder or infection at or near the site of administration.

BOX 8-2 Analgesic Equivalency Chart

All analgesics are compared with 10 mg (IM) of morphine to determine an analgesic dosage equivalent. **Equianalgesic** information, that is, the dose of one drug that produces approximately the same analgesic effect as the dose of another drug, is very useful information for the healthcare professional who is considering drug alternatives.

Analgesic	*IM dose (mg)*	*Oral dose (mg)*
morphine	10	20-60*
hydromorphone	1.5	7.5
oxycodone	Not available	15-30
levorphanol	2	4
methadone	10	20
meperidine	75	300

Suppository Dosage Form

Hydromorphone, 3 mg, is approximately equivalent to 1.5 mg IM dosage.
Morphine, 10-30 mg, is considered equivalent to the oral dosage.
Individualize dosage according to patient response.
Oxymorphone, 5-10 mg, is approximately equivalent to 1 mg of IM oxymorphone.

*For a single dose or intermittent use. Chronic administration may decrease oral dose to 20 or 30 mg equivalent.

Dosage and administration

See Table 8-2 for dosing information for opioid analgesics for infants, children, and adults. The analgesic equivalency chart shown in Box 8-2 may be used to determine drug equivalencies when a prescriber changes a patient's drug from one route of administration to another or from one drug to another opioid medication.

Continuous Infusion of Opioids

Continuous opioid infusions may be used when traditional routes of administration are inappropriate or have failed to provide satisfactory pain relief. Examples include intractable vomiting or severe local bruising after IM or SC injection, severe pain that is not relieved by oral, rectal, or intermittent parenteral opioid dosing, or pain management in the post-operative period. Intravenous opioids are helpful for short-term treatment of severe pain.

Opioids may be infused by a microdrip infusion set and pump or by a patient-controlled analgesia (PCA) infusion

A

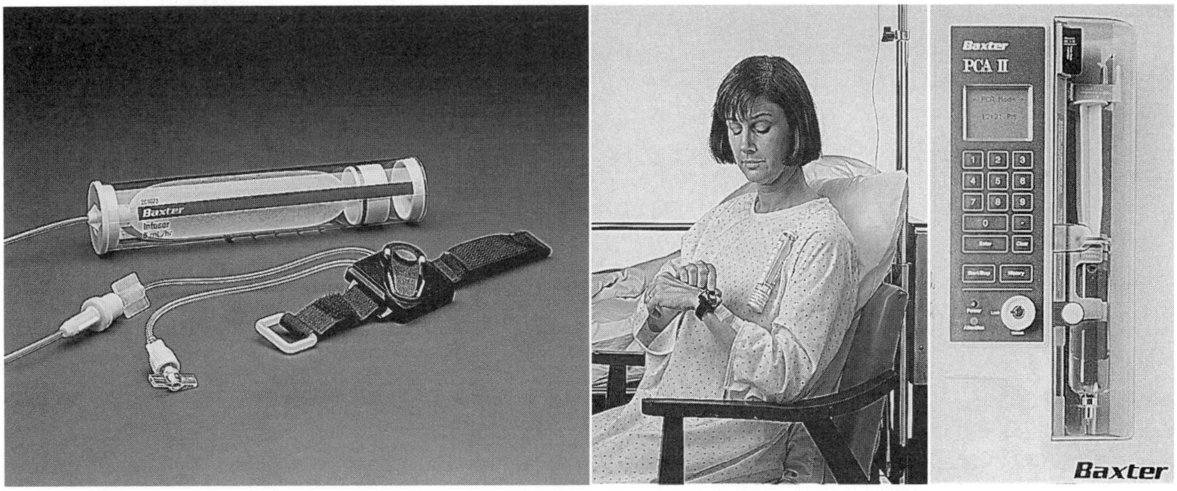

B

FIGURE 8-10
Examples of continuous infusion pumps. **A,** Portable wrist mode. **B,** Patient-controlled analgesia (PCA) pump is designed for patient- or clinician-activated medication delivery. *(Courtesy of Baxter Healthcare Corporation, Deerfield, Ill.)*

pump unit. The PCA unit is commonly ordered in a hospital setting, usually after surgery. It is programmed to deliver a predetermined IV opioid dose when the patient triggers the pump mechanism. This dose is based on the prescriber's order of a specific analgesic dose and a lockout interval (from 5 to 20 minutes). The lockout mechanism protects the patient from excessive releasing of the medication; thus it prevents overdosing. Fig. 8-10, *A* illustrates a portable wrist model of a PCA unit, and Fig. 8-10, *B* shows the CADD PCA pump that can be programmed for continuous drug administration, patient-activated drug release, or clinician-activated drug release. This unit also records all patient bolus attempts so that the prescriber can evaluate the individual's need for the analgesic. The units are usually lightweight and can be worn by ambulating patients in selected settings.

Astramorph/PF and Duramorph are morphine sulfate solutions that are preservative free. They are commonly prescribed for intravenous, epidural, or intrathecal use. Morphine's relatively poor lipid solubility delays the onset of analgesia when morphine is administered by epidural or intrathecal injection (see Table 8-4). Thereafter additional "breakthrough" analgesics may be prescribed. The risk of inducing respiratory depression is reportedly greater by the intrathecal route than by epidural administration (USP DI, 1998).

Opium Preparations

Opium contains several alkaloids that include morphine and small amounts of codeine and papaverine. The effects of opium result from the presence of morphine in the preparations. The mechanism of action and pharmacokinetics are the same as or similar to those of morphine.

Opium tincture contains 10 mg of morphine/mL and is used as an antidiarrheal agent and, when diluted, for the treatment of neonatal opioid dependence.

Camphorated tincture of opium (paregoric) contains 2 mg of morphine/5 mL. It is an antidiarrheal agent. In some instances, it has been used to treat neonatal opioid dependence, but this use is controversial. Paregoric contains camphor, which can cause serious toxicity including seizures and respiratory depression, and benzoic acid, which can displace bilirubin from albumin. Both substances may increase the typical problems seen in such infants (such as convulsions and hyperbilirubinemia); therefore many prescribers seem to prefer the use of diluted opium tincture to paregoric.

Opium alkaloid hydrochloride 🍁 injection (Pantopon) contains 10 mg of morphine/mL. This product is only available in Canada. Opium and belladonna suppositories (B & O Supprettes, No. 15A) contain 30 mg of powdered opium (10% morphine and other alkaloids) and 16.2 mg of powdered belladonna alkaloid (the principal belladonna alkaloids are atropine and scopolamine). Number 16A contains 60 mg of powdered opium and 16.2 mg of belladonna extract. The preparations are used to relieve moderate-to-severe pain reported with ureteral spasms and have also been prescribed for breakthrough pain between injections of opioids. For warnings, contraindications, side effects and adverse reactions, and significant drug interactions, see the discussion on morphine.

The adult dosage of opium tincture is 0.3 to 1 mL PO four times daily up to a maximum of 6 mL daily. The adult dosage for paregoric (camphorated tincture of opium) is 5 to 10 mL PO one to four times daily up to a maximum of 10 mL four times daily. The pediatric dose of paregoric for children 2 years of age and older is 0.25 to 0.5 mL/kg of body weight one to four times daily.

codeine (koe′ deen) (Paveral ♣)

Codeine is available in sulfate and phosphate salts and marketed as oral tablets, oral solution, and injectable dosage forms. Codeine is absorbed well after either oral or parenteral administration and is excreted by the kidneys. Oral administration is used for analgesic, antitussive, and antidiarrheal effects. Codeine may also be injected for treatment of mild-to-moderate pain. See Tables 8-2 and 8-4 for dosing data and pharmacokinetic overviews for opioid analgesics.

hydrocodone bitartrate (hye droe koe′ doen) (Hycodan)

Hydrocodone is marketed in combination with homatropine in the United States. But in Canada, Hycodan is hydrocodone bitartrate only. Although the product name is the same in both countries, the formulation is not identical. Hydrocodone bitartrate is used as an analgesic and antitussive. See Tables 8-2 and 8-4 for additional information.

hydromorphone (hye droe mor′ fone) (Dilaudid, Dilaudid HP)

Hydromorphone is a semisynthetic opioid that has a faster onset of action but a shorter duration of action than morphine. It is prescribed for its analgesic and antitussive effects. See Tables 8-2 and 8-4 for additional information.

meperidine (me per′ i deen) (Demerol, Pethidine)

Meperidine is an effective analgesic for short-term use but is considered "the least potent of the common opioid analgesics, and is administered in the largest doses" (Mather, Denson, 1992, p. 81). A commonly prescribed opioid, it has a pharmacologic profile similar to that of morphine with the following noted differences:

1. Meperidine is less apt to release histamine or to increase biliary tract pressure than morphine; thus it is often prescribed for patients with acute asthma, biliary colic, and pancreatitis (Sinatra, Savarese, 1992).
2. Its duration of action is shorter than morphine's, thus a more frequent dosing schedule is necessary (see Table 8-4).
3. Meperidine has poor oral bioavailability. To achieve an approximate analgesic equivalency to a 75 mg intramuscular dose requires an oral dose of 300 mg (USP DI, 1998). Because the largest oral form of meperidine marketed is a 100 mg tablet, this preparation is often prescribed in dosages that may be less effective than the injectable dosage form. See Table 8-2 for dosing data.
4. Meperidine is metabolized in the liver to normeperidine, a CNS neurotoxic metabolite. Normeperidine has a half-life between 15 and 20 hours in persons with normal renal function. Prolonged administration, use of high doses, or use in older adults or in persons with impaired renal or hepatic function has resulted in normeperidine-induced CNS toxicity. This neurotoxicity may produce significant mood changes such as sadness, anger, restlessness and apprehension, increased irritability, nervousness, tremors, agitation, quivering, convulsions, and myoclonus (AHFS, 1998; Jacox et al, 1994). Neurotoxicity has also been reported in patients with sickle cell anemia, burn injuries, or cancer who had normal renal and hepatic function but were receiving repeated large doses of meperidine (AHFS, 1998).
5. Meperidine produces a vagolytic effect, resulting in significant tachycardia; therefore its use should probably be avoided or closely monitored in patients with dysrhythmias or myocardial infarction.
6. Review the drug interaction section, especially for concurrent use of MAO inhibitors with meperidine. It is contraindicated for use in patients taking MAO inhibitors as very severe, unpredictable life-threatening reactions may result.

methadone (meth′ a done) (Dolophine, Methadose)

Methadone is an effective analgesic with properties similar to those of morphine, with the exception of its extended half-life. The duration of action for methadone is usually listed at 4 to 6 hours, but with repeated oral dosing, the half-life may extend from 22 to 48 hours (perhaps even longer in the elderly and in patients with renal dysfunction). This extended half-life is *not* related to its analgesic effect. To control pain methadone is administered every 6 to 8 hours, based on the individual's response. See Table 8-2 for dosing information.

Because of its extended half-life, methadone is approved by the FDA for use in state-approved detoxification and maintenance treatment programs. In Canada, it is available through specially authorized physicians. Oral administration is preferred for detoxification and required for maintenance programs. Methadone dependence is substituted in individuals who are physiologically dependent on heroin, opium, or other opioids. See Chapter 6 for information on methadone treatment programs. The mechanism of action of methadone is similar to that of morphine, as are the pharmacokinetics (see Table 8-4). Side effects and adverse reactions are also similar to those for morphine, although methadone's miotic and respiratory depressant effects may be present for more than 24 hours. Excessive sedation is reported in some patients after a regular dosing schedule.

levorphanol (lee vor′ fa nole) (Levo-Dromoran)

Levorphanol is an opioid analgesic used for moderate-to-severe pain. This drug has a longer analgesic duration of effect than morphine or meperidine (AHFS, 1998) and a half-life of 12 to 16 hours (Olin, 1998). Therefore the use of large or too frequently administered doses, chronic dosing to children or small adults, or even average doses in medically compromised patients may result in a drug accumulation and overdose (PDR, 1998). Closely monitor patients receiving levorphanol. See Tables 8-2 and 8-4 for additional information.

oxycodone (ox i koe′ done) (Roxicodone)

Oxycodone is approximately 10 times more potent than codeine. It is available alone and in combination with aspirin (Percodan) or acetaminophen (Tylox, Percocet) and in an extended-action dosage form (OxyContin). See Tables 8-2 and 8-4 for additional information. The suppository dosage form is not available in the United States but is available in Canada.

oxymorphone (ox i mor′ fone) (Numorphan)

Oxymorphone is pharmacologically similar to morphine with the following exceptions: in **equianalgesic** dosages, oxymorphone usually causes more nausea, vomiting, and psychic effects (euphoria) than morphine; and it may also be less constipating and cause less suppression of the cough reflex than morphine. Oxymorphone is a potent analgesic used for moderate-to-severe pain, for preoperative medication, for obstetric analgesia, and as adjunct therapy for the treatment of anxiety caused by dyspnea resulting from pulmonary edema associated with left ventricular failure. It is available in parenteral and rectal suppository dosage form. See Tables 8-2 and 8-4 for additional information.

fentanyl (fen′ ta nil)

Fentanyl is an opioid analgesic available in a preservative-free solution (Sublimaze), in combination with droperidol (Innovar), and as a topical transdermal patch (Duragesic). Fentanyl solution and fentanyl with droperidol are used parenterally (IV) for analgesia as a premedication, as an adjunct to anesthesia, and in the immediate postoperative period. Parenteral administration of fentanyl should be restricted to those experienced with this product and with the management of fentanyl-induced respiratory depression. Fentanyl and the fentanyl derivative sufentanil (Sufenta), if given rapidly in large doses, may cause chest wall muscle rigidity, which then requires supportive respiratory ventilation and perhaps a rapid-acting muscle relaxant. This depression is dose related (USP DI, 1998).

Fentanyl is metabolized in the liver and excreted in urine. Drug interactions and side effects and adverse reactions are similar to those for the other opioids. The patch system is available in 25, 50, 75, and 100 μg/hr dosage forms. The manufacturer publishes an equianalgesic potency chart and a morphine to fentanyl conversion chart that should be used to determine the fentanyl dose. See Box 8-3 for additional tips for transdermal administration of fentanyl.

BOX 8-3 Tips for Transdermal Administration of Fentanyl

- Fentanyl is used to provide continuous opioid administration through the skin.
- Water should be used to clean the skin area before application. Do not use soap, oil, lotion, alcohol, or other products because they may alter absorption of this product.
- The patch should be applied intact (do not cut or damage the system) to a flat nonhairy body surface, preferably the upper torso, front or back. Avoid exposing the patch site to direct heat sources such as a heating pad, electric blanket, heat lamp, or hot tub because increased fentanyl release, absorption, and toxicity may result.
- This transdermal patch has a slow onset of action; therefore other shorter-acting analgesics should be administered as ordered when therapy is initiated.
- Fentanyl has a long duration of action (up to 72 hours); therefore side effects and adverse reactions are not easily reversed.
- Fentanyl is *contraindicated* for the treatment of mild, acute, postoperative, or intermittent pain.
- Fentanyl serum levels may increase by one third in patients with a body temperature of 40° C (102° F).
- Fentanyl should not be administered to children younger than 12 years of age or to patients younger than 18 years of age who weigh less than 50 kg (110 lb).
- Fentanyl should not be used in nursing women because it is excreted in human milk.
- Patches should be kept away from children. To discard used patches or patches no longer needed, fold on the adhesive side and flush down the toilet

From PDR, 1998.

propoxyphene (proe pox′ i feen) (Darvon)
propoxyphene napsylate combinations (Darvocet-N)

Propoxyphene is a synthetic analgesic structurally related to methadone that is indicated for the treatment of mild-to-moderate pain. Controlled studies have reported that propoxyphene 65 mg is equivalent to or less effective than acetaminophen 650 mg, aspirin 650 mg, codeine 32 mg, pentazocine (Talwin) 30 mg, or meperidine (Demerol) 50 mg (McCaffery, Pasero, 1999). When combined with aspirin or acetaminophen, propoxyphene combinations usually provide analgesia greater than either medication alone.

Propoxyphene binds to opioid receptors and produces an analgesic effect similar to that of codeine and the opioids. The hydrochloride dosage form is more rapidly absorbed than the water-insoluble napsylate formulation, although peak serum levels are approximately equivalent. The bioavailability of propoxyphene hydrochloride 65 mg is equivalent to that of propoxyphene napsylate 100 mg. The duration of action of propoxyphene is 4 to 6 hours. Propoxyphene crosses into the CNS and is believed to cross the placenta

Metabolism occurs mainly in the liver where approximately one fourth of the dose is metabolized to norpropoxyphene, a toxic metabolite with a half-life of 30 to 36 hours (USP DI, 1998). Norpropoxyphene is a toxic metabolite with a half-life of 30 to 36 hours; this product is also more apt to cause convulsions than most of the other opioid analgesics. See Table 8-4 for pharmacokinetic information.

The usual adult dose for propoxyphene and propoxyphene napsylate is 65 or 100 mg every 4 hours when needed. The pediatric dose is not established.

tramadol (tram′ a doe) (Ultram)

Tramadol is a central-acting synthetic analgesic that is not chemically related to the opioids. This product appears to bind to the mu opioid receptors and also inhibits the reuptake of norepinephrine and serotonin. It is indicated for the treatment of moderate-to-moderately severe pain.

Although this product was initially believed to have a lesser potential for respiratory depression and drug dependency, in 1996 the manufacturer sent a letter to healthcare professionals to warn them of potential seizures, anaphylactoid reactions, and drug abuse associated with tramadol (FDA News and Product Notes, 1996). Therefore this product is not recommended for use in persons with a history of opioid allergy, dependence, or a past or present history of addiction.

Pharmacokinetics

Tramadol is well absorbed orally with an onset of action within 60 minutes, a peak effect in 2 hours, and a half-life of approximately 6 to 7 hours. It is metabolized in the liver to inactive and active metabolites and primarily excreted in urine.

Drug interactions

The following effects may occur when tramadol is given with the drugs listed below:

Drug	Possible Effect and Management
Alcohol, anesthetics, and CNS depressants	Concurrent administration with tramadol may result in an increase in CNS-depressant effects. An increased risk of seizures may result if tramadol is given with a tricyclic antidepressant, fluoxetine, or sertraline. A dosage reduction is highly recommended.
carbamazepine (Tegretol)	Increases the metabolism of tramadol. A dosage increase in tramadol may be necessary.
MAO inhibitors (furazolidone [Furoxone], procarbazine [Matulane],phenelzine [Nardil], tranylcypromine [Parnate])	Monoamine oxidase is necessary for serotonin metabolism while tramadol inhibits the reuptake of serotonin. Serotonin is suspected to be responsible for this drug's toxic effects; therefore concurrent use may lower the seizure threshold, resulting in an increase in toxic effects. If drugs are administered concurrently, monitor closely.

Side effects and adverse reactions

These include abdominal distress, anorexia, increased anxiety, weakness, constipation, confusion, dizziness, insomnia, sweating, visual disturbances, and urinary retention and frequency.

Warnings

Use with caution in patients with seizure disorders, head trauma, renal or liver impairment, acute abdominal problems, and a history of drug abuse and in children and the elderly with increased intracranial pressure.

Contraindications

Avoid use in patients who are hypersensitive to tramadol or someone intoxicated with alcohol or other CNS-depressant drugs.

Dosage and administration

The usual adult dose is 50 to 100 mg every 6 hours. The maximum daily dose is 400 mg.

OPIOID ANTAGONISTS

Naloxone, naltrexone, and nalmefene are opioid antagonists that competitively displace opioid analgesics from their receptor sites, thus reversing their effects. Nalmefene is a chemical analog of naltrexone and at full dosages it has a longer duration of action than naloxone. Nalmefene and naloxone are administered parenterally, whereas naltrexone is available in a oral dosage formulation.

Antagonists block subjective and objective opioid effects and can precipitate withdrawal symptoms in individuals physically dependent on opioids. These products are used to reverse the adverse or overdosage effects of opioids (codeine, diphenoxylate, fentanyl, heroin, hydromorphone, levorphanol, meperidine, methadone, morphine, oxymorphone, opium derivatives, and propoxyphene) and of the partial agonists (agonist-antagonist drugs such as butorphanol, nalbuphine, and pentazocine). Respiratory depression induced by nonopioids (e.g., barbiturates), CNS depression, or disease progression will usually not respond to antagonist drug therapy. It has also been reported that larger drug doses are necessary to antagonize the effects of buprenorphine, butorphanol, nalbuphine, or pentazocine. The effects of a buprenorphine overdose, though, may not be reversed by these agents or, at best, may be only partially reversed (USP DI, 1998).

In an opioid analgesic overdosage, the antagonist drugs will reverse the respiratory depression, sedation, pupillary miosis (constriction), and euphoric effects; they may also reverse the psychotomimetic effects of the agonist-antagonist analgesics (pentazocine and others). The drugs are believed to work at all three receptor sites, but their greatest activity is for mu receptors. See Chapter 6 for management of an opioid overdose.

Side effects and adverse reactions include nausea, vomiting, dizziness, hypertension, tachycardia, sweating, nervousness, abdominal cramps or pain, headache, weakness, joint and muscle pain, insomnia, and postoperative pain.

Pharmacokinetics and dosage

nalmefene (nal′ mah feen) (Revex)

Nalmefene has an onset of action of 2 to 5 minutes (IV) or 5 to 15 minutes (IM or SC). The time to peak levels is 1.5 hours by SC injection and 2.3 hours by IM injection; therefore the time to peak effect and duration of action is dependent on the dose and route of administration. It is metabolized in the liver and excreted primarily by the kidneys.

The adult dose to manage an opioid overdose is 0.5 mg/70 kg IV; a second dose of 1 mg/70 kg IV can be given 2 to 5 minutes later. To reverse a postoperative opioid depression, the dose is 0.25 μg/kg IV at 2- to 5-minute intervals, as necessary.

naloxone (na lox′ one) (Narcan)

Naloxone is inactivated orally, but is very effective parenterally. Its onset of action is 1 to 2 minutes (IV) and 2 to 5 minutes (IM or SC), and its half-life is between 60 and 100 minutes. The duration of action depends on the dose administered and the route of administration. Usually the IM dose results in a prolonged effect. Naloxone is widely distributed throughout the body and also crosses the placenta. It is metabolized in the liver and excreted via the kidneys.

The adult dose of naloxone is 0.4 to 2 mg as a single dose or 0.1 to 0.2 mg for postoperative opioid depression. For continuous infusion, 2 mg of naloxone may be diluted in 500 mL of normal saline or 5% dextrose injection. Because naloxone is shorter acting than most opioids, repeated naloxone injections or a continuous infusion is necessary to prevent the recurrence of respiratory depression.

naltrexone (nal trex′ one) (ReVia)

This drug is indicated for adjuvant treatment in the detoxified opioid-dependent person. Absorption is rapid, but naltrexone undergoes an extensive first-pass metabolism in the liver to the major metabolite 6-beta-natrexol, which also has opioid antagonist effects. The peak serum concentration is reached in 1 hour; elimination half-life for naltrexone is 4 hours and for its metabolite is approximately 13 hours. Its duration of action is dose dependent. Excretion is via the kidneys.

Treatment with naltrexone is started cautiously usually at a dosage of 25 mg orally with close monitoring for withdrawal signs and symptoms for approximately 1 hour. If no withdrawal effects occur, the balance of the daily dosage is given. Maintenance is usually 50 mg orally daily.

OPIOID AGONIST-ANTAGONIST AGENTS

Although the exact mechanism of action of the opioid agonist-antagonist agents is unknown, these agents have both agonist and antagonist effects on the opioid receptors. For example, buprenorphine (Buprenex) is a partial agonist at the mu receptors while butorphanol (Stadol), nalbuphine (Nubain), and pentazocine (Talwin) produce agonist effects at the kappa and sigma receptors and may displace agonists (opioids) from their mu receptor sites, thus inhibiting their effects and perhaps inducing a drug withdrawal reaction in patients physically dependent on agonist opioids. Dezocine (Dalgan) is partial agonist at the mu receptor with some effect at the sigma receptors after high doses. Generally, these drugs are less potent analgesics and have a lower dependency potential than opioids, and withdrawal symptoms are not as severe as those reported with the opioid agonist medications.

The opioid agonist-antagonist agents have pharmacokinetics, adverse effects, and significant drug interactions similar to those of morphine. Table 8-6 lists agonist-antagonist pharmacokinetics, equivalency, and dosing.

butorphanol tartrate (byoo tor′ fa nole) (Stadol)

Butorphanol tartrate is indicated for treatment of moderate-to-severe pain and as an anesthetic adjunct. It is administered parenterally (IM or IV) and in a nasal spray.

Drug interactions

The following effects may occur when butorphanol is given with the drugs listed below:

Drug	Possible Effect and Management
Alcohol or CNS depressants	May increase the potential for CNS depression, respiratory depression, and hypotension. Monitor closely for adverse effects because one or both drugs may need to be reduced.
buprenorphine (Buprenex)	May reduce the therapeutic effects of butorphanol, nalbuphine, or pentazocine at the kappa receptors. Increased respiratory depressant effects may occur when buprenorphine is given with low doses of other mu receptor agonists or kappa receptor agonists. Avoid concurrent administration.
MAO inhibitors	Use opioid analgesics (other than meperidine cautiously in reduced dosages. For safety's safe, one fourth of the usual analgesic dose should be given to determine the patient's response to this combination.

naltrexone (ReVia)	Use of naltrexone will precipitate withdrawal symptoms in the butorphanol-dependent patient. It will also negate any therapeutic use of the drug.

Color type indicates an unsafe drug combination.

Side effects and adverse reactions

These include drowsiness, gastric upset, confusion, constipation, dizziness, nausea, hypotension, psychotomimetic effects (occurs more often with pentazocine), and respiratory depression.

Warnings

Use these agents with caution in patients with a history of drug abuse, increased intracranial pressure, impaired or depressed respiration, and liver or renal impairment. Butorphanol should also be avoided in patients with cardiac disease, that is, congestive heart failure or myocardial infarction.

Contraindications

Avoid use in patients with known drug hypersensitivity.

Dosage and administration

See Table 8-6 for pharmacokinetics and dosing.

butorphanol (byoo tor′ fa nole) (Stadol)

Butorphanol is indicated for the treatment of moderate-to-severe pain and as an anesthetic adjunct. It is administered parenterally (IM or IV).

dezocine (dez′ oh seen) (Dalgan)

Dezocine, a potent parenteral opioid agonist-antagonist comparable to morphine in analgesic potency, onset, and duration of action, is indicated for the treatment of pain. It is administered parenterally (IM, or IV).

When dezocine is used concurrently with other CNS depressants, an additive CNS-depressant effect may occur. It is suggested that the dose of either or both drugs be reduced.

pentazocine (pen taz′ oh seen) (Talwin)

The analgesic pentazocine is not indicated for pain caused from an acute myocardial infarction because of its effects on cardiac function. It increases cardiac workload by increasing systemic and pulmonary arterial pressure, systemic vascular resistance, and left ventricular end-diastolic pressure. It also has a higher incidence of psychotomimetic side effects than the majority of other analgesics, thus limiting its usefulness, especially in terminally ill patients or those who are already anxious or fearful.

Pentazocine tablets are combined with naloxone (Narcan) in the United States because of the high incidence of pentazocine abuse. Naloxone taken orally is not pharmaco-

TABLE 8-6 Agonist-Antagonist Drugs: Pharmacokinetics, Equivalency, and Dosing

Drug	Equivalent Dose* (mg)	Onset (min)	Peak Analgesic Effect (min)	Duration (hr)	Half-Life (hr)	Usual Dose
buprenorphine (Buprenex)						
IV	0.3	<15	<60	6	2-3	0.3 mg q6h
IM	0.3	15	60	6	2-3	
butorphanol (Stadol)						
IV	2	2-3	30	2-4	2-4	0.5-2 mg q3-4h
IM	2	10-30	60	3-4	2-4	
Nasal spray	—	15	30-60	4-5	3-6	1 mg spray in one nostril q3-4h
dezocine (Dalgan)						
IV	10	<15	—	2-4†	2	2.5-10 mg q2-4h
IM	10	<30	60-120	2-4†	2	
nalbuphine (Nubain)						
IV	10	2-3	30	3-6	5	10 mg q3-6h
IM	10	<15	60	3-6	5	
SC	10	<15	—	3-6	5	
pentazocine (Talwin)						
PO	180	15-30	60-90	3	2-3	50 mg PO or 30 mg parenteral q3-4h
IM	60	15-20	30-60	2-3	2-3	
IV	60	2-3	15-30	2-3	2-3	
SC	60	15-20	30-60	2-3	2-3	

*Equivalent to 10 mg of morphine IM dose.
†Dose dependent.

logically active, but if this combination is dissolved and injected, naloxone will block the effects of pentazocine. Significant drug interactions are the same as those for butorphanol. SC administration is to be avoided because of tissue damage at the injection sites; IM sites should be routinely rotated for the same reason. See Table 8-6 for pentazocine pharmacokinetics and dosing.

nalbuphine (na′ byoo feen) (Nubain)

Nalbuphine, an analgesic for moderate-to-severe pain, is also used preoperatively as an adjunct to anesthesia and for obstetric analgesia. Drug interactions are similar to those for pentazocine. See Table 8-6 for pharmacokinetics and dosing.

buprenorphine (byoo pre nor′ feen) (Buprenex)

Buprenorphine dissociates very slowly from the mu receptor; thus it will reduce or block the effect of concurrent or subsequent dosing with opioid agonist drugs. It can precipitate withdrawal symptoms if administered to persons physically dependent on opioids. Buprenorphine-induced respiratory depression and other adverse effects are often difficult to reverse because naloxone is not very effective in treating buprenorphine-induced adverse effects. When naloxone is ineffective, the respiratory stimulant doxapram is recommended (USP DI, 1998). See Table 8-6 for pharmacokinetics and dosing.

Drug interactions

The following effects may occur when buprenorphine is given with the drugs listed below:

Drug	Possible Effect and Management
Other CNS depressants or MAO inhibitors	May result in increased CNS depressant effects, respiratory depression, and hypotension. Monitor closely since one or both drugs may need to be decreased by the prescriber.
Opioid analgesics	The therapeutic effects of the opioid may be reduced. In patients physically dependent on opioids, withdrawal symptoms may be precipitated by coadministration of buprenorphine. Avoid this combination.

Color type indicates an unsafe drug combination.

NONOPIOID ANALGESICS

The nonopioid analgesics are effective for mild-to-moderate pain and are often combined with opioid analgesics to enhance pain control in patients with severe pain. They correspond, in combination with a weak opioid, to step 2 in Fig. 8-9. The major drugs in this classification include acetaminophen, aspirin, nonsteroidal antiinflammatory drugs (NSAIDs), and the adjunct analgesics. These agents are used for the treatment of mild-to-moderate pain, fever, inflammation caused by rheumatoid arthritis, osteoarthritis, and various other acute and chronic musculoskeletal and soft tissue inflammations. The NSAIDs are also used to treat bone pain associated with metastatic cancer, usually in combination with an opioid analgesic (Twycross, 1994). Information about the over-the-counter (OTC) dosage forms of these preparations is given in Chapter 3.

Aspirin (acetylsalicylic acid) may also be prescribed to reduce the risk of transient ischemic attacks, myocardial infarcts, and stroke.

Mechanism of action

Aspirin and the NSAIDs peripherally inhibit the synthesis and release of prostaglandins. This effect on inflamed tissue is believed to be responsible for their analgesic and antiinflammatory action. Salicyates also block the generation of pain impulses and may have a central analgesic action in the hypothalamus. The NSAIDs also inhibit leukocyte migration and the release of the lysosomal enzymes, which contributes to their antiinflammatory effect.

Aspirin also inhibits the formation of platelet aggregation in the blood vessels by inhibiting prostacyclin. Prostacyclin is a platelet aggregation (reversible) inhibitor in blood vessels. Both effects may be dose dependent. Prescription salicylates include controlled-release aspirin 800 mg (Zorprin), salsalate (Disalcid and others), Trilisate, and magnesium salicylate (Magan). Salsalate is converted to salicylate during absorption from the gastrointestinal tract and in the liver. It (as well as Trilisate) has the advantage of producing few, if any, adverse gastrointestinal effects, and does not affect platelet aggregation. Salsalate's analgesic effects are equivalent to those of aspirin. The magnesium from magnesium salicylate may be absorbed, which may result in systemic toxicity in patients with renal impairment.

Acetaminophen appears to produce its analgesic effect by inhibition of prostaglandin synthesis in the CNS (predominant effect) and peripherally (USP DI, 1998). Although its exact mechanisms of action are unknown, antiinflammatory effects are minimal. The antipyretic effect for these agents is mediated centrally, via the hypothalamus. See the boxes for management of acetaminophen and aspirin overdoses.

NONSTEROIDAL ANTIINFLAMMATORY DRUGS

There are approximately 20 different NSAIDs now available in the United States. Although aspirin is also an NSAID, this term most commonly refers to the newer aspirin substitutes on the market. Aspirin and the OTC NSAIDs are reviewed in Chapter 3. The NSAIDs have analgesic, antipyretic, and antiinflammatory effects, although the indications for the individual NSAID may vary according to specific testing and clinical data submitted to the FDA for approval.

MANAGEMENT OF DRUG OVERDOSE

Acetaminophen

- Early symptoms: sweating, anorexia, nausea or vomiting, abdominal pain or cramping and/or diarrhea; usually occur in 6 to 14 hours after ingestion, lasting for approximately 24 hours
- Late symptoms: abdominal area may exhibit swelling, tenderness, or pain in 2 to 4 days after ingestion (hepatotoxicity)
- Treatment: gastric lavage or emesis. Start acetylcysteine administration as soon as possible. Determine acetaminophen serum levels at 4 hours or more, after ingestion. Hepatotoxicity is possible if serum acetaminophen level is more than 150 μg/ml at 4 hours, 100 μg/ml at 6 hours, 70 μg/ml at 8 hours, 50 μg/ml at 10 hours, or 3.5 μg/ml at 24 hours. Administer acetylcysteine orally as soon as possible, within 24 hours of ingestion. See USP DI (1998) for dosage instructions.
- Perform liver, renal, and cardiac function tests. Institute supportive measures as indicated.

The NSAIDs inhibit cyclooxygenase and prevent the synthesis of prostaglandins and thromboxane, which are responsible for the therapeutic effects and some of the adverse reactions of this drug classification (Fig. 8-11). Healthcare professionals should be aware, however, that the inflammatory process has a purpose in the body: it attempts to neutralize, destroy, or prevent the dissemination of the toxic or foreign substances. The cardinal signs of inflammation that result include swelling, pain, redness, and heat at the site. By interfering with prostaglandin synthesis, the NSAIDs tend to reduce the inflammatory process and utimately provide pain relief. It is quite possible that other actions (currently unknown) may also contribute to the therapeutic effects of these medications.

The NSAIDs are indicated for the treatment of acute or chronic rheumatoid arthritis, osteoarthritis, ankylosing spondylitis, and other rheumatic diseases; mild-to-moderate pain, especially when the antiinflammatory effect is also desirable (such as after dental procedures, obstetric and orthopedic surgery, and soft tissue athletic injuries); gouty arthritis; fever; nonrheumatic inflammation; and dysmenorrhea. Refer to a current package insert or to USP DI (1998) for a listing of approved and investigational uses of NSAIDs. The primary NSAIDs include the following:

Acetic acids:

diclofenac (dye kloe′ fen ak) (Voltaren, Voltaren-XR)
etodolac (eh toe′ doe lak) (Lodine)
indomethacin (in doe meth′ a sin) (Indocin)
ketorolac (kee′ toe roe lak) (Toradol)
nabumetone (na byoo′ me tone) (Relafen)
sulindac (sul in′ dak) (Clinoril)
tolometin (tole′ met in) (Tolectin)

MANAGEMENT OF DRUG OVERDOSE

Aspirin

- The treatment of an aspirin overdose may include gastric lavage or emesis followed by the administration of activated charcoal. Close monitoring is necessary to institute appropriate nursing or medical interventions such as correcting hyperthermia, fluid and electrolyte imbalance, acid-base imbalances, hyperglycermia, or hypoglycemia (especially in children).
- Serum salicylate levels are monitored until the concentration is lowered to a nontoxic level. For example, if large amounts of aspirin have been consumed and the salicylate concentration 2 hours after ingestion is 500 μg/mL (50 mg/dL), it would indicate a serious toxicity, whereas a serum level of 800 μg/mL (80 mg/dL) is potentially fatal. Prolonged monitoring of salicylate serum levels is indicated in massive salicylate overdose situations.
- Be aware that serum levels are not reliable for measuring degree of toxicity after consumption of large amounts of the delayed release formulations.
- Exchange transfusion, hemodialysis, peritoneal dialysis, or hemoperfusion may be necessary in patients who have consumed severe salicylate overdoses.

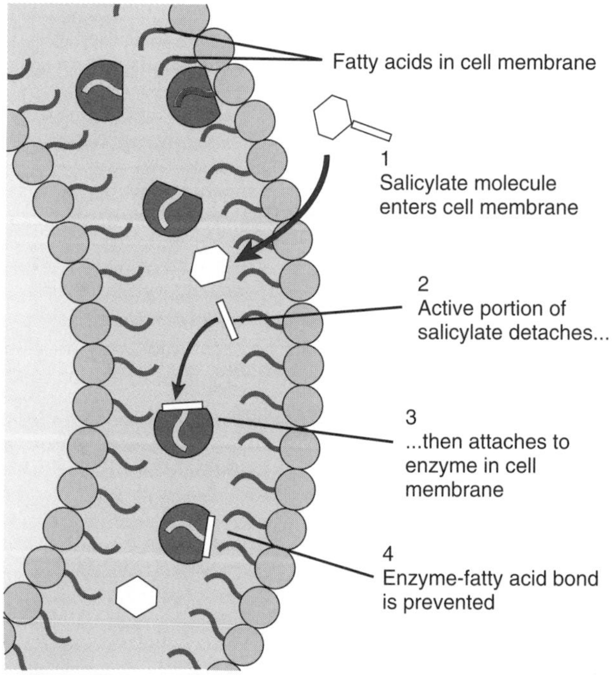
Fatty acids in cell membrane
1
Salicylate molecule enters cell membrane
2
Active portion of salicylate detaches...
3
...then attaches to enzyme in cell membrane
4
Enzyme-fatty acid bond is prevented

FIGURE 8-11
Inhibition of prostaglandin production. Inflammatory diseases and local injuries often lead to increased production of prostaglandins. Nonsteroidal antiinflammatory drugs (NSAIDs) act peripherally by entering the cell membranes (*1*); the active portion (salicylate) detaches (*2*), and attaches to the enzyme (cyclooxygenase) in the cell membrane (*3*). This new complex (*4*) cannot react with fatty acids to induce prostaglandin synthesis, thus reducing inflammation and pain in the affected area.

TABLE 8-7 Nonsteroidal Antiinflammatory Drugs: Pharmacokinetics, Dosing, and Comments

NSAID	***Onset of Action (hr)***	***Half-Life (hr)***	***Usual Adult Dosage (mg/day)***	***Comments****
Acetic Acids				
diclofenac (Voltaren)	0.5	1.2-2	50 mg tid or qid	Has less effect on platelet aggregation that most other NSAIDs (USP DI, 1998). Used to treat arthritis, pain, primary dysmenorrhea, and acute gout attacks.
etodolac (Lodine)	0.5	6-7	200, 300, or 500 mg tid or qid	Also has uricosuric effects. GI distress and ulceration reported less often (Insel, 1996).
indomethacin (Indocin)	0.5	4-6	25 or 50 mg bid to qid	Higher risk for GI effects and renal function impairment than other agents. Use cautiously in persons with epilepsy, depression, and Parkinson's disease because it may aggravate these conditions.
ketorolac (Toradol)	IM: 10 min (dose dependent)	PO: 4 IM: 6	30 mg IM/IV q6h, then 10 mg PO q4-6h	Should not be given by any route for longer than 5 days. Risk of GI bleeding and other severe effects increases with duration of treatment. Do not give preoperatively or intraoperatively if bleeding control is necessary. Severe allergic reactions or anaphylaxis may occur with first dose.
nabumetone (Relafen)	—	22	500, 750, or 1000 mg daily (hs) or in two divided doses	Prodrug (inactive), converted to active metabolite (6-MNA) in liver. Absorption increased by food and milk. Has lower reports of GI ulceration and bleeding than other NSAIDs.
sulindac (Clinoril)	—	8	150-200 mg bid	Renal calculi and biliary obstruction containing sulindac metabolites reported, although it is less likely than most NSAIDs to cause renal toxicity.
tolmetin (Tolectin)	—	5	400 mg tid	High evidence of anaphylactic reactions and may also cause serum sickness or flu-like syndrome (USP DI, 1998).
Fenamates				
meclofenamate (Meclomen)	1	2-3	50 mg tid or qid	Less effect on platelet aggregation than most other NSAIDs. Use cautiously in persons on sodium-restricted diet (USP DI, 1998).
mefenamic acid (Ponstel)	—	2	250 mg q6h	Less effect on platelet aggregation but can prolong prothrombin time. Used for short-term treatment of pain and dysmenorrhea; also for acute gouty attacks and vascular headaches.
Oxicams				
piroxicam (Feldene)	2-4	24	20 mg daily or 10 mg bid	Contraindicated in persons with renal impairment. May cause flu-like syndrome. May accumulate in elderly women (USP DI, 1998).
Propionic acids				
fenoprofen (Nalfon)	—	3	300 to 600 mg tid or qid	Contraindicated in persons with renal impairment. Food decreases absorption and peak serum levels; therefore administer 30 min before or 2 hr after meals unless GI distress occurs, then administer with milk.
flurbiprofen (Ansaid)	—	5.7	100 mg daily bid or tid	Similar to other agents in this category. Currently under study in transdermal patch to treat soft tissue lesions (Insel, 1996).
ibuprofen (Motrin, Advil)	0.5	2	300 to 800 mg tid or qid	Available in tablets, liquid, and OTC. May decrease blood glucose levels (USP DI, 1998). Incidence of GI side effects less than with aspirin (Insel, 1996)
ketoprofen (Orudis)		CAP: 1.6 ERC: 5.4 ERT: 3-4	25 to 75 mg tid or qid	Can cause fluid retention and increase in creatinine levels, especially in persons receiving diuretics and the elderly. Monitor renal function closely (Insel, 1996).
naproxen (Naprosyn)	1	13	250, 375, or 500 mg bid	Available in liquid, tablet, and extended-release tablets. Use tablets and liquid with caution in persons on sodium-restricted diet (USP DI, 1998).
oxaprozin (Daypro)		21-25	600 mg daily or bid	Has a long half-life that accumulates with chronic dosing. Half-life may be 40 to 60 hr or more, which increases with age (Insel, 1996). Discontinue oxaprozin at least 1 to 2 wk before elective surgery because it has a tendency to cause perisurgical bleeding (USP DI, 1998).
Salicylates				
diflunisal (Dolobid)	1	8-12	250-500 mg bid	Higher risk of causing renal impairment but less apt to cause antiplatelet effect than other NSAIDs (USP DI, 1998). Does not have any antipyretic effects (Insel, 1996)

CAP, capsule; ERC, extended-release capsules; ERT, extended-release tablets.
*All oral NSAIDs should be taken with 8 oz of water with person remaining upright for at least 15 to 30 min afterward (USP DI, 1998).

Fenamates:
meclofenamate (me kloe fen am′ ate) (Meclomen)
mefenamic (me fe nam′ ik) (Ponstel)
Oxicams:
piroxicam (peer ox′ i kam) (Feldene)
Propionic acids:
fenoprofen (fen oe proe′ fen) (Nalfon)
flurbiprofen (flure bi′ proe fen) (Ansaid)
ibuprofen (eye byoo proe′ fen) (Motrin, Advil)
ketoprofen (kee toe proe′ fen) (Orudis)
naproxen (na prox′ en) (Naprosyn)
oxaprozin (ox a pro′ zin) (Daypro)
Salicylates (which would also include aspirin and salsalate):
diflunisal (dye foo′ ni sal) (Dolobid)

The following are general pharmacokinetics; for specific NSAID pharmacokinetics, usual adult dose, and comments see Table 8-7.

Oral absorption of these drugs is very good. Food may delay absorption, but it has not been proven to significantly change the total amount absorbed. Protein binding is high (greater than 90%). Sulindac is an inactive substance (prodrug) that is converted by the liver to an active sulfide metabolite. Most of the agents are metabolized by the liver and excreted by the kidneys.

Drug interactions

The following effects may occur when NSAIDs are given with the drugs listed below:

Drug	Possible Effect and Management
Anticoagulants, oral (coumarin or indanedione, heparin, or thrombolytic agents)	May increase the risk of gastrointestinal ulcers or hemorrhage. Monitor closely for signs of these effects. Coumarin or indanedione anticoagulants may be displaced from protein-binding sites, resulting in an increased risk of bleeding episodes. Monitor closely with laboratory coagulation testing. Platelet inhibition may be dangerous for individuals receiving anticoagulant or thrombolytic agents. Avoid concurrent drug administration if possible. If an NSAID is necessary, the usual dosages of diclofenac, diflunisal, meclofenamate, and mefenamic acid reportedly are less likely to significantly affect platelets (USP DI, 1998). With concurrent therapies, monitor closely for potential serious side effects.
Antihypertensives, diuretics (especially triamterene [Dyrenium])	Flurbiprofen, indomethacin, ibuprofen, naproxen, oxaprozin, and piroxicam may reduce the effectiveness of antihypertensive agents. Monitor antihypertensive effect closely whenever an NSAID is used concurrently. Concurrent use of an NSAID and a diuretic may result in a decrease in diuretic, natriuretic, and antihypertensive diuretic effect. Diflunisal has not been reported to decrease furosemide's effectiveness, although diflunisal is reported to increase the serum level of hydrochlorothiazide and decrease the hyperuricemic response to hydrochlorothiazide or furosemide. May increase the risk of inducing renal failure in some patients. Triamterene and indomethacin reportedly caused acute renal failure or renal function impairment; therefore this drug combination should be avoided.
Administration of two NSAIDs concurrently, especially diflunisal (Dolobid) and indomethacin (Indocin) or aspirin	May increase the risk of gastrointestinal side effects, such as duodenal ulcers or hemorrhage. These combinations should be avoided.
cefamandole, (Mandol), cefoperazone Cefobid), cefotetan (Cefotan), picamycin (Mithracin), or valproic acid (Depakene)	These drugs may cause a decrease in prothrombin blood levels and an inhibition of platelet aggregation. Concurrent administration with an NSAID may increase the risk for bleeding episodes, gastrointestinal ulceration, and hemorrhage. Avoid concurrent administration if possible.
cyclosporine, gold compounds, nephrotoxic drugs	Concurrent use with NSAIDs may result in increased serum levels of cyclosporine and possibly gold compounds, resulting in an increased potential for nephrotoxicity. Concurrent use of nephrotoxic drugs and NSAIDs may also increase the risk for nephrotoxicity. Monitor closely during concurrent drug use.

lithium (Lithane)	Diclofenac, ibuprofen, indomethacin, naproxen, and piroxicam may decrease excretion of lithium, which may result in an increased lithium serum level and toxicity. Thus the possibility of inducing this effect with the other NSAIDs exists. Monitor lithium serum levels and for clinical symptoms of lithium toxicity during concurrent therapy and after the NSAID is discontinued.
methotrexate (Mexate)	Concurrent use of methotrexate with low to moderate doses of an NSAID may result in methotrexate toxicity. Adjust methotrexate as necessary according to methotrexate serum levels and the patient's renal function. This reaction can be severe and even fatal; therefore close monitoring is necessary.
probenecid (Benemid)	May result in an increase in serum levels of the NSAIDs and an increased risk of toxicity. Concurrent use with ketoprofen is not recommended, If probenecid is given with an NSAID, monitor closely, since a decrease in NSAID dosage may be indicated.
zidovudine (AZT)	When given concurrently with indomethacin, a decrease in the metabolism of zidovudine may result, leading to increased serum levels and toxicity. It is also possible that an increase in indomethacin serum levels and toxicity may occur. Avoid concurrent use of these medications.

Color type indicates an unsafe drug combination.

Side effects and adverse reactions

These include skin rash, pruritis, heartburn, nausea, vomiting, blurred vision, dizziness, drowsiness, tinnitus, gastric pain, distress and/or ulceration, GI bleeding, perforation, nephrotoxicity, dysuria, and hematuria.

Warnings

Use with caution in elderly and debilitated patients (see Geriatric Implications box), in persons with bleeding disorders, GI disorders, liver and renal impairment, and in patients with compromised cardiac function.

Contraindications

Avoid use in patients with a history of hypersensitivity or a severe allergic reaction to aspirin or to other NSAIDs, asthma, severe renal or liver disease, and ulcer disease.

GERIATRIC IMPLICATIONS

NSAIDS

The incidence of perforated peptic ulcers and/or bleeding is more common in the elderly taking an NSAID than in younger adults. Serious consequences more often occur in this age group.

Patients with renal impairment may be at increased risk for NSAID-induced liver or renal toxicity and often require a dosage reduction to prevent drug accumulation.

Clinicians have recommended that patients 70 years of age or older be started at one half the usual adult dose with close monitoring and careful dosage increases. A dosage increase should be based on the patient's therapeutic response and lack of signs and symptoms of toxicity. Special drug warnings include:

- Flurbiprofen (Ansaid) may result in elevated peak serum levels in women between 74 and 94 years of age. This serum level has not been documented in elderly male patients (USP DI, 1998). Therefore elderly women may need a lower dose to produce a therapeutic response.
- Indomethacin (Indocin) is responsible for a higher incidence of CNS side effects, especially confusion in the elderly.
- Naproxen (Naprosyn) administration in the elderly results in a higher proportion of unbound (free) naproxen, which may not be reflected by the total serum level. The steady-state concentration of unbound naproxen may be nearly double that of a younger adult, which may result in an increase in side/adverse/toxic effects, even with a normal serum level range. The health care professional should be aware of this potential because the prescriber may need to be notified about the possible need for a dosage reduction (USP DI, 1998).

Drug Combination

To reduce the gastrointestinal problems (bleeding, ulcers, and others) associated with NSAIDs, especially in high-risk patients, misoprostol (Cytotec), a gastric mucosa protecting agent, is added to the NSAID therapy. A new combination product was released that contains diclofenac and misoprostol (Arthrotec). It has been reported to lower the risk of ulcers by over 50% (Pharmacist's Letter, 1998). This product is available in two strengths, 50 or 75 mg of diclofenac, with both containing 200 μg of misoprostol. See Chapter 35 for a more thorough review of misoprostol.

Omeprazole (Prilosec) has also been proposed to reduce or prevent the GI problems associated with NSAIDs. This product is also reviewed in Chapter 35.

THROMBOXANE

Thromboxane A_2 is a potent vasoconstrictor that stimulates additional platelet aggregation, therefore inhibiting thromboxane A_2 formation, which decreases platelet aggregation.

Aspirin inhibits thromboxane synthetase, thereby preventing prostaglandin formation. Aspirin irreversibly blocks prostaglandin synthetase, whereas the other NSAIDs are primarily reversible inhibitors (USP DI, 1998).

OTHER DRUGS

Other products, such as the antimalarial agents (Chapter 53), gold salts, and penicillamine, are also used to treat inflammation in patients who have not responded to or cannot tolerate salicylates or NSAIDs. In addition, adjuvant analgesic medications are added to opioid medications to enhance analgesia.

Although in use for over 50 years in the treatment of rheumatoid arthritis, gold compounds are generally much slower acting and more toxic than the other products. Therefore they are reserved for individuals who demonstrate continued or increased disease activity while receiving conservative therapy.

auranofin (au rane′ oh fin) (Ridaura)
aurothioglucose suspension
(aur oh thee oh gloo′ kose) (Solganal)
gold sodium thiomalate injection
(Myochrysine)

Although the exact antiinflammatory mechanism of action is unknown, these drugs appear to suppress the synovitis of the acute stage of rheumatoid disease. Proposed mechanisms of action include inhibition of sulfhydryl systems and various enzyme systems, suppression of phagocytic action of macrophages and leukocytes, and alteration of immune response.

Gold products are indicated for the treatment of rheumatoid arthritis; aurothioglucose and gold sodium thiomalate are also used to treat juvenile arthritis.

Pharmacokinetics

The onset of action after oral administration is in 3 to 4 months, while parenterally it is in 6 to 8 weeks. The half-life of oral gold is 21 to 31 days in blood and 42 to 128 days in body tissues. Auranofin is rapidly metabolized, but the metabolism of aurothioglucose and gold sodium thiomalate is unknown. Excretion is primarily by the kidneys.

Drug interaction

Avoid concurrent use of gold compounds with penicillamine as an increased risk of serious blood dyscrasias and/or renal toxicity may result.

Side effects and adverse reactions

For auranofin these include abdominal distress or pain, gas, diarrhea, nausea, and vomiting. These effects are rare with the other gold products. The most frequent adverse effects include sore, irritated tongue or gums (less with auranofin), allergic skin reaction, and mouth ulcers or fungus.

Warnings

Use with caution in patients with thrombocytopenia or renal or liver impairment, and when cartilage and bone damage is already present. Be aware that elderly patients have difficulty tolerating gold products. Carefully review the benefit to risk ratio before using these products in patients with inflammatory bowel disease, skin rash, or a history of bone marrow depression.

Contraindications

Avoid use in patients with known gold drug hypersensitivity, uncontrolled diabetes, renal or liver disease, uncontrolled congestive heart failure, systemic lupus erythematosus, blood dyscrasias, severe hematologic disease, and marked hypertension, in pregnant patients, and in patients who have recently received radiation.

Dosage and administration

The adult dosage for auranofin is 6 mg daily with a maximum daily dose of 9 mg/day. The pediatric dosage has not been determined. The adult dosage for aurothioglucose suspension and gold sodium thiomalate injection is 10 mg IM the first week, increasing weekly according to the manufacturer's schedule until a total dose of 800 mg to 1 g has been reached. Maintenance dosage is 25 to 50 mg IM every 2 to 4 weeks, according to the manufacturer's schedule. In children 6 to 12 years of age, the dosage is 2.5 mg IM the first week and is increased weekly according to schedule until the total dose of 200 to 250 mg has been reached. Maintenance dosage is 6.25 to 12.5 mg IM every 3 to 4 weeks.

The gold sodium thiomalate pediatric dosage is 10 mg IM the first week, then 1 mg/kg (up to 50 mg/dose) following the adult recommendations for weekly intervals.

penicillamine (pen i sill′ a meen)
(Cuprimine, Depen)

Penicillamine is a chelating agent for heavy metals, such as mercury, lead, copper, and iron. The metals are made more soluble so that they can be readily excreted by the kidneys. The mechanism of action as an antirheumatic agent is unknown, although lymphocyte function is improved, and IgM rheumatoid factor and immune complexes located in the serum and synovial fluids are reduced. The relationship of these effects to rheumatoid arthritis is unknown.

Penicillamine is indicated for the prophylaxis and treatment of Wilson's disease, treatment of rheumatoid arthritis (especially for individuals with severe arthritis who have not responded to other therapies), and treatment of cystinuria.

Pharmacokinetics

The onset of action in Wilson's disease is 1 to 3 months and for rheumatoid arthritis is 2 to 3 months. Penicillamine is metabolized in the liver and excreted renally and in feces.

Drug interactions

Avoid concurrent use of penicillamine with gold compounds or phenylbutazone as very serious blood dyscrasias and/or renal toxicity may occur.

Side effects and adverse reactions

These include anorexia, diarrhea, loss of taste senses, nausea, vomiting, abdominal pain, allergic reactions, and stomatitis.

Warnings

Use with caution in patients with blood dyscrasias, Goodpasture's syndrome, and myasthenia gravis.

Contraindications

Avoid use in pregnancy with the exception of patients with Wilson's disease and certain patients with cystinuria (see current references). Women receiving penicillamine should not breastfeed. Avoid use in patients with renal impairment.

Dosage and administration

The adult dosage of penicillamine as a chelating agent is 250 mg PO, four times daily. As an antirheumatic agent, the dosage is 125 or 250 mg PO daily, increased if necessary at 2- to 3-month intervals, up to a maximum of 1.5 g/day. The dosage as an antiurolithic agent is 500 mg orally 4 times daily. For infants older than 6 months of age and young children, the chelating dosage is 250 mg daily, administered in fruit juice, while the antirheumatic agent has not been determined.

Adjuvant Medications

Adjuvant (coanalgesic) medications are used in combination with other analgesics to enhance pain relief or to treat symptoms that exacerbate pain or in some instances they are used alone to treat specifically identified pain. The NSAIDs are often listed with the adjuvant analgesics, but with this exception: the primary indications for adjuvant medications are not for the treatment of pain. Nevertheless, these agents have been reported to have an analgesic effect in some pain conditions.

Adjuvant analgesic medications include a variety of medications such as anticonvulsants, antidepressants, antihistamines, corticosteroids, local anesthetics, antidysrhythmics, psychostimulants, clonidine, and capsaicin.

Anticonvulsants, antidepressants, anesthetics, and antidysrhythmics are often prescribed for the treatment of neuropathic pain. They are frequently used in combination with opioids for cancer-associated nerve pain (Jacox et al, 1994; Salerno, 1996).

Corticosteroids are beneficial for cancer pain that originates in a fairy restricted area, such as intracranially, alongside a nerve root, or in pelvic, neck, or hepatic areas. Dexamethasone is prescribed for an increase in intracranial pressure and for relief of pain caused by pressure on a nerve. Corticosteroids may also relieve pain by suppressing the release of prostaglandins and thus inhibiting the inflammatory process.

The antihistamine hydroxyzine (Vistaril) is reported to have some analgesic properties (Haddox, 1992). It also has anxiolytic and sedative effects that may be useful in some patients. Psychostimulants, such as methylphenidate (Ritalin) and dextroamphetamine (Dexedrine), potentiate opioid analgesia and also help to increase alertness or reduce persistent, opioid-induced sedation in some patients. The analgesic effects are postulated to occur centrally and in the descending spinal inhibitory pathways. Opioid-induced cognitive impairment patients with cancer and acquired immunodeficiency syndrome (AIDS) has improved with administration of a psychostimulant drug (Bruera, Watanabe, 1994).

The usual approach to opioid-induced persistent sedation is to reduce the opioid dose and increase daily drug frequency. If the patient does not respond appropriately to this method, the opioid should be switched. If the sedation problem persists with these alternative strategies, a psychostimulant may be added to the opioid regimen (Jacox et al, 1994).

Additional useful adjuvant analgesics include clonidine (Catapres) and capsaicin. Clonidine is a centrally acting, alpha$_2$-adrenergic agonist that has been used for the treatment of pain associated with reflex sympathetic dystrophy (Rauck et al, 1993), diabetic neuropathy, postherpetic neuralgia, spinal cord injury, phantom pain, and pain in cancer patients who are opioid tolerant (Portenoy, 1993).

Capsaicin, an alkaloid found in chili peppers, is formulated into a topical cream (Zostrix) that is indicated for the treatment of neuralgia and arthritic pain. On application it causes an initial release and then a depletion of substance P from nerve fibers, which results in a decrease in pain transmission (Salerno, 1996). See the references at the end of this chapter for additional information on adjuvant medications.

SUMMARY

Pain is a major worldwide health problem that, as studies indicate, is often inadequately or inappropriately treated. It is the most common symptom reported that disables and distresses people. The attitude, fear of regulatory bodies, and biases of health care professionals, patients, and family a contribute to the unnecessary undertreatment of pain.

Very effective opioid analgesics that include morphine and other opioid agonists are available for the treatment and/or prevention of pain. Assessment tools, pain scales, and a step-approach as outlined in this chapter are the basic tools necessary for the development of an effective pain management program. The healthcare professional needs to be informed on the pharmacology and pharmacokinetics of these agents, in addition to the agonist-antagonists analgesics, NSAIDs and the opioid antagonists, the antidote for an opioid overdose.

The proper control of pain in the wide variety of patient populations should be the ultimate goal of a healthcare provider.

REVIEW QUESTIONS

1. What are the four primary myths or fears that interfere with healthcare professionals providing adequate pain management?
2. Describe the etiology and recommended drug therapy for bone and neuropathic pain.
3. Mr. Brown is a 59-year-od man with metastatic disease of unknown origin. He reports his pain as a 9 on a scale of 1 (least pain) to 10 (most severe pain). His prescriber ordered Tylenol #3 one or two tablets every 6 hours prn for pain. Two hours after receiving two tablets of this medication, the patient is still in very severe pain. Was this order appropriate for the reported pain level? Which medications would be appropriate for this level of pain? Should adjuvant medications and nonpharmacologic interventions be considered? Why?
4. Name three analgesics that should be avoided for use in the elderly patient. Review at least four potential issues to be considered when selecting an analgesic for a geriatric patient (areas to consider: the individual's current health problems, physiologic changes in the body, and others).

REFERENCES

Acute Pain Management Guideline Panel: *Acute pain management in infants, children, and adolescents: operative and medical procedures. Quick reference guide for clinicians,* AHCPR Pub No 92-0020, Rockville, Md, 1992, Agency for Health Care Policy and Research, Public Health Service, US Department of Health and Human Services.

American Hospital Formulary Service: *AHFS: drug information '98,* Bethesda, Md, 1998, American Society of Hospital Pharmacists.

Beers MH, Ouslander JG, Fingold SF et al: Inappropriate medication prescribing in skilled-nursing facilities, *Ann Intern Med* 117(8):680, 1992.

Bruera E, Watanabe S: Psychostimulants as adjuvant analgesics, *J Pain Sympt Manag* 9(6):412, 1994.

Carr DB, Jacox AK, Chapman CR et al: *Acute pain management: operative or medical procedures and trauma. Clinical practice guideline,* AHCPR Pub No 92-0032, Rockville, Md, 1992, Agency for Health Care Policy and Research, Public Health Service, US Department of Health and Human Services.

Cleeland CS, Gonin R, Hatfield AK et al: Pain and its treatment in outpatients with metastatic cancer, *N Engl J Med* 330:592, 1994.

Cohen F: Postsurgical pain relief: patients' status and nurses' medication choices, *Pain* 9:265, 1980.

Cushing M: Pain management on trial, *Am J Nurs* 92(2):21, 1992.

Eisenach JC: Pain relief in obstetrics. In *Practical management of pain,* ed 2, St Louis, 1992, Mosby.

FDA News and Product Notes: Ultram formulary, 31:450, 1996.

Foley KM: The relationship of pain and symptom management to patient requests for physician-assisted suicide, *J Pain Sympt Manag* 6(5):289, 1991.

Gossel TA, Wuest JR: Control of chronic cancer pain, *Fla Pharm Today* 57(4):21, 1993.

Gu X, Belgrade MJ: Pain in hospitalized patients with medical illnesses, *J Pain Sympt Manag* 8(1):17, 1993.

Haddox JD: Neuropsychiatric drug use in pain management. In Raj PP, editor: *Practical management of pain,* ed 2, St Louis, 1992, Mosby.

Hammack JE, Loprinzi C: Use of orally administered opioids for cancer-related pain, *Mayo Clin Proc* 69:384, 1994.

Insel PA: Analgesic-antipyretic and antiinflammatory agents and drugs employed in the treatment of gout. In Hardman JG, Limbird E, editors: *Goodman & Gilman's the pharmacological basis of therapeutics,* ed 9, New York, 1996, McGraw-Hill.

Jacox A, Carr DB, Payne R et al: *Management of cancer pain: clinical practice guideline no 9* AMCPR Pub No 94-0592, Rockville, Md, 1994, Agency for Health Care Policy and Research, US Department of Health and Human Services, Public Health Service.

Kinzbrunner B, Salerno E: *Vistas pain management formulary,* Miami, 1994, Vistas Healthcare Corp.

Lipman AG: The argument against therapeutic use of heroin in pain management, *Am J Hosp Pharm* 50(5):996, 1993.

Mather E, Denson DD: Pharmacokinetics of systemic opioids for the management of pain. In Sinatra RS, Hord AH, Ginsberg B, Preble M, editors: *Acute pain,* St Louis, 1992, Mosby.

McCaffery M, Pasero C: *Pain: clinical manual,* St Louis, 1999, Mosby.

McCaffery M, Ferrell B: Pain control decisions, *Nursing* 22(8):48, 1992.

McCarthy RL, Montagne M: The argument for therapeutic use of heroin in pain management, *Am J Hosp Pharm* 50(5):992, 1993.

McCombs J: Therapeutic considerations during pregnancy and lactation. In DiPiro JT, Talber R et al, editors: *Pharmacotherapy, a pathophysiologic approach,* ed 2, Norwalk, Conn, 1993, Appleton & Lange.

Melzack R, Wall PD: Pain mechanisms: a new theory, *Science* 150:971 1965.

Olin BR: *Facts and comparisons,* Philadelphia, 1998, JB Lippincott.

Patt RB: Classification of cancer pain and cancer pain syndromes. In Patt RB: *Cancer pain,* Philadelphia, 1993, JB Lippincott.

Pharmacist's Letter: Problems in patients taking NSAIDS (letter), 14(2):7, 1998.

Physicians' desk reference, ed 52, Montvale, NJ, 1998, Medical Economics Co.

Portenoy RK: Adjuvant analgesics in pain management. In Doyle D, Hanks GWC, Macdonald N, editors: *Oxford textbook of palliative medicine,* New York, 1993, Oxford University Press.

Porter J, Jick H: Addiction rare in patients treated with narcotics, *N Engl J Med* 302:123, 1980.

Rauck RL, Eisenach JC, Jackson K et al: Epidural clonidine treatment for refractory reflex sympathetic dystrophy, *Anesthesiology* 79(6):1163, 1993.

Salerno E: Pharmacologic approaches. In Salerno E, Willens JS, editors: *Pain management handbook,* St Louis, 1996, Mosby.

Salerno E, Willens JS: *Pain management handbook,* St Louis, 1996, Mosby.

Sinatra RS, Savarese A: Parenteral analgesic therapy and patient-controlled analgesia for pediatric pain management. In Sinatra RS, Hord AH, Ginsberg B, Preble M, editors: *Acute pain,* St Louis, 1992, Mosby.

Twycross R: *Pain relief in advanced cancer,* Edinburgh, 1994, Churchill Livingstone.

United States Pharmacopeial Convention: *USP DI: drug information for the health care professional,* ed 18, Rockville, Md, 1998, the Convention.
Wallace M: Assessment and management of pain in the elderly, *Medsurg Nurs* 3(4):293, 1994.
Warfield CA, editor: *Principles and practice of pain management,* New York, 1993, McGraw-Hill.
Watt-Watson JH, Donovan MI: *Pain management: nursing perspective,* St Louis, 1992, Mosby.
Weissman DE, Haddox JD: Opioid pseudoaddiction—an iatrogenic syndrome, *Pain* 36(3):363, 1989.
Welk TA: An educational model for explaining hospice services, *Am J Hospice Palliat Care* 8(5):14, 1991.
Willcox SM, Himmelstein DU, Woolhander S: Inappropriate drug prescribing for the community-dwelling elderly, *JAMA* 272(4):292, 1994.
Willens JS: Introduction to pain management. In Salerno E, Willens JS, editors: *Pain management handbook,* St Louis, 1996, Mosby.
Wong D et al: *Whaley and Wong's nursing care of infants and children,* ed 6, St Louis, 1999, Mosby.
World Health Organization: *Freedom from cancer pain: educational lecture for health care professionals.* Geneva, 1990, the Organization.
Zhukovsky DS, Gorowski E, Hausdorff J et al: Unmet analgesic needs in cancer patients, *Pain Sympt Manag* 10(2):113, 1995.

ADDITIONAL REFERENCES

Abramowicz M, editor: Bromfenac for analgesia, *Med Lett Drugs Ther* 39(1011):93, 1997.
Anderson KN et al, editors: *Mosby's medical, nursing, and allied health dictionary,* ed 5, St Louis, 1998, Mosby.
Covington TR, editor: *Handbook of nonprescription drugs,* ed 11, Washington, DC, 1996, American Pharmaceutical Association.
Kenyon J, editor: Fear of adverse effects should not hinder opioid use, *Drugs Ther Perspect* 1(6):13, 1993.
McGrath PA: *Pain in children: nature, assessment, and treatment,* New York, 1990, Guilford Press.
Mosby: *Mosby's GenRx,* St Louis, 1998, Mosby.
Patt RB: Using controlled-release oxycodone for the management of chronic cancer and noncancer pain, *Am Pain Soc Bull* 6(4):1, 1996.
United States Pharmacopeial Convention: *USP DI update: Bromfenac,* vol I and II, Rockville, Md, 1998, the Convention.

CHAPTER 9

Anesthetics

KEY DRUG

halothane (p. 158)

KEY TERMS

balanced anesthesia, (p. 155)
caudal anesthesia, (p. 167)
conduction anesthesia, (p. 167)
dissociative anesthesia, (p. 162)
general anesthesia, (p. 155)
infiltration anesthesia, (p. 155)
local anesthetic agents, (p. 155)
neurolepsis, (p. 161)
neuroleptanesthesia, (p. 163)
regional anesthesia, (p. 164)
saddle block, (p. 167)
spinal anesthesia, (p. 167)

CHAPTER FOCUS

The discovery of anesthesia and the development of new anesthetic drugs have resulted in many advances in modern surgical techniques that would not have been possible without these agents. The use of anesthetics serves to protect patients from pain and the fear and memory of surgery. Anesthetics also reduce surgical muscle damage while providing the surgeon with adequate time to perform advanced procedures.

OBJECTIVES

After reading and studying this chapter, the student should be able to do the following:

1. *Define and discuss the key drug and key terms.*
2. *Describe the four stages of general anesthesia.*
3. *List the most significant drug interactions with suggested management of agents that interact with anesthetic agents.*
4. *Discuss the six special disease states or risk factors that can alter an individual's response to anesthesia.*
5. *Explain the physiologic action of intravenous anesthetics.*
6. *Discuss the use and side effects of local anesthetics, adjunct medications, and the dissociative anesthetic ketamine.*

Anesthetic drugs are central nervous system (CNS) depressants that have (1) an affinity for nerve tissue and (2) a reversible action, that is, cells return to normal when the drug is eliminated from the cells. The two major classifications for these agents are general anesthesia and local anesthesia. **General anesthesia** induces a state of unconsciousness, general loss of sensation, and varying amounts of analgesia, muscle relaxation, and loss of reflexes. **Local anesthetic agents** block nerve conduction when applied locally or topically to nerve tissue. **Infiltration anesthesia** is the use of local anesthetics in an area that circles the operative field.

GENERAL ANESTHESIA

General anesthesia is generally induced by inhalation or intravenous injection of various anesthetic agents. This is an important mode of therapy, especially for surgical procedures.

MECHANISM OF ACTION

General anesthetics affect all excitable tissues of the body at concentrations that produce anesthesia. They vary widely in their chemical structure and individual effects and in the concentration necessary for each to produce a given state of anesthesia. Although many theories of anesthesia have been proposed, none satisfactorily explains the basic mechanisms of action. Indeed, different anesthetics may have different modes of action, and no single theory may suffice.

The pattern of depression is similar for all general anesthetics—irregular and descending. The medullary centers are depressed last. Fortunately the medulla is spared temporarily, since it contains the vital centers concerned with heart action, blood pressure, and respiration. Initially anesthesia produces a loss of the perception of sight, touch, taste, smell, awareness, and hearing. Usually unconsciousness is produced. The two classes of general anesthetics are inhalation anesthetics (gases or volatile liquids) and intravenous agents.

Balanced Anesthesia

A combination of drugs is necessary to produce all the desired effects sought with anesthesia. Analgesia, muscle relaxation, unconsciousness, and amnesic effects are not produced safely by a single anesthetic. The induction of anesthesia by using a combination of drugs, each for its specific effect, rather than by using a single drug with multiple effects, is termed **balanced anesthesia.** For example, anesthesia may be induced by premedication with a short-acting barbiturate or a benzodiazepine and then an opioid analgesic and a skeletal muscle relaxant, followed by administration of an anesthetic gas by the anesthetist. The specific drugs and dosages will depend on the procedure to be done, the physical condition of the patient, and the patient's response to the medications. The advantage of balanced anesthesia is a lower reported incidence of postoperative nausea, vomiting, and pain.

STAGES OF GENERAL ANESTHESIA

General anesthesia generally consists of four stages. The stages of anesthesia vary with the choice of anesthetic, speed of induction, and skill of the anesthetist. The current practice of inducing general anesthesia with an intravenously administered anesthetic before inhalation anesthesia promotes rapid transition from consciousness to surgical anesthesia, and the early stages of anesthesia are not seen. If the drug is given slowly enough, however, usually all stages can be observed. They are most easily seen when an anesthetic gas is used as the only anesthetic. Not all stages occur with all anesthetics.

Stage 1: Analgesia

This stage begins with the onset of anesthetic administration and lasts until loss of consciousness. Smell and pain are abolished before consciousness is lost. Vivid dreams and auditory or visual hallucinations may be experienced. Speech becomes difficult and indistinct. Numbness spreads gradually over the body. The body feels stiff and unmanageable. Hearing is the last sense lost.

The healthcare professional should maintain a quiet area for the patient because low voices and equipment sounds may be interpreted as excessively loud and may be counterproductive to the effects of the anesthetic.

Stage 2: Excitement

This stage varies greatly with individuals. Reflexes are still present and may be exaggerated, particularly with sensory stimulation such as noise. The patient may struggle, shout, laugh, swear, or sing. Autonomic activity, muscle tone, eye movement, and rapid and irregular breathing increase. Irregular respiration may cause uneven absorption of anesthetic; a period of apnea followed by a few deep breaths may produce a high concentration of anesthetic in the blood. Vomiting and incontinence sometimes occur in this stage.

The variability in this stage results from (1) the amount and type of premedication, (2) the anesthetic agent used, and (3) the degree of external sensory stimuli. Since the advent of balanced anesthesia, the signs and duration of this stage have been reduced.

Stages 1 and 2 constitute the stage of induction.

Stage 3: Surgical Anesthesia

The third stage is divided into four planes of increasing depth of anesthesia. Which plane a patient is in is determined by the character of the respirations, eyeball movement, and pupil size, and the degree to which reflexes are present. Most operations are done in plane two or in the upper part of plane three. As the person moves into plane one, the respiratory irregularities of the second stage usually have disappeared and respiration becomes full and regular. As anesthesia deepens, respiration becomes more shallow and more rapid. Paralysis of the intercostal muscles is followed by increased abdominal breathing; finally, only the diaphragm is active. A loss of reflexes occurs in a cephalocaudal direction, from the head downward. The eyelid reflex is lost and the eyeballs, which exhibit a rolling movement at first, gradually move less and then cease to move. Normally, if the pupils were reflexively dilated in the second stage, they now constrict to about their size in natural sleep. The reaction to light becomes sluggish. The pupils dilate as plane four is approached.

The patient's face is usually calm and expressionless and may be flushed or even cyanotic. The musculature becomes increasingly relaxed as reflexes are progressively abolished. Most abdominal surgery cannot be performed until the abdominal reflexes are absent, and the abdominal wall is soft. The body temperature is lowered as the anesthetic state continues. The pulse remains full and strong. Blood pressure may be elevated slightly, but in plane four the blood pressure drops and the pulse weakens. The skin, which was warm, now becomes cold, wet, and pale.

Because each phase of anesthesia is closely monitored by the anesthetist, he or she will give approval to begin the procedure.

Stage 4: Medullary Paralysis (Toxic Stage)

This stage is characterized by respiratory arrest and vasomotor collapse. Respiration ceases before the heart action, so artificial respiration and/or reduction of the gaseous agent may help in the reversal of this stage.

SIGNIFICANT DRUG INTERACTIONS

Among the dangers facing a surgical patient is an unexpected drug interaction occurring in preparation for or during anesthesia. Anesthetists must always be familiar with the interactions between anesthetics and the maintenance drug therapies used in a wide range of illnesses. A serious drug interaction may be underway before surgery, and the surgical anesthesia may complicate the interaction. A critical analysis of the surgical candidate's total drug regimen (prescribed, over-the-counter [OTC], and alternative/complementary medications) should be done in relation to the anesthetic drugs and preanesthetic drugs to be used.

Various pharmacologic classes of medication may result in adverse reactions in patients anesthetized for surgery. For example, anticoagulants such as heparin and coumarin are usually discontinued 48 hours before surgery to reduce the increased risk of hemorrhage, while CNS depressants such as opioids and hypnotics may increase the risk of enhanced CNS-depressant effects.

Antidysrhythmics such as propranolol hydrochloride may induce a decreased cardiac output, decreased heart rate, and bronchospasm. Quinidine, procainamide, and lidocaine may reduce cardiac conduction, increase peripheral vasodilation, and potentiate the effects of neuromuscular blocking agents, such as tubocurarine.

Combining local anesthetic agents with sympathomimetic or vasoconstrictive agents (such as epinephrine, phenylephrine, or methoxamine) can cause ischemia, leading to sloughing of tissue or gangrene in fingers, toes, or areas that have end arteries. If combined with local anesthetics, these agents should be carefully dosed and closely monitored.

Selected antihypertensive agents such as guanethidine (Ismelin) and methyldopa (Aldomet) deplete the synthesis or storage of norepinephrine in the sympathetic (adrenergic) nerve endings and may result in severe hypotension when combined with anesthetics and analgesics. Prescribers may consider reducing or stopping such medications before surgery.

When used as long-term therapy, corticosteroids usually produce adrenal gland suppression, which may result in hypotension during surgery. Because the stress of anesthesia and surgery usually increases the need for and release of endogenous corticosteroids, it is recommended that corticosteroid dosages be increased in the perioperative period.

Cholinesterase inhibitors such as echothiophate iodide (Phospholine Iodide) and demecarium bromide (Humorsol) and exposure to organophosphate insecticides may prolong succinylcholine blockade. Extended apnea and death have been reported with this combination. It is generally recommended that cholinergic eyedrops be stopped approximately 2 weeks before elective surgery.

Antibiotics—particularly aminoglycoside antibiotics (e.g., amikacin and gentamicin), clindamycin, tetracyclines, and polymyxin antibiotics—may potentiate the neuromuscular blocking agent or cause neuromuscular blockade. A reduction in the dose of the neuromuscular blocking agent may be necessary, along with careful titration of the drug. Patients with myasthenia gravis, Parkinson's disease, or other neuromuscular disorders must be monitored carefully.

Many other drugs have the potential for inducing an unwanted effect intraoperatively or postoperatively. Concurrent administration of various drugs with anesthetic agents requires close supervision and monitoring of the surgical patient. As a general guideline, if a drug is needed for treatment preoperatively, it should be continued through surgery. Unnecessary drugs are discontinued for a period at least five times the half-life of the drug before surgery. Drugs having significant interactions with anesthetic agents are replaced, when possible, with an alternative medication before surgery.

SPECIAL ANESTHESIA CONSIDERATIONS

Many disease states and risk factors can alter the individual's response to anesthesia. The preoperative assessment of the patient's health status by the healthcare professional should include acute and chronic medical conditions.

Alcoholism

The alcoholic may have a variety of associated disease states, including liver dysfunction, pancreatitis, gastritis, and

PREGNANCY SAFETY

Category	Drug
B	etidocaine, lidocaine, prilocaine, methohexital, enflurane, propofol
C	alfentanil, bupivacaine, chloroprocaine, dibucaine, etomidate, fentanyl, mepivacaine, methoxyflurane, sufentanil, tetracaine, thiopental
Unclassified	droperidol, halothane, ketamine, isoflurane, procaine, sevoflurane

BOX 9-1 Waste Anesthetic Gases as Occupational Health Hazard

Chronic exposure of healthcare providers in the operating room to waste anesthetic gases may present a significant occupational health hazard. Studies have demonstrated an increased incidence of spontaneous abortions among women exposed to nitrous oxide, as well as among wives of men who are exposed. In addition, neurologic, hepatic, and renal disorders have been seen in the chronically exposed. Healthcare providers should protect themselves by avoiding the area within a foot of the patient's mouth and nose when the breath contains exhaled anesthetic agents. Healthcare providers should be active in establishing exposure monitoring programs to detect unsafe levels caused by faulty equipment and unsafe practices.

esophageal varices. The anesthetic requirements for such a patient may be increased because of the increase in liver metabolizing enzymes and the development of cross-tolerance. The alcoholic patient is monitored closely during the postanesthetic period for alcohol withdrawal syndrome, since its onset may be delayed because of the administration of medications for pain relief. Pharmacologic intervention with diazepam or other agents may be required to prevent the occurrence of withdrawal symptoms.

Obesity

Overweight or obese patients may have cardiac insufficiency, respiratory problems, atherosclerosis, hypertension, or an increased incidence of diabetes, liver disease, or thrombophlebitis. In such patients, obtaining the desired depth of anesthesia and muscle relaxation may be a problem. Generally, fat-soluble anesthetics, especially those with toxic metabolites such as methoxyflurane (Penthrane), should be avoided.

Smoking

Individuals who smoke usually have an increasingly rigid arterial vascular system, adrenal gland stimulation, and perhaps lung disease (e.g., bronchitis, emphysema, or carcinoma). Therefore postoperative complications are six times more common in smokers than in nonsmokers. Smoking also increases the patient's sensitivity to muscle relaxants.

Pregnancy

See the box for Food and Drug Administration (FDA) classifications of anesthetic drug safety during pregnancy. Before any drug is used, the expected drug benefits should be considered against the possible risk to the fetus. Box 9-1 describes risks to healthcare providers.

Young Age

The physical characteristics of a neonate may predispose the infant to upper airway obstruction or laryngospasm during anesthesia or resuscitation. A small mandible and neck, a narrow cricoid ring, and a large body water compartment with a high extracellular water turnover rate, immaturely functioning liver and kidneys, and a rapid metabolic rate all contribute to the need for careful monitoring of the infant or pediatric patient. Drug dosages and administered fluids must be carefully calculated using the body weight or the surface area of the child. Halothane and nitrous oxide are commonly used in pediatrics because the incidence of hepatitis in children is considered rare after halothane usage. Neonates are usually more sensitive to the nondepolarizing muscle-relaxing agents (see Chapter 17).

Advanced Age

Aging results in a generalized decline in organ function (approximately 1% per year after age 30), the existence of chronic disease processes, or both. As the number and complexity of illnesses increase with age, the complexity of drug treatment also increases, which results in greater potential for drug interactions and side effects. Generally, an increased and prolonged drug effect is seen in the elderly. Mortality rates for the aged patient undergoing major surgery may be four to eight times higher than that for younger persons.

TYPES OF GENERAL ANESTHETICS

General anesthetics are usually divided into two groups: (1) the inhalation anesthetics, which include gases and volatile liquids; and (2) intravenous anesthetics, which include barbiturates and nonbarbiturates.

INHALATION ANESTHETICS

Inhalation, or volatile, anesthetics are gases or liquids that can be administered by inhalation when mixed with oxygen. These can effect a concentration in the blood and brain to depress the CNS and cause anesthesia. They have the following characteristics:

- They are complete anesthetics and thus can abolish superficial and deep reflexes.
- They provide for controllable anesthesia, since depth of

anesthesia is easily varied by changing the inhaled concentration.

- Allergic reactions to these agents are uncommon.
- Rapid recovery can occur as soon as administration ceases, since the anesthetic is excreted in expired air.

Although ether and chloroform as volatile liquids and cyclopropane and nitrous oxide as gases were commonly used over the years, only nitrous oxide is still in clinical use today. Chloroform is hepatotoxic, and ether and cyclopropane are highly flammable; thus these agents have been replaced by safer anesthetics. In 1956, halothane (Fluothane), a nonflammable agent, largely replaced the older volatile liquids. Halothane, though, has been associated with hepatic dysfunction and failure. Since then, newer, less toxic, volatile liquids have been developed: desflurane (Suprane), enflurane (Ethrane), isoflurane (Forane), methoxyflurane (Penthrane), and sevoflurane (Ultane).

Gases

nitrous oxide [nye′ trus ox′ ide]

Nitrous oxide, an anesthetic gas, is the most commonly used agent for dental surgery, minor surgery, and obstetric analgesia. It is often combined with other anesthetics to enhance its effects, so it is also used extensively in major surgery. It is excreted 100% unchanged through the lungs. Its few side effects consist primarily of postoperative nausea, vomiting, or delirium, and it has no known significant drug interactions.

For general anesthesia, the recommended dosage is 70% with 30% oxygen inhalation for induction and 30% to 70% with oxygen for maintenance.

At the termination of nitrous oxide anesthesia, the rapid movement of large amounts of nitrous oxide from the circulation into the lungs may dilute the oxygen in the lungs. This dilution may result in a phenomenon known as "diffusion hypoxia." To prevent this, the anesthetist usually administers 100% oxygen to clear the nitrous oxide from the lungs. During recovery the patient should be administered humidified oxygen by mask and encouraged to breathe deeply to promote ventilation.

Volatile Liquid Anesthetics

halothane [ha′ loe thayn] (Fluothane, Somnothane ✤)

Halothane is used primarily as a general anesthetic. Pharmacokinetics, side effects and adverse reactions, and toxicity are detailed in Table 9-1. Postoperative nausea and vomiting may occur in many patients and may be more frequent if nitrous oxide is used to supplement other anesthetics. A rare complication of halothane is liver damage, or "halothane hepatitis," although this belief is controversial. While the mechanism is not known, some experts believe the liver damage to be caused by a hypersensitivity-type reaction to a metabolite of halothane. The diagnosis is made on the clinical findings of unexplained fever, eosinophilia, rashes, and abnormal liver function tests within 2 weeks of exposure, especially after a repeat exposure. The syndrome is more common in older or obese persons and is not seen in children.

Significant drug interactions

Halothane sensitizes the myocardium to the effects of catecholamines (epinephrine, norepinephrine, or dopamine) or sympathomimetic agents (e.g., ephedrine and metaraminol). These agents may produce serious cardiac dysrhythmias in the presence of halothane. Levodopa, which pharmacologically increases the quantity of dopamine in the CNS, should be discontinued at least 6 to 8 hours before halothane is administered. Halothane is the only volatile anesthetic agent that sensitizes the myocardium.

Systemic aminoglycosides, lincomycins, polymyxins, and capreomycin, when given concurrently with any of the volatile anesthetics, may result in skeletal muscle weakness, respiratory depression, or apnea (absence of respiration). Patients usually require mechanical ventilation. If these medications are used, the dosage of the nondepolarizing neuromuscular blocking drugs should be decreased to one third or one half of the usually prescribed dosage.

Dosage and administration

See Table 9-1 for pharmacokinetics and dosing.

desflurane [des floo′ rayn] (Suprane)

Released in late 1992, desflurane is an alternative to halothane and isoflurane. It produces a more rapid induction and emergence from anesthesia than the following agents. The use of desflurane has been associated with a moderately high incidence of airway irritation, coughing, and laryngospasm. For this reason it is not indicated for anesthesia induction in pediatric patients, although it is approved for anesthesia maintenance in infants and young children.

enflurane [en floo′ rayn] (Ethrane)

Enflurane is indicated for induction and maintenance of general anesthesia. It is only slightly metabolized in the body. Its clinical effects are similar to those of halothane, but it is less potent. Enflurane may cause seizures when given at high concentrations; therefore it is not recommended for use with patients who are seizure-prone, such as those with epilepsy or head injuries.

isoflurane [eye soe floo′ rayn] (Forane)

Isoflurane is indicated for induction and maintenance of general anesthesia. It undergoes an extremely low degree of metabolism. Until the release of desflurane, it was promoted as having a more rapid action than the other inhalation agents and causing less cardiovascular depression. Nephrotoxicity is minimal with isoflurane.

TABLE 9-1 Volatile Liquid Anesthetic Agents

Agent	Pharmacokinetics: Absorption	Pharmacokinetics: Metabolism	Pharmacokinetics: Excretion	MAC (%)*	Toxicity	Side Effects and Adverse Reactions
halothane (Fluothane, Somnothane)	By lungs	Up to 20% by liver	60%-80% unchanged by the lungs; remainder excreted or metabolized through kidneys	0.75	May cause "halothane hepatitis"	Hypotension, cardiovascular depression, lowered body temperature, respiratory depression, malignant hyperthermia; emergence delirium—shivering and trembling, confusion, hallucinations, nervousness, increased excitability
desflurane (Suprane)	By lungs	<0.2% by liver	Primarily lungs	7.3	Airway irritation, severe laryngospasm, coughing	See halothane
enflurane (Ethrane)	By lungs	About 2.5% by liver	80% unchanged by lungs; remainder excreted as metabolites through kidneys	1.68		See halothane
isoflurane (Forane)	By lungs	Less than 1% by liver	Almost all through lungs: less than 1% as metabolites through kidneys	1.15		See halothane
methoxyflurane (Penthrane)	By lungs	About 50% by liver	35% unchanged by lungs; remainder excreted as metabolites through kidneys	0.16	Dose-related nephrotoxicity (renal tube damage) from fluoride metabolite	See halothane
sevoflurane (Ultane)	By lungs	—	Primarily lungs	2.1	Cardiac depressant (bradycardia)	See halothane

**MAC*, Minimum alveolar concentration (percent in oxygen) that prevents movement in 50% of patients exposed to painful stimuli. May need higher concentrations in some patients: generally highest in very young children, lowest with increasing age, pregnancy, hypotension, or concurrent CNS depressant use.

methoxyflurane [me thox′ i floo rayn] (Penthrane)

Methoxyflurane is used for anesthesia and analgesic effects. It is a potent anesthetic agent used for obstetric analgesia. It is given in concentrations of 0.3% to 0.8%. Methoxyflurane is highly metabolized, and a by-product of its metabolism is free fluoride, which is toxic to the kidney (nephrotoxic). Because of methoxyflurane's potential for nephrotoxicity, its use is limited to minor surgical procedures and obstetrics.

sevoflurane [sev oe floo′ rayn] (Ultane)

Sevoflurane is indicated for induction and maintenance during surgery. While the induction dose is individualized, the usual adult inhalation dose is between 0.5% to 3% alone or combined with nitrous oxide (USP DI, 1998). Sevoflurane has a faster uptake, distribution, and rate of elimination than isoflurane and halothane. When compared with desflurane, it has a slower uptake and distribution, but the rate of elimination is similar to that of desflurane (Olin, 1998).

INTRAVENOUS ANESTHETICS

Intravenous anesthetic agents are used for induction or maintenance of general anesthesia, to induce amnesia, and as an adjunct to inhalation-type anesthetics. The major groups include ultrashort-acting barbiturates, nonbarbiturates, dissociative anesthetics, and neuroleptanesthesia. Intravenous anesthetics are valuable to allay emotional distress, because many patients dread having a tight mask placed over the face while they are fully conscious. These anesthetics reduce the amount of inhalation anesthetic required. Box 9-2 lists advantages and disadvantages of intravenous anesthetics.

The intravenous anesthetics most commonly used are the ultrashort-acting barbiturates. These drugs are rapidly taken up by brain tissue because of their high solubility. For example, equilibrium between brain and blood occurs within 1 minute after injection of thiopental. Shortness of action results from the drug being quickly redistributed into the fat depots of the body. The amount of body fat affects drug action: the greater the amount of body fat, the briefer the effect of a single intravenous dose. With prolonged administration or large doses, however, prolonged drug action results in delayed recovery. This is caused by saturation of fat depots and the slow rate of drug release (10% to 15% per hour).

BOX 9-2 Advantages and Disadvantages of Intravenous Anesthetics

Disadvantages. Swelling, pain, ulceration, tissue sloughing, and necrosis if drug infiltrates into tissue; thrombosis and gangrene if arterial injection occurs; and hypotension, laryngospasm, and respiratory failure from overdosage or prolonged administration. Muscle relaxation and analgesic effects are minimal.

Advantages. Rapidity with which unconsciousness is induced, amnesic effects, prompt recovery with minimal doses, and simplicity of administration. Intravenous anesthetics are nonirritating to mucous membranes, and use is not accompanied by the hazard of fire or explosion.

Ultrashort-Acting Barbiturates

Ultrashort-acting barbiturates include thiopental sodium (Pentothal) and methohexital sodium (Brevital Sodium). These ultrashort-acting barbiturates are CNS depressants that produce hypnosis and anesthesia without analgesia. They frequently are combined with other drugs for muscle relaxation and analgesia in balanced anesthesia. Their exact mechanism of action for anesthesia, anticonvulsant effects, or the reduction of intracranial pressure (an indication for thiopental) is unknown, although a variety of theories have been proposed. General anesthesia with ultrashort-acting barbiturates is believed to result from suppression of the reticular activating system.

The onset of action for these barbiturates is generally rapid (20 to 60 seconds), and the duration of action is extremely short. They are distributed rapidly throughout the body with accumulation in the fatty tissues, followed by redistribution from brain to lean body mass in emergence from anesthesia. These drugs are metabolized in the liver and excreted through the kidneys.

The most common side effects during the recovery period are shivering and trembling. Less frequently reported are nausea, vomiting, prolonged somnolence, and headache. Serious adverse reactions include emergence delirium (increased excitability, confusion, and hallucinations); cardiac dysrhythmias (tachycardia, bradycardia, or myocardial depression); allergic response (bronchospasm, rash, hives, edema of eyelids, lips, or face, and hypotension); respiratory depression; and thrombophlebitis.

Careful assessment and close monitoring are required when the intravenous barbiturates are used in combination with other CNS depressants, which may result in enhanced depression effects, as well as diuretics, antihypertensive agents, and calcium-blocking drugs, since hypotension may occur.

Dosages for induction of general anesthesia and resultant duration of action vary. Methohexital requires 1 to 2 mg/kg for induction, with a duration of action of 5 to 7 minutes. The dose of thiopental is individualized dosed according to the patient's response.

Nonbarbiturates

Nonbarbiturate intravenous anesthetic agents include the benzodiazepines midazolam, diazepam, and lorazepam; the short-acting hypnotics etomidate and propofol; the opioids fentanyl, sufentanil, and alfentanil; and ketamine, a dissociative anesthetic. Several drugs also may be combined to produce neuroleptanesthesia, a general anesthesia produced by the administration of a neuroleptic agent, a narcotic analgesic, and nitrous oxide in oxygen.

midazolam [mid′ a zoe lam] (Versed)
diazepam [dye az′ e pam] (Valium)
lorazepam [lor az′ e pam] (Ativan)

Benzodiazepines are given intravenously as premedication or for induction of anesthesia. Diazepam and lorazepam are not water soluble; thus their nonaqueous solutions may cause local irritation. Midazolam is water soluble and thus is less irritating locally. In the body midazolam becomes more lipid soluble; therefore it can readily cross the blood-brain barrier. These agents generally have a slower onset of CNS effects than the barbiturates and a more prolonged postanesthetic recovery period, and they often produce an amnesic effect.

Midazolam also causes a decrease in cerebrospinal fluid pressure and thus may be selected for anesthesia induction in patients with intracranial lesions. Intravenously midazolam has a rapid onset of action (1 to 3 minutes) and a short elimination half-life of approximately 2.5 hours. It is metabolized in the liver and excreted by the kidneys.

Concurrent use of benzodiazepines with alcohol or CNS-depressant drugs may result in hypotension, respiratory depression, and possibly respiratory and cardiac arrest. A reduction in drug dosage and close monitoring are indicated if such drugs are used concurrently. Debilitated patients and those 55 years of age and older require a smaller than normal midazolam dose administered at a slower rate. Check a current reference for dosing recommendations. If concurrent CNS-depressant drugs are used, the midazolam dose should be reduced by at least 50% and diazepam dose by 33% (USP DI, 1998).

etomidate [eh toe′ mid date] (Amidate)

Etomidate is a short-acting, nonbarbiturate hypnotic used for the induction of general anesthesia. Etomidate is reported to decrease the activity of the reticular formation in the brainstem (in animals). Its cardiac and respiratory effects are minimal, so use of this product may be advantageous for the patient with impaired cardiac functions, respiratory functions, or both. Etomidate is used intravenously for induction of general anesthesia and in concomitant anesthesia for supplementation of a subpotent anesthetic agent (nitrous oxide in oxygen).

Etomidate (Amidate) induces hypnosis within 1 minute, with a duration of action between 3 and 5 minutes. To reduce recovery time in adults, a 0.1 mg IV dose of fentanyl is administered 1 or 2 minutes before anesthesia induction, thus reducing the amount of etomidate needed. Etomidate is metabolized in the liver and excreted by the kidneys.

The side effects most commonly reported during the recovery period are nausea and vomiting; less often reported are hypotension, hypertension, dysrhythmias, and breathing difficulties. Involuntary muscle movements have been reported, especially when fentanyl is not given before induction with etomidate. Pain at the injection site is also reported. **SPECIAL WARNING:** Etomidate can suppress the adrenal gland's production of steroid hormones (e.g., cortisol), which can result in a temporary gland failure. Electrolyte imbalance, hypotension, and shock may result. Seriously ill or postoperative patients may need adrenal cortex supplementation.

Significant drug interactions

When etomidate is given with other CNS depressants, the patient should be monitored for enhanced CNS depression.

Dosage and administration

See Table 9-2.

propofol [pro poe′ foal] (Diprivan)

Propofol is a rapidly acting, nonbarbiturate hypnotic used for the induction and maintenance of general anesthesia. It has a rapid onset of action of within 40 seconds, and the duration of effect is only from 3 to 5 minutes. Its redistribution from the brain to other body tissues explains the short effect. This agent's elimination half-life is 3 to 12 hours.

This agent is a respiratory depressant and may produce apnea and cardiac depression depending on the dose, rate of administration, and concurrent drugs administered. Bradycardia and hypotension may also occur frequently. Nausea, vomiting, and involuntary muscle movement are commonly reported.

fentanyl [fen′ ta nil] (Sublimaze)
sufentanil [soo fen′ ta nil] (Sufenta)
alfentanil [al fen′ ta nil] (Alfenta)

Adjunct medications for anesthesia include fentanyl (Sublimaze), sufentanil (Sufenta), and alfentanil (Alfenta). These agents have been theorized to produce their effects at the mu receptor. All three are opioid analgesics used for balanced anesthesia (see above) and in combination with oxygen, nitrous oxide, or both for the induction and maintenance of anesthesia. When combined with an agent such as droperidol that produces **neurolepsis** (an altered state of consciousness characterized by quiescence, reduced motor activity and anxiety, and indifference to surroundings), then fentanyl, sufentanil, and alfentanil may be used for neurolepsis or neuroleptanesthesia (see p. 163).

The most commonly reported side effects and adverse reactions are drowsiness, hypotension, bradycardia, and respiratory depression (allergic reaction). Less frequent are chills, nausea, vomiting, increased weakness, dizziness, constipation, depression, pruritus, muscle spasms, and increased excitability (paradoxical reaction). Convulsions are reported with fentanyl; dysrhythmias are reported with sufentanil.

Concurrent use of these drugs with CNS depressants may result in an enhanced CNS-depressant effect, hypotension, and respiratory depression. Dosage adjustment and careful monitoring are required. When other opioid agonist analgesics are used during the recovery phase from fentanyl or sufentanil anesthesia, the dosage should be one fourth

TABLE 9-2 Nonbarbiturates: Dosage and Administration

Agent	*Adults*	*Children*
alfentanil (Alfenta)		
Adjunct to general anesthesia	8-20 μg (0.008-0.02 mg)/kg body weight IV initially. Additional dosages of 3-5 μg/kg as needed for short duration (up to 30 min). For induction anesthesia, may use initial dose of 130-245 μg (0.130-0.245 mg)/kg body weight	Adjunct to anesthesia: IV 30-50 μg (0.03-0.05 mg)/kg body weight initially, then 0.5-1.5 μg/kg body weight by continuous infusion
etomidate (Amidate)		
Anesthesia induction	0.2-0.6 mg/kg body weight administered over 30-60 sec	Children older than 10 yr, 0.2-0.6 mg/kg body weight
fentanyl (Sublimaze)		
Adjunct to general anesthesia		
Minor surgery	2 μg (0.002 mg)/kg body weight IV	Children younger than 2 yr, no established dosage
Major surgery	2-20 μg (0.002-0.02 mg)/kg body weight IV. High doses are used for open-heart surgery, complicated neurosurgery, or orthopedic procedures, i.e., 20-50 μg (0.02-0.05 mg)/kg body weight IV	
Primary agent in major surgery	50-100 μg (0.05-0.1 mg)/kg body weight IV given with oxygen, nitrous oxide, or both and neuromuscular blocking agent	Children 2-12 yr, 2-3 μg (0.002-0.003 mg)/kg body weight IV
Presurgical or postoperative use	0.07-1.4 μg (0.0007-0.0014 mg)/kg body weight IM	
sufentanil (Sufenta)		
Adjunct to general anesthesia	Low dosages, 0.5-1 μg (0.0005-0.001 mg)/kg body weight IV initially. Additional dosages of 10-25 μg may be given as needed. Moderate dosages, 2-8 μg/kg body weight IV initially Additional dosages of 10-50 μg may be given as needed	
Primary agent in major surgery	8-30 μg/kg body weight IV initially with oxygen. Additional dosages of 25-50 μg may be given as needed	Cardiovascular surgery: initially, 10-25 μg/kg body weight IV given with 100% oxygen. Maintenance, up to 25-50 μg IV

From *USP DI*, 1998.

to one third the usually recommended dosage. Naltrexone blocks the effects of opioid analgesics. If an opioid is necessary for elective surgery, naltrexone should be stopped for several days before the scheduled operation. Information on dosage and administration of these drugs appears in Table 9-2.

Fentanyl (Sublimaze), sufentanil (Sufenta), and alfentanil (Alfenta) all cross the blood-brain barrier and are rapidly distributed to various tissues. They are highly protein bound, with a triphasic half-life, that is, distributive phase, redistributive phase, and elimination.

Fentanyl produces an analgesic effect in 7 to 15 minutes when given intramuscularly or 1 to 2 minutes when given intravenously. The rate of loss of consciousness depends on the dose and the rate of administration (usually 4 to 5 minutes at the rate of 0.4 mg/min IV). Its peak effect occurs at 3 to 5 minutes when given IV and at 20 to 30 minutes when given IM. The duration of effect is 0.5 to 1 hour when given IV and 1 to 2 hours when given IM.

Sufentanil has an immediate analgesic effect, with the time until loss of consciousness depending on dose and rate of administration (usually 1 to 1.6 minutes at the rate of 0.3 mg/min). The duration of action is less than 1 hour.

Alfentanil has an immediate analgesic effect, producing a peak effect in 1 to 2 minutes. The duration of action is dose dependent but is usually less than 10 to 15 minutes.

All three drugs are metabolized in the liver, although sufentanil may also have some intestinal metabolism. They are excreted by the kidneys.

DISSOCIATIVE ANESTHETIC

ketamine hydrochloride [keet′ a meen] (Ketalar)

Ketamine is a rapid-acting, nonbarbiturate, intravenous anesthetic. It is a derivative of the psychotomimetic drug of abuse phencyclidine. Ketamine acts on the midbrain within the reticular formation, as do the barbiturates. It produces analgesia and amnesia but not muscular relaxation. The mechanism of action is not fully known. Ketamine blocks afferent transmission of impulses associated with the affective-emotional aspect of pain perception. It may also suppress spinal cord activity. Ketamine produces a **dissociative anesthesia:** an anesthesia characterized by analgesia and amnesia without loss of respiratory function or pharyngeal and laryngeal reflexes. It produces a cataleptic state in which the patient appears to be awake but detached from his or her environment and unresponsive to pain. The person's eyelids usually do not close, nystagmus (rapid, involuntary oscillation of the eyeballs) is common, and slight involuntary and purposeless movements may occur.

Ketamine increases secretions of salivary and bronchial glands; therefore the administration of an anticholinergic agent (such as atropine) may be necessary. Ketamine may increase blood pressure, muscle tone, and heart rate. Respiration is usually not depressed. After recovery, the patient has no recall of events occurring while under the influence of ketamine.

Ketamine is best suited for short diagnostic or surgical procedures not requiring skeletal muscle relaxation. It is also used to induce anesthesia before administration of general anesthetics and as an adjunct to low-potency anesthetics, such as nitrous oxide.

When ketamine is given intravenously, the onset of anesthesia occurs within 30 seconds. When it is administered intramuscularly, the onset of action occurs within 3 to 4 minutes. The duration of action is 5 to 10 minutes for an IV dose of 2 mg/kg of body weight or 12 to 25 minutes for an IM dose of 10 mg/kg.

Ketamine is metabolized in the liver. Termination of anesthetic action occurs with redistribution from the central nervous system and liver biotransformation. Ninety percent is excreted in the kidneys.

The most commonly reported side effects and adverse reactions of ketamine include hypertension and increased pulse rate and an emergence reaction, which may include distortion in body image, delirium, explicit dreams, illusions, and dissociative-type experiences. In some patients, flashbacks of vivid dreams with or without illusions may occur weeks later. Less commonly reported side effects include hypotension, bradycardia, respiratory depression, and vomiting. No significant drug interactions have been reported.

The recommended adult dosage for anesthesia induction is 1 to 2 mg/kg of body weight IV or 5 to 10 mg/kg of body weight IM. The recommended rate for maintenance is 10 to 50 μg/kg of body weight by infusion at a rate of 1 to 2 μg/min. As with any anesthetic, the dosage needs to be carefully assessed and individualized.

NEUROLEPTANESTHESIA

Neuroleptanesthesia is a general anesthesia produced by a combination of a neuroleptic (antipsychotic) such as droperidol (Inapsine), diazepam (Valium), or ketamine (Ketalar) and a narcotic analgesic, most commonly fentanyl but sometimes meperidine (Demerol), morphine, or pentazocine (Talwin). It is used primarily for procedures that require the patient's cooperation.

An example of this classification is droperidol and fentanyl (Innovar injection). Innovar consists of 1 part fentanyl to 50 parts droperidol.

droperidol [droe per′ i dole]
fentanyl [fen′ ta nil] (Innovar injection)

Droperidol is a neuroleptic agent used to induce neuroleptic anesthesia. When used in combination with fentanyl, this product produces a state in which patients are neither asleep nor awake but in a state of profound analgesia and psychomotor sedation. This state permits the patient to undergo short procedures requiring consciousness and cooperation, such as bronchoscopy and cystoscopy, without pain. Droperidol is also used as a premedication for anesthesia and as an adjunct for induction and maintenance of anesthesia. Droperidol has lost some of its earlier popularity, since clinical investigation has demonstrated that the depression of respiratory rate and alveolar ventilation may persist longer than the analgesic effect.

The onset of action for droperidol, when given either intravenously or intramuscularly, is between 3 and 10 minutes, with the peak effect at 30 minutes. The duration of action is 2 to 4 hours. Alteration of consciousness may persist up to 12 hours. Droperidol is metabolized in the liver and excreted in the kidneys.

The most commonly reported side effects and adverse reactions are hypotension, hypertension, dystonia, increased hyperexcitability, anxiety, and sweating. Less frequently reported effects include bronchospasm, emergence delirium (hallucinations), chills, shivering, depression, and nightmares. Respiratory depression has been reported when the drug is used in combination with an opioid analgesic; this can lead to respiratory arrest. Concurrent use should be avoided, but if it is necessary, the dosage of the opioid should be reduced to one fourth to one third of the usual dosage. Concurrent use of other CNS depressants may result in enhanced CNS-depressant effects. Table 9-3 lists dosage and administration recommendations.

PREANESTHETIC AGENTS/ANESTHETIC ADJUNCTIVE AGENTS

Various medications are used as preanesthetic agents or as adjuncts to anesthesia to reduce undesirable effects produced by apprehension or by induction and maintenance of anesthesia. Table 9-4 reviews some of the common agents. Narcotic analgesics not only reduce anxiety and provide analgesia but also allow for a reduction in the dosage of anesthetic administered, because of their additive effects. The administration of muscle relaxants provides surgeons easier access and increased visualization of the abdominal cavity during abdominal surgery or in patients in whom controlled mechanical ventilation is required. Many nondepolarizing neuromuscular blocking agents are available, including atracurium (Tracrium), cisatracurium (Nimbex), doxacurium (Nuromax), mivacurium (Mivacron), pipecuronium (Arduan), rocuronium (Zemuron), and vecuronium (Norcuron) (Olin, 1998).

Box 9-3 discusses remifentanil (Ultiva), a rapid-acting opioid used during general anesthesia.

TABLE 9-3 Droperidol and Fentanyl (Innovar): Dosage and Administration

Use	Adults	Children
Premedication for general anesthesia	0.5 to 2 mL IM given ½-1 hr before surgery	Older than 2 years of age, 0.25 mL/20 lb body weight
General anesthesia adjunct		
Induction	1 mL/20 to 25 lb body weight administered slowly IV. Individualize dosage, since smaller dosages have been found adequate, depending on client's response	
Without general anesthesia for diagnostic procedures	0.5 to 2 mL IM approximately ½-1 hr before procedure	

From *PDR,* 1995.

TABLE 9-4 Preanesthetic Agents

Drug Classification	Agents Most Frequently Used	Desired Effect
Narcotic analgesics	morphine meperidine (Demerol)	Sedation to decrease tension and anxiety; provide analgesia, and decrease amount of anesthetic used
Barbiturates	pentobarbital (Nembutal) secobarbital (Seconal)	Decreased apprehension Sedation Rapid induction
Phenothiazines	promethazine (Phenergan)	Sedation Antihistaminic Antiemetic Decreased motor activity
Anticholinergics	glycopyrrolate (Robinul) atropine scopolamine	Inhibition of secretions, vomiting, and laryngospasms, plus sedation (with scopolamine)
Skeletal muscle relaxants	succinylcholine (depolarizing) (Anectine, Quelicin, Sucostrin) *d*-tubocurarine (nondepolarizing) (Sux-cert)	Promotion of muscular relaxation

BOX 9-3 Rapid-Acting Opioid for Use During General Anesthesia

Remifentanil (Ultiva) is a short-acting analgesic used during induction and maintenance of general anesthesia and also for the immediate postoperative period. This drug should only be administered under the direct supervision of an anesthesiologist or nurse anesthetist.

A mu receptor agonist, remifentanil has a rapid onset of action and is metabolized by nonspecific esterases in blood and tissues; its effects last for between 5 and 10 minutes after the drug is discontinued. To control postoperative pain, adequate analgesia should be instituted before discontinuation of remifentanil (New Ultiva, 1996). Side/adverse effects include hypoxia, apnea, respiratory depression, and muscle rigidity. See current reference or package insert for additional information.

From *New Ultiva,* 1996.

LOCAL ANESTHESIA

Local anesthesia refers to the direct administration of an anesthetic agent to tissues to induce the absence of sensation in a portion of the body. Unlike general anesthesia, consciousness is not depressed with local anesthesia. Local anesthetic agents may be applied to an area or injected into tissues, where they produce their effect in the immediate area only; hence the term "local anesthesia." Local anesthetic drugs may also be injected around a nerve or nerve trunk (spinal, epidural) to produce anesthesia in a large region of the body. This is referred to as **regional anesthesia.**

SURFACE OR TOPICAL ANESTHESIA

The use of surface, or topical, anesthesia is restricted to mucous membranes, damaged skin surfaces, wounds, and burns. The anesthetic is applied in the form of a solution, ointment, gel, cream, or powder to produce loss of sensation

TABLE 9-5 Local Anesthetics: Administration and Use

Method	Tissue Affected	Preparation Used	Examples of Drugs Used	Therapeutic Use
Topical	Sensory nerve endings in mucous membranes and dermis	Solution Ointment Cream Powder	cocaine benzocaine ethyl aminobenzoate lidocaine tetracaine bupivacaine	Relief of pain or itching Examination of conjuctiva
Infiltration	Sensory nerve endings in subcutaneous tissues or dermis	Injection	etidocaine procaine prilocaine lidocaine chloroprocaine mepivicaine	Minor surgery
Block	Nerve trunk	Injection	etidocaine procaine prilocaine lidocaine chloroprocaine mepivacaine	Dental and limb surgry Sympathetic block
Spinal (subarachnoid block)	Spinal roots	Injection	procaine tetracaine lidocaine	Abdominal surgery Surgery of the lower extremities Muscle relaxation

by paralyzing afferent nerve endings. Topical anesthetics do not penetrate unbroken skin. Topical anesthesia is used to relieve pain and itching and to anesthetize mucous membranes of the eye, nose, throat, or urethra for minor surgical procedures. Cocaine in a 4% to 10% solution continues to be one of the most widely used agents for topical anesthesia.

Local anesthesia may also be achieved by freezing. Low temperatures in living tissues produce diminished sensation. This form of anesthesia is sometimes used for minor operative procedures. A caution is that tissues that are frozen too intensely for too long may be destroyed. Ethyl chloride is a local anesthetic that can be used to produce this effect, although it is not used extensively.

LOCAL ANESTHETICS

Local anesthetics are drugs used to abolish pain sensation in a particular part of the body (Tables 9-5 and 9-6). The basic mechanism of action of these drugs is unknown, but most act by stabilizing or elevating the threshold of excitation of the nerve cell membrane without affecting resting potential (blockage of sodium channels). This action is a result of reduction of membrane permeability to all ions; thus depolarization and transmission of nerve impulses are prevented.

Table 9-6 presents some commonly used local anesthetics and their properties. Benzyl alcohol, an aromatic alcohol of low potency, is used topically with procaine to extend procaine's duration of action. The choice of a local anesthetic for a particular procedure depends on the duration of drug action desired. Table 9-7 lists short-, intermediate-, and long-acting local anesthetic drugs. Vasoconstrictors, such as epinephrine and norepinephrine, are used with the local anesthetic to decrease systemic absorption and prolong the anesthetic's duration of action. They are not used for nerve blocks in areas where there are end arteries (fingers, toes, ears, nose, or penis) because ischemia may develop, resulting in gangrene.

A number of local anesthetic agents cannot be injected. However, because they are absorbed slowly, they can be used safely on open wounds, ulcers, and mucous membranes. They occasionally cause dermatitis and allergic sensitization, which necessitate their discontinuance. The ester-type local anesthetics (cocaine, procaine, tetracaine, and benzocaine) are metabolized to *p*-aminobenzoic acid (PABA) metabolites, which are mainly responsible for allergic reactions in some patients. The amide anesthetics (lidocaine, mepivacaine, bupivacaine, etidocaine, and prilocaine) are not metabolized to PABA derivatives; thus allergic reactions induced by these anesthetics are very rare (Katzung, 1992).

Topical anesthetics for skin disorders are used primarily to relieve pruritus, discomfort, pain, and soreness; indications for mucous membranes are similar. The anesthetics are poorly absorbed through the intact skin, but from mucous membranes and skin breaks and sores (e.g., abrasions, trauma, and ulcers) absorption is increased, leading to the possibility of systemic involvement. When they are used in the oral cavity (mouth and pharynx), interference with swallowing may occur, and the patient is at risk for aspiration. The patient is assessed for a returning gag reflex by gentle touching of the back of the pharynx with a tongue blade. All food and fluid are withheld until the reflex returns.

TABLE 9-6 Properties of Commonly Used Local Anesthetics

	Procaine	Cocaine	Benzocaine
Trade names	Novocain	—	Americaine Hurricaine
Potency	—	2-3 times that of procaine	Very low
Onset of action	2-5 min	1 min	Immediate
Duration	½-1 hr	½-1 hr	15-20 min
Dose	0.25%-2%, depending on method of administration 10% for spinal anesthesia Not used topically	1%-4% topically	Variable 5%-20% ointment topically
Toxicity	Least toxic of all local anesthetics	More toxic than procaine when injected subcutaneously	Relatively nontoxic
Precautions	Overdose of rapid injection may cause CNS stimulation	Not recommended for infiltration, nerve block, or spinal anesthesia Repeated use causes psychologic dependence	Suitable for topical use only Sensitization may develop

Local anesthetics are capable of abolishing all sensation, but pain fibers are affected first, probably because they are thinner, unmyelinated, and more easily penetrated by these drugs. Loss of pain is followed in sequence by loss of response to cold, warmth, touch, and pressure. Most motor fibers also can be anesthetized when an adequate concentration of the drug is present over sufficient time.

The parenteral local anesthetics have complete systemic absorption, which is decreased by the addition of a vasoconstrictor such as epinephrine. The half-lives of selected anesthetics are as follows: bupivacaine, 3½ hours; etidocaine, 2¾ hours; lidocaine, 1½ hours; and mepivacaine, 2 hours. Onset of action is a function of the anesthetic technique used, the type of block desired, dosage, and the pK_a (negative logarithm of ionization constant) of each anesthetic. The time it takes for a drug to reach a peak concentration depends on the type of block but ranges from 10 to 30 minutes.

Reactions to Local Anesthetics

Local anesthetics produce vasodilation by direct action on blood vessels and by anesthetizing sympathetic vasoconstrictor fibers. This action can cause rapid absorption of the drug; when the rate of absorption exceeds the rate of elimination, toxic effects can occur. To decrease the rate of absorption and the incidence of toxic effects by allowing more time for metabolic degradation and to prolong local anesthetic effects, epinephrine or other vasoconstrictor drugs are used. The dosages of vasoconstrictors must be carefully determined to prevent ischemic necrosis at the injection site. Because local anesthetics are potentially toxic drugs, a patient's age, weight, physical condition, and liver function must be taken into account in determining drug dosage. Most reactions to local anesthetics result from overdosage, rapid absorption into systemic circulation, or individual hypersensitivity or allergic response.

Central Nervous System

At first, the CNS may be stimulated, which causes anxiety, restlessness, confusion, dizziness, tremors, and even convulsions. Then depression may occur, and unconsciousness and death may ensue.

Cardiovascular System

Myocardial depression, bradycardia, and hypotension can occur because of smooth muscle relaxation and inhibition of neuromuscular conduction. The person suddenly becomes pale, feels faint, and has a drop in blood pressure. Cardiac arrest can be the result of a cardiovascular reaction.

Anesthetics containing a vasoconstrictor are used with caution in patients receiving drugs that may change blood pressure, such as monoamine oxidase inhibitors, phenothiazines, and tricyclic antidepressants. The combination may produce severe hypotension or hypertension. Cardiac dysrhythmias occur when catecholamine vasoconstrictors (e.g., epinephrine) are used in patients receiving cyclopropane, halothane, or trichloroethylene.

Allergic Reaction

True allergic reactions are said to be uncommon. Sometimes a reaction is thought to be allergic when it is really caused by overdosage. However, allergic reactions can occur. They may be relatively mild (hives, itching, or skin rash), or they may be acutely anaphylactic.

The allergic reactions are characteristically manifested by cutaneous lesions, urticaria, or edema. They may result from various factors, such as hypersensitivity, idiosyncrasy, or diminished tolerance. These rare allergic reactions are usually limited to the ester type of anesthetics. The most important risk of local anesthetics is a dose-related CNS toxicity, which may progress from sleepiness to convulsion.

Small test doses are frequently given to gauge the extent of the patient's sensitivity to the anesthetic agent. The anes-

Lidocaine	***Tetracaine***	***Mepivacaine***
Xylocaine	Pontocaine	Carbocaine
2 times that of procaine	10 times that of procaine	2 times that of procaine
2-5 min	3-10 min	Less rapid than procaine
1-3 hr	1->3 hr	1-3 hr
0.5%-4% for injection 2% and 5% topically	1% topically 0.15%-0.25% for injection	1%-2% solution
See procaine	More toxic than procaine, but toxic effects rare because of low dosage used	2 times that of procaine; less than lidocaine
When administered rapidly or in large doses, may cause convulsions and hypotension	Drug interaction with cholinesterase inhibitors and sulfonamides	Combined with vasoconstrictor to delay drug absorption and prolong duration Avoid in pregnancy—may cause constriction of uterine artery

thetic agent chosen, its concentration, the rate of injection, and physical and emotional factors in the patient all influence reactions to local anesthetics.

Anesthesia by Injection

Anesthesia by injection is accomplished by infiltration or by conduction (spinal, caudal, or saddle block).

Infiltration anesthesia is produced by injecting dilute solutions (0.1%) of the agent into the skin and then subcutaneously into the region to be anesthetized. Epinephrine often is added to the solution to intensify the anesthesia in a limited region and to prevent excessive bleeding and systemic effects. Repeated injection will prolong the anesthesia as long as needed. The sensory nerve endings are anesthetized. This method of administration is used for minor surgery such as incision and drainage or excision of a cyst (see Table 9-7).

Conduction (block) anesthesia means a loss of sensation, especially pain, in a region of the body, produced by injecting a local anesthetic into the vicinity of a nerve trunk and thus inhibiting the conduction of impulses to and from the area supplied by that nerve, the region of the operative site. The injection may be made at some distance from the surgical site. A single nerve may be blocked, or the anesthetic may be injected where several nerve trunks emerge from the spinal cord (paravertebral block). A more concentrated solution is required because of the thickness of nerve trunk fibers. This method of anesthesia is often used for foot and hand surgery.

Spinal anesthesia is a type of extensive nerve block sometimes called a subarachnoid block. The anesthetic solution is injected into the subarachnoid space and affects the lower part of the spinal cord and nerve roots.

For low spinal anesthesia, the patient is placed in a flat or Fowler's position. A solution with a specific gravity greater than that of cerebrospinal fluid is used, since it tends to diffuse downward. For high spinal anesthesia, Trendelenburg's position with the head sharply flexed is used, along with an anesthetic solution of lower specific gravity than that of cerebrospinal fluid (which tends to diffuse upward) or a solution with the same specific gravity as cerebrospinal fluid (which may diffuse upward or downward, depending on the position used). Solutions with the same specific gravity as cerebrospinal fluid act primarily at the site of injection.

The onset of anesthesia usually occurs within 1 to 2 minutes after injection. The duration of anesthesia is 1 to 3 hours, depending on the anesthetic used. Spinal anesthesia is used for surgical procedures on the lower abdomen, inguinal area, or lower extremities. It may be the method of choice for patients with severe respiratory problems or with liver, kidney, or metabolic disease. Marked hypotension, decreased cardiac output, and respiratory inadequacy tend to occur during anesthesia and are considered to be disadvantages of this method of anesthesia.

Postoperatively, headache is the most common complaint; this may be accompanied by difficulty in hearing or seeing. Headache may be postural and occur only in the head-up or sitting or standing position. This symptom is the result of the opening in the dura made by the large spinal needle, which may persist for days or weeks, permitting loss of cerebrospinal fluid.

Headache and auditory and visual problems after lumbar puncture result from decreased intracranial pressure. These symptoms usually are alleviated when cerebrospinal fluid pressure returns to normal. Paresthesias such as numbness and tingling may occur after spinal anesthesia; they are usually limited to the lumbar or sacral areas and disappear within a relatively short time. The success and safety of spinal anesthesia depend primarily on the anesthetist's skill and knowledge.

Caudal anesthesia is produced by injecting an anesthetic solution into the caudal canal, the sacral part of the verte-

TABLE 9-7 Selected Injected Anesthetic Drugs: Pharmacokinetic Overview

Name	*Metabolism*	*Use*	*Dosage and Administration*
Short-Acting (½-hr)			
procaine (Novocain)	Ester compound—same as chloroprocaine	Infiltration, never block, spinal anesthesia, epidural block	Usual adult dosage for infiltration: 350-600 mg as 0.25%-0.5% solution Peripheral nerve block: 500 mg as 0.5%, 1%, or 2% solution Spinal and epidural dosage, vary with individual client, procedure, and degree of anesthesia desired Pediatric dosage: not available
chloroprocaine (Nesacaine, Nesacaine-MPF)	Ester compound—metabolized by cholinesterases in plasma and liver to a PABA compound. Excretion: kidneys	Nesacaine—infiltration and regional anesthesia Nesacaine-CE—for caudal and epidural anesthesia	Usual adult dosage for infiltration nerve blocks: 30-800 mg as 1% or 2% solutions, depending on site and length of surgical procedure. Caudal and epidural: 40-500 mg as 2% or 3% solution, without epinephrine Usual pediatric dosage for infiltration nerve blocks: up to 20 mg/kg body weight
Intermediate Duration (1-3 hr)			
lidocaine (Xylocaine, Xylocard 🍁)	Amide compound Metabolism: liver to active and toxic metabolites Excretion: kidneys	Infiltration, nerve block, spinal epidural	Usual adult dosage depends on site and length of surgical procedure Pediatric dosage: same as adult Lidocaine is available with and without epinephrine
mepivacaine (Carbocaine)	Amide compound—see above	Infiltration, nerve blocks, caudal, epidural	Available alone and with levonordefrin (vasoconstrictor). Dosage depends on site and length of surgical procedure Adult maximum dosage: dental, up to 6.6 mg/kg body weight (300 mg maximum per appointment); other usages, up to 7 mg/kg body weight; pediatric, up to 5 or 6 mg/kg body weight
prilocaine (Citanest, Citanest Forte)	Amide compound—see above	Infiltration, peripheral nerve blocks, caudal, epidural	Available alone or with epinephrine (vasoconstrictor). Although dosages vary with site and length of procedure, the adult maximum dosages are as follows: Dental, up to 400 mg as a 4% solution in 2-hr period; other procedures, individualize Pediatric maximum: Dental, children up to 10 yr, 40 mg (4% solution) maximum; other procedures, individualize
Long Duration (3-10 hr)			
bupivacaine (Marcaine, Sensorcaine)	Amide type—see above	Infiltration, caudal, epidural, peripheral nerve blocks	Available alone or with dextrose (Marcaine spinal) or with epinephrine. Dosages vary with site, additional drugs, and length of procedure
etidocaine (Duranest)	Amide type—see above	Infiltration; peripheral nerve blocks, caudal and epidural nerve blocks	Available alone and with epinephrine. Dosages vary with site and length of procedure
tetracaine (Pontocaine)	Ester compound—see above	Saddle block (low spinal), up to costal margin, spinal anesthesia	Available alone and with dextrose. Dosages vary with site and length of procedure

bral canal containing the cauda equina, or the bundle of spinal nerves that innervates the pelvic viscera. It is used in obstetrics and for pelvic or genital surgery. Its advantage over spinal anesthesia is that the anesthetic does not have direct access to the spinal cord and medullary centers. Thus the respiratory muscles and blood pressure are not directly affected, and undesirable effects are less likely to occur.

Saddle block is sometimes used in obstetrics and for surgery involving the perineum, rectum, genitalia, and upper parts of the thighs. The patient sits upright while the anesthetic is injected after a lumbar puncture. The person remains upright for a short time, until the anesthetic has taken effect. The body parts that contact a saddle when riding become anesthetized, hence the name.

Injectable Local Anesthetics

The injectable local anesthetics are listed in Table 9-7. Generally the onset of action for an anesthetic is the result of drug concentration and the targeted nerve-tissue area. Potency and duration of anesthetic action increase with a drug's lipid solubility. For more information on metabolism, indications, and pharmacokinetics, see Table 9-7.

Side effects and adverse reactions

The adverse reactions of injected local anesthetics generally require medical intervention. Cyanosis caused by methemoglobinemia is one of the most common adverse reactions reported with an epidural block or high spinal injection. It has been reported with all local anesthetics but is most prevalent with prilocaine (Citanest). Symptoms may include weakness, breathing difficulties, increased heart rate, dizziness, or collapse.

Other reactions reported with an epidural block or high spinal injection include diaphoresis, hypotension, bradycardia or irregular heart rate, pale skin color (cardiovascular depression), diplopia, seizures, tinnitus, increased excitability, shivering, involuntary shaking (caused by stimulation of CNS), nausea, and vomiting.

Effects most commonly reported with ester compounds include skin rash and an allergic reaction manifested by edema of face, lip, mouth, or throat. Anaphylaxis and severe hypotension are reported rarely.

With central nerve block anesthesia, the most common adverse reactions are in the form of neuropathies or neurologic effects, including headaches. Other adverse reactions include paresthesia or paralysis of lower legs, breathing difficulties, severe hypotension, bradycardia, and backache. Some patients report a reduction or loss of sexual functions, bladder control, or bowel movements.

Meningitis-type effects are most often reported with spinal anesthesia. These include headaches, nausea, vomiting, and stiff or sore neck.

Allergic effects manifested by dental anesthesia are numbing or tingling of lips and mouth, as well as edema of lips or mouth, while sympathomimetic or adrenergic effects are reported with epinephrine or other vasoconstrictors. These most commonly include hypertension, shaking, increased anxiety or nervousness, tachycardia, headache, and chest pain.

Significant drug interactions

The significant drug interactions are limited, but this does not preclude a variety of unexpected responses, thus indicating the need for close observation.

Prior or concurrent administration of CNS-depressant drugs may result in additive CNS depression effects. Adjust dosages and monitor closely.

Vasoconstrictor agents, such as epinephrine, norepinephrine, or phenylephrine, in combination with local anesthetics may cause impaired circulation of the area, resulting in sloughing of tissue. If vasoconstrictor agents are used for end arteries, such as toes or fingers, ischemia resulting in gangrene may develop. Extreme caution is advised.

Dosage and administration

See Table 9-7.

SUMMARY

By altering consciousness or interfering with conduction of nerve impulses to the central nervous system, anesthetic agents have been proven to be invaluable in limiting pain and suffering during surgical procedures. The two major categories of anesthesia are general and regional or local anesthesia. General anesthesia may be achieved either intravenously or by inhalation while regional anesthesia is the injecting of an anesthetic drug near a nerve trunk or specific body site. Local anesthesia is achieved by topical application or by infiltrating the selected operative area. Combination agents are often used to achieve analgesia, muscle relaxation, unconsciousness, and amnesia; this is referred to as balanced anesthesia.

Neuroleptanesthesia is the combined use of a neuroleptic agent and a narcotic analgesic, which is used for procedures in which the individual's cooperation is necessary and desired. Local anesthesia is used to render a specific part of the body, insensitive to pain.

An awareness of drug side effects, adverse effects, toxicity, and potential drug interactions is necessary for the safe and effective use of the various anesthetic agents.

REVIEW QUESTIONS

1. Which eyedrops have been associated with extended apnea and death during surgical procedures? Explain why.
2. Describe the problems reported with the use of systemic aminoglycosides during and after surgery. How can these problems be managed?
3. Discuss the use and advantages of intravenous anesthetics in general anesthesia. What are some of the disadvantages with using intravenous anesthetics?

REFERENCES

Katzung BG: *Basic and clinical pharmacology,* ed 5, Norwalk, Conn, 1992, Appleton & Lange.

New Ultiva, Letter, #ULT037RO, Reserach Triangle Park, NC, 1996, Glaxo Wellcome Inc.

Olin BR: *Facts and comparisons,* Philadelphia, 1998, JB Lippincott.

Physician's desk reference, ed 49, Montvale, NJ, 1995, Medical Economics Co.

United States Pharmacopeial Convention: *USP DI: drug information for the health care professional,* ed 18, Rockville, Md, 1998, the Convention.

ADDITIONAL REFERENCES

American Hospital Formulary Service: *AHFS drug information '98,* Bethesda, Md, 1998, American Society of Hospital Pharmacists.

Anderson KN et al, editors: *Mosby's medical, nursing, and allied health dictionary,* ed 5, St Louis, 1998, Mosby.

Mosby: *Mosby's GenRx,* St Louis, 1998, Mosby.

Riley TN, DeRuiter J: New drugs 1992, *US Pharmacist* 18(3):35, 1993.

CHAPTER 10

Antianxiety, Sedative, and Hypnotic Drugs

KEY DRUGS

diazepam (p. 175)
buspirone (p. 181)

KEY TERMS

anterograde amnesic effect, (p. 176)
antianxiety or anxiolytic agents, (p. 171)
anxiety, (p. 171)
hypnotics, (p. 171)
insomnia, (p. 174)
non-REM sleep, (p. 171)
REM sleep, (p. 171)
sedatives, (p. 171)

CHAPTER FOCUS

Nervousness, anxiety, worry, apprehension, and insomnia are health problems that occur commonly across the life span. When anxiety or fear is the result of a threat or danger, this is a normal physiologic response to a threatening situation. However, excessive anxiety or apprehension that interferes with daily functioning is counterproductive and usually requires medical intervention and treatment. Insomnia is also a common sleep disorder and is often a concern in the elderly. This chapter reviews the antianxiety, sedative, and hypnotic drugs available to treat these disorders.

OBJECTIVES

After reading and studying this chapter, the student should be able to do the following:

1. *Define and discuss the key drugs and key terms.*
2. *Describe the physiology of sleep across the life span.*
3. *Explain the mechanisms of action and indications for the benzodiazepines.*
4. *Discuss nonpharmacologic approaches to sleep and their importance in relation to hypnotic drugs.*
5. *Explain the mechanisms of action, indications, and significant drug interactions for barbiturates.*

The **antianxiety or anxiolytic agents** reduce feelings of excessive anxiety, such as apprehension, fear, nervousness, worry, or panic. **Anxiety** is a state or feeling of apprehension, uneasiness, agitation, uncertainty, and fear resulting from the anticipation of some threat or danger, ually of intrapsychic origin, whose source is generally unknown or unrecognized. It is usually a normal psychologic and physiologic response to a personally threatening situation, such as a threat to one's health, body, loved ones, job, or lifestyle. Generally, this anxiety stimulates the person to take a purposeful or deliberate action to counteract or offset the anxiety-producing state. When a person is unable to cope with a persistently stressful situation because excessive anxiety interferes with daily functioning, help is necessary. Although many nonpharmacologic modalities are available, antianxiety agents are commonly prescribed for the treatment of anxiety. For a proposed site of action for the benzodiazepines, see the discussion of the limbic system in Chapter 7.

Sedatives are central nervous system (CNS)-depressant drugs that were commonly prescribed before the advent of the benzodiazepine family. Their general use today has declined. Sedatives are chemical substances that reduce nervousness, excitability, or irritability by producing a calming or soothing effect. **Hypnotics** are drugs used to induce sleep. The major difference between a sedative and a hypnotic is the degree of CNS depression induced. A small dose may be used for a sedative effect, whereas larger dosages may be used for hypnotic effects. Barbiturates have been used extensively as sedative-hypnotic agents, but because of their low degree of selectivity and safety, they have been largely replaced by the safer benzodiazepines.

PHYSIOLOGY OF SLEEP

Sleep is a recurrent, normal condition of inertia and unresponsiveness during which an individual's overt and covert responses to stimuli are markedly reduced. During sleep a person is no longer in sensory contact with the immediate environment and stimuli that have bombarded the senses of sight, hearing, touch, smell, and taste during waking hours. Such factors no longer attract attention or exert a controlling influence over voluntary and involuntary movements or functions. It is not difficult to understand that everyone needs to escape from constant stimuli.

Research has shown that sleep is not one level of unconsciousness; it consists of two basic stages that occur cyclically:

1. Non-rapid eye movement (non-REM)
2. Rapid eye movement (REM)

During sleep, the individual moves through the four stages of **non-REM sleep** (the first four stages of sleep characterized on an electroencephalogram [EEG] by alpha waves, slow and of low amplitude), with stage 4 considered the deepest level of non-REM sleep, and then through **REM sleep,** the fifth stage of sleep, characterized by rapid eye movement, by dreaming, and by delta waves on an EEG (Fig. 10-1). Alternating periods of REM and non-REM sleep occur throughout the night (McCance, Huether, 1998). It should be kept in mind that REM sleep is not synonymous with light sleep. It takes a more powerful stimulus to arouse a person from REM sleep than from synchronous slow-wave sleep.

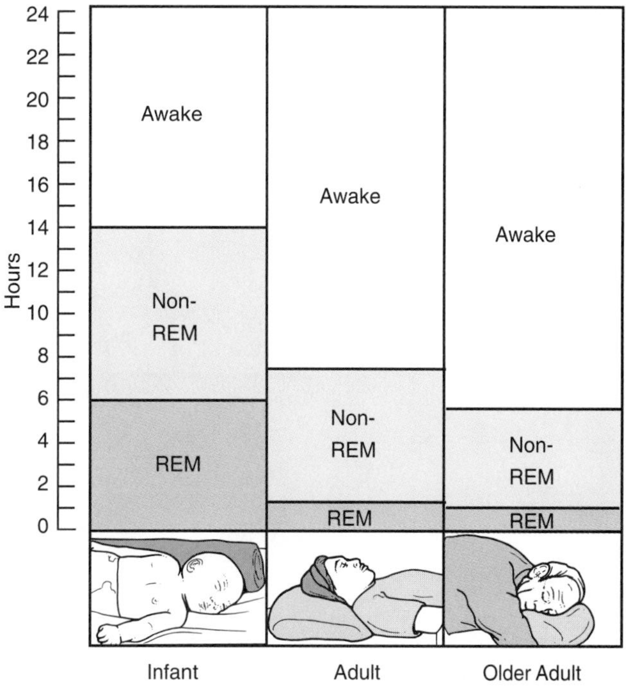

FIGURE 10-1
Sleep-wake cycles across the life span. Infants: approximately 40% of total sleep time is REM. Adults: 20% of total sleep time is REM. Older adults: total sleep time is slightly reduced; REM remains 20% of total. *(From Beare Myers, 1994).*

The stages of sleep are based on electrical activity that can be observed in the brain by means of an EEG. The EEG provides graphic illustrations of brain waves, which are an indication of the electrical activity occurring in the brain (Fig. 10-2).

Sleep research indicates that there are psychologic and physiologic reasons for the body to maintain an equilibrium between the various stages of sleep. The physiologic functions of the body tend to be depressed during nondreaming sleep. For example, it is known that:

1. Blood pressure falls (10 to 30 mm Hg).
2. Pulse rate is slowed.
3. Metabolic rate is decreased.
4. Gastrointestinal tract activity is slowed.
5. Urine formation slows.
6. Oxygen consumption and carbon dioxide production are lowered.
7. Body temperature decreases slightly.
8. Respirations are slower and more shallow.
9. Body movement is minimal.

Dreaming sleep tends to increase most of these parameters. Body movements are more noticeable: turning, jerking, moving of the arms and legs, talking, crying, or laughing,

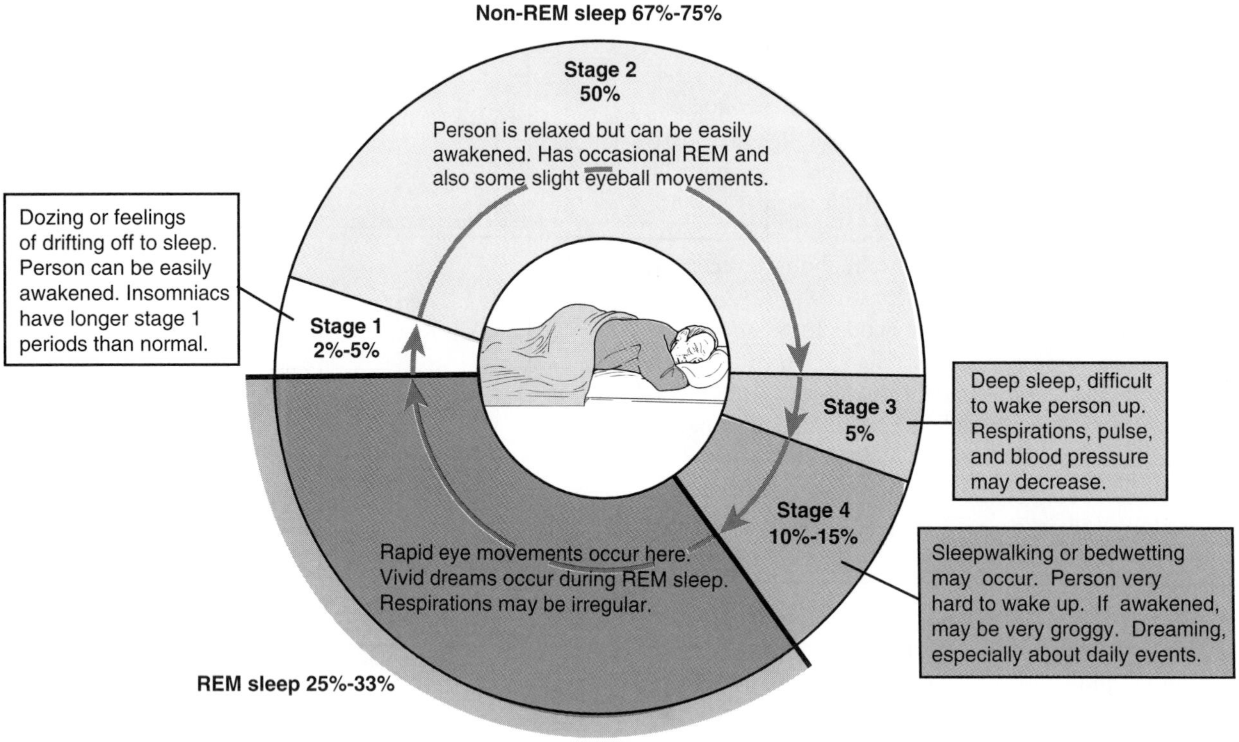

FIGURE 10-2
Stages of sleep.

and, of course, eye movements show under the closed lids. The dynamic physiologic equilibrium of the body continues to be maintained even during sleep. Depression of physiologic functions occurs during deep sleep, and an increase in functions occurs during dreaming. Studies have shown that when individuals are deprived of deep sleep, they become physically uncomfortable, tend to withdraw from their friends and society, are less aggressive and outgoing, and manifest concern over vague physical complaints and changes in bodily feelings. The overall impression made by persons deprived of deep sleep is that of a depressive and hypochondriac reaction.

Dream sleep is also important, as studies indicate that individuals deprived of dreaming sleep (every time the subjects attempted to dream, as evidenced by rapid eye movements, they were awakened and not permitted to dream), experienced a variety of undesirable effects afterward. During waking hours the individuals became less integrated and less effective and exhibited signs of confusion, suspicion, and withdrawal. They appeared anxious, insecure, and irritable; they had greater difficulty concentrating; they had a marked increase in appetite with a definite weight gain; and they were introspective and unable to derive support from other people.

Many psychologists and psychiatrists believe that wish fulfillment finds expression in dreams. Potentially harmful thoughts, feelings, and impulses are released through dreams so that there is no interference with the functioning of the personality during waking hours.

It is also known from dream deprivation studies that the longer dream deprivation continues, the greater the increase in attempts to dream, until the individual begins to dream almost on falling asleep. When subjects are finally allowed to dream, a marked increase in dreaming is noted for the entire night, and as much as 75% of the night may be spent in dreaming. This amount diminishes for each succeeding recovery night until the individual has again established his or her normal sleep pattern.

Research has shown that deep sleep takes priority over dreaming sleep when there has been prolonged sleep deprivation. In other words, deep sleep needs will be met first, after which dreaming sleep needs will be met. The body then attempts to reestablish the normal equilibrium between the sleep stages.

Each individual establishes his or her own normal sleep pattern, which may vary from night to night and which is influenced by the individual's emotional and physical state. For most individuals, any alteration in sleeping habits will cause problems in falling asleep, staying asleep, or both. Because drugs affect physical and emotional states, they also influence an individual's sleep pattern. Box 10-1 lists selected drugs that may cause insomnia.

PEDIATRIC DRUG USE

The use of antianxiety, sedative, or hypnotic agents in children is limited. Because young children are much more sensitive to the CNS-depressant effects of this classification of drugs, counseling and psychotherapy are usually tried first.

BOX 10-1 Drugs Associated with Inducing Insomnia

alcohol
beta-adrenergic blocking agents (Inderal, etc.)
captopril (Capoten)
CNS stimulants (caffeine, Ritalin, etc.)
enalapril (Vasotec)
fluoroquinolones (Cipro, Floxin, Maxaquin, Noroxin, Penetrex)
gemfibrozil (Lopid)
levodopa (Larodopa, etc.)
levothyroxine (Synthroid, etc.)
maprotiline (Ludiomil, etc.)
methyldopa (Aldomet, etc.)
metoclopramide (Reglan, etc.)
metronidazole (Flagyl, etc.)
nicotine
nicotine gum (Nicorette)
oxybutynin (Ditropan, etc.)
pentoxifylline (Trental)
phenylpropanolamine combinations (Contact, Dimetapp, Triaminic, etc.)
protriptyline (Vivactil)
pseudoephedrine combinations (Sudafed, etc.)
quinapril (Accupril)
theophylline (Slo-bid, Theo-24, Theobid, etc.)
thyroid

Withdrawal from CNS Depressants
alcohol
barbiturates
tricyclic antidepressants, such as amitriptyline, imipramine, doxepin, and trimipramine
triazolam (Halcion)
hypnotic drugs

Miscellaneous Drugs with Potential for Inducing Insomnia
contraceptives, oral
phenytoin
corticosteroids
MAO inhibitors

Paradoxical reactions, or reactions contrary to the expected reaction, have been reported with the use of barbiturates in both children and geriatric patients. These reactions include increased excitability, hostility, confusion, hallucinations, and perhaps an acute elevation of body temperature. However, sedation may be indicated for particular situations if the drug and dosage are carefully selected for the individual child (e.g., treatment of severe anxiety associated with an acute attack of asthma, as an adjunct preanesthetic agent, or treatment of convulsive disorders). Close monitoring and assessment by the healthcare provider are required (see Pediatric Implications box).

GERIATRIC DRUG USE

Although they make up approximately 12% of our population, geriatric Americans consume between 35% and 40% of all sedative-hypnotics prescribed. The elderly have more fragmented sleeping patterns; they go to bed earlier and wake up earlier and may take multiple daytime naps. This may in part be due to the changes in the stages of sleep pattern reported in this age group, such as a progressive decline in REM sleep (Gottlieb, 1990).

The Federal guidelines for use of hypnotics in long-term care residents specify that (1) short-acting benzodiazepines should be tried before the long-acting agents are used, (2) hypnotic agents should not be used for more than 10 consecutive days in any 30-day period, and (3) no benzodiazepine should be used longer than 3 to 4 months for treatment of anxiety (Regimen, 1995).

Careful drug selection and dosage are necessary to avoid producing excessive CNS depression in the elderly. The aging process may also be associated with physiologic alterations, including a decline in metabolism and in many or-

PEDIATRIC IMPLICATIONS

Antianxiety Agents and Sedatives

Young children are more susceptible to the CNS-depressant effects of the benzodiazepines. In neonates, profound CNS depression may result because of the lower rate of drug metabolism by the immature liver.

Chronic use of clonazepam may result in impaired physical or mental functions in the developing child, which may not become apparent until years later.

Buspirone use has not been studied in persons under 18 years; therefore it is not recommended for use in this age group.

Although diazepam (Valium) may be used in infants 6 months and older, this drug and other benzodiazepines should not be used to treat a hyperactive or psychotic child.

To reduce or minimize potential adverse CNS-depressant effects, carefully follow the manufacturer's dosage instructions and, whenever possible, avoid concurrent administration of other CNS-depressant types of drugs.

Monitor children for excessive sedation, lethargy, and lack of coordination; if any of these effects are present, dosage adjustments may be necessary.

Paradoxical reactions have been reported in both children and the elderly with the use of barbiturates. (See description under Pediatric Drug Use).

GERIATRIC IMPLICATIONS

Insomnia and Hypnotics

Sleep latency increases while REM and stage 4 sleep may be absent in the geriatric patient. Sleep disturbance is one of the most frequent concerns of the elderly.

Evaluate the individual for preexisting health conditions, since various illnesses such as arthritic pain, hyperthyroidism, cardiac dysrhythmia, and paroxysmal nocturnal dyspnea may alter sleep patterns.

Hypnotics should be reserved to treat acute insomnia and, when prescribed, limited to short-term or intermittent use to avoid the development of tolerance and dependency.

A hypnotic with a short duration of action is preferred. When longer-acting hypnotics are given, daytime sedation, ataxia, and memory deficits may result.

Encourage the older patient to use nonpharmacologic approaches to promote sleep.

Be aware that the elderly, children, and persons with CNS dysfunction may experience a paradoxical reaction (CNS stimulation) to hypnotics and antihistamines.

Common side effects with the antihistamine sleeping aids (which may be prescribed but are also usually in over-the-counter [OTC] drugs) include dizziness, tinnitus, burred or altered vision, gastrointestinal disturbance, and dry mouth.

gan functions, especially liver and kidney functions. Because drug half-lives may be extended, agents with shorter half-lives and no active metabolites may be safer for the geriatric patient. Monitor the elderly patient for paradoxical reactions (i.e., increased excitability, rage, hostility, confusion, and hallucinations), which have been reported with the barbiturates and, in rare instances, the benzodiazepines. The appearance of such adverse reactions requires immediate discontinuance of the medication and consultation with the prescriber. See Chapter 5 for additional information on inappropriate drug use in the elderly.

The short-acting benzodiazepines are much safer than the barbiturates, which are less effective anxiolytic and hypnotic agents. Oxazepam, lorazepam, temazepam, alprazolam, and triazolam have short to intermediate half-lives, and they are usually recommended for an elderly patient who requires a benzodiazepine. Barbiturates should be avoided in the elderly because enhanced CNS depression, confusion, ataxia, and paradoxical reactions are commonly reported.

One of the most frequent concerns of the elderly is **insomnia,** difficulty falling asleep, staying asleep, or early morning awaking. See the Geriatric Implications box for further discussion. Age-related physiologic changes may also contribute to the changes in sleep patterns reported. Many other factors may also result in sleep disturbances, such as retirement, death of a close friend or spouse, social isolation, and increased use of medications.

BOX 10-2 Nonpharmacologic Approaches to Sleep Promotion

1. Restrict use of caffeinated beverages or any caffeine-containing product within 8 hours of bedtime. Read labels because many OTC drugs also contain caffeine.
2. Establish set times for retiring and arising from bed. Avoid daytime napping whenever possible. Try to make the bedroom quiet and dark.
3. Avoid alcohol consumption and smoking cigarettes within 8 hours of bedtime or during the night.
4. Avoid heavy meals several hours before bedtime.
5. Avoid strenuous exercise before bedtime. Exercising during the day is recommended if physical condition permits it.
6. Relax in the evening before retiring by reading, using relaxation techniques, taking a warm bath, listening to relaxing music, or going for a pleasant walk.
7. Try not to worry if unable to sleep because anxiety will add to or cause insomnia. If you cannot sleep, get out of bed and go to another room until sleepy.
8. Do not use the bedroom for wake-time activities, such as eating or watching television.
9. If recurrent and disturbing thoughts interfere with sleep, it may help to write them down and consider a plan of action to solve the problem.
10. Drink warm, noncaffeinated drinks, such as warm milk with honey, before bedtime. Home remedies that help induce sleep include eating a snack high in carbohydrate and low in protein or a few crackers or cookies with a glass of warm malted milk.

From DiPiro et al, 1993.

A study of 430 geriatric persons reported that the most common sleep-related problem was staying asleep (Dopheide, 1995). The three most common reasons for not being able to maintain sleep were respiratory difficulties, pain, and muscle or leg cramps. Appropriate therapy for insomnia should be limited to identification of the cause and treatment of the specific problem.

Gottlieb (1990) indicates that older women report more difficulties with their sleeping patterns than men and are more apt to take hypnotic medications than men and that sleep deprivation in women is more likely to result in mood alterations.

Chloral hydrate and benzodiazepines are usually the agents of choice for treating insomnia in the elderly. When possible, prescribers often suggest that the elderly limit their intake of hypnotic drugs to three or four times a week, allowing patients to select the nights on which they need to take their medication. This schedule usually results in enhanced effectiveness, less daytime drowsiness or sedation, and a decreased potential for inducing tolerance to the medication. Regular and careful assessment, monitoring, and reevaluation of the need for hypnotics are highly recommended. See Box 10-2 for nonpharmacologic approaches to sleep promotion.

PREGNANCY SAFETY

Category	Drug
B	buspirone, zolpidem
C	chloral hydrate, ethchlorvynol, paraldehyde
D	alprazolam, barbiturates, halazepam, lorazepam (parenteral), midazolam (parenteral)
X	quazepam, temazepam, triazolam
Unclassified	other benzodiazepines estazolam, hydroxyzine, meprobamate

It has been reported that many anxiolytic benzodiazepines may also be very effective hypnotic agents. For patients receiving a daytime benzodiazepine (such as alprazolam [Xanax], diazepam [Valium], or lorazepam [Ativan]) who also require temporary use of a hypnotic drug an equivalent hypnotic dose of the anxiolytic agent may be prescribed. For example, 0.5 mg of alprazolam, 5 mg of diazepam, and 1 mg of lorazepam are considered equivalent to 15 mg of flurazepam (Dalmane), 15 mg of temazepam (Restoril), or 0.25 mg of triazolam (Halcion) (Crismon, 1992). See the box for Food and Drug Administration (FDA) pregnancy safety classifications.

BENZODIAZEPINES

The benzodiazepines are among the most widely prescribed drugs in clinical medicine, primarily because of their advantages over the older agents (such as the barbiturates, meprobamate, and alcohol). Their popularity probably results from their anxiolytic and hypnotic dose-related effects, which have the following advantages: (1) lower fatality rates with acute toxicity and overdose, (2) lower potential for abuse, (3) more favorable side and adverse effect profiles, and (4) fewer potentially serious drug interactions reported when administered with other medications.

Diazepam (Valium) is the prototype drug in the benzodiazepine drug family. It was the most commonly prescribed benzodiazepine for many years; that is, until newer and safer (shorter-acting) benzodiazepines were released, such as lorazepam (Ativan) and alprazolam (Xanax). Since the benzodiazepines have similar pharmacologic effects, the following is an overview of their effects with differences illustrated in text, tables, and boxes. See Box 10-3 for benzodiazepine names and pronunciations.

Mechanism of action

Benzodiazepines do not exert a general CNS-depressant effect. Instead a wide range of selectivity is seen with the various members of this class. Some general pharmacologic properties of this class include muscle relaxant, antianxiety, anticonvulsant, and hypnotic effects.

BOX 10-3 Benzodiazepine Names and Pronunciations

alprazolam [al pray' zoe lam] (Xanax)
chlordiazepoxide [klor dye az e pox' ide] (Librium, Libritab, Novoproxide)
clonazepam [kloe na' ze pam] (Klonopin, Rivotril)
clorazepate [klor az' e pate] (Tranxene, Novo-Clopate)
diazepam [dye az' e pam] (Valium, Apo-Diazepam)
estazolam [es tay' zoe lam] (ProSom)
flurazepam [flure az' e pam] (Dalmane, Apo-Flurazepam)
halazepam [hal az' e pam] (Paxipam)
ketazolam [ket az' o lam] (Loftran)
lorazepam [lor a' ze pam] (Ativan, Apo-Lorazepam)
midazolam [mid' ay zoe lam] (Versed)
nitrazepam [nye traz' e pam] (Mogadon)
oxazepam [ox a' ze pam] (Serax, Novoxapam)
prazepam [pra' ze pam] (Centrax)
quazepam [kway' ze pam] (Doral)
temazepam [te maz' e pam] (Restoril)
triazolam [try az' oh lam] (Halcion)

At least two benzodiazepine receptors have been identified, BZ_1 and BZ_2. The BZ_1 receptors are primarily located in the cerebellum and are believed to mediate the antianxiety and sedative effects. BZ_2 receptors are found in the basal ganglia and hippocampus, and so are associated with muscle relaxation and cognitive effects (memory and sensory functions). Both benzodiazepines and barbiturates potentiate the effects of gamma-aminobutyric acid (GABA), the inhibitory neurotransmitter. Benzodiazepines bind to specific benzodiazepine receptors in the brain and spinal cord, which increases the effect of GABA on chloride influx. This results in hyperpolarization of cell membrane and nerve inhibition.

Barbiturates increase GABA binding to receptors sites, and in high concentrations may directly depress calcium-dependent action potentials and increase chloride flux without GABA. Therefore barbiturates result in a broader effect than the benzodiazepines because they also depress excitatory transmitters and nonsynaptic membranes, resulting in a more pronounced CNS-depressant effect.

The limbic system, associated with the regulation of emotional behavior, contains a highly dense area of benzodiazepine receptors in the amygdala that appear to correspond to specific antianxiety effects of certain drugs. These proposed benzodiazepine receptors may share some sites of action with other drugs (alcohol, meprobamate, and barbiturates) and may further explain cross-tolerance to these drugs.

Indications

The most common indications for benzodiazepines include anxiety disorders, alcohol withdrawal, preoperative medication, insomnia, seizure disorders, and neuromuscular disease. They are also used to induce amnesia during cardioversion and endoscopic procedures.

Anxiety disorders. Alprazolam (Xanax), bromazepam (Lectopamo 🍁), chlordiazepoxide (Librium), chlorazepate (Klonopin), diazepam (Valium), halazepam (Paxipam), ketazolam (Loftran 🍁), lorazepam (Ativan), oxazepam (Serax), and prazepam (Centrax) are the benzodiazepines used as antianxiety agents. In addition, alprazolam (Xanax), lorazepam (Ativan) (oral), and oxazepam (Serax) are used as adjunct medications to treat anxiety associated with depression.

Alcohol withdrawal. The benzodiazepines most often used for treatment of alcohol withdrawal syndrome are chlordiazepoxide (Librium), clorazepate (Tranxene), diazepam (Valium), and oxazepam (Serax). These drugs are very useful for the acute agitation, tremors, and other symptoms of acute alcohol withdrawal.

Preoperative medication. Parenteral chlordiazepoxide (Librium), diazepam (Valium), lorazepam (Ativan), and midazolam (Versed) are used preoperatively to reduce anxiety and to help induce general anesthesia; the last three drugs may also decrease the patient's memory of the procedure. These three drugs are also used for endoscopic procedures to decrease anxiety and tension and to produce an **anterograde amnesic effect,** a loss of memory about the procedure.

Sleep disorders. Flurazepam (Dalmane), quazepam (Doral), temazepam (Restoril), and triazolam (Halcion) are usually prescribed for sleep disorders such as insomnia. Generally these drugs are indicated for short-term treatment of insomnia only.

Seizure disorders. Clonazepam (Klonopin) is available orally as an anticonvulsant (see Chapter 11). Parenteral diazepam (Valium) is indicated for intractable, repetitive seizures, such as status epilepticus. Oral diazepam may be used for short-term adjunct therapy (1 to 2 weeks) with other anticonvulsants for the treatment of convulsions.

Neuromuscular disease. Benzodiazepines, especially diazepam (Valium), may be useful as adjunct medications for the treatment of skeletal muscle spasms caused by muscle or joint inflammation or spasticity resulting from upper motor neuron dysfunction, such as cerebral palsy and paraplegia.

Pharmacokinetics

Oral benzodiazepines are readily absorbed from the gastrointestinal (GI) tract. Clorazepate (Tranxene) and diazepam (Valium) are the most rapidly absorbed drugs in this class. Usually the more rapidly absorbed benzodiazepines produce a more prompt and intense onset of action.

The more lipid soluble (lipophilic) benzodiazepines, such as diazepam (Valium), are widely distributed in the body and brain and are also highly protein bound. After multiple doses, benzodiazepines accumulate in the body's fluids and tissues. This saturation of storage sites allows for greater blood concentration and longer action. Accumulation in storage sites also accounts for the prolonged action of benzodiazepines after they have been discontinued.

The GI tract and the liver are the sites of metabolism for either the active drug or metabolite dosage forms of the inactive metabolites. The acid environment of the stomach is the site of conversion of clorazepate (Tranxene) to its active form, desmethyldiazepam. Prazepam (Centrax) also undergoes metabolism in the stomach and liver to the active metabolite desmethyldiazepam. Chlordiazepoxide (Librium), chlorazepate (Tranxene), diazepam (Valium), flurazepam (Dalmane), halazepam (Paxipam), ketazolam (Loftran), and prazepam (Centrax) are converted to active metabolites, notably desmethyldiazepam, a long-acting metabolite (30 to 100 hours) (USP DI, 1998). Therefore long-acting benzodiazepines and their active metabolites are more apt to accumulate, especially in the elderly, resulting in increased risk for falls and hip fractures (USP DI, 1998).

These drugs are highly protein bound and lipid soluble and are excreted by the kidney. Protein binding is reduced in newborns and alcoholic patients and those with cirrhosis or renal insufficiency. Oxazepam (Serax) and lorazepam (Ativan) are metabolized to inactive metabolites; thus they may be preferred agents in elderly patients and persons with liver disease.

The injectable benzodiazepines include chlordiazepoxide (Librium), diazepam (Valium), and lorazepam (Ativan). The onset of anticonvulsant, antianxiety, and muscle relaxant effects of these agents after intravenous administration is approximately 1 to 5 minutes. After intramuscular injection, the onset of action is approximately 15 to 30 minutes. Table 10-1 gives a pharmacokinetic overview of selected benzodiazepine drugs.

Significant drug interactions

Significant drug interactions, such as enhanced CNS-depressant effects, may occur when benzodiazepines are used in combination with alcohol and CNS depressants, opioid analgesics, anesthetics, or tricyclic antidepressants. Close monitoring is necessary because the dosage of one or both drugs may need to be adjusted. Concurrent administration of benzodiazepines with zidovudine (AZT), an antiviral drug, may inhibit zidovudine metabolism, leading to an increased potential for its accumulation and toxicity. If used concurrently, monitor closely for adverse effects.

In 1996, the manufacturers of Halcion and Xanax issued warnings that these benzodiazepines are contraindicated for use in persons receiving ketoconazole and itraconazole. Caution and close monitoring are suggested whenever these drugs are administered in combination with other medications (Drug Product Update, 1996).

Side effects and adverse reactions

Side effects include drowsiness, hiccups (especially with midazolam [Versed]), lassitude, and loss of dexterity. Dry

TABLE 10-1 Pharmacokinetic Overview: Benzodiazepines

Name	Duration of Action*	Time to Peak Plasma Concentration (hr) (Oral)	Half-Life (hr)*	Active Metabolites (Half-Life in hr)
alprazolam (Xanax)	S-I	1-2	11-16	None
chlordiazepoxide (Librium)	L	0.5-4	5-30	desmethylchlordiazepoxide (18) demoxepam (14-95) desmethyldiazepam (30-100) oxazepam (5-15)
clonazepam (Klonopin, Rivotril)	S-I	1-2 (some patients from 4-8 hr)	18-50	None
clorazepate (Tranxene, Novoclopate)	L	0.5-2	Parent drug not active	desmethyldiazepam (30-100) oxazepam (5-15)
diazepam (Valium, Apo-Diazepam)	L	0.5-2	20-70	desmethyldiazepam (30-100) temazepam (9.5-12.4) oxazepam (5-15)
estazolam (ProSom)	S-I	2	10-24	None
flurazepam (Dalmane, Apo-Flurazepam)	L	0.5-1	2.3	desalkylfurazepam (30-100) N-1-hydroxyethylfurazepam (2-4)
halazepam (Paxipam)	L	1-3	14	desmethyldiazepam (30-100)
ketazolam (Loftran)	L	3	2	desmethyldiazepam (30-100) N-methylketazolam (34-52) diazepam (20-70)
lorazepam (Ativan, Apo-Lorazepam)	S-I	1-6	10-20	None
midazolam HCl (Versed)	S	0.25-1	2.5	1-hydroxymethyl and 4-hydroxy midazolam
oxazepam (Serax, Novoxapam)	S-I	1-4	5-15	None
prazepam (Centrax)	L	2.5-6 hr for metabolite desmethyldiazepam (single dose)	Parent drug not active	desmethyldiazepam (30-100) oxazepam (5-15)
quazepam (Doral)	L	2	39	desalkylfurazepam (30-100) 2-oxoquazepam (39)
temazepam (Restoril)	S-I	1-2	8-15	None
triazolam (Halcion)	S-I	within 2	1.5-5.5	None

From USP DI, 1998. S, Short; S-I, short to intermediate acting; L, long acting.
*Elimination half-life.

mouth, nausea, vomiting, headaches, constipation, abdominal cramping, unsteadiness, dizziness, and blurred vision may also occur. Adverse reactions include increased behavioral problems, which are seen mostly with children (anger and decreased ability to concentrate). Neurologic reactions include insomnia, increased excitability, hallucinations, and apprehension (paradoxical reaction). In addition, the patient may experience pruritus, skin rash, sore throat, elevated temperature, increased bruising or bleeding episodes, mental depression, hepatitis, confusion, mouth or throat sores, and muscle weakness. Patients using midazolam (Versed) have also reported muscle tremors, tachycardia, shortness of breath, or breathing difficulties. See the box for the treatment of benzodiazepine overdose.

Warnings

Use with caution in the elderly, in debilitated patients, and in patients with hepatic and renal impairment. See Box 10-4 on triazolam.

MANAGEMENT OF DRUG OVERDOSE

Benzodiazepines

In conscious persons, administer an emetic followed by activated charcoal to adsorb the benzodiazepine. For unconscious persons a gastric lavage with a cuffed endotracheal tube may be used.

Ensure maintenance of an adequate airway, closely monitor vital signs, administer oxygen for depressed respirations, and promote diuresis by the administration of intravenous fluids.

Medications that may be used include IV administration of flumazenil (Romazicon) as a benzodiazepine antagonist and vasopressors such as norepinephrine, metaraminol, or dopamine to treat hypotension. Do not use barbiturates to treat excitation effects as they may exacerbate the condition.

Dialysis is of limited value in treating a benzodiazepine overdose.

BOX 10-4 triazolam [try az' oh lam] (Halcion)

Triazolam is indicated only as a sedative-hypnotic. Although anterograde amnesia may occur with any benzodiazepine, triazolam ". . . may be associated with more frequent psychiatric disturbances than other agents in this class . . ." (McCue et al, 1993). In several European countries, the 0.5 mg dose of triazolam was taken off the market because of the frequency of reports of amnesia and other adverse reactions. In the United States the FDA has required stronger product labeling and patient information. It appears that triazolam reduces the amount of REM sleep, which may contribute to the development or exacerbation of a mental or behavior-type disorder (Jellin, 1991). Effects reported include memory impairment, confusion, depersonalization, and severe anxiety.

Paradoxical rage reactions have also been reported with the benzodiazepines. This reaction is more commonly reported with triazolam according to foreign and domestic studies (Crismon, 1992). The symptoms include depersonalization, increased anxiety and restlessness, agitation, paranoid behavior, rage, panic reactions, and hallucinations. This response may be dose related, since dosages in excess of 0.5 mg/day were recorded in the majority of individuals (Crismon, 1992).

The benzodiazepines have been associated with changes in cognitive function and an increased risk for falls and injuries in the elderly. Altered pharmacokinetics in the geriatric patient may increase the risk for adverse effects; thus close professional supervision along with clear guidelines for benzodiazepine use is necessary. The patient package insert information cautions the patient not to take the medication for more than 7 to 10 days without prescriber consultation, to report any unusual thoughts or behavior during treatment to the prescriber, to avoid the use of alcohol and other drugs including OTC medications unless prescriber approval has been obtained, and also to avoid the use of this product when a full night's sleep is not possible, such as on airline flights of less than 7 or 8 hours (PDR, 1998). Amnesic episodes caused by lack of drug elimination from the body have been reported in such situations. Although many people have taken triazolam (Halcion) without reports of the adverse effects, it may be prudent to avoid the use of this product in the elderly because they generally have an increased susceptibility to memory loss and other adverse drug reactions (Sherman, 1991).

Contraindications

Avoid use in patients who are hypersensitive to benzodiazepines, who have narrow-angle glaucoma or psychosis, or who are pregnant or lactating.

Dosage and administration

See Table 10-2 for approved benzodiazepine indications and dosage and administration information.

New Benzodiazepines Not Available in the United States

Several benzodiazepines currently unavailable in the United States include clobazam (Frisium), an anticonvulsant and anxiolytic similar to diazepam; and nitrazepam (Mogadon), a hypnotic used in Europe and Canada for many years. Both products have long half-lives, which increases the potential for drug accumulation and side effects. They are similar to drugs already marketed in the United States (Olin, 1998). Abecarnil, a partial benzodiazepine-receptor agonist, may have a number of advantages over the currently marketed benzodiazepines. This product initially appears to have less potential for inducing sedation, drug tolerance, ataxia, amnesia, drug dependence, and abuse (Edmonds et al, 1995). Further studies are necessary to clinically validate such claims.

Benzodiazepine Antidote

Flumazenil (Romazicon), a benzodiazepine-receptor antagonist, is indicated for the treatment of a benzodiazepine overdose or to reverse the sedative effects of benzodiazepines after surgical or diagnostic procedures. This drug will not reverse the effects of opioids or other nonbenzodiazepine drugs. Although it can reverse the sedative effects of benzodiazepines, a reversal of the benzodiazepine-induced respiratory depression has not been demonstrated (Abramowicz, 1992; Olin, 1998). Therefore hypoventilation must include the establishment of an airway, assisting ventilation, and interventions to support circulation (USP DI, 1998).

Kirkwood (1991) has suggested using flumazenil to differentiate between accumulation of benzodiazepines or their metabolites in the elderly and physical deterioration from other causes in suspected benzodiazepine overdose situations.

The mechanism of action for flumazenil is that it competes with the benzodiazepine at the receptor sites in the CNS. It is administered intravenously with antagonistic effects occurring within 1 to 2 minutes, peak effect in 6 to 10 minutes, and duration of action of approximately 1 to 3 hours, depending on the dose of benzodiazepine consumed. Because most benzodiazepines have a half-life longer than 1 hour, repeated injections of flumazenil are necessary. Flumazenil is metabolized in the liver and excreted by the kidneys.

Side effects reported with this drug include headache, visual disturbance, excess sweating, increased anxiety, nausea, and lightheadedness. Pain at the injection site can be significantly decreased by infusing the drug through a freely running IV solution into a large vein. Flumazenil may cause convulsions in patients taking benzodiazepines to control epilepsy. Seizures have also been reported in patients who consumed an overdose of a tricyclic antidepressant and a benzodiazepine. Cardiac dysrhythmias have also been reported with the use of flumazenil. Caution is advised when giving flumazenil to patients who are known to use benzodiazepines chronically because moderate to severe withdrawal symptoms may be precipitated in such individuals.

Flumazenil dosage to reverse sedation is an initial intravenous dose of 0.2 mg injected over 15 seconds. This dose may be repeated at 1-minute intervals up to a maximum of

TABLE 10-2 Benzodiazines: FDA-Approved Indications, Dosage, and Administration

Drug	*FDA-Approved Indications**	*Dosage and Administration*
alprazolam (Xanax, generic)	anxiety, panic	*Adults:* antianxiety, 0.25-4 mg/day in divided doses. Antipanic, up to 10 mg/day. *Children up to 18 yr of age:* not recommended.
chlordiazepoxide (Librium, generic)	anxiety, sedative-hypnotic (alcohol withdrawal)	*Adults:* antianxiety, 5-25 mg PO 3 or 4 times a day. Alcohol withdrawal, 50-100 mg PO initially, repeat as needed up to 400 mg/day. Parenteral, 50-100 mg IM or IV 3 or 4 times/day. Preoperative, 50-100 mg IM 1 hr before surgery. *Children:* 6 yr and older, 5-10 mg PO 2 to 3 times a day. Parenteral up to 12 yr, not established; 12 yr and older, 25-50 mg IM or IV.
chlonazepam (Klonopin)	Seizures, panic	See Chapter 17 for information.
clorazepate (Tranxene, generic)	anxiety, seizures, sedative-hypnotic (alcohol withdrawal)	*Adults:* antianxiety, 7.5-15 mg PO 2 to 4 times a day. Alcohol withdrawal, 30 mg initially, then 15 mg 2 to 4 times eventually reduced to 3.75 mg (see current reference for dosing guidelines). Anticonvulsant, 7.5-30 mg 3 times a day per recommended schedule (see current reference for dosing guidelines).
diazepam (Valium, generic)	anxiety, sedative-hypnotic, seizures, skeletal muscle relaxant	*Adults:* antianxiety, 2-10 mg PO 2 to 4 times a day. Sedative-hypnotic (alcohol withdrawal), 5-10 mg 3 or 4 times a day. Anticonvulsant or skeletal muscle relaxant (adjunct), 2-10 mg 3 or 4 times a day. Parenteral, IM, or IV, individualized dose (usually 5 up to 20 mg depending on procedure). See current guidelines.
estazolam (Prosom)	sedative-hypnotic	*Adults:* 1-2 mg PO. *Children up to 18 yr of age:* not recommended.
flurazepam (Dalmane, generic)	sedative-hypnotic	*Adults:* 15-30 mg PO. *Children up to 15 yr of age:* not recommended.
halazepam (Paxipam)	anxiety	*Adults:* 20-40 mg 3 or 4 times a day. *Children up to 18 yr of age:* not recommended.
loraxepam (Ativan, generic)	anxiety, sedative-hypnotic	*Adults:* antianxiety, 1-3 mg 2 or 3 times a day. Sedative-hypnotic, 2-4 mg at bedtime. Parenteral, 0.5 mg/kg IM up to maximum of 4 mg or 0.044 mg/kg or total dose of 2 mg IV (whichever is less). *Children up to 12 yr of age:* PO not recommended. Parenteral not recommended for children up to 18 yr of age.
midazolam (Versed)	preoperative sedation and amnesia, conscious sedation	*Doses are individualized, generally adults:* 70-80 μg/kg ½ to 1 hr before surgery. Also see Chapter 15.
oxazepam (Serax, generic)	anxiety, sedative-hypnotic	*Adults:* antianxiety, 10-30 mg 3 or 4 times a day. Sedative-hypnotic (alcohol withdrawal), 15 or 30 mg 3 or 4 times a day. *Children up to 12 yr of age:* dosage not established.
prazepam (Centrax, generic)	anxiety	*Adults:* 10-20 mg PO 3 times a day or 20-40 mg at bedtime. *Children up to 18 yr of age:* dosage not established.
quazepam (Doral)	sedative-hypnotic	*Adults:* 7.5-15 mg at bedtime. *Children up to 18 yr of age:* dosage not established.
temazepam (Restoril, generic)	sedative-hypnotic	*Adults:* 7.5-15 mg at bedtime. *Children up to 18 yr of age:* dosage not established.
triazolam (Halcion)	sedative-hypnotic	*Adults:* 125-250 μg at bedtime. *Children up to 18 yr of age:* dosage not established.

USP DI, 1998

1 mg. For a benzodiazepine overdose the same initial dose is given, usually over 30 seconds, and then additional doses of 0.3 and 0.5 mg may be given at 1-minute intervals up to a maximum of 3 mg of flumazenil. See current package insert for additional dosing information.

BARBITURATES

The barbiturates were once the most commonly prescribed class of medications for hypnotic and sedative effects. With only a few exceptions, they have been largely replaced by the benzodiazepines. Phenobarbital is generally considered the prototype drug for this classification.

Classification

The barbiturates are classified according to the duration of their action as long-, intermediate-, short-, and ultrashort-acting drugs. The short-acting drugs produce an effect (onset) in a relatively short time (10 to 15 minutes) and peak over a relatively short period (3 to 4 hours). Short-acting barbiturates are used for treating insomnia, for preanesthetic sedation, and in combination with other drugs for psychosomatic disorders.

Long-acting barbiturates require more than 60 minutes for onset and peak over a period of 10 to 12 hours. Long-acting barbiturates are used for treating epilepsy and other chronic neurologic disorders and for sedation in patients with high anxiety.

Ultrashort-acting barbiturates are used as IV anesthetics. Thiopental sodium, which belongs to the ultrashort-acting group of barbiturates, acts rapidly and can produce a state of anesthesia in a few seconds.

Intermediate-acting barbiturates have an onset of 45 to 60 minutes and peak in 6 to 8 hours.

Mechanism of action

The mechanism of action for barbiturates is nonselective depression of the CNS. High doses of the barbiturates may induce anesthesia. Barbiturates similar to the benzodiazepines appear to enhance systems that use GABA as an inhibitory transmitter. In addition, barbiturates may also decrease excitatory neurotransmitter effects. The ascending reticular formation receives stimuli from all parts of the body and relays impulses to the cortex (thus promoting wakefulness and alertness); barbiturate depression of the ascending reticular formation decreases cortical stimuli, reducing the need for wakefulness and alertness.

The extent of barbiturate effect varies from mild sedation to deep anesthesia, depending on the drug selected, method of administration, dosage, and reaction of the individual's nervous system. The barbiturates are not regarded as analgesics and cannot be depended on to produce restful sleep when insomnia is caused by pain. However, when a barbiturate is combined with an analgesic, the sedative action seems to reinforce the action of the analgesic and to alter the patient's emotional reaction to pain.

When used in large doses, all barbiturates depress the motor cortex of the brain, but phenobarbital, mephobarbital (Mebaral), and metharbital (Gemonil 🍁) exert a selective action on the motor cortex, even in small doses. This explains their use as anticonvulsants.

Therapeutic doses have little or no effect on medullary centers, but large doses, especially when administered intravenously, depress the respiratory and vasomotor centers.

Indications

The most common indications for barbiturates include use as adjuncts to anesthesia and treatment of seizure disorders, and several are indicated for treatment of insomnia. However, these agents have generally been replaced by the benzodiazepine family of drugs. Barbiturates are only indicated for short-term use in insomnia because they tend to lose their effectiveness in 14 days or less.

Barbiturates have been used for sedative effects in treating anxiety and nervousness. However, for daytime use the benzodiazepines have largely replaced the barbiturates, primarily because they produce less drowsiness or ataxia.

Short-acting barbiturate anesthetics, such as thiopental and methohexital, are used for selected surgical procedures, especially for surgery of short duration. These barbiturates are discussed more fully in Chapter 9. The short-acting barbiturates, such as pentobarbital (Nembutal), may be used for their preanesthetic effect, to reduce anxiety, and to facilitate anesthesia induction. Diazepam (Valium) and other benzodiazepines are often used today as a preanesthetic agent to help with anesthesia induction, to reduce anxiety, and to induce an amnesic effect.

Anticonvulsant. Barbiturates are also used to prevent or control convulsive seizures associated with tetanus, strychnine poisoning, meningitis, eclampsia, and epilepsy. They may be prescribed alone or in conjunction with other anticonvulsant drugs. Phenobarbital is used in the treatment of epilepsy (generalized tonic-clonic) and for seizures induced by fever, whereas mephobarbital (Mebaral) and metharbital (Gemonil) may be alternative agents for phenobarbital.

Narcoanalysis. Intravenous amobarbital may be used in narcoanalysis, a form of psychotherapy that helps a patient to talk about suppressed feelings and events.

Hyperbilirubinemia. Although not approved for treatment of hyperbilirubinemia, phenobarbital (oral and injectable) is often used to prevent or treat this condition in neonates and in patients with congenital nonhemolytic unconjugated hyperbilirubinemia.

Pharmacokinetics

Barbiturates are readily absorbed after oral, rectal, and parenteral administration. The soluble sodium salts are absorbed faster than the free acids. Most of the barbiturates undergo change in the liver before they are excreted by the kidney. The longer-acting barbiturates are metabolized more slowly than the rapidly acting barbiturates. The slower a barbiturate is altered or excreted, the more prolonged is its action. If excretion is slow and administration prolonged, cumulative effects will result.

Drug interactions

The following effects may occur when barbiturates are given with the drugs listed below:

Drug	Possible Effect and Management
Alcohol and CNS depressants	Enhanced CNS-depressant effects may result. Monitor the patient closely for respiratory pattern changes, and perhaps decrease the dosage of one or both drugs to reduce the possibility of inducing the effect.
Anticoagulants coumarin [Coumadin]	Decrease in anticoagulant effects caused by enhanced metabolism. Prothrombin time tests may be necessary to monitor therapeutic response to anticoagulant and to determine dosage changes of the anticoagulant.

Anticonvulsants carbamazepine [Tegretol]	Monitor serum levels closely whenever carbamazepine or a succinimide is added to or discontinued from a drug regimen. Increased metabolism of the anticonvulsant may occur, leading to decreased serum levels and therapeutic effects.
divalproex sodium (Depakote) or valproic acid (Depakene)	Monitor barbiturate serum levels closely because the metabolism of barbiturates may decrease, leading to elevated levels and an increase in CNS depression and neurologic dysfunction. The half-life of valproic acid may also be reduced, which would also require monitoring of blood levels and dosage adjustments. Phenobarbital may also increase valproic acid hepatotoxicity; monitor closely for jaundice, hepatomegaly, anorexia, abdominal discomfort, clay-colored stools, and dark urine.
Contraceptives, oral	Enhanced metabolism of estrogen (particularly oral estrogen) may result in a decrease in contraceptive effects. The prescriber may need to consider a nonhormonal birth control method or progestin-only oral contraceptive.
Corticosteroids	When given with barbiturates (especially phenobarbital), corticosteroids may enhance metabolism and have decreased therapeutic effects. Dosage adjustments may be necessary. Monitor the patient closely for a lack of therapeutic response to the corticosteroid.

Side effects and adverse reactions

Side effects and adverse reactions include ataxia, drowsiness, dizziness, and hangover effect. Less frequent side effects are nausea, vomiting, insomnia, constipation, restlessness, faintness, headache, and night terrors. If side effects continue, increase, or disturb the patient, inform the prescriber. The most common adverse reactions to these drugs include a hypersensitivity reaction such as skin rash, exfoliative dermatitis, sore throat, fever, edema, serum sickness, apnea, bronchospasms, urticaria, and Stevens-Johnson syndrome. Stevens-Johnson syndrome is a severe, occasionally fatal inflammatory disease of children and young adults, characterized by fever, bullae of the skin, and ulcers of the mucous membranes of mouth, nose, eyes, and genitalia.

Persons of any age, but especially elderly or debilitated patients, may exhibit confusion, disorientation, and mental depression. In children and elderly or debilitated persons, a paradoxical reaction (increased excitability) may occur. Long-term barbiturate use may result in osteomalacia and rickets (bone pain or aching, anorexia, myalgia, and loss of weight). Finally, toxic signs include very severe confusion and persistent irritability. Acute toxic effects may include bradycardia, confusion, respiratory problems (apnea, laryngospasm), ataxia, extreme weakness, and visual disturbances.

Warnings

Use with caution in the elderly, in debilitated patients, in depressed persons or persons with suicidal tendencies, and in patients with liver and renal disease, asthma, hyperkinesis, hyperthyroidism, and severe anemia.

Contraindications

Avoid use in persons with a hypersensitivity to barbiturates, respiratory depression, a history of barbiturate or drug abuse, porphyria, uncontrolled pain, and severe liver or renal impairment.

Dosage and administration

See Table 10-3.

MISCELLANEOUS SEDATIVES AND HYPNOTICS

A number of antianxiety agents/sedatives and hypnotics do not fall into the previously discussed drug classes, but they will be discussed here because they are available for patient use with prescription.

Antianxiety Agents/Sedatives

buspirone [byoo spye' rone] (BuSpar)

Buspirone is not related pharmacologically to the other medications discussed in this chapter. The exact mechanism of action is unknown, but the drug has a high affinity for serotonin receptors and a moderate affinity for brain D_2-dopamine receptors in the CNS. It does not affect GABA, nor does it have any significant affinity to the benzodiazepine receptors.

Indications

Buspirone is indicated for the treatment of anxiety disorders and is considered to be equivalent in efficacy to the benzodiazepines but usually with less sedation.

Pharmacokinetics

Absorption of the drug is very good, but it undergoes extensive first-pass metabolism in the liver. Protein binding is high (95%) and the onset of effect may take 1 to 2 weeks. The drug does not cause muscle relaxation or sedation, so patients may not notice any effects from the medication during this time. The half-life (elimination) is between 2 and 3 hours after a single 10 to 40 mg dose. Buspirone is metabolized in the liver; one of the metabolites is active. It is eliminated through the kidneys and feces.

TABLE 10-3 Selected Barbiturates: Pharmacokinetics, Indications, and Dosage

Name	Onset of Action (min)	Duration of Action (hr)	Indications/Dosage*
Short-Acting			
pentobarbital (Nembutal)	10-15	3-4	*Adults:* hypnotic, 100 mg PO/IV, 150 to 200 mg IM, or 120 to 200 mg rectally at bedtime. Daytime sedative, 20 mg PO or 30 mg rectally 2 to 4 times a day. Preoperative, 100 mg PO or 150 or 200 mg IM. Anticonvulsant, 100 to 500 mg IV. *Children:* sedative-preoperative, 2-6 mg/kg or maximum 100 mg/dose.
secobarbital (Seconal)	10-15	3-4	*Adults:* hypnotic 100 mg PO, 100 to 200 mg IM, or 50 to 250 mg IV at bedtime. Daytime sedative, 30-50 mg 3-4 times daily. *Children:* daytime sedative, 2 mg/kg, preoperative, 2-6 mg/kg or maximum 100 mg/dose given 1-2 hr before surgery.
Intermediate Acting			
butabarbital (Butisol)	45-60	6-8	*Adults:* hypnotic and preoperative, 50-100 mg; daytime sedative, 15-30 mg 3-4 times daily. *Children:* sedative-preoperative, 2-6 mg/kg to maximum of 100 mg/dose.
Long-Acting			
amobarbital (Amytal)	60+	10-12	*Adults:* hypnotic, 65 to 200 mg PO, IM, or IV at bedtime. Daytime sedative, 50-300 mg PO in divided doses or 30 to 50 mg IM or IV 2 or 3 times daily. Anticonvulsant, 65 to 500 mg IV. *Children:* sedative, 2 mg/kg PO 3 times daily; preoperative (6 yr and over), 3-5 mg/kg.
phenobarbital	60+	10-12	*Adults:* hypnotic, 100-320 mg PO or IV hs; daytime sedative, 30-120 mg PO/IM/IV in 2-3 divided doses daily; anticonvulsant, 60-250 mg PO daily or 100 to 320 mg IV. *Children:* anticonvulsant, 1-6 mg/kg/day.

*Barbiturates have generally been replaced by benzodiazepines for daytime sedation and hypnotic effects. See current references for additional information (*USP DI*, 1998).

Drug interaction

Avoid administration of buspirone concurrently with a MAO inhibitor (such as furazolidone, procarbazine, and more than 10 mg a day of selegiline), as hypertension may occur.

Side effects and adverse reactions

Side effects and adverse reactions include headache, nausea, increased nervousness, faintness, tinnitus, abdominal distress, insomnia, nightmares, increased weakness, dry mouth, blurred vision, seizures, muscle pain or spasms, and decreased ability to concentrate. Rarely reported adverse reactions include chest pain, tachycardia, muscle weakness, paresthesia, sore throat, elevated temperature, depression, and confusion.

Warnings

Use with caution in persons with history of drug abuse, in the elderly, and in pregnant and lactating women.

Contraindications

Avoid use of buspirone in persons with drug hypersensitivity and in persons with severe liver or renal impairment.

Dosage and administration

The recommended adult dose is 5 mg orally three times daily, increased by 5 mg/day every 2 to 3 days until the desired response is achieved. The maximum dose is 60 mg/day. No dosage has been established for persons under 18 years old.

hydroxyzine [hye drox' i zeen] (Atarax, Vistaril)

Hydroxyzine, a piperazine antihistamine, is an antianxiety agent, sedative-hypnotic, antihistamine, and antiemetic. The antianxiety effect may be due to hydroxyzine's suppression of activity in selected subcortical areas of the CNS although its full mechanism of action is unknown. Its antihistamine and sedative effects may be due to competition with histamine at H_1 receptor sites. Hydroxyzine's antiemetic, antimotion sickness, and antivertigo effects may be the result of central anticholinergic activity and decreased vestibular stimulation and labyrinthine function. Hydroxyzine may also have an effect on the chemoreceptive trigger zone.

Pharmacokinetics

Absorption of hydroxyzine is good. Onset of action occurs within 15 to 30 minutes after an oral dose. Duration of effect is 4 to 6 hours when the drug is given orally; half-life is 20 to 25 hours. Hydroxyzine is metabolized in the liver and excreted by the kidneys.

Side effect and adverse reactions

Side effects and adverse reactions include sedation, which usually disappears after a few days of therapy or when the dose is reduced. With high drug doses, anticholinergic side effects such as dry mouth are reported. Rare adverse reactions include skin rash, trembling, or seizures (in doses higher than recommended).

Warnings

Use with caution in the elderly, in debilitated patients, and in patients with liver and renal disease, chronic obstructive pulmonary disease (COPD), and prostatic hypertrophy.

Contraindications

Avoid use in persons with known hydroxyzine hypersensitivity.

Dosage and administration

The recommended adult dose of hydroxyzine is 25 to 100 mg orally, three to four times daily as necessary. When the drug is administered to children as an antianxiety agent or sedative-hypnotic, the dosage is 0.6 mg/kg of body weight orally. For antihistamine or antiemetic effects, administer 0.5 mg/kg of body weight orally every 6 hours when necessary. Parenterally the adult dosage is 25 to 100 mg IM every 4 to 6 hours if necessary. When used in children as an antiemetic or adjunct to narcotic medication, hydroxyzine should be administered at 1 mg/kg of body weight IM.

Hypnotics

chloral hydrate [klor al hye′ drate]

(Noctec, Novochlorhydrate ✤)

The CNS-depressant effects produced are believed to be caused by the drug's active metabolite, trichloroethanol, although its exact mechanism of action is unknown.

Indications

Chloral hydrate is indicated as a sedative and as a hypnotic.

Pharmacokinetics

Oral and rectal forms are rapidly absorbed. Chloral hydrate is metabolized in the liver and erythrocytes to its active metabolite, trichloroethanol; further liver metabolism is to inactive metabolites. The onset of action of a hypnotic dose occurs within 30 minutes; the half-life is approximately 7 to 10 hours. The drug is excreted by the kidneys.

Drug interactions

The following effects may occur when chloral hydrate is given with the drugs listed below:

Drug	Possible Effect and Management
Alcohol of other CNS depressants	Enhanced CNS depression effects may result. Monitor closely for respiratory depression and/or lethargy, since the dosage of one or both drugs may need to be reduced.
Anticoagulants (coumarin, indanedone)	Especially within the first few days or weeks, the anticoagulant may be displaced from its protein binding, leading to an enhanced hypoprothrombinemic effect. Monitor closely for bleeding tendencies.

Side effects and adverse reactions

These include nausea, abdominal distress, ataxia, dizziness, drowsiness, confusion, excitability (paradoxical reaction), hallucinations, and skin rash.

Warnings

Use with caution in patients with depression, severe cardiac disease, a history of alcohol or drug abuse, and intermittent porphyria and in the elderly.

Contraindications

Avoid use in patients who are hypersensitive to this drug and in those with severe liver or renal disease, gastritis, esophagitis, or gastric or duodenal ulcers. Also avoid use in pediatric patients with sleep apnea.

Dosage and administration

The adult hypnotic dose is 0.5 to 1 g orally or rectally 15 to 30 minutes before bedtime. The daytime sedative dose is 250 mg three times daily after meals. Use extreme caution with administration of chloral hydrate to children as deaths have occurred with the use of this drug. If administered, the child should be in a healthcare facility that can provide continuous monitoring (USP DI, 1998).

ethchlorvynol [eth klor vi′ nole] (Placidyl)

The CNS-depressant effects are similar to those of chloral hydrate and barbiturates, although the exact mechanism of action is unknown.

Indications

Ethchlorvynol is a sedative-hypnotic.

Pharmacokinetics

Absorption is good from the gastrointestinal tract. The drug's distribution is highly localized in lipid or fat tissues; the drug has also been located in cerebrospinal fluid, brain, bile, liver, kidneys, and spleen. This drug has a half-life of approximately 10 to 20 hours, an onset of action within 15 to 60 minutes, and a duration of action of approximately 5 hours. Ethchlorvynol is metabolized in the liver and excreted by the kidneys.

Side effects and adverse reactions

These include visual disturbances, nausea, vomiting, abdominal distress, increased weakness, facial numbness, unpleasant aftertaste, allergic reactions, paradoxical (increased excitability or nervousness) reaction, and thrombocytopenia. Significant drug interactions are the same as those for chloral hydrate, discussed on p. 183.

Warnings

Use with caution in patients with uncontrolled pain and liver and renal impairment and in the elderly.

Contraindications

Avoid use in patients with known alcohol or drug abuse, mental depression, porphyria, and known sensitivity to ethchlorvynol.

Dosage and administration

The adult sedative-hypnotic dose is 500 to 1000 mg orally at bedtime. The elderly may require lower doses because they are more sensitive to the drug. This drug is not available for use with children.

meprobamate [me proe ba′ mate] (Equanil, Miltown)

Meprobamate functions as a CNS depressant with an unknown mechanism of action.

Indications

Meprobamate is a antianxiety agent.

Pharmacokinetics

Absorption is good; the drug has a half-life of approximately 10 hours. It is metabolized in the liver and excreted by the kidneys.

Side effects and adverse reactions

These include ataxia, drowsiness, visual disturbances, nightmares, muscle twitching, euphoria, headache, and allergic reactions.

Drug interactions

Patients taking meprobamate concomitantly with alcohol or CNS depressants may experience increased alcohol and CNS-depressant effects.

Warnings

Use with caution in patients with epilepsy and liver or renal impairment and in the elderly.

Contraindications

Avoid use in patients with meprobamate hypersensitivity, renal failure, acute intermittent porphyria, and a history of alcohol or drug abuse and in pregnant women.

Dosage and administration

The recommended adult dosage is 400 mg orally three or four times daily or 600 mg twice daily, up to a maximum of 2.4 g/day. Elderly patients may be more sensitive to this drug; their dosage should be lowered, and they should be monitored closely. Meprobamate is not recommended for children younger than 6 years of age. For children 6 to 12 years of age, the dose is 100 to 200 mg orally two or three times daily. The effectiveness of meprobamate beyond 4 months of therapy has not been studied.

paraldehyde [par al′ de hyde] (Paral)

The CNS-depressant effects of paraldehyde, while similar to those of alcohol, barbiturates, and chloral hydrate, have an unknown mechanism of action. It depresses various levels of the CNS, including the ascending reticular activating system.

Indications

Paraldehyde is indicated as an anticonvulsant and in the past has been used as a sedative-hypnotic. The latter is no longer an approved indication as safer and more effective agents are available.

Pharmacokinetics

Absorption is good from the gastrointestinal tract and intramuscular sites; the drug reaches peak serum levels in ½ to 1 hour after oral administration or in 2½ hours after rectal administration. It has a half-life of 3 to 10 hours and is metabolized in the liver (70% to 90%) with trace amounts excreted by the kidneys. The unmetabolized paraldehyde is excreted via exhalation.

Drug interactions

Significant drug interactions are seen when paraldehyde is used in combination with alcohol and CNS depressants (see data on chloral hydrate). The drug also interacts with disulfiram; disulfiram (Antabuse) decreases paraldehyde metabolism, which may lead to increased blood levels of paraldehyde and acetaldehyde. Do not give disulfiram to patients receiving paraldehyde.

Side effects and adverse reactions

These include unpleasant taste, drowsiness, abdominal distress, nausea, vomiting, skin rash, muscle cramps, trembling, and confusion.

Warnings

Use with caution in patients with liver disease and pulmonary disease and asthma and in the elderly.

Contraindications

Avoid use in patients with paraldehyde hypersensitivity and gastroenteritis.

Dosage and administration

The recommended anticonvulsant adult dose is up to 12 ml (diluted to a 10% solution) via gastric tube as needed orally every 4 hours. The rectal dose is 10 to 20 ml. The pediatric anticonvulsant dose is 0.3 ml/kg orally or rectally.

zolpidem tartrate (Ambien)

Zolpidem tartrate is a nonbenzodiazepine that is more selective in its binding to the GABA receptor than the benzodiazepines; thus it has some pharmacologic properties that are similar to those of benzodiazepines. The benzodiazepines bind to $omega_1$, $omega_2$, and $omega_3$ GABA receptors whereas zolpidem only binds to $omega_1$ receptors. Being more selective, it lacks the anticonvulsant, muscle relaxant, and antianxiety properties associated with the benzodiazepines.

Indications

It is the first of a new class, nonbenzodiazepine hypnotics, approved for short-term treatment of insomnia.

Pharmacokinetics

This drug is absorbed well orally; its onset of action is rapid with a time to peak serum level of ½ to 2 hours and a half-life of 1.4 to 4.5 hours. This drug is metabolized in the liver and excreted in urine and feces.

Drug interactions

Avoid concurrent use with alcohol or CNS-depressant medications as an increase in CNS depression may result. If combination therapy is necessary, the dosage of one or both drugs should be reduced.

Side effects and adverse reactions

The most commonly reported side effects are headaches, drowsiness, and myalgia.

Warnings

Use with caution in patients with liver or renal disease, mental depression, severe pulmonary disease, and a history of drug abuse and the elderly.

Contraindications

Avoid use in patients with zolpidem hypersensitivity, acute alcohol intoxication, and sleep apnea.

Dosage and administration

The adult dosage is 10 mg at bedtime. A 5 mg initial dose is recommended for geriatric, debilitated patients and persons with hepatic insufficiency. No dosage has been established for children younger that 18 years of age.

SUMMARY

Benzodiazepines are the most common drugs used to treat anxiety and insomnia today. Because of their safety and effectiveness and the variety of conditions they can be used for, they have largely replaced barbiturates. Antianxiety, sedative, and hypnotic medications may also be used to treat insomnia. As geriatric patients are more sensitive to these agents than the average adult, the use of nonpharmacologic approaches and a limited use of short-acting benzodiazepines should be considered. The healthcare professional should be aware that both the pediatric and geriatric populations are at a greater risk for paradoxical type reactions. It is recommended that prescriptions for these agents be limited with close patient monitoring.

REVIEW QUESTIONS

1. Name and discuss the three Federal guidelines for use of hypnotics in long-term care facilities.
2. Which anxiolytic benzodiazepines are usually recommended for the elderly patient? Why? Can the same medications be used to treat insomnia? What is the usual anxiolytic and hypnotic dose for these agents?
3. Review the mechanisms of action for the benzodiazepines and for flumazenil. Name four patient situations that may become problematic after the use of flumazenil.
4. Explain the major differences in action and effects between a benzodiazepine such as diazepam and zolpidem.

REFERENCES

Abramowicz M, editor: Flumazenil, *Med Lett* 34(874):66, 1992.

Beare PB, Myers JL: *Adult health nursing,* ed 3, St Louis, 1998, Mosby.

Crismon ML: Insomnia. In Koda-Kimble MA, Young LY: *Applied therapeutics,* ed 5, Vancouver, Wash, 1992, Applied Therapeutics, Ltd.

DiPiro JT et al, editors: *Pharmacotherapy,* ed 2, Norwalk, Conn, 1993, Appleton & Lange.

Dopheide JA: Sleep disorders. In Koda-Kimble MA, Young LY: *Applied therapeutics: the clinical use od drugs,* ed 6, Vancouver, Wash, 1995, Applied Therapeutics, Ltd.

Drug Product Update: Halcion, Xanax changes, *ASHP Newslett* 29(10):5, 1996.

Edmonds S et al, editors: Abecarnil shows promise in generalized anxiety disorder, *Drugs Ther Perspect* 5(12):7, 1995.

Gottlieb GL: Sleep disorders and their management—special considerations in the elderly, *Am J Med* 88(suppl 3A):29S, 1990.

Jellin JM, editor: Neurology/psychiatry, *Pharm Lett* 7(11):61, 1990.

Kirkwood CF: Flumazenil—a benzodiazepine receptor antagonist, *P&T* 16(3)243, 1991.

McCance KL, Huether SE: *Pathophysiology: the biologic basis for disease in adults and children,* ed 3, St Louis, 1998, Mosby.

McCue JD et al: *Geriatric drug handbook for long-term care,* Baltimore, 1993, Williams & Wilkins.

Olin BR: *Facts and comparisons,* Philadelphia, 1998, JB Lippincott.

Physicians' desk reference, ed 52, Montvale, NJ, 1998, Medical Economics Co.

Regimen: An update on long-term care drug therapy: monitoring psychoactive drug use in nursing home patients, *NARD* 118(3):1, 1995.

Sherman D: Evaluation and treatment of sleep disorders, *Contemp Long Term Care* 14(12):70, 1991.

United States Pharmacopeial Convention: *USP DI: drug information for the health care professional,* ed 18, Rockville, Md, 1998, the Convention.

Additional References

American Hospital Formulary Service: *AHFS: drug information '98,* Bethesda, Md, 1998, American Society of Hospital Pharmacists.

American Medical Association: *Drug evaluations annual 1995,* Chicago, 1995, the Association.

Anderson KN et al, editors: *Mosby's medical, nursing, and allied health dictionary,* ed 5, St Louis, 1998, Mosby.

Glod CA: Xanax: pros and cons, *J Psychosoc Nurs Ment Health Serv* 30(6):36, 1992.

Grimsley SR: Anxiety disorders. In Koda-Kimble MA, Young LY: *Applied therapeutics: the clinical use od drugs,* ed 6, Vancouver, Wash, 1995, Applied Therapeutics, Ltd.

Hartmann PM: Drug treatment of insomnia: indications and newer agents, *Am Fam Physician* 51(1):191, 1995.

Hoehns JD, Perry PJ: Zolpidem: a nonbenzodiazepine hypnotic for treatment of insomnia, *Clin Pharm* 12(11):814, 1993.

Melmon KL et al: *Clinical pharmacology,* ed 3, New York, 1992, McGraw-Hill.

Morton MR: Managing anxiety disorders in the older adult, *Clin Consult* 11(4):7, 1992.

Mosby: *Mosby's GenRx,* St Louis, 1998, Mosby.

News Capsules: P & T update: new approvals and dosage forms, *Hosp Formulary* 28(3):207, 1993.

Pagel JF: Treatment of insomnia, *Am Fam Physician* 49(6):1417, 1994.

CHAPTER 11

Anticonvulsants

KEY DRUGS

phenobarbital (p. 195)
phenytoin (p. 191)

CHAPTER FOCUS

Epilepsy is a common neurologic illness, second only to stroke in North America. In the United States, between 0.5% to 1% of the population has recurrent epileptic seizures. This chapter discusses seizure classifications, the types of epilepsy, and the various anticonvulsants available to treat this disorder.

OBJECTIVES

After reading and studying this chapter, the student should be able to do the following:

1. *Define and discuss the key drugs and key terms.*
2. *Describe the international classification of seizures.*
3. *Identify the major anticonvulsant drug classifications including drug examples, mechanisms of action, and primary indications.*
4. *Discuss the major drug interactions and management for the hydantoins, succinimides, carbamazepine, and miscellaneous agents.*
5. *Explain the clinical importance of knowledge of a drug's side effects and adverse reactions, warnings, and contraindications to the healthcare professional.*

KEY TERMS

epilepsy, (p. 188)
focal seizure, (p. 188)
generalized absence seizures, (p. 188)
mixed seizures, (p. 189)
partial complex (psychomotor) seizures, (p. 188)
primary or idiopathic epilepsy, (p. 188)
secondary epilepsy, (p. 188)
serum drug half-life, (p. 191)
status epilepticus, (p. 189)
tonic-clonic generalized (grand mal) epilepsy, (p. 188)

Epilepsy is a group of chronic neurologic disorders characterized by sporadic recurrent episodes of convulsive seizures, sensory disturbances, abnormal behavior, loss of consciousness, or all of these symptoms resulting from a brain dysfunction or an abnormal discharge of cerebral neurons. Although nearly 70% of seizures do not have an identifiable cause (**primary or idiopathic epilepsy**), approximately 30% have an underlying cause (**secondary epilepsy**) that is treatable (e.g., head injury, cerebrovascular infarct, or hemorrhage, infection, brain tumor, drug toxicity, or a metabolic imbalance).

CLASSIFICATION OF SEIZURES

The choice of an appropriate anticonvulsant drug for treatment of an individual patient depends on accurate diagnosis and classification of the seizure type. A complete medical history, laboratory tests, a neurologic examination, and an electroencephalogram (EEG) are necessary for classification. Computed tomography (CT) and magnetic resonance imaging (MRI) may also be used to detect anatomic defects or to locate small focal brain lesions. Identifying specific seizure types is critical to the development of a treatment plan.

The terminology currently used with epileptic seizures is illustrated in Box 11-1 on the international classification of seizures. In practice, however, many healthcare providers still use the common terms: grand mal, Jacksonian, psychomotor, and petit mal; therefore the student should be familiar with both seizure classifications. This text will use both classifications.

TYPES OF EPILEPSY

Partial simple motor (Jacksonian) epilepsy is described by some as a type of **focal seizure;** it is associated with irritation of a specific part of the brain. A single body part, such as a finger or an extremity, may jerk, and such movements may end spontaneously or spread over the whole musculature. Consciousness may not be lost unless the seizure develops into a generalized convulsion.

Partial complex (psychomotor) seizures are characterized by brief alterations in consciousness, unusual stereotyped movements (such as chewing or swallowing movements) repeated over and over, changes in temperament, confusion, and feelings of unreality. These seizures are often associated with grand mal seizures and are likely to be resistant to therapy with drugs.

Generalized absence seizures, simple or complex (petit mal), are most often seen in childhood and consist of temporary lapses in consciousness that last for a few seconds. Generally, children appear to stare into space or daydream, are inattentive, and may exhibit a few rhythmic movements of the eyes (slight blinking), head, or hands, but they do not convulse. They may have many attacks in a single day. The EEG records a 3/sec spike wave pattern. Sometimes an attack of generalized absence seizures is followed by a generalized tonic-clonic type of seizure. When the child reaches adulthood, other types of seizures may occur.

BOX 11-1 International Classification of Seizures

Partial Seizures

Simple (No Impairment of Consciousness)

- Motor symptoms (formerly called Jacksonian)
- Sensory (hallucinations of sight, hearing, or taste); somatosensory (tingling)
- Autonomic—autonomic nervous system responses
- Psychic (personality changes)

Complex (Impaired Consciousness)

- Cognitive (memory impairment, confusion)
- Affective (bizarre behavioral effects)
- Psychosensory (automatisms—repetition, purposeless behaviors)
- Psychomotor (complex symptoms that may include an aura, automatism [i.e., chewing, swallowing movements], unreal feelings, bizarre behaviors, and motor seizures)
- Compound (tonic, clonic, or tonic-clonic seizures)

Partial Seizures, Secondarily Generalized

- Unilateral seizures
- Predominantly unilateral seizures

Generalized Seizures (Convulsive or Nonconvulsive)

- Widespread involvement of both cerebral hemispheres
- Tonic-clonic seizures (formerly called grand mal)
- Tonic (sustained contractions of large muscle groups)
- Clonic (various dysrhythmic contractions in the body)
- Myoclonic (unaltered consciousness, isolated clonic contractions)
- Absence (formerly called petit mal—brief loss of consciousness for a few seconds, no confusion, EEG demonstrates 3/sec spike wave patterns)
- Atonic (head drop or falling down symptoms)

Unclassified Seizures

Available data incomplete, inadequate, or lacks classification status (such as neonatal seizures)

Tonic-clonic generalized (grand mal) epilepsy is the type most commonly seen. Such attacks may be characterized by an aura, a sudden loss of consciousness and motor control. The aura is specific to the individual; it may consist of numbness, visual disturbance, or a particular form of dizziness that warns the person of an approaching seizure. The person falls forcefully and has a series of tonic (stiffening, increased muscle tone) and clonic (rapid, synchronous jerking) muscular contractions. The eyes roll upward, the arms flex, and the legs extend. The force of the muscular contractions causes air to be forced out of the lungs, which accounts for the cry that the person may make on falling. Respiration is suspended temporarily, the skin becomes diaphoretic and cyanotic, perspiration and saliva flow, and the person may froth at the mouth and bite the tongue if it gets caught between the teeth. Incontinence may occur.

When the seizure subsides, the individual regains partial consciousness, may complain of aching, and then tends to fall into a deep sleep.

Status epilepticus is a clinical emergency. It is the state of recurrent seizures of more than 30 minutes without an intervening stay of consciousness. A 10% to 20% mortality rate results from anoxia in this state. The major cause of status epilepticus is noncompliance with the drug regimen; other causes include cerebral infarction, central nervous system (CNS) tumor or infection, trauma, or low blood concentration of calcium or glucose.

Mixed seizures are seen in some individuals who have more than one type of seizure disorder. This is significant because different types of seizures respond specifically to certain anticonvulsant drugs. The aim of therapy is to find the drug or drugs that will effectively control the seizures with a minimum of undesirable side effects and restore physiologic homeostasis to arrest convulsive activity.

RELATIONSHIP OF AGE TO SEIZURES

A relationship of age to onset of an epileptic seizure state exists. Most individuals with epilepsy have their initial seizure before the age of 20; however, seizures may have an onset at any age in life. Idiopathic (undefined, unascertainable, or genetic in origin or cause) seizures are often diagnosed between the ages of 5 and 20. Onset before or after this age period is often from nonidiopathic (identifiable, ascertainable) causes and is termed "symptomatic" (acquired, organic) epilepsy.

Neonates

Neonatal seizures occur in newborn children younger than 1 month of age. Among the more common causes of neonatal seizures in this age group are congenital defects or malformation of the brain, abnormality or infections (meningitis, encephalitis, abscess) within the CNS, hypoxia (in utero or during delivery), premature birth, and defects in metabolism. These epileptic seizures are also referred to as organic, symptomatic, or acquired because they may be caused by an identifiable preceding condition or cause.

Infants

In infants younger than 2 years of age, the seizure types most frequently diagnosed include generalized tonic-clonic seizures and partial seizures. The atonic epileptic seizure seen in later development (ages 2 to 5 years) may be preceded by infantile spasms in those younger than 2 years of age. The infantile spasm is not classified as a type of epileptic seizure itself. Among the more common causes of infant seizures are those reported in the neonatal state and, additionally, injury in the perinatal period, infection, exposure to toxins (in utero caused by maternal exposure or drug use, misuse, or abuse), maternal exposure to x-rays, and postnatal trauma.

PEDIATRIC IMPLICATIONS

Anticonvulsants

Chewable phenytoin tablets are not indicated for once-daily administration.

If skin rash develops with use of phenytoin, discontinue drug immediately and notify prescriber.

Avoid intramuscular phenytoin injections.

Be aware that neonates whose mothers received hydantoin drugs during pregnancy may require vitamin K to treat hypoprothrombinemia.

The young person (younger than age 23) is more susceptible to gingival hyperplasia, especially with phenytoin or mephenytoin therapy. Gingivitis or gum inflammation usually starts during the first 6 months of drug therapy, although severe hyperplasia is unlikely at dosages under 500 mg/day. A dental program of teeth cleaning and plaque control started within 7 to 10 days of initiating drug therapy helps to reduce the rate and severity of this condition.

Coarse facial features and excessive body hair growth are more frequently reported in young patients.

Impaired school performance is reported with long-term, high-dose, hydantoin therapy (especially at high or toxic serum levels).

Whenever possible, other anticonvulsants should be considered first because they are less apt to cause the adverse effects induced by the hydantoins.

Children receiving valproic acid, especially those up to 2 years of age or those receiving multiple anticonvulsant drugs, are at a greater risk for developing serious hepatotoxicity. This risk decreases with advancing age.

From USP DI, 1998.

Children

In children 2 to 5 years of age, the seizure types that are frequently diagnosed include generalized tonic-clonic seizures and atonic seizures. The causes are similar to those mentioned in newborns and infants with the addition of chronic diseases involving the CNS. The parents of the child may wrongly believe the child has a behavioral disorder rather than a treatable seizure disorder.

In children aged 6 years and older, brain tumors and vascular disease may cause seizures. Some the convulsive seizure is associated with a brain infection, head trauma, fever, growth of scar tissue, cerebrovascular disease, the presence of a toxin or a poison, or drug withdrawal.

In children 5 to 16 years of age, the seizure types that emerge on diagnosis are absence seizures and generalized tonic-clonic seizures, which may be idiopathic in origin. Seizure types such as partial, myoclonic, and less commonly generalized tonic-clonic may be caused by neurologic diseases, infection, postnatal trauma, or head trauma (accident or sport). See the Pediatric Implications box for more information.

GERIATRIC IMPLICATIONS

Anticonvulsants

If skin rash develops with the use of phenytoin, discontinue drug immediately and notify the prescriber.

Debilitated persons or those with renal or liver disease have a greater risk of developing toxicity with the anticonvulsant agents. Lower doses of the anticonvulsants will help to avoid adverse reactions.

The elderly tend to metabolize anticonvulsants more slowly; thus drug accumulation and toxicity may occur. Monitor closely because dosage adjustments (lower doses) may be necessary.

Serum albumin levels may be lower in geriatric patients, thus resulting in decreased protein binding of bound drugs, such as phenytoin and valproic acid. Monitor closely because lower drug doses may be necessary.

Administer intravenous doses at a rate slower than the recommended rate for an adult. The rate of administration for phenytoin in the elderly should be 5 to 10 mg/min up to a maximum of 25 mg/min.

From USP DI, 1998.

Young Adults

Within the age-group 16 to 25 years, generalized seizures may be idiopathic in origin. The partial seizure and less commonly seen generalized seizures may result from the use of alcohol, social or recreational drug use, drug abuse or misuse, or head injury.

Adults

In patients older than 20 years of age the seizures emerging often are of the generalized type, which may be idiopathic. Also seen are partial seizures and less commonly generalized seizures, which may have been precipitated by trauma to the head or a tumor of the brain.

Elderly

Persons older than age 60 are at greater risk from seizure episodes. In this population osteoporosis and cerebrovascular disease are common, and therefore seizures may lead to fractures, intracranial bleeding, neurologic deficit, cognitive impairment, and severe limitation in daily functioning. Common causes of seizures in the elderly include trauma, brain tumors, vascular disease, embolic stroke, and Alzheimer's disease (Rowan, 1995). See the Geriatric Implications box for more information.

ANTICONVULSANT THERAPY

Although secondary seizures usually respond to correction of the underlying condition and perhaps short-term use of anticonvulsants, primary recurrent seizures require long-term anticonvulsant drug therapy. The primary goal of drug therapy is to control or prevent the recurrence of the seizure disorder. Although there is no ideal anticonvulsant drug, if there were, the following characteristics would be highly desirable:

- The drug should be highly effective but exhibit a low incidence of toxicity.
- The drug should be effective against more than one type of seizure and for mixed seizures.
- The drug should be long acting and nonsedating so that the patient is not inconvenienced by the need for multiple daily drug dosing or excessive drowsiness.
- The drug should be well tolerated by the patient and inexpensive, since the patient may have to take it for years or for the rest of his or her life.
- Tolerance to the therapeutic effects of the drug should not develop.
- The drug should control seizures and permit the patient to function effectively in any environment.

The major drugs used in the treatment of partial seizures and generalized tonic-clonic seizures are phenytoin (Dilantin), carbamazepine (Tegretol), and the barbiturates. Phenytoin is the oldest nonsedating anticonvulsant drug in clinical use and is the most commonly prescribed anticonvulsant in North America. Newer miscellaneous anticonvulsants include felbamate, gabapentin, lamotrigine, tiagabine, and topiramate.

Although the exact modes and sites of action of these drugs are complex and incompletely understood, a major mechanism of action appears to relate to stabilization of the cell membrane by altering cation transport, especially sodium, potassium, and calcium. For example, phenytoin (hydantoins) decreases abnormal seizure discharge by blocking sodium channels and perhaps calcium influx. Thus phenytoin suppresses seizures by stabilizing cell membrane excitability and reducing the spread of seizure discharge. Carbamazepine also enhances inactivation of the sodium channel, which alters neuronal excitability (decreases synaptic transmission).

Thus the two main pharmacologic effects are as follows:

- To increase motor cortex threshold to reduce its response to incoming electric or chemical stimulation
- To depress or reduce the spread of a seizure discharge from its focus or origin by depressing synaptic transport or decreasing nerve conduction.

Anticonvulsants fall into five major classifications: hydantoins, barbiturates, succinimides, benzodiazepines, and a miscellaneous group. The miscellaneous anticonvulsants include carbamazepine (Tegretol), valproic acid (Depakene), primidone (Mysoline), acetazolamide (Diamox), magnesium sulfate, felbamate (Felbatol), gabapentin (Neurontin), lamotrigine (Lamictal), tiagabine (Gabitril), and topiramate (Topamax); these drugs are not chemically similar to one another. For more information see Box 11-2 and the box listing Food and Drug Administration (FDA) pregnancy safety categories.

BOX 11-2 Anticonvulsant Agents for Seizure Disorders

The agents considered most effective with the least toxicity in treatment of seizure disorders are as follows.*

Generalized Tonic-Clonic (Grand Mal)	***Absence Seizures (Petit Mal)***	***Simple or Complex Partial***	***Myoclonic***
valproate phenytoin carbamazepine	ethosuximide valproate	carbamazepine phenytoin valproate	valproate clonazepam

*Listed in order of preference (Lott, 1995).

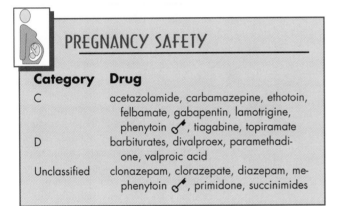

PREGNANCY SAFETY

Category	Drug
C	acetazolamide, carbamazepine, ethotoin, felbamate, gabapentin, lamotrigine, phenytoin, tiagabine, topiramate
D	barbiturates, divalproex, paramethadione, valproic acid
Unclassified	clonazepam, clorazepate, diazepam, mephenytoin, primidone, succinimides

The anticonvulsant therapeutic serum range is used as a guide to therapy. This allows the prescriber to adjust dosages to the individual's requirement, that is, therapeutic response or the development of adverse effects. The time needed to reach a steady drug serum level is usually about four to six times the elimination half-life of the drug. (The **serum drug half-life** is the time necessary for the drug serum level to drop 50% of its initial value when no additional drug is administered; this is a measure of its excretion rate and generally depends on the individual's age as discussed in Chapters 4 and 5.)

DISCONTINUATION OF ANTICONVULSANT THERAPY

A diagnosis of epilepsy no longer implies a lifetime of drug therapy. Studies have indicated that anticonvulsant drugs may be withdrawn from selected patients who are seizure free for at least 2 years. In long-term studies, seizures recurred in 12% to 36% of the patients who were monitored for up to 23 years after complete drug withdrawal. There are some risk factors, though, that may help in predicting which patients may have seizure recurrence after drug withdrawal. They include an onset of seizures after 12 years of age, a family history of seizure activity, a 2- to 6-year range of time before seizures were finally controlled, a large number of seizures before control (>30) or a total of >100 convulsions, an abnormal EEG that was documented even with therapy, the presence of an organic neurologic disorder or moderate-to-severe mental retardation, and perhaps the withdrawal from phenytoin or valproate, drugs that appear to have a higher rate of recurrence when compared with other drugs (Lott, 1995).

Healthcare professionals must be aware that anticonvulsant medications should be tapered down slowly (in an nonemergency situation) to avoid the potential for inducing seizures and status epilepticus. If the patient is taking more than one anticonvulsant, they withdraw each drug separately and slowly.

HYDANTOINS

phenytoin [fen′ i toyn] (Dilantin, Infatabs, various)
phenytoin sodium extended (Dilantin)
fosphenytoin [foss fen′ i toy in] (Cerebyx)

The prototype hydantoin is phenytoin (Dilantin), which was developed from a search for an anticonvulsant that would cause less sedation than the barbiturates. Phenytoin is a drug for the treatment of all types of epilepsy except absence seizures. Fosphenytoin (Cerebyx), a prodrug of phenytoin, was formulated to avoid the problems associated with intravenous administration of phenytoin, i.e., the pain and burning at the site of administration. This product is rapidly converted to phenytoin in the body and has the same pharmacologic profile as phenytoin.

Two other hydantoin drugs are used for their anticonvulsant effects: ethotoin (Peganone) and mephenytoin (Mesantoin). Ethotoin and mephenytoin are usually prescribed only for patients whose symptoms cannot be controlled with other drugs or those who had significant adverse effects from other anticonvulsants. In addition, both drugs are only available in the oral form, which limits their usefulness when a rapid response or parenteral route is needed.

Mechanism of action

See previous paragraph for a complete explanation of the mechanism of action.

TABLE 11-1 Anticonvulsant Therapeutic Plasma Levels and Special Comments

Name	Therapeutic Plasma Levels in Adults (μg/ml)	Special Comments
carbamazepine (Tegretol)	4-12	Take blood sample before morning dose (trough value).
ethosuximide (Zarontin)	40-100	Monitor serum levels as clinically indicated.
methsuximide (Celontin)	10-40	Monitor serum levels as clinically indicated.
phenobarbital (Luminal)	10-40	Monitor serum levels as clinically indicated.
phenytoin (Dilantin)	10-20	Take blood sample before drug dose (trough value). For fosphenytoin, blood samples should be drawn 2 hr after the end of IV infusion or 4 hr after an IM injection. This allows time for fosphenytoin to be converted to phenytoin.
primidone (Mysoline)	5-12	Primidone metabolizes to phenobarbital, so both primidone and phenobarbital levels are monitored.
valproate (Depacon) valproic acid (Depakene)	50-100	Take blood sample in morning before drug dose (trough value). Be aware that trough values >110 μg/ml in females and 135 μg/ml in males significantly increase the potential for thrombocytopenia (USP DI, 1998).

Indications

The hydantoins as a group act to reduce the maximal activity of brainstem centers responsible for the tonic phase of grand mal seizures. Phenytoin is more effective for grand mal than petit mal seizures. It is also frequently prescribed in combination with phenobarbital, and it may be prescribed for patients after surgery on the brain, after head trauma, and for status epilepticus to prevent seizures.

Pharmacokinetics

Oral absorption of phenytoin is slow and variable (poor in neonates); the time to peak serum level is 1.5 to 3 hours, and half-life varies with dose and serum level. It is metabolized in the liver and excreted primarily in urine.

Fosphenytoin is a parenteral drug that reaches peak serum levels in 6 minutes after intravenous administration or 36 minutes after intramuscular injection. Its conversion half-life to phenytoin ranges from 8 to 15 minutes. Metabolism and excretion are the same as for phenytoin. See Table 11-1 for therapeutic plasma levels and special comments.

Drug interactions

The following effects may occur when hydantoins are given with the drugs listed below:

Drug	Possible effect and management
Antacids	Concurrent use may decrease the bioavailability of phenytoin; administer 2 to 3 hours apart.
Anticoagulants warfarin (Coumadin)	A decrease in metabolism may cause an increased serum level and hydantoin toxicity. The anticoagulant effect may be initially increased but will decrease with continuous combined use. Monitor closely for symptoms of thromboembolism.
Adrenocorticoids, corticosteroids, estrogens, or oral contraceptives	An increase in metabolism of these drugs may result from hydantoin's induction of hepatic microsomal enzymes, which may decrease the therapeutic effects of these medications; monitor closely because a dosage adjustment may be necessary. Breakthrough bleeding and an increased risk of conception may occur with estrogen-containing contraceptives.
carbamazepine (Tegretol)	A decrease in therapeutic effect may occur with one or both drugs. Serum drug levels should be closely monitored.
chloramphenicol (Chloromycetin), cimetidine (Tagamet), disulfiram (Antabuse), isoniazid (INH), amiodarone (Cardarone), oral anticoagulants, or sulfonamides	A decrease in metabolism may cause an increased serum level and toxicity of hydantoins. Dosage adjustment may be required.
CNS depressants, alcohol	May result in enhanced CNS depression. Monitor closely for respiratory depression and drowsiness.
calcium	Calcium supplements or calcium sulfate may decrease phenytoin absorption by approximately 20%. Space medications 1 to 3 hours apart.
diazoxide, oral (Proglycem)	May decrease phenytoin effects and decrease the hyperglycemic action of diazoxide. Avoid or a potentially serious drug interaction may occur.
fluconazole (Diflucan)	May decrease phenytoin metabolism, resulting in increased plasma levels of phenytoin and toxicity. Monitor phenytoin serum levels.

TABLE 11-2 Central Nervous System Effects of Selected Anticonvulsants

Drug	*Behavioral Alterations*	*Cognitive Effects*
Barbiturates, especially phenobarbital	May see paradoxical effect, especially in elderly, children, or compromised patients (e.g., increased activity or excitement, irritability, altered sleep patterns, increased tiredness)	Impaired judgment, short-term memory impairment, decreased attention span
carbamazepine	Increased irritability, insomnia, behavioral changes, especially in children, depression	Less than phenytoin, phenobarbital, or primidone
phenytoin	Fatigue, increased clumsiness, confusion, mood alterations	Decreased attention span, decreased ability to problem solve

folic acid	Hydantoins deplete folate from the body. Increased folic acid intake may lower the serum hydantoin levels, leading to a possible loss of seizure control.
lidocaine, propranolol (Inderal), and possible other beta-blocking agents	If given with IV phenytoin, additive cardiac depressant effects may occur. Hydantoins may also increase the metabolism of lidocaine.
methadone	Methadone metabolism may be increased by chronic dosing of phenytoin, which may precipitate an acute withdrawal reaction in patients being treated for narcotic dependence. Methadone dosages may need to be adjusted whenever phenytoin is started or discontinued.
phenacemide (Phenurone)	Increased risk of toxicity when both drugs are used concurrently.
streptozocin (Zanosar)	Phenytoin is reported to protect pancreatic beta cells from streptozocin therapeutic effects. Avoid or a potentially serious drug interaction may occur.
sucralfate (Carafate)	Concurrent use may decrease absorption of hydantoin anticonvulsants. Space medications at least 2 hours apart.
valproic acid (Depakene)	Monitor serum levels of phenytoin (preferably unbound phenytoin) closely, since variable responses have been reported. Adjustments of dosage may be necessary according to patient's clinical response.
Xanthines	Monitor serum concentrations of both drugs. If phenytoin plasma levels are in the therapeutic range, an increase in metabolism of xanthines (except for dyphylline) will occur. Also, if given with xanthines, a decrease in phenytoin absorption may result; monitor closely.

Color type indicates an unsafe drug combination.

Side effects and adverse reactions

These include hirsutism, constipation, nausea, vomiting, drowsiness, dizziness, and gingival hyperplasia (bleeding, sensitive gum tissue, or overgrowth of gum tissue). Signs of overdose or toxicity include blurred or double vision, nausea, vomiting, slurred speech, clumsiness, unsteadiness or staggering gait, dizziness, fatigue, confusion, and hallucinations. In addition, signs of toxicity with intravenous phenytoin include cardiovascular collapse, CNS depression, and hypotension (reported with rapid intravenous administration resulting from propylene glycol solvent). The rate of administration of 25 to 50 mg/min is important, since severe cardiotoxic reactions and fatal outcomes have been reported. See Table 11-2 for CNS effects.

Warnings

Use with caution in persons with drug allergies, diabetes mellitus, systemic lupus erythematosus, and liver or renal impairment.

Contraindications

Avoid use in persons with hydantoin drug hypersensitivity, porphyria, and blood dyscrasias.

Dosage and administration

The usual adult dosage is 100 mg PO three times a day. When the proper dose is established, only the extended phenytoin capsules may be given once a day, depending on the individual's tolerance. For status epilepticus, the dose is 15 to 20 mg/kg IV at a rate of 25 to 50 mg/min (or in the elderly or debilitated, 5 to 25 mg/min). The pediatric dose is 5 mg/kg PO in divided doses initially and then for maintenance dosing is 4 to 8 mg/kg PO in two or three doses daily. For status epilepticus, the dose is 15 to 20 mg/kg administered IV at a rate of 1 mg/kg/min. Do not exceed 50 mg/min (USP DI, 1998).

mephenytoin [me fen′ i toyn] [Mesantoin]

Mephenytoin is chemically similar in structure, activity, and pharmacokinetics to phenytoin, but it is less potent as an anticonvulsant. It produces more sedation than phenytoin, but this side effect is dose related. It also has a greater potential for producing blood dyscrasias and dermatologic effects than the other hydantoins. This product is usually reserved for patients whose seizures are not controlled with safer anticonvulsants.

The usual adult dose is 50 to 100 mg orally daily, increased weekly as necessary up to a 1.2 g/day maximum; for children the dose is 25 to 50 mg daily.

ethotoin [eth' oh toyn] (Peganone)

Ethotoin is similar to phenytoin but less effective and offers little advantage over phenytoin. Side effects of ataxia, hirsutism, and gum hyperplasia are rare, and ethotoin may be substituted for phenytoin to reduce these side effects. Ethotoin is available only for oral administration, with dosage individualized according to response. A maintenance dosage (usually divided into four to six doses) of less than 2 g is usually not effective.

BARBITURATES

Barbiturates, especially phenobarbital, have been used for many years for the treatment of generalized tonic-clonic and partial seizures. This class of medications is relatively inexpensive and efficacious and has a low incidence of side effects. The most commonly prescribed barbiturate is phenobarbital.

Pharmacokinetics

Mephobarbital (Mebaral) is converted by the liver metabolizing enzymes to phenobarbital. Both barbiturates are long-acting compounds, but phenobarbital is the most commonly prescribed barbiturate. See Table 11-1 for therapeutic serum levels and comments.

Drug interactions

The following effects may occur when barbiturates, especially phenobarbital, are given with the drugs listed below:

Drug	Possible effect and management
Adrenocorticoids or corticosteroids (prednisone, etc.)	The effects of these drugs may be decreased because of enhanced metabolism caused by barbiturates. Dosage adjustment may be necessary.
Alcohol, anesthetics, CNS depressants (sedatives, hypnotics, narcotics)	Enhanced CNS depressant effects, respiratory depression; use extreme caution in combining such medications. Usually the dosage of one or both drugs should be reduced.
Anticoagulants warfarin (Coumadin)	Effects may be decreased because of enhanced metabolism produced by barbiturates. Closely monitor prothrombin time. Dosage adjustment of anticoagulants may be necessary.
carbamazepine (Tegretol)	Concurrent drug administration may result in a decrease in the serum level and half-life of carbamazepine. Monitor serum levels whenever carbamazepine is prescribed or discontinued from combination drug therapy.
hydantoin anticonvulsants	Unpredictable effects on hydantoin metabolism may occur. Serum levels should be closely monitored when drugs are given concurrently.
divalproex sodium (Depakote) or valproic acid (Depakene)	Two effects may result from this combination: (1) valproic acid half-life may be decreased, which would require a dosage adjustment to maintain control; or (2) metabolism of barbiturates may be decreased, which can result in elevated barbiturate serum levels and toxicity. Monitor barbiturate levels, since a dosage adjustment may be necessary. Phenobarbital may also increase the potential for valproic acid hepatotoxicity; monitor liver function study results closely.

Side effects and adverse reactions

The adverse effects of apnea, bronchospasm, and respiratory depression may occur after rapidly administered intravenous injections of barbiturates. Severe symptoms of withdrawal may occur in individuals who have a barbiturate dependency from prolonged use at high dosages. Anxiety, trembling, nausea, vomiting, insomnia, orthostatic hypotension, seizures, hallucinations, and even death may result if the drug is withdrawn abruptly.

Gradual withdrawal in a controlled setting is usually recommended for the treatment of dependence. See Table 11-2 for CNS effects.

Warnings

Use with caution in persons with anemia, asthma, hyperkinesis, hyperthyroidism, mental depression, and liver or renal impairment.

Contraindications

Avoid use in patients with a barbiturate hypersensitivity, a history of drug abuse, hepatic coma, acute or chronic pain, or respiratory diseases that include dyspnea or obstruction.

Dosage and administration

The parenteral dosage forms of amobarbital, phenobarbital, and secobarbital have been used in emergency treatment of seizures (Table 11-3). The oral dosage forms are generally not indicated for the treatment of seizure disorders because of their potent sedative-hypnotic effects.

TABLE 11-3 Indications for Parenteral Use of Anticonvulsants

Parenteral Drug	*Use*
barbiturates, especially phenobarbital, also amobarbital, pentobarbital sodium, and secobarbital sodium	Eclampsia, status epilepticus, severe recurrent seizures, tetanus, convulsant drug toxicity, other convulsive states
phenytoin	Status epilepticus, seizure during neurosurgery
magnesium sulfate	Severe toxemias of pregnancy (preeclampsia and eclampsia)
benzodiazepines: diazepam, lorazepam	Status epilepticus, severe, recurrent seizures

phenobarbital [fee noe bar′ bi tal] (Barbita, Luminal)

Phenobarbital is the prototype barbiturate to treat epilepsy. There are many dosage forms (tablets, elixirs, solutions, and parenteral) and strengths available. The healthcare professional must exercise special caution to ensure that the proper dose is given as prescribed.

Several weeks of phenobarbital therapy may be necessary to achieve the maximum anticonvulsant effects. When administered intravenously, 15 to 30 minutes are required to reach the maximum anticonvulsant effect. To avoid excessive barbiturate-induced depression it is important to wait for the anticonvulsant effect to develop before administering additional doses. When administered intravenously, phenobarbital should be administered slowly to avoid respiratory depression; a rate of 60 mg/min should not be exceeded. Resuscitative equipment should be readily available.

The optimal blood concentration of phenobarbital should be determined by seizure control and an absence of toxic effects. A serum concentration of 10 to 40 μg/mL is usually desired. Dosage and administration of phenobarbital are addressed in Table 10-3.

amobarbital [am oh bar′ bi tal] (Amytal)

Amobarbital is indicated for use as a sedative-hypnotic and anticonvulsant. Only the parenteral form is used as an anticonvulsant. Amobarbital should be administered deep intramuscularly to reduce the possibility of sterile abscesses and sloughing of tissue. When administered intravenously to an adult, the rate of injection should not exceed 100 mg/min. Parenteral solutions should be clear and without precipitate when reconstituted. The solution should be used within 30 minutes of reconstitution, since it hydrolyses easily.

mephobarbital [me foe bar′ bi tal] (Mebaral)

Mephobarbital is a barbiturate indicated for use only as an anticonvulsant. Therapy is usually begun with small doses and increased over a period of 4 to 5 days until the optimal dosage has been established. Because mephobarbital is metabolized to phenobarbital, serum levels of phenobarbital may be monitored. Mephobarbital is available in oral dosage forms only.

SUCCINIMIDES

The succinimides include ethosuximide (Zarontin), methsuximide (Celontin), and phensuximide (Milontin). These agents produce a variety of effects, such as increasing the seizure threshold and reducing the EEG spike-and-wave pattern of absence seizures by decreasing nerve impulses and transmission in the motor cortex.

Indications

Ethosuximide and phensuximide are indicated for the treatment of absence seizures, whereas methsuximide is reserved for absence seizures that are nonresponsive to other medications.

Pharmacokinetics

These agents are rapidly absorbed after oral administration and reach peak serum levels as follows: ethosuximide in adults in 2 to 4 hours and in children in 3 to 7 hours; methsuximide and phensuximide in 1 to 4 hours. Half-lives are as follows: ethosuximide 56 to 60 hours in adults and 30 to 36 hours in children; methsuximide 1 to 3 hours; and phensuximide 5 to 12 hours. The drugs are metabolized in the liver (methsuximide to an active metabolite) and excreted in the kidneys. See Table 11-1 for therapeutic serum levels.

Drug interactions

The following effects may occur when succinimides are given in combination with the drugs listed below:

Drug	Possible effect and management
carbamazepine (Tegretol), phenobarbital, or phenytoin (Dilantin)	Results in increased metabolism of succinimide anticonvulsants and decreased serum levels. Monitor serum levels especially when either drug is added, increased, decreased, or deleted from the drug regimen.
haloperidol (Haldol)	May change the pattern or frequency of seizures. Dosage of the anticonvulsant may need to be adjusted. Serum levels of haloperidol may be reduced, which may result in decreased effectiveness.
Phenothiazines, thioxanthenes, antidepressants, loxapine (Loxitane), maprotiline (Ludiomil), or CNS depressants	May decrease the effectiveness of the anticonvulsant, enhance CNS depression, and lower the seizure threshold. Monitor closely for respiratory depression and drowsiness because dosage modifications may be necessary.

Side effects and adverse reactions

These include headache, epigastric pain, anorexia, hiccups, nausea, vomiting, rash, pruritus (possibly Stevens-Johnson syndrome), mood changes, and agranulocytosis.

Warnings

Use with caution in persons with blood dyscrasias, intermittent porphyria, and liver or renal impairment.

Contraindications

Avoid use in persons with succinimide drug hypersensitivity.

Dosage and administration

The ethosuximide dose in adults and children 6 years of age and older is initially 250 mg PO twice daily, increased as necessary in 4 to 7 days. The maximum daily dose is 1.5 g. For children younger than 6 years of age, the initial dose is 250 mg/day, increased by 250 mg at 4- to 7-day intervals. The maximum daily dose is 1 g.

The methsuximide adult dose is 300 mg PO daily initially, increased if necessary by 300 mg increments at weekly intervals until seizures are controlled or the maximum daily dose of 1.2 g is reached. The dosage for children is individualized.

The phensuximide adult and pediatric dose is 500 mg PO two or three times daily, increased by 500 mg at weekly intervals until seizures are controlled or the maximum daily dose of 3 g is reached.

BENZODIAZEPINES

The benzodiazepines include clonazepam (Klonopin), diazepam (Valium), clorazepate (Tranxene), and parenteral lorazepam (Ativan).

Indications

These drugs appear to suppress the propagation of seizure activity produced by foci in the cortex, thalamus, and limbic areas.

Clonazepam (Klonopin) is a long-acting drug used to treat absence seizures and myoclonic seizure disorders. It has been used alone, but more often it is prescribed as an adjunct to other anticonvulsants to establish seizure control. Diazepam (Valium) may be used parenterally for status epilepticus and for severe recurrent convulsive seizures, but the oral dosage form is not effective for maintenance control. The oral form of diazepam has been used as an adjunctive medication for short-term treatment in convulsive disorders. Diazepam is not effective alone and use beyond 4 months has not been clinically evaluated (PDR, 1998).

The usual adult dose is 0.5 mg PO three times daily, increased by 0.5 to 1 mg every third day until seizures are controlled, side effects occur, or the maximum of 20 mg/day is reached. For children younger than 10 years of age or 30 kg the initial dose is 0.01 to 0.03 mg/kg in divided doses (three times a day). Maximum maintenance dose is 0.1 to 0.2 mg/kg daily.

Clorazepate (Tranxene) has been prescribed as an adjunct medication for the treatment of simple partial seizures. See Chapter 10 for the pharmacokinetics and side effects and adverse reactions for these drugs. The usual adult dose is 7.5 mg PO three times daily, increased if necessary by 7.5 mg/wk to a maximum of 90 mg/day. For children 9 to 12 years of age, the dose is 7.5 mg PO twice daily, increased weekly if necessary. The maximum dose is 60 mg daily.

The diazepam adult dose is 5 to 10 mg IV initially, repeated in 10- to 15-minute intervals if necessary to a maximum of 30 mg. Inject the IV drug slowly, at least 1 minute for each 5 mg dose. The oral dose is 2 to 10 mg three to four times daily. See a current reference for pediatric dosing.

Dosage is usually individualized for each patient and increased if necessary. The elderly or debilitated persons and those taking other CNS-depressant-type medications usually receive a smaller dose with a slower dosage increase.

MISCELLANEOUS ANTICONVULSANTS

acetazolamide [a set a zole′ a mide] (Diamox)

Acetazolamide is a carbonic anhydrase inhibitor usually prescribed for the treatment of open-angle glaucoma. It is used in combination with other anticonvulsant agents for the treatment of absence seizures, generalized tonic-clonic seizures, mixed seizures, and myoclonic seizure patterns. Acetazolamide's mechanism of action is unknown. It has been theorized that inhibiting carbonic anhydrase in the CNS may result in an increase in carbon dioxide that retards neuronal activity. Systemic metabolic acidosis may also play a part in its action. See Chapter 28 for pharmacokinetics, side effects, and adverse reactions.

Dosage and administration

Adult and pediatric doses for anticonvulsant therapy is 4 to 30 mg/kg/day PO (initial dose is usually 10 mg/kg/day) in four divided doses (usually 375 to 1000 mg/day).

carbamazepine [kar ba maz′ e peen] (Tegretol)

The exact mechanism of action is unknown, although this drug's effects are somewhat similar to those of phenytoin. Carbamazepine is indicated in the treatment of partial seizures with complex symptomatology, for generalized tonic-clonic seizures, for psychomotor seizures, and for mixed seizure patterns. This drug is also indicated in the treatment of pain associated with true trigeminal neuralgia.

Pharmacokinetics

Oral absorption is slow, and onset of action may range from hours to days, depending on the individual. Due to autoinduction of metabolism, it may take a month to reach a stable therapeutic serum level. Carbamazepine is metabolized in the liver (has one active metabolite) and excreted primarily by the kidneys. See Table 11-1 for therapeutic serum levels.

Drug interactions

The following effects may occur when carbamazepine is given with the drugs listed below:

Drug	Possible effect and management
Anticoagulants, oral warfarin (Coumadin)	Monitor for a decreased anticoagulant effect. Increased hepatic microsomal enzyme activity may increase anti coagulant metabolism, resulting in a decreased half-life and therapeutic effect. Dosage adjustments of anticoagulant may be necessary during and after treatment with carbamazepine.
Anticonvulsants (hydantoin or succinimide); barbiturates, benzodiazepines metabolized by hepatic enzymes, especially clonazepam (Klonopin), primidone (Mysoline), or valproic acid (Depakene)	Concurrent drug administration may result in increased drug metabolism and decreased serum levels and therapeutic effectiveness of these medications. Monitor blood levels whenever any of these medications is added to or discontinued in persons receiving carbamazepine, since dosage adjustment may be necessary. Valproic acid however, may prolong the half-life of carbamazepine.
clarithromycin (Biaxin)	Concurrent use may result in elevated carbamazepine levels. Monitor serum levels closely.
cimetidine (Tagamet), diltiazem (Cardizem), or verapamil (Calan)	May increase plasma levels of carbamazepine, which can result in toxicity. Monitor closely.
Corticosteroids	Concurrent administration may decrease steroidal effect because of an increase in hepatic metabolism. Monitor closely for lack of response to corticosteroid therapy; dosage adjustment may be necessary.
erythromycin	Concurrent use may reduce carbamazepine metabolism, resulting in increased serum levels and toxicity. Avoid this combination and use a different antibiotic with patients taking carbamazepine.
Estrogen-containing contraceptives	Decrease in contraceptive reliability; patients should be advised to use a nonhormonal birth control method or to discuss the possibility of an oral progestin product with their prescriber.
isoniazid (INH)	Carbamazepine may increase liver metabolism of isoniazid, releasing an intermediate metabolite that can lead to hepatotoxicity. Also isoniazid may increase serum concentrations of carbamazepine, which may result in toxicity. Note: concurrent use not recommended or contraindicated because of possible serious outcome.
loxapine (Loxitane), maprotiline (Ludiomil), thioxanthenes, or tricyclic antidepressants	May reduce the convulsive threshold and enhance CNS-depressant effects; dosage adjustment may be necessary to control seizures and reduce side effects. Monitor closely for seizure activity.
Monoamine oxidase (MAO) inhibitors	Hypertensive crisis, elevated temperatures, severe convulsions, and even death have been reported with this combination. When switching from one therapy to another (MAO to carbamazepine or vice versa), a drug-free interval of at least 14 days is recommended. Avoid or a potentially serious drug interaction may occur.
quinidine	Because of increased metabolism, concurrent use may decrease quinidine's therapeutic effects. Monitor closely for cardiac dyshythmias; dosage adjustment may be necessary.
propoxyphene (Darvon, others)	May result in increased carbamazepine serum levels and toxicity. If an analgesic is necessary, it is recommended that another analgesic be selected.

Color type indicates an unsafe drug combination.

Side effects and adverse reactions

These include vertigo, drowsiness, nausea, vomiting, dizziness, blurred vision or other visual disturbances, ataxia, confusion, muscle aches or cramps, allergic reaction, Stevens-Johnson syndrome, systemic lupus erythematosus–type syndrome, and the syndrome of increased release of antidiuretic hormone. See Table 11-2 for CNS effects.

Warnings

Use with caution in persons with alcoholism, coronary artery disease, cardiac, liver or renal disease, diabetes mellitus, glaucoma, and psychosis.

Contraindications

Avoid use in patients with carbamazepine or tricyclic antidepressant hypersensitivity, blood dyscrasias, bone marrow depression, atrioventricular heart block, and absence, atonic, or myoclonic seizures.

Dosage and administration

The adult dose is 200 mg twice daily initially, increased by 200 mg/day weekly in divided doses until response is noted. The maximum dose is 1200 mg/day, with a maintenance range of 800 to 1200 mg/day in divided doses. For children up to 6 years of age, the initial dose is 10 to 20 mg/kg/day in divided doses; increase weekly. Maintenance usually requires between 250 and 350 mg daily. For children 6 to 12 years of age the initial dose is 100 mg twice a day, increased by 100 mg/day weekly until the desired response is obtained. Maintenance is usually between 400 and 800 mg/day in divided dosages. Administer the oral dose with food to reduce gastrointestinal (GI) distress.

felbamate (Felbatol)

Felbamate is an antiepileptic used for the treatment of partial and secondary generalized seizures. It is also used as adjunct therapy for partial and generalized seizures associated with Lennox-Gastaut syndrome in children. Its mechanism of action is unknown although it has some properties in common with the other anticonvulsants: it may increase the seizure threshold, have an inhibitory effect on gamma-aminobutyric acid (GABA) receptor binding, and reduce the spread or progression of a seizure.

Pharmacokinetics

Oral absorption is good; felbamate absorption is not affected by food. The time to peak serum level is 1 to 6 hours; half-life is 13 to 23 hours. Felbamate is metabolized in the liver and primarily excreted in the kidneys.

Drug interaction

When felbamate is given concurrently with carbamazepine, a decrease in the felbamate serum level may occur. If carbamazepine dosage is decreased or discontinued, an elevation in the felbamate serum level may result. Monitor serum levels closely whenever this combination is used or when the carbamazepine dosage is altered.

Side effects and adverse reactions

These include gastric distress, nausea, vomiting, taste alterations, anorexia, constipation, headache, insomnia, dizziness, fever, abnormal gait, and red-purple skin spots.

Warnings

Use with caution in persons with liver impairment.

Contraindications

Avoid use in persons with felbamate hypersensitivity, blood dyscrasias, bone marrow depression, and liver impairment.

Dosage and administration

The usual adult (14 years of age and older) dose is 1200 mg/day in divided doses. Children, 2 to 14 years of age, receive 45 mg/kg/day or 3600 mg/day, whichever is less, in divided doses.

gabapentin (ga ba pen′ ten) (Neurontin)

Gabapentin is an antiepileptic for the treatment of adult partial seizures with or without secondary generalization. It was tested in patients with refractory partial seizures and was reported to significantly reduce seizure frequency. The mechanism for its anticonvulsant action is unknown.

Pharmacokinetics

Gabapentin is absorbed orally, distributed unbound in the circulation, and excreted unchanged by the kidneys.

Side effects and adverse reactions

These include drowsiness, dizziness, tiredness, ataxia, and nystagmus.

Warnings

Use with caution in the elderly and in persons with liver and renal disease.

Contraindications

Avoid use in persons with gabapentin hypersensitivity.

Dosage and administration

The recommended adult dose is 300 to 600 mg three times a day.

lamotrigine (Lamictal)

Lamotrigine is an anticonvulsant whose mechanism of action is unknown. It is believed that lamotrigine stabilizes seizures by blocking sodium channels and thus inhibiting the release of excitatory neurotransmitters (glutamate and aspartate). These substances are believed to have a role in development and spread of epileptic seizures (AHFS, 1998). It is indicated as adjunct therapy for the treatment of partial seizures in adults (16 years of age and older) with epilepsy.

Pharmacokinetics

This drug is well absorbed orally, reaches peak serum levels in 1.4 to 4.8 hours, and has a half-life of 10 to 25 hours if taken with no other medications. If lamotrigine is administered with an enzyme-inducing anticonvulsant, the half-life is 8 to 20 hours; with valproic acid only, the half-life is 59 hours; with both enzyme-inducing and valproic acid anticonvulsants, the half-life is 28 hours. It is metabolized in the liver and excreted primarily by the kidneys.

Drug interactions

The following effects may occur when lamotrigine is given with the drugs listed below:

Drug	Possible effect and management
carbamazepine (Tegretol), phenobarbital, phenytoin (Dilantin), or primidone (Mysoline)	With carbamazepine, an increase in adverse CNS effects (e.g., blurred vision, dizziness, increased excitation, and ataxia) may occur. A reduction in dose of either drug may reduce these effects. Monitor lamotrigine serum levels closely as the clearance of it may increase with combined therapies. Monitor serum levels of other agents also, as dosage adjustments may be necessary.
valproic acid (Depakene)	The half-life and serum levels of lamotrigine may be increased with this drug combination. Monitor serum levels closely as dosage adjustments may be necessary. This drug combination has also resulted in rash and tremors.

Side effects and adverse reaction

These include headache, dizziness, drowsiness, abdominal distress, ataxia, rash, and visual disturbances.

Warnings

Use with caution in persons with liver function impairment, thalassemia, and cardiac disease.

Contraindications

Avoid use in persons with lamotrigine hypersensitivity and severe renal impairment.

Dosage and administration

The usual adult dose if given with enzyme-inducing anticonvulsants is 50 mg daily for 2 weeks, then 50 mg twice a day for 2 weeks. The dose is adjusted according to response. If lamotrigine is administered with enzyme-inducing and valproic acid anticonvulsants, the dose is 25 mg every other day for 2 weeks, then 25 mg daily for 2 weeks. After 2 weeks, the dose is adjusted according to the patient's response.

primidone [pri' mi done] (Mysoline)

Primidone and its metabolites, phenobarbital and phenylethylmalonamide (PEMA), contribute to anticonvulsant activity. The mechanism of action is unknown, but primidone and its metabolites all appear to have active anticonvulsant effects. Primidone is used for control of generalized tonic-clonic (grand mal) and complex seizures.

Pharmacokinetics

Oral absorption is rapid, reaching peak serum levels in 3 to 4 hours. Primidone has a half-life of 3 to 23 hours while its metabolites phenobarbital and PEMA have half-lives of 75 to 126 hours and 10 to 25 hours, respectively. See Table 11-1 for therapeutic serum levels.

Drug interactions

The following effects may occur when primidone is given with the drugs listed below:

Drug	Possible effect and management
Alcohol, CNS depressants	Concurrent therapy may result in increased CNS and respiratory depression effects. Dosage adjustments may be necessary.
Anticoagulants, warfarin (Coumadin); contraceptives with estrogen (oral); corticosteroids; or corticotropin (ACTH)	Primidone may increase the metabolism of these drugs, resulting in a decreased effect. Dosage adjustments may be necessary. Use of a nonestrogen contraceptive may be required during primidone therapy.
Anticonvulsants, other	Altered drug metabolism may result in changes in pattern seizures. Monitor serum levels of both medications as dosage adjustments might be necessary.
MAO inhibitors	Concurrent use may increase primidone effects. Monitor closely as dosage adjustments may be necessary.

Side effects and adverse reactions

These include drowsiness, ataxia, dizziness, allergic reaction, and possibly paradoxical reactions in children and the elderly.

Warnings

Use with caution in patients with hyperkinesis and liver or renal disease.

Contraindications

Avoid use in patients with primidone or barbiturate hypersensitivity, severe respiratory disease, and porphyria.

Dosage and administration

For adults the dose is 100 to 125 mg at bedtime for 3 days, increased by 100 or 125 mg twice a day for days 4

BOX 11-3 Toxemia of Pregnancy

Toxemia of pregnancy is a severe condition that is characterized by elevated blood pressure, edema of the extremities (hands, feet, and ankles) and proteinurea. It occurs in about 5% of all pregnancies in North America. Pregnancy-induced hypertension or hypertension that occurs during pregnancy, is also known as preeclampsia or eclampsia.

Preeclampsia is hypertension that occurs after the 20th week of pregnancy. Its symptoms may range from mild to severe and usually include hypertension, edema, and proteinuria. Preeclampsia can progress to hemolytic anemia, elevated liver enzyme levels, and a decrease in platelet count (HELLP) or eclampsia, that is, seizures or convulsions (Sagraves et al, 1995).

The treatment plan for toxemia of pregnancy is to control the elevated blood pressure, prevent seizures, maintain renal function, and generally, provide optimal conditions for the fetus. This approach is primarily symptomatic because the only real cure for this syndrome is delivery of the baby. The woman should be monitored for up to 2 days after delivery as seizures may still occur in the immediate postpartum period.

through 6, then increased by 100 to 125 mg three times a day until day 9. On day 10, the dose of 250 mg three times a day is established and may be altered according to the patient's needs, up to a maximum of 2 g/day.

For children up to 8 years of age, the initial dose is 50 mg orally at bedtime for 3 days, increased to 50 mg twice a day through day 6, then increased to 100 mg twice daily through day 9. On day 10, maintenance dose is 125 or 250 mg three times a day.

magnesium sulfate [mag nee' zhum]

Magnesium sulfate has a depressant effect on the CNS, which reduces striated muscle contractions. In addition, magnesium sulfate blocks peripheral neuromuscular transmission by reducing acetylcholine release at the myoneural junction, reducing the sensitivity of the motor endplate and lowering the excitability of the motor membrane.

Indications

The drug has three major indications. As an anticonvulsant, it is used in the prevention and control of seizures related to acute nephritis in children and seizures related to toxemias of pregnancy (Box 11-3). As a uterine relaxant, it is used in the treatment of uterine tetany and to inhibit contractions of premature labor. Finally, it is used as replacement therapy for magnesium deficiency.

Pharmacokinetics

About one third of dietary ingested magnesium is absorbed from the GI tract. With intravenous administration, onset of action is immediate, with a duration of action of approximately 30 minutes; with intramuscular administration, onset of action is about 1 hour, with a 3- to 4-hour duration of action. Magnesium undergoes no metabolism and is excreted by the kidneys. See the box above for management of magnesium sulfate overdose.

MANAGEMENT OF DRUG OVERDOSE

Magnesium Sulfate

Signs of hypermagnesemia, which may begin at a serum concentration at or above 5 mEq/L, include flushing, hypotension, sweating, depressed reflexes, reduced respiratory rate, hypothermia, flaccid paralysis, circulatory collapse, slowed heart rate, and CNS depression.

Treatment includes artificial respiration, calcium gluconate IV (5 to 10 mEq of calcium) injected slowly to reverse respiratory depression, and heart block. In patients with reduced renal function, dialysis may be necessary.

Drug interactions

The following effects may occur when magnesium is given with the drugs listed below:

Drug	Possible effect and management
CNS depressants	Dosage of barbiturates, opiates, general anesthetics, or other CNS depressants should be adjusted to avoid additive CNS depressant effects.
Neuromuscular blocking agents	Excessive neuromuscular blockade has occurred when these drugs (blocking agents) are administered with magnesium sulfate. Avoid concurrent use.

Color type indicates an unsafe drug combination.

Warnings

Use with caution in patients with cardiac disease and severe renal impairment.

Contraindications

Avoid use of parenteral magnesium in patients with known magnesium hypersensitivity.

Dosage and administration

For seizures caused by toxemia in pregnancy: administer 4 to 5 g (32 to 40 mEq) IV in 250 ml of 5% dextrose in water or normal saline, administered over ½ hour. In addition, administer IM doses of up to 10 g (maximum 5 g in each buttock).

Pregnancy safety

Magnesium sulfate is used to treat toxemia of pregnancy. The drug crosses the placenta, with fetal blood levels approximately equal to maternal blood levels, and produces similar effects in the neonate and the mother. Decreased reflexes, muscle tone, blood pressure, and respiratory depression may be seen if the mother received magnesium shortly before delivery. It is recommended that magnesium sulfate not be administered during the 2 hours before delivery, if possible.

tiagabine (Gabitril)

Tiagabine is a GABA reuptake inhibitor and is indicated as adjunct therapy in patients with partial seizures.

Pharmacokinetics

Oral absorption in the fasting state is rapid with peak serum levels reached within 45 minutes, elimination half-life is 7 to 9 hours, and steady state is reached in approximately 2 days. This drug is metabolized in the liver and excreted in urine and feces (Olin, 1998).

Drug interactions

The following effect may occur when tiagabine is given in combination with medications such as carbamazepine, phenytoin, primidone, or phenobarbital. It has been reported that tiagabine clearance is increased by nearly 60% when combined with these anticonvulsants; therefore tiagabine dosage adjustment may be necessary (Olin, 1998; Vinson et al, 1998).

Side effects and adverse reactions

These include stomach pain, drowsiness, weakness, memory impairment, headache, dizziness, nausea, vomiting, tremors, diarrhea, and insomnia.

Warnings

Use with caution in persons with liver and renal function impairment and neurologic disorders, such as stroke, dementia, and Alzheimer's disease.

Contraindications

Avoid use in patients with known tiagabine hypersensitivity.

Dosage and administration

The adult dose is 4 mg daily initially increased weekly by 4 to 8 mg until a therapeutic response is achieved or a total of 56 mg/day is reached. This drug should be administered in divided doses (twice or three time a day).

topiramate (Topamax)

Although the exact mechanism of action for topiramate is unknown, it has three properties that may contribute to its anticonvulsant properties. First, it appears to have a sodium channel-blocking action; thus it blocks repetitive depolarization of neurons; second it potentiates the activity of the inhibitory neurotransmitter, GABA; and third, it antagonizes kainate's ability to activate an excitatory glutamate receptor.

Indications

Topiramate is used as therapy for partial onset seizures in adults.

Pharmacokinetics

Topiramate is rapidly absorbed orally; it has a elimination half-life of 21 hours and reaches steady state in approximately 4 days. It is not extensively metabolized in the body and is excreted primarily unchanged by the kidneys.

Drug interactions

The following effects may occur when topiramate is given with the drugs listed below:

Drug	Possible effect and management
Alcohol, CNS depressants	When combined with topiramate, CNS depression, cognitive impairment, and other adverse CNS effects may occur. If possible, avoid this combination.
carbamazepine (Tegretol), phenytoin (Dilantin)	Concurrent therapy may significantly decrease (40% to 50%) topiramate serum concentration. Phenytoin serum levels may also increase by 25% in some patients. Monitor serum drug levels closely as dosage adjustments may be necessary.
Carbonic anhydrase inhibitors	Increases risk for kidney stone formation. Avoid use of this drug combination.
Contraceptives, oral with estrogen	May decrease efficacy of oral contraceptives. Alternative contraceptive methods may need to be considered.

Color type indicates an unsafe drug combination.

Side effects and adverse reactions

These include drowsiness, dizziness, ataxia, speech problems, increased nervousness, paresthesia, tremors, confusion, difficulty with concentration and memory, depression, agitation, nausea, anorexia, visual changes, weight loss, psychomotor slowing, and anxiety.

Warnings

Use with caution in persons with liver and renal impairment.

Contraindications

Avoid use in patients with topiramate hypersensitivity.

Dosage and administration

The adult oral dose is 50 mg/day initially, titrated to effectiveness (see package insert for titration schedule). The usual adjunct dose is 200 mg twice daily. Topiramate can be administered without regard to meals. Encourage increased water or fluid intake to help reduce potential kidney stone formation. This drug is bitter; therefore do not cut or crush this medication before administration.

valproic acid [val proe′ ik] (Depakene [oral]) ***valproate*** [val proe′ ate] (Depacon [parenteral]) ***divalproex sodium*** [dye val′ proe ex] (Depakote)

The mechanism by which valproic acid exerts its anticonvulsant effects has not been fully established. It has been proposed that its activity is related to directly or indirectly increasing or enhancing brain levels of the inhibitory neurotransmitter GABA. By competitive inhibition, it may prevent the reuptake of GABA by glial cells and axonal terminals.

Indications

Valproic acid, valproate, and divalproex sodium are indicated for use as sole and adjunctive therapy in the treatment of absence seizures, including petit mal, and as adjunctive therapy in patients with multiple seizure types, including absence seizures.

Pharmacokinetics

Chemically, valproate sodium is converted in the stomach to valproic acid, which is rapidly absorbed from the gastrointestinal tract. Divalproex sodium is a prodrug, a combination of valproic acid and valproate sodium, in an enteric-coated tablet. Divalproex dissociates into valproate, which is then absorbed in the small intestine. The latter product has nearly replaced the valproic acid dosage form because it produces much fewer gastrointestinal side effects. The term *valproate* has been used to reflect the presence of this drug in the body regardless of its source (valproic acid, divalproex, or valproate).

Valproate has a variable half-life of 6 to 16 hours. The time to peak serum levels varies with the dosage formulation: for example, from 1 to 4 hours for capsules and syrup, from 3 to 4 hours for delayed release capsules and tablets, and at the end of the IV infusion for parenteral administration. Metabolism is primarily in the liver with renal excretion. See Table 11-1 for therapeutic serum level.

Drug interactions

The following effects may occur when valproic acid and divalproex sodium (a drug that contains 50% valproic acid and sodium valproate) are given with the drugs listed below:

Drug	Possible effect and management
Alcohol, anesthetics (general), CNS-depressant–type drugs	May result in potentiated CNS-depressant effects.
Anticoagulants, warfarin (Coumadin), heparin, or thrombolytic agents	Increased risk of bleeding and hemorrhage; monitor closely for early signs if given in combination.
aspirin, dipyridamole (Persantine), or sulfinpyrazone (Anturane)	Increased risk of bleeding and hemorrhage; monitor closely; the prescriber might consider alternative therapeutic agents.
Barbiturates or primidone (Mysoline)	Phenobarbital and primidone serum levels may increase, resulting in increased depression and toxicity. Monitor closely because the prescriber may need to adjust dosage.
carbamazepine (Tegretol) and phenytoin (Dilantin)	Breakthrough seizures may occur because of decreased serum levels of carbamazepine or valproic acid. Phenytoin protein binding may be affected when combined with valproic acid; therefore monitor closely as dosage adjustments may be necessary.
mefloquine (Lariam)	Concurrent use may result in lower valproic acid serum levels and loss of seizure control. Monitor valproic acid levels; dosage adjustments during and after mefloquine therapy may be necessary.

Side effects and adverse effects

These include de tremors, mild gastric distress, diarrhea, weight gain, irregular menses, and hepatotoxicity.

Dosage and administration

The adult dose initially is 5 to 15 mg/kg/day orally or parenterally, increased at weekly intervals as needed. The maximum daily dose is 60 mg/kg/day. The pediatric dose (1 to 12 years old) is 15 to 45 mg/kg/day orally or parenterally, increased at weekly intervals as needed.

SUMMARY

Epilepsy is a symptom of a brain disorder or a discharge of disorganized electrical impulses in the brain that result in seizures. These seizures have various causative factors; thus they are classified by symptoms. The major drug categories used to treat seizures include barbiturates, hydantoins, succinimides, benzodiazepines, and miscellaneous medications.

This chapter reviews the mechanisms of action, primary indications, pharmacokinetics, drug interactions, side effects and adverse reactions, warnings, contraindications, and dosage and administration for these agents. This information is crucial to the healthcare professional providing care for epileptic patients.

REVIEW QUESTIONS

1. Explain the differences between idiopathic and nonidiopathic seizures and their relationship to epilepsy.
2. Discuss the mechanisms of action, indications, and major drug interactions for phenytoin and carbamazepine. Name significant side effects and adverse reactions of these agents for which the healthcare professional should monitor.
3. Name two active metabolites and two indications for primidone. What effect does this drug have on the oral contraceptives with estrogen, warfarin (Coumadin), and other anticonvulsants? Explain the potential for causing a potential paradoxical reaction in children and the elderly.
4. Explain the use of magnesium sulfate in the treatment of toxemia in pregnancy. What are its indications in a clinical setting?
5. What is the pharmacokinetic difference between valproic acid, valproate, and divalproex?

REFERENCES

American Hospital Formulary Service: *AHFS drug information '98,* Bethesda, Md, 1998, American Society of Hospital Pharmacists.

Lott RS: Seizure disorders. In Young LY, Koda-Kimble MA, editors: *Applied therapeutics: the clinical use of drugs,* ed 6, Vancouver, Wash, 1995, Applied Therapeutics, Inc.

Olin BR: *Facts and comparisons,* Philadelphia, 1998, JB Lippincott.

Physicians' desk reference, ed 52, Montvale, NJ, 1998, Medical Economics Co.

Rowan AJ: Recognition and assessment of seizure disorders in the elderly: epidemiology, pathophysiology, and differentiation, *Consult Pharmacist* 10(suppl A):4, 1995

Sagraves, R, Letassy, NA, Barton, TL: Obstetrics. In Young LY, Koda-Kimble MA, editors: *Applied therapeutics: the clinical use of drugs,* ed 6, Vancouver, Wash, 1995, Applied Therapeutics, Inc.

United States Pharmacopeial Convention: *USP DI: Drug information for the health care professional,* ed 18, Rockville, Md, 1998, the Convention.

Vinson MC, Davis WM, Waters IW: The class of 1997: part 2. *Drug Topics* 142(5):97, 1998.

ADDITIONAL REFERENCES

Anderson KN et al, editors: *Mosby's medical, nursing, and allied health dictionary,* ed 5, St Louis, 1998, Mosby.

Carter JR: The use of new antiepileptic medications in pediatric patients with epilepsy, *J Pediatr Health Care* 8(6):277, 1994.

Cloyd J: Pharmacologic considerations of fosphenytoin therapy, *P & T Suppl* 21(55):13s, 1996.

Dichter MA: Deciding to discontinue antiepileptic medication, *Hosp Pract* 27(20):16, 1992.

Drug Update: Pharmacy news, *J Am Pharm Assoc* NS36(10):566, 1996.

Hardman JG, Limbird LE, editors: *Goodman & Gilman's the pharmacological basis of therapeutics,* ed 9, New York, 1996, Macmillan.

Mosby: *Mosby's GenRx,* St Louis, 1998, Mosby.

Steiner JF: Pharmacologic treatment of epilepsy, *J Am Acad Physicians Assist* 7(7):508, 1994.

United States Gabapentin Study Group: The long-term safety and efficacy of gabapentin (Neurontin) as add-on therapy in drug-resistant partial epilepsy, *Epilepsy Res* 18:67, 1994.

Wertz EM: Understanding AEDs . . . anti-epileptic drugs, *Emergency* 27(1):18,23, 1995.

CHAPTER 12

Central Nervous System Stimulants

KEY DRUGS

amphetamine (p. 207)
methylphenidate (p. 209)
caffeine (p. 211)

CHAPTER FOCUS

The central nervous system (CNS) stimulants may produce dramatic effects by increasing the activity of CNS neurons. However, their therapeutic usefulness is limited because of their many general effects and side effects in the body. Chronic use and misuse has occurred with these drugs, which resulted in the patient developing a drug tolerance, drug dependence, and a drug abuse problem. All of the CNS stimulants, if taken in sufficient doses, may cause convulsions. This chapter reviews the central nervous system stimulant drugs that are available for clinical use.

KEY TERMS

amphetamines (p. 205)
analeptics (p. 205)
anorexiants, (p. 205)
attention deficit disorder, (p. 205)
cataplexy (p. 205)
narcolepsy, (p. 205)

OBJECTIVES

After reading and studying this chapter, the student should be able to do the following:

1. *Define and discuss the key drugs and key terms.*
2. *Explain attention deficit disorder (ADD) with hyperactivity and its effects in the child and adult.*
3. *Discuss the CNS-stimulant drugs (methylphenidate, amphetamine, pemoline, and doxapram), including their mechanisms of action, indications, significant drug interactions, and usual adult dosages.*
4. *Describe narcolepsy and the drugs useful in treating this condition.*
5. *Describe the multiple effects of and indications for caffeine in the body and identify the signs of and treatment for a caffeine overdose.*
6. *List the caffeine content in common beverages and OTC medications.*

The classification of stimulants depends on where in the nervous system they exert their major effects—on the cerebrum, on the medulla and brainstem, or on the hypothalamic limbic regions. **Amphetamines** are mainly stimulants of the cerebral cortex, **analeptics** primarily affect the centers in the medulla and the brainstem, and **anorexiants** suppress the appetite, perhaps by a direct stimulant effect on the satiety center in the hypothalamic and limbic regions. Central nervous system stimulants act by increasing the neuronal discharge or by blocking an inhibitory neurotransmitter. These drugs may also affect other parts of the nervous system.

Cerebral stimulants were commonly prescribed in the past for obesity and to counteract central nervous system (CNS)-depressant overdosage, but such use today is considered obsolete. Although the CNS stimulants suppress appetite, tolerance develops to the anorexic effect usually before the weight reduction goal is reached. Treatment of severe CNS depression with stimulants is also discouraged, since close monitoring and supportive measures have been found to be quite successful without the production of undesirable adverse reactions. With their narrow therapeutic index between effectiveness and toxicity, CNS stimulants may induce cardiac dysrhythmias, hypertension, convulsions, and violent behavior. Thus the CNS stimulants have limited use in practice today; they are primarily used for the treatment of attention deficit disorder with hyperactivity and narcolepsy.

The syndrome **attention deficit disorder** (ADD) with hyperactivity is characterized by distractibility, a short attention span, impulsive behavior, hyperactivity, and learning disabilities. Improper functioning of the neurotransmitter systems (noradrenergic, dopaminergic, and serotonergic) have been implicated in this syndrome (Saklad, Curtis, 1995). Stimulant medications tend to decrease the distractibility and hyperactivity, resulting in an increased attention span.

The onset of ADD with hyperactivity usually occurs between the ages of 3 and 7 years, with boys affected more often than girls by a 10:1 ratio (Bolinger et al, 1992). Usually professional intervention is unnecessary until the child enters the school setting. Attention deficit hyperactivity disorder (ADHD) may persist into adulthood. In one report, 31% of young adults who had ADHD in childhood still had the full syndrome. Adults with ADHD may have a higher incidence of substance abuse, antisocial personality disorders, anxiety, and depression when compared with a control group. Children treated with stimulants, however, were reported to have a better outcome as adults (Saklad, Curtis, 1995). Management of this disorder requires a behavioral modification program with use of pharmacologic therapy as an adjunct if necessary.

Approximately 15% to 20% of children do not respond or their symptoms actually increase with the stimulant drugs. Antidepressant therapy (imipramine [Tofranil], desipramine [Norpramin]) should be considered for these individuals, especially if they present with ADHD with anxiety or depression symptoms. Clonidine (Klonopin) has been used, especially for persons who have both ADHD and Tourette's syndrome, but this drug should not be used for children with ADHD and depression, since it can worsen the condition (Saklad, Curtis, 1995).

Although stimulant medications are available in short-acting (4-hour) and long-acting (8- to 10-hour) forms, it is general practice to establish a daily schedule using the short-acting form. The dosage required will be learned from empiric experience. For this reason the prescriber needs to work closely with the child, the parents, and school personnel in evaluating results and planning dosages.

The child's distractibility and hyperactivity must be managed during school hours. However, it may be equally important to contain these symptoms at other times of the day to promote the child's psychosocial development by participation in clubs, religious activities, or social events. Rather than having a continuous approach to dosing, it is more helpful to consider the child's life in 4-hour units and to provide a dose appropriate to the needs of that time block. For example, the child might take 10 mg of a short-acting stimulant at 8 am and again at noon on a school day but add another dose at 4 pm if a music lesson is planned for that evening.

Narcolepsy is a condition characterized by excessive drowsiness and uncontrollable sleep attacks during the daytime. In addition, the patient may exhibit a sleep paralysis (inability to move that occurs immediately on falling asleep or on awakening), **cataplexy** (stress-induced generalized muscle weakness), and hypnagogic illusions or hallucinations (vivid auditory or visual dreams occurring at onset of sleep). CNS stimulants are useful in controlling the daytime drowsiness and excessive sleep patterns, whereas tricyclic antidepressants are being tested in conjunction with the stimulants for cataplexy and sleep paralysis.

The mechanism of action for the cerebral stimulants (amphetamines) includes the release of norepinephrine from storage and also a direct stimulating effect on alpha and beta receptor sites. Although the CNS effects are unknown, the primary action centrally appears to be in the cerebral cortex and possibly the reticular activating system. Stimulation results in an increase in motor function and mental alertness, decreased sense of fatigue, and usually a euphoric effect (AHFS, 1998).

Animal studies indicate that amphetamine blocks reuptake of dopamine and norepinephrine from the synapse, inhibits monoamine oxidase (MAO) action, and also increases the release of catecholamines (USP DI, 1998).

ANOREXIANT DRUGS

Anorexiant or appetite-suppressant drugs include a variety of medications that are used for the short-term treatment of obesity. They are indirect-acting sympathomimetics and with the exception of mazindol, they are phenethylamine- or amphetamine-like drugs. Their exact mechanism of action is unknown, but these agents appear to act on the satiety center in the hypothalamus and limbic areas of the brain.

Benzphetamine (Didrex), diethylpropion (Tenuate), phendimetrazine (Adphen, Bontril) and phentermine (Fastin, Phentride) mainly act on the adrenergic pathways, while mazindol affects both the adrenergic (norephinephrine) and dopaminergic (dopamine) pathways. The newly released drug sibutramine (Meridia) is a serotonin and norephinephrine reuptake inhibitor.

Phendimetrazine affects norepinephrine, and like amphetamine, it produces marked euphoria and stimulation and has an abuse potential. Phentermine and diethylpropion also affects norepinephrine, and they produce mild euphoria and mild to moderate stimulation and have a low abuse potential. Mazindol affects dopamine and adrenergic receptors and has the same CNS effects as diethylpropion, with minimal abuse potential.

Anorexiants have a number of limitations, so careful selection of the clinical choices is necessary to minimize the unwanted effects. As appetite suppressants they are recommended as an adjunct to other regimens, such as physical exercise, behavior modification, and restriction of caloric intake and are prescribed for a short time, since tolerance to the anorectic effect may occur within a few weeks (USP DI, 1998).

Sibutramine (Meridia) was released in 1998 to treat obesity. This product is a serotonin and norepinephrine reuptake inhibitor. Specific guidelines were issued for the use of sibutramine, such as (1) the product is used in conjunction with a reduced-calorie diet and (2) the obese patient is identified as one with an initial body mass index (BMI) of at least 30 kg/m^2 in persons with other risk factors, such as diabetes or hypertension.

Sibutramine does not cause an increased release of serotonin from nerve cells so it is less apt to induce serotonin toxicity, which is the suspected cause of the cardiac adverse effects associated with the previous drugs withdrawn from the market, dexfenfluramine (Redux), and fenfluramine (Pondimin) (Constantine, Scott, 1997).

Pharmacokinetics

The anorexiant drugs are lipid soluble and cross the blood-brain barrier. Orally, the immediate release formulations usually produce their effects for 4 to 6 hours with the exception of mazindol, the effects of which last for 8 to 15 hours. Drugs with longer half-lives include fenfluramine, about 20 hours, and phendimetrazine, from 2 to 10 hours. The drugs and their metabolites are excreted primarily in urine. No pharmacokinetic data are available for sibutramine.

Drug interactions

The following effects may occur when anorexiants are given with the drugs listed below:

Drug	Possible effect and management
Antihypertensive agents, especially clonidine (Catapres), guanadrel (Hylorel), guanethidine (Ismelin), methyldopa (Aldomet), or rauwolfia alkaloids	May decrease the antihypertensive effects; monitor closely.
Alcohol	Concurrent use is not recommended, as the risk increases for adverse CNS effects such as confusion, dizziness, and fainting.
CNS stimulants	Combined use may result in an increase in CNS-stimulant effects. Avoid this combination.
MAO inhibitors	Avoid concurrent use or use within 14 days after the administration of a MAO inhibitor, as a hypertensive crisis may result.

Color type indicates an unsafe drug combination.

In addition to the above drug interactions, use sibutramine very cautiously in patients taking sumatriptan (Imitrex), dihydroergotamine (DHE 45), fentanyl (Duragesic), meperidine (Demerol), pentazocine (Talwin), dextromethorphan, and lithium (Constantine, Scott, 1997). This product can also increase blood pressure in some patients; therefore close monitoring of blood pressure is necessary.

Side effects and adverse reactions

Most frequently reported side effects include euphoria, increased irritability, nervousness, and insomnia. Other less frequent side effects are visual disturbance, diarrhea or constipation, dry mouth, difficulty on urination, tachycardia, impotence, headaches, sweating, and nausea and vomiting.

Adverse reactions include hypertension with all stimulant drugs. Less frequently reported are CNS depression and confusion, allergic rashes or hives, and psychosis. See the box for management of an anorexiant overdose.

Warnings

Use with caution in patients with mild hypertension or cardiovascular disease, a history of seizures, and tartrazine sensitivity.

Contraindications

Avoid use in persons with symptomatic or advanced cardiovascular disease, a history of drug abuse, known hypersensitivity to sympathomimetic agents, and glaucoma, and

MANAGEMENT OF DRUG OVERDOSE

Anorexiants

There is no specific antidote for an overdose of anorexiant drugs. Institute symptomatic and supportive measures according to the individual client's requirement.

Generally, emesis and/or use of gastric lavage is indicated, followed by administration of activated charcoal to adsorb any remaining drug in the gastrointestinal (GI) tract.

Excessive stimulation may be counteracted with barbiturates, chlorpromazine, or haloperidol (to decrease anticholinergic effects). Seizures may be controlled with diazepam or phenobarbital.

Monitor vital signs and respiratory functions frequently. Closely monitor cardiac and respiratory functions. Medications usually used are: for hypertension, IV phentolamine or nitrites; for hypotension, IV fluids; for dysrhythmias, lidocaine IV; and for tachycardia, a beta-adrenergic blocking agent.

Urine acidification and forced diuresis is also recommended.

in agitated patients. Also avoid use during or within 2 weeks after the administration of a MAO inhibitor and concurrent use with other CNS stimulants.

Dosage and administration

See Table 12-1 for the usual adult dose and the Federal Controlled Substances Act schedule for each drug. Be aware that the agents with the greatest abuse potential will be noted by the lower numbers on the scale of II to IV. See the box for Food and Drug Administration (FDA) pregnancy safety categories.

AMPHETAMINES

The mechanism of action was reviewed previously. Amphetamines used over long periods can produce psychologic and physical dependence. Prolonged use of amphetamines leads to the development of tolerance. Because of their potential for abuse, amphetamines are not recommended for use as appetite suppressants; instead they are indicated for the treatment of ADD with hyperactivity and in the treatment of narcolepsy. The have also been classified under the Controlled Substances Act as schedule II, the classification for drugs with a high abuse potential.

Pharmacokinetics

Amphetamines are well absorbed and are distributed to body tissues, with especially high concentrations in the brain and cerebrospinal fluid. The half-life depends on urinary pH. Generally they are as follows: amphetamine, 10 to 30 hours; dextroamphetamine, 10 to 12 hours for adults and 6 to 8 hours in children; and methamphetamine, 4 to 5 hours. These drugs are metabolized in the liver and excreted by the kidneys. Excretion is pH dependent; it is increased in an acidic urine and decreased in a more alkaline urine.

PREGNANCY SAFETY

Category	Drug
B	diethylpropion, doxapram, pemoline
C	amphetamines, caffeine
X	benzphetamine
Unclassified	mazindol, methylphenidate, phendimetrazine, phentermine

The healthcare professional should be aware that long-term amphetamine abuse can lead to chorea, a condition characterized by involuntary, purposeless, rapid motions, which is mediated by alterations in the physiology of the basal ganglia. Chorea is also seen with the administration of cocaine, which reduces dopamine levels.

Drug interactions

The following effects may occur when amphetamines are given with the drugs listed below:

Drug	Possible effect and management
Antidepressants, tricyclic	May result in adverse cardiovascular effects, such as dysrhythmias, tachycardia, or severe hypertension. Avoid or a potentially serious drug interaction may occur.
Beta-adrenergic blocking drugs (systemic and ophthalmic)	May cause unopposed alpha-adrenergic effects resulting in hypertension, bradycardia, and possible heart block. If necessary to use both classifications, labetalol, a beta-blocking agent that also has alpha-blocking effects, may reduce the risk of producing the above effects. Monitor closely for dysrhythmias. Preferably avoid or a potentially serious drug interaction may occur.
CNS stimulants such as appetite suppressants, caffeine, methylphenidate, pemoline, sympathomimetics, theophylline, amantadine	May result in an increase in adverse cardiovascular effects, nervousness, insomnia, and convulsions. Avoid or a potentially serious drug interaction may occur.
Digitalis glycosides	May result in an increase in cardiac dysrhythmias. Avoid or a potentially serious drug interaction may occur.

TABLE 12-1 Anorexiant Medications, Adult Dosages, and CSA Classification*

Drug	*Adult Dosages*	*CSA Classification*
benzphetamine (Didrex)	25-50 mg PO daily, increase if necessary	III
diethylpropion		IV
Tablets (Tenuate)	25 mg 3 times PO daily, 1 hr before meals	
Extended-release tablets (Tenuate Dospan, Tepanil Ten-tab)	75 mg PO daily at midmorning	
mazindol (Mazanor, Sanorex)	1 mg initially PO once a day before breakfast, increase if necessary	IV
phendimetrazine		III
Tablets (Adphen, Bontril)	35 mg PO, 2 or 3 times a day 1 hr before meals	
Capsules (Obalan)	35 mg PO 2 or 3 times a day, 1 hr before meals	
Extended-release (Adipost, Bontril Slow Release)	105 mg PO daily, ½-1 hr before breakfast	
phentermine		IV
Tablets (Phentride)	37.5 mg daily before breakfast	
Capsules (Fastin)	30 mg daily before breakfast	
Resin capsules (Ionamin)	15 or 30 mg PO daily before breakfast	
sibutramine (Meridia)	10 mg PO daily	IV

*Classification under the Federal Controlled Substances Act (CSA) drug schedule (II, III, or IV). See Chapter 2 for further information.

meperidine (Demerol)	Although some investigators believe that the analgesic effect of meperidine might be enhanced, concurrent use should be avoided because it may result in severe respiratory depression, seizures, hyperpyrexia, severe hypotension, cardiovascular collapse, and death in some patients. Avoid or a potentially serious drug interaction may occur.
MAO inhibitors	Avoid concurrent usage because increased release of catecholamines, headaches, dysrhythmias, vomiting, sudden severe hypertension, and possibly a hyperpyretic crisis may result. Avoid or a potentially serious drug interaction may occur. Do not administer during or for 2 weeks after the discontinuance of an MAO inhibitor.
Thyroid hormones	May result in enhanced effects of thyroid or amphetamines. If patient has coronary artery disease, the potential for inducing coronary insufficiency is increased. Avoid or a potentially serious drug interaction may occur.

Color type indicates an unsafe drug combination.

Side effects and adverse reactions

Side effects include euphoria, increased irritability, nervousness, insomnia, restlessness, visual disturbance, excessive sweating, dry mouth, abdominal cramps, impotence, alterations in sexual desire, diarrhea or constipation, dizziness, anorexia, and nausea or vomiting. The most frequently reported adverse reactions include tachycardia or irregular heart rate, allergic reactions including urticaria, hives, angina or chest pain, tremors, hyperreactive reflexes, dyskinesia, and Tourette's syndrome. With high dosage or prolonged consumption, mood changes including depression, increased agitation, and psychosis may occur. Drug dependency and tolerance may also develop.

Treatment of amphetamine overdose consists of symptomatic and supportive care as outlined in the management of an anorexiant overdose, in addition to a saline cathartic if the patient has taken a long-acting dosage form. Monitor vital signs and respiratory functions closely.

Warnings

Use with caution in psychotic patients.

Contraindications

Avoid use in persons with amphetamine hypersensitivity, pregnancy, hyperthyroidism, moderate to severe hypertension, glaucoma, history of drug abuse, cardiovascular disease, severe agitation, severe arteriosclerosis, and Tourette's syndrome.

Dosage and administration

See Table 12-2.

OTHER CENTRAL NERVOUS SYSTEM STIMULANTS

doxapram [dox′ a pram] (Dopram)

At low dosages doxapram stimulates respiration by acting on the peripheral carotid chemoreceptors; at higher dosages the medullary respiratory center is stimulated. This drug is used for the treatment of respiratory depression induced by a drug overdose, chronic obstructive pulmonary disease, or postanesthetic effects.

TABLE 12-2 Amphetamines: Dosage and Administration

Drug	Adults	Children
amphetamine tablets		
Narcolepsy	5-20 mg 1-3 times daily	Children to 6 yr, dosage not determined; 6-12 yr, 2.5 mg orally twice daily, increase by 5 mg/day at 1-wk intervals until therapeutic effect or adult dosage achieved; 12 yr and older, 5 mg twice daily orally, increasing dose by 10 mg/day at weekly intervals until therapeutic effect or adult dosage achieved
Attention deficit disorder	Not applicable	Children up to 3 yr, not recommended; 3-6 yr, 2.5 mg orally, increased by 2.5 mg/day at weekly intervals until therapeutic response achieved; 6 yr and older, 5 mg orally 1 or 2 times/day, increase by 5 mg/day at weekly intervals until therapeutic response achieved
dextroamphetamine tablets		
Narcolepsy	5-60 mg orally 1-3 times daily	Children up to 6 yr, dosage not determined; 6-12 yr, 5 mg daily, increase by 5 mg/day at weekly intervals until therapeutic effect or adult dosage achieved; 12 yr and older, 10 mg daily, increase by 10 mg/day at weekly intervals until therapeutic effect or adult dosage achieved
Attention deficit disorder	Not applicable	Children up to 3 yr, not recommended; 3-6 yr, 2.5 mg orally daily, increase by 2.5 mg/day at weekly intervals until therapeutic response achieved; 6 yr and older, 5 mg orally once or twice/day, increase dosage by 5 mg daily at weekly intervals until therapeutic response achieved Dextroamphetamine extended-release capsules may be used after therapeutic dosage per day is established
methamphetamine tablets (Desoxyn), methamphetamine extended-release tablets (Desoxyn)		
Attention deficit disorder	Not applicable	Children up to 6 yr, not recommended; 6 yr and older, 5 mg orally 1 or 2 times daily, increase by 5 mg/day at weekly intervals until therapeutic effect achieved (usually 20-25 mg/day)

Pharmacokinetics

Doxapram is a parenteral drug administered intravenously. It has an onset of effect at 20 to 40 seconds and a peak effect at 1 to 2 minutes. Doxapram's duration of action is 5 to 12 minutes. It is excreted primarily in the feces.

Drug interactions

Administration of doxapram with MAO inhibitors or vasopressors may result in an increase in blood pressure or a hypertensive crisis. Monitor the vital signs closely.

Side effects and adverse reactions

These include urinary retention or incontinence, headache, diarrhea, dizziness, cough, hiccups, confusion, warm or burning feeling, nausea or vomiting, sweating, chest pains, tachycardia, extrasystoles, hemolysis, thrombophlebitis, dyspnea, and tachypnea. Signs of overdosage are hypertension, convulsions, trembling, tachycardia, and increased deep tendon reflexes.

Warnings

Use with caution in persons with liver impairment, bronchial asthma, and hypertension.

Contraindications

Avoid use in patients with doxapram hypersensitivity, cerebrovascular accidents, advanced coronary artery disease, head injuries, epilepsy, severe hypertension, heart failure, cardiac disease, pheochromocytoma, severe renal impairment, and severe respiratory disease.

Dosage and administration

The adult dose for postanesthesia respiratory depression is 0.5 to 1 mg/kg of body weight IV. Do not exceed 1.5 mg/kg as a single dose. Dose may be repeated every 5 minutes up to maximum of 2 mg/kg of body weight. For acute respiratory insufficiency in persons with chronic obstructive pulmonary disease, the dose is 1 to 2 mg/min by IV infusion; if necessary the dose maybe increased to 3 mg/min. Maximum infusion time is 2 hours.

methylphenidate [meth ill fen′ i date] (Ritalin)

The mechanism of methylphenidate's central action is unknown. Its pharmacologic actions are similar to those of amphetamines, with CNS and respiratory stimulation; sympathomimetic activity is also reported. Sites of action are the cerebral cortex and subcortical areas.

Methylphenidate also appears to block the reuptake of dopamine into the dopaminergic neurons. In persons with ADD with hyperactivity, methylphenidate decreases motor activity and increases the attention span. In narcolepsy it appears to stimulate the cortex and subcortex, including the thalamic area, to increase alertness, lift the spirits, and increase motor activity.

Indications

The drug is indicated for treatment of ADD and narcolepsy.

Pharmacokinetics

Methylphenidate is well absorbed orally. The peak serum concentration of tablets is 1.9 hours in children; the extended-release tablets reach peak serum concentration in 4.7 hours in children. This drug is metabolized in the liver and excreted by the kidneys.

Drug interactions

The following effects may occur when methylphenidate hydrochloride is given with the drugs listed below:

Drug	Possible effect and management
Other CNS stimulants	May result in additive CNS stimulation effects causing increased nervousness, irritability, insomnia, dysrhythmias, and convulsions. Monitor apical pulse, mental status, and behaviors closely.
MAO inhibitors	May result in hypertensive crisis. Do not give drugs concurrently or within 14 days of administration of an MAO inhibitor. Avoid or a potentially serious drug interactions may occur.
pimozide (Orap)	Should not be administered together. Withdraw patient from methylphenidate before starting pimozide therapy. Concurrent use may mask reason for tic development because methylphenidate may also induce tics. Pimozide is indicated for the treatment of tics in patients with Tourette's syndrome.

Color type indicates an unsafe drug combination.

Side effects and adverse reactions

Side effects include anorexia, increased nervousness, insomnia (usually more frequent in children), headache, nausea, abdominal pain, drowsiness, and dizziness. Adverse reactions include hypertension, tachycardia, chest pain, trembling or uncontrolled movement of body, rash, fever of unknown origin, and increased bruising. See the box above for treatment of a methylphenidate overdose.

MANAGEMENT OF DRUG OVERDOSE

Methylphenidate

Signs of overdosage may include confusion, delirium, dry mouth, euphoria, increased fever and sweating, severe headaches, hypertension, tremors, muscle twitching, irregular heartbeats, vomiting, convulsions, and possibly coma.

There is no specific treatment for an overdose of methylphenidate; treatment is symptomatic and supportive. Emesis or gastric lavage is implemented initially in treatment. The patient should be in quiet surroundings and, if necessary, a short-acting barbiturate might be used in severe overdose situations.

Monitor closely and maintain cardiovascular and respiratory function.

Warnings

Use with caution in patients with seizure disorders, a history of drug abuse, and psychosis.

Contraindications

Avoid use in patients with methylphenidate hypersensitivity, Tourette's syndrome, glaucoma, severe anxiety, agitation or depression, hypertension, and motor tics.

Dosage and administration

To treat ADHD in children 6 years of age and older, the dosage is 5 mg twice daily (after breakfast and lunch), increased if needed by 5 to 10 mg weekly, up to 60 mg/day maximum. If no improvement is seen after 30 days, stop the medication. For adults, the dose is 5 to 20 mg two or three times daily, with or after meals. The dosage for the extended release form (Ritalin-SR) in adults is 20 mg one to three times a daily, every 8 hours.

pemoline [pem′ oh leen] (Cylert)

The mechanism of central action is unknown. Pemoline may act by means of dopaminergic mechanisms.

Indications

Pemoline is indicated for treatment of ADD with hyperactivity.

Pharmacokinetics

Pemoline has good absorption and a half-life of 12 hours. The peak serum concentration occurs in 2 to 4 hours with a peak effect reached in 3 to 4 weeks (USP DI, 1998). Pemoline is partially metabolized in the liver and is excreted by the kidneys.

Drug interactions

No significant drug interactions have been reported.

Side effects and adverse reactions

These include anorexia, insomnia, weight loss, dizziness, daytime sedation, irritability, depression, nausea, rash, and abdominal pain.

Signs of overdosage include increased agitation, confusion, euphoria, hallucinations, severe headaches, hypertension, elevated temperatures, increased sweating, convulsions, tachycardia, dilated pupils, vomiting, and uncontrollable muscle movements of eyes.

Warnings

Use with caution in patients with a history of drug abuse, seizure disorders, renal disease, and tics.

Contraindications

Avoid use in patients with pemoline hypersensitivity, severe liver and renal impairment, Tourette's syndrome, and psychosis.

Dosage and administration

For children younger than 6 years of age, dosage is not established; for children 6 years of age or older, dosage is 37.5 mg orally each morning. Dosage may be increased by 18.75 mg daily on a weekly basis until a therapeutic response is noted or a maximum of 112.5 mg/day is reached.

caffeine [kaf feen′]

Caffeine is a stimulant found in many beverages, foods, over-the-counter (OTC) drugs, and prescription drugs (Box 12-1). It is probably the most commonly used stimulant worldwide. It has been estimated that 7 million kg of caffeine are consumed annually in the United States. Many persons do not consider caffeine to be a drug, but this product can produce many therapeutic and adverse effects. For example, a large daily intake of caffeine-containing products may increase alertness but may also induce insomnia and heart dsyrhythmias in some persons, especially the elderly. A withdrawal syndrome of increased irritability, headache, and increased weakness has been reported when users of more than 600 mg/day of caffeine, or approximately 6 cups of coffee, decrease or eliminate this intake. Caffeine has also been implicated in many adverse health effects, such as cancer, fibrocystic breast disease, and birth defects. See Box 12-2 for caffeine-free OTC analgesic medications.

Mechanism of action

The mechanisms of action for caffeine were previously postulated to be an increase in cyclic adenosine monophosphate (cAMP) levels by blocking the enzyme phosphodiesterase. Recent studies, though, indicate that caffeine's effects are primarily due to antagonism of the central adenosine receptors (adenosine is a neurotransmitter that is structurally similar to caffeine). Because caffeine has an effect on many body functions, both its short-term and possible long-term effects are of concern. Following is a discussion of these effects as they involve each body system.

Central nervous system. Although all levels of the CNS may be affected, regular doses of caffeine (100 to 150 mg) will stimulate the cortex to produce increased alertness and decreased motor reaction time to both visual and auditory events. Drowsiness and fatigue generally disappear. Larger doses may affect the medullary, vagus, vasomotor, and respiratory centers, resulting in slowing of the heart rate, vasoconstriction, and increased respiratory rate. Studies attribute such effects to competitive blockade of adenosine receptors. Thus caffeine is still under investigation for the treatment of neonatal apnea, generally as an adjunct to nondrug measures and as an alternative to theophylline.

Analgesic adjunct, vascular effect. Caffeine constricts cerebral blood vessels, resulting in decreased cerebral blood flow and oxygen tension in the brain. Thus caffeine is used in analgesic products and in combination with ergotamine to enhance pain relief and, perhaps, to hasten the onset of action. When caffeine is given with ergotamine, the

BOX 12-1 Caffeine Content in Selected Products

*Analgesics**	*Caffeine per tablet/capsule*
OTC medications	
Anacin	32 mg
Cope	32 mg
Excedrin Extra-Strength	65 mg
Vanquish Caplets	33 mg
Prescription medications	
Cafergot	100 mg
Fiorinal	40 mg
Wigraine	100 mg
Menstrual medications*	
Midol Maximum	60 mg
Beverages	
Brewed coffee, automatic drip	60-180 mg/5 oz
Brewed coffee, percolator	40-170 mg/5 oz
Brewed tea, United States	20-90 mg/5 oz
Instant coffee	30-120 mg/5 oz
Instant tea	25-50 mg/5 oz
Brewed decaffeinated coffee	2-5 mg/5 oz
Chocolate milk	2-7 mg/8 oz
Soft drinks*	
Mountain Dew	54 mg/12 oz
Coca-Cola	45 mg/12 oz
Diet Coke	45 mg/12 oz
Pepsi-Cola	38 mg/12 oz
Diet Pepsi	36 mg/12 oz
Ginger ale	0
7UP	0
Sunkist Orange	0

Modified from American Pharmaceutical Association, 1997.

BOX 12-2 Caffeine-free OTC Analgesic Medications

Aleve	Midol Menstrual Formula
Aspergum	Motrin IB
Bayer Aspirin	Tempra
Bromo-Seltzer	Infants' Tylenol
Bufferin Extra Strength	Tylenol Regular Strength
Bufferin Arthritis Strength	Tylenol Extra Strength
Liquiprin for children	

Modified from American Pharmaceutical Association, 1996.

enhanced effect is believed to be a result of better absorption of the ergotamine in the presence of caffeine.

Respiratory stimulant. Although the mechanism of action is not clearly defined, caffeine appears to stimulate the medullary respiratory center. Thus it may be useful for the treatment of apnea in preterm infants and for Cheyne-Stokes respiration in adults.

Cardiovascular system. Caffeine stimulates the myocardium, increasing both heart rate and cardiac output. This effect is antagonistic to that produced on the vagus center; consequently, a slight slowing of the heart may be observed in some individuals and an increased rate in others. The latter effect usually predominates after large doses. Overstimulation may cause tachycardia and cardiac irregularities.

Depending on the dose, caffeine may cause an increase in systemic vascular resistance, which can cause an increase in blood pressure. This effect may be secondary to stimulation of the sympathetic nervous system and blockade of adenosine-induced vasodilation.

Skeletal muscles. Caffeine affects voluntary skeletal muscles to increase the contractual force and decrease muscle fatigue.

Gastrointestinal tract. Caffeine increases secretion of pepsin and hydrochloric acid from the parietal cells. This is why coffee is restricted in patients who have a gastric or duodenal ulcer.

Renal system. Caffeine produces a mild diuretic effect by increasing renal blood flow and glomerular filtration rate and by decreasing the reabsorption of sodium and water in the proximal tubules.

Additional effects. Caffeine also increases metabolic activity, inhibits uterine contractions, transiently increases glucose levels by stimulating glycolysis, and increases catecholamine levels in plasma and urine.

Indications

Caffeine is used in the treatment of fatigue or drowsiness and as an adjunct to analgesics to enhance relief of pain.

Pharmacokinetics

Caffeine absorption is good, and it is distributed to all body compartments; it will cross the blood-brain barrier and enter the CNS and readily through the placenta. Caffeine is metabolized in the liver.

In adults, caffeine is metabolized to theophylline and theobromine, whereas in the neonate only a small portion is metabolized to theophylline. Caffeine's half-life is 3 to 7 hours in adults and 65 to 130 hours in neonates. The peak plasma level is achieved within 50 to 75 minutes, with therapeutic plasma levels at 5 to 25 μg/ml. In adults, caffeine is excreted by the kidneys, with only 1% to 2% excreted unchanged; in neonates it is excreted by the kidneys, with approximately 85% excreted unchanged.

Drug interactions

The following effects may occur when caffeine is taken with the drugs listed below:

Drug	Possible effect and management
Other CNS-stimulating drugs, other caffeine-containing medications or drinks	May result in increased CNS stimulation and undesirable side effects such as increased nervousness, irritability, insomnia, dysrhythmias, and seizures. Monitor patient's apical pulse and behaviors closely.
MAO inhibitors	Concurrent use with caffeine may result in severe hyper tension or dangerous dysrhythmias. Small amounts of caffeine may induce increased heart rate. Avoid or a potentially serious drug interaction may occur.

Color type indicates an unsafe drug combination.

Side effects and adverse reactions

Side effects include increased nervousness or jittery feelings and irritation of the GI tract resulting in nausea. More frequent adverse reactions in neonates include abdominal swelling or distention, vomiting, body tremors, tachycardia, jitters, or nervousness.

Signs of overdose include increased temperature, headache, increased irritability and sensitivity to pain or touch, increased urination, confusion, dehydration, abdominal pain, agitation, muscle twitching, nausea and vomiting, tinnitus, insomnia, and convulsions. See the box for management of a caffeine overdose.

Warnings

Use with caution in persons with insomnia, nervousness, and tachycardia.

Contraindications

Avoid use in patients with caffeine or xanthine hypersensitivity, severe anxiety including agoraphobia, panic attacks, severe cardiac disease, liver function impairment, and hypertension.

MANAGEMENT OF DRUG OVERDOSE

Caffeine

Institute symptomatic and supportive measures according to the individual client's requirement.

If treatment is started within 4 hours of overdose, induce emesis with ipecac syrup and/or gastric lavage followed by activated charcoal. A magnesium sulfate (Epsom salts) laxative should also be considered.

Maintain fluid and electrolyte balance, ventilation, and oxygenation.

For hemorrhagic gastritis, administer antacids and iced saline lavage; for seizures, give IV diazepam, phenobarbital, or phenytoin.

Dosage and administration

The adult dose is 100 to 200 mg orally, repeated in 3 to 4 hours if necessary to a maximum of 1000 mg daily. The extended-release dosage form (200 to 250 mg) has the same recommendations as the tablets. Caffeine is not recommended for use in children up to 12 years of age (USP DI, 1998).

SUMMARY

The CNS-stimulant drugs have limited use in clinical practice today. The stimulant drugs were commonly prescribed for obesity in the past, but today with their narrow therapeutic index and rapid development of tolerance and adverse effects, their usage has declined or is very limited. When used as appetite suppressants, they are usually recommended as a part of an adjunct to other regimens that include physical exercise, behavior modification, diet, and exercise. Today the primarily indications for these agents are attention deficit disorder and narcolepsy.

Caffeine is also a CNS stimulant that is contained in many beverages and medications. The healthcare professional who has a knowledge of the benefits and risks associated with these agents can actively advise and supervise patients who are taking CNS stimulants.

REVIEW QUESTIONS

1. Differentiate between the mechanisms of action for the amphetamines, anorexiants, and analeptics. Name two other conditions that usually respond to central nervous system stimulant therapy.
2. Sibutramine has been promoted as being advantageous over the previous anorexiant drugs that were removed from the market. Why? What safety guidelines were issued with the release of this product?
3. Select three contraindications for the anorexiant agents and explain why the CNS stimulants should not be used in these conditions.
4. Explain why the stimulant drugs should not be used to treat patients who are currently taking (a) Demerol, (b) timolol ophthalmic drops, and (c) Parnate.
5. When taking a medication history, why is the amount of caffeine consumed daily by the patient a concern? Name three illnesses or conditions that may be induced or exacerbated by the chronic consumption of large amounts of caffeine.

REFERENCES

American Hospital Formulary Service: *AHFS drug information '98,* Bethesda, Md, 1996, American Society of Hospital Pharmacists.

American Pharmaceutical Association: *Nonprescription products: formulations and features '96-'97,* Washington, DC, 1996, the Association.

Bolinger AM et al: General pediatric therapy. In Koda-Kimble MA, Young LY, editors: *Applied therapeutics: the clinical use of drugs,* ed 5, Vancouver, Wash, 1992, Applied Therapeutics, Inc.

Constantine LM, Scott S: Just-approved antiobesity drug awaits DEA scheduling. *Pharmacy Today* 3(12):1, 1997.

Saklad JJ, Curtis JL: Psychiatric disorders in children, adolescents, and people with developmental disabilities. In Young LY, Koda-Kimble MA, editors: *Applied therapeutics: the clinical use of drugs,* ed 6, Vancouver, Wash, 1995, Applied Therapeutics, Inc.

United States Pharmacopeial Convention: *USP DI: drug information for the health care professional,* ed 18, Rockville, Md, 1998, the Convention.

ADDITIONAL REFERENCES

Anderson KN et al, editors: *Mosby's medical, nursing, and allied health dictionary,* ed 5, St Louis, 1998, Mosby.

Bray GA: Use and abuse of appetite-suppressant drugs in the treatment of obesity, *Ann Intern Med* 119(7)707, 1993.

Covington TR, editor: *Handbook of nonprescription drugs,* ed 11, Washington, DC, 1996, American Pharmaceutical Association.

Klein RG, Mannuzza S: Hyperactive boys almost grown up: methylphenidate effects on ultimate height, *Arch Gen Psychiatry* 45(12):1131, 1988.

Leung AKC et al: Attention-deficit hyperactivity disorder: getting control of impulse behavior, *Postgrad Med* 95(2):153, 1994.

Mosby: *Mosby's GenRx,* St Louis, 1998, Mosby.

Newcomb P: Tricyclic antidepressants and children, *Am J Primary Health Care* 16(5):26, 1991.

Olin BR: *Facts and comparisons,* Philadelphia, 1998, JB Lippincott.

Theesen KA, Stimmel GL: Psychiatric disorders. In DiPiro JT et al, editors: *Pharmacotherapy,* ed 2, Norwalk, Conn, 1993 Appleton & Lange.

CHAPTER 13

Psychotherapeutic Drugs

KEY DRUGS

chlorpromazine (p. 218)
haloperidol (p. 222)
imipramine (p. 231)
risperidone (p. 225)

KEY TERMS

affective disorders, (p. 228)
endogenous depression, (p. 229)
exogenous depression, (p. 228)
mania, (p. 238)
psychotic symptoms, (p. 216)
tardive dyskinesia (TD), (p. 215)
Tourette's syndrome, (p. 222)
tranquilizer, (p. 217)

CHAPTER FOCUS

To properly care for patients with psychosis, mental depression, or mania, the healthcare provider must be informed about the central nervous system and emotions, as well as the various roles and uses of different drug therapies. As these medications are very potent substances with the potential for inducing serious adverse reactions, a thorough knowledge of the different medications is required.

OBJECTIVES

After reading and studying this chapter, the student should be able to do the following:

1. *Define and discuss the key drugs and key terms.*
2. *Discuss the interrelationship between the brain and body functions.*
3. *Review the purpose of the OBRA Regulations for psychotropic medications in long-term care.*
4. *Name one drug from each category (phenothiazine, the various antidepressant categories, and lithium) and discuss indications, mechanisms of action, significant drug interactions, warnings, and contraindications.*
5. *Discuss the signs, symptoms, and management of the extrapyramidal adverse effects reported with the psychotherapeutic agents.*
6. *Name four common tyramine-containing substances and describe the interaction reported when administered concurrently with MAO inhibitor drugs.*

Various medications are available to treat psychoses and affective disorders, especially schizophrenia (antipsychotic agents), depression (antidepressants), and mania (lithium and others). Refer to Chapter 7 for a review of the physiology and functions of the various components of the central nervous system (CNS). A review of the CNS functional systems (i.e., reticular activating system [Fig. 13-1]), limbic and extrapyramidal systems, plus acetylcholine and catecholamines is necessary to understand this chapter.

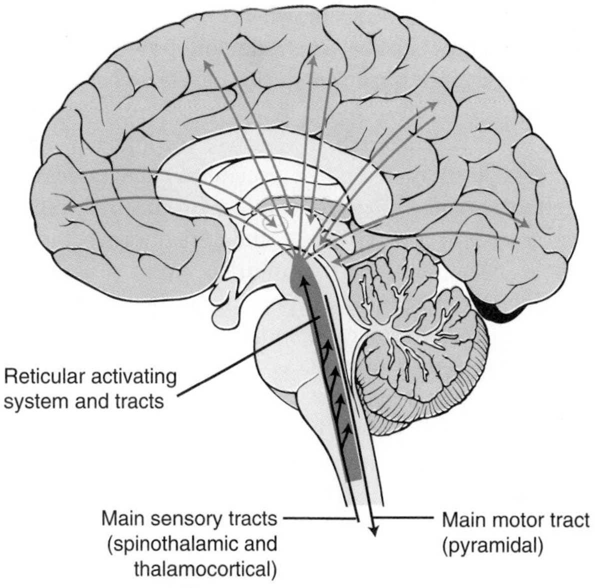

FIGURE 13-1
Reticular activating system.

CENTRAL NERVOUS SYSTEM AND EMOTIONS

To understand the action of drugs in treating the symptoms of mental illness, the healthcare professional must have a knowledge of the functioning of the nervous system. In practice today, it has become more and more difficult to separate the functions of the mind from the body. The CNS is responsible for consciousness, behavior, memory, recognition, learning, and the more highly developed attributes such as imagination, abstract reasoning, and creative thought. In addition, it serves to coordinate vital regulatory functions such as blood pressure, heart rate, respiration, salivary and gastric secretions, muscular activity, and body temperature.

The interrelationships among the various circuits in the brain produce patterns of behavior that can be modified by external situations or by internal autonomic adjustments. This allows the individual to adapt to changes in both the external and the internal environments.

Autonomic Regulation

The functions of the sympathetic and parasympathetic visceral nervous systems are discussed in Chapter 14. These systems play an important role in the production of behavior. An understanding of these mechanisms is the basis for learning the actions and side effects of the drugs that affect mood and behavior.

Biochemical Mechanisms

The functions of the CNS depend on the actions of certain neurohormonal agents located in the brain and peripheral tissues. These neurohormones are stored in inactive forms and at the right moment nerve impulses release their free forms to stimulate transmission of appropriate reactions. The neurotransmitter exerts its action by interacting with the receptor (a specialized protein), located on the outermost part of the postsynaptic cell, which produces both electric and biochemical changes within the postsynaptic cell.

The neurotransmitters, acetylcholine, norepinephrine, and serotonin, have been found in the CNS. Two other normal constituents of the brain, tyrosine and dopamine, are known precursors of norepinephrine synthesis. High concentrations of norepinephrine are located in the hypothalamus, medulla, limbic system, and cranial nerve nuclei. Dopamine is found in high concentrations in the striatum and caudate nucleus. It is believed that both norepinephrine and dopamine function as transmitters. They have widespread inhibitory and excitatory effects on a wide variety of centrally mediated functions, such as sleep and arousal, affect, and memory. Thus some central synapses are adrenergic.

Areas rich in serotonin include the hypothalamus, pineal gland, midbrain, and spinal cord. Alterations of serotonin levels in the nervous system are associated with changes in behavior. Many drugs mimic or block the action of serotonin on peripheral tissues and produce changes in mood and behavior, which suggests that they interfere with the action of serotonin and norepinephrine in the brain.

The relationship of dopamine to the major psychoses has received much attention. There are a variety of dopamine receptors in the brain, especially in the basal ganglia and limbic areas, but D_1 and D_2 receptors are the primary ones involved with the antipsychotic agents. Although both receptors are involved with movement disorders in the basal ganglia, blockade of the D_2 receptors (causing supersensitivity) in animals has resulted in **tardive dyskinesia**. Thus further research in this area may result in the development of more specific treatment agents that have less adverse effects (Ereshefsky, Richards, 1992). Antipsychotic agents with a low affinity for D_2 receptors, such as clozapine, are less apt to cause extrapyramidal side and adverse effects (Hardman, Limbird, 1996).

ROLE OF DRUG THERAPY IN PSYCHIATRY

Drugs play an important role in contemporary approaches of psychiatric care. Clinically, drug therapy reduces or alleviates symptoms and allows the patient an opportunity to participate more easily in other forms of treatment. Drugs temporarily modify behavior, whereas other therapies such as psychotherapy can shape behavior and produce a permanent change. However, any enduring effects on behavior are more likely to result from the individual's concurrent interaction with the environment. Because incoming information must be translated into biochemical changes before it can affect nervous system function, environmental transactions, as with drugs, may affect similar pathways before influencing behavior. The effects of drugs can be additive, potentiating, or antagonistic, depending on their nature and direction. The milieu may potentiate the effectiveness of the drug or may detract from it.

Generally, prescribers select psychotherapeutic agents on the basis of the diagnostic category: schizophrenia, manic-depressive syndrome, or psychoneurosis. The prescriber will try to match a particular drug's therapeutic advantages to the patient's symptoms, assuming the person's diagnosis warrants the use of a psychotropic agent. Since their introduction the antipsychotic and other psychotropic agents have been widely prescribed and in many instances in the elderly, inappropriately used. Inappropriate prescriptions expose the older person to an increased risk of an adverse or serious drug reaction that is often detrimental to the person's cognitive and functional health status. Such studies have resulted in regulations governing Medicare and Medicaid recipients in long-term care facilities.

In 1992, the OBRA Long Term Care Requirements Act for long-term care facilities was implemented. Although this act applies to all the drugs a patient receives, the Health Care Financing Administration's surveyors initially focused their attention on the major CNS drug categories: antipsychotics, antianxiety agents, sedatives, hypnotics, and benzodiazepines. The purpose of this law was to review the indication, dosage (including duplicate-type drug orders), duration, and monitoring parameters to determine if the drugs were given in the presence of side or adverse effects. The surveyors may cite a facility for deficiencies in these areas (Carley, 1992).

For prescription of antipsychotic drugs to a nursing home resident, an appropriate specific condition must be documented, such as schizophrenia, schizoaffective disorder, delusional disorder, psychotic mood disorder, acute psychotic episode, brief reactive psychosis, schizophreniform disorder, atypical psychosis, Tourette's disorder, or Huntington's disease, all of which are organic mental syndromes that have associated psychotic or agitation features. The latter features are defined as (1) specific behaviors that can be quantitatively and objectively documented (e.g., biting, kicking, or scratching) and that cause patient to present a danger to themselves or others and actually interfere with the nursing staff's ability to provide care; or (2) the presence of **psychotic symptoms** (delusions, hallucinations, or paranoid behavior) that are not a result of a previously mentioned disorder but cause the resident extreme distress (Box 13-1). To treat the symptoms of hiccups, nausea, vomiting, or pruritus, short-term therapy of 1 week is permissible.

BOX 13-1 Positive and Negative Symptoms in Schizophrenia

Patients with schizophrenia have a wide variety of symptoms that range from the most responsive (or positive) to less responsive (or negative) to the antipsychotic agents. Most antipsychotic agents produce an effect on the following positive symptoms: agitation, anxiety, hallucinations, poor hygiene and dress, hyperactivity, delusions, paranoia, and hostility, while the negative symptoms of flat affect, social inadequacy, diminished speech patterns, judgment, insight, and others are usually less responsive to drug therapy.

The target symptoms are used as monitoring parameters to evaluate the individual's response to the medication. The atypical antipsychotic drugs such as clozapine and risperidone appear to be more effective than other neuroleptic agents against negative symptoms (Marken, Stanislav, 1995).

The purpose of the regulations was to eliminate or reduce the inappropriate prescribing of such potent medications for behaviors that may be controlled by nonpharmacologic approaches. For example, insomnia, pacing, wandering, restlessness, crying spells or screaming episodes, deficient memory, uncooperativeness, nervousness, or depression alone would not warrant the use of an antipsychotic agent. Such symptoms would have to be associated with an appropriate diagnosis as mentioned previously for an antipsychotic drug to be indicated.

Drug Selection

Once the prescriber establishes the need for drug therapy, the next decision is what agent or combination of agents is best suited for the individual. This selection requires a knowledge of the behavioral actions, pharmacologic effects, and potential adverse reactions of the drugs, as well as an awareness of the many individual and environmental factors present.

The additional effect or side effect profile of a drug is a useful tool to help the prescriber select an appropriate antipsychotic agent (Table 13-1). If a drug with a strong sedation property is desired, chlorpromazine (Thorazine) or thioridazine (Mellaril) might be prescribed. If extrapyramidal side effects are troublesome, thioridazine, with the greatest anticholinergic effect, has less potential for inducing extrapyramidal side effects.

If anticholinergic side effects such as dry mouth, blurred vision, constipation, and urinary retention continue and are disturbing to the patient, the prescriber could select an agent with less potential for inducing such effects, such as fluphenazine (Prolixin, Permitil), thiothixene (Navane), or haloperidol (Haldol). Thereafter the patient is closely monitored for continued drug effectiveness and the development of side effect(s) and adverse reaction(s).

TABLE 13-1 Selected Antipsychotic Agents, Potency, and Major Side Effects

		Frequency of Selected Effects and Side Effects†				
Chemical, Generic Name (Trade Name)	**Equivalent* PO Dose (mg)**	**Antiemetic**	**Sedation**	**Hypotension‡**	**Anticholinergic**	**EPS§**
Phenothiazines						
Aliphatic						
chlorpromazine (Thorazine)	100	3	3	3	2	2
Piperidine						
thioridazine (Mellaril)	100	1	3	3	3	1
mesoridazine (Serentil)	50	1	3	3	3	1
Piperazine						
fluphenazine (Permitil, Prolixin)	2	1	1	1	1	3
perphenazine (Trilafon)	10	3	1	1	1	3
prochlorperazine (Compazine)	15	3	2	1	1	3
trifluoperazine (Stelazine)	5	3	1	1	1	3
Thioxanthenes						
thiothixene (Navane)	4	—‖	1	1	1	3
Other Compounds						
Butyrophenone						
haloperidol (Haldol)	2	2	1	1	1	3
Dihydroindolone						
molindone (Moban)	10	—	1	1	1	3
Dibenzoxapine						
loxapine (Loxitane)	15	—	2	2	1	3
Atypical Agents						
clozapine (Clozaril)	50	1	3	3	3	1
risperidone (Risperdal)	—	—	1	1	1	0/1

Olin, 1998; USP DI, 1998.
*Equivalent dosages are from low potency (50 to 100 mg) to intermediate potency (10 to 49 mg) to high potency (1 to 9 mg).
†Grading: 1, low; 2, moderate; 3, high.
‡Orthostatic hypotension.
§*EPS,* extrapyramidal side effects include akathisia, dystonia, parkinsonism, and tardive dyskinesia.
‖Undocumented or unknown

ANTIPSYCHOTIC OR NEUROLEPTIC AGENTS

Historical Background

Between 1900 and 1950, the population of the United States doubled while the population in public mental hospitals quadrupled. During this time the average length of confinement was usually years, and the trend was definitely toward an increase in admission of patients to such institutions yearly. In addition, patient and employee injuries caused by combative or abusive patients led to the common use of physical restraints and patient isolation.

Before the advent of the antipsychotic agents the treatment of mentally disturbed persons consisted of isolation (i.e., hidden in cellars or attics in their homes), or if they came to the attention of local authorities, they were transferred to jails or homes for the insane. Actual therapies used before antipsychotic agents were water or ice pack therapies, strait-jackets or other physical restraints, shock therapy with insulin or electricity, lobotomy, and the use of a few drugs such as paraldehyde, chloral hydrate, and the barbiturates.

The first antipsychotic agent, which is also the prototype phenothiazine, was chlorpromazine (Thorazine). This was the first **tranquilizer** (a drug prescribed to calm an agitated or anxious individual) released in the early 1950s. However, the term "tranquilizer" had been used approximately 200 years ago by Dr. Benjamin Rush. Dr. Rush, an early pioneer in the mental health field and a signer of the Declaration of Independence, invented a restraining chair named the "tranquilizer chair" (Lyons, Petrucelli, 1978). This chair was modified by the addition of a pulley system, so that the extremely agitated person would be seated and restrained in the chair, and the chair was raised off the ground and rocked back and forth until the person was quieted (Fig. 13-2).

The student should be aware that neither the tranquilizer chair nor the tranquilizing (antipsychotic) agents cure mental illness. They have been and are used to control the symp-

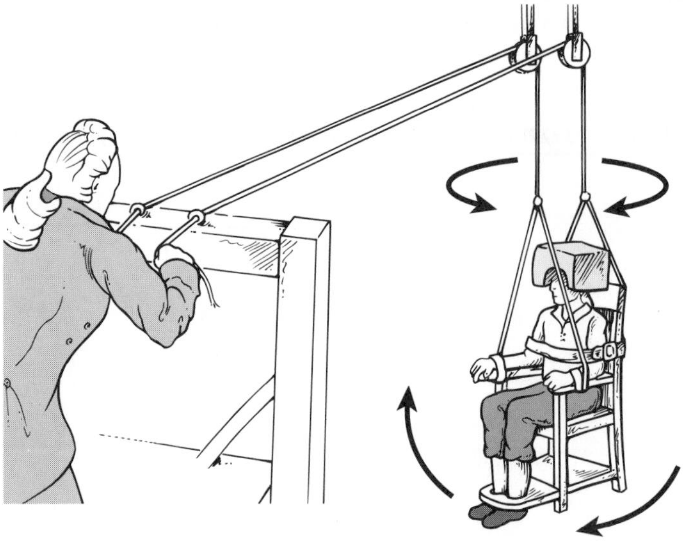

FIGURE 13-2
Tranquilizer or restraining chair used in the eighteenth century to "tranquilize" the agitated patient.

toms associated with this disease state; the chair provided physical and eventually physiologic restraints, whereas the antipsychotic and tranquilizing agents constitute a chemical control of the symptoms.

The use of the antipsychotic drugs proved to be a revolutionary force in the psychiatric field. The duration of institutionalization decreased from years to months for many patients, and others live at home and are treated at community mental health centers. The reported incidence of injuries declined along with the closing of many large public mental health facilities.

This chapter reviews the antipsychotic agents, antidepressant therapy, and antimanic medications.

ANTIPSYCHOTIC AGENTS

The discussion of antipsychotic medications will be divided into phenothiazines, thioxanthenes, and other compounds.

PHENOTHIAZINE DERIVATIVES

The first phenothiazine, chlorpromazine (Thorazine) 🔑, was widely accepted for the treatment of mental illness. Since then, many other drug products have been developed so that phenothiazines now comprise the largest group of psychotropic agents. Phenothiazines are divided chemically into the following three subgroups: (1) the aliphatic compound s(e.g., chlorpromazine), (2) the piperidine compounds (e.g., thioridazine), and (3) the piperazine compounds (e.g., fluphenazine).

Aliphatic phenothiazine derivatives include chlorpromazine (Thorazine and others), methotrimeprazine (Levoprome, Nozinan 🍁), promazine (Sparine), and triflupromazine (Vesprin).

Piperidine phenothiazine derivatives include mesoridazine (Serentil) and thioridazine (Mellaril, Apo-Thioridazine 🍁).

Piperazine phenothiazine derivatives consist of fluphenazine (Prolixin, Permitil), perphenazine (Trilafon, Apo-Perphenazine, prochlorperazine (Compazine, Stemetil 🍁), and trifluoperazine (Stelazine, Novo-Flurazine 🍁) (see Table 13-2 for phenothiazine dosing).

Classification

Antipsychotic medications have been classified as low-potency, intermediate-potency, and high-potency drugs. The basis for the classification is the quantity of medication necessary to produce an equivalent effect when compared with other agents in the same category. For example, 100 mg of chlorpromazine (Thorazine) is considered to be approximately equivalent to 50 mg of mesoridazine (Serentil) or 2 mg of haloperidol (Haldol). Thus chlorpromazine is a low-potency agent, mesoridazine is an intermediate-potency agent, and haloperidol is a high-potency drug (see Table 13-1 for antipsychotic equivalency dosages). The student is cautioned not to confuse potency with effectiveness; potency refers to the quantity of a drug necessary to produce an equivalent effect compared with another drug in the same classification. Effectiveness measures the therapeutic response to various agents, and this may range from less effective, to equivalent in effectiveness, to more effective, depending on the individual drugs being studied.

Although the exact mechanism of action for the antipsychotic effects is unknown, the major therapeutic effects and side and adverse effects are the result of dopamine blockade in specific areas of the CNS. Phenothiazines also produce an alpha-blocking effect (hypotension), inhibit or block dopa-

TABLE 13-2 Phenothiazine Indications and Dosage Range*

Chemical Classification Generic (Trade Name)	*Indication*	*Routes*	*Dosage Range (mg/24 hr)*	
			Adults	*Children*
Phenothiazines				
Aliphatic				
chlorpromazine (Thorazine)	Antipsychotic	PO, IM, R	PO 20-800	6 mo and older, 0.55 mg/kg: q4-6h
	Antiemetic	PO, IM, R	PO 60-150	Same as above
	Hiccups or porphyria	PO, IM	PO 75-200	●●●●
	Tetanus	IM	IM 75-200	IM 0.55 mg/kg q6-8h
Piperidine				
thioridazine (Mellaril)	Antipsychotic	PO	PO 100-800	2-12 yr, 0.25-3 mg/kg 4 times daily
mesoridazine (Serentil)	Antipsychotic	PO, IM	PO 30-400	<12 yr, not available; >12 yr, see adult dosage
Piperazine				
fluphenazine (Permitil, Prolixin)	Antipsychotic	PO, IM	PO 2.5-20	250-750 μg 1-4 times daily
perphenazine (Trilafon)	Antipsychotic	PO, IM	PO 8-64	<12 yr, not available; >12 yr, see adult dosage
	Antiemetic	PO, IM	PO 8-16	<12 yr, not available; >12 yr, see adult dosage
prochlorperazine (Compazine)	Antipsychotic	PO, IM, R	PO 15-40	PO 2-12 yr, 2.5 mg 2-3 times/day; >12 yr, see adult dosage
trifluoperazine (Stelazine)	Antipsychotic	PO, IM	PO 4-40	>6 yr, 1-2 mg daily

*Doses are titrated as needed and tolerated by the individual.

mine at the chemoreceptor trigger zone, and peripherally inhibit the vagus nerve in the gastrointestinal tract (antiemetic effect). They also produce an antianxiety effect by depression of the brainstem reticular system. Most phenothiazines and haloperidol increase prolactin release, which infrequently results in swelling of the breast and milk secretion. Methotrimeprazine (Levoprome) is a phenothiazine with primarily analgesic and sedative effects. It is not used as an antipsychotic drug in the United States.

Indications

Various phenothiazine derivatives are used in the treatment of psychosis, nausea and vomiting, pain, and sedation and as adjuncts to the treatment of tetanus, acute intermittent porphyria, and intractable hiccups.

Pharmacokinetics

Phenothiazines are well absorbed orally with an onset of action between ½ and 1 hour; IM onset of action is within 30 minutes with the exception of the long-acting parenteral forms. The onset of antipsychotic effect is achieved gradually, usually requiring several weeks, while peak therapeutic effect is between 6 weeks and 6 months. Duration of action for these products ranges from 6 to 24 hours or more, depending on dosage and frequency of drug administration. Phenothiazines are metabolized in the liver and excreted primarily by the kidneys. Table 13-3 lists side effects and adverse reactions.

Drug interactions

The following effects may occur when antipsychotic agents are given with the drugs listed below:

Drugs	Possible effect and management
Alcohol, CNS depressants	May result in enhanced CNS depression, respiratory depression, and increased hypotensive effects. The drug dosage should be reduced to one fourth to one half the usual dose. Titrate according to patient's response. Concurrent alcohol use may increase the risk of inducing a heat stroke. Avoid or a potentially serious drug interaction may occur. Barbiturates may decrease chlorpromazine serum levels through an increase in the metabolizing enzymes in the liver. Thioridazine (Mellaril) may decrease serum phenobarbital serum levels. Monitor closely for loss of therapeutic effect of barbiturates, since a dosage adjustment may be necessary.
Anticholinergic drugs	Concurrent drug use may result in an increase in anticholinergic side effects.

Antihypertensive agents	Concurrent drug use with the phenothiazines may result in an increase in hypotensive side effects.
Antithyroid medications	Increase the risk for agranulocytosis when phenothiazines are given concurrently.
epinephrine	Antipsychotic agents block alpha-adrenergic receptors; thus administration of epinephrine to treat phenothiazine-induced hypotension may result in severe hypotension. With the alpha receptors blocked, epinephrine stimulates beta receptors, which can result in severe lowering of blood pressure (BP) and in tachycardia. Avoid or a potentially serious drug interaction may occur.
Extrapyramidal effect-inducing medications (such as amoxapine [Asendin], metoclopramide [Reglan], and reserpine [Serpalan, etc.])	May result in increased frequency and severity of extrapyramidal effects.
guanadrel (Hylorel) or guanethidine (Ismelin)	Concurrent use with antipsychotic agents, especially loxapine and thiothixenes, may reverse the hypotensive drug effectiveness. Closely monitor blood pressure of patients receiving this drug combination.
levodopa (L-dopa)	Concurrent use with the antipsychotic agents may render levodopa ineffective in controlling Parkinson's disease.
lithium (Eskalith)	(1) May decrease gastrointestinal (GI) absorption of chlorpromazine (Thorazine) by as much as 40%; (2) may result in an increase in extrapyramidal symptoms; and (3) may increase the risk of seizures, confusional states, neuroleptic malignant syndrome, and dyskinesia. (4) Phenothiazines may increase the rate of lithium excretion in the kidneys, and (5) phenothiazines and molindone may mask nausea and vomiting, which are early signs of lithium toxicity. Haloperidol (Haldol) may also increase extrapyramidal side effects. Although controversial, there are reports of irreversible neurologic and brain damage when both drugs are given for longer periods than several weeks. If both drugs are given concurrently, monitor patients closely for neurologic changes, since dosage reduction or drug discontinuation may be necessary.
metrizamide (Amipaque)	When given concurrently with phenothiazines, may lower the seizure threshold. Discontinue phenothiazines at least 2 days before and also for 1 day after a myelogram.
quinidine	When given concurrently with the thioxanthenes (chlorprothixene, thiothixene), an increase in cardiac effects may occur. Avoid or a potentially serious drug interaction may occur.

TABLE 13-3 Antipsychotic Medications: Side Effects and Adverse Reactions

*Side Effects**	*Adverse Reactions†*
More frequent: sleepiness, dizziness, dry mouth, constipation, and nasal congestion reported with aliphatic and piperidine phenothiazines and thioxanthenes; incidence less with the piperazine phenothiazines, with the exception of perphenazine thioxanthenes: sun sensitivity loxapine: most often seen are blurred vision, confusion, dizziness, dry mouth, and increase in body weight haloperidol: usually blurred vision, constipation, dry mouth, and increase in body weight molindone: usually sedation, blurred vision, dry mouth, and constipation clozapine: may cause sedation, dizziness, constipation, insomnia, headaches, tremor, and nausea risperidone: nausea, dizziness, sedation, insomnia, and headache	Visual changes and hypotensive episodes (more common with aliphatic and piperidine phenothiazines, thioxanthenes, and possibly, molindone) Dystonia and/or parkinson-type effects including shuffle in walk, arm or leg stiffness, tremors, masklike facial expression, dysphagia, imbalance, and muscle spasms or unusual twisting effects of face, neck, or back (more common with aliphatic and piperazine phenothiazines, thioxanthines, loxapine, molindone, resperidone, and haloperidol) Akathisia (abnormal restlessness and agitation), increased pacing, and insomnia (more often reported with haloperidol, loxapine, and thioxanthene) Tardive dyskinesia, a very serious adverse reaction; although rare, neuroleptic malignant syndrome may occur Clozapine can cause agranulocytosis, hypotension, tachycardia, and seizures Hyperkinesia, agitation, and aggressive behavior

*If side effects continue, increase or disturb the patient, inform the prescriber.
†If adverse reactions occur, contact the prescriber, since medical intervention may be necessary.

Tricyclic antidepressants, monoamine oxidase inhibitors, and procarbazine (Matulane)	Concurrent use may increase the duration and intensify the sedative and anticholinergic side effects of these medications. Metabolism of the phenothiazines and the antidepressants may be inhibited. May enhance the risk of inducing neuroleptic malignant syndrome, hyperthermia, dehydration, cardiovascular instability, hypoxemia, and muscular rigidity. Avoid or a potentially serious drug interaction may occur.

Color type indicates an unsafe drug combination.

Side effects and adverse reactions

Neuroleptic extrapyramidal adverse effects such as akathisia, dystonia, drug-induced parkinsonism, and tardive dyskinesia are often seen during treatment with these potent medications. See Boxes 13-2 and 13-3 for a description and treatment of these disorders. Note that tardive dyskinesia has no known effective treatment; therefore early assessment and diagnosis are crucial for prevention. Also see Table 13-3 for additional side effects and adverse reactions.

Warnings

Use with caution in patients with angina pectoris, breast cancer, cardiac disease, Parkinson's disease, chronic respiratory disease, and epilepsy, in pregnant women (see the box for Food and Drug Administration [FDA] pregnancy safety categories), in children (see Pediatric Implications box), and in the elderly (see Geriatric Implications box).

Contraindications

Avoid use in patients with phenothiazine hypersensitivity, blood dyscrasias, severe liver impairment, severe cardiac disease, severe CNS depression, and Reye's syndrome and in alcohol abusers.

The dosage of antipsychotic agents varies according to the individual, the reason for treatment, and the patient's response to the medication. It is best to titrate from a low dose, increasing when necessary to produce a therapeutic response, which usually occurs within days to several months. Continue at this dosage for 14 days and then gradually decrease dosage to the lowest amount that produces a therapeutic response. See Table 13-2 for phenothiazine indications and dosage.

When stopping antipsychotic therapy, gradually reduce the dosage over 2 or 3 weeks. When antipsychotic agents have been given to patients in high doses or for a long time and are suddenly discontinued, nausea, vomiting, dizziness, tremors, and dyskinesia have been reported.

Acetophenazine (Tindal), promazine (Sparine), and triflupromazine (Vesprin) are available on the market but are not commonly used today.

PREGNANCY SAFETY

Category	Drugs
B	bupropion, clozapine, fluoxetine, maprotiline, sertraline
C	amitriptyline, amoxapine, clomipramine, desipramine, haloperidol, loxapine, mirtazapine, nefazodone, nortriptyline, olsalazine, pimozide, phenelzine, quetiapine, risperidone, trazodone, trimipramine, venlafaxine
D	lithium
Unclassified	doxepin, imipramine, isocarboxazid, molindone, phenothiazines (although not recommended during pregnancy), protriptyline, thiothixene, tranylcypromine

PEDIATRIC IMPLICATIONS

Psychotherapeutic Agents

Children are at a greater risk of developing neuromuscular or extrapyramidal side effects, especially dystonias. Monitor closely if antipsychotic agents are administered.

Pediatric patients with chickenpox, CNS infections, measles, dehydration, gastroenteritis, or other acute illnesses will be at special risk of developing adverse reactions and possibly Reye's syndrome. Avoid use of phenothiazine antiemetic therapy in such patients.

The tricyclic antidepressants are usually not recommended for the treatment of depression in children younger than 12 years of age. Some agents, though, such as amitriptyline (Elavil), desipramine (Norpramin), and imipramine (Tofranil) have been used in children older than age 6 for major depressions. Several of these agents are also used in the treatment of enuresis and attention deficit disorder. Be aware that children are very sensitive to an acute overdose, which should always be considered very serious and potentially fatal. Adolescents often require a decreased dose because of their sensitivity to this drug category.

Adverse effects reported in children receiving tricyclic antidepressants include changes in electrocardiogram patterns, increased nervousness, sleep disorders, complaints of tiredness, hypertension, and mild stomach distress.

Lithium may decrease the bone density or bone formation in children. If necessary to use, closely monitor serum levels and for signs of toxicity.

From *USP DI*, 1998.

BOX 13-2 Neuroleptic Extrapyramidal Adverse Effects

Akathisia

Description:

Motor restlessness; person unable to sit or stand still, feels urgent need to move, pace, rock, or tap foot.

May also present as apprehension, irritability, and general uneasiness and may be mistaken for agitation.

More common in females than males; usually occurs in 5 to 30 days (up to 90 days) of starting drug therapy.

Treatment:

Lower dose of neuroleptic agent, switch to a different drug, or administer an antiparkinson drug, such as benztropine (Cogentin).

Dystonia

Description:

Acute reaction requiring immediate intervention. Patient exhibits muscle spasms of face, tongue, neck, jaw, and/or back. Hyperextension of neck and trunk and arching of back.

Tongue may protrude; facial grimaces; exaggerated posturing of head, neck, or jaw; difficulty swallowing and/or talking. Person may have a fixed upward gaze and/or eye muscle spasms. May be accompanied by excessive salivation.

Commonly occurs after large doses of neuroleptics, usually within an hour up to a week of drug therapy. Occurs more often in males than females.

Treatment:

Depending on the severity of reaction, one or more of the following may be necessary; lower neuroleptic dose, administer benztropine (Cogentin) IM or IV, or diphenhydramine (Benadryl) IM.

Drug-Induced Parkinsonism

Description:

Symptoms similar to Parkinson's disease; shuffling gait, drooling, tremors, increased rigidity (cogwheel). Bradykinesia (slow movements) and akinesia (immobility) also reported.

Treatment:

Add antiparkinson drug, such as benztropine (Cogentin), diphenhydramine (Benadryl), etc.

Physician may switch to a neuroleptic less likely to induce this effect, such as thioridazine (Mellaril).

Tardive Dyskinesia

Description:

Oral/facial dyskinesias, i.e., abnormal involuntary muscle movements around the mouth, lip smacking, tongue darting, constant chewing movements, or tics.

Person may also have involuntary movements of arms or legs. More common in older women but has been reported in younger persons.

Treatment:

Prevention is vital, may be irreversible. No effective treatment.

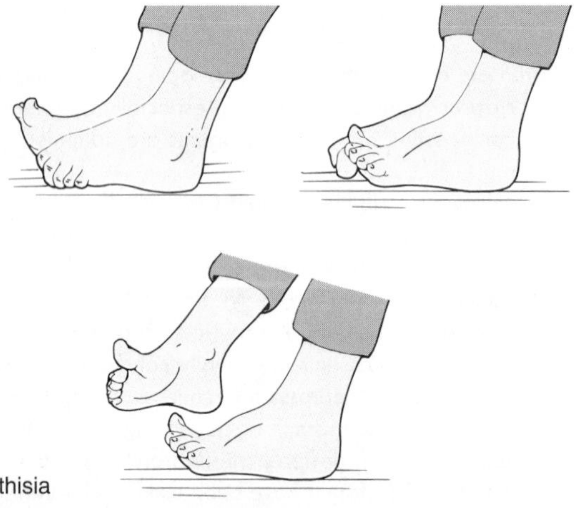

Akathisia

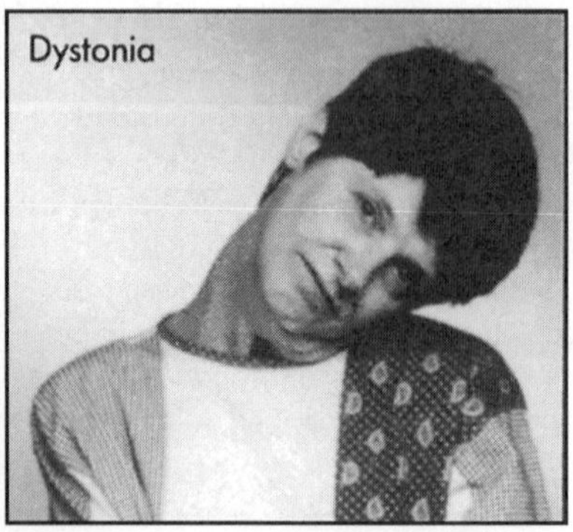

Dystonia

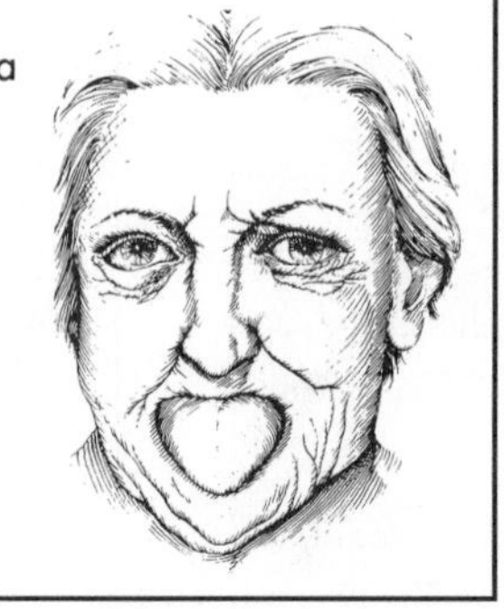

Tardive dyskinesia

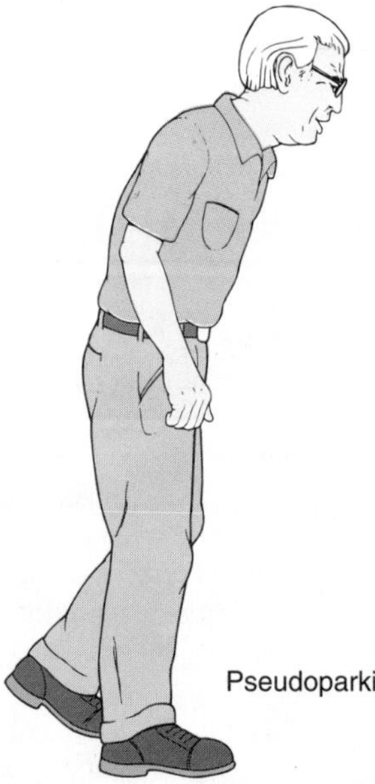

Pseudoparkinsonism

GERIATRIC IMPLICATIONS

Psychotherapeutic Agents

The elderly tend to have higher serum levels of antipsychotic and antidepressant drugs because of changes in drug distribution resulting from a decrease in lean body mass, less total body water, less serum albumin, and usually an increase in body fat. Therefore, these patients require a lower drug dose and a more gradual drug dose titration than the younger adult patient.

Geriatric patients are more prone to have orthostatic hypotension, anticholinergic side effects, extrapyramidal side effects, and sedation. They should be carefully evaluated before starting such potent medications, and if the antipsychotic agents are necessary, close supervision and the prescribing of the lowest dose possible are recommended.

The elderly person generally should receive half the recommended adult dose. The patient with organic brain syndrome should only receive 33% to 50% of the usual adult dose with increases in dosage at 7- to 10-day periods. When clinical improvement is noted, attempts at tapering and discontinuing the drug should be instituted.

The tricyclic antidepressants may cause increased anxiety in the geriatric patient. If the patient has cardiovascular disease, the use of tricyclic antidepressants increases the risk of inducing dysrhythmias, tachycardia, stroke, congestive heart failure, and myocardial infarction.

Lithium is more toxic in the geriatric patient; therefore lower lithium dosages, a lower lithium serum level, and very close monitoring is critical in this age group. The elderly are more prone to develop CNS toxicity, lithium-induced goiter, and clinical hypothyroidism than the average adult. Generally, excessive thirst and elimination of large volumes of urine may be early side effects of lithium toxicity frequently seen in the elderly.

From *USP DI, 1998.*

THIOXANTHENES

chlorprothixene [klor proe thix′ een] (Taractan)
flupenthixol [floo pent′ ole]
(Fluanxol ♣, Fluanxol Depot ♣)
thiothixene [thye oh thix′ een] (Navane)

Thioxanthenes resemble the piperazine phenothiazines in their antipsychotic effects, including the high incidence of extrapyramidal adverse effects (see Table 13-1). Their antipsychotic indications, side effects, precautions, and drug interactions are similar as those for the phenothiazines. Thiothixene is the drug most commonly prescribed in this category. The usual thiothixene adult dose is 2 mg PO three times a day. The oral dose is not established for children up to 12 years of age. For children 12 years and older, see the adult dose. The parenteral dose is 4 mg IM, two to four times a day.

BOX 13-3 Tardive Dyskinesia

Tardive dyskinesia (TD) is a potentially irreversible neurologic disorder that primarily involves the bucco-lingual and masticatory muscles. This adverse effect to the antipsychotic agents may occur within a few months or after years of treatment or after these agents have been discontinued. The risk of inducing TD increases with total dosage of the drug given and the length of the treatment period.

Incidence: Although 0.5% to 65% of the treated population may develop this syndrome, recent reports place the percentage of patients at risk at 10% to 20%.

Presenting features:
- Facial: grimacing or scowling expression, facial tics, arching of the eyebrows
- Ocular: blinking, eyelid spasms (blepharospasm)
- Oral/buccal: lip smacking, lower lip thrusting, sucking, puffing of cheeks, chewing of the cheeks (the inside of the mouth should be checked for this)
- Lingual/masticatory: lateral jaw movements, tongue protrusion or thrusting such as "fly catching movements," tongue in lip or cheek resulting in an observable bulge in the specific area
- Systemic effects: foot tapping; rocking from side to side; arms, hands, and fingers displaying a jerking and/or a writhing motion (choreoathetoid motion); pelvic thrusting motions

Treatment: Prevention only. Early assessment and diagnosis are crucial in preventing the development of an irreversible disorder. Decreasing or discontinuing the antipsychotic agent if possible is the recommended procedure. At present, there is no known effective treatment for TD.

From Kalachnik, 1983; *USP DI,* 1998.

OTHER ANTIPSYCHOTIC COMPOUNDS

Butyrophenone Derivatives

haloperidol [ha loe per′ i dole] (Haldol) 🔑

The butyrophenones, while structurally different from the other antipsychotic agents, have similar properties in terms of antipsychotic efficacy. Haloperidol appears to have a selective CNS effect; it competitively blocks D_2 receptors in the mesolimbic system and also causes an increased turnover of brain dopamine to produce its antipsychotic effect. It has less effect on the norepinephrine and epinephrine receptors and is associated with a significant degree of extrapyramidal effects.

Indications

Haloperidol has both antiemetic and antipsychotic effects. This drug is used to treat psychotic disorders, severe behavioral problems in children, and **Tourette's syndrome,** a rare central nervous system disorder that results in involuntary, rapid, and repetitive motor movements of muscle groups that are usually accompanied by involuntary vocalizations. This syndrome is more common in males, usually appearing before the age of 14, and may present initially as tics (facial grimaces and blinking). Other symptoms include vocal tics or noises, such as grunting, barking, shouting, sniffing, compulsive swearing (coprolalia), and movement disorders (involuntary, purposeless movements). The individual's intellectual functions are normal. The symptoms may peak and wane throughout the person's life. Although there is no cure for Tourette's syndrome, haloperidol (Haldol) and pimozide (Orap) have produced dramatic improvement in some patients.

Drug interactions

The following effects may occur when haloperidol is given with the drugs listed below:

Drug	Possible effect and management
Alcohol, CNS depressants	Combined use may result in enhanced CNS depression, respiratory depression, and hypotensive effects. Concurrent use with alcohol may increase alcohol intoxication. Avoid or a potentially serious drug interaction may occur.
epinephrine	Antipsychotic agents block alpha-adrenergic receptors; thus administration of epinephrine to treat phenothiazine-induced hypotension may result in severe hypotension. With the alpha receptors blocked, epinephrine stimulates beta receptors, which can result in severe lowering of blood pressure and tachycardia. Avoid or a potentially serious drug interaction may occur.
Extrapyramidal effect-inducing medications	May increase the quantity and severity of extrapyramidal effects. Monitor closely.
levodopa (L-dopa)	Haloperidol's blocking of dopamine receptors decreases the effectiveness of levodopa in controlling Parkinson's disease. Avoid concurrent drug administration.
lithium (Eskalith)	Concurrent use may result in an increase in extrapyramidal side effects and in some patients, irreversible neurologic and brain damage. When both drugs are used concurrently, monitor patients closely for neurologic changes since dosage reduction or discontinuation of drug may be necessary.

Color type indicates an unsafe drug combination.

Side effects and adverse reactions

See Tables 13-1 and 13-3 and Boxes 13-2 and 13-3 for detailed information.

Warnings

Use with caution in patients with glaucoma, liver, and pulmonary or renal function disease, and in current alcohol abusers.

Contraindications

Avoid use in patients with haloperidol hypersensitivity, severe angina pectoris, severe cardiac disease, epilepsy, Parkinson's disease, and urinary retention.

Dosage and administration

The usual adult dose is 0.5 to 5 mg PO two to three times a day. The parenteral dose is 2 to 5 mg IM every 2 to 4 hours initially, then every 4 to 8 hours thereafter. Dosage is not established for children. In addition, very low doses of haloperidol have also been found to be useful for the treatment of severe agitation, combativeness, and psychosis in the demented patient. Generally, divided doses of 0.5 to 2 mg/day are sufficient for the elderly patient.

Dihydroindolone Derivative

molindone [moe lin′ done] (Moban)

Molindone is an antipsychotic agent representing a new chemical class.

Mechanism of action

In theory, molindone blocks dopamine receptors in the reticular activating and limbic systems, with activity similar to that of major tranquilizers such as phenothiazines.

Pharmacokinetics

Molindone is well absorbed orally and reaches peak serum levels in 1.5 hours. Its duration of action is 24 to 36 hours. It is believed to be metabolized in the liver and excreted as metabolites in the urine and feces.

Drug interactions

The following effects may occur when molindone is given with the drugs listed below:

Drug	Possible effect and management
Alcohol, CNS depressants	May result in enhanced CNS depressant-effects. Monitor CNS depressants closely.
Extrapyramidal effect-inducing medications	Concurrent use may result in an increase in the quantity and severity of extrapyramidal effects.

lithium	May result in neurotoxic effects, such as confusion, delirium, convulsions, extrapyramidal symptoms, and abnormal electroencephalogram (EEG) alterations. The use of an alternative medication should be considered.

Color type indicates an unsafe drug combination.

Side effects and adverse reactions

Similar to haloperidol, molindone causes little sedation and few anticholinergic and cardiovascular adverse effects, but it reportedly has a high incidence of causing extrapyramidal symptoms.

Warnings

Use with caution in individuals with glaucoma, liver impairment, urinary retention, Parkinson's disease, prostatic hypertrophy, brain tumor, or intestinal obstruction.

Contraindications

Avoid use in patients with severe drug-induced depression and in patients with molindone hypersensitivity.

Dosage and administration

In adults, the initial dose is 50 to 75 mg PO daily in divided doses. Dosages may increase to 100 mg daily in 3 or 4 days up to a maximum of 225 mg/day. The dosage for the elderly patient is lower than the adult dosage and titrated to response or the development of side effects. This drug is not recommended for children younger than 12 years of age.

Dibenzoxapine Derivative

loxapine succinate [lox′ a peen] (Loxitane, Loxapac ♣)

Loxapine, while structurally similar to the phenothiazines, is a member of a distinct chemical class of antipsychotic drugs, the dibenzoxapines. It causes a moderate degree of sedation and orthostatic hypotension, has few anticholinergic effects, and causes a high incidence of extrapyramidal symptoms.

The loxapine adult oral dose (liquid or capsule) is 10 mg twice daily, increased slowly during the first 7 to 10 days as necessary. The maintenance dose is 15 to 25 mg orally two to four times daily. The maximum dosage is 250 mg/day. Dosage for the elderly is 3 to 5 mg twice daily initially. Dosage for children younger than 16 years of age has not been established. Injectable loxapine is administered to adults at 12.5 to 50 mg IM every 4 to 6 hours as necessary, up to a maximum of 250 mg/day.

Atypical Antipsychotic Agents

clozapine [kloe′ za peen] (Clozaril)

Clozapine is considered an "atypical" antipsychotic agent. It differs from the other neuroleptics by being active at the limbic dopamine receptors, affecting both receptors but with less affinity for D_2 receptors, thus it is less apt to induce extrapyramidal side effects. It binds more to serotonin ($5\text{-}HT_2$), $alpha_1$, and histamine (H_1) receptors than dopamine receptors. Because it has the potential for causing agranulocytosis, a potentially life-threatening effect, this drug is reserved for treatment-resistant schizophrenia or for when the adverse effects of other drugs preclude their continued use. Treatment resistance has been defined as the patient not responding to an appropriate course of standard antipsychotic agents after trying at least two antipsychotic medications (USP DI, 1998).

Treatment with clozapine is closely monitored, with the manufacturer recommending dispensing of only weekly supplies and the performance of weekly white blood cell count testing. The adult dose is 25 mg once or twice daily increased by 25 to 50 mg/day until 300 to 450 mg/day is reached by the end of the second week of therapy. Thereafter increases should not exceed 100 mg once or twice a week. The maximum daily dose is 900 mg. Patients should be closely monitored because high doses may result in an increase in adverse effects, such as seizures (USP DI, 1998).

risperidone [ris peer′ i dohn] (Risperdal)

Risperidone is the first benzisoxazole from a new chemical class of antipsychotic drugs that blocks both serotonin and dopamine receptors.

Indications

It is indicated for the treatment of psychotic disorders and improves both the positive and negative symptoms of schizophrenia.

Pharmacokinetics

This drug is well absorbed orally. The peak serum level occurs within 1 to 2 hours, and it is metabolized in the liver to 9-hydroxyrisperidone, an active metabolite that is therapeutically active. Elimination half-life is 20 to 24 hours with excretion primarily via the kidneys.

Drug interactions

The following effects may occur when risperidone is given with the drugs listed below:

Drug	Possible effect and management
Alcohol, CNS depressants	May enhance CNS-depressant effects. Monitor closely as dosage adjustments may be necessary.
Antihypertensive medications	May enhance hypotensive effects; monitor closely.
bromocriptine (Parlodel), levodopa, or pergolide (Permax)	Risperidone may block the effects of these drugs. May need to consider use of another antipsychotic agent.

carbamazepine (Tegretol)	Chronic carbamazepine administration may decrease serum levels of risperidone. Monitor as dosage adjustments may be necessary.
clozapine (Clozaril)	Chronic clozapine administration may result in increased serum levels of risperidone. Monitor closely.

Side effects and adverse reactions

These include fatigue, cough, constipation or diarrhea, dry mouth, increase in dreaming, nausea, weight gain, insomnia, visual changes, sexual dysfunction, agitation, increased anxiety, and extrapyramidal reactions.

Dosage and administration

The usual adult dose is 1 mg twice daily, increasing by 1 mg twice daily on the second and third day if tolerated. Thereafter dosage increases may be instituted at weekly intervals. In the elderly, the dosage is 0.5 mg twice daily, titrated according to response. Safety in children up to 18 years of age is not established.

pimozide [pi′ moe zide] (Orap)

Pimozide is indicated for the treatment of severe motor and vocal tics in persons with Tourette's syndrome who have failed to respond to haloperidol (Haldol).

Mechanism of action

Although the mechanism of action is unknown, pimozide blocks dopamine in the central nervous system. Pimozide is administered orally, is metabolized in the liver to two major metabolites, produces its peak effect in 6 to 8 hours, and has a half-life of 29 hours. Within a week about 50% is excreted, primarily by the kidneys.

Drug interactions

The following effects may occur when pimozide is given with the drugs listed below:

Drug	Possible effect and management
Alcohol, CNS depressants	May enhance CNS depressant effects. Monitor closely.
Amphetamines, methylphenidate (Ritalin), pemoline (Cylert)	These drugs may cause tics; therefore they should be discontinued before pimozide therapy is begun.
Anticholinergic drugs	May result in enhanced anticholinergic side effects, such as dry mouth, constipation, blurred vision, and excitability.
Antidepressants, tricyclic; disopyramide (Norpace), maprotiline (Ludiomil), phenothiazines, procainamide (Pronestyl), or quinidine	May enhance or potentiate cardiac dysrhythmias. Avoid or a potentially serious drug interaction may occur.
Extrapyramidal effect-causing medications, including phenothiazines	May result in an increase in the extrapyramidal side effects of both medications. May also increase the anticholinergic and CNS-depressant effects.

Color type indicates an unsafe drug combination.

Side effects and adverse reactions

These include dry mouth, orthostatic hypotension, skin rash, pruritus, visual disturbances, constipation, sedation, breast soreness, milk secretion, akathisia, behavioral alterations, ventricular dysrhythmias, and drug-induced parkinsonian and extrapyramidal effects. With the exception of mood or behavioral changes, the other adverse effects occur most commonly during the first few days of therapy. Less frequent reactions include intense, irregular muscle spasms (dystonia), tardive dyskinesia, jaundice, neuroleptic malignant syndrome, and blood dyscrasias.

Warnings

Use with caution in patients with liver and renal impairment.

Contraindications

Avoid use in patients with pimozide hypersensitivity, cardiac dysrhythmias, severe CNS depression, motor or vocal tics (other than Tourette's), a history of breast cancer, and hypokalemia.

Dosage and administration

In adults and children 12 and older, administer 1 to 2 mg orally in divided doses, titrated every other day as necessary. For children younger than 12 years of age, the dosage has not been established. The maximum daily dosage is 20 mg in divided doses.

Thienobenzodiazepine

olanzapine (Zyprexa)

Olanzapine is the first agent from the thienobenzodiazepine classification and was approved for the treatment of schizophrenia.

Mechanism of action

Olanzapine is a monoaminergic antagonist that binds with $alpha_1$-adrenergic, dopamine, histamine, serotonin, and muscarinic receptors in the body. While its mechanism of action is unknown, its effectiveness has been proposed to be due to its dopamine and serotonin type 2 blocking action. Action at the other receptors may account for some of olanzapine's other effects and side effects. This product appears to control both positive and negative symptoms with a low incidence of adverse reports (Stat/Gram, 1996).

Pharmacokinetics

Olanzapine is well absorbed orally, reaching peak serum levels in 6 hours. Its half-life is between 21 and 54 hours. It is metabolized and excreted in urine and feces.

Drug interactions

The following effects may occur when olanzapine is given with the drugs listed below:

Drug	Possible effect and management
carbamazepine (Tegretol)	Concurrent use may decrease olanzapine levels (by up to 50%) which may require an dosage adjustment. Monitor closely.
Antihypertensive agents	May result in an increase in hypotension; monitor closely.
levodopa and other dopamine agonists	The effects of levodopa and dopamine agonists may be antagonized by olanzapine.

Side effects and adverse reactions

These include headache, agitation, constipation, orthostatic hypotension, sedation, weight gain, and somnolence.

Warnings

Use with caution in persons with seizures.

Contraindications

Avoid use in patients with olanzapine hypersensitivity, Alzheimer's dementia, breast cancer, cardiac disease, cerebrovascular disease, dehydration, glaucoma, paralytic ileus, prostatic hypertrophy, and liver impairment.

Dosage and administration

The usual adult dose is 5 to 10 mg once daily, titrating weekly as necessary. Antipsychotic efficacy was reported at dosage ranges of 10 to 15 mg/day (Eli Lilly, 1996).

quetiapine (Seroquel)

Quetiapine is an antagonist at many CNS neurotransmitter receptors, such as serotonin ($5\text{-}HT_{1A}$ and $5\text{-}HT_2$), dopamine (D_1 and D_2), histamine (H_1), adrenergic ($alpha_1$ and $alpha_2$) receptors. It is indicated for the treatment of psychotic disorders.

Mechanism of action

The mechanism of action is unknown, but it has been theorized that quetiapine produces its antipsychotic action by its effect on dopamine (D_2) and serotonin ($5\text{-}HT_2$). Its blockade at the other receptors may explain some of its side effects such as, histamine receptor antagonist (sedation) and $alpha_1$ receptor blockade (orthostatic hypotension).

Pharmacokinetics

Quetiapine is well absorbed orally and reaches a peak serum level in 1.5 hours. Food increases its bioavailability. It has a half-life (elimination) of approximately 6 hours. It is metabolized in the liver and primarily excreted by the kidneys.

Drug interactions

The following effects may occur when quetiapine is given with the drugs listed below:

Drug	Possible effect and management
Alcohol, CNS depressant	Alcohol's cognitive and motor effects may be potentiated. Monitor closely.
Liver enzyme cytochrome P450 3A inhibitors such as erythromycin, fluconazole (Diflucan) itraconazole (Sporanox), and ketoconazole (Nizoral)	Use caution when administering quetiapine with these drugs. These drugs inhibit the primary route of metabolism for quetiapine. Monitor closely.
Liver enzyme inducers (cytochrome P450) such as phenytoin (Dilantin)	May need to increase quetiapine dose as concurrent administration with these agents can increase its clearance from the body. Monitor closely.

Side effects and adverse reactions

These include sedation, dry mouth, GI distress, dizziness, weight gain, hypotension, constipation, dyspnea, extrapyramidal symptoms, Parkinson effects, peripheral edema, rash, and flu-like symptoms.

Warnings

Use with caution in patients with Alzheimer's disease, hypothyroidism, a history of seizures, or drug abuse.

Contraindications

Avoid use in individuals with quetiapine hypersensitivity, breast cancer, and cardiac, liver or cerebrovascular disease and in patients with any conditions that may predispose them to hypotension, such as dehydration and hypovolemia.

Dosage and administration

The usual adult dose is 25 mg PO twice daily, increased as necessary by 25 to 50 mg as needed. The maximum dose is 800 mg/day.

ANTIDEPRESSANT THERAPY

AFFECTIVE DISORDERS

Affective disorders, or mood disturbances, include depression, which is the most common affective disorder, and mania or elation. Mania is discussed later in this chapter.

Etiology of Affective Disorders

No single factor has been identified as the cause of affective disorders. Psychiatrists who believe in psychosocial therapies will probe to identify stressful events or mental conflicts that preceded the onset of depression, while others adhering to the biologic theory tend to explain affective disorders by the monoamine theory (i.e., catecholamine [norepinephrine, dopamine, epinephrine] and indolamine [serotonin] levels in the CNS). Many practitioners today believe that both psychosocial and biologic factors lead to a common pathway that results in an affective disorder.

Many factors are involved with affective disorders; some of these are genetics, psychosocial events (divorce or death of a mate), physiologic stress (illness, infection, or childbirth), and personality traits. Any combination of these factors may also affect the CNS's biochemical mechanisms, lending weight again to the theory that affective disorders have a common pathway.

Monoamine Theory in Affective Disorders

Centrally acting monoamines, especially norepinephrine and serotonin, have been theorized to be the cause of depression and mania. A deficiency in central norepinephrine has been associated with depression, whereas an excess of norepinephrine is believed to be related to mania.

The tricyclic antidepressants may block the reuptake of one or both monoamines into the adrenergic neuron. This blockade will lead to elevated levels of norepinephrine and serotonin in the synapse areas. Monoamine oxidase (MAO), an enzyme found in the mitochondria of nerve cells, is responsible for metabolizing norepinephrine within the nerve. Monoamine oxidase inhibitors block this enzyme, leading to increased levels of norepinephrine available for release to the synapse area.

Although the mechanism of action of many antidepressants is inhibition of the reuptake of norepinephrine or serotonin or inhibition of the MAO enzyme system, not all antidepressants have this effect. Therefore it is believed that the full range of the antidepressant activity of these medications is probably unknown (Figure 13-3).

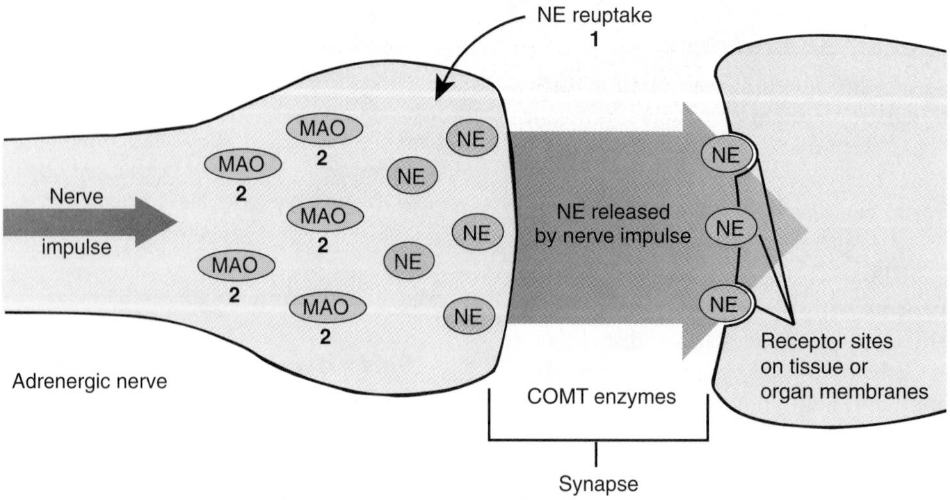

FIGURE 13-3
Proposed action of antidepressant drug therapy. Normally norepinephrine (NE) is released from storage sites within the adrenergic nerve by the arrival of a nerve impulse. The released NE may be metabolized within the nerve by MAO enzyme or after the activity of NE at the receptor sites by catechol O-methyltransferase (COMT) enzymes located in the synaptic cleft. Most NE is taken back into the nerve and stored by way of the reuptake mechanism. Antidepressant drug therapy: *1,* tricyclic antidepressants block the reuptake of released NE and prevent it from reentering the adrenergic nerve; *2,* MAOIs block MAO located on the surface of the cell mitochondria. The result is move NE available for release or available in the synaptic area.

DEPRESSION

Over the years many classifications of depression have been used, such as the time during life that depression occurred (childhood, adolescent, or senile depression) or the reason for the depression, such as exogenous (reactive or secondary) depression or endogenous depression. **Exogenous depression** is often a person's response to a loss (loss of pleasure or interest in activities and everyday living caused perhaps by the loss of a loved one or the presence of a debilitating illness) or disappointment (e.g., from not meeting one's expectations or loss of a job, pet, or friend). This is usually referred to as "the blues" or normal depression, which generally remits in several months without the use of antidepressant medications. The mobilization of support systems and, if necessary, psychotherapy are useful adjuncts in exogenous depression.

Unipolar or **endogenous depression** is characterized by the absence of external causes for depression. This type of depression may be caused by genetic determination and biochemical alterations (Katzung, 1992). Antidepressant medications are very useful in the treatment of this type of depression.

The current classification of depressive disorders has eliminated the use of this terminology. Instead major affective disorders are defined as bipolar disorders (mixed type and manic) and major depression as unipolar (single episode or recurrent episodes), along with atypical affective disorders, which include depression. Psychiatrists have debated over whether the new classification is an improvement over the previous types of classification, since it is important for the clinician to have a diagnostic framework from which to work.

Criteria for major depression include the presence of mood changes (sadness, despondency, anxiety, crying spells, guilt feelings, self-pity, pessimism, and loss of interest in life and social activities), psychologic symptoms (low self-esteem, poor concentration, hopeless or helpless feelings, and suicidal tendencies or increased focus on death), physiologic manifestations (sleep disturbances that may range from insomnia to hypersomnia, decreased interest in sex, complaints of fatigue, loss of energy, menstrual dysfunction, headaches, palpitations, constipation, loss of appetite, and weight loss or weight gain), and thought alterations (a decrease in concentration or attention span, complaints of poor memory, confusion, delusions relating to health, persecution, or religion, and hallucinations if the patient is also psychotic). Mood variations are usually diurnal and often worse in the morning.

Measures to treat depression include electroshock therapy, psychotherapy, reduction of environmental stressors, and milieu therapy. In a number of patients, antidepressant drug therapy in combination with one or more adjunct measures is more effective than drug therapy alone.

Selection of an Antidepressant

The primary antidepressants available include the tricyclic antidepressants, second-generation (tetracyclic) antidepressants, selective serotonin reuptake inhibitors (SSRIs), monoamine oxidase inhibitors (MAOIs), and other miscellaneous antidepressants. The therapeutic response rate is similar with all antidepressants; thus selection is often dependent on the side effect profile of the individual drugs (Table 13-4).

In the past, the tricyclic antidepressants were usually the first drugs prescribed for depression. Today, second-generation drugs, SSRIs, and miscellaneous antidepressants are often more commonly prescribed. The mechanism of action for the tricyclic and MAOI antidepressants was discussed previously and is illustrated in Figure 13-3. The SSRIs selectively block the reuptake of serotonin into the nerve terminal while the actions of the atypical antidepressants are less well defined.

Selection of an antidepressant is empiric, taking into consideration the side effect potential of each antidepressant compared with the medical problems of the individual patient. For example, prescribers might select a sedating antidepressant (amitriptyline [Elavil], doxepin [Sinequan], or fluoxetine [Prozac]) for the agitated depressed person or the potent blockers of norepinephrine reuptake (desipramine [Norpramin], nortriptyline [Aventyl]) for a withdrawn depressive patient. The Agency for Health Care Policy and Research (Depression Guideline Panel, 1993) issued tables on the selection and side effect profiles of antidepressant medications (Box 13-4 and Table 13-4).

Plasma levels of the tricyclic antidepressants can vary widely between different individuals and, with the possible exceptions of nortriptyline (Aventyl), imipramine (Tofranil), and desipramine (Norpramin), they often do not correlate with dose or therapeutic response. Prescribers may order serum level measurements to monitor and help identify the noncompliant patient. A low plasma level should initially indicate the need to interview the person to verify adherence to the prescribed schedule. The reason for the patient's ineffective management of the therapeutic medication regimen (intolerable side effects, misunderstanding of directions, potential drug interaction, or inadequate finances to purchase prescriptions) can then be identified and perhaps resolved (Laird, Benefield, 1995).

If compliance is verified and serum levels still remain low, dosage adjustments may be necessary or the prescriber might consider switching to a different antidepressant. If the person is nonresponsive to a predominantly norepinephrine-potentiating medication, a serotonin-potentiating agent might be indicated (Table 13-5) as the individual may have biochemical differences that would indicate a trial with the opposite reuptake blocking agent.

The elderly often have reduced levels of liver drug metabolizing enzymes and thus higher serum drug levels and a greater potential for side effects exist. Many prescribers start geriatric patients at one third to one half the usual adult

TABLE 13-4 Side Effect Profiles of Antidepressant Medications

	Side Effect						
		Central Nervous System		Cardiovascular			Other
Drug	**Anticholinergic**	**Drowsiness**	**Insomnia/ Agitation**	**Orthostatic-Hypotension**	**Cardiac Arrhythmia**	**Gastrointestinal Distress**	**Weight Gain (Over 6 kg)**
amitriptyline	4+	4+	0	4+	3+	0	4+
desipramine	1+	1+	1+	2+	2+	0	1+
doxepin	3+	4+	0	2+	2+	0	3+
imipramine	3+	3+	1+	4+	3+	1+	3+
nortriptyline	1+	1+	0	2+	2+	0	1+
protriptyline	2+	1+	1+	2+	2+	0	0
trimipramine	1+	4+	0	2+	2+	0	3+
amoxapine	2+	2+	2+	2+	3+	0	1+
maprotiline	2+	4+	0	0	1+	0	2+
trazodone	0	4+	0	1+	1+	1+	1+
bupropion	0	0	2+	0	1+	1+	0
fluoxetine	0	0	2+	0	0	3+	0
paroxetine	0	0	2+	0	0	3+	0
sertraline	0	0	2+	0	0	3+	0
MAO inhibitors	1	1+	2+	2+	0	1+	2+

Adapted from Depression Guideline Panel, 1993.
0 = absent or rare
1+
2+ = in between
3+
4+ = relatively common

BOX 13-4 Selecting Among Antidepressant Medications for Depressed Outpatients

I. First- and Second-line Choices

A. Secondary amine tricyclics (e.g., nortriptyline, desipramine)*
B. bupropion
C. fluoxetine
D. paroxetine
E. sertraline
F. trazodone

II. Alternative Agents for Patients with Special Presentations or Needs

A. Tertiary amine tricyclics (e.g., amitriptyline, imipramine)
Special considerations:
Absence of serious medical illnesses, including cardiac disease, that preclude use
Need for rapid sedation

B. Monoamine oxidase inhibitors (MAOIs)
Special considerations:
Nonresponse or intolerance to at least one tricyclic and one heterocyclic
Family or personal history of MAOI response
Atypical symptom features

C. Selected anxiolytic medications†
Special considerations:
Medical contraindications to FDA-approved antidepressant medications
No adverse cardiovascular effects
Low side effect profile
Substantial withdrawal with long-term use
Limited exposure time expected (<3 months)
Patient has no history of substance abuse
Quick action needed

Adapted from Depression Guideline Panel, 1993.
*Other first- and second-line choices are recommended for patients with dysrhythmias, cardiac conduction defects, ischemic heart disease, cardiomyopathy, or cardiac valve disease.
†Evidence is clearest for alprazolam. Not recommended for severely depressed patients because studies reveal reduced efficacy. Not recommended for prolonged care because no studies longer than 12 weeks are available. Not recommended when FDA-approved antidepressant medications can be used safely. For buspirone, efficacy is suggested in those with primary anxiety disorders and mild associated depressive symptoms.
Note: Evidence for efficacy with severely depressed inpatients is more abundant for the standard tricyclics than for newer agents.

TABLE 13-5 Pharmacology of Antidepressant Medications

Drug	*Therapeutic Dosage Range (mg/day)*	*Average (Range) of Elimination Half-Lives (hr)**	*Potentially Fatal Drug Interactions*
Tricyclics			
amitriptyline (Elavil, Endep)	75-300	24 (16-46)	Antidysrhythmics, MAOIs
clomipramine (Anafranil)	75-300	24 (20-40)	Antidysrhythmics, MAOIs
desipramine (Norpramin, Pertofrane)	75-300	18 (12-50)	Antidysrhythmics, MAOIs
doxepin (Adapin, Sinequan)	75-300	17 (10-47)	Antidysrhythmics, MAOIs
imipramine (Janimine, Tofranil)	75-300	22 (12-34)	Antidysrhythmics, MAOIs
nortriptyline (Aventyl, Pamelor)	40-200	26 (18-88)	Antidysrhythmics, MAOIs
protriptyline (Vivactil)	20-60	76 (54-124)	Antidysrhythmics, MAOIs
trimipramine (Surmontil)	75-300	12 (8-30)	Antidysrhythmics, MAOIs
Second Generation			
amoxapine (Asendin)	100-600	10 (8-14)	MAOIs
bupropion (Wellbutrin)	225-450	14 (8-24)	MAOIs (possibly)
maprotiline (Ludiomil)	100-225	43 (27-58)	MAOIs
mirtazapine (Remeron)	15	30 (20-40)	MAOIs
trazodone (Desyrel)	150-600	8 (4-14)	—
Selected Serotonin Reuptake Inhibitors (SSRIs)			
fluoxetine (Prozac)	10-40	168 (72-360)†	MAOIs
paroxetine (Paxil)	20-50	24 (3-65)	MAOIs‡
sertraline (Zoloft)	50-150	24 (10-30)	MAOIs‡
Monoamine Oxidase Inhibitors (MAOIs)§			For all 3 MAOIs:
isocarboxazid (Marplan)	30-50	Unknown	Vasoconstrictors‖, decongestants,‖ meperidine, and possibly other narcotics
phenelzine (Nardil)	45-90	2 (1.5-4)	
tranylcypromine (Parnate)	20-60	2 (1.5-3)	
Miscellaneous Antidepressants			
nefazodone (Serzone)	200-600	16 (11-24)	MAOIs
venlafaxine (Effexor)	75-225	4 (3-5)	Hypertensive crisis with MAOIs

Adapted from Depression Guideline Panel, 1993.
*Half-lives are affected by age, sex, race, concurrent medications, and length of drug exposure.
†Includes both fluoxetine and norfluoxetine.
‡By extrapolation from fluoxetine data.
§MAO inhibition lasts longer (7 days) than drug half-life.
‖Including pseudoephedrine, phenylephrine, phenylpropanolamine, epinephrine, norepinephrine, and others.

dosage, adjusting as necessary according to therapeutic response or presence of undesirable side effects.

Tricyclic Antidepressants

Tricyclic antidepressants are indicated for the treatment of depression, enuresis (imipramine), and obsessive-compulsive disorder (clomipramine).

Pharmacokinetics

These agents are well absorbed orally. The onset of the antidepressant effect occurs within 2 to 3 weeks, and they are metabolized primarily in the liver and excreted by the kidneys. Active metabolites produced in the liver have in some instances resulted in the marketing of new antidepressants, which are noted in parentheses.

generic (brand name): active metabolite (brand name if marketed)
amitriptyline (Elavil): nortriptyline (Aventyl, Pamelor)
amoxapine (Asendin): 7- and 8-hydroxyamoxapine
desipramine (Norpramin): 2 hydroxydesipramine
doxepin (Sinequan): desmethyldoxepin
imipramine (Tofranil): desipramine (Norpramin)
fluoxetine (Prozac): norfluoxetine

For half-life, dosage, and additional information, see Table 13-5.

Drug interactions

The following effects may occur when tricyclic antidepressants are given with the drugs listed below:

Drug	Possible effect and management
Alcohol, CNS depressants	May result in enhanced CNS-depressant effects; avoid concurrent use if possible, or reduce dosage of one or both drugs and monitor closely.

Antithyroid drugs	May increase risk of inducing agranulocytosis. Avoid or a potentially serious drug interaction may occur.
cimetidine (Tagamet)	May inhibit metabolism of tricyclic agent, leading to increased serum levels and toxicity; lower tricyclic dosage by 20% to 30% and monitor closely.
clonidine (Catapres), guanadrel (Hylorel), or guanethidine (Ismelin)	May decrease the antihypertensive effects of these drugs; monitor BP closely because dosage changes or alternate antihypertensive agents may be necessary. Clonidine and tricyclic antidepressants may increase risk of CNS depression; monitor closely for lethargy, confusion, and respiratory depression.
Contraceptives, oral	May increase or decrease tricyclic serum levels. Monitor closely for decreased therapeutic response or drug toxicity; dosage adjustments may be necessary.
Extrapyramidal effect-inducing medications; amoxapine (Asendin), phenothiazines, haloperidol (Haldol), metoclopramide (Reglan), reserpine (Serpalan), thioxanthenes	May increase risk and severity of extrapyramidal adverse effects. With phenothiazines, sedative and anticholinergic side effects may be enhanced; monitor closely.
metrizamide intrathecal (Amipaque)	Concurrent use of tricyclic antidepressants increases risk of inducing seizures because of a lowered seizure threshold. Discontinue tricyclic agents at least 2 days before and 1 day after a myelogram.
MAOIs	Should be contraindicated in outpatient settings; hypertensive crises, severely elevated temperatures, convulsions, and death have been reported with concurrent administration of MAOIs and tricyclic antidepressants. Before switching from one classification to the other, at least a 2-week period free of drugs from either category should be instituted. If concurrent use is prescribed in an inpatient setting, it would require strict supervision and close monitoring because of the potentially serious adverse effects. See current USP DI for dosing recommendations.
Sympathomimetics	May increase possibility of potentiating cardiovascular toxicities (severe hypertension, dysrhythmias, and tachycardia) or severely elevated body temperatures. If this combination cannot be avoided, monitor very closely. Avoid or a potentially serious drug interaction may occur.

Color type indicates an unsafe drug combination.

Side effects and adverse reactions

See Table 13-4.

Warnings

Use with caution in suicidal patients, seizure disorders, prostatic hypertrophy, psychosis, urinary retention, cardiac, liver or renal disease, and glaucoma. See the box for management of a tricyclic antidepressant overdose.

Contraindications

Avoid use in persons with tricyclic antidepressant hypersensitivity and during the recovery period after a myocardial infarction.

Dosage and administration

See Table 13-5.

clomipramine [kloe mi′ pra meen] (Anafranil)
Clomipramine, an analog of imipramine, is a potent inhibitor of serotonin reuptake, and its active metabolite inhibits norepinephrine reuptake. It is indicated for the treatment of obsessive-compulsive disorders.

Pharmacokinetics

It is well absorbed orally, reaching the peak plasma level within 2 to 4 hours. It has a half-life of 19 to 37 hours and reaches steady-state levels in 1 to 2 weeks. Metabolism is via the liver, and excretion is in the urine.

Side effects and adverse reactions

Side effects and adverse reactions and drug interactions are similar to those for the other tricyclic antidepressant agents.

Dosage and administration

The initial adult dose is 25 mg daily gradually increased as necessary and tolerated, to 100 mg during the first 14 days, administered in divided doses to reduce the gastrointestinal side effects. After 2 weeks the dose may be increased over several more weeks if necessary, to a maximum dose of 250 mg/day. After the dose is established, the total daily dose may be given at bedtime to reduce daytime sedation effects. In children and adolescents the initial dose is 25 mg/day; increased as necessary during the first 14 days, to a daily maxi-

MANAGEMENT OF DRUG OVERDOSE

Tricyclic Antidepressants

Tricyclic antidepressant (TCA) overdose can be life-threatening, resulting in serious adverse reactions such as heart block, cardiac dysrhythmias, hypotension, seizures, coma, and in some instances fatalities. In the United States, the third most common drug-induced death is due to TCA overdoses (Montano, 1994).

Montano (1994, p 32) also states that "70% to 80% of people who take overdoses of TCAs do not reach the hospital alive." Therefore, it is critically important that healthcare professionals know how to deal with a tricyclic overdose.

SIGNS AND SYMPTOMS

The signs and symptoms of a TCA overdose may vary in severity, depending on numerous factors including the amount ingested and absorbed, the age of the individual, and the interval between ingestion and initiation of a treatment modality. Any acute overdose or unwarranted ingestion of a TCA in children or adults must be considered serious and potentially fatal.

CNS abnormalities include agitation, ataxia, choreoathetoid movements, drowsiness, hyperactive reflexes, muscle rigidity, restlessness, stupor, seizures, and coma. Cardiac abnormalities may include dysrhythmia, electrocardiogram evidence of impaired conduction, signs of congestive heart failure, and tachycardia. Quinidine-like adverse effects are common in poisonings with tricyclic antidepressants.

TREATMENT

Symptomatic and supportive measures are instituted according to the individual patient's requirements. They may include:

- Emesis and/or use of gastric lavage to empty stomach followed by administration of activated charcoal to absorb any remaining drug in the GI tract.
- Close monitoring of cardiovascular functioning for at least 5 days. Cardiac dysrhythmias have occurred up to 6 days after massive TCA doses, which may require treatment with lidocaine or phenytoin.
- Maintenance of body temperature and respiratory and cardiac functions.
- For all tricyclics except amoxapine, physostigmine salicylate may need to be administered. This product is used for persons with life-threatening signs such as coma with respiratory depression, very serious cardiac dysrhythmias, severe hypertension, or uncontrollable convulsions. Physostigmine salicylate is not administered for amoxapine overdoses because it has the potential of increasing seizure activity.
- Administration of anticonvulsants such as diazepam (Valium), phenytoin (Dilantin), paraldehyde, or an inhalation anesthetic to control seizures.

Be aware that hemodialysis, peritoneal dialysis, forced diuresis, and exchange transfusions are not successful for treating a TCA overdose (USP DI, 1998).

mum of 3 mg/kg or 100 mg (whichever is the smaller dose). The dose may later be increased to 3 mg/kg or 200 mg (whichever is smaller) as necessary. Once the titrated dose is established, the entire daily dose may be administered at bedtime.

Second-Generation Antidepressants

The second-generation antidepressants include amoxapine (Asendin), bupropion (Wellbutrin), maprotiline (Ludiomil), mirtazapine (Remeron), and trazodone (Desyrel). Generally, these agents have fewer long-term side effects (such as weight gain) than the tricyclic antidepressants; in addition, they have other advantages and disadvantages that need to be considered.

Amoxapine (Asendin), an active metabolite of loxapine (an antipsychotic agent), inhibits the reuptake of norepinephrine and is a potent dopamine-blocking agent. The latter effect may result in extrapyramidal side effects and neuroleptic malignant syndrome (Olin, 1998). With therapeutic doses, amoxapine and maprotiline have fewer cardiovascular side effects than the tricyclic agents (Laird, Benefield, 1995). An amoxapine overdose, though, may result in seizures and status epilepticus within 12 hours of ingestion. Renal failure has also been reported with an amoxapine overdose.

Bupropion's (Wellbutrin) mechanism of action is unknown although it weakly blocks the reuptake of dopamine, serotonin, and norepinephrine. This drug and the newer agents are used for persons who are nonresponsive to other antidepressants. Bupropion has fewer anticholinergic effects, rarely produces hypotension or sexual dysfunction, but is reported to cause agitation, insomnia, tremors, and dose-related seizures (Abramowicz, 1994).

Maprotiline (Ludiomil) is similar to the tricyclic antidepressants except it is associated with an increased risk of skin rash (redness, swelling, and pruritus) and seizures. Seizures have been reported with therapeutic daily doses of maprotiline in persons without any history of seizures (Wells, 1994). Therefore this product is contraindicated in anyone with a history of seizures.

Trazodone (Desyrel) is chemically different from the other antidepressants. It blocks serotonin reuptake and also produces changes in the binding at serotonin receptors. Trazodone has few if any anticholinergic effects and thus has minimal effects on cardiac conduction. The prescriber should still use caution in using this drug with persons with a history of cardiac disease because several cases of ventricular dysrhythmia have been reported with its use. It can cause gastric distress, postural hypotension early in treatment especially in the elderly, and priapism (Laird, Benefield, 1995).

Mirtazapine (Remeron) is a potent serotonin receptor antagonist, especially the 5-HT_2 and 5-HT_3 receptors. It is also a potent histamine receptor antagonist which is related to its sedative or drowsiness properties.

Drug interactions

The following interactions may occur when maprotiline is administered with the following drugs (1993):

Drug	Possible effect and management
Anticholinergic agents	May cause additive anticholinergic side effects. Monitor closely.
guanethidine (Ismelin)	The antihypertensive effects of guanethidine may be blocked or decreased. Monitor closely.
Phenothiazines	Concurrent use increases the risk of seizures. Monitor closely.

Side effects and adverse reactions

Side effects and adverse reactions for maprotiline and mirtazapine includes the following: dry mouth, constipation, nausea, dizziness, and tremors. In addition, mirtazapine may cause weakness, flu-like syndrome, weight gain, somnolence, and unusual dreams. See Table 13-4 for its side effect profile.

Warnings

See discussion of tricyclic antidepressants.

Contraindications

See discussion of tricyclic antidepressants.

Dosage and administration

See Table 13-5.

Monoamine Oxidase Inhibitor Antidepressants

MAOIs are indicated as second- or third-line antidepressants for the treatment of depression that does not respond to other safer antidepressants (Depression Guideline Panel, 1993). These agents have numerous drug interactions with prescription and over-the-counter (OTC) medications, caffeine, and tyramine-containing foods and beverages. The major adverse reaction with these agents is the occurrence of sudden and possibly very severe hypertension that if untreated can progress to vascular collapse and fatality.

MAO, an enzyme found in nerve terminals, the liver, and the brain, is necessary to the inactivation and degradation of tyramine, catecholamines, serotonin, and various medications. The MAOIs interfere with this inactivation, which may result in a potentiation of vasopressor effects and serious adverse effects.

Two types of MAO enzymes have been identified and named: MAO-A and MAO-B. MAO-A appears to have a preference for serotonin and is located throughout the body, with high concentrations located in the human placenta. MAO-B is mainly contained in human platelets, but approximately equal amounts of both types are found in the liver and brain. The MAOIs in current use are nonselective.

The MAOIs are capable of blocking or diminishing the activity of MAO, resulting in a net increase in brain amine levels. Current research indicates that the MAOIs produce desensitization of the $alpha_2$ or beta and serotonin receptors (down-regulation). During early clinical trials of MAOIs as antidepressants, orthostatic hypotension was encountered as a common but inconsistent side effect; thus many MAOIs were produced and studied specifically as antidepressant and antihypertensive agents.

The MAOIs discussed in this section are those used as antidepressants: the hydrazines, isocarboxazid (Marplan) and phenelzine (Nardil), and the nonhydrazine, tranylcypromine sulfate (Parnate). The MAOIs are indicated primarily in resistant depression and anxious and hostile depression, especially if panic attacks or phobic symptoms are also involved.

MAOIs can increase the concentration of all central amines, although different effects on the individual amines are possible. For example, some of the MAOIs may increase dopamine or norepinephrine concentrations to a more extensive degree than serotonin concentrations, whereas other MAOIs may raise the level of serotonins to a greater degree than those of norepinephrine and dopamine. The increase in amine concentration is associated with behavioral hyperactivity (amphetamine-like psychomotor stimulation with large doses) produced by the MAOIs and, in some cases, with the exacerbation of psychotic symptoms. In lower doses antiphobic and antidepressant activities are seen. In general these compounds are most effective in reversing the dysphoric state and its attendant vegetative disturbances in patients with depressive syndromes.

Therapeutic doses of the MAOIs take from days to weeks to attain a maximal effect. MAOIs produce an irreversible inactivation of MAO by forming a stable complex with the enzyme; recovery from the effect of MAOIs thus depends on enzyme regeneration, which may occur over several weeks. Inhibition occurs only in very high doses and may be responsible for some of the toxic effects of MAOIs. The mechanism of action of MAOIs was discussed in the previous section. The MAOIs are well absorbed orally; onset of action in some individuals occurs in 7 to 10 days while the full effect usually takes 4 to 8 weeks of therapy. These agents irreversibly bind MAO activity; recovery may take 10 days to 2 weeks. MAOIs are metabolized in the liver and excreted primarily by the kidneys.

Side effects and adverse reactions are listed in Table 13-4.

Drug interactions

The following effects may occur when MAOIs are given with the drugs listed below:

Drug	Possible effect and management
Alcohol, CNS depressants	May enhance CNS-depressive effects. If alcohol contains tyramine, may result in severe hypertensive reaction. Avoid or a potentially serious drug interaction may occur.
Local anesthetics containing epinephrine or cocaine	May result in very severe hypertensive reaction. Cocaine should not be administered during or within 2 weeks after an MAOI. Avoid or a potentially serious drug interaction may occur.
Antidepressants, tricyclics, carbamazepine (Tegretol), maprotiline (Ludiomil), other MAO inhibitors, furazolidone (Furoxone), selegiline (Eldepryl), or procarbazine (Matulane)	May result in severely elevated temperatures, hypertensive crises, severe seizures, and death. Avoid a potentially serious drug interaction may occur. Before switching from one of these medications to an MAOI or vice versa, a 2-week drug-free period should be instituted. Several studies have used tricyclic antidepressants with an MAOI for refractory depression. See current USP DI for explicit instructions on proper dosing and monitoring of this combination.
Antidiabetic agents (oral or insulin)	Enhanced hypoglycemic effects reported. Reduction in oral hypoglycemic agent may be required during or even after concurrent drug therapy.
bupropion (Wellbutrin)	Concurrent use increases the risk of bupropion toxicity. A 2-week interval is recommended from the discontinuance of MAOIs and the start of bupropion therapy.
buspirone (BuSpar)	May cause hypertension. Avoid or a serious drug interaction may occur.
caffeine (e.g., drug products, coffee, tea, chocolate, cola), carbamazepine (Tegretol), cyclobenzapine (Flexeril), maprotiline (Ludiomil), or other MAO inhibitors	May result in severe cardiac dysrhythmias or hypertension. Avoid or a serious drug interaction may occur. May result in severe hypertensive crises, convulsions, and death. At least a 2-week drug-free interval is recommended to avoid this reaction.
dextromethorphan (Benylin DM, Robitussin DM)	May result in increased excitability, hyperpyrexia, and hypertension. Avoid or a serious drug interaction may occur.
doxapram (Dopram)	Enhanced and severe hypertensive effects may result. Avoid or a potentially serious drug interaction may occur.
fluoxetine (Prozac)	May result in agitation, restlessness, gastrointestinal distress, or seizures and hypertensive crises. Avoid or a potentially serious drug interaction may occur. For patient safety, a minimum of a 2-week drug-free period should be instituted when switching from an MAOI to fluoxetine. When switching from fluoxetine to an MAOI, a 5-week drug-free period should be implemented.
guanadrel (Hylorel), guanethidine (Ismelin), rauwolfia alkaloids	May result in severe hypertension. Withdraw MAOIs at least 7 days before starting therapy with these agents. Rauwolfia alkaloid: if an MAOI is added to a medication schedule already containing a rauwolfia alkaloid, serious CNS depression may result. If a rauwolfia alkaloid is added to a medication schedule that already includes an MAOI, hypertension and increased excitability may result. Avoid or a potentially serious drug interaction may occur.
levodopa (L-dopa)	Avoid this combination. Severe and sudden hypertensive crisis reported. Before starting levodopa therapy, MAOIs should be withdrawn with at least a 2- to 4-week drug-free period.
meperidine (Demerol) and perhaps other opioid narcotics	Severe hypertension, increased excitability, sweating and rigidity reported with concurrent use. Also in some individuals, hypotension, seizures, elevated temperature, respiratory depression, cardiovascular collapse, coma, narcotics, and death reported, which may be caused by serotonin accumulation from the MAOI. Avoid or a potentially serious drug interaction may occur. Do not use meperidine for at least 14 to 21 days after an MAOI is stopped. Such a severe reaction has not been reported with morphine and other narcotics, but it is recommended that the opioid dosage be reduced to one-fourth (test dose) the usual dosage. Monitor closely whenever opioids or anesthesia adjuncts (fentanyl [Sublimaze], sufentanil [Sufenta]) are given to persons who have received MAOIs in the previous 2 or 3 weeks.
methyldopa (Aldomet)	Severe headache, hypertension, hallucinations, and increased excitability have been reported. Avoid or a serious drug interaction may occur.

methylphenidate (Ritalin)	Concurrent use may result in a hypertensive crisis. Avoid or a serious drug interaction may occur. At least a 2-week drug-free period should be allowed before instituting methylphenidate therapy.
Sympathomimetics, systemic	Direct-acting (dopamine, mephentermine, metaraminol, dobutamine, methoxamine, and phenylephrine) or indirect-acting (amphetamines, phenylpropanolamine, and pseudoephedrine) or combination effects (ephedrine) should not be given during or within 2 weeks of an MAOI. Severe hypertensive crisis, elevated temperatures, cardiac dysrhythmias, headaches, and vomiting have been reported. Avoid or a serious drug interaction may occur.
Tryptophan and tranylcypromine (Parnate)	May result in hyperventilation, increased temperature, shivering, disorientation, mania, or hypomania. If necessary to use both drugs, start tryptophan in low doses and increase dose slowly. Monitor mental status and BP closely.
tyramine or foods and beverages containing high amounts of pressors (see Box 13-5)	Sudden, severe hypertensive crisis has been reported. Avoid or a potentially serious drug interaction may containing occur. Patient teaching is important for any persons receiving MAOIs. MAOIs and tyramine must be avoided during therapy and for a minimum of 2 weeks after therapy is discontinued.

Color type indicates an unsafe drug combination.

Dosage and administration

See Table 13-5. See the box on p. 221 for FDA pregnancy safety categories.

Selective Serotonin Reuptake Inhibitors

SSRIs are safer and as effective as the other antidepressants. Fluoxetine (Prozac), the first SSRI released in this category, was followed by fluvoxamine (Luvox), paroxetine (Paxil), and sertraline (Zoloft). All except fluvoxamine are used to treat depression, while fluoxetine and fluvoxamine are used to treat obsessive-compulsive disorders. Unlike the tricyclic agents that often cause weight gain, the SSRIs, with the exception of paroxetine, may cause anorexia and weight loss (Olin, 1998).

Pharmacokinetics

The SSRIs are absorbed orally, reaching a peak serum level in 3 to 8 hours. Half-lives vary: for example, fluoxetine, from 1 to 384 hours (which includes active metabolites); fluvoxamine, 77 to 80 hours; paroxetine, 21 hours; sertraline, between 26 to 104 hours (including active metabolites).

BOX 13-5 Tyramine-Containing Substances

Tyramine content of foods varies according to the references reviewed. This variation may result from different conditions or preparation of the foods, different food samples, or different producers or manufacturers. The major goal should be to advise the client to avoid foods and drinks with reported moderate to high tyramine content as follows:

Cheese: aged (blue, Boursault, natural brick, Brie, Camembert, cheddar, Emmenthaler, Gruyère, mozzarella, Parmesan, Romano, Roquefort, Stilton)

Meat and fish: beef and chicken liver, unrefrigerated, fermented; caviar, fish, unrefrigerated, fermented; fish, dried; herring, dried, salted, and pickled; fermented sausages (bologna, pepperoni, salami, summer sausage) and any other unrefrigerated, fermented meats

Vegetables: overripe avocado and overripe fava beans

Fruit: overripe figs, bananas, and raisins

Alcoholic beverages: red wines, especially Chianti; sherry; beer; liquors

Other foods may contain tyramine or high amounts of pressor amines but when eaten in moderation and only when fresh, they are said to be less apt to cause a serious reaction (*USP DI*, 1998). Such foods include yogurt, sour cream, cream cheese, cottage cheese, chocolate, and soy sauce.

Fluoxetine's primary route of excretion is hepatic, while elimination for the other three drugs is mainly renal and hepatic.

Drug interactions

The following effects may occur when fluoxetine is given with the drugs listed below:

Drug	Possible effects and management
Alcohol, CNS depressants	Concurrent use may result in increased CNS depressant effects. Monitor closely.
Highly protein-bound drugs such as oral anticoagulants, digitalis, or digitoxin	Combined use may displace medications from the protein binding sites, resulting in an increased serum level and toxicity. Monitor closely.
MAOIs	May result in serotonin syndrome that is, confusion, hyperreflexia, diaphoresis, chills, tremors, diarrhea, ataxia, myoclonus, restlessness, and/or fever.
phenytoin (Dilantin)	Concurrent use may result in elevated phenytoin serum levels. Monitor closely.
tryptophan	Combined use may result in agitation, increased restlessness, and GI distress. Monitor closely.

Side effects and adverse reactions

These include headache, weakness, insomnia, sedation, anxiety, dizziness, tremors, nausea, vomiting, constipation, diarrhea, GI distress, dry mouth, anorexia, gas, visual disturbance, sexual dysfunction, and excessive sweating. See Table 13-4 for the side effect profile.

Warnings

Use fluoxetine with caution in patients with diabetes mellitus and seizure disorders.

Contraindications

Avoid use in patients with fluoxetine hypersensitivity and severe liver and renal impairment. See Table 13-5 for additional pharmacology and dosing information.

Other Miscellaneous Antidepressants

The miscellaneous antidepressants include nefazodone (Serzone) and venlafaxine (Effexor). Although the mechanism of action for nefazodone is unknown, it does inhibit serotonin and norepinephrine reuptake and also is a serotonin receptor antagonist. The greatest effect of venlafaxine and its active metabolite is interference with the reuptake of serotonin. To a lesser degree it also interferes with reuptake of norepinephrine and dopamine.

Pharmacokinetics

Both products are well absorbed orally. The half-life of nefazodone is 2 to 4 hours; half-lives for venlafaxine and its active metabolite are 3 to 5 hours and 9 to 11 hours, respectively. With both drugs, the onset of antidepressant effects is several weeks. They are metabolized in the body and liver and excreted primarily by the kidneys.

Drug interactions

The following effects may occur when nefazodone or venlafaxine is given with the drugs listed below:

Drug	Possible effect and management
MAOIs	Concurrent use may result in a serious reaction, such as confusion, increased agitation, GI distress, severe convulsions, hyperthermia, myoclonus, hypertensive crisis, or the serotonin syndrome. Such reactions may, at times, be fatal. Concurrent drug use should be avoided and at least 2 weeks should elapse between the stopping of an MAOI and the start of either of these medications.

Color type indicates an unsafe drug combination.

The following effects may occur when nefazodone is given with the following drugs:

Antihistamines, nonsedating such as astemizole (Hismanal)	Concurrent use may result in increased astemizole serum levels, resulting in severe cardiac dysrhythmias. Avoid or a serious drug interactions may occur.
Benzodiazepines, such as alprazolam (Xanax), and triazolam (Halcion)	Significant increases in the benzodiazepine serum levels have occurred. Be aware that this interaction is not reported with lorazepam (Ativan) (Olin, 1998).

Color type indicates an unsafe drug combination.

Side effects and adverse reactions

Side effects and adverse reactions for nefazodone include nightmares, constipation or diarrhea, sedation, dry mouth, agitation, an increase in appetite and cough, insomnia, nausea, vomiting, paresthesia, peripheral edema, tremors, ataxia, blurred vision or visual disturbances, lightheadedness, skin rash, pruritus, and tinnitus.

Venlafaxine side effects and adverse reactions include nightmares, anorexia and weight loss, weakness, chills, constipation or diarrhea, lightheadedness, dry mouth, dyspepsia, sweating, insomnia, nausea, vomiting, abdominal gas or pain, taste alterations, tremors, rhinitis, sexual dysfunction, visual disturbances, and headaches. Some of these effects, such as sexual dysfunction, nausea, vomiting, anorexia, tremors, and chills, may be dose related.

Warnings

Use venlafaxine with caution in patients with a history of drug abuse, mania, mental retardation, and seizures, and in children. Use nefazodone with caution in patients with seizure disorders and cardiovascular disease, in children, and in the elderly.

Contraindications

Avoid venlafaxine use in persons with hypersensitivity, problems with blood pressure, and cardiac, liver, or renal function disease or impairment. Avoid nefazodone in patients with hypersensitivity.

Dosage and administration

The usual adult dose for nefazodone is 100 mg bid and for venlafaxine is 25 mg tid with food. Doses may be increased according to the individual's response and tolerance for the product. See the box on p. 221 for pregnancy safety information.

ANTIMANIC THERAPY

Mania is characterized by the presence of speech and motor hyperactivity, reduced sleep requirements, flight of ideas, grandiosity, elation, poor judgment, aggressiveness, and possibly hostility. The manic state is seen with recurrent manic symptoms with little or no depression, whereas bipolar affective disorders have both an acute manic phase and a hypomanic state or alternating periods of mania and depression. Counseling, psychotherapy, and drug therapy are useful for the treatment of bipolar disorders. Although lithium is considered the drug of choice for this disorder, carbamazepine (Tegretol) and valproic acid (Depakene) have been used investigationally for persons who are not responsive or are unable to take lithium (USP DI, 1998; Love, Grothe, 1995). These agents are approved as anticonvulsants and are reviewed in Chapter 11. The following is a list of lithium products:

lithium carbonate capsules [lith′ ee um] (Eskalith, Carbolith ✤)
lithium carbonate tablets (Eskalith, Lithane)
lithium carbonate extended-release tablets (Lithobid, Eskalith CR)
lithium citrate syrup (Cibalith-S)

Lithium's mechanism of action has not been established. It is theorized that lithium accelerates the presynaptic destruction of catecholamines (serotonin, dopamine, and norepinephrine), inhibits transmitter release at the synapse, and decreases postsynaptic receptor sensitivity with the result that the presumed overactive catecholamine systems in mania are corrected.

Sodium in the cells has been reported to increase as much as 200% in manic patients. Lithium and sodium are both actively transported across cell membranes, but lithium cannot be as effectively pumped out of the cell as sodium. Thus lithium may stabilize cell membranes.

An additional mechanism is lithium blockade of the inositol tri- and diphosphate system in the CNS, that is, its effects on the second messengers necessary for alpha-adrenergic and muscarinic transmission. At the current time, the latter is the most accepted theory (Katzung, 1992).

Indications

The drug is indicated in the treatment of manic-depressive illness, although it is being investigated for other uses.

Pharmacokinetics

With the exception of the slow-release dosage form, lithium is completely absorbed in 6 to 8 hours and has a half-life in adults of 24 hours, in adolescents of 18 hours, and in geriatric patients of up to 36 hours. Times to peak serum levels are: syrup, 30 minutes; capsules/tablets, 1 to 3 hours; and extended-release tablets, 4 hours. Therapeutic serum levels for the treatment of bipolar disorder are: acute, 0.8 to 1.2 mEq/L; and maintenance, 0.5 to 1 mEq/L. A clinical response is usually reported in 1 to 3 weeks. Lithium is not metabolized and is excreted primarily unchanged by the kidneys.

Drug interactions

The following effects may occur when lithium is given with the drugs listed below:

Drug	Possible effect and management
Antithyroid drugs, calcium iodide, potassium iodide, or iodinated glycerol	May enhance the hypothyroid goitrogenic effects of lithium or these medications; monitor closely for lethargy, intolerance to cold, etc.
Antiinflammatory analgesics, nonsteroidal	May decrease excretion of lithium, leading to increased lithium levels and toxicity; monitor closely for blurred vision, confusion, and dizziness.
chlorpromazine (Thorazine), possibly other phenothiazines	Concurrent use has reduced absorption of chlorpromazine (and possibly other phenothiazines) up to 40%. Reduced serum levels may lead to treatment failure. Also, an increased rate of lithium excretion has been reported. Adverse effects, especially neurotoxic and extrapyramidal, and delirium are reportedly increased in the elderly. Nausea, vomiting, and other signs of lithium toxicity may be masked by the phenothiazines. Monitor physical symptoms and drug serum levels closely.
Diuretics	Decreased lithium excretion results in an increased lithium level and toxicity. A reduction in lithium dosage may be indicated. Monitor closely (see Box 13-6 for other factors affecting lithium serum levels).
fluoxetine (Prozac)	Lithium serum levels may be altered. Monitor closely.
haloperidol	Concurrent use in early therapy has been associated with irreversible neurologic toxicity and brain damage in some persons, who usually had organic brain syndrome or another CNS impairment. However, this interaction is controversial within the professions. Be aware that extrapyramidal signs and symptoms may be increased with this combination, and patients should be closely monitored whenever this combination is used.
molindone (Moban)	Concurrent use may result in neurotoxicity, as evidenced by confusion, convulsions, delirium, or abnormal EEG changes. Avoid concurrent administration.

Color type indicates an unsafe drug combination.

BOX 13-6 Factors Affecting Lithium Serum Levels

	Excretion:
Increased by:	
Diarrhea	Decreased
Diuretics or dehydration	Decreased
Low-salt diets	Decreased
High fevers or strenuous exercise	Decreased
Decreased by:	
High salt intake	Increased
High intake of sodium bicarbonate	Increased
Pregnancy	Increased

Side effects and adverse reactions

These include tremors of hands (slight), thirst, nausea, increased urination, diarrhea, tachycardia, increased weakness, weight gain, respiratory difficulties (on exertion), fainting, and irregular pulse rate. Early signs of toxicity include diarrhea, anorexia, muscle weakness, nausea, vomiting, tremors, slurred speech, and drowsiness. Later signs are blurred vision, convulsions, severe trembling, confusion, ataxia, and increased production of urine.

Warnings

Use with caution in patients with diabetes mellitus, hypothyroidism, goiter, hyperparathyroidism, schizophrenia, and psoriasis and severely debilitated patients or patients on a sodium restricted diet (see Box 13-6 for factors that affect lithium serum levels).

Contraindications

Avoid use in persons with a history of lithium hypersensitivity, leukemia, severe dehydration, cardiovascular disease, epilepsy, Parkinson's disease, severe infections, renal impairment, and urinary retention.

Dosage and administration

The usual adult dose for acute mania for lithium is 300 to 600 mg three times daily, adjusted according to patient's response and tolerance up to a maximum dose of 2.4 g/day. The maintenance dose is 300 mg three or four times a day. Geriatric patients usually require a lower dosage. The dose for children up to 12 years old is 15 to 20 mg/kg in two or three divided doses, adjusted according to response.

SUMMARY

To treat mental illness, the healthcare professional should understand the effects of the mind on the body and the primary medications used to treat the symptoms of psychoses, mental depression, and mania. As the medications used are very potent, the drug selected should be appropriate for the individual's specific disorder or condition.

Since the discovery of tranquilizers in the 1950s, there has been a reported decrease in the length of institutionalization for psychiatric disorders. Many individuals are now treated as outpatients at various community mental health centers as a result of the availability of these agents.

Phenothiazine derivatives are divided into three subgroups: aliphatic, piperidine, and piperazine compounds. Although the exact mechanism of their antipsychotic effect is unknown, a primary effect is dopamine blockade in specific areas of the CNS. Antidepressant drug therapy is used for the treatment of affective disorders or mood disturbances, while lithium is usually the drug of choice for mania or bipolar affective disorders.

All psychotherapeutic medications can produce undesirable side effects or adverse reactions. Therefore patient teaching and close monitoring is necessary to improve clinical outcome and avoid or reduce the potential for unwanted and potentially serious adverse effects.

REVIEW QUESTIONS

1. Review Table 13-1: "Selected antipsychotic agents, potency, and major side effects" and answer the following questions:
   a. If a patient is receiving chlorpromazine (Thorazine) 100 mg tid and the prescriber wants to change to mesoridazine (Serentil) or perphenazine (Trilafon), what would be the equivalent dose for each drug?
   b. Name four drugs on this chart with a high antiemetic effect.
   c. If the prescriber wants to change from chlorpromazine (as in a) to an antipsychotic agent with an equivalent antiemetic effect but less sedation, less hypotension, and fewer anticholinergic effects, which drug would he or she select?
2. Discuss the use of antipsychotic and antidepressant drugs in the elderly. Address usual dosages, pharmacokinetics, and side effects and adverse reactions.
3. Explain the warning about cautiously using antipsychotic agents in patients with Parkinson's disease.
4. List several reasons why the selective serotonin reuptake inhibitors are preferred over the tricyclic antidepressants for the treatment of depression.
5. Describe the various theories for the mechanism of action of lithium in the treatment of mania.

REFERENCES

Abramowicz M, editor: Drugs for psychiatric disorders, *Med Lett* 36(933):89, 1994.

Carley M: Unnecessary drug requirements, *Contemp Long Term Care* 15(12):68, 1992.

Depression Guideline Panel: Depression in primary care. *Treatment of major depression,* vol 2, Clinical practice guideline no 5, AHCPR Pub No 93-0551, Rockville, Md, 1993, US Department of Health and Human Services, Public Health Service, Agency for Health Care Policy and Research.

Eli Lilly Industries, Inc: *Zyprexa, package insert #PV2960,* Indianapolis, Ind, 1996, the Company.

Ereshefsky L, Richards AL: Psychoses. In Koda-Kimble MA, Young LY, editors: *Applied therapeutics: the clinical use of drugs,* ed 5, Vancouver, Wash, 1992, Applied Therapeutics, Inc.

Hardman JG, Limbird LE, editors: *Goodman & Gilman's the pharmacological basis of therapeutics,* ed 9, New York, 1996, McGraw-Hill.

Kalachnik JE, Tardive dyskinesia, *Minn Pharmacist* 37(4):14, 1983.

Katzung BG: *Basic and clinical pharmacology,* ed 5, Conn, 1992, Appleton & Lange.

Laird LK, Benefield WH: Mood disorders. I: major depressive disorders. In Young LY, Koda-Kimble MA, editors: *Applied therapeutics: the clinical use of drugs,* ed 6, Vancouver, Wash, 1995, Applied Therapeutics, Inc.

Love RC, Grothe DR: Mood disorders. II: bipolar affective disorders. In Young LY, Koda-Kimble MA, editors: *Applied therapeutics: the clinical use of drugs,* ed 6, Vancouver, Wash, 1995, Applied Therapeutics, Inc.

Lyons AS, Petrucelli RJ: *Medicine: an illustrated history,* New York, 1978, Harry N Abrams.

Marken PA, Stanislav SW: Schizophrenia. In Young LY, Koda-Kimble MA, editors: *Applied therapeutics: the clinical use of drugs,* ed 6, Vancouver, Wash, 1995, Applied Therapeutics, Inc.

Montano CB: Recognition and treatment of depression in a primary care setting, *J Clin Psychiatry* 55(12 suppl):18, 1994.

Olin BR: *Facts and comparisons,* Philadelphia, 1998, JB Lippincott.

Stat/Gram: Letter, OL-0077, Indianapolis, Ind, 1996, Eli Lilly and Company.

United States Pharmacopeial Convention: *USP DI: drug information for the health care professional,* ed 18, Rockville, Md, 1998, the Convention.

ADDITIONAL REFERENCES

Abrams WB, Berkow AB, editors: *The Merck manual of pediatrics,* Rahway, NJ, 1990, Merck Sharp & Dohme Research Laboratories.

American Hospital Formulary Service: *AHFS: drug information '98,* Bethesda, Md, 1998, American Society of Hospital Pharmacists.

Anderson KN et al, editors: *Mosby's medical, nursing, and allied health dictionary,* ed 5, St Louis, 1998, Mosby.

Bond WS: Ethnicity and psychotropic drugs, *Clin Pharm* 10:467, 1991.

Harrington C et al: Psychotropic drug use in long-term care facilities: a review of the literature, *Gerontology* 32(6):822, 1992.

Keltner NL, Folks DG: *Psychotropic drugs,* ed 2, St Louis, 1997, Mosby.

Lin T: Multiculturalism and Canadian psychiatry: opportunities and challenges, *Can J Psychiatry* 31(7):681 1986.

Maxmen JS, Ward NG: *Psychotropic drugs: fast facts,* ed 2, New York, 1995, WW Norton.

Medicare and Medicaid: *OBRA requirements for long-term care facilities.* Section 483.60 Level A Requirement: Pharmacy services; Section 483.10 Level A Requirement: Resident rights; Section 483.20 Level A Requirement: Resident assessment; Section 482.25 Level A Requirement: Quality of Care and Interpretive Guidelines. Washington, DC, 1989, Health Care Financing Administration.

Mosby: *Mosby's GenRx,* St Louis, 1998, Mosby.

Physicians' desk reference, ed 52, Montvale, NJ, 1998, Medical Economics Co.

Stramek R et al: Prevalence of tardive dyskinesia among three ethnic groups of chronic psychiatric patients, *Hosp Commun Psychiatry* 42:590, 1991.

Wells BG, editor: *Therapeutic options in the treatment of depression: a special report,* Washington, DC, 1994, American Pharmaceutical Association.

Zal HM: Depression in the elderly: differing presentations, wide choice of therapies, *Consultant* 34(3):354, 1994.

UNIT IV

Drugs Affecting the Autonomic Nervous System

CHAPTER 14

Overview of the Autonomic Nervous System

CHAPTER FOCUS

The autonomic nervous system is responsible for the regulation of internal viscera such as the heart, blood vessels, digestive organs, kidneys, and reproductive organs. A basic understanding of the autonomic nervous system in health and when dysfunctional is necessary to understand the pharmacologic agents used in treatment.

OBJECTIVES

After reading and studying this chapter, the student should be able to do the following:

1. *Define and discuss the key terms.*
2. *Describe the major differences between the parasympathetic and sympathetic divisions of the autonomic nervous system.*
3. *Explain the reflex control system and blood pressure control in the body.*
4. *Name and describe the synthesis, function, and disposition of the primary neurotransmitters for each system.*
5. *Identify the three different kinds of postganglionic neurons in the sympathetic nervous system.*

KEY TERMS

adrenergic, (p. 251)
autonomic nervous system (ANS), (p. 244)
catecholamine, (p. 248)
cholinergic, (p. 251)
conduction, (p. 246)
feedback control mechanism, (p. 244)
muscarinic (M) receptors, (p. 247)
neuroeffector junction, (p. 246)
neurohumoral transmission, (p. 246)
nicotinic (N) receptors, (p. 247)
reflex arc, (p. 244)
somatic nervous system, (p. 244)
synaptic junction, (p. 247)

The **autonomic nervous system** (ANS) functions primarily as a regulatory or self-governing system for maintaining the internal environment of the body at an optimal level (homeostasis). This system automatically controls the function of smooth muscle, cardiac muscle, and glandular secretions, which interact in many vital physiologic tasks. Digestion of a meal, maintenance of the pressure of circulating blood, and many other processes are internally regulated by the ANS.

REFLEX CONTROL SYSTEM

The nervous system is the important control and communication system within the body. It collects information about conditions inside and outside of the body. The simplest means by which the nervous system responds to environmental change is through the action of the reflex arc. The **reflex arc** is the automatic motor response to sensory stimuli. In any reflex a nerve fiber conducts a nerve impulse; these impulses are the basis of communication of information through the nervous system.

The reflex act consists of two major functional processes: the sensory input and the motor output. The first component of the reflex arc is the receptor, which detects environmental changes such as temperature, pressure in blood vessels, and distention in the viscera. These changes are responsible for producing a stimulus in the receptor. Information from the sensitized receptor is then transmitted as a nerve impulse along the afferent neuron to the central nervous system (CNS), the site of integration. The CNS then issues instructions as an altered motor nerve impulse along the efferent neuron to the effector, which produces the appropriate movements of muscles and glands.

The information carried to the CNS (sensory input) and instructions sent from the CNS (motor output) constitute a **feedback control mechanism.** Information fed back to the CNS from a receptor is modulated so that nerve impulses may vary in frequency and pattern according to the degree of activity required of the effector. The control of visceral function is involuntary, so the feedback mechanism must include all the components of a control system essential for performing the reflex act. Therefore reflex action functions as a feedback mechanism, operating from a receptor to an effector. Its purpose is to prevent extreme changes in function that may create a disturbance in the internal environment.

A good example of feedback control is the blood pressure-regulating reflex. Again, the sequence of events follows the pattern of the reflex arc. The carotid sinus in the carotid artery and the aortic sinus in the aortic arch serve as pressure receptors (baroreceptors) that are highly sensitive to stretch, and the degree of wall stretching is determined by the amount of pressure within these vessels. Thus any increase in blood pressure stimulates the baroreceptors, and this information is conveyed as nerve impulses along the afferent neuron to the vasomotor center in the medulla.

The medulla is the CNS site for integration of blood pressure. After the appropriate neuronal connections, a decrease in sympathetic discharge is conducted along the efferent neuron to the effectors, which produces relaxation of arteriolar smooth muscles. This relaxation causes dilation of the arteries and a reduction in blood pressure. This is only a partial explanation of blood pressure regulation, since a decrease in arterial pressure produces the opposite response in the same neuronal pathway. In addition, this control mechanism operates in coordination with cardiac function.

NERVOUS SYSTEM CLASSIFICATION

The nervous system is classified on the basis of the reflex arc. The two main divisions are the central nervous system and the peripheral nervous system. The central nervous system consists of the brain and spinal cord and performs the important integrative functions from the peripheral sources. The peripheral system has two divisions: the **somatic nervous system,** which innervates voluntary or skeletal muscles; and the autonomic nervous system, which influences the involuntary activities of smooth muscles, cardiac muscles, and glands. The afferent fibers of both systems are the first link in the reflex arc by carrying sensory information to the central nervous system. After integration at various levels in the brain, the outflow from the central nervous system is conducted along either the somatic efferent system or the autonomic efferent system. Both of these systems constitute the final link in the reflex arc (Fig. 14-1).

Several centers in the central nervous system integrate all autonomic nervous system activities. There is evidence that the hypothalamus, in particular, performs such integrating

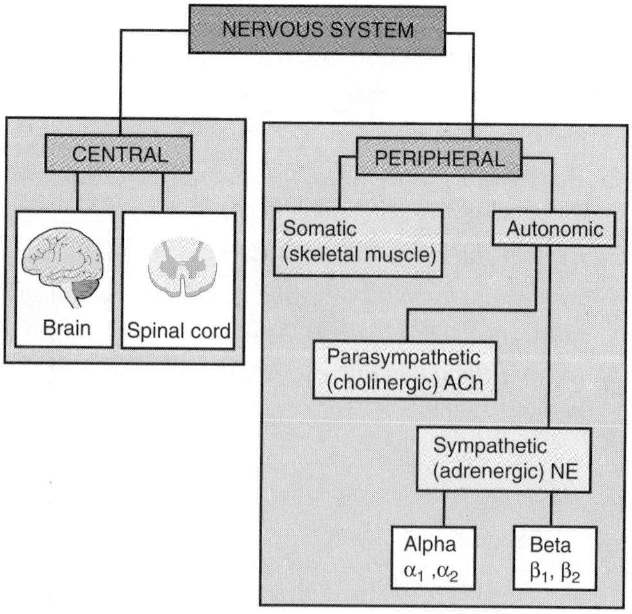

FIGURE 14-1
Divisions of the nervous system. *ACh*, Acetylcholine; *NE*, norepinephrine.

activities. It contains centers that regulate body temperature, water balance, and carbohydrate and fat metabolism. It also integrates mechanisms concerned with emotional behavior, the waking state, and sleep. The medulla oblongata integrates the control of blood pressure, respiration, and cardiac function. A series of "vital centers," including the vasomotor center, respiratory center, and cardiac center, respectively, coordinate these activities. The midbrain, limbic system, cerebellum, and cerebral cortex are all involved in the control of and in physiologic functions regulated by the autonomic nervous system.

DIFFERENCES BETWEEN THE PARASYMPATHETIC AND SYMPATHETIC SYSTEMS

The autonomic nervous system is organized into two subdivisions: (1) the parasympathetic system and (2) the sympathetic system (Box 14-1). The anatomic arrangement of each system consists of two motor nerves, a preganglionic nerve and a postganglionic nerve, with a ganglion (group of nerve cell bodies) connecting the two neurons (Fig. 14-2).

Physiologic Differences

Since the parasympathetic system and the sympathetic system simultaneously innervate many of the same organs, the opposing actions of the two systems balance one another. The parasympathetic system functions mainly to conserve energy and restore body resources of the organism, otherwise known as the system of rest and digestion. These include cardiac deceleration, a rise in gastrointestinal activity associated with increased digestion and absorption, and an increase in excretion. In contrast, the sympathetic system mobilizes the organism during emergency and stress situations, and so it is called the "fight or flight" system. These functions involve expenditure of energy and increases in the blood sugar concentration, heart activity, and blood pressure (Table 14-1).

BOX 14-1 ANS Terminology

Over the years, various terminology has been used to describe the division of the autonomic nervous system. The anatomic names are sympathetic and parasympathetic, and the corresponding functional terms, which relate to the primary neurotransmitters for each system, are adrenergic and cholinergic, respectively. Generally, the terms are used interchangeably—that is, sympathetic or adrenergic and parasympathetic or cholinergic nervous systems. It is important to understand the terms parasympatho*mimetic* and sympatho*mimetic*, which mean to mimic or produce an effect similar to activation of either system. Parasympatho*lytic* or sympatho*lytic* implies blocking of the normal effects seen with activation of either system. Anticholinergic is synonymous with parasympatholytic.

Anatomic	*Functional*	*Primary neurotransmitter*
Sympathetic	Adrenergic	norepinephrine (NE)
Parasympathetic	Cholinergic	acetylcholine (ACh)

Anatomic Differences

The parasympathetic or cholinergic system's preganglionic fibers emerge with the cranial nerves III, VII, IX, and X and at the sacral spinal levels from about S3 through S4. The tenth cranial nerve or vagus nerve has extensive branches that supply fibers to the heart, lungs, and almost all the abdominal organs.

The sympathetic (adrenergic) system is also called the thoracolumbar system because its preganglionic fibers originate in the spinal cord from the thoracic segment T1 to the lumbar segment at L2 level (Fig. 14-3 and Table 14-2).

NEUROHUMORAL TRANSMISSION

There is general agreement that information in the nervous system is transmitted both electrically and chemically. This phenomenon occurs because nerve cells have two special characteristics:

1. They can conduct electrical signals. The passage of a nerve impulse or an action potential along a nerve fiber or a muscle fiber is called **conduction.**
2. They have intercellular connections with other nerve cells and with innervated tissues such as muscles and glands. The presence of a specific chemical at these connections determines the type of information a neuron can receive and the range of responses it can yield in return. The passage of a nerve impulse across a synaptic or neuroeffector junction with the use of a chemical is called **neurohumoral transmission.**

Although each nerve fiber may conduct an impulse along the neuron, it is solely the chemical substance called the neurotransmitter or neurohormone that permits the action potential of a neuron to cross (1) the **synaptic junction** from one neuron to another neuron or (2) the **neuroeffector junction** from a neuron to an effector organ. In this mechanism the arrival of an action potential at a nerve terminal starts the release of the neurotransmitter. The hormone or mediator then acts as a messenger by which nerve cells communicate information to the structures they innervate. The neurotransmitter exerts its influence primarily at the junctional spaces (synaptic junction or neuroeffector junction) to facilitate the transmission of impulses to their final destination. Many drugs may also act selectively at these junctions.

Types of Neurohumoral Transmission

The neurohormones acetylcholine and norepinephrine are responsible for neurohumoral transmission. Nerves that contain acetylcholine are called cholinergic neurons, and they are involved in cholinergic transmission. Nerves that

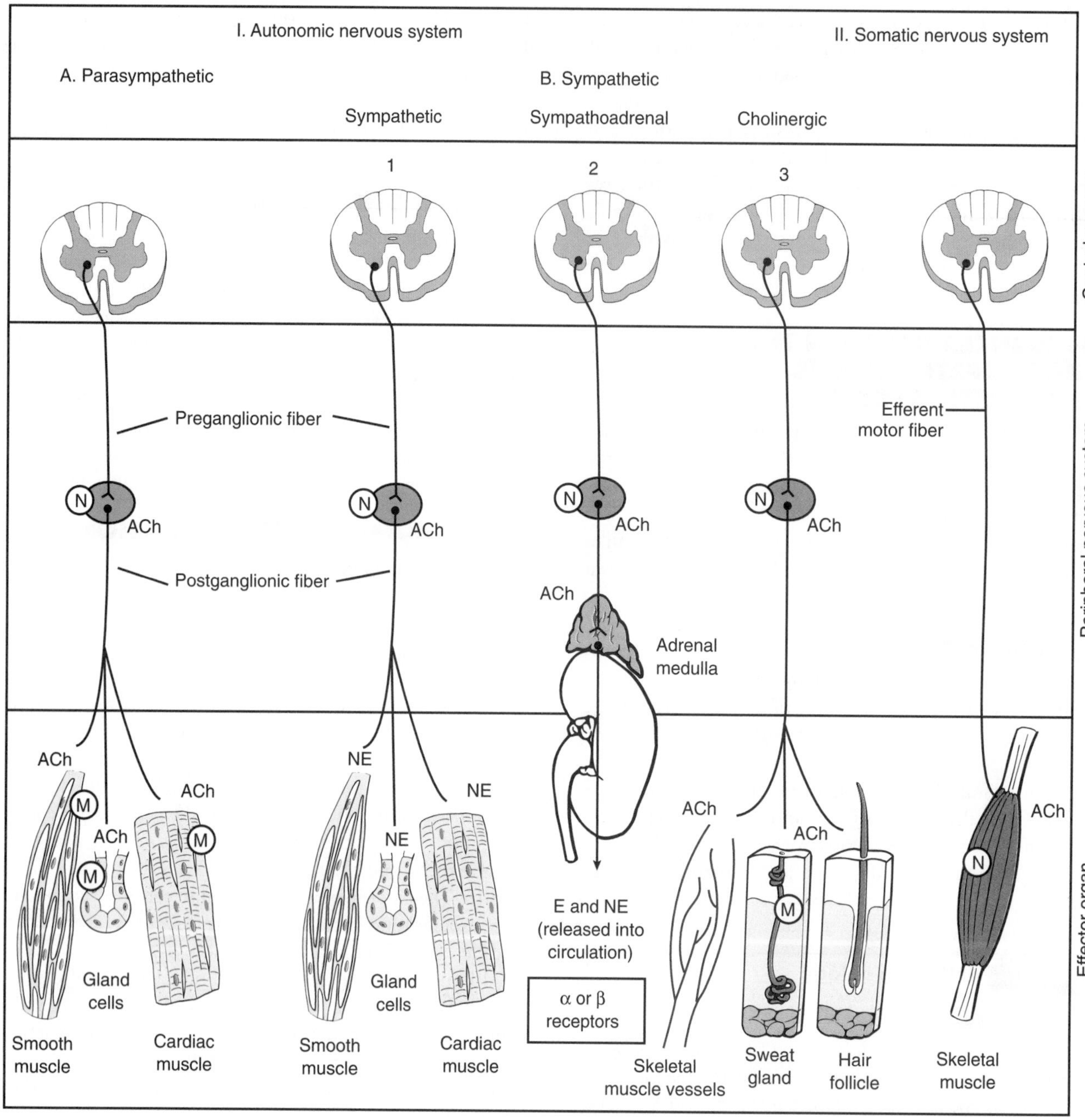

FIGURE 14-2
Schema of receptor sites for neurohumoral transmission. *I*, Autonomic nervous system, where preganglionic fibers of both parasympathetic and sympathetic nerves synapse in the ganglia. *II*, Somatic motor nervous system. *N*, Nicotinic sites; *M*, muscarinic sites; *ACh*, acetylcholine; *E*, epinephrine; *NE*, norepinephrine.

contain norepinephrine or epinephrine (from adrenal medulla) are known as adrenergic neurons, and they are associated with adrenergic transmission.

In neurohumoral transmission, the sequence of events includes (1) biosynthesis, (2) storage, (3) release, (4) action, and (5) inactivation of the mediator (Figs. 14-4 and 14-5). Many autonomic drugs affect one of these individual events, so it is essential to understand the basic mechanisms involved in this complicated process. These drugs have been useful in treating many persons afflicted with autonomic disorders.

Cholinergic Transmission

Synthesis and storage

Acetylcholine is synthesized in the cytoplasm of the nerve terminal. Once synthesized, the acetylcholine is stored in packets called synaptic vesicles or granules, which are located in the nerve terminal (Fig. 14-4, *A-2*).

TABLE 14-1 Classification of the Effector Organ Responses to Autonomic Nerve Impulses

		Response to Sympathetic (Adrenergic) Impulses	
Effector Organs	**Responses to Parasympathetic (Cholinergic) Impulses**	**Receptor**	**Response**
Cardiovascular system			
Heart			
Sinoatrial node	Decreased heart rate	$Beta_1$	Increased heart rate
Atrioventricular node	Decreased conduction velocity	$Beta_1$	Increased automaticity and conduction velocity
Ventricles	No innervation	$Beta_1$	Increased force of contraction and conduction velocity
Arterioles (smooth muscle)			
Coronary	Dilation	Alpha, $beta_2$, dopaminergic	Constriction and dilation
Skin and mucosa	Dilation	Alpha	Constriction
Skeletal muscle	No innervation	Cholinergic	Dilation
Cerebral	Dilation	Alpha	Slight constriction
Mesenteric	None	Alpha, $beta_2$, dopaminergic	Constriction and dilation
Renal	None	Alpha, $beta_2$, dopaminergic	Constriction and dilation
Veins	None	Alpha, $beta_2$	Constriction and dilation
Lung			
Bronchial muscle	Bronchoconstriction	$Beta_2$	Relaxation (bronchodilation)
Bronchial glands	Stimulation		Inhibition
Gastrointestinal tract			
Motility	Increased motility	Alpha, $beta_2$	Relaxation (decreased motility)
Sphincters	Relaxation	Alpha	Contraction
Exocrine glands	Increased secretion	?	Decreased secretion
Salivary glands	Dilation: copious, watery secretion	Alpha	Constriction: thick, viscous secretion
Gallbladder and ducts	Contraction		Relaxation
Kidney	None	$Beta_2$	Renin secretion
Urinary bladder			
Detrusor muscle	Contraction	$Beta_2$	Relaxation
Sphincter	Relaxation	Alpha	Contraction
Eye			
Radial muscle	Contraction of sphincter muscle	Alpha	Contraction of radial muscle
Iris	(miosis, pupillary constriction)		(mydriasis)
Ciliary muscle	Contracted for near vision		Relaxed for far vision
Liver	Glycogen synthesis	Beta	Glycogenolysis, gluconeogenesis
Pancreas	Secretion	Alpha	Decreased secretion
Skin	None	$Beta_2$	Increased secretion
Sweat glands	No innervation	Cholinergic	Increased sweating
Pilomotor muscle	No innervation		Contraction (gooseflesh)
Lacrimal glands	Increased secretion		No innervation
Nasopharyngeal glands	Increased secretion		No innervation
Male sex glands	Erection		Ejaculation

Release and action

The arrival of an action potential at the nerve ending causes the vesicle to approach the membrane and release acetylcholine molecules into the synaptic cleft or space. Calcium ions must be present for an efficient release. Once free, acetylcholine diffuses across the synaptic or junctional cleft and attaches to specialized receptors (postjunctional sites) on the membrane of the next neuron or neuroeffector. The binding of acetylcholine to the receptor increases the permeability of the membrane to sodium and potassium ions; thus a depolarizing action results in excitation or inhibition of neural, muscular, or glandular activity (Fig. 14-4, *A-3*).

Cholinergic receptors

The cholinergic receptor sites that are stimulated by the acetylcholine are either nicotinic or muscarinic. **Nicotinic (N) receptors** appear in the ganglia of both the parasympathetic and sympathetic fibers, the adrenal medulla, and the skeletal (striated) muscle that is supplied by the somatic motor system. **Muscarinic (M) receptors** (postganglionic sites) are located in the smooth muscle, cardiac muscle, and glands of the parasympathetic fibers and the effector organs of thecholinergic sympathetic fibers. The nicotinic and muscarinic receptors are shown in Fig. 14-2.

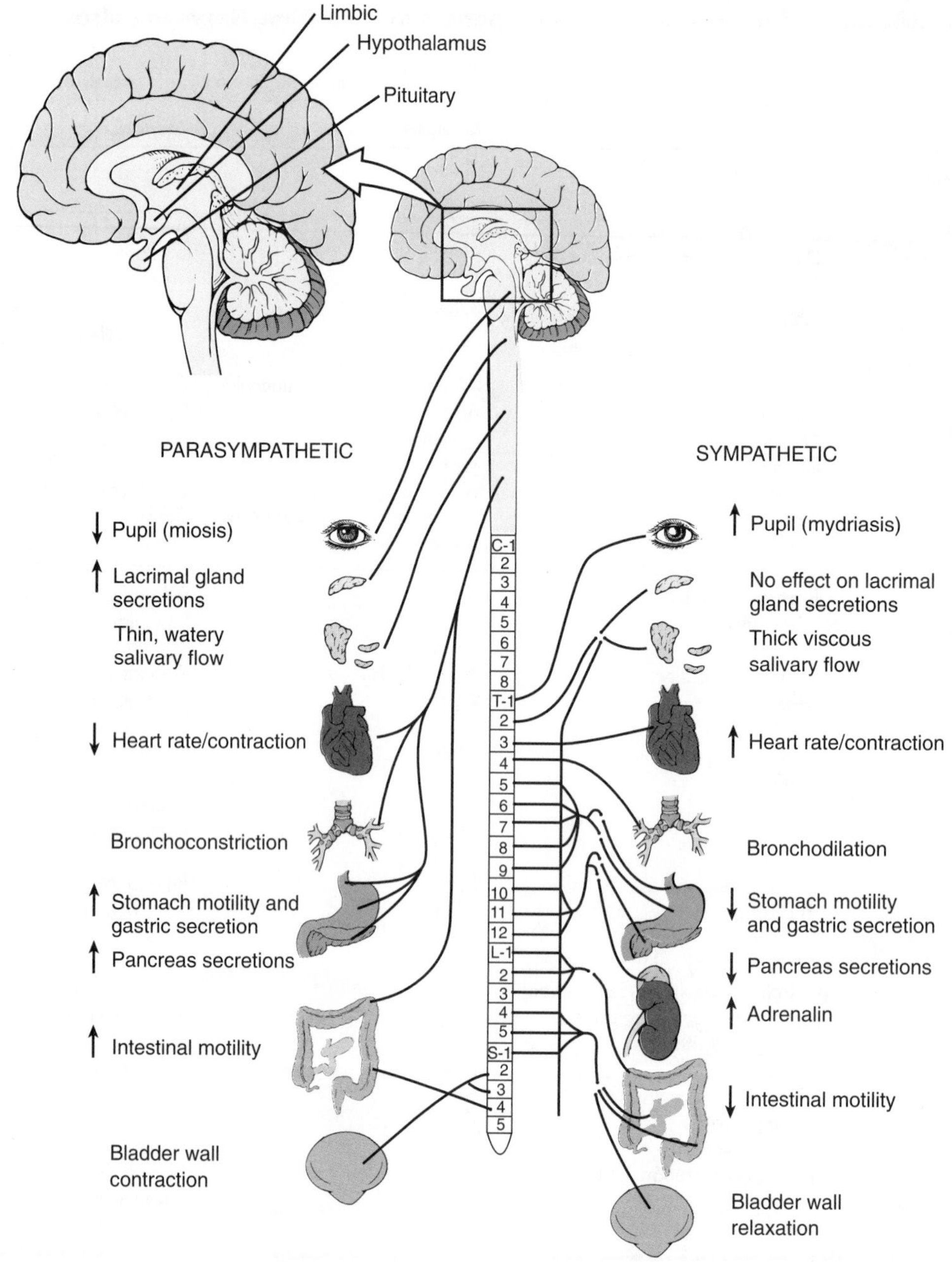

FIGURE 14-3
Diagram of the autonomic nervous system.

Inactivation

Once acetylcholine has exerted its effect on the postjunctional sites, the excess amount is inactivated rapidly by the enzyme acetylcholinesterase. The metabolites formed in this reaction are chemically inactive and are the same compounds from which acetylcholine is formed. Inactivation of this neurohormone is shown as a reverse action in Fig. 14-4, *A-5*.

Adrenergic Transmission

The term **catecholamine** refers to a group of chemically related compounds: norepinephrine (noradrenalin), epinephrine (adrenaline), and dopamine. They are all involved in some aspect of adrenergic transmission.

Synthesis and storage

The catecholamines produced by the sympathetic nervous system include norepinephrine and epinephrine. The complex pathway for synthesis of these neurotransmitters is mediated by different enzymes located in the postganglionic nerve terminals and in the chromaffin cells of the adrenal medullary glands.

The formation of norepinephrine is initiated by tyrosine, which is an amino acid derived from proteins in the diet.

TABLE 14-2 **Differentiating Characteristics Between the Parasympathetic and Sympathetic Nervous Systems**

Characteristic	*Parasympathetic Nervous System*	*Sympathetic Nervous System*
Origin	Craniosacral	Thoracolumbar
Structure innervation	Cardiac muscle Smooth muscle Glands Viscera	Cardiac muscle Smooth muscle Glands Viscera
Ganglia	Near the effector (vagus, atria of heart)	Near central nervous system
Length of fibers	Preganglionic (long) Postganglionic (short)	Preganglionic (short) Postganglionic (long)
Ratio of preganglionic to postganglionic fibers	Branching is minimal (1:2), very discrete, fine responses	High degree of nerve branching (1:11, 1:17)
Response	Discrete	Diffuse
Ganglion transmitter	Acetylcholine	Acetylcholine
Transmitter substance (postganglionic nerve endings)	Acetylcholine	Norepinephrine (most cases); epinephrine and norepinephrine (adrenal medulla) Acetylcholine for sweat glands and blood vessels of skeletal muscles
Blocking drugs (postganglionic nerve endings)	Cholinergic blocking agents (atropine)	Adrenergic blocking agents Alpha: phentolamine Beta: propranolol

When tyrosine enters the cytoplasm of the nerve terminal, it is converted into dopa, which in turn is decarboxylated to dopamine. Dopamine is then taken up into the storage vesicles, or granules, where it is transformed into the neurotransmitter norepinephrine by the enzyme dopamine β-hydroxylase. Fig. 14-5 shows the steps of the synthetic process.

In the adrenal medullary gland, the enzyme methyl transferase converts norepinephrine to epinephrine. On stimulation, both epinephrine and norepinephrine are released from the adrenal medulla and carried by the circulation to all parts of the body.

Release

The arrival of an action potential at the nerve terminal of the postganglionic fibers causes the vesicles to fuse with the cell membrane and release the stored supply of norepinephrine into the junctional cleft. Calcium ions must be present to enhance the release of norepinephrine from the vesicles. The free form of norepinephrine then diffuses across the cleft to the receptor sites on the postjunctional membrane of neuroeffector cells (smooth muscle, cardiac muscle, or glands) (Fig. 14-5).

Action

Once the norepinephrine combines with either the alpha or beta receptor sites on the membrane of the neuroeffector cells, a series of chemical and electrical events produces either an excitatory or an inhibitory effect. The alpha receptor activation is primarily responsible for an excitatory response, although it results in intestinal relaxation. By contrast, beta receptor activation is usually inhibitory except in the myocardial cells, where norepinephrine produces an excitatory effect.

Adrenergic receptors

The adrenergic receptor sites that are stimulated by the endogenous catecholamines—norepinephrine, epinephrine, and dopamine—are classified as alpha and beta receptors. Both classes have two subtypes. The alpha receptors are identified by neuronal location: (1) $alpha_1$ sites are located on the postsynaptic effector cells, and (2) $alpha_2$ sites appear on the presynaptic nerve terminals, controlling the amount of norepinephrine release that operates through a negative feedback mechanism. By contrast, the beta receptors are designated by organ location: (1) $beta_1$ receptors are located primarily in the heart, and (2) $beta_2$ receptors appear in the smooth muscle of the bronchioles, arterioles, and various other visceral organs in the body. At least five types of dopamine receptors have been identified in the CNS. D_1 and D_2 receptors are associated with the antipsychotic medications and movement disorders, such as Parkinson's disease. Stimulation of D_2 receptors is primarily responsible for antiparkinson drug activity, and the D_1 receptors may play a similar, although smaller, role in this area.

Inactivation

Once norepinephrine has performed its adrenergic function, its action must be rapidly stopped to prevent prolongation of its effects, which could lead to a loss of regulatory control of visceral function. The inactivation of norepinephrine occurs by (1) enzymatic transformation, (2) reuptake of the norepinephrine into nerve terminals, and (3) diffusion.

Catecholamines are metabolized by two enzymes, monoamine oxidase (MAO) and catechol O-methyltransferase (COMT). Free norepinephrine within the cytoplasm of the nerve terminal is metabolized by MAO, which is stored in

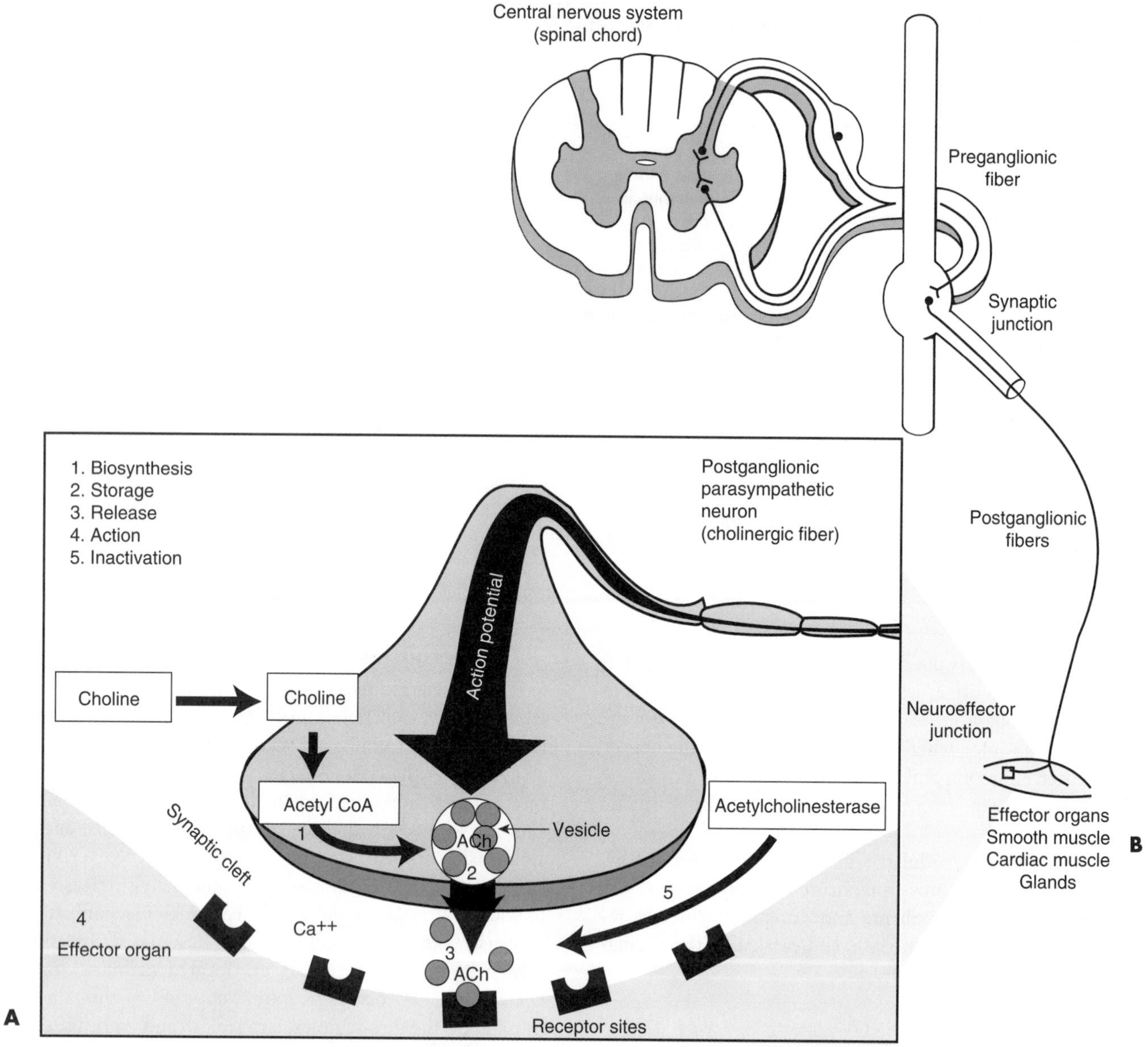

FIGURE 14-4

A, Cholinergic transmission. Schematic diagram of parasympathetic postganglionic neuron, showing steps in cholinergic transmission at the neuroeffector junction. *1,* Biosynthesis of acetylcholine (ACh): choline is taken up by the nerve terminal, and it interacts with acetyl coenzyme A (CoA) to synthesize ACh. *2,* Storage: following synthesis, ACh is stored in the vesicle until the arrival of a nerve impulse. *3,* Release: an action potential of the nerve terminal causes the vesicle to attach itself to the membrane and release ACh. The neurohormone then diffuses across the synaptic cleft and combines with the receptors on the effector cell. *4,* Action: the interaction of ACh with the receptor sites results in a motor response. *5,* Inactivation of ACh: at the synaptic cleft, ACh is hydrolyzed by the enzyme acetylcholinesterase. **B,** Schematic representation to show the relationship between a neuron in the central nervous system, a neuron in the peripheral ganglion, and an effector organ supplied by the parasympathetic nerve.

the mitochondria of sympathetic neurons. COMT, which is located outside the neuron or at the synaptic cleft, participates in the inactivation or metabolism of norepinephrine outside the neuron.

The mechanism of norepinephrine reuptake plays a more significant role than enzymatic transformation in catecholamine inactivation. In the reuptake process, norepinephrine is removed by the active transport ("amine pump") from the junctional sites (synaptic and neuroeffector junctions) and is returned to the sympathetic nerve terminal and storage vesicles. In this way, an adequate supply of norepinephrine is provided by reuptake, as well as by the process of synthesis.

Finally, a small portion of norepinephrine released at the

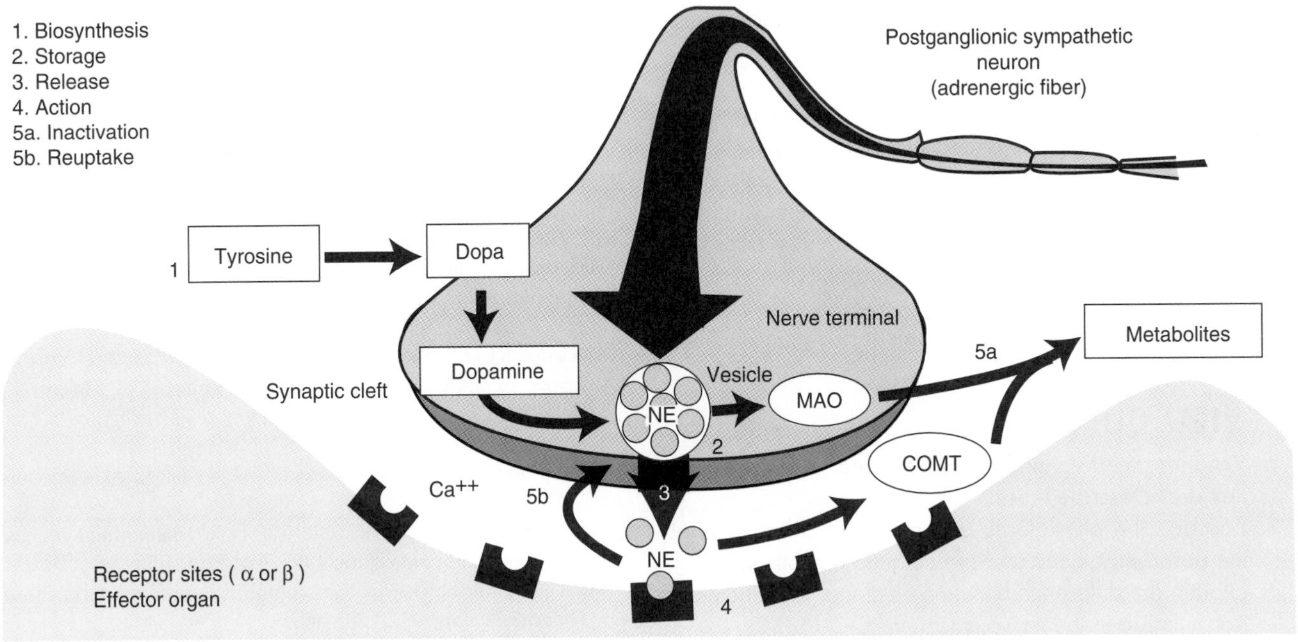

FIGURE 14-5
Adrenergic transmission at the neuroeffector junction. *NE,* Norepinephrine.

synaptic cleft may be picked up by the circulation and metabolized elsewhere in the body. This is known as the diffusion process. Fig. 14-5 portrays the steps in adrenergic transmission.

General Actions of Autonomic Transmitters

In 1933 Dale and co-workers determined the chemical differences between fibers that release acetylcholine (**cholinergic** fibers) and those that release norepinephrine and epinephrine (**adrenergic** fibers). In the autonomic nervous system, all the preganglionic fibers originate in the CNS and synapse with the ganglia of the postganglionic fibers. The terminals of all the preganglionic fibers release acetylcholine and interact with nicotinic receptors in the membrane of the postganglionic fibers or the adrenal medulla.

In the parasympathetic system the terminals of the postganglionic fibers also release acetylcholine and interact with muscarinic receptors in the membrane of the smooth muscle, cardiac muscle, and glands.

In the sympathetic nervous system there are three different kinds of postganglionic neurons. (1) The sympathetic neuron, the major type, releases norepinephrine and activates either alpha or beta receptors in the membrane of the smooth muscle, cardiac muscle, and glands. (2) The sympathoadrenal neuron, in which the preganglionic fiber synapses with a modified sympathetic ganglion, the adrenal medulla, releases mostly epinephrine and a small amount of norepinephrine, which are secreted into the circulation and carried to all parts of the body. (3) The cholinergic sympathetic neuron releases acetylcholine and stimulates muscarinic receptor sites on the sweat glands to produce sweating and on the blood vessels in skeletal muscle to increase vasodilation and enhance blood flow.

In the somatic (sensory) nervous system a single neuron, the efferent (motor) fiber, releases acetylcholine and interacts with the nicotinic sites on the skeletal muscle membrane. The autonomic drugs play an important role by enhancing or inhibiting physiologic activity at these sites of neurohumoral transmission (see Fig. 14-2 and Table 14-2).

SUMMARY

This chapter reviews the primary functions of the autonomic nervous system, that is, a regulatory system to maintain homeostasis within the internal body environment. Its functions include collecting information about conditions inside and outside the body and communicating this information to several centers in the CNS, such as the hypothalamus, medulla oblongata, midbrain, limbic system, cerebellum, and cerebral cortex. These centers along with the vital centers (vasomotor center, respiratory center, and cardiac center) are all involved in controlling the physiologic functions regulated by the autonomic nervous system. The autonomic nervous system innervates the smooth muscles, cardiac muscles, and glands and is composed of two divisions, the parasympathetic and the sympathetic nervous system. These systems usually innervate the same organs and have opposing actions; in other words, they balance each other. Their function involves the following:

1. Only one system predominates at any given time.
2. When one nervous system function is blocked, the opposite effect will take precedence.
3. Medications are available to act on either system, that is, to stimulate or block the system.

Parasympathetic nervous system functions include essentially the system of rest and digestion while the sympathetic system prepares the person for emergency and stress situations (whether physical or emotional). The latter require expenditure of energy and increases in blood sugar, heart activity, and blood pressure to meet the situation.

The chemical neurotransmitters acetylcholine and the catecholamines are necessary for nerve impulse transmission. The nerve fibers that synthesize and release acetylcholine are known as cholinergic fibers; those that synthesize and secrete norepinephrine and epinephrine are called adrenergic fibers.

REVIEW QUESTIONS

1. What are the two major functional processes of the reflex arc? Describe these.
2. Describe the physiologic and anatomic differences of the parasympathetic and sympathetic nervous system.
3. Explain the difference between electrical and chemical transmission in the nervous system.
4. Describe the functioning of the somatic nervous system.

REFERENCES

Anderson KN et al, editors: *Mosby's medical, nursing, and allied health dictionary,* ed 5, St Louis, 1998, Mosby.

Guyton AC: *Textbook of medical physiology,* ed 8, Philadelphia, 1990, WB Saunders.

Hardman JG, Limbird LE, editors: *Goodman & Gilman's the pharmacological basis of therapeutics,* ed 9, New York, 1996, McGraw-Hill.

McCance KL, Huether SE: *Pathophysiology: the biologic basis for disease in adults and children,* ed 3, St Louis, 1998, Mosby.

Seeley RR, Stephens TD, Tate P: *Anatomy & physiology,* ed 3, New York, 1995, McGraw-Hill.

Thibodeau GA, Patton KT: *Anatomy and physiology,* ed 4, St Louis, 1999, Mosby.

Van Wynsberghe D, Noback CR, Carola R: *Human anatomy and physiology,* ed 3, New York, 1995, McGraw-Hill.

Vinik AI, Vinik E: The diabetes complication no one talks about, *Diabetes Forecast* 45(7):70, 1992.

CHAPTER 15

Drugs Affecting the Parasympathetic Nervous System

KEY DRUGS

atropine (p. 257)
bethanechol (p. 255)
nicotine (p. 262)

CHAPTER FOCUS

The autonomic nervous system is composed of the parasympathetic component and sympathetic nervous system. This system innervates various organs and their functions to control body functions that occur without conscious thought. This chapter reviews the autonomic drugs that may mimic, intensify, or block the effects of acetylcholine in the parasympathetic system.

OBJECTIVES

After reading and studying this chapter, the student should be able to do the following:

1. *Define and discuss the key drugs and key terms.*
2. *Name two major effects of acetylcholine on the nervous system.*
3. *Explain the difference between a direct-acting and indirect-acting cholinergic drug.*
4. *Describe the major drug interactions and side effects and adverse reactions of cholinergic, cholinergic blocking, and synthetic antispasmodic agents.*
5. *List the primary pharmacologic effects of nicotine.*
6. *Discuss the pharmacologic effects and limitations associated with the use of ganglionic blocking drugs.*

KEY TERMS

adrenergic, (p. 254)
adrenergic blocking, (p. 254)
anticholinergic, (p. 257)
antimuscarinic, (p. 257)
cholinergic, (p. 254)
cholinergic blocking, (p. 254)
direct-acting cholinergic drugs, (p. 254)
indirect-acting cholinergic drugs, (p. 254)
muscarinic effect, (p. 254)
parasympatholytic, (p. 254)
parasympathomimetic, (p. 254)
sympatholytic, (p. 254)
sympathomimetic, (p. 254)

AUTONOMIC DRUGS

Autonomic drugs may mimic, intensify, or block the effects of the parasympathetic and sympathetic divisions of the autonomic nervous system. The following is a brief review of these agents:

1. **Cholinergic (parasympathomimetic)** drugs (e.g., bethanechol) act like mediators of the parasympathetic nervous system.
2. **Cholinergic blocking (parasympatholytic** or **anticholinergic)** drugs (e.g., atropine) block the action of the parasympathetic nervous system.
3. **Adrenergic (sympathomimetic)** drugs (e.g., norepinephrine) act like mediators of the sympathetic nervous system.
4. **Adrenergic blocking (sympatholytic)** drugs (e.g., propranolol, a beta blocking agent) block the action of the sympathetic nervous system.

CHOLINERGIC DRUGS

As discussed in Chapter 14, acetylcholine plays an important role in the transmission of nerve impulses in both the parasympathetic and sympathetic divisions of the autonomic nervous system.

Acetylcholine has two major actions on the nervous system: (1) it has stimulant effects on the ganglia, adrenal medulla, and skeletal muscle, and (2) it has stimulant effects at postganglionic nerve endings in cardiac muscle, smooth muscle, and glands. The first action resembles the effects of nicotine, such as tachycardia, elevated blood pressure, and peripheral vasoconstriction, and is referred to as the "nicotine effect" of acetylcholine. The second action of acetylcholine at the postganglionic nerve endings is like that of muscarine (an alkaloid obtained from the toadstool *Amanita muscaria*) and is referred to as the **muscarinic effect** or cholinergic effect of acetylcholine. These receptors may be selectively blocked by atropine (Table 15-1). See Fig. 14-2 to review nicotinic and muscarinic sites.

Cholinergic drugs are agents that bring about effects in the body similar to those produced by acetylcholine. These agents are also called parasympathomimetics because they mimic the action produced by stimulation of the parasympathetic nervous system.

Cholinergic fibers are widespread: they are present in heart, spleen, uterus, vas deferens, colon, and the vessels of the skin and muscles. Cholinergic fibers probably are present in many more tissues of the body. In the gastrointestinal tract, parasympathetic innervation predominates: it stimulates both motor and secretory action.

Although acetylcholine is important physiologically, it has no therapeutic value because (1) its actions are very brief owing to rapid hydrolysis by acetylcholinesterase, and (2) no selective purpose can be achieved through its use, since it has numerous sites of action.

Cholinergic drugs may be obtained from natural (plant) or synthetic sources. The synthetic drugs are more stable and have a more selective action on particular organs. The two groups of cholinergic drugs available are (1) direct-acting and (2) indirect-acting. **Direct-acting cholinergic drugs** combine directly with the cholinergic receptors in postsynaptic membranes innervated by parasympathetic neurons and evoke effects similar to those produced by acetylcholine. By contrast, instead of a direct effect on receptors, **indirect-acting cholinergic drugs** act primarily on the enzyme inhibiting the action of cholinesterase (acetylcholinesterase) that normally degrades acetylcholine. This results in an accumulation of acetylcholine at all the sites where it is liberated (see Fig. 14-4, *A-5*). By rendering the enzymatic action ineffective, the anticholinesterase drugs

TABLE 15-1 Acetylcholine: Sites for Muscarinic and Nicotinic Actions

Site	Muscarinic Action*	Nicotinic Actions
Cardiovascular		
Blood vessels	Dilation	Constriction (with large doses after atropine)
Heart rate	Slowed	Increased (with large doses after atropine)
Blood pressure	Decreased	Increased (with large doses after atropine)
Gastrointestinal		
Tone	Increased	Increased
Motility	Increased	Increased
Sphincters	Relaxed	—
Glandular secretions	Increased salivary, lacrimal, intestinal, and sweat secretion	Initial stimulation, then inhibition of salivary and bronchial secretions
Skeletal muscle	—	Stimulated
Autonomic ganglia	—	Stimulated
Eye	Pupil constriction Decreased accommodation	—
Blocking agent	Atropine	Tubocurarine
Remarks	Above effects increase as dosage increases	Increased dosage inhibits effects and causes receptor blockade

*Usual sites for therapeutic effects.

cause a prolonged and intensified cholinergic response at the various effector sites.

Cholinergic drugs may be used for the following:

1. Stimulate the intestine and bladder postoperatively thus increasing peristalsis and urination
2. Lower intraocular pressure in patients with glaucoma
3. Promote salivation and sweating
4. Terminate curarization (neuromuscular blockade used as an adjunct to general anesthesia)
5. Treat myasthenia gravis symptomatically*

The therapeutic effectiveness of cholinergic drugs depends primarily on their muscarinic action, but some of them also possess nicotinic action. This nicotinic action usually requires doses much larger than those used therapeutically. However, some drugs may exhibit more nicotinic than muscarinic effects (Table 15-1).

The ideal cholinergic or anticholinesterase drug would do the following:

1. Mimic or inhibit the effect of acetylcholine on a particular structure or organ
2. Be effective when administered orally
3. Be more stable and less easily inactivated than the drugs now available
4. Produce a therapeutic effect with minimal side effects

Although these ideal drugs are not yet available, progress is being made in this direction. Cholinergic drugs used primarily to lower intraocular pressure are discussed in Chapter 36. These include pilocarpine and carbachol. Table 15-2 lists the prominent cholinergic and anticholinesterase drugs.

Direct-Acting Cholinergic Drugs (Choline Esters)

Drugs that are chemically similar to the neurotransmitter acetylcholine include bethanechol, carbachol, and methacholine. All compounds in this group are quaternary amines, so they are poorly absorbed orally. Their actions are comparable although longer acting then those of the physiologic mediator acetylcholine. The side effects of these drugs, which include bradycardia, hypotension, sweating, salivation, vomiting, diarrhea, and intestinal cramps, are a consequence of parasympathetic stimulation.

*Cholinergic, but not parasympathomimetic, action involves the somatic nervous system, innervating skeletal muscle.

bethanechol [be than′ e kole] (Urecholine, Duvoid ✱) ⚷

Bethanechol is a synthetic choline ester with actions similar to those of acetylcholine. It produces the effects of stimulation of the parasympathetic nervous system. Its action is predominantly muscarinic with particular selectivity on the detrusor muscle of the urinary bladder and smooth muscle of the gastrointestinal tract. Hence, contraction of the smooth muscle of the bladder is sufficiently strong to initiate micturition and empty the urinary bladder. In the gastrointestinal tract, the drug stimulates gastric motility, increases gastric tone, and often restores impaired peristaltic activity of the esophagus, stomach, and intestine. It also promotes defecation. Unlike acetylcholine, bethanechol is not destroyed by cholinesterase; Therefore its effects are more prolonged than that of the natural neurotransmitter. Therapeutic test doses in normal human subjects have little effect on heart rate, blood pressure, or peripheral circulation.

Indications

Bethanechol has generally been replaced by more effective drugs, but it is available in the United States for the treatment of postoperative and postpartum nonobstructive urinary retention and for neurogenic atony of the urinary bladder associated with retention. Although not indicated on its U.S. product labeling, it has also been used to relieve postoperative abdominal distention and gastric atony or stasis and reflux esophagitis associated with decreased pressure of the lower esophageal sphincter.

Pharmacokinetics

Despite being poorly absorbed from the gastrointestinal tract, bethanechol chloride is effective orally. It is widely dis-

TABLE 15-2 Cholinergic Agents: Direct-Acting and Indirect-Acting (Anticholinesterase) Agents

Generic Name (Trade Name)	*Action**	*Usual Adult Dose (24 hr)*	*Usual Route of Administration*
ambenonium (Mytelase)	I	5 mg tid to qid	PO
bethanechol ⚷ (Urecholine)	D	10-50 mg tid to qid	PO
		5 mg tid or qid	SC
isoflurophate (Floropryl)	I	Thin strip (0.5 cm) of 0.025%, variable instructions	Topical (eye) ointment
neostigmine bromide (Prostigmin)	I	15 mg q3-4h	PO
neostigmine methylsulfate (Prostigmin)	I	0.5 mg dose variable	IM or SC
physostigmine (Eserine)	I	1 drop, 0.25%-0.5% solution bid or tid	Topical (eye)
physostigmine (Antilirium)	I	0.5-2 mg (maximum)	IM or IV
pilocarpine	D	1 drop, 0.5%-4% qid	Topical (eye)
pyridostigmine (Mestinon)	I	Highly variable	PO

**D*, direct acting; *I*, indirect acting.

tributed to organs innervated by the parasympathetic nervous system. Onset of action is within 30 to 90 minutes after oral administration, peak effect occurs within 1 hour, and duration of action is up to 6 hours, depending on the dose administered. If administered subcutaneously, the onset of action is within 5 to 15 minutes, peak effect occurs within 15 to 30 minutes, and the duration of action is approximately 2 hours. The route of excretion is currently unknown.

Drug interactions

The following effects may occur when bethanechol is given with the drugs listed below:

Drug	Possible effect and management
Other cholinergic or anticholinesterase medications	Enhanced cholinergic effects and perhaps toxicity. Monitor closely for adverse effects or, if possible, avoid this combination of medications (Table 15-3).
Ganglionic blocking agents	May result in severe abdominal distress followed by a precipitous fall in blood pressure. Avoid or a potentially serious drug interaction may occur.
procainamide or quinidine	Cholinergic effects may be antagonized. Monitor closely for dry mouth, urinary retention, blurred vision, confusion, and ataxia.

Color type indicate an unsafe drug combination.

Side effects and adverse reactions

See Table 15-3.

Warnings

Use with caution in patients with Parkinson's disease, vagotonia, hypertension, seizure disorders, and atrioventricular conduction defects.

Contraindications

Avoid use in patients with bethanechol hypersensitivity, asthma, severe bradycardia, hypotension, gastrointestinal (GI) obstruction, coronary artery disease, hyperthyroidism, and peptic ulcer.

Dosage and administration

The oral dosage for adults is 10 to 50 mg orally, three to four times daily; for children the dosage is 0.6 mg/kg of body weight in three or four divided doses per day. The parenteral adult dose is 5 mg subcutaneously, three or four times per day when needed, and for children (subcutaneous use only) the dose is 0.2 mg/kg of body weight in three or four divided doses per day.

TABLE 15-3 Drugs Affecting the Parasympathetic Nervous System: Side Effects and Adverse Reactions

Drugs	*Side Effects and Adverse Reactions*
Cholinergic	
bethanechol (Urecholine, Duvoid)	Abdominal pains or upset, increased salivation and sweating, nausea or vomiting, flushed skin, blurred or disturbed vision, unsteadiness, headache, and diarrhea.
Anticholinergic	
atropine scopolamine	Inhibition of sweating, constipation, dry mouth, throat, and skin, blurred vision, urinary retention, headache, photophobia, drowsiness, weakness, nausea or vomiting, urticaria, dermatitis, and eye pain from increased intraocular pressure. In addition, euphoria, amnesia, and insomnia are reported more often with scopolamine. Dilated and fixed pupil has been reported on the side where the transdermal disk is applied. To avoid extensive neurologic examinations, unconscious individuals appearing with the above symptoms should be checked first for the use of a disk behind the ear. If disk is removed, this syndrome usually abates within weeks.
Synthetic Antispasmodics	
clidinium (Quarzan) dicyclomine (Bentyl, Antispas) glycopyrrolate (Robinul)	Abdominal distention, headache, dizziness, constipation, nausea, vomiting, sedation, dry mouth, nose, throat and skin, blurred or disturbed vision, dysuria, weakness, hypotension, and decreased sexual ability.
Ganglionic Blocking Agents	
trimethaphan camsylate (Arfonad)	Side effects are dose related: anorexia, nausea, vomiting, constipation, dilated pupils, dry mouth, impotency, pruritis, hives, hypotension, tachycardia, angina, and urinary retention.

Indirect-Acting Cholinergic Drugs

The indirect-acting cholinergic drugs are anticholinesterases or cholinesterase inhibitors because they inhibit the action of the enzyme cholinesterase, thereby prolonging the effect of acetylcholine. Anticholinesterase agents (e.g., neostigmine and physostigmine) exert their influence on both muscarinic and nicotinic sites. They are used in the treatment of myasthenia gravis and glaucoma (see Chapters 17 and 36, respectively). Physostigmine salicylate is used for overdosage and anticholinergic substance toxicity. (See the discussion about treatment of tricyclic antidepressant overdosage in Chapter 13.)

Drugs Used to Treat Myasthenia Gravis

Myasthenia gravis is a condition characterized by weakness of the skeletal muscles innervated by the somatic efferent fibers. Because the disease affects cholinergic transmission, the anticholinesterase drugs are used because they elevate the concentration of acetylcholine at the myoneural junctions. The prolonged activity of the neurohormone at these sites results in a dramatic increase in muscle strength and function. There is a more extensive discussion of myasthenia gravis and its treatment in Chapter 17. (See also Fig. 14-2 for site of action.)

CHOLINERGIC BLOCKING DRUGS

MUSCARINIC BLOCKING DRUGS

The cholinergic blocking, or parasympatholytic, drugs have many important uses in medicine. More specifically, these agents are called **antimuscarinic** or **anticholinergic** drugs because they block the muscarinic effects of acetylcholine. When the nerve fiber is stimulated, the acetylcholine liberated from the terminal is unable to bind to the receptor site and fails to produce a cholinergic effect. Thus these agents also are referred to as anticholinergic drugs. (See Fig. 14-2 for muscarinic receptor sites.)

Belladonna Alkaloids

The best known muscarinic or cholinergic blocking drugs are the belladonna alkaloids. The major drugs in this class are atropine, hyoscyamine, and scopolamine (Table 15-4). A number of plants belonging to the potato family (Solanaceae) contain similar alkaloids. *Atropa belladonna* (deadly nightshade), *Hyoscyamus niger* (henbane), *Datura stramonium* (Jimson weed), and several species of *Scopolia* also contain belladonna alkaloids. The principal alkaloids of these plants are atropine, scopolamine (hyoscine), and hyoscyamine. Atropine is the prototype of the antimuscarinic drugs. It has been in use for over half a century and continues to be a popular drug because of its therapeutic effectiveness.

TABLE 15-4 Selected Anticholinergic Agents Containing Specific Alkaloids*

Trade Name	*Alkaloid Formation†*
Anaspaz	hyoscyamine
Cystospaz	
Cystospaz-M	
Levsin	
Buscopan	scopolamine
Transderm-Scop	
Transderm-V	
Barbidonna	atropine, hyoscyamine, scopolamine, and phenobarbital
Barophen	
Donnatal	
Donnatal Extentabs	
Antrocol	atropine and phenobarbital
Butibel	belladonna and butabarbital
Chardonna-2	belladonna and phenobarbital
Levsin-PB	hyoscyamine and phenobarbital

*Specific alkaloids include the active alkaloids of belladonna, such as hyoscyamine, atropine, and scopolamine.
†The alkaloid formulation lists the active ingredients as marketed under the various trade names. Individual salts, strengths, and dosing intervals may vary according to the manufacturer's instructions.

atropine sulfate [a′ troe peen]
(Atropine, Isopto Atropine)

Mechanism of action

As a competitive antagonist, atropine acts by occupying the muscarinic (M) receptor sites, thereby preventing or reducing the muscarinic response of acetylcholine (see Fig. 14-2). The drug-receptor complex is formed at the neuroeffector junctions of smooth muscle, cardiac muscle, exocrine glands, and eye.

Atropine has very little effect on the actions of acetylcholine at nicotinic receptor sites. So at the autonomic ganglia, where transmission normally involves the action of acetylcholine, relatively high doses of atropine are required to produce even a partial block. At the neuromuscular junctions of the somatic nervous system, where the receptors are exclusively nicotinic, extremely high doses of atropine are required to produce any degree of block. See Fig. 14-2 for nicotinic (N) receptor sites on the ganglia or parasympathetic and sympathetic nerve divisions, and for nicotinic sites on effector organ (skeletal muscle) of the somatic motor system.

Atropine can produce a wide range of pharmacologic effects because a vast distribution of parasympathetic cholinergic nerves normally exists in the body. Furthermore, drug activity is dose dependent. Small doses depress salivary and bronchial secretions and sweating. Large doses dilate the pupils, inhibit accommodation of the eyes, and increase heart rate by blocking vagal effects of the heart. Larger doses inhibit micturition and decrease the tone and motility of the gut by inhibiting parasympathetic control of both the urinary bladder and the gastrointestinal tract. In addition, still larger doses are required to inhibit gastric secretion and motility.

Pharmacologic properties

Eye. The pupil is dilated (mydriasis), and the ciliary muscle (muscle of accommodation) is relaxed (cycloplegia). The sphincter muscle of the iris and the ciliary muscle are both innervated by cholinergic nerve fibers and therefore are affected by atropine. Because the sphincter muscle is unable to contract normally, the radial muscle of the iris causes the pupil to dilate.

Pupil dilation may reduce outflow of aqueous humor, causing a rise in intraocular pressure. This is a hazardous situation for persons with glaucoma (angle closure). These effects in the eye are brought about by both local and systemic administration of atropine, although the usual single therapeutic dose of atropine given orally or parenterally has little effect on the eye. After the pupil is dilated, photophobia occurs, and when the drug has reached its full effect, the usual reflexes to light and accommodation disappear.

Systemic absorption of ophthalmic medications resulting in undesirable side effects or adverse reactions have been reported with atropine and a number of other eye preparations. Therefore ophthalmic preparations should be included in the review of the patient's current medications because an ophthalmic preparation may be an offending agent (USP DI, 1998).

Skin and mucous membranes. Because the sweat glands of the skin are supplied by sympathetic cholinergic nerves, atropine decreases or abolishes their activity. This causes the skin to become hot and dry. Furthermore, since the flow of secretions from glands lining the respiratory tract is reduced, drying of the mucous membranes of the mouth, nose, pharynx, and bronchi occurs. Patients who have been given atropine, particularly for preoperative preparation, often complain of a dry mouth and thirst.

Respiratory system. Secretions of the nose, pharynx, and bronchial tubes are decreased. The muscles of the bronchial tubes relax, and the airway widens to ease breathing. Atropine and scopolamine are less effective than epinephrine as bronchodilators and are seldom used for asthma.

Cardiovascular system. When low doses are given or an intravenous dose is administered slowly, the cardiac rate is temporarily and slightly slowed because of the central action of the drug on the cardiac center in the medulla (paradoxical bradycardia). Larger intravenous doses given rapidly will block the vagal effect on the sinoatrial node node and atrioventricular junction and cause an increased heart rate.

In therapeutic doses atropine has little or no effect on blood pressure. This is expected because most vascular beds lack significant cholinergic innervation. However, large (and sometimes ordinary) doses cause vasodilation of vessels in the skin of the face and neck. This may result from a direct dilator action or from histamine release. Reddening of the face and neck is seen, especially after large or toxic doses.

Gastrointestinal tract. It appears that the amount and character of the gastric secretion are little affected by atropine given in ordinary therapeutic doses. The secretion of acid in the stomach is presumably less under vagal control than under hormonal or chemical control. The effect of atropine on the secretion of the pancreas and intestinal glands is not therapeutically significant. Atropine and other belladonna alkaloids decrease tone and peristalsis in the stomach and small and large intestines. Atropine does not affect the secretion of bile, but it exerts a mildly antispasmodic effect in the gallbladder and bile ducts.

Urinary tract. The drug relaxes the ureter, especially when it has been in a state of spasm. Therapeutic doses decrease the tone of the fundus of the urinary bladder. When the detrusor muscle is hypertonic, it is relaxed by atropine. It also causes constriction of the internal sphincter, which can produce urinary retention.

Central nervous system. Atropine has prominent effects on the central nervous system and in large doses causes excitement and maniacal behavior. These behavioral effects suggest the existence of important cholinergic pathways and receptors within the central nervous system.

Small or moderate doses of atropine have little or no cerebral effect. Large or toxic doses cause the patient to become restless, wakeful, and talkative. This condition may develop into delirium and finally stupor and coma. The exalted, excited stage has sometimes been called a "belladonna jag." A rise in temperature is sometimes seen, especially in infants and young children. This is probably the result of suppression of sweating rather than action on the heat-regulating center.

Atropine has been used to diminish tremor in Parkinson's disease, perhaps due to the reduction in cholinergic synaptic transmission. Therapeutic doses of atropine stimulate the respiratory center and make breathing faster and sometimes deeper. When respiration is seriously depressed, atropine is not always reliable as a stimulant; in fact, it may deepen the depression. Large doses stimulate respiration, but they can also cause respiratory failure and death.

Small doses stimulate the vagus center in the medulla, causing primary slowing of the heart. The vasoconstrictor center is stimulated briefly and then depressed. Because depression follows soon after stimulation, atropine has been called a borderline stimulant of the central nervous system.

Topical effects. There is a slight amount of absorption when atropine or belladonna is applied to the skin, especially if it is an alcoholic preparation or in the form of a transdermal patch.

Indications

Atropine is indicated for the treatment of irritable bowel syndrome, spastic biliary tract disorders, and genitourinary disorders and as an antidote for cholinergic toxicity from excessive amounts of cholinesterase inhibitors, muscarinic drugs, or organophosphate pesticide poisoning. Atropine is also used to treat sinus bradycardia and Parkinson's disease, to prevent excessive salivation and respiratory tract secretions as a preanesthetic agent, and as an adjunctive medication for peptic ulcers and for gastrointestinal radiography.

Pharmacokinetics

Atropine is readily absorbed after oral and parenteral administration; it is also absorbed from mucous membranes. After oral administration, the maximum effect is reached within 1 hour; the duration of action is 4 to 6 hours. It is widely distributed in fluids of the body and easily passes the placental barrier to the blood of the fetus and the blood-brain barrier. Atropine is metabolized primarily in the liver; approximately 30% to 50% of atropine is excreted unchanged in the urine.

Drug interactions

The following effects may occur when atropine (and other belladonna alkaloids) are given with the drugs listed below:

Drug	Possible mechanism of action
Antacids or antidiarrheal agents	May reduce absorption and therapeutic effectiveness of atropine. Space medications at least 2 to 3 hours apart.
Other anticholinergic drugs	Increase in anticholinergic effects reported. Monitor for symptoms such as decreased perspiration, dry mouth, blurred vision, and confusion because dosage adjustment may be necessary.
cyclopropane	The concurrent administration with anticholinergic drugs may result in ventricular arrhythmias. With glycopyrrolate, this potential adverse effect may be reduced if glycopyrrolate is carefully dosed in increments of 100 μg or less.
ketoconazole (Nizoral)	Increase in gastrointestinal pH by atropine may result in reduced absorption of ketoconazole. Atropine should be administered preferably 2 hours after ketoconazole.
potassium chloride, especially wax matrix formulations	Increased contact with gastrointestinal tract may result in mucosal irritation and lesions. Liquid formulations of potassium should be considered a replacement for the wax matrix formulation in this situation.

For additional atropine preparations, see Chapters 35 and 36.

Side effects and adverse reactions

See Table 15-3.

Warnings

Use with caution in children with brain damage, spastic paralysis, Down's syndrome, fever, liver and renal disease, hypertension, hyperthyroidism, urinary retention, toxemia of pregnancy, and zerostomia and in the elderly.

Contraindications

Avoid use in persons with atropine hypersensitivity, esophageal reflux, severe cardiac disease, GI obstructive disease, glaucoma, acute hemorrhage, hiatal hernia, myasthenia gravis, prostatic hypertrophy, urinary retention, pyloric obstruction tachycardia, or ulcerative colitis and in debilitated patients with intestinal atony or paralytic ileus.

Dosage and administration

The oral anticholinergic adult dose for atropine sulfate is 0.3 to 1.2 mg PO, every 4 to 6 hours. The pediatric dose is 0.01 mg/kg, not exceeding 0.4 mg, every 4 to 6 hours. The adult oral dose to prevent excessive salivation and respiratory tract secretions during anesthesia is 0.4 to 0.6 mg, titrated as necessary. The adult parenteral anticholinergic dose is 0.4 to 0.6 mg IM, IV, or SC every 4 to 6 hours. The pediatric anticholinergic dose is 0.01 mg/kg IM, IV, or SC, not exceeding 0.4 mg repeated every 4 to 6 hours if necessary. The adult parenteral dose to treat bradycardia (dysrhythmia) is 0.4 to 1 mg IV, every 1 to 2 hours, up to a maximum of 2 mg; the pediatric dysrhythmic dose is 0.01 to 0.03 mg/kg.

scopolamine [skoe pol′ a meen] (Transderm-Scop, Transderm-V ✤)
scopolamine hydrobromide

See the preceding discussion of atropine for mechanism of action. Scopolamine's peripheral effects are similar to those of atropine, but its effects on the central nervous system (CNS) differ. At therapeutic doses, it depresses the CNS and causes drowsiness, euphoria, memory loss, relaxation, sleep, and relief of fear. It does not increase blood pressure or respiration.

It is used in the treatment of irritable bowel syndrome and renal and ureteral colic and for dysrhythmias induced during surgery owing to increased vagal stimulation. Because of its depressant action on vestibular function, it is used for motion sickness to prevent nausea and vomiting. It is used as an adjunct medication with general anesthesia to check secretions, to prevent laryngospasm, and for its sedative (twilight sleep) and amnesic effects.

Scopolamine's pharmacokinetics are the same as those of atropine. The transdermal dosage form produces its antiemetic effects for up to 72 hours. For side effects and adverse reactions, see Table 15-3.

An oral dosage form is not available in the United States. The anticholinergic and antiemetic parenteral adult dose is 0.3 to 0.6 mg as a single dose. As an adjunct to anesthesia or for sedation-hypnosis, the dose is 0.6 mg IM, IV, or SC, three or four times daily. For amnesia effects, the dose is 0.32 to 0.6 mg IM, IV, or SC. Lower doses are recommended for the elderly. The antiemetic dose in children is 6 μg (0.006 mg)/kg IM, IV, or SC as a single dose. A transdermal scopolamine patch is applied behind the ear for 3 days. For an antiemetic effect, apply 4 hours before desired effect is required. As the elderly are more sensitive to this drug at adult dosage; monitor closely for hyperpyrexia, confusion, blurred vision, and ataxia. The transdermal patch is not recommended for children.

Synthetic Substitutes for Atropine

The usefulness of atropine is limited by the fact that it is a complex drug that produces effects in a number of organs or tissues simultaneously. When it is administered for its antispasmodic effects, it also produces prolonged effects in the eye, causing dilated pupils and blurred vision. It also causes dry mouth and possibly rapid heart rate. When the antispasmodic effect is desired, other effects become side effects, which may be distinctly undesirable.

A large number of drugs have been synthesized in an effort to capture the antispasmodic effect of atropine without its other effects. Drugs of this type are frequently used to relieve hypertonicity and hypersecretion in the stomach.

Many products are marketed as antispasmodic and anticholinergic agents, but their formulations are either modifications of a belladonna alkaloid or include one or more of the natural alkaloids as their active ingredients. The pharmacologic properties are therefore similar to previously reviewed substances and will not be repeated here (see Table 15-4). The more commonly used or newer systemic agents—dicyclomine (Bentyl), glycopyrrolate (Robinul), and clidinium bromide (Quarzan)—will be discussed.

dicyclomine [dye sye′ kloe meen]
(Bentyl, Bentylol ✤, and others)

Dicyclomine produces both a direct effect on smooth muscle, resulting in a decreased tone, and motility of the gastrointestinal, biliary, and urinary tracts. It only appears to produce the typical anticholinergic (antimuscarinic) effect when administered in large doses.

Indications

Dicyclomine is indicated for the treatment of the irritable bowel syndrome.

Pharmacokinetics

Little has been determined about the pharmacokinetics of this product. It is rapidly absorbed after oral or parenteral administration; about 50% of the dose is excreted by the kidneys and the other 50% in the feces. Its half-life is 1.8 hours initially and 9 to 10 hours for the second phase.

Side effects and adverse reactions

See Table 15-3.

Drug interactions, warnings, and contraindications

See discussion of atropine.

Dosage and administration

The adult oral dose is 10 to 20 mg three or four times daily, titrated if necessary to a maximum of 160 mg/day. For children 6 months to 2 years of age, the dose is 5 to 10 mg (syrup dosage form) PO three or four times daily; for children 2 years of age and older the dose is 10 mg PO three or four times daily. The parenteral adult dose is 20 mg IM every 4 to 6 hours. *Do not administer intravenously.* For children, the dosage is not established.

glycopyrrolate [glue koe pye′ roe late]
(Robinul, Robinul Forte)

This is a synthetic anticholinergic product with effects similar to those atropine. Unlike atropine, it is unable to easily cross lipid membranes (such as the blood-brain barrier); Therefore it has minimal central nervous system side effects. It also appears to be less likely to produce pupillary or ocular eye effects.

Glycopyrrolate is indicated as an anticholinergic (antimuscarinic) drug to prevent or reduce hypersecretion or reduce dysrhythmias induced during anesthesia and to prevent or reduce toxicities induced by cholinesterase inhibitors (neostigmine or pyridostigmine). It is administered PO, IV, IM, or SC.

Pharmacokinetics

The onset of action of an IV dose occurs within 1 minute. For IM or SC routes, onset of action is 15 to 30 minutes. Vagal blocking action lasts from 2 to 3 hours, while the antisialagogue effect, the inhibition of the flow of saliva, may last up to 7 hours. Glycopyrrolate is excreted by the kidneys.

Side effects and adverse reactions

See Table 15-3.

Drug interactions, warnings, and contraindications

See discussion of atropine.

Dosage and administration

The adult dose to treat peptic ulcer is 1 to 2 mg PO two or three times daily and if necessary 2 mg at bedtime; afterward reduce the dose to 1 mg twice daily or adjust the dosage according to the patient's response and tolerance. The elderly may be more sensitive to this glycopyrrolate dosage, so a lower dosage schedule should be considered. For children, the dosage is not established.

The parenteral anticholinergic adult dose of glycopyrrolate for peptic ulcer is 0.1 to 0.2 mg IM or IV every 4 hours (up to a maximum of 4 doses per 24 hours). To prevent or reduce excessive salivation and respiratory tract secretions or gastric hypersecretory during anesthesia, the dose is 4.4 μg/kg of body weight parenterally, 30 to 60 minutes before anesthesia. For dysrhythmias during anesthesia or surgery, 0.1 mg IV is given at 2- to 3-minute intervals as necessary. As a cholinergic adjunct medication, glycopyrrolate 0.2 mg IV is given for each 1 mg of neostigmine or 5 mg of pyridostigmine and may be administered in the same syringe.

Parenteral dosages for children with peptic ulcer have not been determined. To prevent or reduce excessive salivation and respiratory tract secretions or gastric hypersecretory situations during pediatric anesthesia, 4.4 to 8.8 μg/kg of body weight IM is given 30 to 60 minutes before anesthesia. For children with dysrhythmias during anesthesia or in surgery, the dose is 4.4 μg/kg of body weight IV given every 2 or 3 minutes as necessary. As a cholinergic adjunct medication with children, glycopyrrolate 0.2 mg IV is given for each 1 mg of neostigmine or 5 mg of pyridostigmine and may be administered in the same syringe.

clidinium [kli di′ nee um] (Quarzan)

Clidinium is a synthetic product related to the belladonna alkaloids, especially atropine. It competitively antagonizes acetylcholine at the postganglionic parasympathetic receptor sites in both smooth muscles and the secretory glands, thus reducing GI motility and gastric acid secretion. Ganglionic blockade may be produced if high doses of clidinium are given. Unlike atropine, it produces few, if any, CNS side effects or alterations on the eye.

Clidinium is indicated as an adjunctive treatment for peptic ulcers. After oral absorption the onset of action occurs within 1 hour; the duration of action lasts up to 3 hours. Clidinium is metabolized in the liver and excreted primarily by the kidneys. For side effects and adverse reactions, see Table 15-3.

Drug interactions, warnings, and contraindications

See discussion of atropine.

Dosage and administration

The adult dose is 2.5 to 5 mg PO three or four times daily, before meals and at bedtime. Dosage for the elderly or debilitated patient is 2.5 mg orally three times a day before meals. The pediatric dosage has not been determined.

GANGLIONIC DRUGS

The major neurotransmitter of all autonomic ganglia is acetylcholine. As postganglionic fibers produce specific effects on smooth muscle, cardiac muscle, and glands (see Fig. 14-2), nonselective drugs, agents that stimulate or block in this area, can result in a broad range of pharmacologic effects. This section will address drugs that affect nicotinic or cholinergic receptor sites on autonomic ganglia, that is, (1) ganglionic stimulating drugs and (2) ganglionic blocking drugs.

GANGLIONIC STIMULATING DRUGS

NICOTINE

Nicotine is a liquid alkaloid, freely soluble in water. It turns brown on exposure to air and is the chief alkaloid in tobacco. Nicotine has no therapeutic use but is of great pharmacologic interest and toxicologic importance. Its use in experiments performed on animals has helped to increase the understanding of the autonomic nervous system. Nicotine is readily absorbed from the gastrointestinal tract, respiratory mucous membrane, and skin.

Pharmacologic Effects

Nicotine may produce a variety of complex and often unpredictable effects in the body. Many actions are dose related, with generally small doses inducing activation or stimulation and larger doses producing a decreased or depressed response. Because nicotine acts on multiple systems within the body, the ultimate response may be the sum of the different stimulation and depressant actions of this chemical.

At the autonomic ganglia, nicotine temporarily stimulates all sympathetic and parasympathetic ganglia. This is followed by depression, which tends to last longer than the period of stimulation. Its effects on skeletal muscle are similar to its effects on the ganglia: a depressant phase follows stimulation. During the depressant phase, nicotine exerts a curare-like action on skeletal muscle.

Nicotine stimulates the central nervous system, especially the medullary centers (respiratory, emetic, and vasomotor). Large doses may cause tremor and convulsions. Stimulation is followed by depression. Death may result from respiratory failure, although it may be caused more by the curare-like action of nicotine on nerve endings in the diaphragm, rather than by action on the respiratory center.

The actions and effects of nicotine on the cardiovascular system are complex. Heart rate is frequently slowed at first but later may be accelerated above normal. Various disturbances in rhythm have been observed. The small blood vessels in peripheral parts of the body constrict but later may dilate, and the blood pressure will fall; this occurs in nicotine poisoning. Nicotine also has an antidiuretic action. Repeated administration of nicotine causes development of tolerance to some of its effects.

Toxicity

Nicotine has both short- and long-term toxic effects that are extremely important to the healthcare professional. Nicotine toxicity has resulted from misuse of insecticides containing nicotine, which at times has led to the death of farm workers. And because nicotine is a major ingredient in tobacco products, both acute toxicity (with ingestion of such products by small children) and chronic toxicity are well documented. See the box for management of a nicotine overdose.

Tobacco Smoking and Nicotine

Burning of tobacco can generate approximately 4000 compounds in a gaseous and a particulate or particle phase and 60 carcinogens (Environmental Tobacco Smoke, 1998). Gas phase substances include carbon monoxide, carbon dioxide, hydrogen cyanide, ammonia, volatile nitrosamines, and many other substances. The particulate phase contains mainly nicotine, water, and tar. Known carcinogens such as tar, formaldehyde, hydrogen cyanide, benzene, carbon monoxide, and others have been identified as etiologic factors in a variety of neoplastic diseases, such as cancer of the blad-

MANAGEMENT OF DRUG OVERDOSE

Nicotine

SIGNS AND SYMPTOMS

Increased flow of saliva, nausea and vomiting, abdominal cramps, diarrhea, confusion, cold sweat, headache, fainting, hypotension, tachycardia, prostration, and collapse. Convulsions may occur; death usually results from respiratory failure.

GENERAL APPROACH

Nicotine gum: To decrease absorption, induce vomiting in conscious patient with ipecac syrup. If person is unconscious, a gastric lavage followed by an activated charcoal suspension left in the stomach is used. A saline laxative will aid in elimination from the gastrointestinal tract.

Transdermal system: Remove patch and flush area with water. Do not use soap as it may enhance nicotine absorption. If patch was swallowed, an activated charcoal suspension is administered and repeated for as long as the patch is in the GI tract. A saline laxative or sorbitol may be added to the first activated charcoal dose to increase the passage of the patch.

SPECIFIC APPROACH

Treat medical complications as necessary. For example,

- Give respiratory support and interventions for respiratory failure
- Treat hypotension and cardiovascular collapse aggressively
- Use anticonvulsants (diazepam or barbiturates) for convulsions
- Use atropine for excessive bronchial secretions

Closely monitor and treat other side and adverse effects as necessary.

der, lung, buccal cavity, esophagus, and pancreas. Other smoking-related illnesses include pulmonary emphysema, chronic bronchitis, coronary heart disease, and myocardial infarction. Chronic dyspepsia may develop in heavy smokers; patients with gastric ulcer are usually advised to avoid smoking. Of considerable importance is the fact that smokers absorb sufficient nicotine to exert a variety of effects on the autonomic nervous system.

In individuals with peripheral vascular disease such as thromboangiitis obliterans (Buerger's disease), nicotine is generally believed to be a contributing factor in the disease. It may cause spasms of the peripheral blood vessels thus reducing the blood flow through the affected vessels. Vasospasm in the retinal blood vessels of the eye, associated with smoking of tobacco, is thought to cause serious disturbance of vision.

Passive smoking (involuntary smoking or second-hand smoke) refers to the inhalation of cigarette smoke by nonsmokers. Even though this exposure is less concentrated than inhaled smoke, the health risk and harmful effects to the nonsmoker can be significant. Reports from the U.S. Surgeon General and the Expert Committee on Passive Smoking indicate that (1) environmental smoke can cause lung cancer in healthy nonsmokers; (2) children of parents who smoke often have a greater incidence of respiratory tract symptoms and infections than children from a nonsmoking family; (3) environmental smoke may be a risk factor for cardiac disease; and (4) studies have linked environmental smoke exposure to cancers other than lung (Environmental Tobacco Smoke, 1998).

In addition, mothers who smoke may deliver infants with low birth weights and increased incidence of congenital abnormalities. Children of parents who smoke have an increased incidence of sudden infant death syndrome, an increased incidence of respiratory infections and allergic reactions, and an increased likelihood of becoming smokers. Special effort should be made to assist women to stop smoking, particularly during the childbearing years.

The addictive component of tobacco is nicotine. Many drugs are reported to interact with nicotine. See the following section on drug interactions for additional information.

nicotine gum [nik' oe teen] (Nicorette)
nicotine transdermal systems
(Habitrol, Nicoderm, Nicotrol, Prostep)
nicotine nasal spray (Nicotrol NS)

Nicotine is available in gum (resin) and transdermal systems (patches) for use in smoking cessation programs. The nicotine resin is in the form of chewing gum and provides a source of nicotine for the nicotine-dependent patient who is undergoing acute cigarette withdrawal. When the person has a strong urge to smoke, a stick of gum is chewed instead, which relieves the physical symptoms of nicotine withdrawal. The number of pieces of gum chewed is gradually reduced over a 2- to 3-month period. For mechanism of action, see the discussion of pharmacologic effects of nicotine.

Pharmacokinetics

Nicotine gum is indicated for adjunct treatment of nicotine dependence. It is absorbed through buccal mucosa, slower than if inhaled while smoking. It is metabolized primarily by the hepatic route, with smaller amounts metabolized in the kidney and lung. The half-life is 1 to 2 hours. Elimination is primarily renal with 10% excreted unchanged and the remainder as metabolites; the drug is excreted in breast milk.

Nicotine transdermal systems (patches) are also available to aid a person in withdrawing from smoking. Three of the patches (Habitrol, Nicoderm, and Prostep) are worn for 24 hours whereas Nicotrol was formulated to be worn for 16 hours a day. The latter patch was designed to mimic the individual's natural smoking pattern, which usually has higher nicotine serum levels during the day with lower nicotine levels overnight. Thus a decrease in nicotine serum levels will theoretically not affect the patient's sleeping

BOX 15-1 Nicotine Transdermal Systems

Brand Name	Dosage Per Patch	Recommended Duration of Use
Habitrol	21 mg/24 hr	4-8 wk
	14 mg/24 hr	2-4 wk
	7 mg/24 hr	2-4 wk
Nicotrol	15 mg/16 hr	4-12 wk
	10 mg/16 hr	2-4 wk
	5 mg/16 hr	2-4 wk
Nicoderm	21 mg/24 hr	6 wk
	14 mg/24 hr	2-4 wk
	7 mg/24 hr	2-4 wk
Prostep	22 mg/24 hr	4-8 wk
	11 mg/24 hr	2-4 wk

patterns. A potential disadvantage is that the drug-free period may result in early morning craving for a cigarette. Box 15-1 lists products and dosage forms. To achieve long-term smoking abstinence, all four products should be used in conjunction with a behavioral modification program.

Nicotine nasal spray administers 1 mg of nicotine per two sprays to the nasal membrane. The spray is comparable in efficacy to the gum and patches, but it has a faster onset of action. The patient should be instructed to stop smoking before using the spray and not to use any other nicotine products while using this product. The Food and Drug Administration (FDA) recommends that the spray be used for at least 3 months but not longer than 6 months because it is possible to become dependent on the spray (New Drugs/Drug News, 1996).

Drug interactions

The following effects may occur when nicotine is taken with the drugs listed below:

Drug	Possible effect and management
acetaminophen, caffeine, oxazepam (Serax), pentazocine (Talwin), propranolol (Inderal), propoxyphene (Darvon), and theophylline	Smoking increases drug metabolism, which may result in lower blood levels of these medications. Thus some persons may require higher or more frequent drug dosing. Smoking cessation will generally reverse this effect.
Adrenergic agonists or blocking agents, catecholamines, and cortisol	Smoking and nicotine increase cortisol and catecholamine levels; therefore therapy with the adrenergic agonists or blocking agents may require dosage adjustment based on the individual's response.
furosemide (Lasix)	When used in combination with nicotine (smoking), a decrease in diuretic effect and cardiac output has been reported. These effects may be reversed if the person stops smoking.
insulin	Smoking cessation may result in an increased insulin effect; dosage reduction may be necessary. Monitor closely for symptoms of hypoglycemia.

Side effects and adverse reactions

Side effects include belching, fast heart beat, mild headache, increased appetite, increased watering of mouth, sore mouth or throat, coughing, dizziness or lightheadedness, dry mouth, hiccups, hoarseness, irritability, indigestion, and difficulty in sleeping. Transdermal patches may cause pruritus and/or erythema under the patch, a generalized rash, nausea, dizziness, myalgias, coughing, difficulty in sleeping, and nightmares. Adverse reactions with nicotine gum include injury to mouth, teeth, or dental work. Early signs of overdose are nausea and vomiting, severe increased watering of the mouth, severe abdominal pain, diarrhea, cold sweat, severe headache, severe dizziness, disturbed hearing and vision, confusion, and severe weakness while advanced overdose signs include fainting, hypotension, difficult breathing, fast, weak, or irregular pulse, and convulsions.

Warnings

Use with caution in persons with angina pectoris, cardiac dysrhythmias, insulin-dependent diabetes mellitus, hypertension, hyperthyroidism, Buerger's disease, a history of myocardial infarction, peptic ulcer disease, and pheochromocytoma.

Contraindications

Avoid use in patients with nicotine hypersensitivity, severe angina pectoris, and life-threatening cardiac dysrhythmias, and after myocardial infarction.

Dosage and administration

The oral dosage is 2 mg as a chewing gum, repeated as needed to curb the person's urge to smoke, with up to 30 pieces of gum per day maximum. The gum should be chewed intermittently and very slowly when the individual has the urge to smoke. Most patients require about 10 pieces of gum per day during the first month of treatment. Transdermal systems: patches are reapplied every 24 hours except in the case of Nicotrol, which is worn for 16 hours each day.

GANGLIONIC BLOCKING DRUGS

Ganglionic blocking agents block the action of acetylcholine on the ganglion cells by competing with acetylcholine at the synapse of autonomic ganglia. This results in reduced impulse transmission from preganglionic to postganglionic fibers in both sympathetic and parasympathetic nerves. A blockade of sympathetic ganglia abolishes vasoconstrictor tone; the blood vessels dilate and arterial blood pressure falls (antihypertensive effect).

In 1950 the methonium derivatives were introduced, and hexamethonium chloride became the drug of choice to treat severe and malignant hypertension. Despite the difficulties in managing individuals receiving hexamethonium because of its erratic absorption and action and severe side effects, its use demonstrated that severe hypertension could be controlled. Since 1961, the ganglionic blocking agents have been rarely used as newer antihypertensive drugs that have more selective action and fewer severe side effects are preferred.

However, the student should be aware of these products because some prescribers may select trimethaphan as an alternative for patients who are resistant to the effects of sodium nitroprusside. Other prescribers may use a ganglionic blocking agent such as trimethaphan for the treatment of a hypertensive crisis in individuals with an acute dissecting aortic aneurysm. The two ganglionic blocking agents available are mecamylamine hydrochloride (Inversine tablets) and trimethaphan camsylate (Arfonad injection). Because mecamylamine has many side effects and is not considered a first-line drug in the treatment of hypertension, the healthcare professional is referred to the package insert or current USP DI for additional information on this product.

trimethaphan camsylate [trye meth′ a fan] (Arfonad)

Trimethaphan camsylate is used in the treatment of hypertension and is administered by intravenous infusion. It is also used to produce controlled hypotension during surgery.

Pharmacokinetics

The onset of action is immediate, and the duration of effect is 10 to 15 minutes. Metabolism is probably by pseudocholinesterase. The drug is excreted mostly unchanged by the kidneys.

Drug interactions

The following effects may occur when trimethaphan is given with the drugs listed below:

Drug	Possible effect and management
ambenonium (Mytelase), neostigmine (Prostigmin), or pyridostigmine (Mestinon)	The antimyasthenic effects of these drugs will be blocked, which may result in increased weakness and inability to swallow. Avoid or a potentially serious drug drug interaction may occur.

Color type indicate an unsafe drug combination.

Side effects and adverse reactions

See Table 15-3.

Warnings

Use with caution in persons with prostatic hypertrophy, glaucoma, urethral stricture, chronic pyelonephritis, and a history of allergies.

Contraindications

Avoid use in patients with a trimethaphan hypersensitivity, Addison's disease, anemia, hypovolemia, cerebrovascular, coronary or respiratory insufficiency, diabetes mellitus, and liver or renal function impairment and in debilitated patients.

Dosage and administration

For a hypertensive emergency in adults, the dosage is 0.5 to 1 mg/min by intravenous infusion, adjusting as necessary. The maintenance dosage is 1 to 5 mg/min by intravenous infusion. To control blood pressure during surgery, the dosage is 3 to 4 mg/min initially, adjusted as necessary. The maintenance dose is 0.2 to 6 mg/min by intravenous infusion.

The elderly may be more sensitive to trimethaphan, so a lower dosage with close monitoring of the blood pressure is indicated. With children, the dosage is initially 0.05 to 0.15 mg/min by intravenous infusion, adjusting the dosage as necessary.

SUMMARY

This chapter reviews the drugs that may mimic, intensify, or inhibit the effects of the parasympathetic nervous system. The cholinergic receptor sites that are stimulated by acetylcholine are either nicotinic or muscarinic, that is, nicotinic receptors appear in the ganglia of both the parasympathetic and sympathetic fibers, adrenal medulla, and skeletal muscle (somatic motor system) while the muscarinic receptors are located at postganglionic sites in smooth muscle, cardiac muscle, and glands. Therefore drugs that affect acetylcholine at either site can produce profound effects in the human system. Cholinergic (parasympathomimetic) medications are used primarily to stimulate the intestine and bladder postoperatively, terminate curarization, lower intraocular pressure, promote salivation and sweating, dilate peripheral blood vessels, and treat myasthenia gravis. Conversely, the anticholinergic (parasympatholytic) drugs are used to treat illnesses with spasms, such as irritable bowel syndrome, spastic biliary disorders, and urinary disorders. They are also used as preanesthetic drugs to decrease respiratory secretions. Ganglionic blocking drugs are indicated for the management of severe and malignant hypertension, but the advent of more selective and effective antihypertensive drugs has limited their use.

REVIEW QUESTIONS

1. Bethanechol (Urecholine) is contraindicated for use in patients with asthma, severe bradycardia, GI obstruc-

tion, and peptic ulcer. Discuss why this drug has these contraindications by reviewing cholinergic stimulation effects on these diseases/illnesses.

2. Discuss the effects of atropine in the body, particularly on smooth muscle, cardiac muscle, exocrine glands, and the eye. Name four indications for atropine.
3. Review the pharmacologic, toxic, and passive smoking effects of nicotine. Discuss the potential problems that may result from smoking during pregnancy. As a health-care professional, how would you address this problem?

REFERENCES

Environmental Tobacco Smoke: *Cancer facts, 3.90,* http://rex.nci.nih.gov/INFO__CANCER/Cancer__facts/Section3/FS3__90.html (May 5, 1998).

New Drugs/Drug News: Nasal spray smoke cessation approved, *P&T* 21(6):303, 1996.

United States Pharmacopeial Convention: *USP DI: drug information for the health care professional,* ed 18, Rockville, Md, 1998, the Convention.

ADDITIONAL REFERENCES

Abramowicz M, editor: Nicotine patches, *Med Lett* 34(868):37, 1992.

American Hospital Formulary Service: *AHFS: drug information '98,* Bethesda, Md, 1998, American Society of Hospital Pharmacists.

American Medical Association: *AMA drug evaluations 1995,* Chicago, 1995, the Association.

Anderson KN et al, editors: *Mosby's medical, nursing, and allied health dictionary,* ed 5, St Louis, 1998, Mosby.

Geiger-Bronsky MJ: Anticholinergic therapy in the critically ill patient with bronchospasm, *AACN Clin Issues Adv Pract Acute Crit Care* 6(2):287, 1995.

Hardman JG, Limbird LE, editors: *Goodman & Gilman's the pharmacological basis of therapeutics,* ed 9, New York, 1996, McGraw-Hill.

Mosby: *Mosby's GenRx,* St Louis, 1998, Mosby.

Strecher WJ et al: Evaluation of a minimal contact smoking cessation program in a health care setting, *Patient Educ Counsel* 7(4):395, 1985.

CHAPTER 16

Drugs Affecting the Sympathetic (Adrenergic) Nervous System

CHAPTER FOCUS

The sympathetic (adrenergic) nervous system is the second major subdivision of the autonomic nervous system. This system regulates the heart, secretory glands, and smooth muscles and is responsible for the "fight or flight" reaction in the body. Drug therapies that interact with the adrenergic receptors are very common in clinical practice today. Therefore healthcare professionals must be well informed on drugs that affect the adrenergic nervous system.

OBJECTIVES

After reading and studying this chapter, the student should be able to the following:

1. *Define and discuss the key drugs and key terms.*
2. *Explain the major effects of the alpha$_1$-, alpha$_2$-, beta$_1$-, and beta$_2$ adrenergic effects.*
3. *Name and describe the three types of adrenergic drugs.*
4. *Discuss epinephrine's mechanism of action, indications, significant drug interactions, and side effects and adverse reactions.*
5. *Describe the effects of the three naturally occurring catecholamines on the body.*
6. *Name the three categories of the alpha-adrenergic blocking agents and list a drug example for each.*

KEY DRUGS

dopamine (p. 275)
epinephrine (p. 270)
norepinephrine (p. 373)

KEY TERMS

alpha-adrenergic blocking agents, (p. 279)
beta-adrenergic blocking agents, (p. 282)
calorigenic effect, (p. 270)
chronotropic effect, (p. 269)
dromotropic effect, (p. 269)
inotropic effect, (p. 269)
sympathomimetic drugs, (p. 267)

ADRENERGIC DRUGS

Sympathomimetic drugs are medications that enhance or mimic the effects of sympathetic nerve stimulation. These drugs are designed to produce actions similar to those of the neurotransmitters, such as increasing cardiac output, vasoconstriction of arterioles and veins, regulation of body temperature, bronchial dilation, and a variety of other effects. (For additional information on adrenergic effects, see Chapter 14.) The sympathomimetic drugs are also called adrenergic drugs. There are three types of adrenergic drugs: (1) direct-acting, (2) indirect-acting, and (3) dual-acting (direct and indirect) agents.

Direct-Acting Adrenergic Drugs

Catecholamines

The three naturally occurring catecholamines in the body—dopamine, norepinephrine, and epinephrine—are synthesized by the sympathetic nervous system. While dopamine is a precursor of norepinephrine and epinephrine, it also has a transmitter role of its own in certain portions of the central nervous system. (For information on adrenergic transmission, see Fig. 14-5 and the discussion in Chapter 14.)

Epinephrine is primarily an emergency hormone, while norepinephrine is an important transmitter of nerve impulses. The latter is also an intermediary in epinephrine biosynthesis. Catecholamines, which depend on their ability to interact directly with adrenergic receptors (alpha and beta), are called direct-acting drugs. Thus the response of these agents is mediated by directly stimulating the adrenergic receptors. In the sympathetic nervous system, the adrenergic effector cells contain two distinct receptors, the alpha (α) and beta (β) receptors.

There is evidence that the alpha receptors appear on two primary locations. The alpha$_2$ receptors are found on the presynaptic nerve terminals, platelets, and smooth muscle; thus they are called presynaptic (prejunctional) receptor sites. The presynaptic receptor controls the amount of transmitter released per nerve impulse, which can be regulated by a feedback mechanism. Thus when the concentration of transmitter released from the nerve terminal into the synaptic cleft reaches a high level, it stimulates the presynaptic receptors and prevents further release of the transmitter. This kind of feedback prevents excessive and prolonged stimulation of the postsynaptic cell. The postsynaptic receptors, which are located on the effector organs, are known as alpha$_1$ receptors (eye, arterioles, veins, male sex organ, and bladder neck).

The beta receptors are subdivided on the basis of their responses to drugs. Beta$_1$ receptors are primarily located in the heart, whereas beta$_2$ receptors mediate the actions of catecholamines on smooth muscle, especially bronchioles, arterial smooth muscle, and skeletal muscle.

Norepinephrine acts mainly on alpha receptors causing vasoconstriction. Epinephrine acts on both alpha and beta receptors, producing a mixture of vasodilation and vasoconstriction. Isoproterenol, a synthetic catecholamine, acts only on beta receptors. For a discussion of receptor sensitivity, see Box 16-1.

The most important alpha-adrenergic activities in humans include the following: (1) vasoconstriction of arterioles in the skin and splanchnic area, resulting in a rise in blood pressure; (2) pupil dilation; and (3) relaxation of the gut. Beta-adrenergic activity includes (1) cardiac acceleration and increased contractility, (2) vasodilation

BOX 16-1 Overview of Adrenergic Receptor Stimulation

Receptor	*Effect*
Alpha$_1$	Contraction or vasoconstriction of peripheral blood vessels
	Dilation (contraction) of pupil
	Increased contractibility of heart
Alpha$_2$	Limits or controls transmitter release
	Aggregation of platelets
	Contraction of smooth muscle
Beta$_1$	Increased acceleration of heart rate (chronotropic)
	Increased contractibility of heart (inotropic)
Beta$_2$	Dilation of bronchial smooth muscle
	Relaxation of uterus
	Activation of glycogenolysis

Location

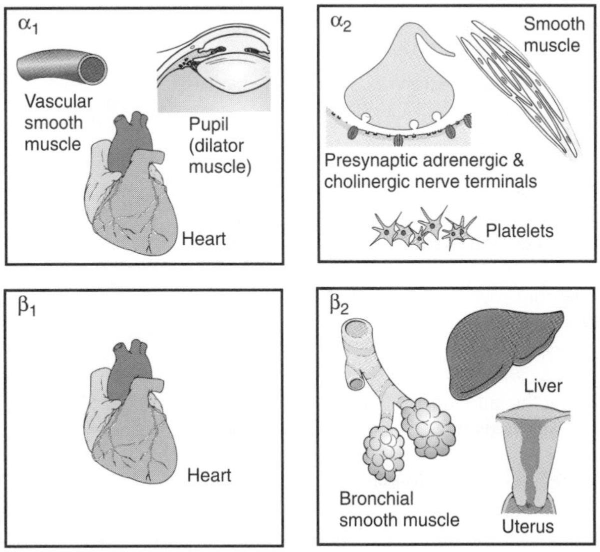

of arterioles supplying skeletal muscles, (3) bronchial relaxation, and (4) uterine relaxation. The effects of both alpha and beta stimulation result from a summation of action where they are interrelated. That is, a change in blood pressure will depend on the degree of vasoconstriction in the skin and splanchnic area and the extent of vasodilation in skeletal muscles, along with changes in heart rate. Large arteries and veins contain both alpha and beta receptors; the heart contains only beta receptors (Table 16-1).

Specific drugs that stimulate or block alpha and beta receptors are available. With the exception of central $alpha_2$ receptors, which are discussed in Chapter 21, these agents work at peripheral autonomic sites.

As catecholamines, norepinephrine and epinephrine are important neurohormones in neural and endocrine integration. They are always present in arterial blood, although the amount varies widely during any one day. Certain physiologic stimuli such as stress and exercise significantly increase blood levels of catecholamine. Studies indicate that the major sources of circulating norepinephrine are stimulated sympathetic nerve endings. Organs such as the heart and blood vessels receive a large fraction of blood and possess large numbers of sympathetic nerve endings; thus they contain the greatest amount of catecholamines. The number of sympathetic nerve endings or adrenergic nerves to various organs determines the magnitude of response of these organs to increased levels or injections of catecholamines.

TABLE 16-1 Adrenergic Receptor Stimulation

Effector Organs	*Receptor Type*	*Adrenergic Response*
Heart		
Cardiac muscle (atria, ventricles)	$beta_1$	Increased force of contraction (inotropic action)
Sinoatrial node	$beta_1$	Increased heart rate (chronotropic action)
Atrioventricular node	$beta_1$	Increased automaticity and conduction velocity; shortened refractory period (chronotropic action)
Blood vessels		
Arterioles		
Coronary	$alpha_1$, $beta_2$, dopaminergic	Constriction, dilation*
Cerebral	$alpha_1$	Constriction
Pulmonary	$alpha_1$, $beta_2$	Constriction,* dilation
Mesenteric visceral	$alpha_1$, $beta_2$	Constriction,* dilation
Renal	$alpha_1$, $beta_2$, dopaminergic	Constriction,* dilation
Skin, mucosa	$alpha_1$, $alpha_2$	Constriction
Skeletal muscle	$alpha_1$, $beta_2$	Constriction, dilation
Veins	$alpha_1$, $beta_2$	Constriction, dilation
Lung		
Bronchial smooth muscle	$beta_2$	Bronchodilation
Bronchial glands	$alpha_1$, $beta_2$	Inhibition
Gastrointestinal tract		
Smooth muscle (motility, tone)	$alpha_1$, $alpha_2$, $beta_2$	Decreased
Sphincter	$alpha_1$	Contraction
Secretion	?	Inhibition
Gallbladder and ducts	—	Relaxation
Liver	$beta_2$	Glycogenolysis
Spleen capsule	$alpha_1$, $beta_2$	Contraction,* relaxation
Pancreas: insulin secretion	$alpha_2$	Decreased
Adipose tissue	$beta_1$	Lipolysis
Urinary bladder		
Detrusor muscle	$beta_2$	Relaxation
Sphincter	$alpha_1$	Contraction
Kidney ureter	$alpha_1$	Contraction
Kidney secretion (renin)	$beta_1$	Increased
Uterus		
Pregnant	$alpha_1$	Contraction
Nonpregnant	$beta_2$	Relaxation
Sex organs, male	$alpha_1$	Ejaculation
Skin		
Pilomotor muscles	$alpha_1$	Contraction
Sweat glands	$alpha_1$, cholinergic	Increased secretion
Eye		
Radial muscle, iris (pupil size)	$alpha_1$	Contraction: pupil dilation (mydriasis)
Ciliary muscle	$beta_2$	Relaxation for far vision

*Predominant response.

Pharmacologic effects

Catecholamines produce a variety of physiologic responses.

Cardiac. Epinephrine and norepinephrine produce almost the same cardiac responses when injected. A significant increase in myocardial contraction (positive **inotropic effect**) is the result of increased influx of calcium into cardiac fibers. The strong myocardial contractions result in more complete emptying of the ventricles and an increase in cardiac work and oxygen consumption. Strong contractions brought about by isoproterenol and epinephrine also increase cardiac output, or volume. Norepinephrine, on the other hand, may not alter cardiac output and may even decrease it slightly. This effect of norepinephrine is believed to result from its potent vasoconstriction action, which increases resistance to ejection of blood from the heart. The increased work of the heart to move the blood against increased pressure is "pressure work" rather than "volume work."

It has been shown experimentally and clinically that 0.5 mg of epinephrine injected into arterial or venous blood and circulated by cardiac compression or massage may stimulate spontaneous and vigorous cardiac contractions. Even though the heart is in ventricular fibrillation, epinephrine increases fibrillation vigor and frequently promotes successful electric defibrillation of the individual. In these situations the drug may be injected repeatedly. However, epinephrine cannot be used repeatedly to improve the function of a failing heart (congestive heart failure), because it increases oxygen consumption by cardiac muscle. It can also cause anginal pain in patients with angina pectoris because it increases cardiac oxygen demand. Therefore although it increases coronary blood flow, its use is contraindicated for persons with angina. The production of strong contractions provides the rationale for the use of epinephrine in cardiac arrest.

A significant increase in cardiac rate (positive **chronotropic effect**) is the result of the increased rate of membrane depolarization in the pacemaker cells in the sinus node during diastole. Action potential threshold is reached sooner, pacemaker cells fire more often, and heart rate increases.

Norepinephrine, with its predominantly alpha-adrenergic activity, may not produce as severe a tachycardia as epinephrine. The increased vasoconstriction and increased blood pressure may cause a reflex bradycardia. Isoproterenol usually produces a tachycardia, since its direct and reflex effects act in the same direction. Dosage and patient variables affect these responses.

An increase in atrioventricular conduction (positive **dromotropic effect**) is another physiologic response. Because epinephrine increases atrioventricular conduction, some cardiologists use it in the treatment of heart block.

Catecholamines may also produce spontaneous firing of Purkinje fibers, which may cause them to exhibit pacemaker activity. This effect may cause ventricular extrasystoles and increase the susceptibility of ventricular muscle to fibrillation. These effects are more likely to occur with epinephrine than norepinephrine.

Vascular. Vascular effects of the catecholamines depend on the dose and the vascular bed affected. Low doses of epinephrine may decrease total peripheral vascular resistance and decrease blood pressure. In large doses epinephrine activates alpha receptors in the greater peripheral vascular system, which increases resistance and increases blood pressure. Norepinephrine elevates blood pressure by increasing peripheral resistance and decreasing blood flow through skeletal muscles.

Norepinephrine, a vasoconstrictor, increases total peripheral resistance. Isoproterenol is not a vasoconstrictor but a pure vasodilator; epinephrine is both a vasoconstrictor and vasodilator, with vasodilation being greater in its overall net effects. For example, during great stress, the release of epinephrine from the adrenal medulla constricts blood vessels in the skin and splanchnic areas but dilates those of skeletal muscles, thus shunting blood to the areas needed for "fight or flight" responses.

Renal artery constriction and resistance is greater with epinephrine than with norepinephrine. In large doses, epinephrine may actually stop blood flow through some nephrons and stimulate release of antidiuretic hormone, thereby reducing urinary excretion.

Central nervous system. In sufficient amounts, epinephrine and isoproterenol can lead to alertness, tremors, respiratory stimulation, and anxiety. Norepinephrine is less likely to cause anxiety and tremors. Beneficial cerebral effects from epinephrine and norepinephrine in persons with hypotension are thought to be the result of increased systemic pressure with a resultant improvement in cerebral blood flow.

Smooth muscle. Generally the catecholamines relax nonvascular smooth muscles. When smooth muscle of the gastrointestinal (GI) tract is relaxed, the amplitude and tone of intestinal peristalsis are reduced. In theory, this may retard propulsion of food and gastrointestinal emptying; however, this effect is rare in humans with therapeutic doses of catecholamines.

In some situations smooth muscle of some organs reacts like vascular smooth muscle and contracts. For example, radial and sphincter muscles of the iris contract, and the smooth muscle of the lids may contract, giving rise to the widened, staring eyes seen in sympathetically stimulated individuals.

In the urinary bladder epinephrine causes trigone and sphincter constriction and detrusor relaxation with a delay in the desire to void.

Respiratory. Catecholamines dilate bronchial smooth muscle. Isoproterenol is a more active bronchodilator than epinephrine, while epinephrine is a stronger bronchodilator than norepinephrine.

Glandular. Epinephrine may increase the amount of viscid saliva excreted; however, as a rule, sympathomimetics

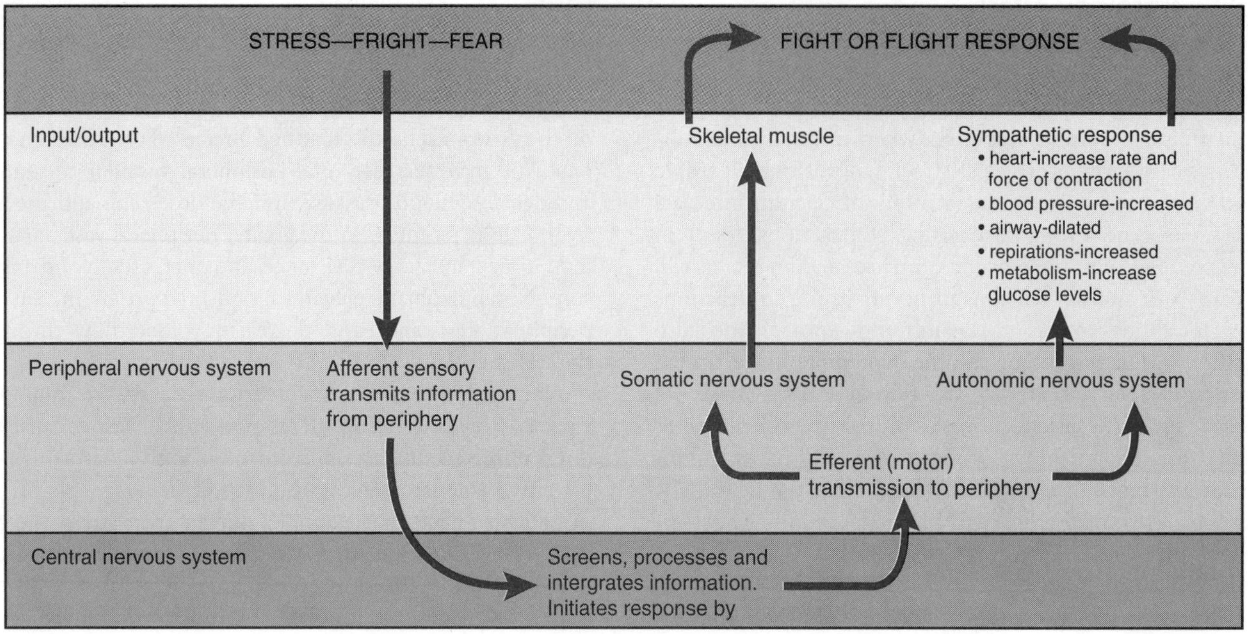

FIGURE 16-1
Nervous system response to severe fright or stress.

decrease secretion and produce a dry mouth. Catecholamines may produce local sweating on the palms of the hands and in the axillary and genital areas. The exact mechanism for these effects is not clear.

Metabolic. Epinephrine inhibits insulin secretion. Catecholamines have antagonistic effects on gluconeogenesis, and they decrease liver and skeletal muscle glycogen and increase lipolysis in adipose tissue. The result of these effects is a rise in blood glucose and an increase in free fatty acids. Thus in response to stress ("fight or flight" response), there can be an abundant supply of fuel and energy (Fig. 16-1).

Catecholamines also have a **calorigenic effect** (capable of generating heat, which increases oxygen consumption) resulting from the sum of the preceding effects. Norepinephrine's action in relation to these effects is weaker than that of epinephrine or isoproterenol.

epinephrine [ep i nef′ rin] (Adrenalin)

Epinephrine is available in solutions for inhalation and nebulization and parenteral and ophthalmic administration. Many bronchodilator aerosols are available over the counter in solutions containing up to 1% of the epinephrine base. For example:

- epinephrine inhalation aerosol (Bronkaid Mist, Bronkaid Mistometer ♣)
- epinephrine bitartrate inhalation aerosol (Asthmahaler, Medihaler-Epi)
- racepinephrine inhalation solution (AsthmaNefrin, Vaponefrin)

Parenteral dosage forms and ophthalmic solutions include the following:

- epinephrine injection (Adrenalin, EpiPen Auto-Injector)
- sterile epinephrine suspension (Sus-Phrine)

Ophthalmic epinephrine is discussed in Chapter 36.

Mechanism of action

Epinephrine is a direct-acting catecholamine which is naturally released from the adrenal medulla in response to sympathoadrenal stimulation. It also is prepared synthetically. Epinephrine stimulates alpha and beta receptors although its primary action is on the beta receptors of the heart, the smooth muscle of the bronchi, and the blood vessels. The $beta_1$ action stimulates the heart by increasing heart rate, force of myocardial contraction, and cardiac output. The $beta_2$ action on the smooth muscle of the bronchioles produces bronchodilation, thereby increasing tidal volume and vital capacity of the lung. Stimulation of alpha receptors constricts arterioles of the bronchioles and inhibits histamine release, thus reducing nasal congestion and edema. In contrast, $beta_2$ adrenergic activity of the smooth muscle of arterioles causes vasodilation.

Another effect of epinephrine is alpha activity, which results in contraction of the radial muscle in the iris ($alpha_1$), causing dilation of the pupil (mydriasis). Constriction of the blood vessels in the skin is also activated by alpha activity. The detrusor muscle in the urinary bladder contains beta receptors and is relaxed by epinephrine (Table 16-1).

Indications

1. Used for symptomatic treatment of bronchial asthma and other obstructive pulmonary diseases, such as

chronic bronchitis and emphysema, which cause bronchospasm.

2. Used for symptomatic relief of acute hypersensitivity reactions. Indicated in the emergency treatment of acute anaphylactic shock and severe acute reactions to drugs, animal serums, insect stings, and other allergens to relieve bronchospasm, urticaria, hives, angioneurotic edema, and swelling of nasal mucosa. Pulmonary congestion is also alleviated by constriction of mucosal blood vessels.
3. Used as an adjunct with local anesthetics. Concurrent administration of epinephrine with local anesthetics reduces circulation to the site, which results in a slowing of vascular absorption. This promotes a local effect of the anesthetic and also prolongs its duration of action, thus reducing the risk of anesthetic toxicity.
4. Administered as a hemostatic agent to control superficial bleeding from arterioles and capillaries in the skin, mucous membranes, or other tissues.
5. Used in ocular surgery to control bleeding, induce mydriasis and conjunctival decongestion, and decrease intraocular pressure.
6. Used to treat cardiac arrest or cardiac standstill. On occasion it may be given by intracardiac injection in acute attacks of ventricular standstill after physical measures and electrical defibrillation have failed.

Pharmacokinetics

Epinephrine should not be given orally because it is rapidly metabolized in the mucosa of the GI tract and liver; serum levels achieved would be inadequate. It is well absorbed after IM or SC injection.

Epinephrine has a rapid onset of action, from 3 to 5 minutes by inhalation or between 6 and 15 minutes after SC injection. The duration of action of epinephrine is 1 to 3 hours by inhalation and 1 to 4 hours after IM or SC injection. In severe anaphylaxis, asthma, or cardiac arrest, epinephrine doses may need to be repeated every 5 to 20 minutes, depending on dosage used and patient's response. Epinephrine is metabolized in the liver and excreted in the kidneys.

Drug interactions

The following interactions may occur when epinephrine is given with the drugs listed below:

Drug	Possible effect and management
Anesthetics, such as cyclopropane, halothane (Fluothane), enflurane (Ethrane), isoflurane (Forane), trichloroethylene, etc.	May sensitize the heart, increasing risk of severe dysrhythmias. Monitor closely because a reduction in epinephrine (sympathomimetics) is usually necessary.
Local parenteral anesthetics	When used in end artery areas, such as fingers, toes, or penis, the reduced blood supply to the area may result in ischemia and gangrene. Use very cautiously in such areas and monitor closely.
Beta-adrenergic receptor blocking agents, including ophthalmics	Therapeutic effects of both agents may be inhibited. With bronchodilators having both alpha and beta stimulating effects (epinephrine) with beta receptor blockade, stimulation of alpha receptors may result in hypertension, severe bradycardia, and possibly heart block. Avoid or serious drug interaction may occur.
Digitalis glycosides	Digitalis sensitizes the myocardium to the effects of epinephrine; the additive effect of the catecholamine may precipitate ectopic pacemaker activity. Avoid or serious drug interaction may occur.
ergotamine or vascular ergoloid mesylates (Hydergine)	Concurrent use may produce severe hypertension, peripheral vascular ischemia, and gangrene. Avoid or serious drug interaction may occur.
maprotiline (Ludiomil), tricyclic antidepressants, monoamine oxidase (MAO) inhibitor antidepressants, or cocaine	Concurrent use may result in dysrhythmias, tachycardia, and hypertension or hyperpyrexia. Avoid or serious drug interaction may occur.

Color type indicates an unsafe drug combination.

Side effects and adverse reactions

These include increased nervousness, restlessness, insomnia, tachycardia, tremors, sweating, increased blood pressure, nausea, vomiting, pallor, and weakness. With inhalation devices, side effects and adverse reactions include bronchial irritation and coughing (with high doses), dry mouth and throat, headaches, and flushing of face and skin.

Warnings

Use with caution in patients with diabetes mellitus, angle-closure glaucoma, hyperthyroidism, Parkinson's disease, and pheochromocytoma.

Contraindications

Avoid use in persons with known hypersensitivity to epinephrine (or sympathomimetics), organic brain damage, cardiovascular disease, and shock.

Dosage and administration

See Table 16-2.

TABLE 16-2 Epinephrine: Dosage and Administration

Indication	*Adults*	*Children*
Parenteral		
Bronchodilator	SC 0.2-0.5 mg every 20 min up to 4 hr as needed, with dosage increase to max. 1 mg/dose if needed.	SC 0.01 mg/kg every 15 min for 2 doses, then every 4 hr if needed. Max. dose 0.5 mg/dose.
Anaphylaxis	IM/SC 0.2-0.5 mg repeated every 10-15 min as needed, with dosage increase to max. of 1 mg/dose if needed.	SC 0.01 mg/kg repeated every 15 min for 2 doses, then every 4 hr as needed; severe cases: dosage may increase to 0.5 mg/dose.
Cardiac stimulant	IV or intracardiac injection 0.1-1 mg (base) diluted to 10 ml with sodium chloride injection given to restore myocardial contractility. After intracardiac administration, external cardiac massage should be applied to enhance drug entry into coronary circulation. May repeat every 5 min if needed. Endotracheal tube instillation dosage is 1 mg (base) for cardiac resuscitation.	IV or intracardiac, 0.005-0.01 mg/kg; repeat every 5 min or follow with IV infusion at initial rate of 0.001 mg/kg/min. May be increased in increments of 0.0001 mg/kg/min if necessary to max. of 0.0015 mg/kg/min.
Anesthetic (local) adjunct	Intraspinal 0.2-0.4 mg added to anesthetic spinal mixture. With local anesthetic: 0.1 to 0.2 mg in a 1:200,000 to 1:20,000 solution.	See adult dosing.
Auto-injection		
Auto-injector for emergency self-treatment of anaphylaxis (EpiPen Auto-Injector)	Available in 0.5 and 1 mg/ml.	
Suspension (Sus-Phrine)		
Bronchodilator	SC 0.5 mg initially, followed by 0.5-1.5 mg every 6 hr as necessary.	SC 0.025 mg/kg. May be repeated in 6 hr. If child weighs 30 kg, max. single dose is 0.75 mg.
Inhalation		
Bronchodilator 1:100 (1%) solution	Proper dose automatically dispensed by metered nebulizer. Allow 1-5 min between inhalations. Use fewest possible inhalations.	
Topical		
Nasal decongestant	1-2 drops (0.1% solution) every 4-6 hr.	
Antihemorrhagic	0.002%-0.1% (1:50,000 to 1:1000) solution of epinephrine applied locally.	

isoproterenol hydrochloride

[eye soe proe ter′ enole] (Isuprel)

isoproterenol sulfate (Medihaler Iso)

Isoproterenol, a synthetic catecholamine, is a nonselective beta-adrenergic drug; it stimulates $beta_1$- and $beta_2$-adrenergic receptors. The $beta_1$ receptor activity produces an increase in the force of myocardial contraction and heart rate. The $beta_2$ receptor response of the smooth muscle of the bronchi, skeletal muscle, GI tract, and blood vessels of the splanchnic bed causes a relaxation of these organs. More importantly, isoproterenol can greatly relax the smaller bronchi and may even dilate the trachea and main bronchi. This drug also stimulates insulin secretion and releases free fatty acid.

Hemodynamically, the $beta_1$ activity of the heart increases cardiac output and venous return to the heart. Moreover peripheral vascular resistance is reduced, and in normal individuals it may cause a significant drop in blood pressure with excessive dosage.

Indications

Isoproterenol is used as a cardiac stimulant in cardiac arrest, Adams-Stokes syndrome, atrioventricular block, and carotid sinus hypersensitivity. It also may be used as adjunct therapy in treatment of cardiogenic shock, and it relieves bronchospasm associated with bronchial asthma, pulmonary emphysema, and bronchitis.

Pharmacokinetics

Isoproterenol is readily absorbed when given parenterally or by inhalation. Absorption of sublingual isoproterenol is erratic and unreliable. Its duration of action is usually up to 2 hours after oral inhalation or subcutaneous administration and less than 1 hour after IV administration. Isoproterenol is metabolized in the GI tract, liver, and lungs and is excreted in the urine.

Drug interactions

See epinephrine. Also avoid concurrent administration of isoproterenol with epinephrine as an increase in adverse effects and cardiotoxicity may result.

Side effects and adverse reactions

The effects of isoproterenol are similar to those for epinephrine with the following exceptions: inhalation and sublingual dosage forms may induce a pink to red discoloration of saliva, which is an expected alteration.

Warnings

Use with caution in patients with seizures, diabetes mellitus, hyperthyroidism, and pheochromocytoma.

Contraindications

Avoid use in persons with known hypersensitivity to isoproterenol and cardiovascular disease.

Dosage and administration

Cardiac standstill and dysrhythmias. The adult isoproterenol IV dose is 0.02 to 0.06 mg initially, then 0.01 to 0.2 mg if necessary. The IM dose is 0.2 mg initially, then 0.02 to 1 mg if necessary. For IV infusion, intracardiac, and subcutaneous dosing, see a current drug reference. Dosage in children has not been determined and is individualized by prescriber.

Bronchodilator. The sublingual dose for adults is 10 to 15 mg three to four times per day; for children the dose it is 5 to 10 mg three times per day.

Inhaler. Follow individual manufacturer's instructions carefully when administering isoproterenol by inhalation. Generally, with a metered-dose nebulizer, one inhalation is administered, which may be repeated in 1 to 5 minutes if necessary, four to six times daily. For bronchospasm of chronic obstructive pulmonary disease (COPD), the second dose should be given 3 to 4 hours after the initial dose. When treating acute asthma in children, give oral inhalation of a 0.5% nebulized solution (5 to 15 deep inhalations). If necessary, repeat in 5 to 10 minutes. Dosage may be repeated up to five times daily.

norepinephrine bitartrate [nor ep i nef′ rin] (Levophed)

Norepinephrine is a direct-acting sympathomimetic amine identical to the body catecholamine synthesized in the postganglionic nerve ending of the sympathetic nervous system. This agent has a high affinity for the alpha receptors. Because the blood vessels of the skin and mucous membrane contain only alpha receptors, norepinephrine produces a powerful constriction in these tissues. In addition, the blood vessels (both arteriolar and venous beds) in the visceral organs, including the kidneys, contain predominantly alpha receptors. Consequently, norepinephrine causes vasoconstriction and a reduced blood flow through the kidneys and other visceral organs. This agent also activates beta$_1$ receptors in the heart and exerts an increase in the force of myocardial contraction, resulting in an increase in cardiac output.

The main therapeutic effect of norepinephrine results from peripheral arteriolar vasoconstriction in all vascular beds. Both systolic and diastolic pressures are elevated, causing an increase in mean arterial pressure. Of importance during shock is constriction of the venous capacitance vessels, which reduces splanchnic and renal blood flow. This is brought about by severe restriction of tissue perfusion in these regions. In persistent hypotension after blood volume deficit has been corrected, norepinephrine helps to raise the blood pressure to an optimal level and establishes a more adequate circulation.

Indications

Norepinephrine is selectively used for restoring blood pressure in certain acute hypotensive states such as sympathectomy, myocardial infarction, pheochromocytomectomy, and blood transfusion reaction. When it is used to treat hypotension associated with an acute myocardial infarction, an increase in cardiac output and oxygen demand plus the possibility of inducing dysrhythmias may offset the benefits of using the drug to increase blood pressure. This would have to be carefully considered when selecting norepinephrine for use in such conditions.

Norepinephrine is also used as adjunct therapy in cardiac arrest and profound hypotension. Since the advent of dopamine, the use of norepinephrine to treat shock has declined significantly. It is usually prescribed for patients whose shock produces severe hypotension and vasodilation of the peripheral blood vessels.

Pharmacokinetics

Norepinephrine is administered only by intravenous infusion because oral norepinephrine is destroyed in the GI tract and subcutaneous norepinephrine is poorly absorbed. Onset of action is immediate or rapid by intravenous infusion and distribution mainly concentrates in sympathetic tissues; duration of action is approximately 1 to 2 minutes after an intravenous infusion is discontinued. The drug is metabolized in the liver and other tissues, and by reuptake into the sympathetic nerves and is excreted in the kidneys.

Drug interactions

Norepinephrine's drug interactions are similar to epinephrine's with hydrocarbon inhalation anesthetics, beta-adrenergic blocking agents, digitalis glycosides, maprotiline (Ludiomil), tricyclic antidepressants, MAO inhibitors, cocaine, and ergotamine. In addition, when norepinephrine is given concurrently with doxapram (Dopram), an increase in central nervous system stimulation and blood pressure may occur. Monitor closely because dosage adjustments may be required.

BOX 16-2 Sulfite Sensitivity

Sulfite is contained in the commercially available formulations of:

amrinone (Inocor)
dobutamine (Dobutrex)
dopamine ⚷ (Intropin)
epinephrine ⚷ (Adrenalin)
metaraminol (Aramine)
methoxamine (Vasoxyl)
norepinephrine ⚷ (Levophed)
phenylephrine (Neo-Synephrine)

These drugs should not be administered to individuals with a known sensitivity to sulfite agents (sulfur dioxide, potassium or sodium bisulfite, potassium or sodium metasulfite, sodium sulfite).

Symptoms of sulfite sensitivity include:

Skin: clamminess, flushed, pruritus, urticaria, cyanosis
Respiratory: bronchospasm, shortness of breath, wheezing, laryngeal edema, respiratory arrest
Cardiovascular: hypotension, syncope
Central nervous system: severe dizziness, loss of consciousness
Other: anaphylaxis, death

Side effects and adverse reactions

These include anxiety, dizziness, pallor, tremors, insomnia, headache, pounding heart rate, and sometimes swelling of thyroid gland in neck.

Warnings

Use with caution in patients with arterial embolism, atherosclerosis, and other occlusive vascular diseases, metabolic acidosis, hypoxia, atrial fibrillation, narrow-angle glaucoma, and pulmonary hypertension.

Contraindications

Avoid use in persons with hypersensitivity to norepinephrine, hypovolemia, myocardial infarction, and ventricular dysrhythmias.

Dosage and administration

Stimulation of alpha and $beta_1$ receptors with norepinephrine is dose-related. At low doses (<2 μg/min), $beta_1$ receptors are stimulated thus producing an inotropic and chronotropic response. Doses higher than 4 μg/min result in stimulation of the alpha receptors or increased total peripheral resistance. Determine if the patient is sulfite sensitive, as Levophed contains a sulfite preservative (Box 16-2).

When norepinephrine is used in the treatment of hypotension in adults, an IV infusion of 0.5 to 1 μg/min is given; the dosage is adjusted as necessary to raise and maintain the desired pressure. The maintenance dose ranges from 2 to 12 μg/min with dosage adjustment as necessary to raise and maintain the desired pressure.

Drugs Used for Circulatory Shock

In any instance of shock, treatment must be directed to the cause. A main concern is the need to improve circulation so that enough oxygen is available for tissue perfusion. Hypoxia that denotes impaired tissue perfusion may result from inadequate pumping action of the heart, decreased blood volume, decreased peripheral resistance of arterial vessels, or increased size of the venous bed.

During circulatory shock the autonomic nervous system plays an essential compensatory role in an attempt to restore normal circulation. Therefore many sympathomimetic drugs are used to manage this condition. Although there are other agents, the five drugs that are widely used for circulatory shock are dopamine, epinephrine, and norepinephrine, which are all vasopressors, and dobutamine and isoproterenol, which possess cardiogenic activity. Amrinone (Inocor), which has positive inotropic and vasodilator effects, can also be used for persons with congestive heart failure who are not responsive to standard therapy. Milrinone (Primacor), an analog of amrinone, is also available for short-term use in congestive heart failure (see Chapter 19).

Vasopressors have strong alpha activity, and dopamine produces less vasoconstriction than epinephrine and norepinephrine. Dobutamine and isoproterenol are important for improving cardiac output because of their capability to stimulate $beta_1$ receptors in the heart. Most of the agents are nonselective beta acting drugs, but norepinephrine lacks $beta_2$ activity. Also, with the exception of isoproterenol and amrinone, all of these agents stimulate alpha receptors (Table 16-3).

dobutamine [doe byoo′ ta meen] (Dobutrex)

Dobutamine is a synthetic catecholamine that acts directly on the heart muscle to increase the force of myocardial contraction. This response is attributed to the direct stimulation of the $beta_1$-adrenergic receptors of the heart. At the same time, dobutamine produces comparatively little increase in heart rate or peripheral vascular resistance. By enhancing stroke volume, this agent is an effective positive inotropic drug. Because of its minimal influence on heart rate and blood pressure (both major determinants of myocardial oxygen demand), it is valuable for use in individuals with low cardiac output syndrome.

Indications

Dobutamine is administered intravenously in the short-term management of patients requiring inotropic support, as in those with congestive heart failure or after cardiac surgery. It is used to strengthen the decompensated heart in individuals with low cardiac output syndrome. Its beneficial effects include a progressive increase in cardiac output and a decrease in pulmonary capillary wedge pressure, thereby improving ventricular contraction.

In patients with congestive heart failure or after an acute myocardial infarction, the concomitant use of sodium nitroprusside and dobutamine is sometimes beneficial. It re-

TABLE 16-3 Vasopressor Effects in Shock

	Receptor Site Effects*			Organ Response†		
Drug	**$beta_1$**	**$beta_2$**	**$alpha_1$**	**Kidneys**	**Cardiac**	**BP**
epinephrine	+++	+/++	+++	D	I	D
dobutamine	+++	+	0/+	0	I	
dopamine	+++	0/+	++	I		0/I
isoproterenol	+++	+++	0	I/D	I	#
norepinephrine	++	0	+++	D	0/D	I

*Receptor site effects: $beta_1$, inotropic effects; blood vessel effects; $beta_2$, vasodilation; $alpha_1$, vasoconstriction.
†Organ response: kidneys—renal perfusion; cardiac—cardiac output; BP—blood pressure.
+, minimal effect; ++, moderate effect; +++, greatest effect; 0, no effect; I, increased; D, decreased; # usual doses maintain or increase systolic pressure.

sults in a higher cardiac output and a lower pulmonary capillary wedge pressure than when either drug is used alone. Because of the vasodilating effect of nitroprusside, the decrease in peripheral resistance lessens the workload on the heart.

Pharmacokinetics

Dobutamine is administered by IV infusion with an onset of action within 1 to 2 minutes. Its plasma half-life is 2 minutes as it is rapidly metabolized by the liver and is excreted in the urine.

Drug interactions

See discussion of norepinephrine.

Side effects and adverse reactions

These include nausea, headache, angina, respiratory distress, palpitation, increased heart rate and blood pressure, and sometimes premature ventricular beats.

Warnings and contraindications

See discussion of norepinephrine.

Dosage and administration

Adult dosage is by IV infusion, 2.5 to 15 μg/kg/min. For children, the dosage ranges from 5 to 20 μg/kg/min.

dopamine [doe′ pa meen] (Intropin)

Dopamine is a catecholamine that occurs as an immediate precursor of norepinephrine (see Fig. 14-5). It acts both directly and indirectly by releasing norepinephrine. It stimulates dopaminergic receptors, $beta_1$ receptors, and in high doses, alpha receptors. Actually, receptor activity is dose dependent; it depends on the amount of drug administered.

Unlike norepinephrine, in low doses (0.5 to 2 μg/kg/min), dopamine is unique because it acts mainly on dopaminergic receptors to cause vasodilation of the renal and mesenteric arteries. Renal vasodilation increases renal blood flow usually with a greater amount of urine and sodium excretion. This prevents kidney failure secondary to shock.

In low to moderate doses (usually 2 to 10 μg/kg/min), dopamine acts directly on the $beta_1$ receptors on the myocardium and indirectly by releasing norepinephrine from its neuronal storage sites in the sympathetic neuron. These actions increase myocardial contractility and stroke volume, thereby increasing cardiac output. Systolic blood pressure and pulse pressure may increase with either no effect or a slight elevation in diastolic blood pressure. Nevertheless, total peripheral resistance is usually unchanged. Coronary blood flow and myocardial oxygen consumption increase. However, heart rate increases only slightly at low doses.

With higher doses of dopamine (10 μg/kg/min or more), alpha-adrenergic receptors are stimulated, increasing peripheral resistance. Because of a rise in cardiac output, blood pressure increases. As a consequence, a high dose level may reduce urinary output, eliminating the benefit of vasodilation because the renal artery becomes constricted. From the therapeutic standpoint, it is important to note that dopamine in low to moderate doses causes vasodilation in the renal, mesenteric, coronary, and cerebral blood vessels. These vasodilator properties suggest the presence of specific dopamine receptors.

Therefore unlike norepinephrine, dopamine helps alleviate inadequate tissue perfusion through the vital splanchnic organ systems. The combination of cardiac and circulatory effects has led to dopamine's successful use in the treatment of circulatory shock and refractory heart failure. Dopamine is used to correct hemodynamic imbalances associated with shock syndrome caused by myocardial infarction, trauma, endotoxin septicemia, open heart surgery, renal failure, and chronic cardiac decompensation (as in congestive heart failure).

Pharmacokinetics

Dopamine is administered by IV infusion. The drug has rapid onset of action (2 to 5 minutes) and a short duration of action (5 to 10 minutes). It is widely distributed by the body but does not cross the blood-brain barrier. Dopamine is rapidly metabolized by the liver, kidney, and plasma to inactive substances. The drug is excreted in the urine.

Side effects and adverse reactions

These include headaches, nausea, vomiting, angina, respiratory difficulties, and decreased blood pressure and less frequently, hypertension, irregular or ectopic heart beats, tachycardia, and palpitations.

Drug interactions, warnings, and contraindications

See discussion of norepinephrine.

Dosage and administration

For vasopressor effects, the adult dose, administered by IV infusion, ranges by effect desired (see previous section). The pediatric IV infusion rate ranges from 5 to 20 μg/kg/min.

Indirect- and Dual-Acting Adrenergic Drugs

The direct-acting adrenergic (catecholamines) drugs act directly on alpha and beta receptors to stimulate adrenergic response. The indirect-acting adrenergic drugs act indirectly on receptors by first triggering the release of the catecholamines, norepinephrine and epinephrine, from their storage sites; these neurotransmitters then activate the alpha and beta receptors.

Finally, the dual-acting adrenergic drugs have both indirect and direct effects. These drugs have many and varied uses in medicine.

ephedrine [e fed′ rin] (Ephed II)

Ephedrine has both a direct and an indirect sympathomimetic action. It acts indirectly by stimulating release of norepinephrine from presynaptic nerve terminals and also acts directly on both alpha and beta receptors. Like epinephrine and norepinephrine, ephedrine has positive inotropic (myocardial stimulation) and chronotropic (increased heart rate) activities, but it is a less effective vasoconstrictor. However, it does raise the blood pressure and is used for this purpose during spinal anesthesia and to treat orthostatic hypotension.

Indications

Parenteral ephedrine has been used in hypotensive patients who do not respond to fluid replacement, position changes, and specific antidotes in the case of drug overdosage. However, be aware that if severe peripheral vasoconstriction is present, ephedrine may be ineffective and may actually worsen the situation (Table 16-4).

Ephedrine has been used to produce bronchodilation in the treatment of milder forms of bronchial asthma, but generally more $beta_2$-selective drugs are preferred, such as albuterol, metaproterenol, and terbutaline. It is also used to relieve nasal mucosal congestion.

Ephedrine is also used as a pressor agent in hypotensive states during spinal anesthesia or after sympathectomy.

Pharmacokinetics

Absorption of the drug is rapid after oral, IM, or SC administration. Onset of action for bronchodilation occurs within 15 to 60 minutes with the oral dosage form and within 10 to 20 minutes with the intramuscular dosage form. Duration of action is 3 to 5 hours after oral dosage and 30 to 60 minutes after IM or SC injections of 25 to 50 mg doses. The pressor effects and cardiac responses after parenteral administration of ephedrine usually occur within 60 minutes. The drug is metabolized in the liver and excreted in the kidneys.

Drug interactions

See discussion of norepinephrine.

Side effects and adverse reactions

These are similar to those for epinephrine although norepinephrine is not available in aerosol form so coughing and local irritation are not reported. In addition, ephedrine may cause mood changes and hallucinations.

Warnings and contraindications

See discussion of norepinephrine.

Dosage and administration

For vasopressor effects, the adult ephedrine dose IM or SC is 25 to 50 mg, repeated if necessary. If a faster effect is desired, it may be administered IV. For bronchodilator or decongestant effects, the dose is 25 to 50 mg orally or 12.5 to 25 mg SC, IM, or slow IV every 3 or 4 hours as needed. For decongestion, several drops of a 0.5% to 1% ephedrine solution may be applied topically and repeated every 4 hours if necessary.

phenylephrine systemic [fen ill ef′ rin] (Neo-Synephrine injection)
phenylephrine nasal (Neo-Synephrine, Alconefrin)

Phenylephrine is primarily a direct-acting agent. Its main effects are stimulation of the alpha receptors, resulting in vasoconstriction and an increase in both diastolic and systolic blood pressures. The drug has little effect on the $beta_1$ receptors of the heart. Its vasoconstricting action is more prolonged than that of norepinephrine; thus, it may be used for acute hypotension that occurs from spinal anesthesia. It is not effective in shock caused by loss of blood volume. Phenylephrine is also contained in many combination cough-cold, antihistamine and decongestant, and ophthalmic preparations.

It is a synthetic adrenergic drug chemically related to epinephrine, norepinephrine, and ephedrine. Phenylephrine exhibits fewer side effects than epinephrine and has longer-lasting therapeutic effects. It has little or no effect on the central nervous system.

Indications

When applied topically to mucous membranes, phenylephrine reduces swelling and congestion by constricting the small blood vessels. It is useful in the treatment of sinusitis, vasomotor rhinitis, and hay fever. It is sometimes com-

TABLE 16-4 Indirect- and Dual-Acting Adrenergic Drug Effects

Receptors, Action Sites	***Ephedrine***	***Phenylephrine***	***Mephentermine***	***Metaraminol***	***Methoxamine***
Trade names	Ephedrine Sulfate	Neo-Synephrine	Wyamine	Aramine	Vasoxyl
Mode of action					
Alpha receptors	Stimulates	Stimulates	Stimulates	Stimulates	Stimulates
Beta receptors	Stimulates More prolonged but less intense action than epinephrine	NS*			
Effects					
Cardiovascular					
Myocardium	Variable	NS Bradycardia may occur reflexively	Increases contractility and rate May cause bradycardia	Some increase in contractility Bradycardia may occur	— Reflex bradycardia may occur
Pacemaker cells	NS	NS	NS	—	—
Coronary vessels	Dilates: increases blood flow	Dilates: increases blood flow	Dilates: increases blood flow	—	—
Blood pressure	Increases	Increases	Increases	Increases	Increases
Bronchi	Dilates	Dilates but less than epinephrine	Dilates but less than epinephrine	NS	—
Cerebral effects	Stimulating action	NS	NS	—	—
Blood vessels					
Skeletal muscle	NS	—†	NS	NS	Decreases blood flow
Kidney	Constricts	Constricts	Constricts but less than ephedrine	Constricts: decreases blood flow	
Gastrointestinal tract	Decreases peristalsis	Decreases motility	Relaxes smooth muscle: inhibits	Some inhibition	Inhibits
Metabolic	Increases metabolic rate	Some increase in metabolic rate	NS	NS	NS
Remarks	Serious dysrhythmias may occur if used with digitalis Can be given orally			Prolonged duration of action; cumulative effects may occur; give drug slowly May cause tissue sloughing; do not give subcutaneously	
Uses	Vasopressor Allergic states Nasal decongestant Enuresis Myasthenia gravis	Nasal decongestant Vasopressor Paroxysmal atrial tachycardia Mydriatic	Vasopressor	Vasopressor	Vasopressor Paroxysmal atrial tachycardia

*NS, Not significant.
†Effect is slight, nonexistent, or unknown in humans.

bined with local anesthetics to retard their systemic absorption and to prolong their action.

Phenylephrine is used as a mydriatic for certain conditions in which dilation of the pupil is desired without cycloplegia paralysis of the ciliary muscle and may be applied intranasally for congestion caused by colds, hay fever, sinusitis, or allergies.

Pharmacokinetics

Administered IV, phenylephrine produces an immediate effect with a duration of action of 5 to 20 minutes. The drug is metabolized partially in gastrointestinal tract tissues and in the liver by the enzyme MAO. The route of excretion is not identified.

Drug interactions

The following interactions may occur when phenylephrine is given with the drugs listed below:

Drug	Possible effect and management
Alpha receptor blocking agents	May reduce or block the vasopressor effect of phenylephrine, resulting in hypotension.
Anesthetics, inhalation of hydrocarbons such as chloroform, enthrane, halothane, and others, plus digitalis glycosides	Increases risk of inducing serious cardiac dysrhythmias. If necessary to use concurrently, monitor closely with electrocardiogram (ECG) readings because therapeutic interventions may be necessary. Avoid or serious drug interaction may occur.
Beta blocking agents	Therapeutic effects of both drugs may be inhibited. This can occur with both oral and ophthalmic beta-adrenergic blocking drugs. Avoid concurrent use.
ergotamine and ergoloid mesylates	Increases vasoconstriction; severe hypertension and peripheral vascular ischemia and gangrene may occur. This combined use is not recommended. Avoid or serious drug interaction may occur.
doxapram (Dopram)	The vasopressor effects of either or both drugs may increase. Monitor blood pressure closely since dosage adjustments may be necessary.
cocaine, maprotiline (Ludiomil), or tricyclic antidepressants	May potentiate cardiovascular effects of phenylephrine, such as dysrhythmias and increased heart rate, and cause severe hypertension and elevated body temperature. Avoid or serious drug interaction may occur
MAO inhibitors	May cause increased release of accumulated neurotransmitters into the synapse area, resulting in severe headaches, dysrhythmias, vomiting, severe hypertension, and/or high fevers. Avoid or a serious drug interaction may occur. Phenylephrine should not be given during or within 2 weeks after the administration of an MAO inhibitor.

Color type indicates an unsafe drug combination.

Side effects and adverse reactions

Side effects and adverse reactions, while uncommon, include anxiety, restlessness, dizziness, tremors, difficult breathing, pallor, increased weakness, angina, and allergic reactions with preparations that contain sulfites (Box 16-2).

Warnings and contraindications

See discussion of norepinephrine.

Dosage and administration

The adult hypotensive dose is 2-5 mg (IM or SC) of 1% solution, repeated if necessary. The IV dose is 0.2 mg, repeated in 15 minutes if necessary; IV infusion is 100 to 180 μg/min until the blood pressure stabilizes, then 40 to 60 μg/min.

mephentermine [me fen′ ter meen] (Wyamine)

Mephentermine's effects are similar to those of ephedrine, but it produces more cerebral stimulation. Mephentermine is a dual-acting (primarily) sympathomimetic agent. It releases catecholamines from storage sites in the heart and other tissues (indirect action). Therefore it tends to bring about both alpha and beta stimulating effects, including inotropic and chronotropic effects on the heart. Because mephentermine improves cardiac contraction and mobilizes blood from venous pools, thereby increasing cardiac output, it acts as a peripheral vasoconstrictor (see Table 16-4).

Indications

This drug is used as a pressor agent in the treatment of hypotension secondary to spinal anesthesia and as adjunct therapy for hypotension secondary to hemorrhage, medications, and shock due to brain tumor or trauma.

Pharmacokinetics

Administered IM, the onset of action occurs within 5 to 15 minutes; its duration of action is 1 to 4 hours. Administered IV, mephentermine is nearly immediate in action; the duration of action is 15 to 30 minutes. The drug is metabolized in the liver and excreted in the kidneys.

Drug interactions

See discussion of norepinephrine.

Side effects and adverse reactions

These include anxiety, nervousness, restlessness, and tachycardia.

Warnings and contraindications

See discussion of norepinephrine.

Dosage and administration

For hypotension, the adult mephentermine dosage is 30 to 45 mg IV in a single injection. Repeat doses of 30 mg are given as needed to maintain blood pressure. Dosage for children has not been established.

metaraminol [met a ram′ i nole] (Aramine)

Metaraminol is a vasopressor agent with both direct (primarily) and indirect effects on the sympathetic system. It acts indirectly by releasing norepinephrine from tissues and storage sites and directly on alpha receptors as a neurohormone.

Metaraminol has positive inotropic effects. Because it constricts blood vessels, increases peripheral resistance, elevates both systolic and diastolic blood pressure, and improves cardiac contractility and cerebral, coronary, and renal blood flow, the drug is used for the treatment of shock.

Since metaraminol exhibits beta- and alpha-adrenergic activity, it is often effective in raising blood pressure when alpha-adrenergic agents are ineffective. This may be because of its ability to bring about more effective venous flow. It does not appear to cause dysrhythmias. It generally lacks central nervous system (CNS) stimulatory effects, and its side effects are rare and often related to rapid drug administration. Although similar to norepinephrine in action, it is generally considered a less potent drug.

Indications

Metaraminol is used for acute hypotensive states occurring with spinal anesthesia. It is also administered for the prevention and treatment of acute hypotension associated with surgery, drug-induced reactions, and shock.

Pharmacokinetics

The drug is administered parenterally only. When given IV, the onset of action is within 1 to 2 minutes; when given SC or IM, the onset of action is within 10 minutes. The duration of action is between 20 to 60 minutes, and it is metabolized in the liver and excreted in the bile and kidneys.

Drug interactions

See discussion of norepinephrine.

Warnings and contraindications

See discussion of norepinephrine.

Dosage and administration

The metaraminol adult dose is 2 to 10 mg given SC or IM to prevent acute hypotension and by IV infusion to treat hypotension. By IV infusion, the dose is 15 to 100 mg in 500 ml of sodium chloride injection (0.9%) or 5% dextrose in water at rate determined by the prescriber to maintain the desired blood pressure response. The drug is given by direct IV injection for severe shock, 0.5 to 5 mg followed by the infusion described previously. The pediatric dosage has not been established.

methoxamine [meth ox′ a meen] (Vasoxyl)

Methoxamine is an alpha-adrenergic stimulator devoid of beta receptor activity, except in high doses. The direct-acting sympathomimetic agent is pharmacologically related to phenylephrine. Because it has no stimulating effect on the heart, the rise in blood pressure causes a reflex bradycardia. This effect makes it useful in treating paroxysmal supraventricular tachycardia and in restoring or maintaining blood pressure during anesthesia (Table 16-4).

Pharmacokinetics

Intravenously administered, the effects of methoxamine are immediate; its duration of action as a vasopressor is 5 to 15 minutes. After IM administration the effects are seen within 15 to 20 minutes, with duration of effects between 60 and 90 minutes. Metabolism and excretion routes are unknown.

Drug interactions

See discussion of norepinephrine.

Side effects and adverse reactions

These are infrequent and include sweating, severe headaches, hypertension, vomiting, and urinary urgency with high doses.

Warnings and contraindications

See discussion of norepinephrine.

Dosage and administration

The adult vasopressor dose is 10 to 15 mg IM or 3 to 5 mg given slowly by direct IV. The dose for children is not established.

See Box 16-3 for information about midodrine (ProAmatin), an alpha agonist used to treat orthostatic hypotension.

ADRENERGIC BLOCKING DRUGS

ALPHA-ADRENERGIC BLOCKING DRUGS

Most **alpha-adrenergic blocking agents** are competitive blockers; they compete with the catecholamines at receptor sites and inhibit adrenergic sympathetic stimulation. They are more effective against the action of circulating cat-

BOX 16-3 Midodrine (ProAmatin)

Midodrine (ProAmatine) is indicated for the treatment of symptomatic orthostatic hypotension. It is a prodrug that is converted to an active metabolite desglymidodrine, and $alpha_1$ agonist that activates arteriolar and venous receptors to increase blood pressure. It can raise systolic blood pressure by 15 to 30 mm Hg in 1 hour after a 10 mg dose.

Pharmacokinetics

Midodrine metabolite peaks in 1 to 2 hours; half-life is 3 to 4 hours with metabolism in many tissues including the liver. It is excreted renally.

Side and adverse effects include paresthesia, pruritus, dysuria, and supine hypertension. Adult dose is 10 mg PO three times daily during daytime hours (every 4 hours but not later than 6 PM). Because of the risk of supine hypertension, do not give midodrine after evening meal or less than 4 hours before retiring (Olin, 1998).

echolamines than against catecholamines released from storage sites in the neurons. These drugs may be obtained from natural sources, such as ergot and its derivatives, or they may be synthesized.

The alpha-adrenergic blocking agents fall into three categories:

1. Noncompetitive, long-acting antagonists (e.g., phenoxybenzamine [Dibenzyline]): action persists for several days or weeks because a stable bond is formed between a specific component of the drug and the alpha receptor site.
2. Competitive, short-acting antagonists (e.g., phentolamine [Regitine] and tolazoline [Priscoline]): the blocking action is reversible and competitive at the alpha receptor site and the effects last only several hours.
3. Ergot alkaloids: usually act as partial alpha-adrenergic antagonists. However, the drugs produce primarily a spasmogenic effect on smooth muscle of blood vessels, thereby causing vasoconstriction.

Noncompetitive, Long-Acting Antagonists

phenoxybenzamine [fen ox ee ben′ za meen] (Dibenzyline)

Phenoxybenzamine is a long-acting, irreversible alpha-adrenergic blocking agent that abolishes or decreases the receptiveness of alpha receptors to adrenergic stimuli. Because phenoxybenzamine competes with the catecholamines, it is also useful in decreasing the blood pressure of patients with pheochromocytoma. It does not block sympathetic impulses on the heart, and therefore does not directly impair cardiac output.

All $alpha_1$ blockers are also used to relieve symptoms of benign prostatic hyperplasia, although this indication is not included in the U.S. product labeling. By noncompetitively blocking alpha-adrenergic receptors of the bladder neck and proximal urethra, the internal sphincter is relaxed, improving voiding efficiency in patients with functional outlet obstruction.

Indications

Phenoxybenzamine is used in the management of pheochromocytoma, preparation of patients for surgery, and chronic treatment of individuals with malignant pheochromocytoma. It is also used to treat individuals for whom surgery of pheochromocytoma is contraindicated. However, because a 2-year study in rats using large doses of phenoxybenzamine demonstrated basal cell growth in the stomach, the manufacturer recommends only emergency, short-term use, such as preoperative management of patients with pheochromocytoma (AMA, 1995).

Pharmacokinetics

Oral absorption of the drug is variable. Onset of action occurs in 2 hours. The drug can persist for 3 or 4 days since it forms a stable bond with the receptor. The half-life is about 24 hours with metabolism in the liver and excretion in the kidney and bile.

Drug interactions

Avoid concurrent use with other sympathomimetics, such as dopamine, ephedrine, epinephrine, metaraminol, methoxamine, and phenylephrine, because a decrease in therapeutic effects (vasopressor effect) may occur. With epinephrine, a block of the alpha receptors by phenoxybenzamine may result in tachycardia and severe hypotension.

Side effects and adverse reactions

These include dizziness (postural hypotension), miosis, tachycardia, nasal congestion, confusion, dry mouth, headache, and inhibition of ejaculation.

Warnings

Use with caution in patients with cerebrovascular insufficiency, heart failure, coronary artery disease, respiratory infections, and kidney impairment.

Contraindications

Avoid use in persons with known hypersensitivity to phenoxybenzamine.

Dosage and administration

The adult dose initially is 10 mg twice daily orally, increased by 10 mg every other day until the desired effect is noted. The maintenance dose is 20 to 40 mg two or three times daily. the initial pediatric dose is 0.2 mg/kg PO up to a maximum of 10 mg, administered once daily. Dosage may be increased every 4 days until the desired effect is noted. Maintenance dose is 0.4 to 1.2 mg/kg body weight, given in three or four divided doses.

Competitive, Short-Acting Antagonists

phentolamine mesylate [fen tole′ a meen] (Regitine, Rogitine ✦)

Phentolamine is an alpha-adrenergic blocking agent that competitively blocks $alpha_2$ (presynaptic) and $alpha_1$ (postsynaptic) receptors. The action occurs at both arterial and venous vessels. This direct relaxation of vascular smooth muscle lowers total peripheral resistance. Accordingly, hypertension is inhibited when there are excessive levels of epinephrine and norepinephrine. It also decreases pulmonary vascular resistance.

Indications

This drug is used to prevent or control hypertensive episodes in the individual with pheochromocytoma. It is also used to reverse the vasoconstrictive action of an overdose or excessive response to IV administration or extravasation of norepinephrine (Levophed) or dopamine. The SC injection of phentolamine (Regitine) after extravasation of intravenous norepinephrine or dopamine will prevent tissue necrosis if prompt action is taken.

Pharmacokinetics

Parenteral phentolamine is administered IV; its half-life is approximately 19 minutes. Metabolism and excretion sources are unknown, because only 13% (approximately) of the drug is found in urine after parenteral administration.

Drug interactions

See discussion of phenoxybenzamine.

Side effects and adverse reactions

These include diarrhea, dizziness (postural hypotension), nausea, vomiting, abdominal pain, and tachycardia.

Warnings

Use with caution in patients with gastritis and peptic ulcers.

Contraindications

Avoid use in persons with a history of phentolamine hypersensitivity or myocardial infarction, angina pectoris, and coronary insufficiency.

Dosage and administration

The phentolamine adult dose is 5 mg IV administered 1 to 2 hours before surgery; dosage may be repeated if necessary during surgery. As an antiadrenergic preoperative medication in children, 1 mg (IM or IV) is administered 1 to 2 hours before surgery and repeated if necessary.

tolazoline [toe laz′ a leen] (Priscoline)

Like phentolamine, tolazoline produces a moderately effective competitive alpha-adrenergic blocking action, although tolazoline is considerably less potent. It acts as a vasodilator by a direct relaxant effect on vascular smooth muscle. It usually reduces pulmonary arterial pressure and peripheral vascular resistance.

Indications

The drug is used to treat persistent pulmonary hypertension in the newborn when systemic arterial levels of oxygen cannot be maintained by oxygen supplementation and/or mechanical ventilation machines.

Pharmacokinetics

Parenterally, the onset of action is within ½ hour of initial dose. The half-life in neonates is 3 to 10 hours. Tolazoline is excreted in the kidneys, mainly unchanged.

Drug interactions

No clinically significant interactions are reported (USP DI, 1998), although concurrent use with other sympathomimetics such as dopamine and epinephrine may reduce the effectiveness of these agents.

Side effects and adverse reactions

These include GI bleeding, systemic alkalosis, hypotension, thrombocytopenia, and oliguria or acute renal failure.

Warnings

Use with caution in patients with metabolic acidosis.

Contraindications

Avoid use in children with known hypersensitivity to tolazoline, hypotension, mitral stenosis, and kidney impairment.

Dosage and administration

The parenteral dose for children is 1 to 2 mg/kg (IV) initially via a scalp vein over a 5- to 10-minute period. The maintenance dose is 0.2 mg/kg for each 1 mg/kg loading dose by IV infusion. When arterial blood gases appear to be stable, the drug may be gradually withdrawn.

Ergot Alkaloids

Ergot is a fungus that grows on rye, and when it is hydrolyzed, many of its derivatives dissociate to yield lysergic acid diethylamide (LSD). The ergot alkaloids have diverse and somewhat contradictory effects. They are partial agonists or antagonists at alpha-adrenergic receptors. The primary effect of the ergot alkaloids used to treat or prevent migraine and other vascular headaches is alpha-adrenergic blockade. Only ergoloid mesylates are not used to treat headaches; they are indicated as adjunct therapy to treat dementia symptoms (USP DI, 1998). The mechanism of action is reviewed below. The following are examples of ergot preparations:

- dihydroergotamine mesylate [dye hye droe er got′ a meen] (D.H.E. 45)
- ergoloid mesylates [er′ goe loid mess′ i lates] (Hydergine)
- ergotamine tartrate [er got′ a meen] (Ergomar, Gynergen)

- ergotamine tartrate and caffeine (Cafergot)
- ergotamine tartrate inhalation (Medihaler Ergotamine)
- ergotamine, belladonna alkaloids, and phenobarbital (Bellergal-S, Bellergal)
- methysergide maleate [meth i ser′ jide] (Sansert)

The exact mechanism of action of ergoloid mesylates is unknown, but they may increase nerve cell metabolism which can result in improved oxygen uptake and cerebral metabolism. Thus lowered neurotransmitter levels may increase to normal. The other ergot alkaloids stimulate smooth muscle, especially of the blood vessels and the uterus, so they decrease the cerebral blood supply.

The early phase of a migraine attack is associated with constriction of the cranial blood vessels. It is characterized by visual symptoms and malaise and appears as a warning or "aura" of an oncoming attack. This is followed by the painful phase of a migraine headache, which results in cranial vasodilation. The increase in blood flow in the vessels produces pulsations, which appear to be the source of the pain. The ergot alkaloids act as alpha-adrenergic blocking agents and depress the central vasomotor center. They cause direct vasoconstriction of cranial blood vessels during the vasodilation phase, thereby reducing the pulsation thought to be responsible for the headache. These drugs also possess antiserotonin activity.

Abnormalities in serotonin metabolism may play a role in the migraine syndrome. Evidence exists that the drugs which act favorably in alleviating migraine influence serotonin metabolism. Methysergide is a serotonin inhibitor and also acts as a potent vasoconstrictor. (See Chapter 33 for serotonin information.) Ergotamine tartrate inhalation is used to abort or reduce a migraine attack, whereas ergotamine, belladonna alkaloids, and phenobarbital are used in combination to prevent vascular headaches. Some of these drugs are used for treatment of vascular headaches, such as migraine and cluster headaches. The drug (dihydroergotamine mesylate or ergotamine tartrate) must be given early in the attack; it does not prevent migraine attacks.

Dihydroergotamine is administered parenterally. The ergoloid mesylates and ergotamine tartrate (and its combinations without caffeine) are slowly and erratically absorbed from the GI tract. Caffeine is said to aid oral absorption. The aerosol dosage form, like methysergide, is well absorbed. Rectal suppositories of ergotamine tartrate (available in combination products) produce higher plasma concentrations than oral administration and may be used if other routes are ineffective.

Pharmacokinetics

The onset of action for dihydroergotamine mesylate (IM, SC, or IV) is fairly rapid: IM, 15 to 30 minutes; IV within minutes. The half life is 1.4 to 15 hours. The duration of action for an IM dose is 3 to 4 hours, and if is mainly excreted in the bile. Ergotamine tartrate and its combinations have onset of action within 1 to 2 hours and a half-life of about 2 hours. Methysergide maleate has an onset and duration of action of 24 to 48 hours. The half-life of ergoloid mesylates is 3.5 hours. The ergot alkaloids are metabolized in the liver. Dihydroergotamine mesylate and methysergide maleate are both excreted in the kidney.

Drug interactions

Beta receptor blocking agents and the macrolide (azithromycin, clarithromycin, erythromycin, and others) antibiotics may interact with ergot alkaloids to produce peripheral ischemia. Concurrent use with nitrates may result in drug antagonism while concurrent ergot use with vasodilators has resulted in severe hypertension (Olin, 1998). If possible, avoid concurrent drug use.

Side effects and adverse reactions

Side effects and adverse reactions of ergot alkaloids include dizziness, nausea, vomiting, headache, diarrhea, pruritus, edema of lower extremities, and peripheral vasoconstriction or vasospasms (dose-related), which may result in cold hands or feet, leg weakness, and pain in arms, legs, or lower back. Long-term use of methysergide may result in retroperitoneal fibrosis; therefore this product should not be routinely administered for longer than 6 months.

Warnings

Monitor usage closely, as excessive use may result in ergotism, gangrene, and drug dependence.

Contraindications

Avoid use in persons with hypersensitivity to ergot preparations, peripheral vascular disease, severe liver or renal impairment, and psychosis, in pregnant or lactating women, and in children. Ergoloid mesylates should also not be administered to individuals with hypotension or bradycardia.

Dosage and administration

The dose for dihydroergotamine mesylate is 1 mg IM at the start of an attack, repeated in 1 hour if needed up to 3 mg maximum per day, 6 mg maximum per week. The IV dose is 0.5 mg initially with an antiemetic, repeated once in 1 hour if needed. The dose for ergoloid mesylates is 1 to 2 mg PO three times per day. For ergotamine the dose is 1 to 2 mg PO initially, repeated in ½ hour if needed to a maximum of 6 mg/day and no more than twice weekly at least 5 days apart. For ergotamine aerosol use one inhalation at the beginning of an attack and repeat every 5 min if needed to maximum of 6 sprays per day. Methysergide dose is 4 to 6 mg PO in divided doses, taken with milk or after meals.

Beta-Adrenergic Blocking Agents

Beta blocking agents inhibit beta receptors by competing with the catecholamines at the receptor site. **Beta-**

adrenergic blocking agents are differentiated into two subclasses: $beta_1$ and $beta_2$ blockers. Drugs that selectively inhibit only one type of receptor, $beta_1$ or $beta_2$, are called selective. $Beta_1$-selective blocking agents are frequently referred to as cardioselective blockers because these agents block the $beta_1$ receptors in the heart. Drugs that inhibit both types of receptors, $beta_1$ and $beta_2$, are referred to as nonselective beta-adrenergic blocking agents.

A further differentiation often identifies beta-adrenergic blocking agents that have intrinsic sympathomimetic activity (ISA). The ISA property was initially believed to be advantageous when compared with agents that only possess beta blocking effects. It was projected that fewer serious side effects would occur with such agents, but clinically the significance of this property has not been proven. Intrinsic sympathomimetic activity causes partial stimulation of the beta receptor although this effect is less than that of a pure agonist. For example, if the patient has a slow heart rate at rest, the partial agonists may help to increase the heart rate by their partial agonist property. But if the person has a rapid heart rate or tachycardia from exercise, these agents may help to slow down the heart rate secondary to the predominate beta blocking effect. It is believed that the only role for the ISA property might be to treat patients who experience severe bradycardia from the non-ISA medications (Carter et al, 1995). These drugs should also not be used to prevent myocardial infarction because of their partial agonist properties.

Examples of adrenergic blocking drugs by classification include the following (Carter et al, 1995; Olin, 1998):

1. $Beta_1$ antagonist effects:
   a. Selective $beta_1$-adrenergic blocking agents (cardioselective) include atenolol (Tenormin), betaxolol (Kerlone), bisoprolol (Zebeta), esmolol (Brevibloc), and metoprolol (Lopressor).
   b. Selective $beta_1$-adrenergic blocking agents with ISA effects include acebutolol (Sectral).
2. $Beta_1$ and $beta_2$ antagonist effects
   a. Nonselective beta-adrenergic blocking agents include labetalol* (Normodyne), nadolol (Corgard), propranolol (Inderal), sotalol (Betapace), and timolol (Blocadren).
   b. Nonselective beta-adrenergic blocking agents with ISA effects include carteolol (Cartrol), carvedilol* (Coreg), penbutolol (Levatol), and pindolol (Visken).

The key or prototype beta-adrenergic blocking drug is propranolol.

Mechanism of action

Beta-adrenergic blocking agents compete with beta-adrenergic agonists (e.g., catecholamines) for available beta receptor sites located on the membrane of cardiac muscle, smooth muscle of bronchi, and smooth muscle of blood vessels. Cardiac muscle contains $beta_1$ receptors while the smooth muscle sites contain primarily $beta_2$ receptors. Pharmacologically, the $beta_1$ adrenergic blocking action in the heart decreases heart rate, conduction velocity, myocardial contractility, and cardiac output.

The antiangina effects produced by the beta blockers are primarily caused by their ability to lower the myocardial oxygen requirements. Their antihypertensive actions are not specifically identified, but these effects may result from a decrease in cardiac output, a diminished sympathetic outflow from the vasomotor center in the brain to the peripheral blood vessels, and an inhibition of renin release by the kidney. The result is a decrease in peripheral vascular resistance, which lowers blood pressure.

To prevent a recurrence of a myocardial infarction, beta blockers (without ISA properties) are used for their antidysrhythmic effect plus their ability to decrease the myocardial oxygen demands on the heart. The latter effect may reduce the progression of ischemia and its severity on the heart.

Various mechanisms may be involved in the prevention of vascular headaches, such as prevention of arterial vasodilation, inhibition of platelet aggregation, and increased oxygen release to tissues.

Indications

Beta-adrenergic blocking agents are used to treat chronic angina pectoris, hypertension, hypertrophic cardiomyopathy, tremors and anxiety; to prevent or treat cardiac dysrhythmias, a second myocardial infarction and vascular headaches; as an adjunct to thyrotoxicosis and pheochromocytoma therapy; and to treat mitral valve prolapse syndrome. Esmolol (Brevibloc) is a parenteral agent indicated for treatment of supraventricular tachycardia and noncompensatory sinus tachycardia.

Pharmacokinetics

For the pharmacokinetics and usual adult dose of the beta-adrenergic blocking agents, see Table 16-5. Propranolol, metoprolol, and penbutolol are highly lipid soluble; therefore they have a larger volume of distribution in the body, a greater first-pass liver metabolism, and also a wider range of effective doses (individual variability) than the other agents. For example, the range for propranolol is 10 to 640 mg/day (Table 16-5) compared with a drug with a less-lipophilic (more water-soluble) profile, such as atenolol (50 to 100 mg), betaxolol (10 to 20 mg), and others. The less-lipophilic agents are not as affected by liver metabolism and are excreted more unchanged by the kidneys, therefore requiring dosage adjustments in persons with renal impairment (Carter et al, 1995).

When these agents are discontinued, they should be slowly withdrawn to avoid inducing a potentially serious withdrawal syndrome. See Box 16-4 for information on withdrawal of a beta blocking agent.

*Also $alpha_1$-antagonists.

TABLE 16-5 Beta-Adrenergic Blocking Agents: Pharmacokinetics and Adult Dosing

Drug	Time to Peak Effect (hr)	Half-Life (hr)	Metabolism/Excretion (%)*	Usual Adult Dose (Range)
acebutolol (Sectral)	2.5-3.5	3-8	Liver/renal (30-40) Bile/feces (50-60)	200 mg twice daily (600-1200 mg/day)
atenolol (Tenormin)	2-4	6-7	Renal (85-100)	50 mg daily (50-100 mg/day)
betaxolol (Kerlone)	3-4	14-22	Liver/renal (>80)	10 mg daily (10-20 mg/day)
bisoprolol (Zebeta)	N/A	9-12	Liver/renal (50)	5 mg daily (2.5-20 mg/day)
carteolol (Cartrol)	1-3	6	Liver/renal (50-70)	2.5 mg daily (2.5-10 mg/day)
carvedilol (Coreg)	N/A	7-10	Liver renal (2) Metabolites primarily in bile/feces (no value available)	6.25 mg twice daily (6.25-50 mg/day)
labetalol (Normodyne)	PO: 2-4 IV: 5 min	6-8 5.5	Liver/renal (55-60)	PO: 100 mg twice a day (400-1200 mg/day) IV: 20 mg intravenously
metoprolol (Lopressor)	PO: 1-2	3-7	Liver/renal (3-10)	100 mg daily (50-450 mg/day)
nadolol (Corgard)	4	20-24	Renal (70)	40 mg daily (40-240 mg/day)
penbutolol (Levatol)	1.5-3	5	Liver/renal (90)	20 mg daily (10-40 mg/day)
pindolol (Visken)	1-2	3-4	Liver/renal (40)	5 mg twice daily (5-45 mg/day in Canada; 60 mg/day in US)
propranolol (Inderal)	1-1.5	3-5	Liver/renal (<1)	40 mg twice daily (10-640 mg/day)
sotalol (Betapace)	2-3	7-18	Liver/renal (75)	80 mg twice daily (80-320 mg/day)
timolol (Blocadren)	1-2	4	Liver/renal (20)	10 mg twice daily (10-60 mg/day)

*Percent excreted unchanged (Olin, 1998; *USP DI*, 1998).

BOX 16-4 Withdrawal of a Beta Blocking Agent

It is recommended that the dose of a beta-adrenergic blocking agent be slowly tapered or lowered over approximately 14 days.

The patient should be advised to avoid vigorous physical exercises or activity during this time to decrease the risk of a reinfarction or cardiac dysrhythmia.

If withdrawal signs occur (angina or chest pain, sweating, rebound hypertension, dysrhythmias, tremors, tachycardia, or respiratory distress), temporarily reinstitute the beta blocking agent to stabilize the patient. Then slowly lower the dose with close supervision.

Drug interactions

The following interactions are possible when beta-adrenergic blocking agents are given with the drugs listed below:

Drug	Possible effect and management
Allergen immunotherapy or allergic extracts for skin testing	Use of these agents place patient at risk for serious systemic reaction; another drug should be substituted for the beta-adrenergic blocking agent. Avoid or a potentially serious drug interaction may occur.
Antidiabetic agents, oral hypoglycemic agents, or insulin	May cause hyperglycemia or hypoglycemia. Symptoms of hypoglycemia, such as increased heart rate and decreased blood pressure, may be blocked, thus making it difficult to monitor. Monitoring of blood glucose levels and dosage adjustments of the hypoglycemic agent may be necessary.
Calcium channel blocking agents, clonidine (Catapres), or guanabenz (Wytensin)	May result in potentiated antihypertensive effects; monitor blood pressure closely. If therapy with a beta-adrenergic blocking agent, clonidine, or guanabenz is to be discontinued, taper the dose of the beta blocker gradually over several days. When it is discontinued, the clonidine or guanabenz may then be tapered and discontinued also over several days. Monitor blood pressure closely throughout this procedure. Use caution when high doses of calcium channel blocking agents are given concurrently with a beta-adrenergic blocking agent. Nifedipine (Procardia, Adalat) may, in some instances, result in excessive hypotension in patients receiving concurrent therapy.

cocaine	May reduce or cancel the effects of the beta-adrenergic blocking agents. Also, whereas beta blocking agents are used to treat symptoms induced by cocaine (i.e., increased heart rate, cardiac dysrhythmias, etc.), an increased risk of inducing hypertension, severe bradycardia, and heart block can occur. If a beta blocker is necessary, labetalol may present less risk than the other beta-adrenergic blocking agents (because of its alpha-adrenergic blocking effect).
MAO inhibitors	This combination is not to be used; severe hypertension may result, even up to 14 days after the MAO inhibitor is discontinued. Avoid or a potentially serious drug interaction may occur.
Sympathomimetics	The effects of both drugs may be reduced or blocked (sympathomimetics with beta activity). With sympathomimetics having both alpha and beta activity, beta blockade may result in increased alpha effects, i.e., hypertension, severe bradycardia, and possibly heart block. Avoid or a potentially serious drug interaction may occur. Labetalol may be used if combination therapy is necessary because it has alpha blocking effects.
Xanthines (aminophylline or theophylline)	Therapeutic response of both drugs may be reduced or blocked. May also result in theophylline accumulation in the body. Monitor vital signs closely when this drug combination is prescribed.

Color type indicates an unsafe drug combination.

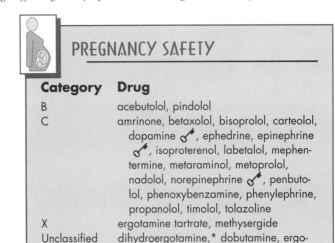

PREGNANCY SAFETY

Category	Drug
B	acebutolol, pindolol
C	amrinone, betaxolol, bisoprolol, carteolol, dopamine, ephedrine, epinephrine, isoproterenol, labetalol, mephentermine, metaraminol, metoprolol, nadolol, norepinephrine, penbutolol, phenoxybenzamine, phenylephrine, propanolol, timolol, tolazoline
X	ergotamine tartrate, methysergide
Unclassified	dihydroergotamine,* dobutamine, ergoloid mesylates, phentolamine

*Not recommended.

Side effects and adverse reactions

These include drowsiness, weakness, trouble sleeping, anxiety, nasal congestion, abdominal distress, dizziness, bradycardia, nausea, vomiting, depression, cold hands and feet, and difficulty breathing (bronchospasm).

Warnings

Use with caution in patients with liver or renal function impairment, myasthenia gravis, pheochromocytoma, and psoriasis.

Contraindications

Avoid use in persons with drug hypersensitivity, heart failure, cardiogenic shock, heart blocks, bradycardia, a history of allergies, bronchial asthma, diabetes mellitus, hyperthyroidism, and depression.

Dosage administration

For pregnancy safety, see the box above.

Serotonergic Drug

sumatriptan [soo ma trip′ tan] (Imitrex)

Sumatriptan is an antimigraine product that is believed to produce its effects at one serotonin receptor subtype ($5\text{-}HT_{1d}$) selectively, which results in a binding and stimulation of these receptors located on cranial blood vessels. The receptors' response is constriction of blood vessels, and perhaps, cerebral blood vessel constriction, which results in the reduction of pulsation associated with pain from vascular headaches (USP DI, 1998). Sumatriptan may also decrease mediators of inflammation, which are somehow involved with serotonergic mechanisms. This product has no effect on other receptors in the body.

Pharmacokinetics

Sumatriptan is available in oral and parenteral dosage forms. Orally it is rapidly, although incompletely absorbed; has an onset of action within ½ hour, reaches its peak effect in 2 hours (in 50% to 75% of patients), is metabolized in the liver, and is excreted renally. Parenterally it is administered subcutaneously with an onset of action (relief of headache pain) within 10 minutes; peak serum level within 1 hour, metabolism in the liver, and excretion via the kidneys.

Drug interactions

Avoid concurrent drug administration with MAO inhibitors as a dangerous hyperserotonergic situation may occur. The MAO inhibitor inhibits MAO-A isoenzyme, which is necessary for the metabolism of sumatriptan, thus resulting in a decrease in elimination and an increased potential for toxicity. Do not take oral sumatriptan during or within 2 weeks after administration of an MAO inhibitor.

Side effects and adverse reactions

These include nausea, vomiting, dizziness, weakness, drowsiness, and fatigue. As these symptoms also occur during and after a migraine headache, it is difficult to determine sumatriptan's contribution to these effects. Chest pain, difficulty swallowing, and tightness in chest and neck may also occur. Several deaths have resulted 3 hours or more after its administration (from stroke and cerebral hemorrhage), and it is not certain if they were due to underlying disease or directly related to sumatriptan. Individuals with migraines are at increased risk for cerebrovascular accidents or a transient ischemic attack, and it has been postulated that maybe a cerebrovascular attack rather than a migraine caused the symptoms that resulted in the administration of sumatriptan (USP DI, 1998).

Warnings

Use with caution in patients with hypertension.

Contraindications

Avoid use in persons with sumatriptan hypersensitivity, liver or renal function impairment, cardiac dysrhythmias, coronary artery disease, a history of cerebrovascular disease, and uncontrolled hypertension.

Dosage and administration

The adult antimigraine oral dose is 100 mg. If the person responds, this dose may be repeated if the headache pain returns or increases in intensity. The maximum dosage is a 100 mg dose, three times in 24 hours. Parenterally, 6 mg SC is injected in the outer thigh or outer upper arm. If the patient responds to this dose in 1 to 2 hours, an additional dose may be given if the headache pain returns or increases.

SUMMARY

A comprehensive understanding of the autonomic nervous systems is necessary to understand the (1) principal functions of each system, (2) primary receptor effects, and (3) pharmacologic agents that enhance, mimic, or block therapeutic response. The sympathetic nervous system is responsible for major physiologic changes in the body to prepare the individual for emergency responses, that is, the "fight or flight" response. Drugs that affect this system are either adrenergic (sympathomimetic) drugs (i.e., mimic the effects of sympathetic nerve stimulation) or adrenergic blocking (sympatholytic) drugs (i.e., drugs compete at receptor sites to inhibit adrenergic sympathetic stimulation). These agents may be direct-acting, indirect-acting, or dual-acting (direct and indirect) agents affecting alpha and/or beta receptors.

Epinephrine is an important drug (a direct-acting catecholamine) that stimulates alpha, $beta_1$, and $beta_2$ receptors. It is commonly used in the treatment of asthma, emergency treatment of anaphylactic shock and cardiac arrest, treatment of local hemostasis, and management of simple open-angle glaucoma.

Norepinephrine (Levophed) has a high affinity for alpha receptors; thus, it is a potent peripheral arteriolar vasoconstrictor. It raises both systolic and diastolic pressure. (Whereas dobutamine is used for patients with low cardiac output because it directly stimulates the $beta_1$-adrenergic receptors of the heart and dopamine effects are dose related.) In the lower dose range, it causes vasodilation of the renal and mesenteric arteries. All of these agents have been used for the treatment of circulatory shock.

The adrenergic blocking agents (sympatholytic) are classified by their receptor activity, that is, alpha and/or beta receptor competitive blocking effects. Three categories of antagonists are reviewed in this chapter. In addition, four classifications of beta-adrenergic blocking agents including selective $beta_1$ or cardioselective agents, selective $beta_1$ with ISA effects, and nonselective beta-adrenergic blocking agents with and without ISA effects are discussed.

REVIEW QUESTIONS

1. Discuss the three usual dopamine dosage ranges and the principal effects produced with each. Name a clinical situation when each range might be appropriately applied.
2. Describe the pharmacologic effects of norepinephrine in the treatment of acute hypotensive episodes. What receptors are affected? What dosage ranges?
3. Explain the proposed mechanisms of action for the use of the ergot alkaloids and sumatriptan in the treatment of migraine and the use of ergoloid mesylates in dementia. Name four major drug interactions associated with the ergot alkaloids.
4. Discuss the potential mechanisms of action for the beta-adrenergic blocking agents when used to treat angina pectoris, hypertension, and vascular headaches, and as a prophylactic treatment for myocardial infarction.

REFERENCES

American Medical Association: *AMA drug evaluations 1995,* Chicago, 1995, the Association.

Carter BL, Furmaga EM, Murphy CH: Essential hypertension. In Young LY, Koda-Kimble MA, editors: *Applied therapeutics: the clinical use of drugs,* ed 6, Vancouver, Wash, 1995, Applied Therapeutics, Inc.

Olin BR: *Facts and comparisons,* Philadelphia, 1998, JB Lippincott.

United States Pharmacopeial Convention: *USP DI: drug information for the health care professional,* ed 18, Rockville, Md, 1998, the Convention.

ADDITIONAL REFERENCES

American Hospital Formulary Service: *AHFS drug information '98,* Bethesda, Md, 1996, American Society of Hospital Pharmacists.

Anderson KN et al, editors: *Mosby's medical, nursing, and allied health dictionary,* ed 5, St Louis, 1998, Mosby.

Hardman JG, Limbird LE, editors: *Goodman & Gilman's the pharmacological basis of therapeutics,* ed 9, New York, 1996, McGraw-Hill.

Jackson G: The management of stable angina, *Hosp Pract* 28(1):59, 1993.

Katzung BG: *Basic and clinical pharmacology,* ed 5,. Norwalk, Conn, 1992, Appleton & Lange.

CHAPTER 17

Drugs for Specific Central-Peripheral Nervous System Dysfunctions

KEY DRUGS

baclofen (p. 303)
benztropine (p. 290)
levodopa (p. 291)
selegiline (p. 296)
tacrine (p. 301)

CHAPTER FOCUS

This chapter reviews the etiology and treatment of Parkinson's disease, myasthenia gravis, dementia, and Alzheimer's disease. Skeletal muscle relaxants are also discussed. As central-peripheral nervous system dysfunctions are often progressive and incapacitating, an understanding of the disease process and appropriate interventions are vitally important for the healthcare professional.

OBJECTIVES

After reading and studying this chapter, the student should be able to do the following:

1. *Define and discuss the key terms and key drugs.*
2. *Name the two neurotransmitters that centrally affect motor function and balance. Explain the neurotransmitter balance theory in Parkinson's disease.*
3. *Discuss the primary agents used to treat Parkinson's disease and myasthenia gravis, including mechanisms of action, pharmacokinetics, drug interactions, and primary side effects and adverse reactions.*
4. *Review medications used to treat dementia, Alzheimer's disease, and muscle spasm/spasticity.*
5. *Compare the mechanisms of action of central-acting and direct-acting skeletal muscle relaxants. Name and present one example of each.*

KEY TERMS

akinesia, (p. 290)
Alzheimer's disease, (p. 300)
anticholinesterase agents, (p. 297)
bradykinesia, (p. 289)
dementia, (p. 299)
dystonia, (p. 303)
myasthenia gravis, (p. 297)
on-off syndrome, (p. 292)
Parkinson's disease, (p. 289)
spasms, (p. 302)
spasticity, (p. 302)

The need to develop and monitor rational pharmacologic interventions for the progressively deteriorating conditions of Parkinson's disease, myasthenia gravis, dementia, and Alzheimer's disease is apparent. Currently there are no cures available; therefore drug therapies are the primary methods utilized to minimize the symptoms of these illnesses.

Spasticity of the skeletal muscles can also be debilitating, but these muscles are affected by many pharmacologic substances. Agents with an effect at the neuromuscular junction or at different levels in the central nervous system (CNS), i.e., at the brain or the spinal cord, will also be discussed in this chapter.

PARKINSON'S DISEASE

Parkinson's disease is a progressively debilitating disorder of the CNS characterized by tremors at rest, **bradykinesia** (abnormal slowing of all voluntary movements and speech), forward flexion of the trunk, muscle rigidity, and weakness. It occurs usually between the ages of 50 to 80, affecting both sexes equally. Approximately 1% of the American population, or 1 million persons, currently have Parkinson's disease (Flaherty, Gidal, 1995). While the cause is unknown, genetic factors, viral influences, and environmental contaminants have been suspected. The disease is caused by a disorder of the extrapyramidal system in the brain, particularly the basal ganglia area. Degeneration of the dopamine-producing neurons in this area produces a dopamine/acetylcholine imbalance, a progressive loss of dopamine (inhibitory neurotransmitter), and an increase in acetylcholine (excitatory neurotransmitter). It has also been induced by designer drugs (Box 17-1). The correct balance of dopamine and acetylcholine is important in regulating posture, muscle tone, and voluntary movement (Fig. 17-1). The amounts of other neurotransmitters such as norepinephrine and serotonin are also decreased in the brain of a person with Parkinson's disease.

BOX 17-1 Parkinson's Disease Induced by Designer Drugs

Designer drugs, or chemical variations of illegal or controlled substances, are an ever-increasing problem in North America. Such products are usually not illegal but generally are produced to induce the psychoactive effects of selected illegal products. Often the user consumes an unknown substance that may or may not be the desired product. Reports indicate that MPTP, a chemical produced as an analog of meperidine in clandestine laboratories, has been sold on the streets as heroin, cocaine, or a contaminant of other products.

MPTP has reportedly induced a degenerative CNS disorder characterized by tremors and muscle paralysis similar to the symptoms of Parkinson's disease. In a number of patients the paralysis reported has been permanent.

The central nervous system has two major types of dopamine receptors: D_1 and D_2 receptors. The D_1 receptor role is not currently known, but D_2 and especially D_{2A} receptors are involved with the effects of levodopa and the other dopamine agonists (Flaherty, Gidal, 1995). Drug therapy is focused on correcting this dopamine/acetylcholine imbalance by increasing dopamine levels and blocking acetylcholine levels. The classes of drugs used in treatment include: (1) drugs with central anticholinergic activity (anticholinergics and antihistamines) and (2) drugs that affect brain dopamine levels to enhance dopaminergic mechanisms.

DRUGS WITH CENTRAL ANTICHOLINERGIC ACTIVITY

Symptoms of Parkinson's disease caused by an excess of cholinergic activity include muscle rigidity and muscle tremor. The muscle rigidity or increased tone appears as "ratchet resistance," or "cogwheel rigidity," wherein the affected muscle moves easily, then meets resistance or remains fixed in the new position. The muscle tremors appear to have a "to-and-fro" movement caused by the sequence of contractions of agonistic and antagonistic muscles involved. The tremors are usually worse at rest and are commonly manifested as a "pill-rolling" motion of the hands and a

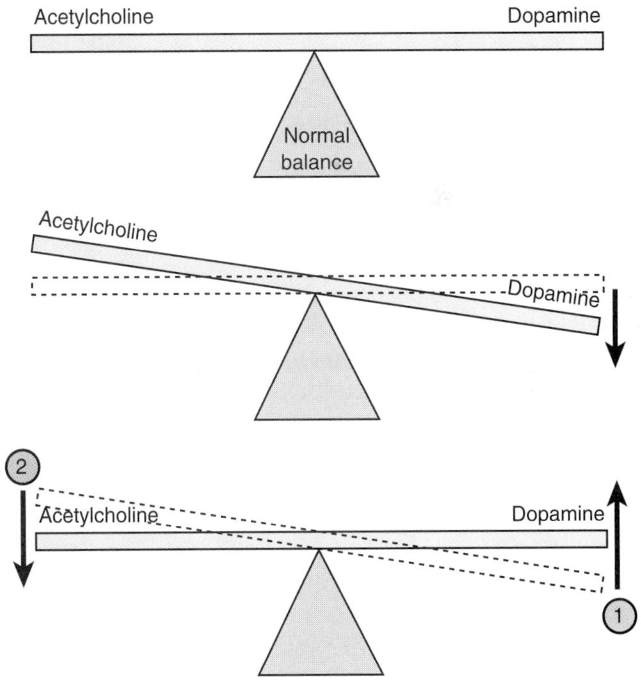

FIGURE 17-1
Central acetylcholine/dopamine balance. **A,** Normal "balance" of acetylcholine and dopamine. **B,** In Parkinson's disease, a decrease in dopamine results in an acetylcholine/dopamine imbalance. **C,** Drug therapy for Parkinson's disease focuses on increasing the dopamine level, which restores the acetylcholine/dopamine balance toward normal by (1) increasing the supply of dopamine or (2) blocking or lowering acetylcholine levels.

bobbing of the head. Anticholinergics are more useful early in the course of this disease because the dopamine depletion side effects are not prominent at this stage.

Various drugs with central anticholinergic activity are used to treat Parkinson's disease, such as benztropine (Cogentin), trihexyphenidyl (Artane), and diphenhydramine (Benadryl). These agents are used in the treatment of mild Parkinson's disease and as an adjunct to dopamine replacement.

ANTICHOLINERGIC AGENTS

benztropine [benz troe′ peen] (Cogentin, Apo-benztropine ✤) 🔑
biperiden [bye per′ i den] (Akineton)
procyclidine [proe sye′ kli deen] (Kemadrin, Procyclid ✤)
trihexyphenidyl [trye hex ee fin′ i dill] (Artane)

Drugs that inhibit or block the effects of acetylcholine are referred to as anticholinergic drugs. The belladonna alkaloids, atropine and scopolamine, were the first centrally active (i.e., crossing the blood-brain barrier) anticholinergic agents used to treat parkinsonism; for many years these were the only drugs available for such treatment. These drugs have been supplanted by synthetic anticholinergics, which were developed in an effort to produce drugs as effective as the belladonna drugs but with fewer side effects. In this group benztropine is the key drug.

The anticholinergics, which readily cross the blood-brain barrier, can produce some improvement in functional capacity. The usefulness of these drugs is limited because of their side effects and their tendency to be less effective with continued use. Some anticholinergics are also used to control extrapyramidal reactions, such as rigidity, **akinesia** (difficulty in or lack of ability to initiate muscle movement), tremor, and akathisia, which are caused by antipsychotic drugs such as the phenothiazines.

Anticholinergic drugs block central cholinergic excitatory pathways, returning the dopamine/acetylcholine balance in the brain (especially in the basal ganglia) to normal. The effects of the anticholinergic agents include decreased salivation and relaxation of smooth muscle with a decrease in tremors. Decreased rigidity and akinesia (in nearly 50% of the patients) are also reported.

Indications

Anticholinergic agents are indicated for use as antidyskinetics and for treatment of Parkinson's disease and drug-induced extrapyramidal reactions.

Pharmacokinetics

These drugs are very well absorbed, and the onset of action for specific drugs is as follows: benztropine oral, 1 to 2 hours; benztropine IM/IV, within minutes; biperiden IM, within 10 to 30 minutes; biperiden IV, within minutes; and trihexyphenidyl oral, 1 hour. For the onset of action for diphenhydramine, see the section on antihistamines in Chapter 38. The duration of effect for specific agents is as follows: benztropine (Cogentin) oral, IM, or IV, 24 hours; biperiden (Akineton) IV, 1 to 8 hours; procyclidine (Kemadrin, Procyclid ✤) oral, 4 hours; and trihexyphenidyl (Artane) oral, 6 to 12 hours. Metabolism of the anticholinergics is undetermined. They are most likely excreted by the kidneys.

Drug interactions

The following effects may occur when anticholinergics are given with the drugs listed below:

Drug	Possible effect and management
Alcohol and CNS depressants	May result in enhanced CNS-depressant effects. Monitor closely for hypoventilation, sedation, confusion, and ataxia.
Antacids	Concurrent administration may reduce absorption and therapeutic effects of anticholinergic agents. Separate administration of antacids and anticholinergics by at least 1 to 2 hours.
Anticholinergic or other antimuscarinic* medications	May result in enhanced anticholinergic effects. Monitor for constipation because bowel impaction and paralytic ileus may be produced. Increased fluid intake, exercise, stool softeners, and laxatives may be necessary.
ketoconazole (Nizoral)	Anticholinergics may increase gastrointestinal (GI) pH, resulting in a marked reduction in the absorption of ketoconazole. Patients should be advised to take the drugs 2 hours apart.

*Drugs that block cholinergic receptors at postganglionic parasympathetic synapses and a small number of postganglionic sympathetic synapses (atropine and scopolamine) (see Chapter 15).

See the discussion of atropine in Chapter 15 and the Pediatric and Geriatric Implication boxes for additional information.

Side effects and adverse reactions

These include blurred vision, mydriasis, constipation, dry skin, anhidrosis, urinary hesitancy, pain on urination, nausea, vomiting, photophobia, drowsiness, xerostomia, and dysphagia.

Warnings and contraindications

Same as atropine in Chapter 15. See the box for Food and Drug Administration (FDA) pregnancy safety categories.

PEDIATRIC IMPLICATIONS

Anticholinergics

Infants and young children are very susceptible to side and adverse effects of anticholinergic drugs.

Closely monitor pediatric patients with spastic paralysis or brain damage, since they generally have an increased reaction to these agents, thus requiring a dosage reduction.

Anticholinergics, especially at high doses, may cause a paradoxical type reaction of increased nervousness, confusion, and hyperexcitability.

Children receiving these agents where hot weather prevails or environmental temperatures are high have an increased risk of developing a rapid body temperature increase (anticholinergic drugs suppress sweat gland activity).

Dosage adjustments are often necessary for infants, patients with Down's syndrome, and blonds since they generally have an increased response to this drug category. Flushing, increased temperature, irritability, and increased pulse and respiratory rate may occur.

Start with low doses and increase gradually, as needed and tolerated.

GERIATRIC IMPLICATIONS

Anticholinergics

The elderly are highly susceptible to side effects of anticholinergic drugs, especially constipation, dry mouth, and urinary retention (usually in men).

Avoid use of these agents in persons with narrow-angle glaucoma or a history of urinary retention.

Memory impairment has been reported with continuous administration of these agents, especially in older persons.

When usual adult doses are administered, some elderly may have a paradoxical reaction: hyperexcitability, agitation, confusion, and sedation.

Chronic use decreases or inhibits the flow of saliva, which may contribute to oral discomfort, periodontal disease, and candidiasis.

Overheating resulting in heat stroke has been reported in persons receiving anticholinergic drugs during vigorous exercise or periods of hot weather.

Blurred vision and/or increased sensitivity to light may occur.

Anticholinergic dosing in the elderly should begin at the lowest dose with gradual increases until maximum improvement is noted or intolerable side effects occur.

Dosage and administration

The adult benztropine dose for Parkinson's disease (PD) is 1 to 2 mg PO, IM, or IV daily, adjusted as necessary. For drug-induced extrapyramidal reactions (DIE), the dose is 1 to 4 mg PO, IM, or IV once or twice a day up to a maximum of 6 mg/day. The biperiden adult dose for PD is 2 mg PO three to four times daily or 2 mg IM or slow IV. The procyclidine adult dose for PD or DIE is 2.5 mg PO three times daily after meals, and the trihexyphenidyl adult dose is 1 to 2 mg initially, adjusted at 3- to 5-day intervals as needed for PD. For DIE, the dose is 1 mg PO initially, adjusted as necessary.

PREGNANCY SAFETY

Category	Drug
B	bromocriptine, pergolide
C	amantadine, biperiden, carbidopa/levodopa, edrophonium, neostigmine, selegiline
Unclassified	ambenonium, benztropine, levodopa, procyclidine, pyridostigmine, trihexyphenidyl

DRUGS AFFECTING BRAIN DOPAMINE

Three classifications of drugs affect brain dopamine: those that release dopamine, those that increase brain levels of dopamine, and dopaminergic agonists. The drugs of choice in the treatment of Parkinson's disease are those that increase the brain levels of dopamine. The other two classifications are used as adjuncts or when normal therapy is contraindicated.

The drugs affecting brain dopamine have their major effect on the akinesia seen in Parkinson's disease. Akinesia is the difficulty in or the lack of ability to initiate muscle movement caused in Parkinson's disease by decreased levels of brain dopamine. The person with akinesia exhibits a masklike facial expression, impairment of postural reflexes, and eventually an inability for self-care. Drugs affecting brain dopamine increase the level of brain dopamine, thus creating a balance between dopamine and acetylcholine in the brain, especially in the basal ganglia area.

DRUGS THAT INCREASE BRAIN LEVELS OF DOPAMINE

levodopa [lee voe doe' pa]
(l-Dopa, Dopar, Larodopa)

A small percentage of levodopa crosses the blood-brain barrier intact. It is decarboxylated to dopamine, stimulates dopamine receptors, and helps to balance dopamine/acetylcholine concentrations.

Indications

Levodopa is indicated for treatment of Parkinson's disease (idiopathic, postencephalitic, or symptomatic) or parkinsonism associated with cerebral atherosclerosis.

Pharmacokinetics

This product is absorbed by active transport; approximately 30% to 50% reaches the systemic circulation. The drug is distributed to most body tissues; the CNS receives less than 1% of the dose because of peripheral metabolism. The enzyme decarboxylase converts levodopa (95%) to dopamine in the stomach, the intestines, and also the liver. Levodopa has a half-life of 1 to 3 hours.

Usually improvement is seen within 2 to 3 weeks (although other patients may require levodopa for up to 6 months to obtain a therapeutic effect). The peak concentration is achieved in 1 to 3 hours. The duration of action is up to 5 hours per dose. The drug is excreted by the kidneys.

Drug interactions

The following effects may occur when levodopa is given with the drugs listed below:

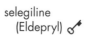

Drug	Possible effect and management
Anesthetics, hydrocarbon	May result in dysrhythmias. Discontinue levodopa 6 to 8 hours before hydrocarbon anesthetics, especially halothane.
Inhalation anticonvulsants, haloperidol (Haldol), or phenothiazines	May result in decreased levodopa effects, because hydantoin anticonvulsants increase levodopa metabolism and haloperidol and phenothiazines block dopamine receptors in the brain. When hydantoin and levodopa are given concurrently, monitor closely, as increased doses of levodopa may be necessary. If at all possible, avoid the combination of haloperidol or phenothiazines with levodopa.
cocaine	May result in increased risk of dysrhythmias. If medically necessary to give both drugs concurrently, reduce doses and monitor closely with electrocardiogram (ECG).
monoamine oxidase (MAO) inhibitors	This combination may result in a hypertensive crisis. Avoid or a potentially serious drug interaction may occur. MAO inhibitors should be discontinued 2 to 4 weeks before starting levodopa therapy.
pyridoxine (vitamin B_6)	Dosages of 10 mg or more may reverse the antiparkinsonian effect of levodopa. Monitor closely.
selegiline (Eldepryl)	Although this combination may be used, it may result in increased levodopamine-induced nausea, dyskinesias, confusion, hypotension, and hallucinations. If this combination is used, the dose of levodopa should be reduced within several days of starting the selegiline.

Color type indicates an unsafe drug combination.

Side effects and adverse reactions

These include anxiety, nervousness, confusion (especially in the elderly), constipation, nightmares, difficult urination, depression, orthostatic hypotension, mood changes, increased aggressiveness, irregular heart rate, severe nausea or vomiting, and choreiform and involuntary movements of the body (face, arms, hands, tongue, head, and upper body). See Box 17-2 for more information.

Dosage and administration

The levodopa (Dopar, Larodopa) dose for children 12 years of age and older and adults is 250 mg orally 2 to 4 times daily, increased by 100 to 750 mg/day at 3- to 7-day intervals until a therapeutic response is achieved. The maximum dose is 8 g/day. Elderly and postencephalitic patients may require lower doses because they are more sensitive to this medication. Dosage for children younger than 12 years of age has not been established.

BOX 17-2 Levodopa On-Off Syndrome

On-off syndrome refers to a complication following prolonged levodopa therapy (2 years or more). The patient fluctuates from being symptom free ("on") to demonstrating full-blown Parkinson's symptoms ("off") during therapy. These effects may last from minutes to hours and may be due to a decrease in delivery of dopamine centrally, an alteration in sensitivity of the dopamine receptors, a variation in the amount and rate of drug absorption, a dopamine metabolite interference, or a combination of effects.

Treatment may require more frequent administration of levodopa or levodopa-carbidopa and perhaps the addition of a direct-acting dopamine agonist, bromocriptine. After a drug holiday (drug withdrawal) of several days to a week, some persons may demonstrate an improved response to the drug therapy. This may be because of the reestablishment of dopamine receptor sensitivity to levodopa, which is usually only temporary. Because symptoms may worsen during the drug-free period, this approach should be instituted in a hospital setting (Flaherty, Gidal, 1995).

levodopa-carbidopa

[lee voe doe′ pa/kar bi doe′ pa] (Sinemet)

Sinemet and Sinemet CR (control or extended release) are combinations of levodopa with the dopa decarboxylase inhibitor, carbidopa. Carbidopa competes for the enzyme dopa decarboxylase, thus retarding the peripheral breakdown of levodopa. Carbidopa does not cross the blood-brain barrier like levodopa; therefore it does not interfere with the intracerebral transformation of levodopa to dopamine. Because carbidopa prevents much of the peripheral conversion of levodopa to dopamine, the incidence of systemic side effects of levodopa, such as nausea, vomiting, and cardiac dysrhythmias, is decreased. The CNS effects of levodopa are a greater risk with this combination because more levodopa is reaching the brain to be converted to dopamine.

The addition of carbidopa to levodopa reduces the required dose of levodopa to approximately 20% to 25% of the original levodopa dosage. The available levodopa-carbidopa combination dosage forms include 10/100 (10 mg of carbidopa and 100 mg of levodopa), 25/100 (25 mg of carbidopa and 100 mg of levodopa), and 25/250 (25 mg of carbidopa and 250 mg of levodopa). To obtain the peripheral inhibitor effect of carbidopa, a minimum of 75 mg (range, 75 to 100 mg) per day is necessary. Saturating peripheral dopa decarboxylase requires between 75 to 100 mg/day of carbidopa (Flaherty, Gidal, 1995). Nausea and vomiting are reported in persons receiving dosages lower than 75 mg/day of carbidopa. Therefore three combination dosage forms are available to permit greater flexibility in prescribing sufficient amounts of both levodopa and carbidopa for the individual. The manufacturer recommends that not more than 200 mg/day of carbidopa be prescribed. As with levodopa alone, the decarboxylation to dopamine replaces the missing brain dopamine and restores a balance to dopamine/acetylcholine concentrations.

Indications

Levodopa-carbidopa is indicated for the treatment of idiopathic, postencephalitic, and symptomatic Parkinson's disease.

Pharmacokinetics

For levodopa's pharmacokinetics, see above. Between 40% and 70% of an oral dose of carbidopa is absorbed. The drug is distributed widely to many body tissues with the exception of the CNS. The drug's metabolism is insignificant. It is excreted by the kidneys.

Drug interactions

These are the same as for levodopa, with the exception of the pyridoxine interaction. The interaction between levodopa and pyridoxine does not occur in the presence of carbidopa.

Side effects and adverse reactions

These are similar to those for levodopa. Eyelid spasms or closing may be an early sign of drug overdose. Mental or mood changes may also occur earlier and may be dose related.

Warnings and contraindications

See levodopa.

Dosage and administration

For persons not previously receiving levodopa therapy, start oral dosage at 10/100 or 25/100 three times daily. Increase dose as needed every 1 or 2 days until the desired response is obtained. For patients previously receiving levodopa therapy, discontinue levodopa at least 8 hours before instituting combination therapy. If the individual is receiving less than 1.5 g of levodopa daily, start with 10/100 or 25/100 of carbidopa/levodopa three or four times daily; increase at 1- or 2-day intervals until the desired response is obtained. If the person is receiving more than 1.5 g of levodopa daily, the dose is usually 25/250 carbidopa/levodopa PO three or four times daily, increasing if necessary at 1- or 2-day intervals until the desired response is obtained.

Be aware that conversion from levodopa to combination levodopa-carbidopa requires only 25% of the original dosage of levodopa initially, with a maximum of up to 200 mg of carbidopa and 2 g of levodopa daily. If additional levodopa is necessary, give as a single agent.

Geriatric and postencephalitic patients may require a lower dose because they are more sensitive to this combination. Dosage for children under 18 years of age has not been established.

DOPAMINE-RELEASING DRUG

amantadine [a man′ ta deen] (Symmetrel)

Amantadine is a synthetic antiviral compound. Although its exact mechanism of its action is not completely known, it is postulated that amantadine releases dopamine and other catecholamines from neuronal storage sites. It also blocks the uptake of dopamine into presynaptic neurons, thus permitting peripheral and central accumulation of dopamine. Amantadine may also give the person a sense of well-being and elevation of mood. It is less effective than levodopa but produces more rapid clinical improvement and causes fewer untoward reactions.

Indications

Amantadine is indicated for use as an antidyskinetic (treatment of Parkinson's disease) and as an antiviral (systemic agent).

Pharmacokinetics

Amantadine is well absorbed; it is not metabolized. The drug has a half-life of 11 to 15 hours. The peak serum levels are reached within 2 to 4 hours, with onset of antidyskinetic action within 48 hours. A steady state is reached within 2 to 3 days with daily drug administration; the drug serum level is 0.2 to 0.9 μg/mL. Levels above 1 μg/mL are considered toxic. Amantadine is excreted by the kidneys.

Drug interactions

The following effects may occur when amantadine is given with the drugs listed below:

Drug	Possible effect and management
Alcohol	Increased CNS side effects, such as confusion, lightheadedness, orthostatic hypotension, and fainting spells reported. Avoid or a potentially serious drug interaction may occur.
Anticholinergics	May enhance anticholinergic side effects, such as confusion, hallucinations, and frightening dreams. Dosage adjustments may be necessary. Also monitor for paralytic ileus.
CNS stimulants	Additive CNS stimulation reported; side effects include increased nervousness, irritability, difficulty sleeping, and, at times, seizures and cardiac dysrhythmias. Closely monitor patients receiving concurrent stimulant therapy.

Color type indicates an unsafe drug combination.

Side effects and adverse reactions

These include impaired concentration, dizziness, increased irritability, anorexia, nausea, nervousness, purple-red skin spots (livedo reticularis, usually seen with chronic therapy), confusion, hallucinations, mental or mood variations, orthostatic hypotension, and difficult urination. Symptoms of overdose include severe confusion, insomnia, nightmares, and seizures.

Warnings

Use with caution in psychotic patients and in persons with a history of or current eczema-type rash.

Contraindications

Avoid use in persons with congestive heart failure, seizure disorders, and kidney function impairment.

Dosage and administration

The adult antidyskinetic dose is 100 mg PO once or twice daily. The maximum dosage is 400 mg/day. The elderly are given a dose of 100 mg daily to start, titrating to two or three times a day as necessary.

DOPAMINERGIC AGONISTS

bromocriptine [broe moe krip′ teen] (Parlodel)

Bromocriptine is an ergot alkaloid derivative marketed as the first agonist of dopamine receptor activity. It activates postsynaptic dopamine receptors, stimulating the production of dopamine and correcting the brain dopamine/acetylcholine imbalance.

Indications

The drug is indicated as an antidyskinetic, growth hormone suppressant, antihyperprolactinemic, and prophylactic for lactation after second or third trimester pregnancy loss.

Pharmacokinetics

Approximately 28% of a dose is absorbed, but only 6% reaches the systemic circulation. Bromocriptine's half-life is biphasic: alpha, 4 to 4½ hours; beta, 15 hours. Its onset of activity from a single dose used for antiparkinsonism is 30 to 90 minutes, reaching a peak concentration at 2 hours. The drug is metabolized in the liver. Metabolites of bromocriptine are excreted primarily in bile.

Drug interactions

The following effects may occur when bromocriptine is given with the drugs listed below:

Drug	Possible effect and management
Alcohol	Concurrent use may result in a disulfiram-like reaction, i.e., tachycardia, flushing, increased sweating, nausea, vomiting, severe headache, blurred vision, confusion, and chest pain. Avoid or a potentially serious drug interaction may occur.
erythromycin	A vast increase (more than 200%) in bromocriptine's serum level may occur. Monitor closely for bromocriptine toxicity. It has been proposed that this interaction may also occur with clarithromycin and troleandomycin (USP DI, 1998).
risperidone (Risperdal)	May increase prolactin serum levels and also interfere with bromocriptine's effects. Monitor closely as dosage adjustments may be needed.
ritonavir (Norvir)	Bromocriptine's serum levels may increase by 300% in combination with ritonavir. It is recommended that the dose of bromocriptine be decreased by 50% when this combination is used (USP DI, 1998).

Color type indicates an unsafe drig combination.

Side effect and adverse reactions

These include drowsiness, headache, nausea, hypotension, and, less frequently, confusion, hallucinations, and uncontrolled movements of body, face, tongue, arms, hands, and head.

Warnings

Use with caution in patients with psychosis, hypertension, and liver function impairment.

Contraindications

Avoid use in persons with a known hypersensitivity to bromocriptine or to other ergot alkaloids.

Dosage and administration

The adult antidyskinetic dose is 1.25 to 2.5 mg PO daily, titrated as necessary. The maintenance dosage may range from 2.5 to 100 mg daily in divided doses. Dosage for children younger than 15 years of age has not been established.

pergolide [per′ go lide] (Permax)

Pergolide is a dopamine agonist usually used in conjunction with levodopa or levodopa-carbidopa to treat the signs and symptoms of Parkinson's disease. It is more potent and longer-acting than bromocriptine and directly stimulates both D_1 and D_2 receptors (Flaherty, Gidal, 1995). In combination the dose of levodopa or levodopa-carbidopa is often reduced. According to Flaherty and Gidal, up to 75% of patients who did not respond to levodopa improved with the addition of pergolide to levodopa. Also, clinical fluctuations reported in persons receiving levodopa-carbidopa may be reduced; that is, the "on" period was prolonged while the "off" period was decreased in most of the patients studied.

Pergolide stimulates dopamine receptors in the nigrostriatal area, but unlike bromocriptine its action is independent of dopamine synthesis or dopamine storage sites. It also inhibits prolactin secretion.

Indications

Pergolide is indicated as an adjunct treatment for Parkinson's disease.

Pharmacokinetcs

Pergolide is well absorbed, and its serum protein binding is high (about 90%). The drug is excreted in the kidneys.

Drug interactions

No significant drug interactions are reported to date, but be aware that dopamine antagonists, such as the phenothiazines, loxapine (Loxapac, Loxitane), methyldopa (Aldomet), metoclopramide (Reglan), thioxanthenes, and haloperidol (Haldol), may decrease the effects of pergolide. Also, drugs that produce hypotension may have an additive hypotensive effect when administered concurrently with pergolide.

Side effect and adverse reactions

These include stomach distress/pain, constipation, lightheadedness, sedation, hypotension, cold-type symptoms, nausea, lower back pain, confusion, dyskinesias such as uncontrollable body movements, and hallucinations.

Warnings

Use with caution in patients with dysrhythmias and psychosis.

Contraindications

Avoid use in persons with known pergolide or other ergot alkaloid hypersensitivity.

Dosage and administration

The recommended adult dose is 0.05 mg PO daily for 2 days, increased by 0.1 to 0.15 mg every 3 days over the next 12 days. The dose may then be increased by 0.25 mg every 3 days until maximum therapeutic effect is reached. Doses should be divided and given three times daily. The maximum dose is 5 mg/day. The pediatric dosage has not been established.

DOPAMINE AGONISTS, NON-ERGOT

pramipexole [pra mi pex′ ol] (Mirapex)
ropinirole [roh pin′ a rohl] (Requip)

Pramipexole and ropinirole are non-ergot dopamine receptor agonists for Parkinson's disease. Although their exact mechanism of action is unknown, they are postulated to stimulate dopamine receptors in the striatum.

Pharmacokinetics

These agents are rapidly absorbed orally, reaching peak serum levels in 1 to 2 hours. The half-life of pramipexole is 8 hours (12 hours in geriatric patients); ropinirole's half-life is 6 hours. Ropinirole is extensively metabolized with only 1% to 2% excreted unchanged by the kidneys. Pramipexole is not metabolized and is primarily excreted unchanged in the urine.

Drug interactions

The following effects may occur when pramipexole is given the drugs listed below:

Drug	Possible effect and management
cimetidine (Tagamet)	Increases serum level of pramipexole by up to 50% and also extends pramipexole's half-life. Monitor closely as dosage adjustments may be necessary or preferably consider switching to a different histamine antagonist.

Other renally excreted drugs, i.e., cimetidine (Tagamet), ranitidine (Zantac), diltiazem (Cardizem), triamterene (Dyrenium), verapamil (Calan), and quinidine.	Concurrent drug administration of drugs eliminated by the same system may result in a decrease in pramipexole elimination (by approximately 20%). Monitor closely.

The following effects may occur when ropinirole is given with the drugs listed below:

Drug	Possible effect and management
ciprofloxacin (Cipro)	Concurrent use may increase ropinirole serum levels (by up to 80%). Monitor closely as dosage adjustment or alternate antibiotic may be necessary.
Liver metabolism (CYP1A2) inhibitors, i.e., cimetidine (Tagamet), ciprofloxacin (Cipro), dilitazem (Cardizem), enoxacin (Penetrex), erythromycin, fluvoxamine (Luvox), mexiletine (Mexitil), norfloxacin (Noroxin), and tacrine (Cognex)	Ropinirole's metabolism and excretion may be altered if it is given concurrently with these medications. Monitor patient closely, especially if one of these agents is added or discontinued from therapy.

Side effects and adverse reactions

These include nausea, constipation, dizziness, sedation, dyskinesia, hallucinations, confusion, and dystonia. Ropinirole has a higher reported incidence of dizziness, sedation, nausea, vomiting, stomach pain, and dyspepsia.

Warnings

Use with caution in patients with hypotension, the elderly (greater risk of hallucinations), and those with impaired kidney function.

Contraindications

Avoid use in persons with drug hypersensitivity.

Dosage and administration

The pramipexole adult dose ranges from 0.375 to 4.5 mg/day, in divided doses. The ropinirole adult dose is 0.25 to 1 mg tid with dosages adjusted weekly as necessary.

MONOAMINE OXIDASE INHIBITOR

selegiline [sel ee' jell een]
(Eldepryl, SD-Deprenyl)

Selegiline is used in combination with levodopa or levodopa-carbidopa to treat Parkinson's disease. There are two types of monoamine oxidase in the body: monoamine oxidase A is necessary to metabolize norepinephrine and serotonin; monoamine oxidase B metabolizes dopamine. Selegiline irreversibly inhibits monoamine oxidase B, thus preventing the breakdown of dopamine. As a result it will enhance or prolong levodopa's antiparkinson effect, which may result in a lowering of the daily dose of levodopa.

Pharmacokinetics

Selegiline is well absorbed orally, reaches its peak serum level in ½ to 2 hours, and has three active metabolites (with half-lives of 2 to 20 hours). It readily crosses the blood-brain barrier and is excreted slowly via the kidneys.

Drug interactions

The following effects may occur when selegiline is given with the drugs listed below:

Drug	Possible effect and management
fluoxetine (Prozac), fluvoxamine (Luvox), nefazodone (Serzone), paroxetine (Paxil), sertraine (Zoloft), and venlafaxine (Effexor)	Concurrent use may result in mania and a reaction similar to the serotonin syndrome (confusion, restlessness, hyperreflexia, sweating, shivering, tremors, diarrhea, ataxia, and fever) when administered with these selective serotonin reuptake inhibitors (SSRIs). Avoid or a potentially serious drug interaction may occur. The SSRIs should not be initiated until at least 2 weeks after selegiline is discontinued. However, in persons taking fluoxetine, selegiline should not be initiated for at least 5 weeks after fluoxetine has been discontinued (USP DI, 1998).
levodopa (L-dopa)	Although it is indicated to be given concurrently with levodopa, be aware that this combination may increase levodopa-induced side effects such as dyskinesias, nausea, hypotension, confusion, and hallucinations. To reduce this potential, the dose of levodopa should be lowered within 2 to 3 days after selegiline therapy is initiated.

meperidine (Demerol)	Concurrent drug administration may result in severe adverse reactions such as severe hypertension, respiratory depression, sweating, excitation, rigidity, seizures, hyperpyrexia, vascular collapse, coma, and death. Avoid or a potentially serious drug interaction may occur. Avoid administration of meperidine for at least 2 to 3 weeks after use of an MAO-inhibiting drug. Although the use of other opioids, such as morphine, are not as likely to cause such a severe reaction, they should also be used very cautiously in lowered doses in any person receiving a MAO inhibitor.
tyramine	The use of tyramine or foods and beverages that contain tyramine or high pressor amines should be avoided, or if consumed in very small quantities, should be carefully monitored. This combination may result in an immediate, severe hypertensive episode requiring medical attention. Avoid or a potentially serious drug interaction may occur. It is recommended that dietary restrictions be continued for at least 2 to 3 weeks after the discontinuance of a MAO inhibitor.

Color type indicates and unsafe drug combination.

Side effects and adverse reactions

These include dry mouth, nausea, vomiting, insomnia, dizziness, stomach distress or pain, dyskinesias, and mood alterations.

Warnings

Use with caution in patients with tremors, dementia, psychosis, and tardive dyskinesia.

Contraindications

Avoid use in persons with selegiline hypersensitivity and a history of peptic ulcer disease.

Dosage and administration

The usual adult dose of selegiline is 5 mg at breakfast and lunch.

MYASTHENIA GRAVIS

Myasthenia gravis is a progressive, incurable disease characterized by the loss of or decrease in acetylcholine receptors caused by an autoimmune process, resulting in skeletal muscle weakness and fatigue. Because of its involvement with the production of antibodies, the thymus gland is believed to have a role in the causation of myasthenia gravis. Nearly 15% of all myasthenia gravis patients have a thymoma, or tumor of the thymus gland.

Symptoms of myasthenia gravis usually become worse with exertion and are less noticeable with rest. Stress, infection, menses, surgery, and other factors may also increase the symptoms. The most common early reported symptoms are ptosis and diplopia. Dysarthria, dysphagia, and limb weakness, especially of the upper extremities, also occur in the advanced stages. The person may complain of shoulder fatigue after shaving or combing the hair or of hand weakness, finding it difficult to open doors or kitchen jars or to perform repetitive tasks, such as lawn work or playing the piano (Fig. 17-2).

The most serious effects of myasthenia gravis are dysphagia and respiratory muscle weakness, since these may result in aspiration pneumonia or respiratory failure. Treatment of this disease state may include thymectomy, cholinesterase inhibitors, plasmapheresis, and, at times, corticosteroids. The mainstay, though, is cholinesterase-inhibitor drugs such as the anticholinesterase agents.

ANTICHOLINESTERASE AGENTS

The **anticholinesterase agents** (antimyasthenics or cholinesterase inhibitors) are drugs that enhance cholinergic action by blocking the effect of cholinesterase. These drugs act by inactivating or inhibiting cholinesterase at the sites of acetylcholine transmission, permitting the accumulation of acetylcholine.

Indications

Because anticholinesterase agents increase the amount of acetylcholine at the myoneural junction, the cholinesterase inhibitors are primarily used for the diagnosis and treatment of myasthenia gravis and for their local effects in the eye (see Chapter 36). These drugs are used also for urinary retention and paralytic ileus and as an antidote for the curariform effects of the nondepolarizing skeletal muscle relaxants, such as tubocurarine (Tubarine) and pancuronium (Pavulon).

Pharmacokinetics

Orally, all are poorly absorbed from the GI tract. The onset of action of these drugs is as follows: ambenonium (Mytelase), within 30 minutes; edrophonium (Tensilon), IM within 2 to 10 minutes and IV within 30 to 60 seconds; neostigmine (Prostigmin), orally within 45 to 75 minutes, IM within 30 minutes, and IV within 4 to 8 minutes; and pyridostigmine (Mestinon) oral tablet or syrup within 30 to 45 minutes, extended-release tablet, 30 to 60 minutes, IM within 15 minutes, and IV within 2 to 5 minutes.

The duration of effect of each is as follows: ambenonium, 3 to 8 hours; edrophonium IM within 5 to 30 minutes and IV approximately 10 minutes; neostigmine oral

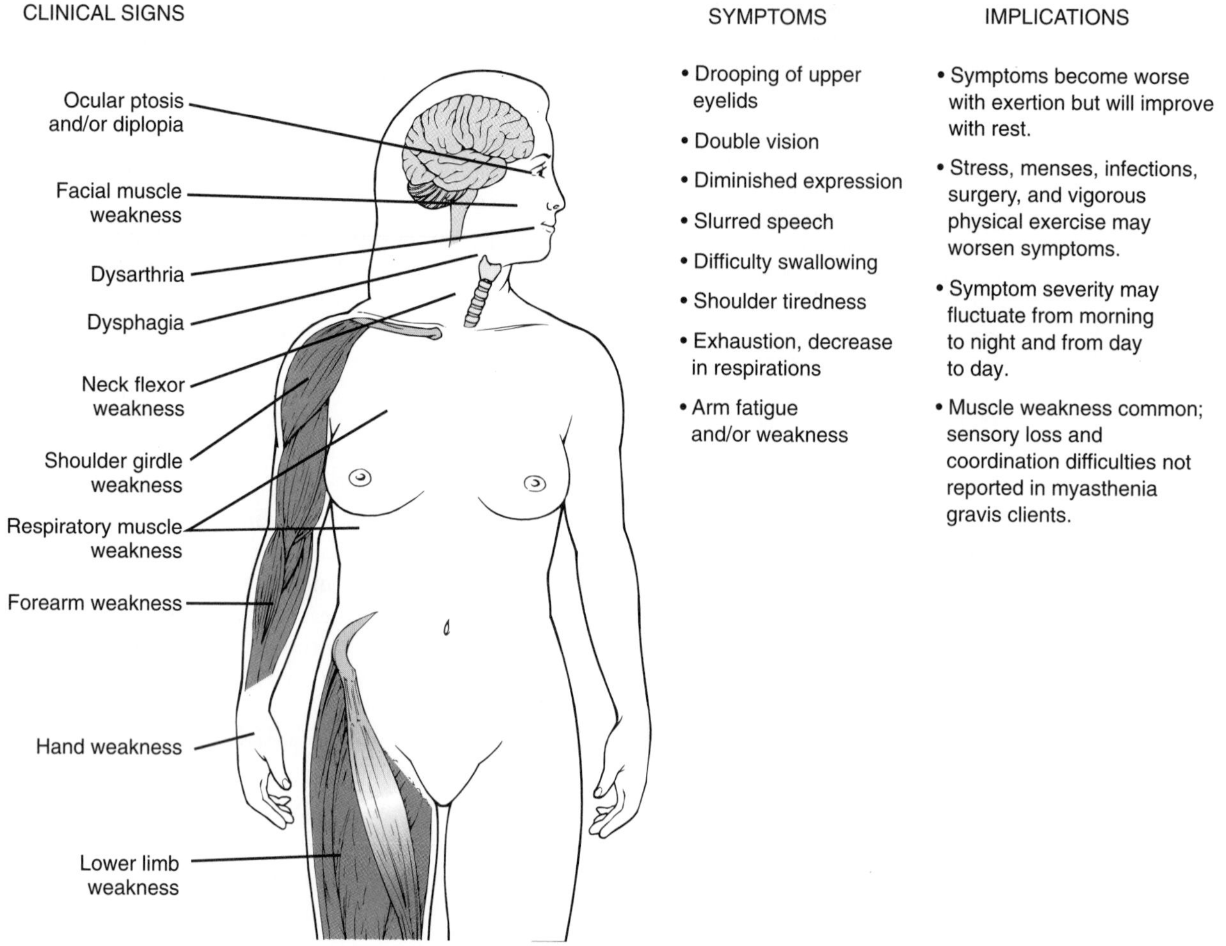
CLINICAL SIGNS
Ocular ptosis and/or diplopia
Facial muscle weakness
Dysarthria
Dysphagia
Neck flexor weakness
Shoulder girdle weakness
Respiratory muscle weakness
Forearm weakness
Hand weakness
Lower limb weakness
SYMPTOMS
• Drooping of upper eyelids
• Double vision
• Diminished expression
• Slurred speech
• Difficulty swallowing
• Shoulder tiredness
• Exhaustion, decrease in respirations
• Arm fatigue and/or weakness
IMPLICATIONS
• Symptoms become worse with exertion but will improve with rest.
• Stress, menses, infections, surgery, and vigorous physical exercise may worsen symptoms.
• Symptom severity may fluctuate from morning to night and from day to day.
• Muscle weakness common; sensory loss and coordination difficulties not reported in myasthenia gravis clients.

FIGURE 17-2
Signs, symptoms, and implications of myasthenia gravis.

and parenteral, 2 to 6 hours; and pyridostigmine oral syrup or tablets, 3 to 6 hours; extended-release tablet, 6 to 12 hours; and parenteral, 2 to 4 hours. Neostigmine and pyridostigmine are metabolized mainly in the liver and are excreted in the kidneys.

Drug interactions

The following effects may occur when cholinesterase inhibitors are given with the drugs listed below:

Drug	Possible effect and management
Other cholinesterase inhibitors such as demecarium (Humosol), echothiophate (Phospholine). and isoflurophate (Floropryl)	This combination of drugs is not recommended. Avoid or a potentially serious drug interaction may occur.
guanadrel (Hylorel), guanethidine (Ismelin), mecamylamine (Inversine), or trimethaphan (Arfonad)	These are ganglionic blocking agents that may antagonize the action of the cholinesterase-inhibitor drugs, resulting in increased muscle weakness, respiratory muscle weakness, and difficulty in swallowing. Avoid or a potentially serious drug interaction may occur.
procainamide (Pronestyl) or quinidine	The neuromuscular blocking action and possibly antimuscarinicpossibly antimuscarinic effect of procainamide may antagonize the action of the quinidinthe cholinesterase inhibitor drugs. If used concurrently, monitor patient closely.

Color type indicates an unsafe drug combination.

Side effects and adverse reactions

These include nausea, vomiting, diarrhea, abdominal cramps, increased sweating, drooling, increased urge to urinate, pinpoint pupils, eye watering, and increased bronchial secretions. Overdose effects include blurred vision, severe diarrhea, increased salivation, increase in bronchial secretions, severe nausea or vomiting, respiratory difficulties, severe abdominal pain, bradycardia, increased weakness, ataxia, confusion, slurred speech, and muscle weakness.

Warnings

Use with caution in patients with asthma, postsurgical atelectasis, pneumonia, and cardiac dysrhythmias.

Contraindications

Avoid use in persons with drug hypersensitivity, urinary tract or gastrointestinal tract obstruction, and urinary tract infections.

Dosage and administration

The neostigmine adult dose is 15 mg PO every 3 to 4 horrs as necessary. The parenteral antimyasthenic dose is 0.5 mg IM or SC. The children's dose is 2 mg/kg divided into six or eight doses. The parenteral antimyasthenic dose is 0.01 to 0.04 mg/kg IM or SC. The pyridostigmine adult dose is 30 to 60 mg PO every 3 to 4 hours, as needed. The dose in extended release tablets is 180 to 540 mg one to two times daily. The parenteral dose is 2 mg IM or IV every 2 to 3 hours. the children's antimyasthenic dose is 7 mg/kg PO divided in five or six doses daily.

Ambenonium (Mytelase) is a slowly reversible cholinesterase inhibitor; therefore it may accumulate at cholinergic synapses and produce increased prolonged effects. Because of the narrow margin between first appearance of side effects and serious toxicity, ambenonium is usually reserved for patients who have not responded adequately to neostigmine or pyridostigmine or for patients who are hypersensitive to the bromide component in both drugs. The usual adult dose is 5 mg PO 3 or 4 times daily, as necessary. Children's dose is 0.3 mg/kg in divided doses.

Edrophonium chloride injection (Tensilon) is used to diagnose myasthenia gravis. Because of its short duration of action, it is not indicated for the treatment of myasthenia gravis

DEMENTIA

Dementia, a progressive mental disorder characterized by chronic personality disintegration, confusion, and deterioration of intellectual capacity and impulse control, affects 3% to 16% of Americans older than age 65. Alzheimer's disease accounts for approximately 50% to 60% of dementia, while vascular dementia (including multi-infarct dementia, formerly known as cerebrovascular arteriosclerosis), Pick's disease, Parkinson's disease dementia, and other forms comprise the balance (Williams, 1995). It has been estimated that irreversible dementias occur in about 90% of persons with dementia (Bravyak, Schechter, 1992).

Reversible dementias may be caused by drugs, emotion, metabolic or endocrine alterations, nutrition, trauma, infection, alcoholism, and systemic illness. The medications most associated with this type of dementia include anticholinergic agents, cardiac drugs, selected antihypertensives, and psychotropics. Box 17-3 lists selected potentially reversible causes of dementia.

BOX 17-3 Potentially Reversible Causes of Dementia

Drugs, chemicals, or toxins
- a. Bromides
- b. Mercury
- c. Drugs such as butyrophenones, phenothiazines, diuretics, and sedatives

Emotional problems
- a. Depression
- b. Chronic alcoholism

Metabolic disorders
- a. Hyperglycemia
- b. Hypothyroidism
- c. Hypopituitarism

Eye/ear deprivation
- a. Blindness
- b. Deafness

Nutritional deficits
- a. Vitamin B_{12} deficiency
- b. Folic acid deficiency
- c. Niacin deficiency

Tumors/trauma, acute
- a. Subdural hematoma
- b. Brain metastasis
- c. Brain tumors

Infections and/or fever
- a. Viral infections
- b. Bacterial (tuberculosis)
- c. Bacterial (endocarditis)

Arteriosclerotic events
- a. Vascular occlusion
- b. Stroke

Modified from Lamy, 1980.

The syndrome of dementia usually develops slowly. Early signs include depression, loss of ability to concentrate, and increased anxiety, irritability, and agitation. Intellectual ability is usually the first to decline and then recent memory (such as names of acquaintances or recent events) followed by the loss of orientation to time, place, and person. Personal habits will change. The person may become loud or obscene, or some personality characteristics that were present might become magnified.

Helplessness, total dependency, and loss of manual skills may occur next. In the final stages, the person may be bedridden with loss of sphincter control and eventually will die, usually of bronchopneumonia.

The prescriber should rule out all the possible reversible causes of dementia first. Then treatment should be instituted to try to prevent or reduce the ongoing damage and to support the patient and family in managing this disease process. Drug treatment is only indicated for symptom control, that is, the use of low-dose antipsychotic agents for treating severe agitation, delusions, and hallucinations, or antidepressants for severe depression. Supportive care should include proper nutrition, moderate exercise if permitted, vitamins if indicated, and the use of environmental aids in a consistent fashion, such as night lights and daily calendar reminders.

ALZHEIMER'S DISEASE

Alzheimer's disease is a presenile dementia characterized by confusion, memory failure, disorientation, restlessness, speech disturbances, and hallucinosis, and is tragically incurable. It affects approximately 4 million Americans with about 250,000 new cases diagnosed annually (Lamy, 1992). It has been estimated to be the major underlying reason for over 50% of all nursing home admissions (Miller, 1995). It has been estimated that approximately 3% of Americans older than age 65 have Alzheimer's disease, which increases with age to 19% of persons between 75 and 84 years of age and 47% of elders 85 years and older (Miller, 1995).

Clinically, a progressive decline in intellectual functions is noted, such as memory loss, loss of logic thinking or judgment, time and space disorientation, and an increased tendency to wander as a result of progressive disorientation. As the disease progresses, profound memory loss, personality changes, hyperactivity, hostility, and paranoia may be present. This middle phase in Alzheimer's disease is also characterized by the presence of aphasia (loss of speech or ability to express oneself), apraxia (loss of complex or intentional movements), and anomia (loss of ability to remember names of persons and objects). In the terminal phase, nearly all higher mental functioning is lost, and the person needs assistance with activities of daily living; thus the person requires continuous nursing care.

In this final period patients may be unable to speak intelligibly, walk, sit up in bed, eat or groom themselves, smile, or recognize simple objects or familiar persons. Table 17-1 explains the staging of cognitive decline.

In the terminal or last phase, the person wants to touch or examine all objects with the mouth (hyperorality), exhibits a decrease or loss in emotions, may be bulimic, and may also have a compulsion to touch everything in sight. Insomnia, nighttime wandering, and restlessness have also been reported. The progressive deterioration of brain cells may lead to increased dependency for all needs, decreased mobility to the point of being bedridden, and eventually death.

While researchers are still searching for the cause of Alzheimer's disease, many theories have been proposed. Currently the theories under study include: (1) a deficiency in acetylcholine, a major neurotransmitter, and perhaps other neurotransmitters in the brain; (2) a slow virus or infection that attacks selected brain cells; (3) a genetic predisposition; (4) an autoimmune theory (that the body fails to recognize host tissue and attacks itself); and (5) beta-amyloid protein accumulation in the CNS (Williams, 1995). A primary hypothesis is that Alzheimer's disease results from the loss of related cholinergic nerves in the CNS (Miller, 1995).

Current pharmacotherapy is focused on improving cognitive functioning or limiting disease progression and symptom control. Unfortunately no known current medication cures, retards, or prevents Alzheimer's disease. Three medications, the ergoloid mesylates (Hydergine), tacrine (Cognex), and donepezil (Aricept) have been approved by the FDA to treat memory deficits. The ergoloid mesylates have been used to treat early dementia, but their use is con-

TABLE 17-1 Staging of Cognitive Decline

Stage	*Clinical Phase*	*Symptoms*
1	Normal	No change in cognition
2	Very mild	Forgets object location, some deficit in word finding
3	Mild (early confusion)	Early cognitive decline in one or more areas: memory loss, decreased ability to function in work situation, name-finding deficit, some decrease in social functioning, recall difficulties, and anxiety
4	Moderate	Unable to perform complex tasks such as managing personal finances, planning a dinner party, concentration, and knowledge of current events
5	Moderately severe (early dementia)	Usually needs assistance for survival; reminders to bathe, help in selecting clothes, and other daily functions; may be disoriented as to time and recent events although this can fluctuate; may become tearful
6	Severe (dementia)	Needs assistance with dressing, bathing, and toilet functions (flushing, etc.); may forget spouse's, family's, and caregivers' names and details of personal life and generally be unaware of surroundings; may have incontinence of urine and feces; shows an increase in CNS disturbances such as agitation, delusions, paranoia, obsessive anxiety, and increased potential for violent behavior
7	Very severe (late dementia)	Unable to speak (speech limited to 5 words or less); may scream or make other sounds; unable to ambulate, sit up, smile, or feed themselves; unable to hold head erect, will ultimately slip into stupor or coma

troversial in Alzheimer's disease. One study reported no improvement with their use and instead some worsening of cognitive ability and behaviors (USP DI, 1998).

tacrine [tack' rin] (Cognex)

Tacrine, a centrally acting cholinesterase inhibitor, has a longer duration of action than physostigmine. This product appears to improve cognitive function in a limited number of persons with mild-to-moderate Alzheimer's disease.

Indications

Tacrine is used as an adjunct treatment for dementia symptoms.

Pharmacokinetics

Tacrine is rapidly absorbed orally and reaches its peak serum level in 0.5 to 3 hours with a half-life of 1.5 to 4 hours. It is metabolized in the liver with one major metabolite having central cholinergic effects.

Drug interactions

The following effects may occur when tacrine is given with the drugs listed below:

Drug	Possible effect and management
cimetidine (Tagamet)	May increase serum levels of tacrine. Monitor closely to avoid the potential for tacrine toxicity.
Neuromuscular blocking agents, i.e., succinylcholine (Anectine) and mivacurium (Mivacron)	Tacrine may inhibit the metabolizing enzyme (cholinesterase) of these agents, resulting in increased or prolonged muscle relaxation. Monitor closely or, if possible, avoid concurrent drug administration.
Nonsteroidal antiinflammatory drugs (NSAIDs)	Tacrine may increase gastric acid secretion which in combination with a NSAID, may increase the potential for GI irritation and bleeding. Monitor closely for occult GI bleeding.
Smoking tobacco	Tacrine serum levels are approximately 67% lower in smokers than in nonsmokers. The effectiveness of tacrine may be decreased in persons who are current smokers.
theophylline	Concurrent use increases theophylline levels to approximately double the normal values, thus increasing the potential for theophylline toxicity. Monitor theophylline plasma levels as dosage adjustments may be necessary.

Color type indicates an unsafe drug combination.

Side effects and adverse reactions

These include nausea, vomiting, loss of appetite, diarrhea, headache, ataxia, muscle aches, and hepatotoxicity. See current literature for recommended schedule for routine testing of serum alanine aminotransferase for liver toxicity.

Warnings

When discontinuing tacrine, use a tapered schedule under medical supervision. It is recommended that tacrine be discontinued at least 3 days before any surgery that involves general anesthesia.

Contraindications

Avoid use in patients with known tacrine hypersensitivity, asthma, cardiac disease (bradycardia, hypotension, and sick sinus syndrome), epilepsy, head injuries or intracranial lesions, metabolic disorders, obstruction of GI or urinary tract, Parkinson's disease, peptic ulcers, and liver function impairment.

Dosage and administration

The oral adult dose is 10 mg four times daily, increased at 6-week intervals as necessary. The maximum daily dose is 160 mg. For better absorption, this medication should be taken on an empty stomach (1 hour before meals or 2 hours after). However, if stomach upset occurs, it may be taken with food.

The benefits from tacrine have been limited; therefore many other drugs are under investigation. These agents include the NSAIDs (piracetam [Nootropil], oxiracetam, and indomethacin [Indocin]); velnacrine maleate (Mentane), a centrally acting cholinesterase inhibitor; nimodipine (Nimotop) a calcium antagonist; and selegiline (Eldepryl), a MAO-B inhibitor that may have antioxidant effects and also increases serotonin and norepinephrine concentrations (Eggert, Crismon, 1994; Bravyak, Schechter, 1992). It has also been reported that postmenopausal women treated with estrogen were less likely to get Alzheimer's disease than those who were untreated (Williams, 1995). Serotonin antagonists and angiotensin-converting enzyme inhibitors are also under investigation.

donepezil (Aricept)

Donepezil is the second drug released for the treatment of Alzheimer's disease. This drug inhibits the enzyme acetylcholinesterase, which permits an increased accumulation of acetylcholine in the brain.

Pharmacokinetics

Donepezil is well absorbed orally, reaches peak serum levels between 3 to 4 hours, and has a elimination half-life of 70 hours. It is metabolized in the liver to four major metabolites (two of which are active metabolites) and excreted primarily by the kidneys.

Drug interactions

No significant drug interactions are noted.

Side effects and adverse reactions

These include muscle cramping, nausea, vomiting, diarrhea, and insomnia.

Warnings

Use with caution in patients with history of asthma or chronic obstructive pulmonary disease, convulsions, liver impairment, and urinary tract obstruction.

Contraindications

Avoid use in persons with donepezil hypersensitivity, cardiac disease (sick sinus syndrome and supraventricular conduction alterations), and peptic ulcer disease.

Dosage and administration

The usual adult dose for Alzheimer's dementia is 5 mg daily, taken in the evening.

SYMPTOM MANAGEMENT

Symptom management includes small dosages of antipsychotic agents such as haloperidol (Haldol), 0.5 to 5 mg/day, for delusions and hallucinations. However, two precautions exist: first, start with a low dosage and only gradually increase it if necessary. Monitor the person closely for side effects. Second, be aware that antipsychotic agents or any medications with a high anticholinergic potential could worsen the cognitive functioning of the patient.

For depression, antidepressants with a low anticholinergic profile, such as desipramine (Norpramin) or trazodone (Desyrel, Trazon), have been used. Start at one third to one half the usual adult dose for persons with Alzheimer's disease and increase slowly as necessary. The antianxiety agents, especially those with a short-to-intermediate half-life such as lorazepam (Ativan), oxazepam (Serax), or alprazolam (Xanax), are generally selected for patients who exhibit severe anxiety. Be aware that if such agents are used to treat agitation in patients with dementia (or specifically, Alzheimer's disease), the potential for inducing a paradoxical reaction is present. Such persons may respond with an increase in activity, restlessness, and agitation. So it is important for the prescriber to differentiate between agitation and anxiety. If the benzodiazepine antianxiety agents are used, they should be closely monitored because symptoms change with time. Short-term use or reevaluation at least every 3 to 6 months is necessary.

SKELETAL MUSCLE RELAXANTS

Most muscle strains and spasms are self-limited and respond to rest and physical therapy and short-term skeletal muscle relaxants. However, **spasticity** (a form of muscular hypertonicity with increased resistance to stretch) as the result of stroke, closed head injuries, cerebral palsy, multiple sclerosis, spinal cord trauma, and other neurologic disorders requiring long-term use of these agents will challenge the nurse's rehabilitative skills and knowledge. In both short- and long-term care, the nurse's role, in addition to medication administration, is to provide comfort and rehabilitative measures in collaboration with physical therapists and other members of the healthcare team.

Neuromuscular Junction

Skeletal muscles are striated (striped) muscles attached to the skeleton. They are usually under voluntary control. These muscles produce body movements, maintain body position against the force of gravity, and counteract environmental stressors such as wind. A muscle is made of numerous muscle cells or muscle fibers. Each muscle cell is connected to only one motor nerve fiber, but each of the nerve fibers is connected to several muscle cells. Therefore stimulation of one nerve fiber will cause stimulation and activation of a group of muscle cells. The region where a motor nerve fiber makes functional contact with a skeletal muscle fiber (synaptic contact) is known as the neuromuscular junction.

Skeletal Muscle Spasm and Spasticity

Skeletal muscle **spasms** result when there is an involuntary contraction of a muscle or group of muscles that is accompanied by pain or limited function. Most skeletal muscle spasms are caused by local injuries, but some may result from low calcium levels or epileptic myoclonic seizures. Each type of spasm is treated according to its cause.

Skeletal muscle injuries are usually self-limiting and can be treated with rest; physical therapy; immobility by use of casts, neck collars, crutches, or arm slings; or whirlpool baths. With tissue damage and edema, however, antiinflammatory drugs may be used.

Central skeletal muscle relaxants are used mainly for conditions in which muscle spasms do not quickly respond to other forms of therapy. Such conditions include musculoskeletal strains and sprains, trauma, and cervical or lumbar radiculopathy as a result of degenerative osteoarthritis, herniated disk, spondylosis, or laminectomy. Unlike diazepam (Valium), the centrally acting drug, baclofen (Lioresal), which is used for skeletal muscle spasticity, has not been found useful in the treatment of muscle spasms.

Skeletal muscle spasticity, characterized by skeletal muscle hyperactivity, occurs when gamma motor neurons (which tonically control muscle spindle contractile activity) become hyperactive. There are two primary types of muscle spasticity: spinal and cerebral. Spinal spasticity can be identified by a marked loss of inhibitory influences with hyperactive tendon stretch reflexes, clonus (alternate contraction and relaxation of muscles), primitive flexion withdrawal reflexes, and a flexed posture. Varying degrees of spasticity of the bladder and bowel can also be seen. Cerebral spasticity has less reflex excitability, increased muscle tone, and no primitive flexion withdrawal reflexes or flexed posture. **Dystonia,** an impairment of muscle tone, may also be present in individuals with cerebral spasticity.

Muscle spasticity is most commonly seen in patients with central nervous system injuries and strokes. Moderate to severe spasticity can be seen in two thirds of patients with multiple sclerosis. Individuals with cerebral palsy and rare neurologic disorders can also have muscle spasticity, but it is seen less frequently in these instances.

Central-acting and direct-acting skeletal muscle relaxants are the drugs of choice in the treatment of muscle spasticity. These drugs include baclofen (Lioresal), diazepam (Valium), and dantrolene (Dantrium). They are more effective in the treatment of spinal spasticity than cerebral spasticity. However, optimal therapy cannot be achieved in the treatment of either unless physical therapy is given concurrently.

Central-Acting Skeletal Muscle Relaxants

The exact mechanism of action of the central skeletal muscle relaxants is not known. Action results from CNS depression in the brain (brainstem, thalamus, and basal ganglia) and spinal cord that results in relaxation of striated muscle spasm. Removal of the central nervous depressive action from the skeletal muscle relaxation action of the central-acting skeletal muscle relaxants is not possible currently. As a result, these drugs create the side effects of drowsiness, blurred vision, lightheadedness, headache, and feelings of weakness, lassitude, and lethargy that make their long-term use undesirable. The drugs used primarily as antispastic agents are baclofen, diazepam, and dantrolene. Dantrolene, a direct-acting skeletal muscle relaxant (peripheral action) is discussed below.

baclofen [bak′ loe fen] (Lioresal)

Baclofen, a gamma-aminobutyric acid (GABA) inhibitory neurotransmitter, inhibits transmission of monosynaptic and polysynaptic reflexes. Although its exact mechanism of action is unknown, it is a spasmolytic agent at the spinal level, where it inhibits transmission.

Indications

It is used in the treatment of spasticity resulting from multiple sclerosis or from injuries to the spinal cord. Baclofen may reduce pain in spastic patients by inhibiting substance P release in the spinal cord (Katzung, 1992).

Pharmacokinetics

Absorption is generally good but may vary with different individuals. The time to peak concentration is 2 to 3 hours. The onset of action is variable and may occur in hours or up to weeks. Baclofen has a half-life of 2.5 to 4 hours and a therapeutic serum level of 80 to 400 ng/mL. Baclofen is metabolized in the liver and excreted in the kidneys.

Drug interactions

Enhanced CNS-depressant and hypotensive effects may occur when baclofen is given concurrently with other CNS-depressant medications or with MAO inhibitors. Use caution as one or both drugs may need a dosage reduction.

Side effects and adverse reactions

These include transient drowsiness, vertigo, confusion, sleepiness, muscle weakness, nausea, hallucinations, depression, tinnitus, painful urination, edema, anorexia, and GI upset.

Warnings

Use with caution in patients with cerebral lesions, cerebrovascular accident, diabetes mellitus, seizure disorders, kidney impairment, and a history of psychiatric problems and in the elderly.

Contraindications

Avoid use in persons with known baclofen hypersensitivity.

Dosage and administration

The adult dose is 5 mg orally three times daily, increased by 5 mg per dose every 3 days until the desired response is achieved, not to exceed 80 mg/day. The dosage for children has not been determined.

diazepam [dye az′ e pam]
(Valium, Apo-Diazepam 🍁)

Although the mechanism of action for diazepam is unknown, it appears to act primarily by inhibiting afferent spinal polysynaptic (and possibly monosynaptic) pathways. It may also directly suppress muscle function at the neuromuscular synapse. Diazepam is used in the treatment of skeletal muscle spasm caused by reflex spasm to local pathologic conditions, such as inflammation of muscle and joints or secondary to trauma. It is also used to treat spasticity caused by upper motor neuron disorders (cerebral palsy and paraplegia), athetosis, tetanus, and stiff-man syndrome (to overcome the widespread chronic muscular rigidity, pain, and skeletal muscle spasms). See Chapter 10 for more information on diazepam.

carisoprodol [kar eye soe proe′ dole] (Soma)
chlorphenesin carbamate [klor fen′ e sin] (Maolate)
chlorzoxazone [klor zox′ a zone] (Paraflex)
cyclobenzaprine [sye kloe ben′ za preen] (Flexeril)
metaxalone [met ax′ ah lone] (Skelaxin)
methocarbamol [meth oh kar′ ba mole] (Robaxin, Marbaxin)
orphenadrine [or fen′ a dreen] (Disipal)
orphenadrine extended-release (Norflex)

Muscle spasms are treated with central-acting skeletal muscle relaxants that are analogs to various antianxiety

TABLE 17-2 Other Central-Acting Skeletal Muscle Relaxants: Pharmacokinetics

Drug	Onset of Action	Time to Peak Concentration (hr)*	Peak Serum Concentration*	Duration of Action (hr)	Half-Life (hr)	Metabolism/Excretion
carisoprodol	30 min	4 (350 mg)	4-7 μg/ml	4-6	8	Liver/kidneys
chlorphenesin	N/A	1 to 3	3.8-17 μg/ml (800 mg)	N/A	2.5-5	Liver/kidneys
chlorzoxazone	Within 60 min	1 to 2	10-30 μg/ml (750 mg)	3-4	1-2	Liver/kidneys
cyclobenzaprine	Within 60 min	3 to 8	15-25 ng/ml (10 mg)	12-24	24-72	GI tract and liver/kidneys
metaxalone	60 min	2 (800 mg)	295 μg/ml (800 mg)	N/A	2-3	Liver/kidneys
methocarbamol	PO, within 30 min	2 (2 g)	16 μg/ml (2 g)	N/A	0.9-2.2	May be liver/kidneys and feces
	IV, immediate	Nearly immediate	19 μg/ml (1 g)	N/A		
orphenadrine						
extended release	Within 60 min	6 to 8 (100 mg)	60-120 ng/ml (100 mg)	12	14†	Liver/kidneys and feces
IM	5 min	½ (60 mg)				
IV	Immediate	Immediate				
orphenadrine HCl	Within 60 min	3 (50 mg)	110-210 ng/ml (100 mg)	8	14†	Liver/kidneys and feces

N/A, not available.
*Single dose.
†Parent drug half-life. Half-lives of metabolites may range between 2 and 25 hours.

medications. The exact mechanism of action of these drugs has not been determined, but it is believed the muscle relaxant effects of many of these drugs may be related to this CNS-depressant activity. Carisoprodol interferes with nerve transmission in the descending reticular formation and spinal cord while chlorzoxazone produces its effects in the spinal cord and subcortical brain areas. In addition to skeletal muscle relaxant effects, orphenadrine is also an analgesic.

Indications

These drugs are used in adjunct treatment for skeletal muscle spasms along with rest and physical therapy.

Pharmacokinetics

For information see Table 17-2.

Drug interactions

Increased CNS depression effects may occur if a skeletal muscle relaxant is given concurrently with alcohol or with other CNS depressants. Use caution as one or both drugs may need a dosage reduction.

Side effects and adverse reactions

These include drowsiness, dizziness, dry mouth, and abdominal distress. In addition, metaxalone (Skelaxin) may cause nausea, vomiting, increased excitability, and restlessness while methocarbamol (Robaxin) and orphenadrine (Disipal) may cause visual disturbances.

Warnings

Use with caution in patients with allergies, depression, and liver and kidney function impairment.

Contraindications

Avoid use in persons with known drug hypersensitivity. For orphenadrine, avoid use in individuals with glaucoma, myasthenia gravis, prostate hypertrophy, obstructions in the bladder neck, pyloric or duodenum, and peptic ulcers.

Dosage and administration

See Table 17-3. See the Pregnancy Safety box for FDA classification of the skeletal muscle relaxants.

Direct Acting Skeletal Muscle Relaxant

dantrolene [dan′ troe leen] (Dantrium)

Dantrolene is used in the prophylaxis and treatment of malignant hyperthermia that occurs during surgery and spasticity, especially upper motor neuron disorders, such as multiple sclerosis, cerebral palsy, spinal cord insults, and cerebrovascular accident. Dantrolene acts directly on skeletal muscles to produce skeletal muscle relaxation by inhibiting the release of calcium from the sarcoplasmic reticulum to the myoplasm. This results in a decreased muscle response to the action potential and decreased muscle contraction. As an antispastic agent, dantrolene's direct effect on skeletal muscle dissociates the excitation-contraction coupling. This effect is probably induced by the interference with calcium ion release from the sarcoplasmic reticulum. Dantrolene reduces both monosynaptic- and polysynaptic-induced muscle contractions.

Pharmacokinetics

Dantrolene is available orally and parenterally. The drug's oral absorption is fair; the onset of action when dan-

TABLE 17-3 Central-Acting Muscle Relaxants: Dosage and Administration

Drug	*Adults*	*Children*
carisoprodol (Soma)	350 mg PO 4 times daily	Under 5 yr, not recommended; 5-12 yr 6.25 mg/kg 4 times daily.
chlorphenesin (Maolate)	800 mg PO 3 times daily initially; later decreased to 400 mg 4 times daily	Not determined
chlorzoxazone (Paraflex)	250-750 mg PO 3-4 times daily, adjusted as necessary	20 mg/kg in 3 or 4 divided doses daily
cyclobenzaprine (Flexeril)	20-40 mg daily in divided doses	Not determined
metaxalone (Skelaxin)	800 mg PO 3-4 times daily	Not determined
methocarbamol (Robaxin)	1.5 g PO 4 times daily for 2-3 days, increased if necessary; parenteral: 1-3 g IM or IV daily for 3 days	Not determined
orphenadrine (Disipal, Norflex)	50 mg PO 3 times daily or 100 mg twice daily for extended-release dosage; parenteral: 60 mg IM or IV every 12 hr	Not determined

PREGNANCY SAFETY

Category	Drug
B	cyclobenzaprine
C	donepezil
Unclassified	baclofen, diazepam,* carisoprodol, chlorphenesin, chlorzoxazone, metaxalone, methocarbamol, orphenadrine, dantrolene

*To be avoided during pregnancy, especially during the first trimester.

trolene is used to treat the spasticity of upper motor neurons is 1 week or more. The drug has a half-life (orally) of 8.7 hours (100-mg dose); the IV half-life is 4 to 8 hours. The time to peak concentration is 5 hours (oral dose). It is metabolized in the liver and excreted in the kidneys.

Drug interactions

When dantrolene is given concurrently with other CNS depressants, an increase in CNS-depressant effects may result. Monitor closely as dosage reduction of one or both drugs may be necessary. When dantrolene is used chronically, be aware that concurrent use of hepatotoxic medications increases the potential risk for hepatotoxicity.

Side effects and adverse reactions

These include diarrhea, dizziness, sleepiness, uncomfortable feelings, unusual fatigue, muscle weakness, nausea, vomiting severe diarrhea, respiratory difficulty, and respiratory depression.

Warnings

Use with caution in patients with myopathy, liver or pulmonary function impairment, and neuromuscular diseases and in individuals older than 35 years of age (especially women) as they present an increased potential for hepatotoxicity.

Contraindications

Avoid use in persons with dantrolene hypersensitivity and active liver diseases, such as hepatitis or cirrhosis.

Dosage and administration

See Table 17-4.

SUMMARY

This chapter reviews the etiology and treatment of Parkinson's disease, myasthenia gravis, dementia, Alzheimer's disease, and muscle spasticity. These are all progressive diseases that often incapacitate the individual. Use of pharmacologic agents is essential for symptom control, which allows the patient to function as independently as possible for as long as possible.

Persons with Parkinson's disease usually require correction of the disorder's imbalance of dopamine/acetylcholine. Therefore they are treated with drugs that have a central effect, anticholinergics and antihistamines, and also dopaminergic agents to increase brain levels of dopamine.

Myasthenia gravis, which is characterized by skeletal muscle weakness and fatigue, is also a debilitating disease. The drugs of choice in treatment are the anticholinesterase drugs. While several drugs are available to treat Alzheimer's disease, there really is no known current medication to cure or prevent Alzheimer's disease and dementia. Pharmacotherapy is often used for symptom control and to control agitation, delusions and hallucinations.

The skeletal muscle relaxants affect skeletal muscle at the neuromuscular junction or at different levels in the central nervous system, such as the spinal cord or the brain. They are usually the drugs of choice in the treatment of muscle spasticity.

REVIEW QUESTIONS

1. Describe the three classifications of drugs that affect brain dopamine. Name one drug from each category

TABLE 17-4 Dantrolene: Dosage and Administration

Adults	*Children*
Antispastic	
25 mg PO daily initially, increased by 25 mg as necessary every 4-7 days until adequate response or 100 mg 4 times a day is reached.	0.5 mg/kg PO twice daily, increased by 0.5 mg/kg/day as necessary every 4-7 days until adequate response or a 3 mg/kg 4 times a day until dosage is reached. Do not exceed 400 mg/day.
Prophylaxis for Malignant Hyperthermic Crisis	
4-8 mg/kg PO in 3 or 4 divided doses daily for 24-48 hr before surgery. Last dose is given 3-4 hr before surgery, with minimum water. IV infusion: 2.5 mg/kg is given over 1 hr before anesthesia.	Not available
Acute Malignant Hyperthermic Reaction	
IV push of minimum of 1 mg/kg; continue this dose until symptoms abate or maximum cumulative dose of 10 mg/kg is reached. After IV therapy, 4-8 mg/kg PO in four divided doses daily is given for 1-3 days.	See adult dose

and identify and describe the classification that contains the drug of choice.

2. A patient is receiving levodopa 1 g qid for Parkinson's disease. Calculate the equivalent conversion to levodopa-carbidopa (Sinemet), which is available in 10/100, 25/100 and 25/250. Which combination of Sinemet would be appropriate for this dose?
3. What is the mechanism of action for selegiline (Eldepryl) when used to treat Parkinson's disease? Name three potentially serious drug interactions with selegiline.
4. What is myasthenia gravis? Describe the action, side effects and adverse reactions, and overdose effects of the anticholinesterase drugs.
5. Discuss the mechanisms of action for the skeletal muscle relaxants baclofen (Lioresal), diazepam (Valium), and dantrolene (Dantrium). Name two major drug interactions with baclofen and dantrolene.

REFERENCES

Bravyak JAT, Schechter BR: *Alzheimer's disease management,* Philadelphia, 1992, Philadelphia College of Pharmacy and Science.

Eggert A, Crismon ML: Current concepts in understanding Alzheimer's disease, *Clin Pharm Newswatch* 1(1):1-8, 1994.

Flaherty JF, Gidal BE: (1995). Parkinson's disease. In Young LY, Koda-Kimble MA, editors: *Applied therapeutics: the clinical use of drugs,* ed 6, Vancouver, Wash, 1995, Applied Therapeutics, Inc.

Katzung BG: *Basic and clinical pharmacology,* ed 5,. Norwalk, Conn, 1992, Appleton & Lange.

Lamy PP: Alzheimer's disease: 1906-1991, *Elder Care News* 8(4):27, 1991.

Lamy PP: *Prescribing for the elderly,* Littleton, Colo, 1980, PSG Publishing.

Miller S: Management strategies for the Alzheimer's disease patient, *Clin Consult* 14(1):1, 1995.

United States Pharmacopeial Convention: *USP DI: drug information for the health care professional,* ed 18, Rockville, Md, 1998, the Convention.

Williams BR: Geriatric dementias. In Young LY, Koda-Kimble MA, editors: *Applied therapeutics: the clinical use of drugs,* ed 6, Vancouver, Wash, 1995, Applied Therapeutics, Inc.

ADDITIONAL REFERENCES

American Hospital Formulary Service: *AHFS drug information '98,* Bethesda, Md, 1996, American Society of Hospital Pharmacists.

American Medical Association: *AMA drug evaluations 1995,* Chicago, 1995, the Association.

Anderson KN et al, editors: *Mosby's medical, nursing, and allied health dictionary,* ed 5, St Louis, 1998, Mosby.

Cutson TM et al: Pharmacological and nonpharmacological interventions in the treatment of Parkinson's disease, *Phys Ther* 75(5):363, 1995.

Lopate G, Pestronk A: Autoimmune myasthenia gravis, *Hosp Pract* 28(1):109, 1993.

Mosby: *Mosby's GenRx,* St Louis, 1998, Mosby.

Schneider LS et al: Emerging drugs for Alzheimer's disease: mechanisms of action and prospects for cognitive enhancing medications, *Med Clin North Am* 78(4):911, 1994.

Waldman HJ: Centrally acting skeletal muscle relaxants and associated drugs, *J Pain Sympt Manage* 9(7):434, 1994.

Whitehouse PJ et al: Pharmacotherapy for Alzheimer's disease, *Clin Geriatr Med* 10(2):339, 1994.

Young LY, Koda-Kimble MA, editors: *Applied therapeutics: the clinical use of drugs,* ed 6, Vancouver, Wash, 1995, Applied Therapeutics, Inc.

UNIT V

Drugs Affecting the Cardiovascular System

CHAPTER 18

Overview of the Cardiovascular System

CHAPTER FOCUS

Cardiovascular disease is the leading cause of death in the United States. According to 1995 statistics, approximately 58 million Americans have one or more types of cardiac illness (American Heart Association, 1998). In 1995, cardiovascular diseases were responsible for over 960,000 deaths, which equals approximately 42% of all deaths reported that year. One third of all deaths of women annually is due to heart disease. In fact, "Heart disease kills more women each year than cancer, accidents, and diabetes combined" (Sifton, 1994, p. 127). As life expectancies increase, it is anticipated that more people will be coping with acute and chronic cardiovascular conditions. A thorough knowledge of the anatomy and physiology of the cardiovascular system is essential for the healthcare professional providing care for this population.

OBJECTIVES

After reading and studying this chapter, the student should be able to do the following:

1. *Define and discuss the key terms.*
2. *Describe the heart's anatomy and physiology and the role of electrical excitation in myocardial contractions.*
3. *Name and describe the three major tissues of the heart.*
4. *Explain the ion exchange during an action potential of a myocardial cell.*
5. *Describe the events that occur in a normal heart during systole and diastole.*
6. *Describe the autonomic nervous system effects on the heart.*
7. *Describe the coronary blood vessels and their basic functions.*

KEY TERMS

action potential, (p. 312)
atria, (p. 310)
automaticity, (p. 314)
AV junction, (p. 314)
cardiac output, (p. 310)
conduction system, (p. 314)
conductivity, (p. 315)
depolarization, (p. 312)
diastole, (p. 314)
electrocardiogram (ECG), (p. 315)
electrophysiologic properties, (p. 314)
myocardium, (p. 310)
refractoriness, (p. 315)
repolarization, (p. 312)
rhythmicity, (p. 315)
sarcomere, (p. 310)
stroke volume, (p. 314)
systole, (p. 314)
ventricles, (p. 310)

Advances in science and technology have resulted in new technical knowledge and treatment for cardiac disease. For example, the American Heart Association reported in 1998 that the death rate from heart attack dropped nearly 29% from 1985 to 1995. This expansion in anatomic, electrophysiologic, and pharmacologic information has resulted in improvements in the diagnosing and treatment of cardiac disease, particularly the dysrhythmias. Along with these advances has come the increased use of electrocardiographic monitoring of acutely ill patients and those with known or suspected cardiovascular disorders. Microelectrode techniques have grown increasingly sophisticated and have helped provide greater understanding of the electrical properties of cardiac fibers and the causes of various cardiac disorders. Fortunately, these advances have led to the discovery of new drugs that are useful for treating cardiac conditions.

Cardiac drugs primarily affect three major tissues of the heart: cardiac muscle (myocardium), conduction system, and coronary vessels. In this chapter, the normal function of these structures is discussed. The physiologic properties of these structures and the drug groups used therapeutically are summarized in Table 18-1.

THE HEART

The heart is a hollow muscular organ that consists of two main pumping chambers: the right ventricle, which is linked with the pulmonary circulation, and the left ventricle, which is connected to the systemic circulation. The cardiac muscle or myocardium is the largest and most important structure of the heart. As a contractile muscle, under normal conditions it can adapt its performance by adjusting the cardiac output according to the body's needs. **Cardiac output** is the volume of blood expelled by the ventricles of the heart, equal to the amount of blood ejected at each beat multiplied by the number of beats in the time used in computation. However, when the heart cannot produce a variable output, the therapeutic use of digitalis or cardiac glycosides (i.e., the digitalis drugs) produces changes at the cellular level. The following description of myocardial ultrastructure and the contractile process facilitates an understanding of the basic mechanisms in cardiac glycoside action.

Cardiac Muscle

The pumping action of the heart depends on the ability of the cardiac muscle to contract. The **myocardium,** the thick, contractile, middle layer of the heart, is composed of many interconnected branching fibers or cells that form the walls of the two **atria,** the upper chambers of the heart, and the two **ventricles,** the lower chambers of the heart. Each individual myocardial fiber contains a nucleus in the middle and a plasma membrane (cell membrane), the sarcolemma (Figs. 18-1, *2* and *3*). By joining end to end, the cells form a long fiber, with each cell separated from the other by a plasma membrane called the intercalated disk. This disk is believed to provide sites of low electrical resistance to permit the spread of exciting impulses throughout the cardiac muscle.

Each individual muscle fiber (cell) comprises a group of multiple parallel myofibrils, and each myofibril is arranged end to end in a series of repeating units called the sarcomere (Figs. 18-1, *4*). By light microscope examination, the muscle fiber reveals its most characteristic feature, alternating light and dark bands. These bands result from crossing of the multiple parallel myofibrils, which are aligned in register with one another (Figs. 18-1, *3*). At the level known as the Z line, the sarcolemma of the muscle fiber interlocks (invaginates) at its end with the sarcomere to form the transverse sarcotubule or T system, which penetrates deeply into the cell. Furthermore, internal membranes form an extensive network called the sarcoplasmic reticulum. This structure encircles groups of myofibrils and makes contact with the sarcotubules. The tremendous energy requirements for cardiac muscle contraction may be seen by the great numbers of mitochondria lined up in long chains between the myofibrils (Figs. 18-1, *3*). Fig. 18-1, *4* shows the **sarcomere,** which is the basic unit of contraction in the heart. It lies between two successive Z lines and in part of the myofibril. The sarcomere consists of dark bands called A bands and lighter I bands. The end unit of the myofibril is the myofilament. The darkness of the A band results from the thicker

TABLE 18-1 Effect of Cardiac Drug Groups on Cardiac Tissues

Cardiac Tissue	*Physiologic Property*	*Drug Group*	*Pharmacologic Action*
Cardiac muscle (myocardium)	Force of myocardial contraction (Frank-Starling's law)	Cardiac glycosides	Positive inotropic effect—increases cardiac output
Sarcomere (functional unit)	Contractility and conductivity		
Cardiac conduction system	Automatically (rhythm and rate)	Antidysrhythmic drugs	Converts to normal sinus rhythm or abolishes dysrhythmia
	Conductivity	Calcium channel blockers	
Coronary arteries	Nutritional blood flow to myocardium and other cardiac structures	Antianginal drug Calcium channel blockers	Coronary vasodilation or lessens work of the heart

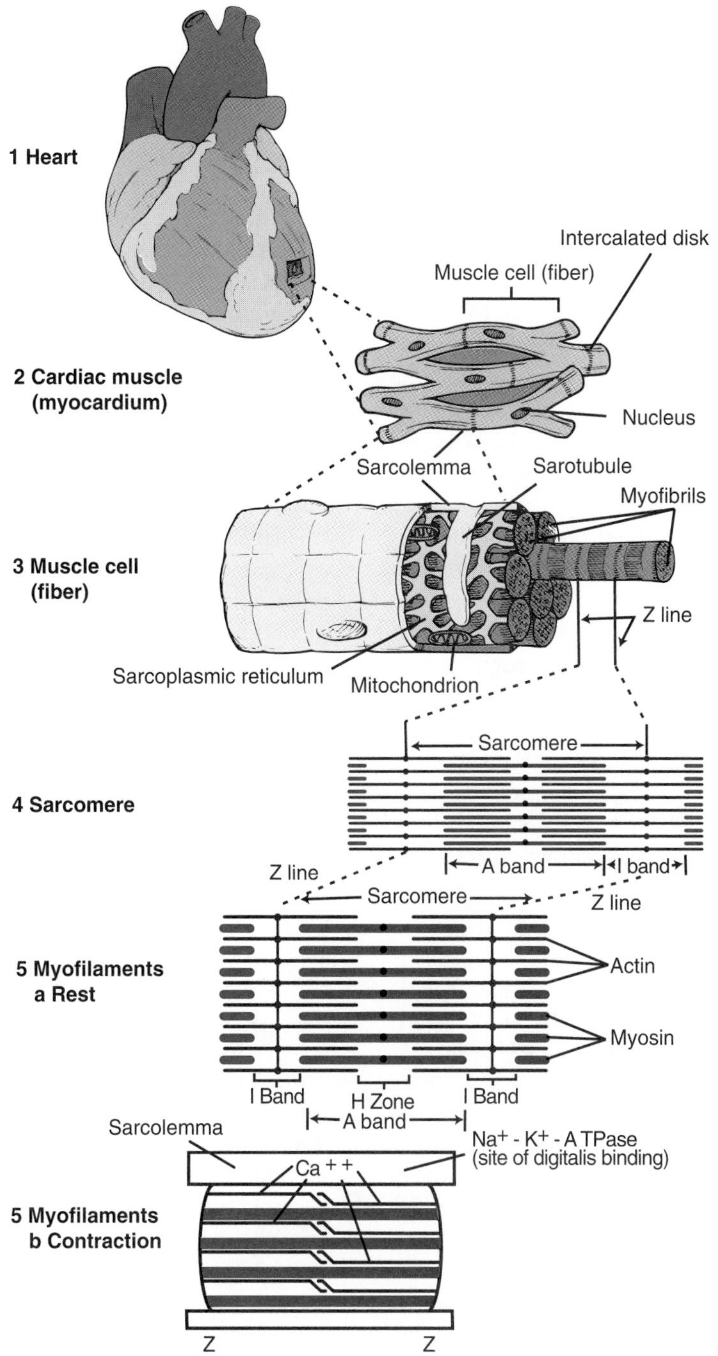

FIGURE 18-1

Structure of heart and cardiac muscle cell fibers. The heart *(1)* is mainly a muscular organ. The enlargement of the square illustrates a portion of the cardiac muscle (myocardium) *(2)*, which is composed of myocardial cells. Each cell contains a centrally located nucleus and a limiting plasma membrane (sarcolemma), which forms the intercalated disk at the termination of each cell. An individual muscle cell (fiber) *(3)* consists of multiple parallel myofibrils. Each myofibril is arranged longitudinally in a series of light and dark repeating units, and the content of a unit is called a sarcomere. At the Z line, the sarcolemma invaginates to form the transverse sarcotubules or T system. An extensive network, called the sarcoplasmic reticulum, encircles groups of myofibrils and makes contact with the sarcotubules. The sarcoplasmic reticulum contains a high concentration of calcium ions. The mitochondria appear in long chains between the myofibrils. The sarcomere *(4)* is the unit of muscle contraction. It is composed of two types of bands, the A band and the I band. The latter is divided by the Z line. Myofilaments *(5)* of the sarcomere include the thin filament, actin, and the thick filament, myosin. The dark appearance of the A band is caused by the myosin and the lighter appearance of the I band by the actin. Here, the sarcomere is at rest *(a)*. On contraction *(b)* the sarcomere shortens so that the thick filaments approach the Z line and the width of the H zone narrows between the thin filaments. Calcium ions are needed for systolic contractions.

myosin filaments, and the lightness of the I bands reflects the thinner actin filaments. Crossbridges, which are small projections that extend from the sides of the myosin filament, appear along the entire length of the thick filament. The interaction between these crossbridges of myosin and the active sites of actin produces contraction. In the sarcomere, the H zone represents the middle, less dense portion of the A band, and the myosin filament runs the entire length of this band. The I band, on the other hand, is divided by the Z line. The actin filament runs through the whole I band and terminates at the H zone. This arrangement is shown in Figs. 18-1, *5*.

Myocardial Contraction

Throughout the past decade, our understanding of the fundamental mechanisms governing contraction of cardiac muscle in both normal and pathologic states has increased tremendously. Yet some aspects of this complicated process are still unknown. Cardiac muscle contraction begins with a rapid change in the cell membrane's electrical charge. This electrical current spreads to the interior of the cell where it causes release of calcium ions from the sarcoplasmic reticulum. The calcium ions then initiate the chemical events of contraction. The overall process for controlling cardiac muscle contraction, called excitation-contraction coupling, involves electrical excitation, mechanical activation, and contractile mechanisms.

Electrical Excitation

Cardiac muscle contraction begins with electrical excitation or stimulus of the myocardial fiber. The source of electricity in the heart is found in the charges of ion concentration—mainly sodium, potassium, and calcium ions—across the cardiac cell membrane of the sarcolemma. The **action potential,** the difference in electrical charge, which produces the rapid ion changes, occurs in the membrane of the myocardial cell and results in a self-propagating series of polarization and depolarization. The resting state of an inactive muscle cell in the ventricle is created by the difference in electrical charge across the sarcolemma. In this case the inside of the cell is negative with respect to the cell's outside, which is positively charged. Because the sarcolemma separates these opposite charges, the membrane in effect is polarized. At rest, the extracellular environment is rich in sodium ions (Na^+) and the intracellular environment in potassium ions (K^+), with a rich calcium ion (Ca^{++}) concentration in the region of the sarcolemma and where it invaginates on the sarcotubule (Fig. 18-2, *B*).

The cardiac action potential is divided into two stages: **depolarization** (the stage in which an electrical impulse results in contraction of the ventricular muscle represented by the QRS interval on the electrocardiogram) and **repolarization** (the recovery phase after muscle contraction represented by the T wave). These stages are subdivided into five phases of ionic changes. The resting potential of an inactive myocardial cell is called phase 4; in this phase the membrane is polarized with a charge of approximately −90 millivolts (mv). At this voltage the interior of the cell is negative with respect to the cell's exterior. During this time the membrane cannot be penetrated by ions. However, any stimulus that changes the resting membrane potential to a critical value, called the threshold, can generate an action potential. Follow Fig. 18-2, *A* for steps of the action potential.

Threshold may be reached by normal pacemaker activity or by propagation of an electrical impulse from a nearby cell, which opens the sodium channels. The fast inward current of sodium ions (fast channel), results in a membrane that is positively charged to +20 mv. This difference in membrane potential results in depolarization and is designated as phase 0 of the action potential. Phase 0 in the ventricular muscle is the contraction phase and is represented by QRS on the surface electrocardiogram. Soon after, the repolarization period occurs in three phases. The beginning of phase 1 is the overshoot, and it makes a brief change toward repolarization. Phase 2 is a slow period that forms a plateau with a slow inward current of calcium ions (slow channel) and outward flow of potassium ions. Calcium ion entry into the cell is essential for the excitation-contraction coupling mechanism, which will be explained later.

Phase 3 is accomplished by rapid potassium ion efflux from the cell. After repolarization, phase 4 recovery or a resting period ensues, represented by the T wave, whereby the cell membrane actively transports sodium ions outside and potassium ions inside, returning the cell membrane to a state of rest or polarization. These cation exchanges during recovery require the energy-utilizing transport mechanism of the Na^+-K^+ pump, or Na^+-K^+-adenosine triphosphatase (ATPase). ATPase, which is powered by oxygen, is an enzyme that is located in the cell membrane or sarcolemma; it furnishes the energy needed for active transport to return sodium ions and potassium ions to their original resting positions at the membrane. Digitalis plays a key role at this site. By binding to the sarcolemma Na^+-K^+-ATPase, digitalis inhibits the return of sodium ions and potassium ions to their resting positions. Consequently, digitalis allows more sodium ions and calcium ions to enter the cell to strengthen myocardial contraction. However, it is also thought that if an excessive amount of these ions appears intracellularly, digitalis toxicity may occur.

Mechanical Activation

As previously stated, the unit that contracts is the sarcomere. It consists of two contractile proteins, actin and myosin. Myosin, the thicker filament, contains the ATPase enzyme system that is needed to hydrolyze adenosine triphosphate (ATP). Hydrolysis is required to provide the energy for contraction. ATP is synthesized in the mitochondria, which are normally abundant in cardiac muscle. Actin, the thin filament, is involved with calcium ion activity. These two filaments combine to help effect cardiac contraction.

Contraction is initiated when the nerve impulse reaches the myocardial cell and travels along the sarcolemma of the

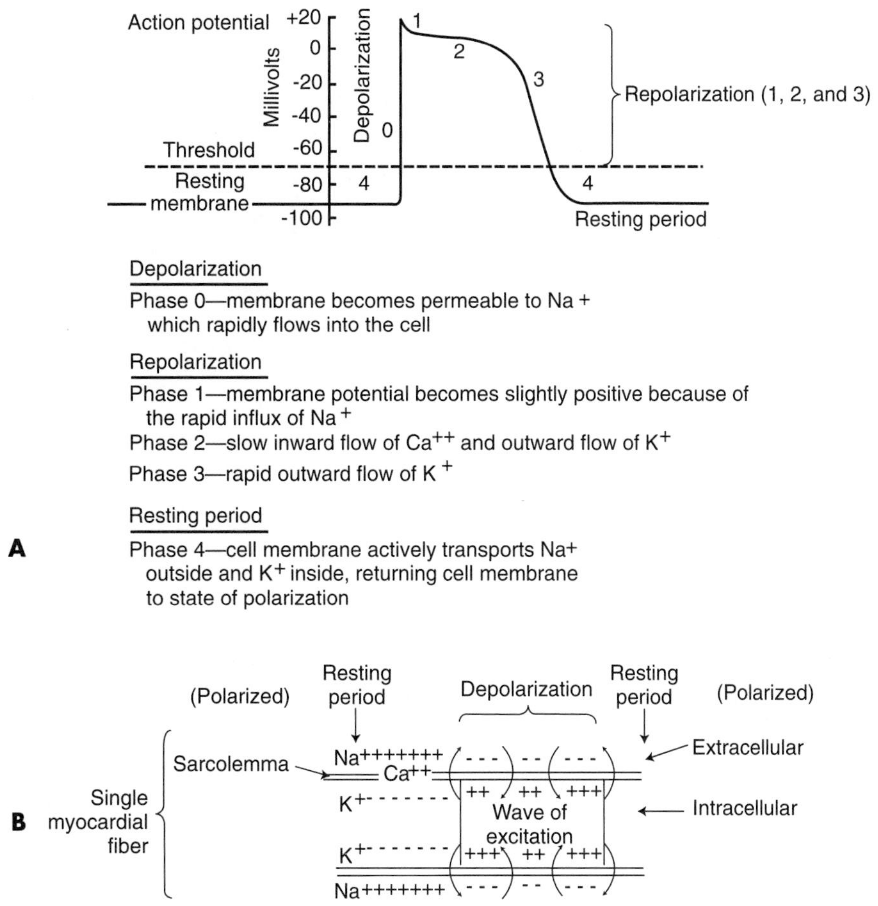

FIGURE 18-2

A, Action potential of a single myocardial fiber (cell). **B,** Ionic exchanges that occur across the cell membrane of a single myocardial fiber during an action potential.

muscle fiber. As the depolarization wave spreads along the sarcotubules, it arrives at the sarcoplasmic reticulum, causing the release of its large quantities of calcium ions. These ions then bind to special receptors on the actin filaments. Hence the plateau, which is phase 2 of the action potential, is reached through the slow inward calcium current flow (slow channel). Calcium ion movement is the chief component that links or couples electrical excitation of the sarcolemma with muscle activation of the myofilaments in the sarcomere. Thus mechanical activation finally is accomplished when calcium ions bind to troponin, a regulator protein located on the actin filaments. This in turn mediates the interaction of actin and myosin.

Contractile Mechanism

As soon as the actin filaments are activated by the calcium ions, the myosin filaments become attracted to the active sites of the actin filament. This interaction pulls the actin along the immobile myosin filaments toward the center of the A band, thus shortening the sarcomere and producing muscle contraction. In this process the lengths of individual filaments remain unchanged. The I band narrows as the thick filaments approach the Z line, and the H zone narrows between the ends of the thin filaments when they meet at the center of the sarcomere (Figs. 18-1, *5a* and *5b*). The greater the quantity of calcium ions delivered to troponin, the faster the rate and numbers of interactions between actin and myosin. As a result of this response, the development of tension and contractility is increased.

When magnesium is present, ATP is cleaved by myosin ATPase. This reaction releases the energy needed to perform work. The conversion of chemical energy to mechanical energy by ATP plays an essential role in energizing muscle shortening. In other words, it provides the energy so the actin-myosin filaments move and produce muscle contraction. Although this is a somewhat simplified explanation of the contractile mechanism, it illustrates the important events pertinent to understanding cardiotonic drug action.

Finally, muscle relaxation depends on removing calcium ions from the sarcomere. The calcium ATPase (located in the walls of the sarcoplasmic reticulum) actively returns calcium ions to the sarcoplasmic reticulum and the sarcolemma, thereby allowing the actin-myosin filaments of the sarcomere to return to their resting positions.

In the normal heart, the Frank-Starling relationship holds true. This relationship means that the longer the muscle fibers are at the end of **diastole** (period of heart relaxation), the more forceful the contraction will be during **systole** (the period of contraction). This mechanism applies only when the muscle fiber is lengthened within physiologic limits. If a diseased heart is dilated and the fibers are stretched to a critical point beyond their limits of extensibility, the forces of contraction and cardiac output are both diminished and ineffective. Thus the functional significance of the Frank-Starling relationship is that effective cardiac output can be brought about only by adequate relaxation and refilling of cardiac chambers after each myocardial contraction.

Cardiac Conduction System

The effective pumping action of the heart depends on the regularity of events occurring in the cardiac cycle. Each cycle consists of a period of relaxation, diastole, followed by a period of contraction, systole. The rhythm and rate of the cardiac cycle are regulated by the conduction system, specialized tissue that has the ability to initiate and transmit the electrical impulses needed to stimulate contraction of the cardiac muscle.

The **conduction system** is made up of the following structures: (1) sinoatrial (SA) node, (2) internodal pathways, (3) atrioventricular (AV) node, (4) bundle of His, (5) right and left bundle branches, and (6) Purkinje fibers. The Purkinje fibers penetrate the endocardium and end in the myocardial cells. The AV node and the His area form the **AV junction,** which extends from the atrial fibers through the AV node to the bifurcation of the bundle of His. When referring to this region, the term AV junction is considered to be more accurate than AV node (Fig. 18-3).

In the normal heart, the SA node initiates the heartbeat. The impulses generated here are then conducted through the internodal pathways to the "working" fibers of the atrial myocardium, producing atrial contraction. When the impulses move through the AV junction, electrical conduction is delayed. However, at the bundle of His, conduction speeds up and the impulses travel through the right bundle branch and the left bundle branch, then through the posteroinferior and anterosuperior fascicles of the left bundle branch. The transmission of impulses at the Purkinje fibers, which consist of tiny fibrils that spread around the ventricles and connect directly with the myocardial cells, is very rapid. Finally, the simultaneous depolarization of both ventricles produces ventricular contraction, resulting in **stroke volume,** the volume of blood being propelled through the pulmonary artery and aorta by the ventricles.

Electrophysiologic Properties

The coordinated pumping action of the heart is initiated and regulated by the specialized fibers of the conduction system. The individual fibers of this system possess three basic **electrophysiologic properties:** (1) automaticity, (2) conductivity, and (3) refractoriness.

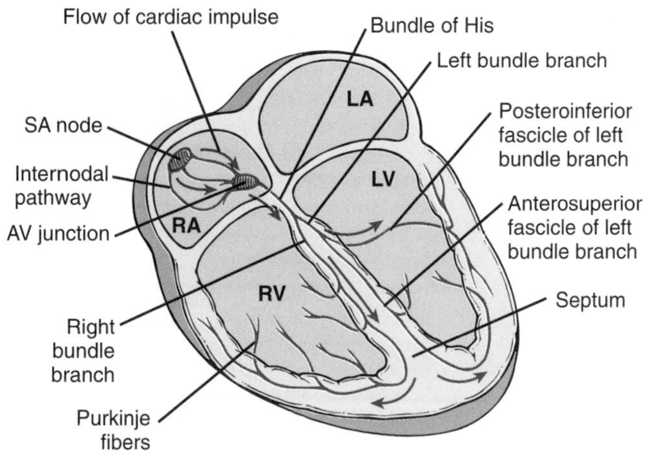

FIGURE 18-3
Conduction system of the heart. The cardiac impulse is initiated at the SA node and is transmitted through the internodal pathways to the two atria, resulting in atrial contraction. At the AV node, the electrical impulse is delayed. Conduction then speeds up at the bundle of His, with the impulse traveling through the right bundle branch and the left bundle branch and continuing through the posteroinferior fascicle and anterosuperior fascicle of the latter bundle branch. Finally, the arrival of impulses at the Purkinje fibers results in their distribution to all parts of both ventricles, where, upon excitation, ventricular contraction is produced. *RA,* Right atrium; *RV,* right ventricle; *LA,* left atrium; *LV,* left ventricle.

Automaticity

The specialized fibers of the conduction system have the inherent ability to spontaneously initiate an electrical impulse without any external stimuli. This is the most fundamental mechanism of impulse formation, and the cells that possess this property of **automaticity,** the ability to initiate an impulse, are called pacemaker cells. They are found in specialized conducting tissues such as the SA node, the AV junction, and the His-Purkinje system. Normally, the impulse of the heart is spontaneously and regularly initiated at the pacemaker cells of the SA node. During resting potential (phase 4), the membrane of the cell depolarizes itself, spontaneously and gradually, until it reaches threshold and an action potential occurs. The slow depolarization of the membrane in the resting state is called spontaneous diastolic depolarization, or phase 4 depolarization, and defines automaticity. Thus the membrane of pacemaker cells is never at rest, and this property is attributed to the continuous influx of sodium ions into the interior of the cells, which readily drives the membrane to threshold. The resting potential of automatic pacemaker cells differs from that of the nonautomatic myocardial cells. After full repolarization, the membrane of myocardial cells maintains a steady resting potential until an external stimulus causes it to achieve threshold. To summarize, automaticity is a property of fibers of the conduction system that normally controls heart rhythm; it is not a feature of "working" muscle (atria and ventricles). However, under pathologic conditions, myocardial cells do have the potential to exhibit spontaneous depolarization.

The spontaneous excitation of pacemaker cells establishes the normal rhythm of the heart. The regularity of such pacemaking activity is termed **rhythmicity.** Under normal circumstances, only one functional pacemaker, the SA node, predominates because it has the highest frequency of depolarization. The normal rate of impulse formation is about 72 beats/min. If the SA node decreases its rate of impulse formation to a level below the AV junction (40 to 60 beats/min), then the AV junction becomes the primary pacemaker of the heart and will drive the heart at about 40 beats/min.

Conductivity

Conductivity refers to the ability to transmit an action potential or nerve impulse from cell to cell. The property of conductivity therefore exists not only in the cells of the conduction system but also in the cardiac musculature. The speed of impulse conduction varies as it passes from one tissue to another in the heart. It is slowest in the AV junction and fastest in the Purkinje fibers. The significant delay of conduction at the AV junction allows more time for ventricular filling. On the other hand, the rapid depolarization of Purkinje fibers creates an instantaneous spread of impulses from the terminals to the ventricular muscles. Simultaneous activation of the musculature is essential for producing powerful ventricular contraction.

Velocity of Conduction

The speed with which electrical activity is spread within the sinus node is quite slow, about 0.05 m/sec. The impulse then spreads out rapidly over the atrial musculature at a rate of about 1 m/sec. When the impulse reaches the AV node, a delay of about 0.05 m/sec occurs, and atrial systole takes place. The impulse then spreads rapidly, 2 to 4 m/sec, along the right and left bundle branches and Purkinje fibers. Studies indicate that no more than 22 sec may elapse during this time. This rapid activation of contractile elements evokes a synchronous contraction of the ventricles.

The velocity of conduction is determined by the size of the resting potential of the cell membrane and the rate of rise of phase 0 of the action potential. This defines membrane responsiveness. Antidysrhythmic drugs may affect conduction by slowing phase 0 depolarization rate, thereby decreasing membrane responsiveness.

Refractoriness

Cardiac tissue is nonresponsive to stimulation during the initial phase of systole (contraction). This is known as **refractoriness,** and it determines how closely together two action potentials can occur. Throughout most of repolarization, the cell cannot respond to a stimulus. The effective refractory period represents that period in the cardiac cycle during which a stimulus, no matter how strong, fails to produce an action potential. Antidysrhythmic drugs can lengthen or shorten the refractory period of cardiac tissues by influencing the level of responsiveness of the cell membrane. After the effective refractory period and as repolarization nears completion, a relative refractory period occurs. This is defined as that period during which a propagated action potential can be elicited, provided the stimulus is stronger than normally required in diastole. When this happens, the fiber is stimulated to contract prematurely.

AUTONOMIC NERVOUS SYSTEM CONTROL

Although the conduction system possesses the inherent ability for spontaneous, rhythmic initiation of the cardiac impulse, the autonomic nervous system has an important role in the regulation of the rate, rhythm, and force of myocardial contraction of the heart. The heart is innervated by both the parasympathetic and sympathetic nerves. Vagal nerve fibers of the parasympathetic branch are found primarily in the SA node, atrial muscles, and AV junction, whereas the sympathetic fibers innervate the SA node, AV junction, and the atrial and ventricular muscles.

Vagal stimulation to the heart is mediated by the release of acetylcholine, a neurohormone that acts on the muscarinic receptors to decrease heart rate and is also believed to decrease ventricular contraction. The main effect of acetylcholine on the AV junction is to slow the rate of conduction and lengthen the refractory period. By contrast, sympathetic fiber stimulation is mediated by the release of norepinephrine, which acts specifically on the $beta_1$ receptors in the cardiac tissue. Circulating epinephrine from the adrenal medulla may also elicit cardiac responses. By acting on the beta-adrenergic receptors, norepinephrine and epinephrine increase both heart rate and force of myocardial contraction. They also increase conduction velocity and shorten the refractory period of the AV junction. Epinephrine has a very potent effect on the heart. In large doses its direct effect on the electrophysiologic properties of cardiac tissue can create cardiac dysrhythmias (Box 18-1). Normally the heartbeat is under the continuous influence of both parasympathetic and sympathetic control, so that the resting heart rate is the result of their opposing influences.

ELECTROCARDIOGRAMS

An **electrocardiogram** (ECG) is a graphic representation of electrical currents produced by the heart, which is a useful tool in determining the therapeutic effectiveness of certain drugs. Drugs used to treat cardiovascular disease may alter the electric activity of the heart. The ECG may provide the earliest objective evidence of a drug's effectiveness or its toxic manifestations.

Electrical activity always precedes mechanical contraction. Immediately after a wave of electrical activity moves through atrial muscle, the muscle contracts and blood flows from the atria into the ventricles. (Fig. 18-4 shows an illustration of the normal ECG.) The P wave is produced by a wave of excitation through the atria (atrial depolarization).

BOX 18-1 Common Cardiac Dysrhythmias

Heart block—impaired impulse conduction through the heart; usually the impaired conduction occurs between atria and ventricles
First-degree heart block—conduction time is prolonged, but all impulses are conducted from atria to ventricles
Second-degree heart block—some but not all atrial impulses are conducted to ventricles
Third-degree heart block—no atrial impulses are conducted to ventricles
Ectopic beats—a contraction of the heart that originates some place other than the sinoatrial node
Extrasystole "premature beat"—a premature contraction of the heart that arises independent of the normal rhythm
Tachycardia—unusually rapid heart rate (usually over 100 beats/min in adult)
Bradycardia—unusually slow heart rate (usually less than 60 beats/min in adult)
Atrial flutter—extremely rapid rate of atrial contraction; may be 200 to 350 beats/min
Atrial fibrillation—rapid and incoordinated contraction of the atria
Ventricular fibrillation—rapid and incoordinated contraction of the ventricles; because of the incoordination of contractions, there is little or no effective pumping of blood; death will result if not immediately treated

The onset of the P wave follows the firing of the SA node. After the P wave, a short pause or interval (P-R interval) occurs while the electrical activity is transmitted to the AV junction, conduction tissue, and ventricles. Repolarization, or recovery, of the ventricles is indicated by the T wave. Atrial recovery or repolarization does not show on the ECG because it is hidden in the QRS complex.

PHYSIOLOGY OF FAST AND SLOW CHANNELS OF CARDIOVASCULAR FIBERS

To understand the clinical application of calcium channel blockers, it is necessary to review the normal physiology of the fast and slow channels that exist in the membrane of the cardiovascular fibers. The cell membrane is composed of two types of channels that are controlled by "gates." When opened, they allow the movement of an inward current of (1) sodium ions through the fast channels and (2) calcium ions through the slow channels into the cell, depending on the type of fibers involved. These channels appear in the cell membrane of three types of cardiovascular fibers. The heart contains two types: fast-channel fibers, which appear in the myocardial cells of the atria and ventricles and the Purkinje fibers, and slow-channel fibers, which occur in the SA node and the AV junction. The third type, slow fibers, are present in the smooth muscle of the coronary and peripheral arterial vessels.

In this mechanism, the role of calcium ions is essential in affecting three physiologic processes: (1) increasing the strength of myocardial contraction (fast fibers); (2) enhancing automaticity and conduction speed (slow fibers); and (3) vasoconstricting coronary arteries and peripheral arterioles (slow fibers).

As previously described, the action potential that generates excitation-contraction coupling in the fast fibers consists of five phases. Depolarization (phase 0) results from an electrical stimulus that produces a fast inward current of sodium ion (fast channel). This is then followed by repolarization, which begins with a short phase 1, but, more importantly, phase 2, the plateau phase, produces a slow inward current of calcium ions into the cell (slow channel). The influx of calcium ions is responsible for linking electrical excitation to myocardial contraction (excitation-contraction coupling) required to promote the sliding of actin and myosin filaments for myocardial contraction (positive inotropic effect). Rapid repolarization occurs during phase 3, and, finally, phase 4 reestablishes the resting state. (See configuration of action potential in Fig. 18-2, *A*.) In the slow fibers of the SA and AV nodes, the action potential consists of only three phases. The principal distinguishing feature of the pacemaker fiber resides in phase 4. A slow spontaneous depolarization occurs that requires no external stimulus and is termed "diastolic depolarization." This is responsible for automaticity. Also, unlike the fast fibers of the myocardium, depolarization (or phase 0) is achieved by the slower current carried by both calcium ions and sodium ions through the slow channels of nodal cells. Thus phase 0 results in a slower conduction velocity in nodal cells than in myocardial cells. Calcium channel blockers inhibit these slow channels. Repolarization is more gradual and involves only phase 3. The membrane then finally returns to phase 4 (Fig. 18-5). The smooth muscle of blood vessels depends primarily on the presence of calcium ions to initiate and sustain contraction. The main source of calcium ions in cardiac muscle cells is the sarcoplasmic reticulum. In the action potential for smooth muscle, it is believed that the onset of depolarization (phase 0) is caused mainly by calcium ions rather than by sodium ions. Calcium ions enter the smooth muscle cell through slow channels, and it is the rise in free calcium ion concentration that is considered to be the primary event in excitation-contraction coupling that is responsible for increasing muscle tone and vasoconstriction. In addition, activation of smooth muscle can reduce the caliber of small vessels markedly, as is apparent from the "spasm" that may occur in coronary vessels. The calcium channel blockers (specifically verapamil, nefidipine, and diltiazem) are capable of blocking the slow calcium ion influx in smooth muscle of blood vessels, thereby producing relaxation.

CORONARY VASCULAR SUPPLY OF THE HEART

The entire blood supply to the myocardium is provided by the right and left coronary arteries, which arise from the base of the aorta (Fig. 18-6). The right atrium and ventricle

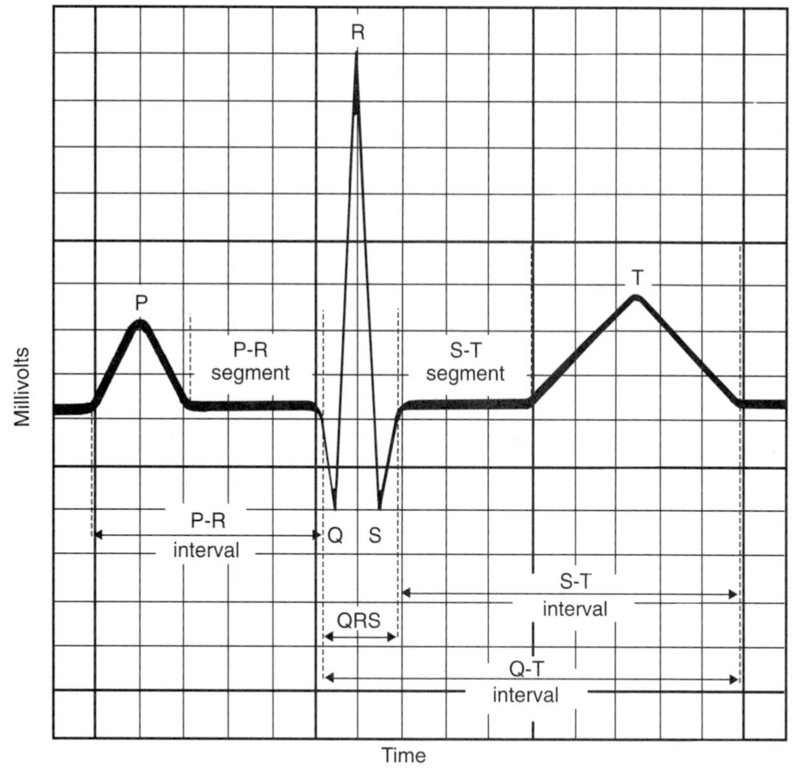

FIGURE 18-4

Graphic representation of the normal electrocardiogram. Vertical lines represent time, each square represents 0.04 second, and every five squares (set off by heavy black lines) represents 0.20 second. The normal P-R interval is less than 0.20 second; the average is 0.16 second. The average P wave lasts 0.08 second, the QRS complex is 0.08 second, the S-T segment is 0.12 second, the T wave is 0.16 second, and the Q-T interval is 0.32 to 0.40 second if heart rate is 65 to 95 beats/min. Each horizontal line represents voltage; every five squares equals 0.5 mv.

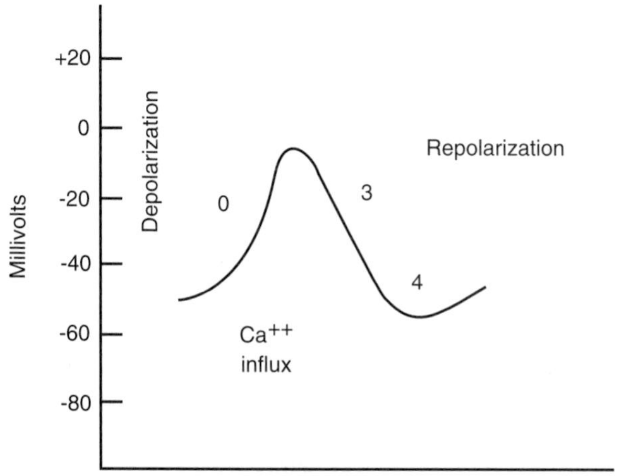

FIGURE 18-5

Action potential of slow channel fiber, the SA node. It consists of three phases. Unlike the fast fibers of myocardial cells, depolarization (phase 0) is attributed primarily to Ca^{++} inflow through slow channels of the cell membrane. Repolarization involves only phase 3, which is followed by phase 4.

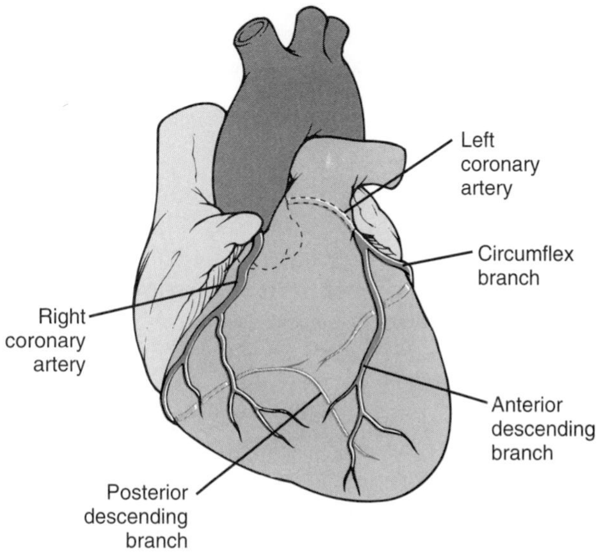

FIGURE 18-6

Coronary blood supply to the heart. Dark shaded vessels are those located on the external surface of the ventricles; light shaded vessels show penetration of arterial branches toward the endocardial surface.

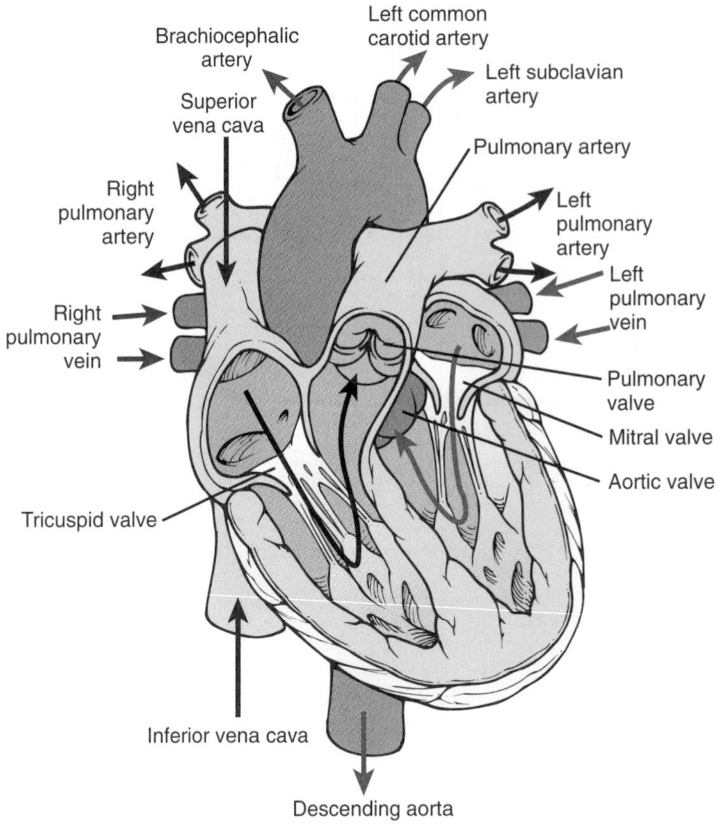

FIGURE 18-7
Overview of heart, blood flow, and valves.

are supplied with blood from the right coronary artery. The left coronary artery divides into the anterior (descending) branch and the circumflex branch and supplies blood to the left atrium and ventricle. These main coronary vessels continue to divide, forming numerous branches. The result is a profuse network of coronary vessels. The major arterial vessels are located on the external surface of the ventricles. Arterial branches penetrate the myocardium toward the endocardial surface.

Increased oxygen delivery to the myocardium is supported almost exclusively by increased coronary blood flow. When the demand for oxygen and nutrients by body tissues is increased, the heart must increase its output. At the same time, the heart muscle itself must be supplied with enough oxygen and nutrients to replace the energy expended. In other words, a balance must be maintained between energy expenditure and energy restoration. During systole the myocardial contraction compresses the coronary vascular bed. This restricts coronary inflow but increases coronary outflow. Coronary inflow in the left ventricle occurs primarily during diastole when the ventricles have relaxed and the coronary vessels are no longer compressed. Blood is driven through the coronary arteries by aortic pressure perfusing the myocardium.

A change in heart rate is accomplished by shortening or lengthening diastole. With tachycardia the increased number of systolic contractions per minute reduces the time available for diastole and coronary inflow. An increase also occurs in the metabolic needs of the rapidly beating heart. Normally, coronary dilation occurs in an attempt to meet increased metabolic demand and to overcome restricted blood inflow. With bradycardia, the decreased number of systolic contractions per minute prolongs the diastolic period. Resistance to coronary flow and metabolic requirements of the myocardium are reduced.

Whenever the delivery of oxygen to the myocardium is inadequate to meet the heart's oxygen consumption needs, myocardial ischemia occurs. One of the major causes of ischemia is coronary artery disease. Fig. 18-7 shows an overview of heart, blood flow, and valves.

SUMMARY

To understand the drug therapies used to treat cardiovascular disease, the healthcare professional must have a solid understanding of the anatomy, physiology, and electrical properties of the heart. The medications in current use may produce their effects on the myocardium, the conduction system, and the coronary vessels. The cardiac action potential is divided into two stages, depolarization and repolarization, which include five phases of ionic changes. The overall process of controlling cardiac muscle contractions involves electrical excitation, mechanical activation, and contractile mechanisms. The cardiac conduction system involves automaticity, conductivity, and refractoriness, processes necessary for the initiation and transmission of electrical impulses necessary for the myocardium contraction. Electrocardiograms are graphic representations of electrical currents produced by the heart. This is a useful tool for monitoring cardiac activity.

REVIEW QUESTIONS

1. Discuss myocardial contraction by addressing the electrical excitation, mechanical activation, and contractile mechanisms.
2. Describe the Frank-Starling relationship in a normal heart.
3. Describe the cardiac conduction system, including heart structures and electrophysiologic properties of the heart.
4. Describe the cardiac effects of the parasympathetic and sympathetic nervous system.

REFERENCES

American Heart Association: *Cardiovascular disease statistics* (http:www.amhrt.org/Heart__and__Stroke__A__Z__Guide/cvds.html), 1998.

Sifton DW: *The PDR family guide to women's health and prescription drugs,* Montvale, NJ, 1994, Medical Economics.

ADDITIONAL REFERENCES

Anderson KN et al, editors: *Mosby's medical, nursing, and allied health dictionary,* ed 5, St Louis, 1998, Mosby.

Gilman AG et al, editors: *Goodman & Gilman's the pharmacological basis of therapeutics,* 8th ed., New York, 1990, Macmillan.

Guyton AC: *Human physiology and the mechanism of disease,* ed 4, Philadelphia, 1987, WB Saunders.

Martini F et al: *Fundamentals of anatomy and physiology,* ed 2, Englewood Cliffs, NJ, 1992, Prentice Hall.

Seeley RR, Stephens TD, Tate P: *Anatomy and physiology,* ed 3, New York, 1995, McGraw-Hill.

Thibodeau GA, Patton KT: *Anatomy and physiology,* ed 4, St Louis, 1999, Mosby.

Van Wynsberghe D, Noback CR, Carola R: *Human anatomy and physiology,* ed 3, New York, 1995, McGraw-Hill.

CHAPTER 19

Cardiac Glycosides

KEY DRUG

digoxin (p. 324)

KEY TERMS

chronotropic, (p. 321)
congestive heart failure, (p. 321)
digitalization, (p. 327)
dromotropic, (p. 321)
inotropic, (p. 321)

CHAPTER FOCUS

The digitalis glycosides were discovered more than 400 years ago and are still used today for the treatment of congestive heart failure (CHF). In the past decade, other drugs have also been found to be useful in treating CHF; therefore the digitalis glycosides are no longer the single first-line drug in treatment. Digoxin is often used in combination with other therapies and, perhaps, alone in chronic heart failure. Therefore the healthcare professional must be informed about this product, a drug with a narrow therapeutic range and potentially life-threatening toxicities.

OBJECTIVES

After reading and studying this chapter, the student should be able to do the following:

1. *Define and discuss the key terms and key drug.*
2. *Name three major signs and symptoms of right- and left-sided heart failure.*
3. *Describe the etiology and name two major risk factors of congestive heart failure.*
4. *Name and describe the two primary mechanisms of action for digitalis glycosides.*
5. *Describe the two potentially serious drug interactions with digitalis.*
6. *Discuss at least three other drug interactions with the digitalis glycosides.*
7. *Describe the initial symptoms of digitalis toxicity and the different dysrhythmias usually seen in young children and in adults.*
8. *Review the use of digoxin immune Fab in digitalis glycoside toxicity.*
9. *Discuss the fast (rapid) and slow method of digitalization.*

Various medications may change the force of myocardial contraction and the rate and rhythm of the heart. Pharmacologic terms that have specific meaning for the actions of drugs on the cardiovascular system include the following: inotropic, chronotropic, and dromotropic effects.

Drugs with an **inotropic** effect influence myocardial contractility. Drugs with a positive inotropic effect strengthen or increase the force of myocardial contraction (e.g., digitalis, dobutamine, dopamine, epinephrine, and isoproterenol) while drugs with a negative inotropic effect weaken or decrease the force of myocardial contraction (e.g., lidocaine, quinidine, and propranolol).

Drugs with **chronotropic** action affect heart rate. A positive chronotropic effect is produced if the drug accelerates the heart rate by increasing the rate of impulse formation in the sinoatrial (SA) node (e.g., norepinephrine). A negative chronotropic drug has the opposite effect and slows the heart rate by decreasing impulse formation (e.g., acetylcholine).

Dromotropic effect refers to drugs that affect conduction velocity through specialized conducting tissues. A drug having a positive dromotropic action speeds conduction (e.g., phenytoin) while a negative dromotropic action drug delays conduction (e.g., verapamil).

Drugs in the digitalis group are among the oldest drugs known as therapeutic agents for treatment of heart failure. The effects of digitalis glycosides are twofold: they increase the strength of contraction (positive inotrope) and alter the electrophysiologic properties of the heart by slowing the heart rate (negative chronotrope) and slowing conduction velocity (negative dromotrope). Other agents may produce varying effects with the same objective of treating heart failure. To better understand the beneficial and toxic effects of the digitalis glycosides and other agents, the mechanisms of heart failure will first be described.

HEART FAILURE

Congestive heart failure (CHF) affects more than 2 million Americans with 400,000 new cases diagnosed annually. It is primarily a disease of the elderly with 10% of the patients dying within a year while the 5-year mortality rate is 50% (AHCPR, 1994; Hsu, 1996). Heart failure accounted for 1 million hospitalizations and approximately 7 billion dollars in hospital costs annually in 1990 (Hsu, 1996). Because CHF adversely impacts quality of life and has a high mortality rate, an understanding of its etiology and appropriate interventions is important.

Etiology

Congestive heart failure or pump failure is a pathologic state in which the weakened myocardium is unable to pump sufficient oxygenated blood from the ventricles (i.e., cardiac output) to sustain normal circulation required to meet the metabolic demands of the body organs. Hypertension and coronary artery disease, which are more prevalent in the elderly, are considered to be important risk factors for heart failure. See Table 19-1 for etiology of heart failure. There are multiple factors that may contribute to the development of CHF, many of which are reversible. They include the administration of excessive amounts of intravenous fluids, poor patient compliance with medications and sodium restriction, dysrhythmias, anemia, infection, hypoxia, hyperthyroidism, stress, and medications (e.g., cardiac-depressant drugs such as beta receptor antagonists and selected antineoplastics and sodium retaining medications). See Box 19-1 for drugs that may precipitate or exacerbate heart failure. Also, many drugs contain sodium; the avoidance of their use must be considered in those consuming a salt-restricted diet (Table 19-2).

Despite the etiologic factors, depressed myocardial contractility is primarily the underlying cause of heart failure. Therefore in patients with heart failure, it is important to identify and remove the cause and correct the problem whenever possible and then treat the heart failure state.

TABLE 19-1 Etiology of Heart Failure

Organic Heart Disorders	*Other Causes*
Cardiac dysrhythmia	Alcoholism
Hypertension	Anemia
Infective endocarditis	Hyperthyroidism
Valvular disorders (mitral valve stenosis, regurgitation etc.).	Liver disease
Myocardial infarction	Nutritional deficiency
Pulmonary embolism	Renal disease

BOX 19-1 Drugs That May Precipitate or Exacerbate Heart Failure

1. Drugs that cause sodium and water retention or expand intravascular volume:
   albumin
   androgens
   corticosteroids (cortisone, hydrocortisone, fludrocortisone [Florinef], etc.)
   diazoxide (Proglycem, Hyperstat)
   estrogens
   guanethidine (Ismelin)
   mannitol
   methyldopa (Aldomet)
   minoxidil (Lonitin)
   nonsteroidal antiinflammatory drugs (NSAIDs)
   urea
2. Drugs that inhibit myocardial contractility (negative inotropic or cardiotoxic agents):
   beta blocking agents
   calcium channel blockers (especially verapamil)
   disopyramide (Norpace)
   doxorubicin (Adriamycin)
   quinidine

TABLE 19-2 Sodium Content of Selected Prescription and Over-the-Counter Medications

Medications	*Sodium/Unit*	*Sodium/Maximum Daily Dose (Adult)*
Antibiotics		
carbenicillin disodium (Geopen, Pyopen)	108-150 mg/g	4.5 to 6 g/40 g
ticarcillin injection (Ticar)	120-150 mg/g	2.9 to 3.6 g/24 g
ampicillin sodium (Polycillin-N, Omnipen-N, and others)	62-78 mg/g	1 to 1.2 g/16 g
cephalosporins		
cefamandole naftate (Mandol)	77 mg/g	0.9 g/12 g
ceftriaxone sodium (Rocephin)	83 mg/g	0.33 g/4 g
cephradine injection (Velosef)	136 mg/g	1 g/8 g
Over-the-Counter Medications		
Alka-Seltzer Effervescent Pain Reliever and Antacid Tablets	0.5 g/tablet	
Alka-Seltzer, Lemon-Lime	506 mg	
Alka-Seltzer, Original	567 mg	
Bellans	144 mg	
Bromo-Seltzer powder	0.76 g/capful	
Eno powder	0.8 g/tsp	
Rolaids	53 mg/tablet	
Soda mint tablets	90 mg/tablet	
Food Supplements		
Ensure	844 mg/L	
Meritene	880-1078 mg/L	
Osmolite	549 mg/L	
Sustacal	924-940 mg/L	

Pathogenesis

On a cellular level, heart failure may be associated with a defect in the excitation-contraction coupling, and in some individuals dysfunction of contractile proteins may occur as an additional abnormality. Ineffective calcium pumping by the sarcoplasmic reticulum may alter the normal relaxation process. Furthermore, the mitochondria, not the sarcoplasmic reticulum, may act as the dominant calcium uptake storage site. If so, less calcium is available for release from the sarcoplasmic reticulum to activate contraction. Thus the amount of coupling is reduced and depressed myocardial contractility ensues.

With regard to dysfunction of contractile proteins in heart failure, attention has been focused on abnormal energy utilization. Some researchers have shown that the activity of myosin adenosine triphosphatase (ATPase) is decreased. When the activity of this enzyme is reduced in heart failure, the interaction between actin-myosin filaments is reduced in intensity, and thus the force of contractility is lowered.

An important consequence of inadequate performance of the myocardium is hemodynamic alterations. Compensatory mechanisms are activated, and incomplete emptying of the heart during ventricular systole eventually allows blood to accumulate inside the heart chambers, causing dilation or enlargement of the heart; this is referred to as low output, systolic dysfunction. During this process, blood backs up into the atria.

In the left atrium, this can lead to pulmonary congestion; in the right atrium, systemic congestion, including ascites, may occur. During the interim, the heart attempts to pump the blood forward in the circulation, but instead the increased fluid in the left ventricle produces stretching of the myocardial fibers and dilation of the ventricles.

Athletes commonly have cardiac hypertrophy, which is an enlargement of cardiac muscle and of the ventricular chambers. Thus the overall effectiveness of the heart as a pump is increased. Frank-Starling's law states that an increase in the length of the heart's muscle fibers results in increased contraction and cardiac output. This stretching of cardiac muscle results from increased preload, an increased amount of blood returned to the heart and entering the heart chambers. Therefore the more the cardiac muscles are stretched during diastole, the greater the contraction in systole.

CHF is a myocardial dysfunction resulting in a decreased cardiac output. Regardless of the primary cause, the result is that preload can increase until a massive overload results. The ventricles are unable to meet the needs for contraction or pumping. Mechanisms to compensate, involving adrenergic (sympathetic).stimulation, may occur as the body attempts to maintain an adequate cardiac output. But the increased heart rate and peripheral vascular resistance also elevate the heart's demand for oxygen, thus further contributing to myocardial dysfunction. The inability to obtain adequate cardiac output is referred to as myocardial insufficiency or cardiac decompensation. Furthermore, chronic

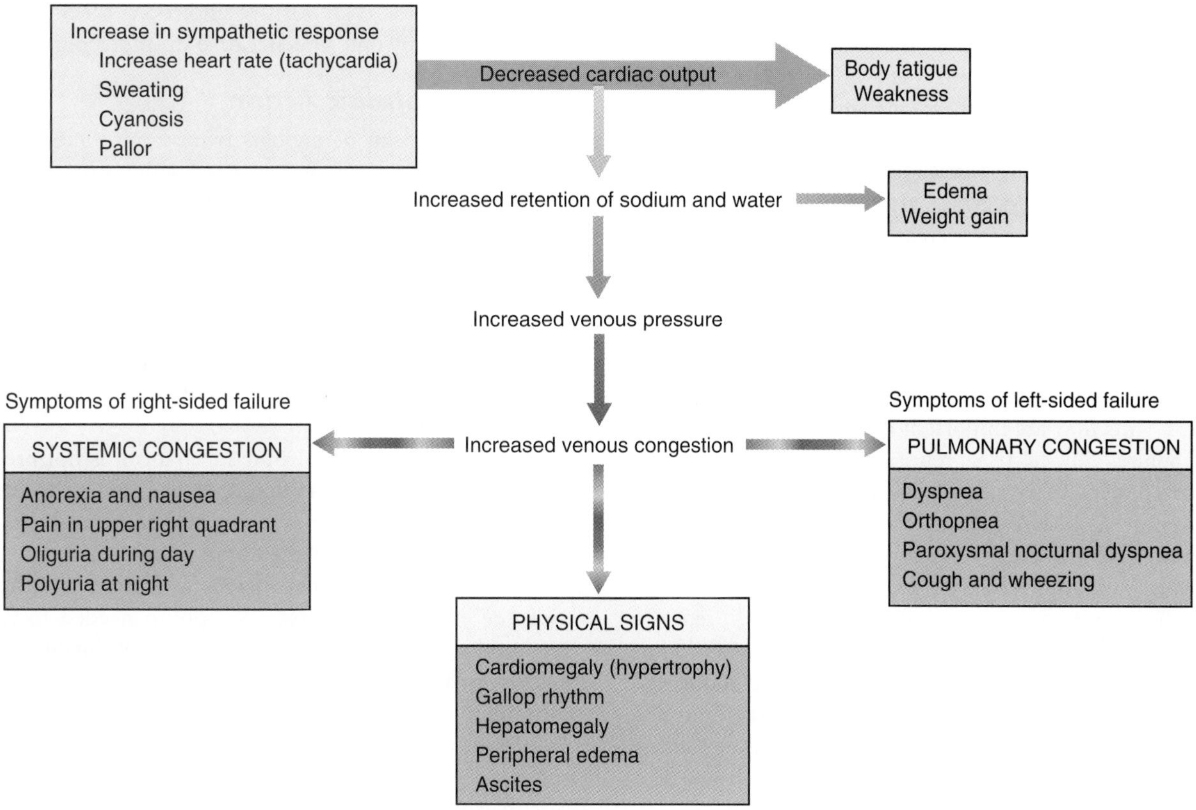

FIGURE 19-1
Signs and symptoms of heart failure.

progressive ventricular failure generally leads to congestive heart failure, which means that the heart's ability to contract decreases to the extent that the heart pumps out less blood than it receives. Subsequently, myocardial infarction produces circulatory failure.

A decrease in cardiac output means less blood is in the blood vessels, and the body's various organs are receiving less blood. The kidneys respond by retaining more water and electrolytes, producing fluid retention and electrolyte disturbances. Excess fluid accumulates behind the affected ventricle. In right-sided heart failure; the right ventricle is initially affected (usually by pulmonary hypertension or stenosis) and the clinical signs and symptoms include jugular vein distention, hepatomegaly, ascites, abdominal distention, cyanosis, and peripheral edema. Left ventricle heart failure, which is most common, leads to fluid accumulation in the lungs—pulmonary edema—producing dyspnea, tachypnea, and orthopnea (person needs to sit up or stand to breath comfortably), as well as interference with oxygen and carbon dioxide exchange. Failure of one side of the heart is usually followed by failure of the other side, which produces total heart failure. See Fig. 19-1 for the signs and symptoms of heart failure.

In summary, the failing heart may show increases in both preload (increased blood volume return to the heart chambers) and afterload (the increased pressure in the aorta, which the ventricle muscles must overcome to open the aortic valve and push blood through). The decrease in renal perfusion just described may activate the renin-angiotensin-aldosterone (RAA) feedback mechanism. Then sodium and water are retained, and intravascular volume and blood flow back to the heart increase. In less serious situations, this is usually enough to maintain arterial blood pressure, thus turning off the RAA system. But in individuals who have conditions bordering on heart failure, this can produce a frank decompensation or acute heart failure. The increase in circulatory blood volume increases the demands on the heart, which may result in acute pulmonary edema.

General Treatment Goals

The overall goals of therapy are to treat any correctable underlying causes of the heart failure, such as hypertension or dysrhythmias; to institute recommendations for nondrug approaches such as dietary changes (low sodium consumption restricted to 2 to 3 g/day; limiting alcohol consumption to one drink per day; avoidance of excessive fluid intake) and activity (exercise, when appropriate during the treatment program); and to counsel the patient and family members on the signs and symptoms of heart failure and the need for compliance with the nonpharmacologic and pharmacologic treatments as prescribed.

Pharmacologically, the following drugs are prescribed: diuretics to reduce the increase in blood volume and edema; an angiotensin-converting enzyme (ACE) inhibitor (such as enalapril, captopril, and others) for left-ventricular systolic dysfunction; vasodilators (nitrates that pool blood in the extremities, thus reducing blood return or preload, and arterial vasodilators that decrease arterial resistance, reducing afterload); dobutamine to increase myocardial contractility (see Chapter 16); and the cardiotonic drugs such as digitalis glycosides (to increase contractility).

The ACE inhibitors decrease peripheral vascular resistance (afterload), pulmonary capillary wedge pressure (preload), pulmonary vascular resistance, and secretion of aldosterone. Thus they are important drugs in the treatment of heart failure. Clinical trials report that the ACE inhibitors improve patient survival, even in persons with severe congestive heart failure. While digoxin improves some patient symptoms, there is conflicting or no evidence that it alone improves patient survival. (AHCPR, 1994, Kienle, 1995). The ACE inhibitors are used with digitalis and diuretics to treat CHF unresponsive to other therapies. The ACE inhibitors will be discussed in Chapter 21. In this chapter, the discussion will focus on digitalis glycosides, digoxin immune Fab (Digibind), amrinone (Inocor), and milrinone lactate (Primacor).

DIGITALIS GLYCOSIDES

The story of the origin of digitalis is interesting in that it demonstrates an herbal remedy that was used for hundreds of years by common people (it was called "housewife's recipe"), which was prepared by farmers and housewives for dropsy (fluid accumulation). More than 400 years ago Dr. Leonhard Fuchs recommended that physicians use it "to scatter the dropsy, to relieve swelling of the liver, and even to bring on menstrual flow" (Silverman, 1942). Dr. Fuchs was a botanist-physician, and at that time, the medical profession paid little attention to a "mere flower picker."

In the mid-1700s, a female patient shared an old family recipe for curing dropsy with Dr. William Withering, which he then used for his dropsy patients, and after spending 10 years studying digitalis, he published his conclusions in "An Account of the Foxglove." This remarkable publication stressed instructions that are still valid today: the necessity of individualizing dosage according to the patient's response. Digitalis was finally admitted to the London Pharmacopeia in 1722.

The digitalis glycosides belong to many different botanical families. The action of each is fundamentally the same, so that the description for digoxin, with minor differences, applies to all. The principal forms are discussed here.

digitoxin [di ji tox′ in] (Crystodigin)
digoxin [di jox′ in] (Lanoxin, Lanoxicaps)

Digoxin is the most commonly used digitalis glycoside and is generally considered the prototype drug in this classification. Digitalis affects cardiac function through two important mechanisms: (1) positive inotropic action and (2) negative chronotropic and negative dromotropic actions.

Positive Inotropic Action

The main function of digitalis is inotropic. The increased myocardial contractility is associated with more efficient use of available energy. If the failing heart is enlarged, the positive inotropic action of digitalis can cause the myocardium to beat more forcefully, thereby increasing cardiac output and decreasing oxygen use. Thus the improved pumping action of the heart in individuals with congestive heart failure may reach levels that approach normal because the net effect is not only reduced heart size but also decreased venous pressure to relieve edema.

While the positive inotropic mechanism is not precisely known, one theory asserts that digitalis is bound to sites on the myocardial cell membrane (sarcolemma), where it inhibits the action of the membrane-bound enzyme, Na^+-K^+-ATPase. Normally, this enzyme hydrolyses ATP to provide the energy for the Na^+-K^+ pump needed to release Na^+ and transport K^+ into the cardiac cell during repolarization. By binding specifically to Na^+-K^+-ATPase, digitalis inhibits the active transport of Na^+ and K^+ (see Fig. 18-1, *5b*). Then intracellular Na^+ accumulates, which stimulates the release of large quantities of free calcium ion from the sarcoplasmic reticulum. The free calcium ion is essential for linking the electrical excitation of the cell membrane to the mechanical contraction of the myocardial cell, a mechanism known as excitation-contraction coupling.

Thus more free calcium ion produces a greater degree of coupling of actin and myosin to form actinomyosin, which results in more forceful myocardial contraction with a concomitant increase in cardiac output. Therefore inhibition of Na^+-K^+-ATPase activity is projected to be the mechanism by which the cardiac glycosides increase myocardial contraction without causing increased oxygen consumption. (See Chapter 18.)

Negative Chronotropic and Negative Dromotropic Actions

Digitalis has negative chronotropic (decreased heart rate) and negative dromotropic (slowed conduction velocity) effects because it can alter three electrophysiologic properties of cardiac tissues:

1. *Automaticity.* Cardiac tissue has the inherent ability to initiate and propagate an impulse without external stimulation. This property affects the rate and rhythm of the heart. Low to moderate doses of digitalis slow the heart rate because the SA node depolarizes less frequently. On the other hand, toxic concentrations of digitalis can directly increase automaticity. This increases the rate of both action potentials and spontaneous depolarization and is one of the mechanisms responsible for digitalis-induced ectopic pacemakers. Toxic doses of digitalis may significantly increase impulse formation in latent or potential pacemaker tissue, causing dysrhythmia.

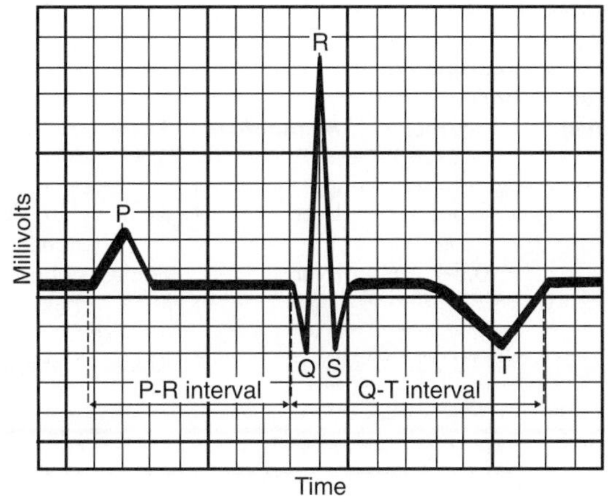

FIGURE 19-2
Representation of typical effects of digitalization on the electric activity of the heart as shown on the electrocardiogram. Note the prolonged P-R interval, the shortened Q-T interval, and the T wave inversion.

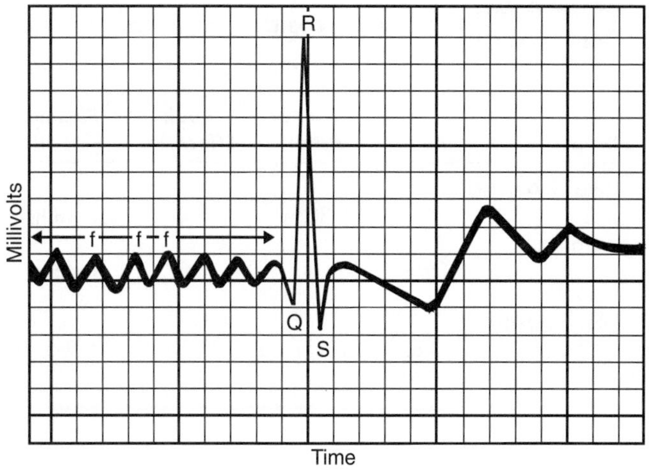

FIGURE 19-3
Graphic representation of atrial fibrillation as seen on the electrocardiographic monitor or tracing paper. No true P waves are noted; but f (fibrillation) waves consisting of rapid, small, and irregular waves are noted. The QRS complex is normal in configuration and duration but occurs irregularly.

2. *Conduction velocity.* All concentrations of digitalis decrease conduction velocity. The atrioventricular (AV) conduction velocity is slowed both by the direct action of digitalis and by increased vagal action. The electrocardiogram (ECG) shows a prolonged P-R interval, and in toxic doses the drug can lead to increased heart block (Fig. 19-2).
3. *Refractory period.* The refractory period effects of digitalis vary in different parts of the heart. If the refractory period in the ventricles is reduced, nearly toxic amounts of digitalis are required. A prolonged refractory period occurs in the AV conduction system, which is very sensitive to digitalis action. This action is partly direct and partly caused by increased vagal tone. Toxic doses of digitalis may prolong the refractory period and depress conduction in the AV conduction system until complete heart block may occur.

Congestive Heart Failure

A heart in failure is no longer capable of supplying body tissue with adequate oxygen and nutrients or of removing metabolic waste products. The positive inotropic effect of digitalis, which results in increased myocardial contractility, benefits the person with a failing heart. The increased force of systolic contraction causes the ventricles to empty more completely. Also, a slower heart rate permits more complete filling, which results in the following:

1. Venous pressure falls, and the pulmonary and systemic congestion and their accompanying signs and symptoms are either diminished or completely abolished.
2. Coronary circulation is enhanced, myocardial oxygen demand is reduced, and the supply of oxygen and nutrients to the myocardium is improved.
3. Heart size is often decreased toward normal.

Some cardiac glycosides have a true, but mild, diuretic effect. However, marked diuresis in the edematous patient primarily results from improved heart action, improved circulation to all body tissues, and improved tissue and organ function including renal function. When digitalis is effective, the patient shows noticeable improvement and has an increased sense of well-being.

Atrial Fibrillation

During atrial fibrillation several hundred impulses originate from the atria, but only a fraction of them are transmitted through the AV junction. (Fig. 19-3 shows the electrocardiographic pattern of atrial fibrillation.) Digitalis is ideal for slowing the ventricular rate because it increases the refractory period of the AV junction and also slows conduction at this site. It is important to know that the purpose of using digitalis in atrial fibrillation is to slow the ventricular rate to reduce the possibility of inducing ventricular tachycardia. It also may prevent or eliminate cardiac failure. Digitalis does not convert the fibrillating atria into normally contracting ones.

Indications

These drugs are used in the treatment of congestive heart failure and in the treatment or prevention of cardiac dysrhythmias, especially atrial fibrillation, atrial flutter, and paroxysmal atrial tachycardia. These agents are more effective in low-output heart failure (depressed ventricular function) than in high-output failure (anemia, AV fistula, or bronchopulmonary insufficiency).

Pharmacokinetics

Digoxin's bioavailability is approximately 60% to 80% with tablets, 70% to 85% with the elixir, and 90% to 100%

TABLE 19-3 Cardiac Glycosides: Pharmacokinetic Parameters

Drug	Route	Onset of Action	Peak Effect (hr)	Plasma Half-Life	Duration of Action (days)	Therapeutic Plasma Level (ng/mL)	Metabolism	Excretion
Rapid Acting								
digoxin (Lanoxin)	IV	5-30 min	1-4	36-48 hr	6	0.5-2	Liver	Kidney (50%-70% unchanged)
	Oral	½-2 hr	2-6	36-48 hr	6	0.5-2	Liver	Same as above
Long Acting								
digitoxin (Crystodigin)	Oral	1-4 hr	8-14	5-9 days	14	13-25	Liver	Kidney (metabolites)

with the capsule dosage form. Digitoxin is very lipophilic, so it is almost completely absorbed orally. The cardiac glycosides can be categorized into two main groups: rapid-acting agents and long-acting agents. Table 19-3 lists specific pharmacokinetic information.

Drug interactions

The following interactions may occur when digitalis glycosides are given with the drugs listed below:

Drug	Possible effect and management
amiodarone (Cordarone)	May increase digoxin serum levels (possibly other digitalis glycosides also) to toxic levels. Reduce dosage of digitalis preparation and monitor serum digoxin levels closely.
Antacids (especially aluminum and magnesium types)	May decrease digitalis glycoside absorption 25% to 35%. Space medications apart, preferably giving digitalis glycoside 1 to 2 hours before antacids.
Antidysrhythmic agents, injectable calcium salts, succinylcholine, or sympathomimetics	Concurrent administration may enhance risk of cardiac dysrhythmias. Avoid or a potentially serious drug interaction may occur.
Antidiarrheal adsorbents (kaolin, pectin, etc.), cholestyramine (Questran), colestipol (Colestid), or large quantities of dietary fiber (bran)	May reduce absorption of digitalis glycosides, resulting in a decreased therapeutic response. Administer digitalis products 1 to 2 hours before these agents, then monitor closely for digitalis effectiveness.
Calcium channel blocking agents (verapamil [Calan, Isoptin], diltiazem [Cardizem])	Concurrent use may require reduced digitalis glycoside dosages. Monitor closely for digitalis-related dysrhythmias.
indomethacin (Indocin)	Renal excretion of digitalis glycosides is reduced, leading to increased serum levels and possibly toxicity. Reduce digitalis glycoside dosage by 50% when indomethacin is started. Monitor closely for both therapeutic and toxic effects and make dosage adjustments accordingly.
magnesium sulfate injection	Use with extreme caution in individuals receiving digitalis. Alterations in cardiac conduction and heart block may result. Avoid or a potentially serious drug interaction may occur.
Potassium-depleting drugs, such as amphotericin B (parenteral), corticosteroids, or potassium-depleting diuretics	The potential for inducing hypokalemia with these medications, if used concurrently with digitalis preparations, may increase the possibility of digitalis toxicity. Monitor potassium levels closely and the patient for signs and symptoms of hypokalemia.
Potassium salts	Although potassium salts are commonly prescribed to treat hypokalemia, especially when patients are also taking a digitalis glycoside, potassium salts are not indicated in persons with severe heart block who are receiving digitalis. Hyperkalemia may be very dangerous in such individuals.
propafenone (Rythmol)	Concurrent use may increase digoxin levels by 25% to 85%, resulting in digitalis toxicity. Careful monitoring of serum digoxin levels and dosage adjustments may be necessary.
quinidine	May result in an increased serum level of digoxin and digitoxin. Monitor serum levels and patient's response closely; dosage reductions may be necessary.
spironolactone (Aldactone)	Concurrent administration may increase half-life of digoxin. Monitor closely; dosage reduction may be needed.

sucralfate (Carafate)	Concurrent use decreases absorption of digoxin; space apart by at least 2 hours.

Color type indicates an unsafe drug combination.

Side effects and adverse reactions

These include anorexia, nausea, bradycardia, stomach upset or pain, and dysrhythmias. The dysrhythmias seen with digitalis toxicity are premature ventricular beats, paroxysmal atrial tachycardia with AV block, progressing AV blocks, and ventricular dysrhythmias such as ventricular tachycardia (USP DI, 1998). Usually loss of appetite is the first sign of toxicity while nausea and vomiting and abdominal distress usually occur several days after the anorexia.

Warnings

Use caution in patients with hepatic impairment (especially digitoxin), renal impairment (digoxin), hypothyroidism, hyperthyroidism, and chronic constrictive pericarditis, and in debilitated patients or persons with cardiac pacemakers.

Contraindications

Avoid use in persons with digitalis hypersensitivity, Stokes-Adams attacks, glomerulonephritis, hypercalcemia, hyperkalemia, hypocalcemia, hypokalemia, hypomagnesemia, acute myocardial infarction, myxedema, severe respiratory disease, premature ventricular contractions, ventricular tachycardia, sick sinus syndrome, and Wolff-Parkinson-White syndrome.

Dosage and administration

Digoxin has a narrow therapeutic range for its effect, and sometimes patients within the higher end of the normal range or just slightly above it can display toxic effects. See Box 19-2 for serum digoxin concentration determinations. Although glycoside serum levels are of limited value in establishing therapeutic serum levels, they are sometimes helpful as an indicator of toxicity. Be aware that the elderly population may have age-related, renal, or hepatic impairment and a decreased volume of distribution for digitalis; thus lower doses are necessary to avoid digitalis toxicity. See the Geriatric Implications box for more information about cardiac glycosides.

Digitalization

Digitalization is the saturation of body tissues with a loading dose of digoxin to achieve maximum effects rapidly. Although nomograms and formula calculations are available to estimate digoxin dosage based on lean body weight and renal function, most prescribers still calculate digoxin dosage according to the body weight of the patient. There are two methods of digitalization: the rapid (fast) method, which requires hospitalization of the patient, and the slow method, which is usually prescribed in an ambulatory setting.

BOX 19-2 Serum Digoxin Concentration Determinations

The therapeutic serum digoxin concentration is 0.5 to 2 ng/mL, but be aware that serum levels do not clearly delineate patients with toxic levels from those with nontoxic levels. It has been reported that 38% of individuals with actual digoxin toxicity had a digoxin serum level 2 µg/mL. Some patients with hypokalemia had digoxin toxicity with serum levels of 1.5 ng/mL (Kradjan, 1995). Therefore use serum levels only as a guide; clinical impressions or evaluations are best in measuring therapeutic outcome.

Criteria for use of serum digoxin levels:

1. Suspected toxicity
2. Individual's compliance questionable or unreliable
3. Patient not responding appropriately to therapy
4. Presence of impaired renal function
5. Use of drugs with documented interference (e.g., quinidine, calcium channel blocking agents, etc.)
6. Confirmation of unusual or seriously abnormal digoxin serum level

The time that a blood sample is drawn for a digoxin serum level is critical. Serum levels obtained 6 to 8 hours after the last oral dose, 2 hours after an intravenous dose, or just before a dose is scheduled are the most reliable.

GERIATRIC IMPLICATIONS

Cardiac Glycosides

- Digoxin, one of the most commonly prescribed drugs in the world, must be closely monitored as the treatment dose is approximately 60% of the toxic dose (Long, Rybacki, 1995). Elderly persons often have a reduced tolerance for the cardiac glycosides, and thus lower doses may be necessary to reduce the potential for drug toxicity.
- Early toxic signs often include anorexia, nausea, and vomiting; difficulty with reading, which may appear as visual alterations such as green and yellow vision, double vision, or seeing spots or halos; headaches; dizziness; fatigue; weakness; confusion; depression; increased nervousness; and diarrhea. Decreased libido and impotency have been reported in approximately 35% of men as a result of digoxin's estrogen-type effects. Also, male breast enlargement and breast tenderness have been reported (Long, Rybacki, 1995).
- Be aware that exercise reduces serum digoxin levels because of increased uptake in skeletal muscles.
- Research indicates that bisacodyl (Dulcolax, Fleet Laxative) may reduce absorption of Lanoxin (digoxin) (Graedon, Graedon, 1995). Do not administer these drugs concurrently.

The rapid digitalization (loading) method is reserved for the patient in acute distress from heart failure. If the patient has not previously received any digitalis glycoside, then intravenous digoxin is given in divided doses in a 24-hour period. The goal of treatment is to obtain the maximum therapeutic effect of the glycoside as rapidly as possible. With this method, the drug toxicities will quickly become evident, while the patient is in the controlled environment of the hospital unit. An advantage is that the toxicities can be easily correlated to a specific drug concentration. For example, the prescriber decides to intravenously administer to an individual a total dose of 1 mg of digoxin. Digoxin may be prescribed as 0.5 mg IV now and 0.25 mg IV every 6 hours for two doses for a total of 1 mg. If the patient demonstrates digitalis toxicity after the 1 mg dose, the prescriber would know that this person was not able to tolerate a 1 mg total dose and in the future would avoid any dosage regimen that might reach this level.

The slow method of digitalization is generally used in less acute situations in the ambulatory setting. The length of time before an individual has reached full digitalization is approximately 1 week, which is longer than with the rapid method. For example, a typical dose of 0.25 mg daily is administered, and digoxin, which has a 36-hour half-life, would take approximately 7 days for digitalization, whereas digitoxin (with a half-life of 7½ days) would require more than a month. The advantages of the slow method include: (1) the individual may be treated on an outpatient basis; (2) it is a safer method; (3) close monitoring is not required; and (4) the doses may be taken orally. The disadvantages are (1) the extended length of time before the individual is digitalized, and (2) the difficulty of determining when digitalis toxicity occurs, since the onset of symptoms may be very gradual. However, according to the Clinical Practice Guidelines (AHCPR, 1994), loading doses of digoxin are usually unnecessary.

The maintenance adult digoxin dose is usually 0.125 mg or 0.25 mg PO daily, and the digitoxin adult dose is 0.05 to 0.3 mg PO daily. The pediatric dose is usually one fifth to one third of the total digitalization dose, once daily or an alternate dose is 17 μg/kg/daily (see Pediatric Implications box).

PEDIATRIC IMPLICATIONS

Cardiac Glycosides

A fall in serum potassium levels enhances the effect of digitalis and increases the risk of digitalis toxicity. Monitor serum potassium levels closely.

Early signs of CHF include tachycardia (especially during rest and minimum activity), increased fatigue and irritability, a sudden weight gain, respiratory distress, and profuse scalp sweating especially noted in infants.

Individualize dosing with very close monitoring, especially in infants. Be extremely careful in calculating digitalis dosages; one decimal point placement error can increase the dose 10-fold. Double check all calculations with another health care professional (nurse, pharmacist, or physician).

Common signs of digoxin toxicity in children include nausea, vomiting, anorexia, bradycardia, and dysrhythmias.

Give digoxin on a regular time schedule, either 1 hour before or 2 hours after feedings.

From Wong, 1999.

Additional Dosing Considerations

Digoxin bioavailability and patient electrolyte imbalances can alter the effects of the digitalis glycosides.

Bioavailability (discussed in more detail in Chapter 4) refers to the amount of the administered drug that is usable in the target tissue. Bioavailability must be considered when a change is made in the patient's dosage form; a dosage adjustment may be required to compensate for the pharmacokinetic differences of the dosage form. A 100 μg (0.1 mg) dose of the injection or of the digoxin-solution capsule is bioequivalent to a 125 μg (0.125 mg) dose of the tablet or elixir. When a patient's dosage form is switched from capsules to tablets (or vice versa), this difference in bioavailability must be kept in mind.

Electrolyte Imbalances

Hypokalemia and hypomagnesemia increase the risk for digitalis toxicity whereas hypocalcemia may reduce the effectiveness of a digitalis glycoside. See Box 19-3 for information on digitalis toxicity.

ANTIDOTE FOR DIGITALIS GLYCOSIDES

digoxin immune Fab (ovine) for injection

(Digibind)

This drug is an antidote for severe digitalis glycoside toxicity. Digoxin immune Fab (ovine) binds and makes complex molecules with digoxin or digitoxin in the serum. These molecules are then excreted by the kidneys. As more tissue digoxin is released into the serum to maintain an equilibrium, it will be bound and removed by this product, which results in lower levels of digoxin in serum and body tissues.

Indications

The drug is indicated for treatment of life-threatening digoxin or digitoxin overdose (see Box 19-3).

Pharmacokinetics

The onset of action takes place in less than 1 minute, and the drug's half-life is 15 to 20 hours. Initial signs of improvement in digitalis toxicity may be seen in 15 to 30 minutes after administration but can take up to several hours. Dysrhythmias and hyperkalemia are usually reversed first, whereas the inotropic effect reversal may take several hours. The drug is excreted in the kidneys.

BOX 19-3 Digitalis Toxicity

Almost every type of dysrhythmias can be produced by digitalis toxicity. The type of dysrhythmia produced varies with the age of the client and other factors. Premature ventricular contractions and bigeminal rhythm (two beats and a pause) are common signs of digitalis toxicity in adults, whereas children tend to develop ectopic nodal or atrial beats. Digitalis-induced dysrhythmias are caused by depression of the SA and AV nodes of the heart. This results in various conduction disturbances (first- or second-degree heart block or complete heart block). Digitalis may also cause increased myocardial automaticity, producing extrasystoles or tachycardias.

Healthcare professionals must be aware of the predisposing factors to digitalis toxicity. The presence of any of these factors in patients indicates the need for close observation for signs and symptoms of digitalis intoxication:

1. Potassium loss. Hypokalemia (low potassium levels) can increase digitalis cardiotoxicity. Since potassium inhibits the excitability of the heart, a depletion of body or myocardial potassium increases cardiac excitability. Low extracellular potassium is synergistic with digitalis and enhances ectopic pacemaker activity (dysrhythmias). The following are causes of potassium loss:
   a. Hypokalemia occurs if large amounts of body fluids are lost as a result of vomiting, diarrhea, and gastric suctioning.
   b. The use of various diuretic agents (carbonic anhydrase inhibitors, ammonium chloride, furosemide, and thiazide preparations) induces potassium diuresis along with sodium and water diuresis.
   c. Poor dietary intake or severe dietary restrictions that decrease electrolyte intake can cause loss of potassium.
   d. Adrenal steroids cause potassium loss and sodium retention.
   e. Surgical procedures associated with severe electrolyte disturbances such as abdominoperineal resection, colostomy, ileostomy, colectomy, and ureterosigmoidostomy can cause loss of potassium.
   f. Use of potassium-free intravenous fluids can cause hypokalemia.
2. Hypercalcemia. Excess calcium in the presence of digitalis may cause sinus bradycardia, atrioventricular conduction block, and ectopic dysrhythmia.
3. Pathologic conditions. Kidney, liver, and severe heart disease are major factors in digitalis toxicity. Approximately 80% of digoxin is excreted by the kidneys, whereas approximately 90% of digitoxin is first metabolized by the liver. Therefore in a clinical setting, the physician may choose digitoxin as the drug of choice for a person in renal failure, because of its mode of excretion, i.e., liver metabolism. For a patient with liver impairment, the physician may select digoxin as the drug of choice, mainly because it does not rely on the liver for metabolism before excretion. The long half-life of digitoxin is a disadvantage in treatment. If the individual should develop digitalis toxicity, the half-life of digoxin may increase from 36 hours to 120 hours, whereas the half-life of digitoxin increases from 120 to 210 hours.

Drug interactions

No significant drug interactions have been reported.

Side effects and adverse reactions

Close monitoring is necessary, as withdrawal of digitalis may result in a decrease in cardiac output, congestive heart failure, and hypokalemia. An increase in ventricular rate may be seen in persons with atrial fibrillation.

Warnings

Use with caution in patients with kidney function impairment and a history of allergies.

Contraindications

Avoid use in persons with known drug hypersensitivity.

Dosage and administration

The adult dose may be calculated on the amount of digoxin or digitoxin consumed, or it may be based on steady-state serum levels. Usually a 38 mg dose of digoxin immune Fab (ovine) for injection will bind approximately 0.5 mg of digoxin or digitoxin. The formulas in Box 19-4 may be applied to determine the dose of the antidote.

BOX 19-4 Formulas for Digoxin ⚷ Immune Fab (ovine)

For digoxin tablets, oral solution, or IM injection:

$$\text{Dose (mg)} = \frac{\text{dose ingested (mg)} \times 0.8}{0.5} \times 38$$

For digitoxin tablets, digoxin capsules, or IV digoxin:

$$\text{Dose (mg)} = \frac{\text{dose ingested (mg)}}{0.5} \times 38$$

When the amount of digitalis ingestion is unknown and the steady-state serum level is also not available, then 760 mg of digoxin immune Fab (ovine) is usually administered because it is reportedly sufficient to treat most life-threatening ingestions.

MISCELLANEOUS AGENTS

amrinone (Inocor)

The mechanism of action of amrinone has not been fully identified. Amrinone increases force and velocity of myocardial tissues, resulting in a positive inotropic effect. Experiments indicate that amrinone inhibits phosphodiesterase activity, which in turn increases cellular cyclic adenosine monophosphate (cAMP) concentration and cardiac contractility. Amrinone appears to produce a direct relaxant effect on the vascular smooth muscle (vasodilation) and reduced preload and afterload.

Indications

It is used to treat congestive heart failure in individuals who do not respond to standard therapies such as digitalis glycosides, diuretics, and vasodilators.

Pharmacokinetics

Administered intravenously, amrinone's time to peak action is within 10 minutes. The duration of effect is dose-related. If 0.75 mg/kg is administered, the duration of action is approximately 30 minutes. If 3 mg/kg is administered, the duration is approximately 120 minutes. The half-life when administered in CHF is between 5 to 8.3 hours. The drug is metabolized in the liver and excreted primarily via the kidneys.

Drug interactions

No significant drug interactions are reported.

Warnings

Use with caution in patients with liver or renal function impairment.

Contraindications

Avoid use in persons with amrinone hypersensitivity, cardiomyopathy (hypertrophic), and advanced aortic or pulmonary valvular disease.

Side effects and adverse reactions

These are infrequent and include nausea, vomiting, abdominal pain, fever, taste alterations, hypotension, dysrhythmias, chest pain, and thrombocytopenia. Inotropic effects are additive to those of digitalis.

Dosage and administration

The adult dose is 0.75 mg/kg IV slowly over 2 to 3 minutes, repeated in 30 minutes if necessary. The maintenance dose by IV infusion is 5 to 10 μg/kg/min, individualized according to response. The maximum dosage is 10 mg/kg/day, but in several reports, dosages up to 18 mg/kg/day were given for short time periods.

For neonates and infants, the initial dose is 3 to 4 mg/kg, in divided doses; the maintenance dose is 3 to 5 μg/kg/min for neonates and 10 μg/kg/min for infants. See the box for Food and Drug Administration (FDA) pregnancy safety categories.

milrinone injection (Primacor IV)

Milrinone is a selective inhibitor of cAMP isozymes in cardiac and vascular muscle; thus it improves cardiac function, contractility and vasodilation, without increasing myocardial oxygen consumption and heart rate. It is a positive inotrope and vasodilator with very little chronotropic activity.

Indications

Milrinone is indicated for the short-term treatment of CHF.

Pharmacokinetics

Administered IV, milrinone has a half-life of 2.5 hours and a duration of action between 3 to 6 hours. It is excreted by the kidneys.

Drug interactions

No significant drug interactions are reported, but its administration with other hypotension-producing drugs may have an additive effect.

Side effects and adverse reactions

These include headaches, hypotension, ventricular dysrhythmias, and, rarely, angina and thrombocytopenia.

Dosage and administration

The adult dose for CHF is 50 μg/kg initially, administered over 10 minutes. The maintenance dose is 0.375 to 0.75 μg/kg/min for up to 5 days.

PREGNANCY SAFETY

Category	Drugs
C	amrinone, digoxin, digitoxin, digoxin immune Fab (ovine), milrinone

SUMMARY

The digitalis glycosides are used in the treatment of congestive heart failure because of their pharmacologic properties in increasing the strength of cardiac contraction and altering the electrophysiologic properties of the heart by slowing conduction velocity. Rapid digitalization is not as common now as in the past, but if it is prescribed, the patient should be hospitalized. The slower oral method of digitalization is often prescribed in an ambulatory setting. Digitalis toxicity is common because of the drug's narrow therapeutic index. Therefore healthcare professionals must be aware of the signs of toxicity, the major drug interactions, and appropriate interventions, such as the proper dosing and use of digoxin immune Fab (ovine) as an antidote for severe digitalis glycoside toxicity.

The miscellaneous agent amrinone (Inocor) is available for individuals who do not respond to the standard drug therapies, whereas milrinone (Primacor IV) is used for the short-term treatment of congestive heart failure.

REVIEW QUESTIONS

1. Review the treatment goals for a patient with congestive heart failure.
2. Compare the effects of the ACE inhibitors and digitalis glycosides in heart failure and patient survival.
3. Describe the use of digoxin immune Fab (ovine) in digitalis toxicity. How is the dose calculated?
4. Name four drugs that may precipitate or exacerbate heart failure. What effect do they produce that can result in this failure?
5. Name three over-the-counter medications and/or food supplements with high sodium content. As a healthcare professional, what recommendations might you suggest to the patient on a restricted-sodium diet?

REFERENCES

Agency for Health Care Policy and Research: *Heart failure: evaluation and care of patients with left-ventricular systolic dysfunction,* Clinical Practice Guideline, Number 11, Rockville, MD, 1994, US Department of Health and Human Services.

Graedon J, Graedon T: *The people's guide to deadly drug interactions,* New York, 1995, St Martin's Press.

Hsu, I: Optimal management of heart failure, *J Am Pharm Assoc,* NS236(2):92, 1996.

Kienle, PC: *Interventions to optimize management of congestive heart failure in long-term care,* Application of the AHCPR Guidelines, An Inservice Kit, 1995, Medical Education Systems, Inc.

Kradjan WA: Congestive heart failure. In Young LY, Koda-Kimble MA, editors: *Applied therapeutics: the clinical use of drugs,* ed 6, Vancouver, Wash, 1995, Applied Therapeutics, Inc.

Long JW, Rybacki JJ: *The essential guide to prescription drugs,* New York, 1995, HarperCollins.

Olin BR: *Facts and comparisons,* Philadelphia, 1998, JB Lippincott.

United States Pharmacopeial Convention: *USP DI: drug information for the health care professional,* ed 18, Rockville, Md, 1998, The Convention.

ADDITIONAL REFERENCES

American Hospital Formulary Service: *AHFS drug information '98,* Bethesda, Md, 1996, American Society of Hospital Pharmacists.

American Medical Association: *Drug evaluations: annual 1995,* Chicago, 1995, The Association.

American Pharmaceutical Manufacturers Association: *New medicines: 107 medicines in testing for two leading causes of death in Americans,* 1995, The Association.

Anderson KN et al, editors: *Mosby's medical, nursing, and allied health dictionary,* ed 5, St Louis, 1998, Mosby.

Cawley M: The role of digoxin in the treatment of atrial fibrillation, *J Cardiopulm Rehabil* 14(6):373-375, 1994.

Covington TR, editor: *Handbook of nonprescription drugs,* ed 11, Washington, DC, 1996, American Pharmaceutical Association.

Marcus FI: Digitalis: how well are you using it? *Patient Care* 25(17):21, 1991.

Mosby: *Mosby's GenRx,* St Louis, 1998, Mosby.

Semla TP, Beizer JL, Higbee MD: *Geriatric dosage handbook,* Hudson, Ohio,1993, Lexi-Comp.

Silverman M (1942). *Magic in a bottle.* New York: Macmillan.

Wong D et al: *Whaley and Wong's nursing care on infants and children,* ed 6, St Louis, 1999, Mosby.

CHAPTER 20

Antidysrhythmics

KEY DRUGS

lidocaine (p. 338)
procainamide (p. 337)
quinidine (p. 335)

KEY TERMS

Adams-Stokes syndrome, (p. 339)
automaticity, (p. 333)
conductivity, (p. 333)
dysrhythmia (arrhythmia), (p. 333)
sinus bradycardia, (p. 333)
sinus tachycardia, (p. 333)
Wolff-Parkinson-White syndrome, (p. 339)

CHAPTER FOCUS

While the number of antidysrhythmic agents has increased over the past decade, these drugs are very potent, with as much potential for life-saving properties as for drug toxicities. Careful drug selection, along with close patient monitoring, is crucial for achieving the goal of safe and effective antidysrhythmic therapy.

OBJECTIVES

After reading and studying this chapter, the student should be able to do the following:

1. *Define and discuss the key terms and key drugs.*
2. *Describe the two primary disorders in cardiac electrophysiology.*
3. *Discuss the different mechanisms of action for group I, II, III, and IV drugs.*
4. *Identify the medications most commonly used as antidysrhythmic agents by individual classification.*
5. *List the most distinguishing side effects of or adverse reactions to disopyramide, procainamide, lidocaine, mexiletine, and moricizine.*

A cardiac **dysrhythmia (arrhythmia)** is defined as any deviation from the normal rhythm of the heartbeat. Dysrhythmia may be caused by a disorder that modifies the electrophysiologic properties of the cells of the conduction system or cardiac muscle cells. For a review of the electrophysiologic events of a normal action potential, see Chapter 18.

Antidysrhythmic drugs are used for the treatment and prevention of disorders of cardiac rhythm. Dysrhythmias often develop in individuals about 4 to 72 hours after myocardial infarction ("heart attack"). In addition, abnormal rhythm may occur in those recovering from cardiac surgery, in patients with coronary artery disease, and in individuals with extracardiac disorders such as pheochromocytoma, electrolyte imbalance, or thyroid disease.

DISORDERS IN CARDIAC ELECTROPHYSIOLOGY

Disorders of cardiac rhythm arise as a result of (1) abnormality in spontaneous initiation of an impulse, or **automaticity,** or (2) abnormality in impulse conduction, or **conductivity.** With some conditions, a combination of both processes may occur.

Abnormality in Automaticity

A disturbance in automaticity may alter the heart's rate, rhythm or site of origin of impulse formation. When the rate of pacemaker activity is affected, a decrease in automaticity of the sinoatrial (SA) node produces **sinus bradycardia** (an abnormal condition in which the myocardium contracts steadily but at a rate less than 60 contractions per minute). An increase in automaticity of the SA node results in **sinus tachycardia** (an abnormal condition in which the myocardium contracts regularly but at a rate greater than 100 beats per minute). On the other hand, a shift in the site of origin of impulse formation can generate an abnormal pacemaker or an ectopic focus, resulting in activation of some part of the heart other than the SA node. This is called an ectopic pacemaker, and it may discharge at either a regular or an irregular rhythm. It occurs because the cardiac fibers depolarize more frequently than the SA node.

Consequently, abnormal automaticity may develop in cells that usually do not initiate impulses (for example, atrial or ventricular cells). Clinical disorders such as hypoxia or ischemia can activate sympathetic receptors, which in turn become centers to initiate impulses. In addition, ischemic sites can cause impulse disturbances in automaticity and also in conductivity, and both manifestations are responsible for ectopic beats. The ectopic beats are classified as escape beats, premature beats or extrasystoles, and ectopic tachydysrhythmia.

Abnormality in Conductivity

Altered conduction of the cardiac impulse probably accounts for more dysrhythmias than a change in automaticity. A disturbance in conductivity may be caused by (1) a delay or block of impulse conduction or (2) the reentry phenomenon.

Delay or Block of Impulse Conduction

Normally, the SA node and atrioventricular (AV) junction are poor conductors of impulse transmission. Under abnormal circumstances, conduction of an atrial impulse to the ventricles may be delayed or blocked in the AV junction or structures beyond this region in the conduction pathway. However, impaired impulse transmission generally appears in the AV junction and occurs in varying degrees of block. In first-degree AV block, the impulses from the SA node pass through to the ventricles very slowly; this is noted by a prolonged P-R interval on the electrocardiogram (ECG). In second-degree block, some atrial beats fail to pass into the ventricles through the AV junction. Finally, in third-degree block or complete heart block, no impulses reach the ventricle, in which case the Purkinje fibers initiate their own spontaneous depolarization at a very slow rate. This results in independent ventricular and atrial rhythms referred to as ventricular "escape."

Reentry Phenomenon

Reentry phenomenon is the mechanism responsible for initiating ectopic beats. A necessary condition for reentry is unidirectional block. Normally, when an impulse travels down the Purkinje fiber, it spreads along two branches and when it enters the connecting branch, impulses are extinguished at the point of collision in the center (Fig. 20-1, *A*). At the same time, other impulses that begin laterally from the Purkinje fibers activate ventricular muscle tissue. In an abnormal situation the impulse descending from the central Purkinje fiber travels down the right branch normally but encounters a block in the left branch as a result of ischemia or injury (Fig. 20-1, *B*). This is a unidirectional block, because the impulse is capable of passing in one direction but not in the other. As a result, in the left branch, where the impulse is blocked in the forward direction at the site of injury, a retrograde or reverse impulse from the ventricular tissue penetrates or reenters the depressed region from the other direction, provided that the pathway proximal to the block is no longer refractory. When the effective refractory period of the blocked area is over, reentry of the impulse from the ventricular muscle into this site causes the impulse to circulate or recycle repetitively through the loop, resulting in a circus-type movement that produces dysrhythmia.

As shown in Fig. 20-1, *C*, reentry is abolished by certain drug groups, which are explained below. Drugs that decrease or slow conduction velocity can convert unidirectional block to a two-way or bidirectional block. As the impulses traveling in the antegrade or forward direction and those appearing in a retrograde or reverse direction are blocked at the injured site, the reentry pathway is interrupted, thereby abolishing the ectopic beats. In Fig. 20-1, *D*, the conditions required for preventing reentry by another

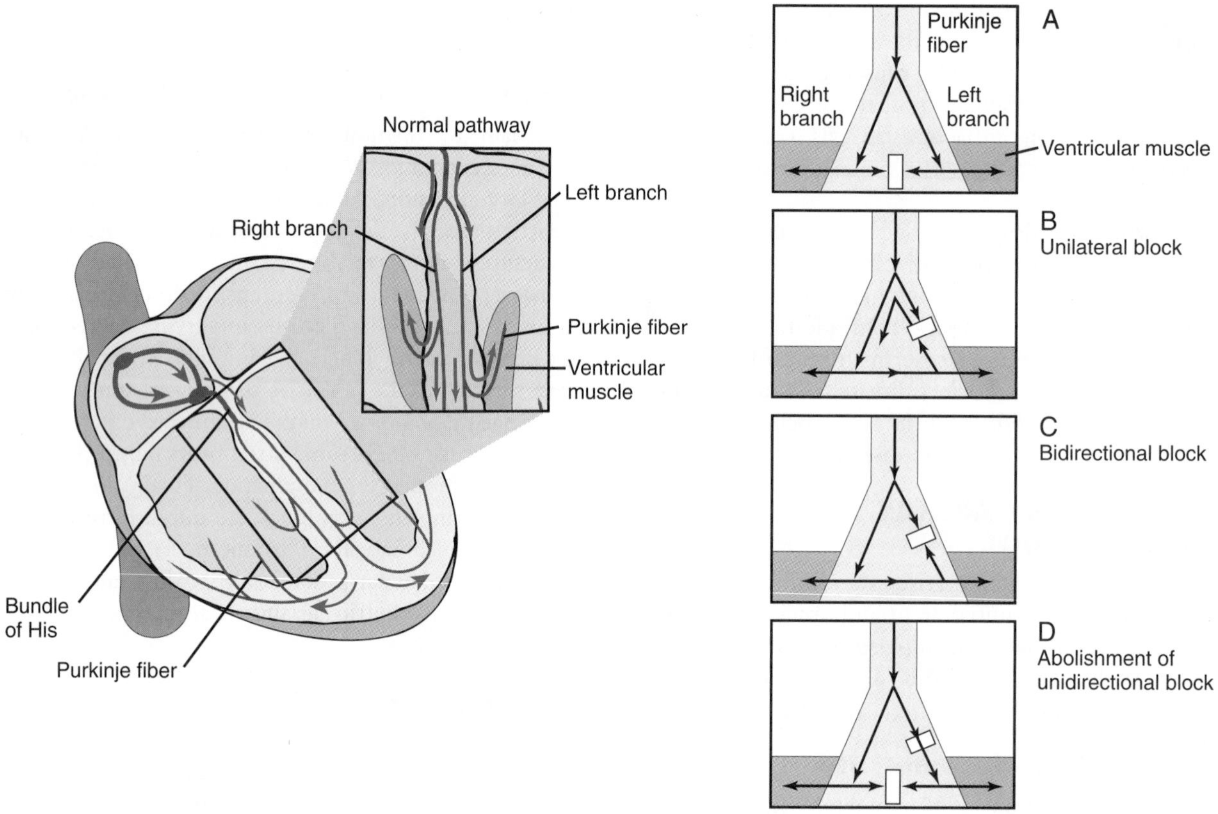

FIGURE 20-1
Reentry phenomenon. Illustration of a branched Purkinje fiber that activates ventricular muscle.

mechanism are also illustrated. Group I-B drugs have no effect on conduction velocity; thus they eliminate reentry by stopping unidirectional block entirely. Consequently the normal impulse conduction along the right and left branches of the Purkinje fibers is again restored.

In recent years, an increasing number of antidysrhythmic drugs have required classification into categories based on their fundamental mode of action on cardiac muscle. Such a grouping of antidysrhythmic mechanisms should prove of value in predicting the drug's therapeutic efficacy, although all drugs belonging to a particular class do not necessarily possess totally identical actions. In some cases a given agent may have subsidiary properties (extracardiac effects) that alter the basic electrophysiologic actions on the cardiac muscle. The currently available antidysrhythmic drugs are classified into four categories according to their mechanisms of action (Box 20-1). However, these drugs have one major electrophysiologic property in common: they all have the ability to suppress automaticity.

Group I compounds are subdivided into groups I-A, I-B, or I-C to reflect the similar electrophysiologic effects of each subgroup. The only exception to the subcategory division is moricizine. Moricizine (Ethmozine) is listed under group I as it has characteristics of all three groups, 1A, 1B, and 1C (Olin, 1998). Class I drugs bind to sodium channels interfering with sodium influx during phase 0 of the action potential, thus depressing conduction velocity. Group I-A drugs include disopyramide (Norpace), procainamide (Pronestyl), and quinidine; group I-B are lidocaine, mexiletine (Mexitil), phenytoin (Dilantin), and tocainide (Tonocard) while group I-C includes flecainide (Tambocor), and propafenone (Rythmol). Group 1-C drugs, because of their prodysrhythmic effects, should be carefully selected and closely monitored when prescribed.

Propranolol (Inderal), acebutolol (Sectral), and esmolol (Brevibloc) are considered group II drugs because of their beta-adrenergic blocking action.

Group III drugs include bretylium (Bretylol), amiodarone (Cardarone), ibutilide (Corvert), and sotalol (Betapace). The principal action of bretylium is antiadrenergic; it also has a positive inotropic action and prolongs repolarization. Amiodarone increases the refractory period and increases the P-R interval, QRS complex, and Q-T interval, contrary to the typical effects of bretylium.

The last category, which is identified as group IV agents, is characterized by a selective calcium antagonistic action. For this reason, verapamil is classified independently of other conventional compounds and is discussed in Chapter 22. Adenosine is listed under the unclassified antidysrhythmic agents.

BOX 20-1 Antidysrhythmic Classifications

Group I drugs—fast sodium channel blockade in cardiac muscle, resulting in an increased refractory period

(Subclasses I-A, I-B, and I-C further define the differences between the drugs).

Group II drugs—beta-adrenergic blocking agents that reduce adrenergic stimulation on the heart

Group III drugs—generally do not affect depolarization but work by prolonging cardiac repolarization

Group IV drugs—block the slow calcium channel, resulting in depression of myocardial and smooth muscle contraction, decreased automaticity, and, perhaps, decreased conduction velocity

GROUP I-A DRUGS

The pharmacologic effects of procainamide, quinidine, and disopyramide are similar: they bind to sodium channels and interfere with sodium influx during phase 0 of the action potential. The result is depression of conduction velocity. ECG effects of these drugs include widening of the QRS complex and a prolonged Q-T interval. Of these agents quinidine has been most widely used and serves as the key drug for this group.

quinidine gluconate [kwin′ i deen] (Quinaglute) 🔑
quinidine polygalacturonate (Cardioquin) 🔑
quinidine sulfate (Quinora) 🔑

Quinidine stabilizes the cell membrane by preventing ready movement of sodium and potassium across this cellular barrier. This inhibition of cation exchange results in a decrease in the rate of diastolic depolarization from resting potential during phase 4 and an increase in the threshold potential (the voltage shifts toward 0 mv). Therefore quinidine decreases impulse conduction and delays repolarization in the atria, ventricles, and Purkinje fibers. By decreasing impulse generation at ectopic sites, quinidine suppresses or abolishes dysrhythmias. Fortunately, abnormal or ectopic pacemaker tissue appears to be more sensitive to quinidine than normal pacemaker tissue (SA node), thus permitting the SA node to reestablish control over impulse formation in the heart.

Widening of the QRS complex indicates a decrease in intraventricular conduction, and lengthening of the P-R interval represents slower conduction through the AV junction, which are changes observed on the ECG when quinidine is used. Thus caution must be used when the drug is given to individuals with intraventricular conduction disorders.

Perhaps the most significant action of quinidine is its ability to prolong the effective refractory period of atrial and ventricular fibers. A delay in completion of repolarization probably exerts an important antifibrillatory action. The tissue remains refractory for a period of time after full restoration of the resting membrane potential. This property is believed to influence the conversion of unidirectional block to bidirectional block, thereby abolishing the reentry type of dysrhythmia (Fig. 20-1, *C*).

The indirect anticholinergic effect of quinidine inhibits vagal action on the SA node and AV junction. This atropine-like effect permits the sinus node to accelerate and often may provoke a dangerous sinus tachycardia. Therefore digoxin, a beta blocker, or verapamil is usually administered before quinidine to prevent ventricular acceleration, when one is attempting to convert atrial fibrillation to normal sinus rhythm. Finally, the chief noncardiac action of quinidine is peripheral vasodilation, which results from quinidine's alpha-adrenergic blocking effect on vascular smooth muscle. The combined effect of a decrease in peripheral vascular resistance and a reduced cardiac output caused by depressed myocardial contractility contributes to the development of hypotension, a condition that may become a serious problem during quinidine therapy.

Indications

Quinidine is used in the management of ventricular and supraventricular dysrhythmias.

Pharmacokinetics

Quinidine's pharmacokinetics are detailed in Table 20-1. The time to peak concentration is 1 to 4 hours; for quinidine gluconate it is 3 to 4 hours, for quinidine sulfate it is 1 to 1.5 hours, and for IM administration it is 1 hour.

Drug interactions

The following significant drug interactions may occur when quinidine is given with the drugs listed below:

Drug	Possible effect and management
Antidsyrhythmic agents	May result in enhanced response. Monitor ECG tracings closely.
Anticoagulants, such as coumarin (Coumadin) therapy	Monitor for signs of additional anticoagulant effects, such as excessive bruising, bleeding gums, black stools, hematuria, and hematemesis. It may be necessary to adjust anticoagulant dosage both during therapy and after quinidine therapy is discontinued.
Neuromuscular blocking agents	Monitor for increased or enhanced blocking effects, especially in the postsurgical patient.
pimozide (Orap)	May potentiate cardiac dysrhythmias. Monitor closely, preferably with an ECG, as intervention may be necessary.

TABLE 20-1 Selected Antidysrhythmics: Pharmacokinetics

Drug	*Time to Peak Level or Effect (hr)*	*Duration of Action* (hr)*	*Therapeutic Serum Level‡ (μ/mL)*
Group I-A Drugs			
disopyramide	0.5-3	1.5-8.5	2-4
procainamide	1-1.5	3	4-10
quinidine	1-4	6-8	3-6
Group I-B Drugs			
lidocaine	IV: 1 min	10-20 min	1.5-5
	IM: 3-15 min	60-90 min	
tocainide	½-2	8	4-10
mexiletine	2-3	—	0.5-2
Group I-C Drugs			
flecainide	3	—	0.2-1
encainide	0.5-1.5	—	—
propafenone	1-3.5	—	0.2-1.5 (trough)
Group I (A, B, and C)			
moricizine	0.5-2 level 6-14 effect	10-24	—
Group II Drugs			
propranolol	1-1.5	3-5	—
Group III Drugs			
bretylium	IV: 5-10 min† IM: 1†	6-24	0.5-2.5
amiodarone	3-7	Variable	—
sotalol	2-3	7-18	—
Group IV Drugs			
Calcium antagonists (see Chapter 22)			

From Olin, 1998; *USP DI*, 1998; Chow, Kertland, 1995.
*Metabolism/excretion is primarily via the liver/kidneys with the exception of amiodarone, mexiletine, and moricizine, which are mainly excreted via bile.
†To treat ventricular fibrillation.
‡Steady-state plasma level.

Urinary alkalizers, such as carbonic anhydrase inhibitors, citrus fruit juices in large amounts, antacids	May result in increased reabsorption of quinidine and elevated serum levels; dosage adjustments may be necessary.

Side effects and adverse reactions

These include anorexia, diarrhea, bitter taste, nausea, vomiting, abdominal distress, flushing, rash, tinnitus, confusion, and visual changes.

Warnings

Use with caution in patients with asthma, emphysema, hyperthyroidism, hypokalemia, infection, and psoriasis.

Contraindications

Avoid use in persons with quinidine hypersensitivity, incomplete and complete AV block, digitalis glycoside toxicity with AV conduction alterations, severe conduction defects, myasthenia gravis, thrombocytopenia, and liver or kidney function impairment.

Dosage and administration

Because quinidine salts contain different percentages of active drug (quinidine gluconate, 62%; quinidine polygalacturonate, 80%; quinidine sulfate, 83%), they are not interchangeable without an appropriate dosage adjustment. Quinidine sulfate 200 mg is considered equivalent to 275 mg of quinidine gluconate or of quinidine polygalacturonate. The usual adult quinidine sulfate dose is 200 to 300 mg PO three to four times daily; the pediatric dose is 6 mg/kg of body weight in five divided doses.

disopyramide [dye soe peer′ a mide] (Norpace)

Disopyramide's effects are similar to those of quinidine with the exception that its anticholinergic effects are more prominent. This is the reason why a drug that slows AV conduction is administered with disopyramide when it is used in the treatment of atrial flutter or atrial fibrillation (see Box

20-2 for definitions). Reentrant dysrhythmias are abolished by converting a unidirectional block into a bidirectional block (Fig. 20-1).

Indications

Disopyramide is indicated to treat ventricular dysrhythmias.

Pharmacokinetics

See Table 20-1. Disopyramide has an active metabolite with both antidysrhythmic and anticholinergic effects.

Drug interactions

The following interactions may occur when disopyramide is given with the drugs listed below:

Drug	Possible effect and management
Other antidsyrhythmic agents, such as diltiazem (Cardizem), flecainide (Tambocor), lidocaine, procainamide (Pronestyl), beta-adrenergic blocking agents, quinidine, tocainide (Tonocard), or verapamil (Calan)	Monitor closely for prolonged electrophysiologic conduction and decreased cardiac output. Beta-adrenergic blocking agents may exacerbate heart failure, especially in individuals with compromised ventricular function. Avoid or a potentially serious drug interaction may occur. Do not administer disopyramide concurrently or within 48 hours before or 24 hours after verapamil, since fatalities have been reported.
pimozide (Orap)	Concurrent therapy may prolong the Q-T interval, which may result in cardiac dysrhythmias. If used concurrently, monitor closely.

Color type indicates an unsafe drug combination.

Side effects and adverse reactions

These are similar to those of quinidine with the exceptions of tinnitus, visual changes, and rash. In addition, disopyramide may cause dry mouth and throat, difficulty in urination, weight gain, and sexual impotency.

Warnings

Use with caution in patients with obstruction of the bladder neck.

Contraindications

Avoid use in persons with disopyramide hypersensitivity, AV block, cardiogenic shock, cardiac conduction abnormality, cardiomyopathy, heart failure, diabetes mellitus, glaucoma (closed-angle), hyperkalemia or hypokalemia, myasthenia gravis, enlarged prostate, and liver or kidney function impairment.

BOX 20-2 Cardiac Terms and Definitions

Atrial flutter—Atrial tachycardia with heart rates between 230 and 380 beats/min. Two types have been identified.
Atrial fibrillation—A dysrhythmia caused by disorganized electrical activity in the atria, resulting in a fast, irregular ventricular response.
Adams-Stokes syndrome—Incomplete heart block that causes episodes of loss of consciousness.
Cardiomyopathy—Illness/disease that affects heart structure and function.
Cardiogenic shock—A low cardiac output that occurs with myocardial infarctions and congestive heart failure. If not corrected, it can be fatal.
Heart block—Interference with the conduction of electric impulses in heart muscle. This is often further defined, e.g., as a first-degree AV block (atrial impulses reach the ventricles but are delayed) or the delay that occurs in a specific area such as bundle branch block or intraventricular block.
Sick sinus syndrome—Sinus node dysfunction that is characterized by severe sinus bradycardia and symptoms of weakness, dizziness, lethargy, and syncope. Treatment usually requires a pacemaker.
Supraventricular tachycardia—A heart rate that exceeding 100 beats/min that originates above the ventricles, such as in the atria, SA node, or AV junction.
Torades de pointes—A ventricular tachycardia with a prolonged repolarization. It can be drug-induced (usually by the antidysrhythmic agents, tricyclic antidepressants, and other drugs). Contributing factors include hypokalemia, hypomagnesemia, and bradycardia.
Wolff-Parkinson-White syndrome—A disorder in AV conduction that is often seen as two AV conduction pathways.

Dosage and administration

Dosage and administration are individualized according to response and tolerance. The usual adult loading dose is 300 mg for patients weighing 50 kg or greater; the maintenance dose is 150 mg every 6 hours. Elderly patients usually require a reduction in dosage, since they are more sensitive to the effects produced by the usual adult dosage. The pediatric dose varies by age; check a current reference for specific dosing recommendations.

procainamide [proe kane′ a mide] (Pronestyl)

Procainamide's electrophysiologic effects are similar to those of quinidine with the following exceptions:

- Procainamide appears to be less effective for controlling abnormal ectopic pacemaker activity.
- Procainamide has fewer anticholinergic effects.
- Procainamide has more potent negative inotropic effects.

The result is that the direct depressant effect of procainamide on the SA node and AV junction may not be as effectively balanced by vagal blockade as it is with quinidine. In persons with a preexisting ventricular dysfunction, procainamide may also cause severe congestive heart failure.

Indications

The primary indications for procainamide are to treat atrial and ventricular dysrhythmias, such as premature ventricular contractions, ventricular tachycardia, atrial fibrillation, and paroxysmal atrial tachycardia. It is also used to treat cardiac dysrhythmias associated with anesthesia and surgery.

Pharmacokinetics

See Table 20-1. Procainamide has a half-life of 2.5 to 4.5 hours while its active metabolite *N*-acetylprocainamide has a half-life of 6 hours. It is excreted primarily by the kidneys (50% to 60% unchanged).

Drug interactions

The following interactions may occur when procainamide is given with the drugs listed below:

Drug	Possible effect and management
Other antidysrhythmic agents	Monitor for enhanced or additive cardiac effects.
Antihypertensive agents, parenteral	Increased hypotension has been reported, especially when parenteral (intravenous) procainamide is given with antihypertensive agents. Monitor closely, as dosage adjustments may be necessary.
Antimyasthenia agents	The effect of antimyasthenic agents on skeletal muscle may be blocked by the antimuscarinic effects of procainamide. Monitor closely, as dosage adjustments of the antimyasthenic agent may be required.
Neuromuscular blocking agents	Concurrent use may result in enhanced neuromuscular blockade. Monitor closely since reversal of blockade may be prolonged.
pimozide (Orap)	Prolonged Q-T intervals and cardiac dysrhythmias may be reported with concurrent use. Monitor closely, preferably with an ECG, since intervention may be necessary.

Side effects and adverse reactions

These are similar to those of quinidine with the exception of tinnitus and visual changes. In addition, an systemic lupus erythematosus-type reaction may occur, that is, fever, chills, painful joints, and rash.

Warnings

Use with caution in persons with asthma.

Contraindications

Avoid use in persons with procainamide hypersensitivity, AV blocks, Torsades de pointes dysrhythmia, heart failure, digitalis glycoside toxicity, lupus erythematosus, myasthenia gravis, and kidney function impairment.

Dosage and administration

The adult antidysrhythmic dose is 50 mg/kg PO or IM in eight divided doses daily. The pediatric oral dose is 12.5 mg/kg four times daily. Procanbid is an extended-release tablet that is given twice daily.

GROUP I-B DRUGS

The group I-B drugs (e.g., lidocaine [Xylocaine], phenytoin [Dilantin], tocainide [Tonocard], and mexiletine [Mexitil]) differ from group I-A drugs in that they either increase or have no effect on conduction velocity. While not approved by the Food and Drug Administration (FDA), phenytoin is used in the therapy of digitalis-induced dysrhythmias. Lidocaine, tocainide, and mexiletine are related therapeutically and are particularly useful for acute ventricular dysrhythmias. Mexiletine's high incidence of side effects and adverse reactions has limited its use. Tocainide can cause the serious adverse reaction of agranulocytosis; Therefore it is usually reserved for patients who have not responded to other drug therapies.

lidocaine [lye′ doe kane]
(Xylocaine, Xylocard ♣) 🔑

Lidocaine, an agent used extensively as a local and topical anesthetic agent, is also an antidysrhythmic agent, especially for ventricular dysrhythmias seen after cardiac surgery or an acute myocardial infarction. Lidocaine appears to act primarily on the sodium channel, blocking both the activated and inactivated sodium channels, although its greater effect is in depolarized or ischemic tissues. These effects are indicative of the efficacy of lidocaine for suppressing dysrhythmias associated with depolarization (such as ischemia and digitalis-induced toxicity) and its lack of effectiveness in dysrhythmias that occur in normal polarized tissues (atrial fibrillation and atrial flutter). Lidocaine has few electrophysiologic effects in normal cardiac tissue.

Unlike quinidine and procainamide, lidocaine has no vagolytic properties nor does it influence cardiac output and arterial pressure. Also, it does not depress myocardial contractility and thereby provides no potential for the development of congestive heart failure. Because it exerts a limited effect, if any on the SA node and atrial myocardium, the drug has no use in the treatment of supraventricular tachycardias.

BOX 20-3 Adverse Effects Related to Serum Concentrations of Lidocaine

1.5-6 μg/ml	6-8 μg/ml	>8 μg/ml
Anxiety, nervousness, drowsiness, dizziness, sensations of cold, heat, or numbness	Tremors, twitching, blurred or double vision, nausea, vomiting, tinnitus	Dyspnea, severe dizziness, fainting, bradycardia, convulsions

Indications

Because electric activities are primarily limited to the ventricular cells, the major use of lidocaine is for abolishing ventricular dysrhythmias (Fig. 20-1, *D*).

Pharmacokinetics

See Table 20-1. This drug also has active metabolites that, after a 24-hour infusion, may also add to its therapeutic and toxic effects.

Drug interactions

Concurrent drug administration with the hydantoin anticonvulsants may result in increased cardiac depression. The hydantoins may also increase metabolism of lidocaine, reducing its effectiveness. Persons receiving this combination should be monitored closely for drug effectiveness and potential drug toxicity.

Side effects and adverse reactions

These include dizziness, anorexia, nausea, vomiting, chest pain, and breathing difficulties.

Warnings

Use with caution in patients with liver or kidney function impairment and the elderly.

Patients older than 65 years of age should have their infusion reduced by half to lower the potential of inducing adverse effects. See Box 20-3 for adverse effects of lidocaine as related to serum concentration.

Contraindications

Avoid use in persons with lidocaine hypersensitivity, severe heart blocks, congestive heart failure, incomplete heart block, shock, sinus bradycardia, **Adams-Stokes syndrome,** and **Wolff-Parkinson-White syndrome** (see Box 20-2 for definitions).

Dosage and administration

The lidocaine adult dose is given by IV bolus, 1 mg/kg at a rate of 25 to 50 mg/min, which may be repeated in 5 minutes if necessary (maximum dose per hour is 300 mg). Children receive the same 1 mg/kg dose initially, but repeat dosages in 5 minutes should not exceed a total dose of 3 mg/kg. By IV infusion, the dose is usually 20 to 50 μg/kg/min given at a rate of 1 to 4 mg/min for both adults and children.

mexiletine [mex il′ e teen] (Mexitil)
tocainide [toe kay′ nide] (Tonocard)

Mexiletine and tocainide are chemically and therapeutically related to lidocaine. Because they resist first-pass liver metabolism, they may be administered orally. Dysrhythmias that respond to parenteral lidocaine are usually responsive to these drugs.

Indications

These drugs are indicated for the treatment and prevention of ventricular dysrhythmias.

Pharmacokinetics

See Table 20-1.

Side effects and adverse reactions

Side effects and adverse reactions are similar to those for lidocaine. In addition, paresthesia of fingers and toes, rash, tremors, and, with tocainide primarily, pneumonitis and sweating are reported.

Warnings

Use mexiletine with caution in patients with severe heart failure, an acute myocardial infarction, convulsive disorders, hypotension, sinus node or intraventricular conduction dysfunction, and liver function impairment. Use tocainide with caution in patients with atrial flutter or fibrillation, heart failure, and liver or renal function impairment.

Contraindications

Avoid use of mexiletine in persons with drug hypersensitivity, AV blocks, and cardiac shock. Avoid use of tocainide in persons with drug hypersensitivity and AV blocks.

Dosage and administration

The mexiletine adult dose is usually 200 mg PO every 8 hours, titrated as necessary. The tocainide adult dose is 400 mg PO every 8 hours. Geriatric patients should receive smaller doses.

GROUP I-C DRUGS

The group I-C drugs include flecainide (Tambocor) and propafenone (Rythmol), which are used to treat and prevent supraventricular tachydysrhythmias. These agents can cause sinus arrest, AV block, and life-threatening ventricular dysrhythmias. This prodysrhythmic effect is of special concern, especially in persons with poor left ventricular function or sustained ventricular dysrhythmias. The group I-C drugs can also aggravate congestive heart failure.

flecainide [fle kay′ nide] (Tambocor)

Flecainide is a sodium channel blocking agent used to treat ventricular dysrhythmias; it has minimal effects on repolarization and no anticholinergic properties. It suppresses premature ventricular contractions and in high doses may exacerbate dysrhythmias in patients with a preexisting ventricular tachydysrhythmia or in persons with a previous myocardial infarction.

Indications

It is indicated for the treatment of ventricular dysrhythmias and as prophylaxis for supraventricular dysrhythmias, such as AV junction reentrant tachycardia.

Pharmacokinetics

See Table 20-1.

Drug interactions

The administration of flecainide with other antidysrhythmic drugs may result in enhanced adverse cardiac effects; in patients with hypotensive ventricular tachycardia, irreversible ventricular tachycardia or ventricular fibrillation has been reported. Avoid concurrent usage.

Side effects and adverse reactions

These include blurred vision, dizziness, headaches, constipation, nausea, weakness, chest pain, irregular heartbeats, and dysrhythmias.

Warnings

Use with caution in patients with heart failure, hypokalemia or hyperkalemia, kidney impairment, a history of myocardial infarction, and permanent pacemakers.

Contraindications

Avoid use in persons with flecainide hypersensitivity, AV block, cardiogenic shock, and liver impairment.

Dosage and administration

The flecainide adult dose is 50 to 100 mg PO every 12 hours, titrated every 4 days as necessary.

propafenone [proe pa feen′ one] (Rythmol)

Propafenone is similar to flecainide in action and therapeutic uses. It also has some beta blocking and weak calcium channel blocking activity. It prevents the passage of sodium ions into the fast sodium channels (phase 0), resulting in a decrease in depolarization rate. It also prolongs the refractory period in cardiac tissues.

Indications

It is indicated for the treatment of life-threatening ventricular dysrhythmias.

Pharmacokinetics

See Table 20-1. Propafenone has a significant first-pass effect in the liver and is metabolized to two active metabolites (5-hydroxypropafenone and *N*-depropylpropafenone). Its half-life is 2 to 10 hours in active metabolizers and 10 to 32 hours in poor metabolizers.

Drug interactions

When propafenone is administered concurrently with digoxin, digoxin serum levels may increase from 35% to 85%, which increases the potential for digitalis toxicity. Closely monitor digoxin serum levels as dosage adjustment may be necessary. Warfarin serum levels may increase (approximately 40%) with concurrent drug administration. This may result in an increase in prothrombin times by approximately 25%. Monitor prothrombin times closely as dosage adjustment is usually necessary.

Side effects and adverse reactions

These include dizziness, nausea, headaches, constipation, weakness, chest pain, irregular heartbeats, and dysrhythmias. The dysrhythmia most often reported is ventricular tachydysrhythmias.

Warnings

Use with caution in patients with cardiomyopathy, asthma, liver or kidney function impairment, hypokalemia, hyperkalemia, hypotension, a history of myocardial infarction, and permanent pacemakers.

Contraindications

Avoid use in persons with propafenone hypersensitivity, AV block, cardiac shock, sinus bradycardia, heart failure, and sick sinus syndrome

Dosage and administration

The usual adult dose is 150 mg PO every 8 hours, with dosage adjustments at 3- to 4-day intervals as necessary. The pediatric dosage is unknown.

GROUP I DRUGS (A, B, and C)

moricizine [mor′ i siz een] (Ethmozine)

Moricizine (Ethmozine) has properties of all three classes (A, B, and C) and does not belong to one individual classification. It is a fairly potent sodium channel blocking agent that does not prolong the action potential duration. It has local anesthetic action and a membrane-stabilizing effect; thus it decreases AV junction and His-Purkinje conduction.

Indications

Moricizine is indicated for the treatment of life-threatening ventricular dysrhythmias.

Pharmacokinetics

See Table 20-1.

Side effects and adverse reactions

These include lightheadedness or dizziness (dose related), dry mouth, blurred vision, nausea, vomiting, weakness, chest pain, heart failure, and ventricular tachydysrhythmias.

Drug interactions

No significant drug interactions are noted (USP DI, 1998).

Warnings

Use with caution in patients with cardiomegaly, severe heart failure, coronary artery disease, liver or kidney impairment, hypokalemia, hyperkalemia, a history of myocardial infarction, and a pacemaker.

Contraindications

Avoid use in persons with moricizine hypersensitivity, AV block, cardiac shock, and sick sinus syndrome.

Dosage and administration

The adult dose is 200 to 300 mg PO three times daily, every 8 hours, titrated as necessary at 3-day intervals. The maximum daily dose is 900 mg.

GROUP II DRUGS

propranolol [proe pran′ oh lole] (Inderal)
acebutolol [a se byoo′ toe lole] (Sectral)
esmolol [ess′ moe lol] (Brevibloc)

All three drugs are beta-adrenergic blocking agents used to control cardiac dysrhythmias caused by excessive sympathetic nerve activity. Dysrhythmias caused by increased sympathetic discharge (hyperthyroidism) are effectively blocked by the beta-adrenergic blocking action of propranolol. Acebutolol is used to treat ventricular dysrhythmias such as ventricular premature beats, whereas esmolol is indicated for short-term treatment of supraventricular tachycardia induced by atrial fibrillation or atrial flutter (see the drug monographs in Chapter 16).

GROUP III DRUGS

The electrophysiologic properties of drugs in this group differ markedly from the drugs previously discussed. Drugs in this group prolong the effective refractory period by prolonging the action potential (delay repolarization).

bretylium tosylate [bre til′ ee um] (Bretylol, Bretylate ♣)

Unlike the other antidysrhythmics, bretylium does not suppress automaticity and has no effect on conduction velocity. The direct electrophysiologic action on the heart appears to be prolongation of the action potential and lengthening of the effective refractory period. It is believed that this mechanism helps to terminate dysrhythmias caused by the reentry phenomenon. Bretylium is also taken up and concentrated in the adrenergic nerve terminals where, after an initial release of norepinephrine, it prevents any further release. This sympatholytic action significantly increases the threshold, producing an antifibrillatory response in the ventricles. Bretylium produces a positive inotropic effect, increasing myocardial contractility. With long-term treatment, the drug shows increased responsiveness to circulating epinephrine and norepinephrine, which may account for the increased myocardial contractility.

Indications

Bretylium is indicated for the prophylaxis and treatment of ventricular dysrhythmias.

Pharmacokinetics

See Table 20-1.

Drug interactions

Do not administer digitalis glycosides to patients receiving bretylium. The initial release of norepinephrine produced by bretylium may increase digitalis toxicity.

Side effects and adverse reactions

These include anorexia, headaches, nausea, vomiting, bitter taste, impotency, dizziness, cough, breathing difficulties, fever, paresthesia of fingers or toes, hand tremors, and weakness.

Warnings

Use with caution in patients with aortic stenosis, severe pulmonary hypertension, and kidney function impairment.

Contraindications

Avoid use in persons with bretylium hypersensitivity.

Dosage and administration

The usual adult dose for life-threatening ventricular fibrillation or ventricular tachycardia is 5 mg/kg IV of undiluted solution, followed by 10 mg/kg every 15 to 30 minutes as needed. For dosage recommendations for other ventricular dysrhythmias, see a current reference.

amiodarone [a mee′ oh da rone] (Cordarone)

Amiodarone increases the refractory period in all cardiac tissues by a direct effect on the tissues. It decreases automaticity, prolongs AV conduction, and decreases the automaticity of fibers in the Purkinje system. It may block potassium, sodium, and calcium channels and beta receptors. It has the potential of causing a variety of complex effects on the heart and has serious adverse effects.

Indications

Amiodarone is reserved for the prevention and treatment of life-threatening ventricular dysrhythmias in persons not responding to or tolerating other drug therapies.

Pharmacokinetics

See Table 20-1. Amiodarone is widely distributed in the body (e.g., in adipose tissues, liver, and lung), so it is slow to reach steady-state, therapeutic serum levels and has a prolonged elimination time. It has an onset of action between several days and 2 to 3 months, even if loading dosages are administered. It has a biphasic elimination half-life, that is, the initial half-life is 2.5 to 10 days; the terminal half-life is 26 to 107 days. It has one active metabolite (desethylamiodarone), which has a terminal half-life of approximately 60 days.

Drug interactions

The following drug interactions may occur when amiodarone is given with the drugs listed below:

Drug	Possible effect and management
Other antidysrhythmic agents	May increase cardiac effects and the risk of inducing tachydysrhythmias. It also increases serum levels of quinidine, procainamide, flecainide, and phenytoin. If amiodarone must be given with group I antidysrhythmic agents, reduce the dose of the group I antidysrhythmic drug by 30% to 50% several days after starting amiodarone and gradually withdraw the group I drug. If additional treatment with amiodarone is necessary, start therapy at half the usual recommended dosage.
Anticoagulants, coumarin (Coumadin),	May increase anticoagulant effect. The dose of anticoagulant should be reduced by one third to one half when adding amiodarone to the patient's drug regimen. Prothrombin times should also be closely monitored.
Digitalis glycosides	May increase the serum level of digoxin and other digitalis glycosides, resulting in toxicity. Digitalis glycosides should be stopped or the dose reduced to 50% whenever amiodarone is given. Monitor serum levels closely. May also see additive effects of both drugs on the SA node and AV junction.
phenytoin (Dilantin)	May result in increased serum levels of phenytoin, possibly resulting in toxicity. Monitor serum levels of phenytoin.

Side effects and adverse reactions

These include dizziness, bitter taste, headache, flushing, nausea, vomiting, constipation, ataxia, weight loss, tremors, numbness and tingling of fingers and toes, photosensitivity, blue-gray skin discoloration, pulmonary fibrosis or pneumonitis, cough, dyspnea, fever, allergic reaction, and blurred vision.

PREGNANCY SAFETY

Category	Drug
B	lidocaine, moricizine
C	adenosine, bretylium, disopyramide, flecainide, mexiletine, procainamide, propafenone, quinidine, tocainide
D	amiodarone
Unclassified	sotalol

Warnings

Use with caution in patients with heart failure, liver or thyroid function impairment, and hypokalemia.

Contraindications

Avoid use in persons with amiodarone hypersensitivity, AV blocks, bradycardia, and sinus node function impairment.

Dosage and administration

The usual adult dose for ventricular dysrhythmias is 800 mg to 1.6 g PO daily for 1 to 3 weeks until a therapeutic response is noted or side effects appear. The dose is then reduced to 600 to 800 mg daily for 1 month, eventually decreasing to the lowest effective dose. See the box for FDA pregnancy safety categories.

The pediatric dose is 10 mg/kg/day for 10 days or until a therapeutic response is noted or side effects appear. Dose is then decreased and tapered to the lowest effective dose as outlined in the package insert.

ibutilide (Corvert)

Ibutilide has class III effects; it prolongs the action potential and increases atrial and ventricular refractory period. It may produce its effect at the sodium channels by slowing the inward current or by blocking the potassium outward currents.

Indications

It is indicated for the treatment of atrial fibrillation or atrial flutter.

Pharmacokinetics

Ibutilide is administered by IV infusion; it has one active metabolite and a half-life of approximately 6 hours. The time to peak effect (to resume normal sinus rhythm) is 0.5 to 1.5 hours. It is primarily excreted by the kidneys.

Drug interactions

The following drug interactions may occur when ibutilide is given with the following medications:

Drug	Possible effect and management
Other antidysrhythmic agents	Avoid concurrent administration with class Ia or other class III drugs (amiodarone and sotalol) because of their potential additive effects in prolonging the refractory period.
Antidepressants, tricyclic; phenothiazines, disopyramide (Norpace), maprotiline (Ludiomil), procainamide (Pronestyl), and quinidine	Concurrent use with these medications, drugs that induce Q-T prolongation, may increase the potential for dysrhythmias. Avoid concurrent usage.

Color type indicates an unsafe drug combination.

Side effects and adverse reactions

These include headache, nausea, cardiovascular alterations (e.g., AV block, bradycardia, and ventricular extrasystoles), hypotension, and hypertension.

Warnings

Use with caution in patients who are breastfeeding.

Contraindications

Avoid use in persons with ibutilide hypersensitivity, atrial fibrillation, a history of heart failure or ventricular tachycardia, hypokalemia, and hypomagnesemia.

Dosage and administration

The adult dose for persons weighing less than 60 kg is 0.01 mg/kg given over 10 minutes. The dose may be repeated in 10 minutes if the dysrhythmia is still present.

sotalol [soe′ ta lole] (Betapace)

Sotalol is a beta-adrenergic blocking agent that prolongs the action potential duration, increasing the effective refractory period in atrial, ventricular, and AV junction. It is indicated for life-threatening ventricular dysrhythmias. Be aware that sotalol is contraindicated in patients with bronchial asthma, sinus bradycardia, AV blocks, cardiogenic shock, and heart failure, and in patients who have sotalol hypersensitivity. See Chapter 22 for additional information.

GROUP IV: MISCELLANEOUS DRUG GROUP

Calcium antagonists are selective antidysrhythmic agents reviewed in Chapter 22.

UNCLASSIFIED ANTIDYSRHYTHMIC AGENT

adenosine (a den′ o sin)

Adenosine is a natural constituent of muscle tissue used to slow AV node conduction. Thus it is indicated for the conversion of paroxysmal supraventricular tachycardia to normal sinus rhythm. Administered by intravenous bolus, it is nearly immediately taken up by red blood cells and vascular endothelial cells and metabolized in the body to inosine (which is processed to uric acid) and adenosine monophosphate (AMP).

Pharmacokinetics

Adenosine is administered IV, has an immediate onset of action, and a half-life of less than 10 seconds and is primarily eliminated by cellular uptake and metabolism. Its principal metabolite is uric acid, which is excreted via the kidneys.

Drug interactions

No significant drug interactions reported, although caffeine and theophylline may antagonize adenosine's effects whereas dipyridamole (Persantin) may increase its effects. Carbamazepine (Tegretol) may increase the risk of heart block that is caused by adenosine.

Side effects and adverse reactions

These include dyspnea, flushing, cough, dizziness, tingling in arms, nausea, headache, new dysrhythmias such as premature ventricular contractions, sinus bradycardia, sinus tachycardia, skipped beats, and chest pain/pressure.

Warnings

Use with caution in patients with asthma.

Contraindications

Avoid use in persons with adenosine hypersensitivity, AV block, and sick sinus syndrome.

Dosage and administration

The usual dose is 6 mg administered rapidly in an IV bolus over 1 to 2 seconds. If the dysrhythmia is still present 1 to 2 minutes after the injection, then a 12 mg dose may be administered.

SUMMARY

The antidysrhythmic drugs are used to treat and prevent cardiac rhythm disorders. These disorders are usually the result of a abnormality in the electrophysiologic status of the cells in the cardiac conduction system or cardiac muscle cells. The antidysrhythmic drugs are subdivided into group classifications, according to their mechanism of action and therapeutic application. Group I-A, I-B, and I-C suppress automaticity. For example group I-A, which includes disopyramide, procainamide, and quinidine, decreases conduction velocity and prolongs the action potential. Group I-B (lidocaine, phenytoin, tocainide, and mexiletine) may increase or have no effect on conduction velocity. Group I-C drugs (flecainide and propafenone) are indicated to treat or prevent supraventricular tachydysrhythmias. Group II drugs have beta-adrenergic blocking action and are discussed in Chapter 16, while the group III agents (bretylium and amiodarone) are primarily antiadrenergic. Some group IV drugs (miscellaneous agents) have selective calcium antagonistic action, which is discussed in Chapter 22. These are potent medications that require careful patient selection and close monitoring to avoid drug-induced adverse effects or toxicity.

REVIEW QUESTIONS

1. Describe quinidine's pharmacologic effects in the treatment of ventricular and supraventricular dysrhythmias.
2. Why are quinidine and disopyramide contraindicated for use in patients with myasthenia gravis?
3. What are the differences in electrophysiologic effects of procainamide and quinidine?
4. Why is moricizine effective in the treatment of life-threatening ventricular dysrhythmias?
5. Discuss the primary therapeutic effects and adverse effects of amiodarone. Why is it contraindicated for use in patients with AV blocks?

REFERENCES

Chow MSS, Kertland HR: Cardiac arrhythmias. In Young LY, Koda-Kimble MA, editors: *Applied therapeutics: the clinical use of drugs,* ed 6, Vancouver, Wash, 1995, Applied Therapeutics, Inc.

Olin BR: *Facts and comparisons,* Philadelphia, 1998, JB Lippincott.

United States Pharmacopeial Convention: *USP DI: drug information for the health care professional,* ed 18, Rockville, Md, 1998, The Convention.

ADDITIONAL REFERENCES

Abramowicz M, editor: Drugs for cardiac arrhythmias, *Med Lett* 36(937):111, 1994.

American Hospital Formulary Service: *AHFS drug information '98,* Bethesda, Md, 1996, American Society of Hospital Pharmacists.

Anderson KN et al, editors: *Mosby's medical, nursing, and allied health dictionary,* ed 5, St Louis, 1998, Mosby.

Dreifus LS, Longano J, Phibbs BP: Symptomatic arrhythmias, *Patient Care* 26(18):176, 183, 187, 190, 193, 196, 198, 213, 1992.

Formulary Drug Review: A review of propafenone, *Hosp Pharmacy* 25(2):177, 1990.

Mosby: *Mosby's GenRx,* St Louis, 1998, Mosby.

Chapter 21

Antihypertensives

KEY DRUGS

KEY TERMS

CHAPTER FOCUS

High blood pressure, or hypertension, is a chronic cardiovascular disease that affects millions of Americans. It has been estimated that approximately 50 million Americans have hypertension or systolic and/or diastolic blood pressures higher than 140/90 (Oates, 1996). Inadequately treated or undiagnosed hypertension often increases the risk of stroke, cerebral hemorrhage, congestive heart failure, coronary heart disease, and renal failure. The risk factors for essential hypertension include family history, stress, overweight, excess intake of sodium or salt, use of tobacco, sedentary lifestyle, diabetes mellitus, and aging. The nonpharmacologic approaches (lifestyle changes) and pharmacologic medications available, if properly utilized, can control hypertension and reduce the serious and life-threatening complications.

OBJECTIVES

After reading and studying this chapter, the student should be able to do the following:

1. *Define and discuss the key terms and key drugs.*
2. *Discuss the physiologic control of blood pressure.*
3. *Present the JNC VI (1997) classifications for adult hypertension.*
4. *Describe the stepped-care approach that is currently recommended for treatment of hypertension.*
5. *Discuss the three risk stratifications and suggested antihypertensive treatments.*
6. *Present the mechanisms of action for the five major categories of antihypertensive drugs: diuretics, adrenergic inhibitors, vasodilators, ACE inhibitors and antagonists, and calcium antagonists.*
7. *Identify commonly used key antihypertensive drugs as to mechanism of action, pharmacokinetics, side effects and adverse reactions, drug interactions, and dosages.*

The number of persons with the silent killer hypertension is alarming, because while this condition seems relatively harmless, hypertension severely damages an individual's major body organs. Approximately 50 million Americans have been estimated to have hypertension. Untreated hypertension is dangerous, as it may result in the complications of congestive heart failure, renal failure, cerebral hemorrhage, and, ultimately, death. The American Heart Association has reported that 50% of the hypertensive persons in this country are not receiving antihypertensive therapy. Of the hypertensive patients in treatment, however, only 21% are receiving adequate treatment (Portyansky, 1997). The need for improving medical care for hypertensive patients is apparent, as cardiovascular disease has been and still is the number one cause of death in North America.

DEFINITION OF HYPERTENSION

Hypertension is defined as an elevated systolic blood pressure, diastolic blood pressure, or both. The classification for adult hypertension was defined by the Joint National Committee on Prevention, Detection, Evaluation, and Treatment of High Blood Pressure (JNC VI) (Kaplan, 1997) as follows:

HYPERTENSION	SYSTOLIC (mm Hg)	DIASTOLIC (mm Hg)
Normal	<130	<85
High normal	130-139	85-89
Stage 1	140-159	90-99
Stages 2 and 3	≥160	≥100

This classification has also stratified the patients based on blood pressure levels, the presence of risk factors and the degree of target organ damage secondary to hypertension. See Table 21-1 for the implications of risk stratification and antihypertensive treatment.

The major risk factors in hypertensive patients include smoking, diabetes mellitus, high blood cholesterol or lipid levels, age older than 60 years or age, family history of heart disease (i.e., women younger than 65 years of age and men older than age 55), and gender (men and postmenopausal women are at greater risk). The target organ damage or cardiovascular disease in hypertensive patients includes stroke or transient ischemic attacks (TIA), kidney disease, retinopathy, and various heart diseases such as angina, congestive heart failure, left ventricular hypertrophy, and prior myocardial infarction.

Patients with stage 1 hypertension are instructed on lifestyle modifications such as weight loss if overweight, moderate alcohol intake, exercise, sodium restriction (Box 21-1), adequate consumption of dietary potassium, calcium, and magnesium, elimination of tobacco, and reduction of saturated fat intake. Then these patients should be reevaluated in 6 to 12 months. Patients with stages 2 and 3 hypertension, however, require drug therapy.

Obtaining a careful and detailed drug history before diagnosis is also important, as many over-the-counter (OTC) and prescription medications may increase blood pressure or interfere with the effectiveness of an antihypertensive agent. Oral contraceptives (estrogen-containing agents), corticosteroids, nonsteroidal antiinflammatory agents (NSAIDs), antidepressants, nasal decongestants, and appetite-suppressing agents are typical examples of interfering substances. Fig. 21-1 illustrates sites of drug effects that can induce or exacerbate hypertension.

CLASSIFICATION OF HYPERTENSION

In **primary (idiopathic or essential) hypertension,** the specific cause of the hypertension is unknown. This group accounts for approximately 90% of cases.

Secondary hypertension, representing approximately 10% of cases, may be a symptom of pheochromocytoma, toxemia of pregnancy, or renal artery disease or may result

BOX 21-1 Fruits and Vegetables Low in Sodium and Calories and High in Potassium

Artichokes	Cantaloupe	Peaches
Bananas	Carrots	Potatoes
Broccoli	Honeydew melon	Strawberries
Brussels sprouts	Oranges	Tomatoes
	Orange juice	

TABLE 21-1 Risk Stratification and Antihypertensive Treatment

	Treatment*		
Risk Group	***High-Normal 130-139/85-89 (mm Hg)***	***Stage 1 140-159/90-99 (mm Hg)***	***Stages 2 and 3 >160/>100 mm Hg***
A†	Lifestyle	Lifestyle	Drug therapy
B‡	Lifestyle	Drug therapy; lifestyle	Drug therapy
C§	Drug therapy; lifestyle	Drug therapy	Drug therapy

*Lifestyle changes are appropriate in all stages.
†Risk group A: patient has no risk factors or target organ damage.
‡Risk group B: patient has at least one risk factor (not diabetes) with no target organ damage.
§Risk group C: patient has target organ damage and/or diabetes with or without other risk factors.

from use of specific medications. If the cause of secondary hypertension is corrected, the blood pressure will usually return to normal.

PHYSIOLOGIC CONTROL OF BLOOD PRESSURE

Control of blood pressure involves a complex interaction between the nervous, hormonal, and renal systems, since all play a part in regulating arterial blood pressure (Fig. 21-2).

The body has two primary mechanisms to control blood pressure:

1. Adrenergic nervous system or baroreceptor reflex—a rapid-acting system
2. Renin-angiotensin-aldosterone mechanism—a long-acting system

ADRENERGIC NERVOUS SYSTEM

The adrenergic or sympathetic nervous system uses a reflex mechanism, the **baroreceptor reflex,** to maintain blood pressure. The baroreceptors are nerve endings located in the walls of the internal carotid arteries and the aortic arch. These sensory receptors rapidly respond to changes in blood pressure. Any elevation in pressure stretches the receptors, causing an impulse to be transmitted along the afferent neuron (vagus nerve) to the vasomotor center in the brainstem. The vasomotor center responds to the impulse by causing (1) a decrease in heart rate and force of myocardial contraction, which lowers cardiac output, and (2) vasodilation of peripheral vessels, which decreases total peripheral resistance. The subsequent reduction in blood pressure is attributed to the reflex activity of the baroreceptor reflex.

When blood pressure is low, this information is projected to the vasomotor center that then activates sympathetic nerves. The sympathetic nervous system is mediated by two hormones: norepinephrine and epinephrine. Norepinephrine acts mainly on alpha-adrenergic receptors, located in the arterioles, while epinephrine acts on both alpha- and beta-adrenergic receptors. The affinity of norepinephrine for these receptors produces vasoconstriction, with a resultant increase in blood pressure. The $beta_1$-adrenergic receptors prevalent in the heart are also activated by norepinephrine. This response increases both the heart rate and the force of myocardial contraction, thereby indirectly causing an elevation in blood pressure.

Because it produces dilation of skeletal muscle blood vessels, epinephrine does not cause any increase in peripheral resistance. However, epinephrine does produce a considerable increase in heart rate and force of myocardial contraction, so the elevation in cardiac output indirectly raises the blood pressure (Box 21-2).

This reflex functions as a rapidly acting system for short-term control of pressure, both low and high blood pressure. It has been demonstrated that over a prolonged period the rate of firing of the baroreceptors diminishes even if the blood pressure remains elevated. Therefore in hypertension, it has been speculated that these receptors are "reset" to maintain a higher level of blood pressure.

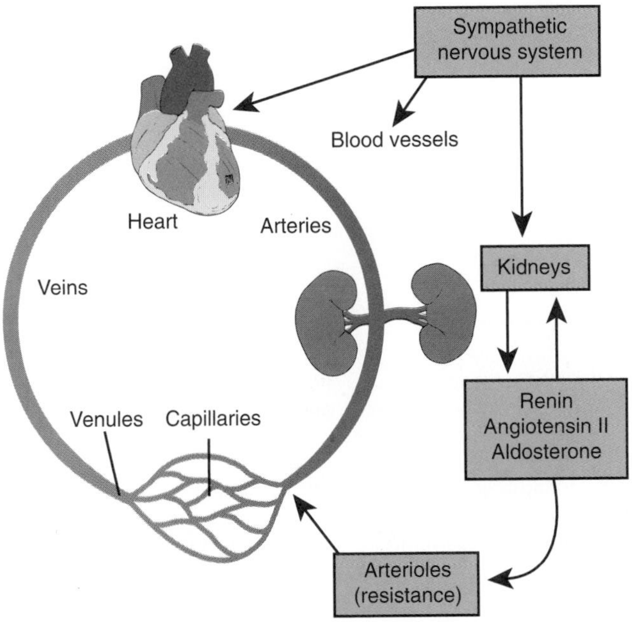

FIGURE 21-1
Sites of drug effects that can induce or exacerbate hypertension. Many drugs can do either. The sympathetic nervous system is affected by many drugs that can increase blood pressure by their action on the heart and blood vessels (i.e., sympathomimetics): cocaine, amphetamine, ergotamine, estrogen, monoamine oxidase (MAO) inhibitors, and NSAIDs, The kidneys are affected by NSAIDs, estrogens, corticosteroids, cocaine, and amphetamine. The renin-angiotensin II-aldosterone system is affected by estrogens, alcohol, and glycyrrhizic acid (licorice). Arterioles are affected by alcohol, sympathomimetics, cocaine, amphetamine, and ergotamine.

RENIN-ANGIOTENSIN-ALDOSTERONE MECHANISM

The **renin-angiotensin-aldosterone mechanism** regulates blood pressure by increasing or decreasing the blood volume through kidney function (Fig. 21-3). The initiating factor is renin, an enzyme secreted from the juxtaglomerular cells located in the afferent arteriolar walls of the nephron. When blood flow through the kidneys is reduced, renal arterial pressure is reduced, which causes release of renin into the circulation. Here renin catalyzes the cleavage of a plasma protein to form angiotensin I, a weak vasoconstrictor. Subsequently, in the small vessels of the lung, angiotensin I is converted by angiotensin-converting enzyme (ACE) to angiotensin II.

Angiotensin II is one of the most potent vasoconstrictors known. It is particularly effective in constricting arterioles, which increases peripheral resistance and raises blood pressure. In addition, angiotensin II acts on the adrenal cortex to stimulate the secretion of aldosterone, a hormone that promotes reabsorption of sodium by the kidneys. The increased sodium elevates the osmotic pressure in the plasma, causing a release of antidiuretic hormone from the hypothalamus.

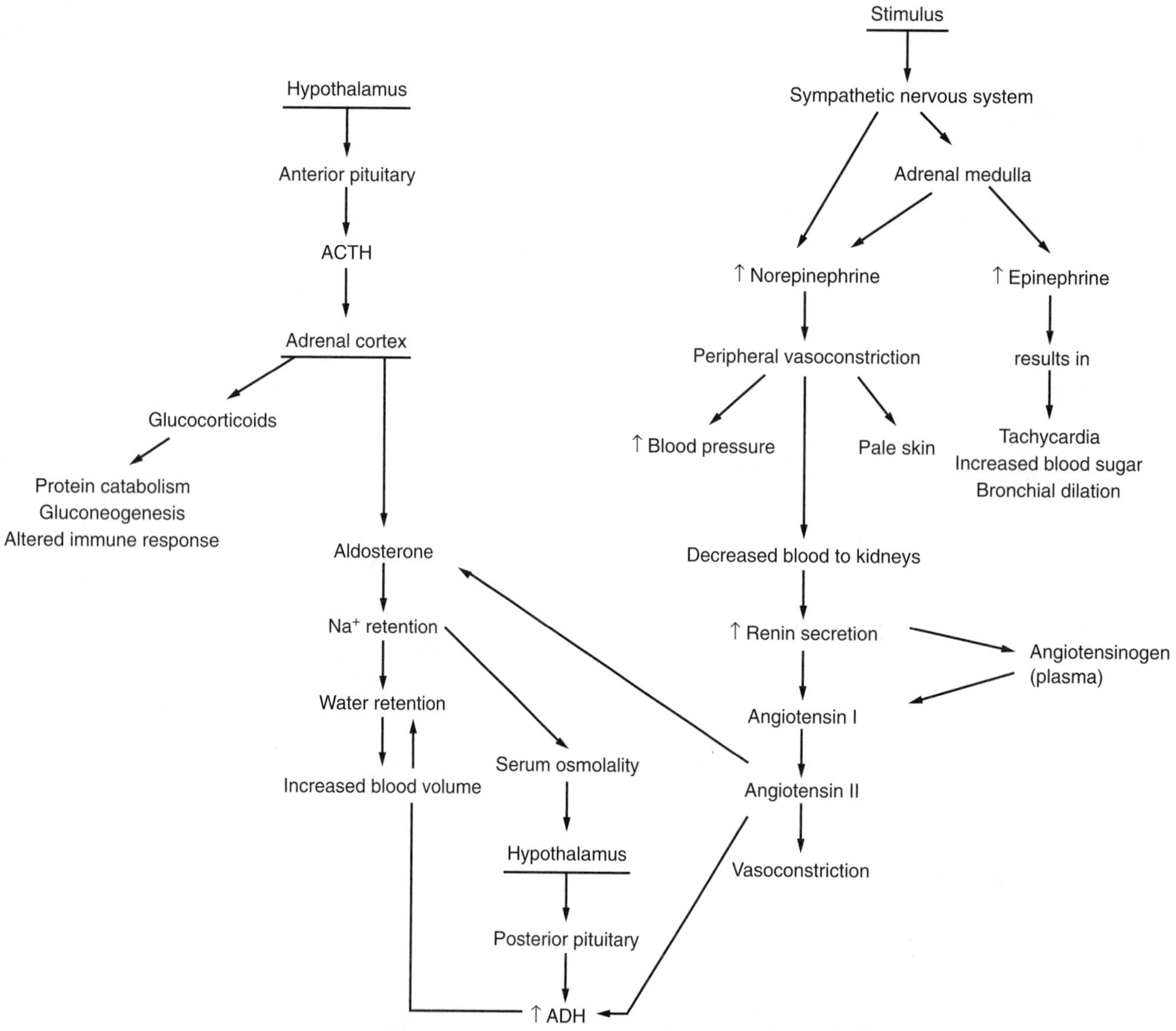

FIGURE 21-2
Physiologic control of blood pressure. Activation of the sympathetic nervous system causes increased release of norepinephrine, resulting in peripheral vasoconstriction and increased blood pressure. Increased release of epinephrine increases heart rate and the force of myocardial contractions, also resulting in elevation of blood pressure. Vasoconstriction results in increased blood supply to the kidneys, which activates the angiotensin system. Ultimately, the release of angiotensin II (a potent vasoconstrictor) results in an increase in aldosterone release from the adrenal cortex, an increase in release of antidiuretic hormone (ADH), and increased blood volume. See the text for a description of mechanisms.

BOX 21-2 Basic Blood Pressure Equations

Blood pressure (mean arterial pressure) = cardiac output × peripheral resistance
Cardiac output = stroke volume × heart rate

Angiotensin II acts on the kidney tubules to promote reabsorption of water.

Excessive fluid retention is controlled by the negative feedback mechanism operating within this system so that fluid balance is restored to a normal level. Thus the renin-angiotensin-aldosterone system involves slow adjustments to changes in fluid volume. The kidneys are by far the most important organs in the body for long-term regulation of blood pressure. When the operation of the urinary system fails, increased peripheral resistance and retention of fluid

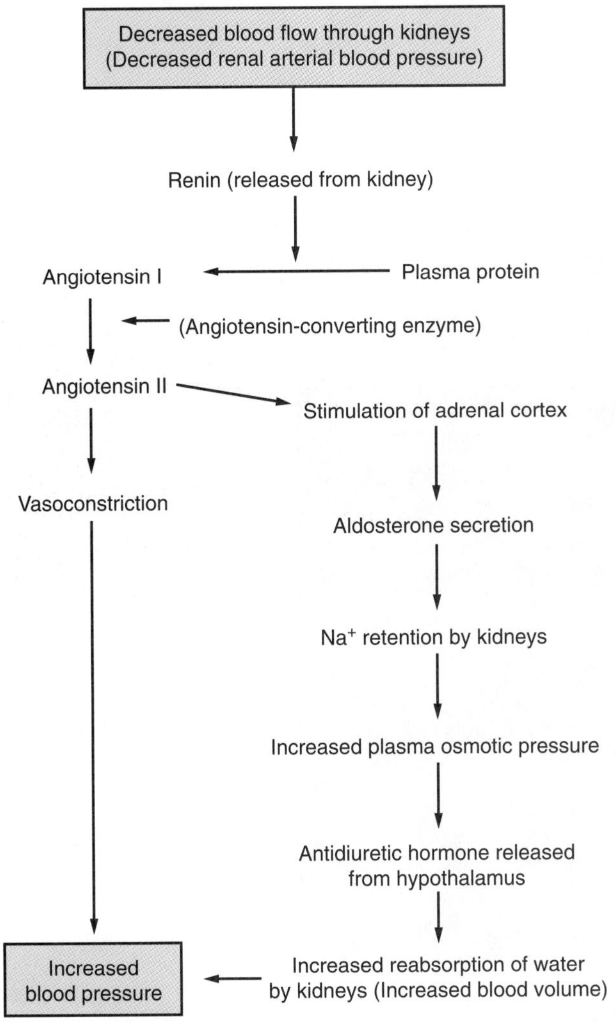

FIGURE 21-3
The renin-angiotensin-aldosterone system.

volume produce a combination of hypertensive effects, which keep blood pressure constantly elevated.

Thus knowledge of the normal mechanisms for blood pressure control has led to the development of the pharmacologic agents. For example, the beta-adrenergic blocking agents suppress renin release while the ACE inhibitors prevent the conversion of angiotensin I to angiotensin II. The mechanism of action for the antihypertensive agents is reviewed in this chapter.

ANTIHYPERTENSIVE THERAPY

Patient participation in antihypertensive therapy is essential for control of blood pressure. The person needs to understand that hypertension is usually asymptomatic and that therapy does not cure but only controls hypertension. Long-term therapy is necessary to prevent the morbidity and mortality that result from primary hypertension. Compliance with an individualized antihypertensive regimen is associated with a good prognosis and healthy lifestyle. The nonpharmacologic approaches are legitimate interventions as previously discussed.

Careful use of antihypertensive drugs can effectively control blood pressure in a majority of hypertensive individuals with less risk of serious complications and intolerable side effects. The JNC VI report (Kaplan, 1997) proposes a new pharmacologic treatment approach for hypertension based on the individual's risk factors and target organ damage. Fig. 21-4 depicts the **stepped treatment approach** for hypertension, a program that is tailored to the individual and becomes more aggressive with each level of treatment.

Special Concerns

Demographics

African Americans generally respond better to diuretics and calcium antagonists than to ACE inhibitors or beta blocking agents. Gender differences in blood pressure response to antihypertensive agents have not been identified. Hypertension has been reported to be two to three times more common in women who have used oral contraceptive agents for 5 years or longer compared with those not taking any oral contraceptives. This risk increases with age, smoking, and higher doses of estrogen and progesterone. If hypertension occurs, the customary treatment is to discontinue the oral contraceptive, and usually blood pressure normalizes in 3 to 6 months. If the blood pressure does not return to normal, lifestyle modifications and antihypertensive drugs should be instituted according to Table 21-1 and Fig. 21-4.

Age Differences

Age differences also affect blood pressure. A significant proportion of persons older than 65 years of age have elevated systolic or diastolic blood pressure or both, which increases their risk of cardiovascular morbidity and mortality. Antihypertensive drugs should be started with smaller than usual doses, increased by smaller than usual amounts, and scheduled at less frequent intervals with the elderly, since they are more sensitive to volume depletion and sympathetic inhibition than younger persons. They commonly have impaired cardiovascular reflexes, which make them more susceptible to hypotension.

Patients with concurrent disease/illness may respond best or, in some instances, adversely to selected medications. For example, if the hypertensive patient also has angina or atrial tachycardia and fibrillation, the beta blocking agents and calcium receptor antagonists are preferred drugs. In patients with type 2 diabetes mellitus, low-dose diuretics are recommended while for preoperative hypertension, the beta blocking agents are usually preferred. The beta blocking agents should be avoided though in patients with asthma, heart blocks, depression, dyslipidemia, congestive heart failure (except carvedilol), and types 1 and 2 diabetes mellitus (Kaplan, 1997).

The antihypertensive drugs currently used to reduce blood pressure are classified into five major categories: diuretics, adrenergic inhibitors (central and peripheral),

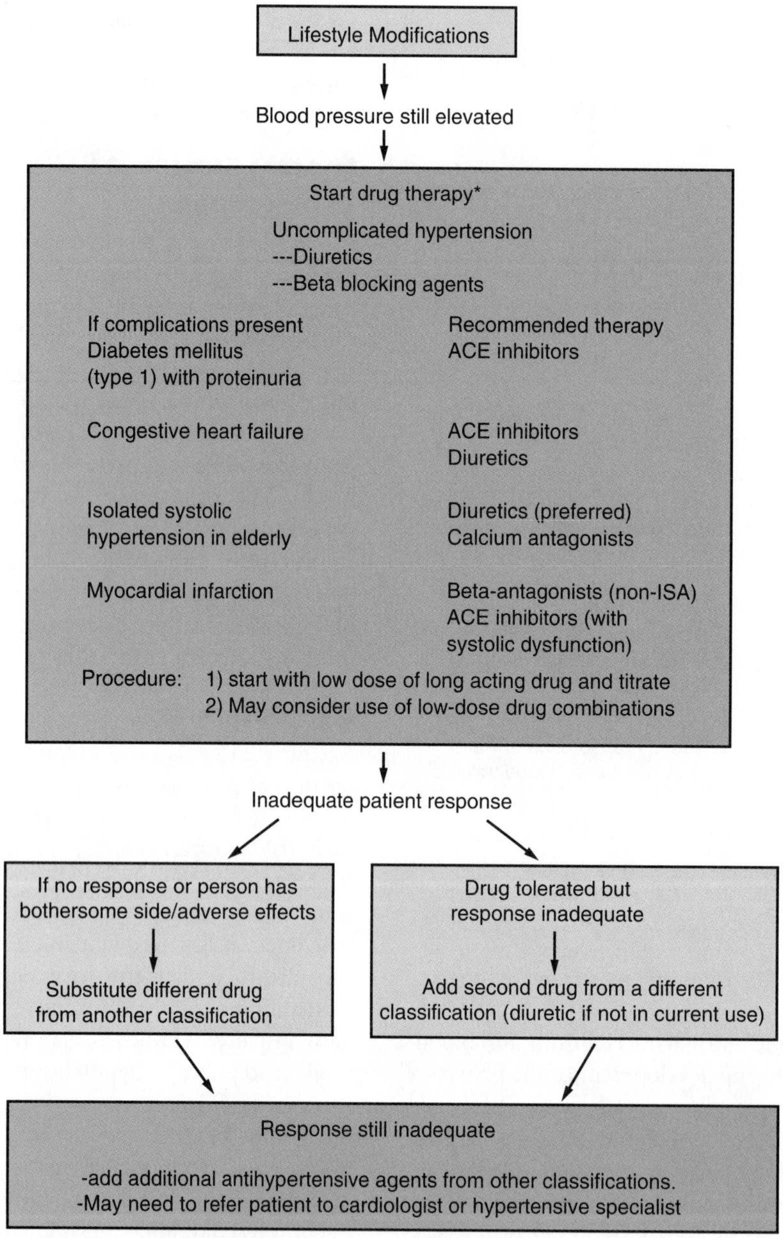

*Unless contraindicated. these are the recommendations.

FIGURE 21-4
Stepped treatment approach for hypertension.

PREGNANCY SAFETY

Category	Drug
B	guanadrel, guanfacine, methyldopa
C	clonidine, diazoxide, doxazosin, hydralazine, prazosin, guanabenz, guanethidine, reserpine, minoxidil, nitroprusside, terazosin, all ACE inhibitors in first trimester, irbesartan, losartan, and valsartan in first trimester
D	all ACE inhibitors in second and third trimesters, trimethaphan, irbesartan, losartan, and valsartan in second and third trimesters

angiotensin-converting enzyme (ACE) inhibitors and antagonists, calcium antagonists, and vasodilators. The use of diuretics or the beta blocking agents in patients with hypertension have resulted in a reduction in morbidity and mortality.

Hypertension during pregnancy is a serious condition that requires early detection and treatment. See the box for Food and Drug Administration (FDA) pregnancy safety classifications.

DIURETIC DRUGS

Diuretic drugs play a vital role in lowering blood pressure. The use of **diuretics,** agents that promote the formation and excretion of urine, results in a loss of excess salt and water from the body by renal excretion. The decrease in plasma and extracellular fluid volume subsequently depresses vascular reactivity to sympathetic stimulation. Thus volume depletion, plus a direct diuretic effect on the arterioles that produces vasodilation, results in lowering of the blood pres sure. This response causes an initial decline in cardiac output, followed by a decrease in peripheral resistance and a lowering of blood pressure (Fig. 21-5).

The **thiazides** and related sulfonamide diuretics, such as chlorthalidone and metolazone, when used in maximum therapeutic doses, are moderately effective in decreasing blood pressure. Therefore these mild diuretics can be used alone for individuals with early stages of hypertension. By contrast, many of the other types of antihypertensive agents, when used alone on a long-term basis, cause a gradual retention of sodium and water and expansion of plasma fluid volume. Thus a low-dose diuretic is often given in combination with ACE inhibitors, alpha blocking agents, vasodilators, or adrenergic inhibitors to prevent fluid retention.

The **potassium-sparing agents** such as spironolactone and triamterene are useful in counteracting potassium loss induced by other diuretics. They promote sodium and water loss without accompanying loss of potassium. These drugs are indicated for management of hyperaldosteronism and renal vascular hypertension when the patient's condition is resistant to other diuretics. See Chapter 28 for information on diuretic drugs.

ADRENERGIC INHIBITING (SYMPATHOLYTIC) AGENTS

Adrenergic inhibitors, the most effective antihypertensive drugs, inhibit the activity of the sympathetic nervous system. The heart, blood vessels, and kidneys influence arterial pressure through various reflex mechanisms. Sympathetic stimulation increases heart rate and force of myocardial contraction, constricts arterioles (resistance vessels) and venules (capacitance vessels), and releases renin from the kidneys. Adrenergic inhibiting agents then are effective in reducing blood pressure and preventing serious cardiovascular complications. The sites at which these drugs modify sympathetic nervous system activity vary widely and usually involve complex mechanisms.

Beta-Adrenergic Blocking Agents

The beta-adrenergic blocking agents decrease cardiac output and inhibit renin secretion, which results in a lowering of blood pressure. By competing with epinephrine for available beta receptor sites, they inhibit typical organ or tissue response to beta stimulation. For additional information about this drug category, see Chapter 16.

The other adrenergic inhibitors are also effective in lowering blood pressure and generally have multiple sites of action or may have unknown mechanisms of action. For clarification, the drugs are characterized by their primary proposed site of action.

Centrally Acting Adrenergic Inhibitors

The centrally acting agents clonidine (Catapres), methyldopa (Aldomet), guanfacine (Tenex), and guanabenz (Wytensin) are effective antihypertensives, especially when combined with a diuretic. When given as a single agent, clonidine and methyldopa (guanfacine and guanabenz to a lesser extent) usually produce sodium and water retention.

clonidine hydrochloride [kloe' ni deen] (Catapres, Catapres-TTS)

Clonidine reduces systolic and diastolic blood pressure by stimulation of central alpha$_2$ receptors, which decreases sympathetic outflow of norepinephrine from the brain to the blood vessels and heart. Blood pressure is lowered by decreasing cardiac output, heart rate, and peripheral vascular resistance. The depressed cardiac output is the result of a reduction in both heart rate and stroke volume. Consequently, this action can cause bradycardia.

Clonidine is also used in the diagnosis of pheochromocytoma; prophylaxis of migraine or vascular headaches; treatment of dysmenorrhea, menopause, and Gilles de la Tourette's syndrome; and nicotine and opioid withdrawal

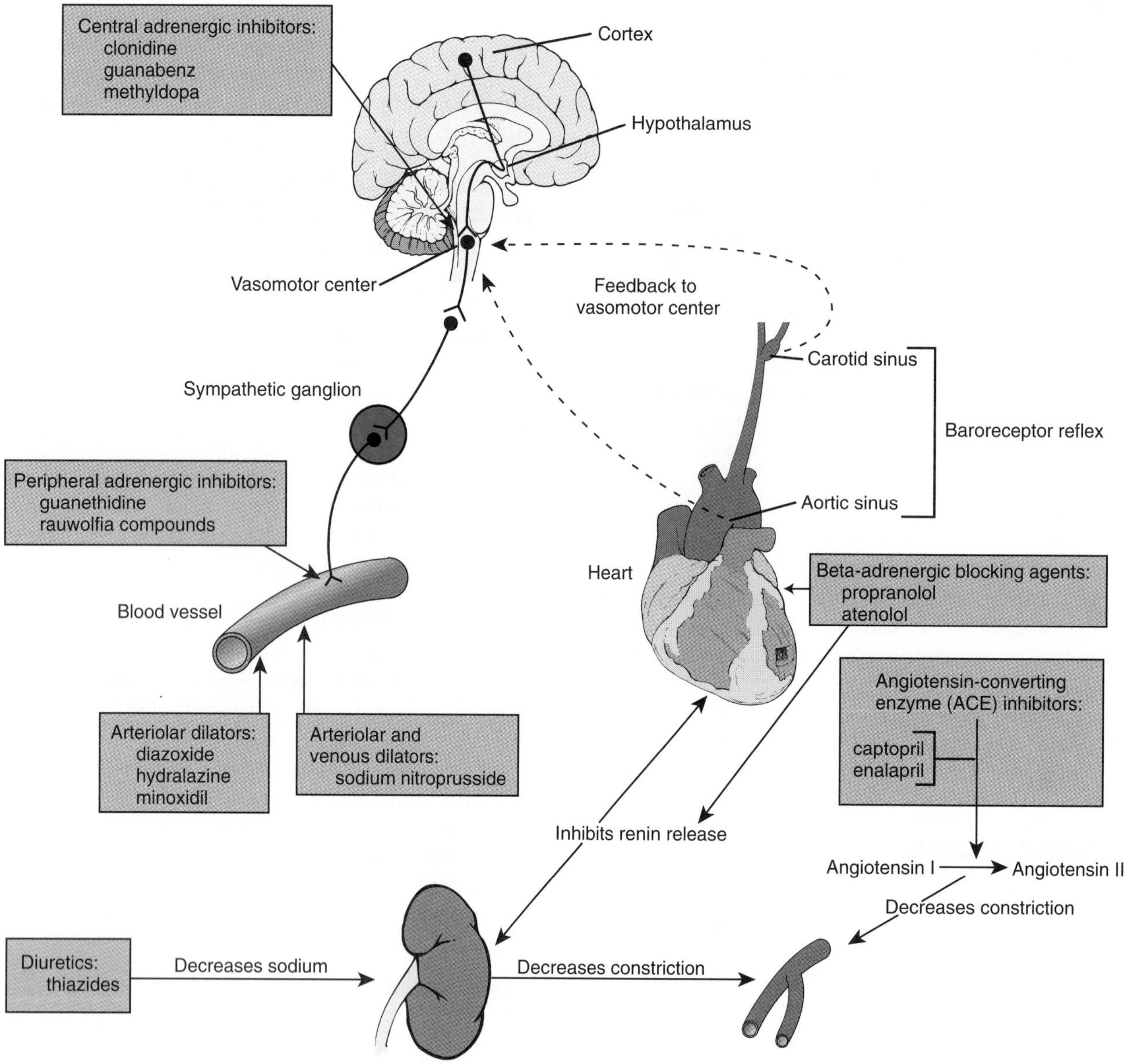

FIGURE 21-5
Site and method of action for various antihypertensive drugs, based on reported clinical and experimental evidence.

(USP DI, 1998). These are not approved indications in the United States.

The decreased sympathetic outflow to the kidneys reduces renal vascular resistance and thus preserves renal blood flow. In some persons, renin activity may be suppressed (Hoffman, Lefkowitz, 1996). With continued clonidine use, a diuretic is prescribed to correct fluid retention.

Pharmacokinetics

Oral clonidine has an onset of action within ½ to 1 hour, a peak effect in 2 to 4 hours, and a duration of action up to 8 hours. The serum half-life is between 12 and 16 hours, and it is metabolized in the liver and excreted primarily by the kidneys. Transdermal clonidine is best absorbed from the chest and upper arm. The onset of action and time to peak effect are 2 to 3 days, while the duration of action is approximately 1 week if the drug is in continuous contact with the body (about 8 hours if removed from the body). Metabolism and excretion are the same as for oral clonidine.

Drug interactions

The following interactions may occur when clonidine is given with the drugs listed below:

BOX 21-3 Rebound Hypertension and Hypertensive Crisis

The abrupt withdrawal of discontinuation of antihypertensive medications may result in rebound hypertension and possibly a hypertensive crisis. **Rebound hypertension** refers to the sudden increase of blood pressure to the pretreatment level or above. Hypertensive crisis or hypertensive emergency is the elevation of diastolic blood pressure above 120 to 130 mm Hg (Hawkins et al, 1993).

Symptoms of rebound hypertension depend on the elevation of the blood pressure. Usually the symptoms involve sympathetic system hyperactivity, such as sweating, anxiety, tachycardia, insomnia, muscle cramps, chest pain, headache, and nausea. In a hypertensive emergency or crisis, the extreme rise in blood pressure may cause target organ damage, e.g., to the eyes (retinal), heart, kidneys, or neurologic system.

In both instances, therapy is instituted to reduce blood pressure as soon as possible (Hawkins et al, 1993).

Drug	Possible effect and management
Beta-adrenergic blocking agents	Concurrent administration with clonidine may lead to loss of blood pressure control. Additive bradycardiac effects may also occur. Monitor pulse rate closely. If the prescriber wants to discontinue both drugs, the beta blocking agent should be stopped first. Discontinuing clonidine first may increase the risk of inducing a withdrawal hypertensive crisis (Box 21-3).
Tricyclic antidepressants	The antihypertensive effectiveness of clonidine may be reduced. This usually occurs in the first or second week of therapy. Monitor closely, since dosage adjustments and/or alternative hypotensive agents may need to be considered by the prescriber.

Side effects and adverse reactions

These include dry mouth, headaches, constipation, weakness, postural hypotension, impotency or decreased sexual drive, insomnia, anxiety, anorexia, nausea, vomiting, and pruritus.

Warnings

Use with caution in the elderly and in patients with impaired atrioventricular (AV) node or sinus node function, coronary insufficiency, depression or a history of depression, Raynaud's syndrome, or a recent myocardial infarction. For the transdermal patch only, use with caution in patients with systemic lupus erythematosus (SLE), scleroderma, polyarteritis nodosa, and skin irritations.

Contraindications

Avoid use in persons with clonidine hypersensitivity.

Dosage and administration

The adult dose is 0.1 mg twice daily initially; increased every 2 to 4 days by 0.1 or 0.2 mg as necessary to control blood pressure. For maintenance, the dose is 0.2 to 0.6 mg daily in divided doses. The dosage for children has not been established.

The clonidine transdermal system (Catapres-TTS) is available in various strengths (0.1, 0.2, or 0.3 mg) programmed to deliver the specified strength daily for 1 week. The system is composed of four layers: a film that contains a drug reservoir of clonidine, a membrane that controls the rate of drug delivery, an adhesive layer that also contains clonidine to initially saturate the skin site, and a top backing or cover layer. The system was formulated for the drug to flow from a higher concentration to the lower concentration in the body, which is limited by the rate-controlling membrane layer. It takes approximately 2 to 3 days to reach a therapeutic clonidine serum level on initial application; replacing the system weekly at a new body site will maintain the therapeutic serum level.

methyldopa [meth ill doe' pa] (Aldomet) ***methyldopate injection*** [meth ill doe' pate] (parenteral Aldomet)

Although the exact hypotensive mechanism is unknown, the theory is that a metabolite of methyldopa (alpha-methylnorepinephrine) stimulates the central $alpha_2$ receptors, which results in a reduction in norepinephrine (sympathetic) outflow to the heart, kidneys, and peripheral vasculature.

Indications

An antihypertensive, methyldopa lowers blood pressure in a way to similar to clonidine.

Pharmacokinetics

Methyldopate is hydrolyzed to methyldopa in the body, which then must undergo the previous theoretical process to produce the hypotensive effect. The antihypertensive effect produced by the parenteral dosage form begins in approximately 4 to 6 hours, so it should not be used as the primary single drug in a hypertensive emergency.

Methyldopa's peak effect occurs in 4 to 6 hours after a single dose or in 48 to 72 hours with multiple dosing. The duration of action is 12 to 24 hours (after a single oral dose), 1 to 2 days (after multiple oral doses), or 10 to 16 hours (after IV administration). Methyldopa is metabolized centrally to alpha-methylnorepinephrine. Excretion is primarily by the kidneys.

Drug interactions

The following interactions may occur when methyldopa is given with the drugs listed below:

Drug	Possible effect and management
Monoamine oxidase (MAO) inhibitors	Hyperexcitability, hallucinations, headache, and hypertension have been reported with this combination. Avoid or a serious drug interaction may occur.
Sympathomimetics (cocaine, epineohrine, norphenylephrine, and others)	A decrease in methyldopa's antihypertensive effect and a possible increase in the pressor effects of these medications may result. Avoid or a serious drug interaction may occur.

Color type indicates an unsafe drug combination.

Side effects and adverse reactions

These include drowsiness, dry mouth, headaches, edema of the feet and legs, fever, postural hypotension, impotency, insomnia, depression, anxiety, and nightmares.

Warnings

Use with caution in patients with severe cerebrovascular disease, bilateral, angina pectoris, depression, Parkinson's disease, and kidney impairment.

Contraindications

Avoid use in persons with methyldopa hypersensitivity, hepatitis, cirrhosis, hemolytic anemia, and pheochromocytoma.

Dosage and administration

The initial adult oral dose is 250 mg two to three times daily for 2 days, titrated as necessary. The maintenance dose is 500 to 2000 mg/day, divided into two to four individual doses (maximum daily dosage is 3 g/day). Children's dose is initially 10 mg/kg PO in two to four divided doses, increased at 2-day intervals as necessary, up to 65 mg/kg or 3 g/day, whichever is less.

The parenteral adult dose is 250 to 500 mg in dextrose 5% solution (100 ml) administered over ½ to 1 hour every 6 hours as needed. Maximum dose is 1 g every 6 to 12 hours. The pediatric IV infusion dose is 20 to 40 mg/kg in dextrose 5% administered over ½ to 1 hour every 6 hours as needed up to 65 mg/kg or 3 g/day, whichever is less.

guanabenz acetate [gwahn′ a benz] (Wytensin)

The mechanism of action of guanabenz acetate is believed to be the same as that for clonidine; it is a centrally acting $alpha_2$ agonist. Cardiac output remains unchanged, and the antihypertensive effect occurs without major changes in peripheral resistance. Nevertheless, peripheral resistance does eventually decrease with continued therapy.

Pharmacokinetics

Guanabenz has an onset of action within 1 hour (for a single dose), the peak effect occurs in 2 to 4 hours, and the duration of action is 12 hours. The serum half-life is 6 hours. The drug is metabolized in the liver, and excretion is via the kidneys and feces.

Drug interactions

When guanabenz is given concurrently with a beta receptor blocking agent or other hypotensive medications, an enhanced hypotensive effect may result. Monitor blood pressure closely as drug dosage adjustments may be necessary. When the prescriber discontinues both drugs, the beta blocking drug should be tapered first to prevent a severe withdrawal hypertensive reaction.

Side effects and adverse reactions

These include drowsiness, headaches, nausea, and impotency or decreased sexual drive.

Warnings

Use with caution in patients with cerebrovascular disease, coronary insufficiency, and liver or kidney disease, and in patients who have had a recent myocardial infarction.

Contraindications

Avoid use in persons with guanabenz hypersensitivity.

Dosage and administration

The initial adult dose is 4 mg given PO twice daily, increased if necessary every 1 to 2 weeks by increments of 4 to 8 mg/day up to a maximum of 32 mg/day. The dosage for children is not established.

guanfacine [gwahn′ fa seen] (Tenex)

Guanfacine (Tenex) is a centrally acting $alpha_2$-adrenergic agonist antihypertensive similar to clonidine. Thus peripheral vascular resistance, heart rate, and blood pressure are lowered.

Pharmacokinetics

Guanfacine is well absorbed orally, with a peak effect in 8 to 12 hours (single dose) or 1 to 3 months (long-term dosing). The onset of action occurs within 7 days of chronic dosing. The duration of effect is 1 day (single dose). Metabolism occurs in the liver with excretion by the kidneys.

Drug interactions

No significant drug interactions are reported, although the professional should monitor for enhanced central nervous system (CNS)-depressant effects if it is administered with other CNS-depressant drugs and enhanced antihypertensive effects if given with other antihypertensive agents.

Side effects and adverse reactions

These include constipation, dry mouth, sedation, lightheadedness, headache, nausea, vomiting, insomnia, impotency, dry or itching eyes, weakness, and depression.

Warnings

Use with caution in patients with cerebrovascular disease, coronary insufficiency, depression, recent myocardial infarction, and liver disease.

Contraindications

Avoid use in persons with guanfacine hypersensitivity.

Dosage and administration

The adult dose is 1 mg PO daily at bedtime, increased if needed in 3 to 4 weeks (to 2 mg/day). The pediatric dosage has not been determined.

Peripheral Adrenergic Inhibitors

The peripherally active adrenergic inhibitors include guanethidine (Ismelin), guanadrel (Hylorel), and reserpine (Serpalan), whereas the alpha-adrenergic blocking agents include doxazosin (Cardura), Prazosin (Minipress), and terazosin (Hytrin).

guanethidine sulfate [gwahn eth′ i deen] (Ismelin)

Guanethidine sulfate is a powerful antihypertensive drug that acts as a postganglionic adrenergic neuron blocking agent. Guanethidine enters the storage vesicles of the adrenergic nerve terminal, where it gradually displaces the stored norepinephrine. The subsequent depletion of norepinephrine inhibits transmission of nerve impulses at the neuroeffector junction. Although there is no significant change in peripheral resistance, the drug reduces blood pressure by decreasing vascular tone, primarily at the venous side and secondarily at the arterial side of the circulatory system.

A lower venous return reduces cardiac output, which consequently decreases cerebral, splanchnic, and renal blood flow. The venous pooling of blood is responsible for the severe orthostatic hypotension that is reported with this drug. This is a limiting factor for the use of this product. The reduction in blood pressure is noticeably greater with the patient in the standing position than in the recumbent position.

The adrenergic blocking action of guanethidine increases gastrointestinal motility, frequently causing diarrhea. The drug does not affect the catecholamines in the adrenal medulla. It is contraindicated for use in patients with pheochromocytoma because it may cause the release of catecholamines, thus producing a hypertensive crisis.

Pharmacokinetics

Guanethidine has a variable absorption orally (3% to 30% absorbed) with long-term dosing. Its peak effect occurs within 8 hours (single dose) or 1 to 3 weeks (with long-term dosing). It has a biphasic half-life; that is, alpha is 1 to 2 days, beta is between 4 and 8 days. When the drug is stopped (with long-term dosing), there is a gradual blood pressure increase to pretreatment levels within 1 to 3 weeks. Guanethidine is metabolized in the liver and excreted by the kidneys.

Drug interactions

The following interactions may occur when guanethidine is given with the drugs listed below:

Drug	Possible effect and management
Oral antidiabetic medications or insulin	May result in an increased hypoglycemic effect. Advise patients to monitor blood glucose levels closely and communicate results with their prescriber as dosage adjustments may be necessary.
minoxidil (Loniten) or hypotension-producing medications	Concurrent use with guanethidine is not recommended, as antihypertensive effects may be potentiated.
Monoamine oxidase (MAO) inhibitors	Severe hypertension may result. Avoid or a serious drug interaction may occur. It is recommended that MAO inhibitors be discontinued for a minimum of 1 week before starting guanethidine.
metaraminol (Aramine), and possibly other sympathomimetics	The antihypertensive effectiveness of guanethidine may be reduced. Concurrent use of metaraminol and guanethidine may result in cardiac dysrhythmias, severe and prolonged hypertension, or a hypertensive crisis. Avoid or a serious drug interaction may occur.

Tricyclic antidepressants, loxapine (Loxitane) thioxanthenes, and possibly other psychotropic medications	May reduce the antihypertensive effect of guanethidine by blocking its access to the adrenergic nerve site. Monitor closely, as dosage adjustments or alternate antidepressant medications may be necessary.

Color type indicates an unsafe drug combination.

Side effects and adverse reactions

These include orthostatic hypotension, weakness, impaired ejaculation, diarrhea, bradycardia, stuffy nose, alopecia, blurred vision, ptosis of eyelids, nausea, vomiting, muscle pain or tremors, dry mouth, headache, edema, and chest pain (angina).

Warnings

Use with caution in patients with asthma, cerebrovascular insufficiency, coronary insufficiency, diabetes mellitus, diarrhea, sinus bradycardia, fever, recent myocardial infarction, peptic ulcer, and liver or kidney impairment.

Contraindications

Avoid use in persons with guanethidine hypersensitivity, heart failure that is severe but not due to hypertension, and pheochromocytoma.

Dosage and administration

For adult ambulatory patients the dose is 10 or 12.5 mg PO daily initially, increased by 10 or 12.5 mg increments at 5- to 7-day intervals as necessary. The maintenance dose is 25 to 50 mg daily. For hospitalized patients, the initial dose is 25 to 50 mg PO daily, increased by 25 to 50 mg increments at daily or every-other-day intervals as necessary.

The pediatric dose is 0.2 mg/kg PO daily, increased at 7- to 10-day intervals as necessary for blood pressure control.

guanadrel [gwahn′ a drel] (Hylorel)

The mechanism of action for guanadrel is the same as that for guanethidine.

Pharmacokinetics

Guanadrel has an onset of action within 2 hours and a peak effect between 4 and 6 hours (after a single dose). The half-life is variable, but generally it is about 10 hours. The duration of effect is about 9 hours. The drug is metabolized by the liver and excreted by the kidneys.

Drug interactions

Metaraminol (Aramine) and other sympathomimetics, MAO inhibitors, tricyclic antidepressants, loxapine (Loxitane) thioxanthenes, and psychotropic agents (especially chlorpromazine [Thorazine]) may cause drug interactions; see guanethidine above. In addition, trimeprazine (Arfonad) may reduce the antihypertensive effect of guanadrel by displacement and blocking guanadrel's access to the adrenergic neuron. Monitor blood pressures closely.

Side effects and adverse reactions

These include hypotension, weakness, impaired ejaculation, increased urination at night, muscle pain or tremors, dry mouth, headache, edema, and chest pain.

Warnings

Use with caution in patients with asthma, cerebrovascular insufficiency, coronary insufficiency, diarrhea, fever, sinus bradycardia, recent myocardial infarction, and peptic ulcer disease.

Contraindications

Avoid use in persons with guanadrel hypersensitivity, heart failure (not due to hypertension), and pheochromocytoma.

Dosage and administration

The initial adult oral dose is 5 mg twice daily, which may be increased at daily, weekly, or monthly intervals as necessary for blood pressure control. The maintenance dosage is 20 to 75 mg/day in two to four divided doses. Pediatric doses have not been established.

Rauwolfia Derivatives

reserpine [re ser′ peen] (Serpalan, Serpasil)

Rauwolfia derivatives are alkaloids obtained primarily from *Rauwolfia serpentina,* a shrub endemic to India and various tropical areas of the world. Reserpine, a rauwolfia alkaloid, lowers blood pressure by depleting the storage sites of norepinephrine in the peripheral postganglionic adrenergic neuron. Without adequate norepinephrine available for release, discharges of nerve impulses from the peripheral sympathetic neurons, which supply the smooth muscle of arterioles, produce little or no effect on these blood vessels. The resultant vascular relaxation decreases peripheral resistance, thereby reducing blood pressure. These compounds also decrease heart rate and thus lower cardiac output. Reserpine also depletes stores of serotonin.

Pharmacokinetics

Reserpine has an onset of antihypertensive action of days to 3 weeks with multiple dosing, and a peak antihypertensive effect within 3 to 6 weeks. The half-life is initially 4.5 hours, but with long-term dosing it is extended to 45 to 168 hours. Reserpine is metabolized in the liver and excreted primarily in the feces.

Drug interactions

The following interactions may occur when reserpine is given with the drugs listed below:

Drug	Possible effect and management
CNS depressants and/or alcohol	Enhanced CNS-depressant effects. Monitor vital signs, level of consciousness, and mental status closely.
MAO inhibitors	May result in hyperpyrexia and hypertension (moderate, severe, or even crisis level). Concurrent administration is not recommended. MAO inhibitors should be discontinued for at least 1 week before a rauwolfia alkaloid is started.

Color type indicates an unsafe drug combination.

Side effects and adverse reactions

These include nausea, vomiting, anorexia, diarrhea, dizziness, dry mouth, stuffy nose, lightheadedness, fluid retention, sexual dysfunction, chest pain, bradycardia, and bronchospasms.

Warnings

Use with caution in patients with cardiac dysrhythmias or cardiac depression, epilepsy, Parkinson's disease, pheochromocytoma, pulmonary disease, and kidney impairment.

Contraindications

Avoid use in persons with rauwolfia alkaloid hypersensitivity, gallstones, peptic ulcers, colitis, and depression.

Dosage and administration

The adult dose is 0.1 to 0.25 mg PO daily.

Alpha-Adrenergic Blocking Drugs

The alpha-adrenergic blocking agents used in the management of hypertension include phenoxybenzamine (Dibenzyline), phentolamine (Regitine), doxazosin (Cardura), prazosin (Minipress), and terazosin (Hytrin). Phenoxybenzamine and phentolamine are alpha blockers that are relatively nonselective because they antagonize responses mediated by both $alpha_1$ and $alpha_2$ receptors. Hence, they lower blood pressure by preventing norepinephrine from activating $alpha_1$ receptors on vascular smooth muscle to produce vasoconstriction. See Chapter 16 for discussions of phenoxybenzamine and phentolamine. Doxazosin, prazosin, and terazosin are more selective in activity and are classed as $alpha_1$-adrenergic blocking agents.

doxazosin [dox ay′ zoe sin] (Cardura)
prazosin hydrochloride [pra′ zoe sin] (Minipress)
terazosin [ter ay′ zoe sin] (Hytrin)

Doxazosin, prazosin, and terazosin are selective $alpha_1$-adrenergic blocking agents that dilate both arterioles and veins. This action results in a decrease in peripheral vascular resistance and lowered blood pressure. With prazosin and terazosin, the lowering of blood pressure is not associated with reflex tachycardia, while doxazosin may cause a small increase in heart rate. Prazosin has been used as adjunct therapy to digoxin and diuretics in the treatment of congestive heart failure. This combination, however, has not resulted in improved survival (USP DI, 1998). While all three drugs have been used to treat benign prostatic hyperplasia (BPH) to improve urinary flow and the symptoms of BPH, only doxazosin and terazosin are FDA-approved for this indication (USP DI, 1998). (Doxazosin may be used in normotensive patients with BPH since it does not appear to significantly lower blood pressure. In individuals with both hypertension and BPH, it is effective in treating both conditions.)

Pharmacokinetics

The onset of action for doxazosin is 1 to 2 hours, the peak effect occurs in 5 to 6 hours, and the duration of action is 24 hours. Prazosin has an onset of action within 0.5 to 1.5 hours and reaches its peak effect within 2 to 4 hours (in congestive heart failure, peak effect is in 1 hour); the duration of effect in patients with hypertension is 7 to 10 hours (single drug dose), whereas with congestive heart failure it is 6 hours. Terazosin is rapidly absorbed orally with onset of action within 15 minutes, peak effect in 2 to 3 hours, and duration of action of approximately 24 hours. Metabolism for all three drugs (active and inactive metabolites) is in the liver with excretion primarily in feces.

Drug interactions

There are no known major drug interactions with these agents to date (USP DI, 1998).

Side effects and adverse reactions

These include weakness, nausea, vomiting, stuffy nose, orthostatic hypotension, angina, edema of lower extremities, headaches, syncope, and shortness of breath.

Warnings

Use doxazosin with caution in patients with liver or kidney function impairment; prazosin with caution in patients with angina pectoris, narcolepsy, and kidney impairment; and terazosin with caution in patients with angina, severe heart disease, and liver or kidney impairment.

Contraindications

Avoid use of these drugs in persons with known drug hypersensitivity and the use of prazosin in persons with severe heart disease.

Dosage and administration

The initial doxazosin adult dose is 1 mg PO daily at bedtime, increased if necessary, every 2 weeks. The maximum

TABLE 21-2 ACE Inhibitors: Pharmacokinetics and Dosing

Drug	Onset of Action (hr)	Duration of Effect (hr)	Active Metabolite	Usual Adult Dosage (mg/day)*
benazepril (Lotensin)	Within 1	24	benazeprilat	5-40
captopril (Capoten)	0.25-1	6-12	—	25-100
enalapril (Vasotec)	1	24	enalaprilat	5-40
fosinopril (Monopril)	within 1	24	fosinprilat	10-40
lisinopril (Prinivil, Zestril)	1	24	—	10-40
moexipril (Univasc)	1	24	moexiprilat	7.5-30
quinapril (Accupril)	within 1	up to 24	quinaprilat	10-80
ramipril (Altace)	1-2	24	ramiprilat	2.5-20

*Oral doses titrated as needed and tolerated (Olin, 1998; *USP DI*, 1998).

daily dose is 16 mg. A pediatric dosage has not been established. The prazosin adult dose is 0.5 mg PO two or three times daily for at least 3 days. If tolerated, the dose may be increased if necessary, according to individual response. The pediatric dose is 0.05 to 0.4 mg/kg/day, administered in two or three divided doses. The terazosin adult oral dose is 1 mg PO daily at bedtime. The maintenance dose is between 1 and 5 mg daily, as needed to control blood pressure. The maximum daily dose is 20 mg. A pediatric dosage has not been established.

ANGIOTENSIN-CONVERTING ENZYME INHIBITORS AND ANTAGONISTS

ACE inhibitors competitively block the angiotensin I-converting enzyme necessary for the conversion to angiotensin II. Angiotensin II is a powerful vasoconstrictor that raises blood pressure and also causes aldosterone release, resulting in sodium and water retention. Thus the inhibition of ACE has the following results: (1) a decrease in vascular tone, thereby directly lowering blood pressure; (2) an inhibition of aldosterone release, reducing sodium and water reabsorption; the resultant excretion of fluid is thought to cause only a secondary reduction in blood pressure (decrease in aldosterone secretion does lead to a slight elevation in serum potassium); and (3) an increase in plasma renin activity, caused by a loss of negative feedback on renin release. See Figs. 21-2 and 21-3 for physiologic blood pressure control and the renin-angiotensin-aldosterone system. Captopril (Capoten) is the key or prototype drug for this category.

captopril [kap′ toe pril] (Capoten)

Indications

ACE inhibitors are used alone or in combination with the thiazide diuretics to treat hypertension. Other indications for the ACE inhibitors include the following:

- Captopril, enalapril, and lisinopril are also used in combination with digoxin and diuretics for the treatment of congestive heart failure not responsive to standard therapies.
- Captopril has been used to treat diabetic nephropathy and also left ventricular dysfunction after a myocardial infarction. It has been reported to increase survival and decrease the incidence of heart failure in such persons (USP DI, 1998).

It is apparent that a disturbance of the basic function of the renin-angiotensin-aldosterone system can cause increased vascular resistance or hypertension (Hawkins et al, 1993). Furthermore, a damaged kidney that cannot regulate its renin release through normal feedback mechanisms may easily cause an elevation in blood pressure in certain individuals. This evidence has led to the development of the angiotensin II inhibitors. Benazepril (Lotensin), captopril (Capoten), enalapril (Vasotec), fosinopril (Monopril), lisinopril (Prinivil, Zestril), moexipril (Univasc), quinapril (Accupril), ramipril (Altace), and trandolapril (Mavik) are angiotensin-converting enzyme inhibitors. Enalapril is a prodrug that is converted to an active metabolite, enalaprilat, by the liver. Many of the other ACE inhibitors have active metabolites (Table 21-2).

Blood pressure is lowered to about the same extent in patients in supine and upright positions. Although orthostatic hypotension and tachycardia are uncommon, they have been reported in volume-depleted individuals.

Combination drug therapies for hypertension are sometimes necessary to maintain blood pressure control. Products have been formulated that contain several active drugs in one tablet or capsule to help improve patient compliance with prescribed therapy. Examples of combination drugs include benazepril and the calcium blocking agent amlodipine marketed as Lotrel, trandolapril with verapamil as Tarka, enalapril with diltiazem as Teczem, and others.

For pharmacokinetics and adult dosage, see Table 21-2.

Drug interactions

The following interactions may occur when ACE inhibitors are given with the following drugs:

Drug	Possible effect and management
Alcohol or diuretics	Concurrent administration with an ACE inhibitor may result in a sudden, very severe hypotensive episode. Avoid or a potentially serious drug interaction may occur. To reduce this reaction, either discontinue the diuretic for approximately 1 week before starting ACE inhibitor therapy, increase the salt intake of the patient for 1 week before, or start the ACE inhibitor at low dosages. Generally, this reaction does not recur with continued dosing, and the diuretic may be given later if necessary.
Potassium-sparing diuretics, low-salt milk, potassium supplements, or potassium-containing medications and salt substitutes	Closely monitor serum electrolytes, especially potassium, because of the high risk for hyperkalemia.

Color type indicates an unsafe drug combination.

Side effects and adverse reactions

These include dry cough, headaches, diarrhea, loss of taste, weakness, nausea, dizziness, hypotension, rash, fever, and joint pain. See the box for management of ACE inhibitor overdosage.

Warnings

Use with caution in patients with SLE, scleroderma, bone marrow depression, cerebrovascular insufficiency, coronary insufficiency, diabetes mellitus, and liver function impairment (the latter warning is for all ACE inhibitors with the exception of lisinopril and quinapril).

Contraindications

Avoid use in persons with ACE inhibitor hypersensitivity, angioedema, hyperkalemia, and renal artery stenosis, transplant, or impairment.

ANGIOTENSIN II RECEPTOR ANTAGONISTS

A more recent discovery is the angiotensin II receptor antagonists drug category: losartan potassium (Cozaar), valsartan (Diovan), and irbesartan (Avapro). These agents block the receptors for angiotensin II; thus they block the vasoconstriction and an increase in aldosterone release, but they have very little effect on serum potassium. Losartan is considered the key drug in this category.

MANAGEMENT OF DRUG OVERDOSE

ACE Inhibitors

- For hypotension, institute fluid volume expansion.
- If angioedema of face, mucous membranes of mouth, lips, and extremities occurs, an antihistamine may be useful. If the angioedema affects the tongue, glottis, or larynx, then withdraw the ACE inhibitor and hospitalize the patient. Epinephrine SC, IV diphenhydramine, and IV hydrocortisone may be necessary.
- Hemodialysis will remove captopril, enalaprilat, and lisinopril

losartan potassium [lo zar′ tan] (Cozaar)

Losartan is indicated for the treatment of hypertension alone or in combination with other antihypertensives.

Pharmacokinetics

Losartan is orally administered and reaches peak effect in 6 hours. It undergoes substantial first-pass metabolism in the liver and is converted to at least six metabolites with one very active one (carboxylic acid metabolite) that is between 10 to 40 times more potent than the parent drug. The half life of losartan is 2 hours and for the carboxylic acid metabolite is between 6 to 9 hours. The duration of action is at least 24 hours with metabolism in the liver and excretion in bile (approximately 60%) and kidneys (35%).

Drug interactions

When losartan is administered with a diuretic, a hypotensive effect may result. Usually a lower losartan dose is necessary with close monitoring.

Side effects and adverse reactions

These include headache, tiredness, back or muscle pain, diarrhea, nasal congestion, dizziness, and upper respiratory infection. Dry cough and insomnia are considered rare effects.

Warnings

Use with caution in patients with kidney impairment. Use extreme caution in administering losartan to patients who are volume or sodium depleted as severe hypotension may result. Correct the deficiency first or start at a smaller drug dose.

Contraindications

Avoid use in persons with losartan hypersensitivity, liver impairment, and stenosis of the renal artery.

Dosage and administration

The initial adult dose is 50 mg PO daily; the maintenance dose is 25 to 100 mg daily. The pediatric dose has not been established.

valsartan [val zar′ tan] (Diovan)
irbesartan [irbe zar′ tan] (Avapro)

Valsartan and irbesartan are the second and third angiotensin II receptor antagonists available in the United States. Both drugs are approved for the treatment of hypertension, alone or in combination with other antihypertensive agents.

Pharmacokinetics

Valsartan and irbesartan are metabolized in the liver to inactive metabolites. The time to peak serum levels is 1.5 to 2 hours for irbesartan and 2 to 4 hours for valsartan while half-life (elimination) is 11 to 15 hours for irbesartan and 6 hours for valsartan. Both drugs are primarily excreted in feces.

Drug interactions

Same interaction with diuretics as losartan; see losartan potassium on p. 359.

Side effects and adverse reactions

Side effects and adverse reactions with valsartan are usually mild and infrequent, such as dizziness, headache, and fatigue. Irbesartan effects are also infrequent and may include stomach pain and/or distress, increased anxiety, diarrhea, dizziness, nausea, vomiting, chest pain, edema, muscle pain, and rash.

Warnings

For both drugs, use caution in patients with dehydration, renal artery stenosis, and kidney function impairment. For valsartan, use with caution in patients with severe liver disease.

Contraindications

For both drugs, avoid use in persons with drug hypersensitivity and severe heart failure.

Dosage and administration

The usual adult dose for irbesartan is 150 mg PO daily, titrated as necessary to maximum 300 mg/day. The valsartan adult dose is 80 mg daily, titrated as necessary to maximum or 320 mg/day. The pediatric dosage has not been established.

CALCIUM ANTAGONISTS

Calcium channel blocking agents are used for the treatment of hypertension, angina pectoris, supraventricular tachycardia, and vascular headaches. See Chapter 22 for additional information.

VASODILATORS

Vasodilators exhibit a direct action on the smooth muscle walls of the arterioles and veins, thereby lowering peripheral resistance and blood pressure. Although various theories have been proposed, the mechanism of action, at least in part, involves the direct relaxation of vascular smooth muscle by stimulation of the calcium-binding process. The drop in blood pressure stimulates the sympathetic nervous system and activates the baroreceptor reflexes, increasing heart rate and cardiac output. This also increases renin release. Therefore combined therapy is recommended. To inhibit sympathetic reflex response, use of a beta-adrenergic blocker such as propranolol (Inderal) has been advocated, along with a diuretic to alleviate the sodium and water retention that occurs during vasodilator therapy.

There are two types of vasodilators: (1) arteriolar dilators, such as diazoxide (Hyperstat IV), hydralazine (Apresoline), and minoxidil (Loniten), which exert a selective effect on arterioles, and (2) arteriolar and venous dilators, such as sodium nitroprusside (Nipride, Nitropress), which lower blood pressure by acting on both arteriolar resistance vessels and venous capacitance vessels.

Arteriolar Dilator Drugs

diazoxide [dye az ox′ ide] (Hyperstat IV)

The antihypertensive action results from direct relaxation of smooth muscles in the peripheral arterioles, which causes a decrease in peripheral resistance. As blood pressure is reduced, a reflex increase in heart rate and cardiac output occurs, with resultant maintenance of coronary and cerebral blood flow. This cardiovascular reflex mechanism also inhibits the development of orthostatic hypotension.

When administered intravenously, diazoxide is a potent antihypertensive agent. However, the oral form (Proglycem) produces only a slight decrease in blood pressure. Its main action is to stimulate hyperglycemia and decrease plasma insulin levels by suppressing insulin release (see Chapter 42).

Diazoxide is administered intravenously to reduce blood pressure promptly in hypertensive emergencies such as malignant hypertension and hypertensive crisis. Intravenous diazoxide is ineffective in reducing elevated blood pressure in patients with MAO-induced hypertension or pheochromocytoma. Because of its adverse effects, the drug is not used for treatment of chronic hypertension.

Pharmacokinetics

Administered by IV push, the onset of action is 1 minute, the peak effect occurs within 2 to 5 minutes, the half-life is approximately 28 hours, and the duration of effect is 2 to 12 hours. Diazoxide is metabolized in the liver and excreted by the kidneys.

Drug interactions

Concurrent use with other antihypertensives or peripheral vasodilators may result in an additive and, perhaps, severe hypotensive effect. Monitor closely for several hours after drugs are administered, as the prescriber may need to adjust the drug dosages.

Side effects and adverse reactions

These include nausea, vomiting, tachycardia, anorexia, headache, constipation, abdominal cramps, changes in taste perception, and edema.

Warnings

Use with caution in patients with gout, hypokalemia, and liver or kidney function impairment.

Contraindications

Avoid use in persons with diazoxide hypersensitivity, coronary or cerebral insufficiency, diabetes mellitus, heart failure, and aortic dissection. Before use in patients with these conditions, the prescriber should carefully evaluate risk to benefit for the individual patient.

Dosage and administration

The adult dose is up to 150 mg IV administered within 10 to 30 seconds and repeated in 5 to 15 minutes if necessary, up to a maximum of 1.2 g/day. After the emergency period, give diazoxide as needed for several days, until an oral hypertensive agent is effective. The pediatric dosage is 1 to 3 mg/kg IV, repeated if necessary in 5 to 15 minutes.

hydralazine [hye dral′ a zeen] (Apresoline)

Hydralazine hydrochloride is believed to produce its hypotensive effects by direct relaxation of vascular smooth muscle, particularly the arterioles, with little effect on veins, which results in a reduction in peripheral resistance. Consequently, renal blood flow is increased, providing an advantage to patients with renal failure. Hydralazine also maintains cerebral blood flow and produces sodium and water retention. However, the resultant hypotension is thought to stimulate the baroreceptor reflex, causing an increase in heart rate and cardiac output. Unfortunately, this response offsets the antihypertensive effects of the drug.

Tolerance to the antihypertensive action may be offset by the addition of a diuretic to the drug regimen. The diuretic enhances the antihypertensive effect and reduces the potential for increased cardiac output and fluid retention. Hydralazine decreases diastolic pressure more than systolic. It also increases plasma renin activity.

Pharmacokinetics

An oral dose of hydralazine has an onset of action in 45 minutes; by IV administration the onset is within 10 to 20 minutes. Its peak effect is within 1 hour (orally) or 15 to 30 minutes (IV). The half-life is between 3 and 7 hours, and duration of action is 3 to 8 hours. It is metabolized in the liver and excreted by the kidneys.

Drug interactions

Concurrent drug administration with diazoxide or other antihypertensives may result in severe hypotension. Monitor patients closely for several hours if drugs are given concurrently.

Side effects and adverse reactions

These include diarrhea, nausea, vomiting, tachycardia, anorexia, headache, facial flushing, stuffy nose, edema, angina, rash, peripheral neuritis, and an SLE-like syndrome. The SLE-like syndrome may include myalgia, arthralgia, arthritis, weakness, fever, and skin changes.

Warnings

Use with caution in patients with aortic aneurysm, cerebrovascular disease, heart failure, and kidney function impairment.

Contraindications

Avoid use in persons with hydralazine hypersensitivity, aortic dissection, coronary artery disease, and rheumatic heart disease. Before use in patients with these conditions, the prescriber should carefully evaluate risk to benefit for the individual patient.

Dosage and administration

The adult oral dose is 40 mg daily PO for 2 to 4 days, then 100 mg in divided doses for the remainder of the first week. The maintenance dose is 50 mg four times a day or the lowest effective dosage. Children receive 0.75 mg/kg divided into two to four doses, increased slowly over 1 to 4 weeks as necessary to a maximum of 7.5 mg/kg. Parenterally, the adult dose is 5 to 40 mg IM or IV, repeated if necessary. Pediatric dosage is 1.7 to 3.5 mg/kg divided into four to six daily doses.

minoxidil [mi nox′ i dill] (Loniten)

Minoxidil (Loniten) is an orally effective direct-acting peripheral vasodilator. It reduces blood pressure by decreasing peripheral vascular resistance in the arteriolar vessels with little effect on veins. It does not cause orthostatic hypotension. It is a potent vasodilator and also causes a reflex increase in cardiac output, induces sodium retention, promotes development of edema, and increases plasma renin activity.

Indications

Minoxidil is reserved for severe hypertension that is unresponsive to traditional agents, i.e., severe hypertension that is associated with chronic renal failure. Concomitant administration of a beta-adrenergic blocking agent such as propranolol (Inderal) is necessary to prevent severe reflex tachycardia. Administration of a diuretic agent is also essential to counteract sodium and water retention.

Pharmacokinetics

Minoxidil has an onset of action in 30 minutes and peak effect in 2 to 3 hours (after a single dose). The half-life of the drug and metabolites is 4.2 hours. Its duration of effect is between 1 and 2 days. It is metabolized by the liver and excreted mostly by the kidneys.

Drug interactions

The following interactions may occur when minoxidil is given with the following drugs:

Drug	Possible effect and management
guanethidine (Ismelin)	This combination is not recommended, as antihypertensive effects may be potentiated. Avoid or a potentially serious drug interaction may occur.
diazoxide (Hyperstat IV), nitrates, or nitroprusside (Nitropress)	This combination may result in severe hypotensive reaction. Avoid or a potentially serious drug interaction may occur. If administered, monitor patient closely for several hours.

Color type indicates an unsafe drug combination.

Side effects and adverse reactions

These include nausea, vomiting, tachycardia, anorexia, headaches, excessive hair growth (hypertrichosis), usually on face, arms and back, red flushing of skin, edema, angina, and pericarditis.

Warnings

Use with caution in patients with cerebrovascular disease and myocardial infarction.

Contraindications

Avoid use in persons with minoxidil hypersensitivity, heart failure (not due to hypertension), coronary insufficiency, angina, pericardial effusion, pheochromocytoma, and kidney impairment. Before use for any of these conditions, the prescriber should carefully evaluate the risk to benefit for the individual patient.

Dosage and administration

For children 12 years and older and adults, the dose is 5 mg PO daily, increased in 100% increments as necessary (10 mg, 20 mg, 40 mg, etc.). It is usually recommended that dosage increases be on a minimum 3-day schedule, but in selected patients, increases can be made every 6 hours with close patient monitoring. For children up to 12 years of age the dose is 0.2 mg/kg/day.

Arterial and Venous Dilator Drugs

nitroprusside [nye troe pruss′ ide]
(Nipride, Nitropress)

Nitroprusside is a potent and fast direct-acting vasodilator agent that greatly reduces arterial blood pressure. It relaxes both arterial and venous smooth muscles but is more active on veins. Therefore nitroprusside reduces cardiac load; that is, the decrease in systemic resistance results in a reduction in preload and afterload, improving cardiac output in the patient with congestive heart failure. It is indicated for rapid reduction of blood pressure in hypertensive emergencies, adjunct therapy in myocardial infarction, and valvular regurgitation and also as an antidote for ergot alkaloid toxicity.

Pharmacokinetics

Sodium nitroprusside has an onset of action and peak effect almost immediately (within minutes) after administration by IV infusion. The half-life of nitroprusside is 2 minutes; the half-life of thiocyanate, a possible toxic metabolite, is 3 days. The duration of effect is between 1 and 10 minutes after the discontinuance of the infusion. Metabolism is by erythrocytes (to cyanide) and the liver (cyanide to thiocyanate). The drug is excreted by the kidneys.

Drug interactions

Although no significant drug interactions are noted (USP DI, 1998), the healthcare professional should be aware that concurrent use with other antihypertensives need to be closely monitored as severe hypotension may result. Also, nitroprusside hypotensive effects may be reduced if it is given with estrogens or sympathomimetic agents. Close monitoring and dosage adjustments are necessary.

Side effects and adverse reactions

These include dizziness, excessive sweating, headaches, anxiety, abdominal cramps, tachycardia, hypothyroidism, flushing, rash, and muscle twitching. If the patient has thiocyanate toxicity, ataxia, blurred vision, headache, nausea, vomiting, tinnitus, shortness of breath, delirium, and unconsciousness may occur. For cyanide toxicity, hypotension, metabolic acidosis, pink coloration, very shallow breathing pattern, decreased reflexes, coma, and widely dilated pupils may be observed. See the box for treatment of nitroprusside overdose.

Warnings

Use with caution in patients with anemia, hypothyroidism, fluid and electrolyte imbalance, and lung disease.

Contraindications

Avoid use in persons with nitroprusside hypersensitivity, cerebrovascular or coronary artery disease, encephalopathy, liver disease, kidney disease, and metabolic induced vitamin B_{12} deficiency. Before use in patients with any of these conditions, the prescriber should carefully evaluate the risk to benefit for the individual patient.

Dosage and administration

For adult and pediatric dosage, mix contents of vial in dextrose 5% injection only and administer by IV infusion. The initial dose is 0.3 μg/kg/min, which is slowly increased as necessary. The usual dose is or 3 μg/kg/min.

Solution should be freshly prepared and protected from light by wrapping the container in the supplied opaque sleeve, aluminum foil, or other opaque material. The prepared solution usually has a 24-hour expiration time. A freshly prepared solution has a faint brown tinge; discard if it is highly colored (e.g., blue, green, or dark red).

SUMMARY

Hypertension is a very common cardiovascular disease that affects approximately 50 million Americans. In the vast majority of cases, the cause of hypertension is unknown, or essential, idiopathic, or primary hypertension. To reduce the high risk for cardiovascular complications in this population, lifestyle changes and antihypertensive medications may be indicated as outlined in the latest JNC VI recommendations.

The diuretics and beta blocking agents are still the drugs for initial therapy in uncomplicated hypertension. When complications are present, specific therapeutic agents that take into consideration concurrent diseases/illness as noted in the stepped treatment approach (Fig. 21-4) are recommended.

Lifestyle changes or modifications such as weight reduction, sodium restriction, elimination or limited consumption of alcohol and tobacco, reduction of dietary saturated fats, exercise, and, perhaps, relaxation techniques to reduce stress are advocated.

Five drug classifications to treat hypertension were reviewed in this chapter, including the diuretics, adrenergic inhibitors, angiotensin-converting enzyme inhibitors and antagonists, calcium antagonists, and vasodilators. Depending on the individual's response to therapy, combination drug therapies are often required for good control of hypertension. Such combinations are often based on an understanding of the physiologic control of blood pressure, the sites of action of the drugs involved, and additional pharmacologic information for these medications as presented in this chapter.

REVIEW QUESTIONS

1. Why is hypertension referred to as the "silent" killer?
2. Describe the physiologic effects of two antihypertensives from different classifications (for example, a diuretic and beta blocking agent or a diuretic and calcium antagonist). What is the purpose of combining antihypertensive agents?
3. Discuss the action, metabolism, and toxicities associated with use of nitroprusside.

MANAGEMENT OF DRUG OVERDOSE

Nitroprusside

ACTION AND METABOLISM

The structure of nitroprusside contains five cyanide groups which, when the drug is administered IV, splits off to free cyanide and nitric oxide, the active substance. Nitric oxide then activates the enzyme guanylate cyclase to produce cyclic guanosine monophosphate (GMP) and vasodilation. The free cyanide is converted to hydrogen cyanide (prussic acid), which is metabolized in the liver by rhodanase and a sulfur donor (such as thiosulfate) to convert it to thiosulfate, which is then excreted by the kidneys.

TOXICITY

When the amount of sulfur donors are limited or overwhelmed by high-dose nitroprusside therapy, hydrogen cyanide may accumulate in the body and cause toxicity. Some investigators report that if thiosulfate is mixed in the nitroprusside infusion at a 5 to 10:1 ratio (such as 250 to 500 mg of thiosulfate to 50 mg of nitroprusside) during administration of the nitroprusside, the less toxic thiocyanate will be formed and excreted. This method reduces the potential for cyanide accumulation and toxicity (Michocki, 1995; USP DI, 1998).

Thiocyanate toxicity may occur in patients with chronic therapy and renal impairment. The half-life of nitroprusside in persons with normal renal function is 2.7 days; in those with renal failure it is 9 days. Therefore, depending on the amount of drug administered to the patient, this toxicity is usually more apt to occur than the cyanide toxicity (Michocki, 1995).

TREATMENT

For severe hypotension, slow or discontinue the infusion. Placing the patient supine with the legs elevated on pillows will maximize venous return.

CYANIDE TOXICITY

- Discontinue nitroprusside and administer sodium nitrite (3% solution) in dose of 4 to 6 mg/kg IV over 2 to 4 minutes. If IV sodium nitrite is not immediately available, amyl nitrite inhalation should be used.
- Nitrites buffer the cyanide by converting about 10% of the patient's hemoglobin to methemoglobin.
- After administration of sodium nitrite, administer sodium thiosulfate (150 to 200 mg/kg) IV to convert the cyanide to thiocyanate.
- Thiocyanate is less toxic and rarely a problem, but if thiocyanate toxicity occurs, use hemodialysis. Be aware, however, that hemodialysis does not remove cyanide.
- If necessary, this regimen (nitrite and thiocyanate) may be repeated after 2 hours, at one half the original dose.

4. Describe rebound hypertension. How can it be avoided?

REFERENCES

Hawkins DW et al: Hypertension. In DiPiro JT, Talber R et al, editors: *Pharmacotherapy, a pathophysiologic approach,* ed 2, Norwalk, Conn, 1993, Appleton & Lange.

Hoffman BB, Lefkowitz RF: Catecholamines, sympathomimetic drugs, and adrenergic receptor antagonists. In Hardman JG, Limbird E, editors: *Goodman & Gilman's the pharmacological basis of therapeutics,* ed 9, New York, 1996, McGraw-Hill.

Kaplan NM: Perspectives on the new JNC VI guidelines for the treatment of hypertension, *Formulary* 32(12):1224-1231. 1997.

Michocki R: Hypertensive emergencies. In Young LY, Koda-Kimble MA, editors: *Applied therapeutics: the clinical use of drugs,* ed 6, Vancouver, Wash, 1995, Applied Therapeutics, Inc.

Oates JA (1996). Antihypertensive agents and the drug therapy of hypertension. In Hardman JG, Limbird E, editors: *Goodman & Gilman's the pharmacological basis of therapeutics,* ed 9, New York, 1996, McGraw-Hill.

Olin BR: *Facts and comparisons,* Philadelphia, 1998, JB Lippincott.

Portyansky E: Hypertension, new treatment approaches target organ damage, *Drug Topics* 141(21):78, 81-83, 87, 91, 1997.

United States Pharmacopeial Convention: *USP DI: drug information for the health care professional,* ed 18, Rockville, Md, 1998, The Convention.

ADDITIONAL REFERENCES

American Hospital Formulary Service: *AHFS: drug information '98,* Bethesda, Md, 1998, American Society of Hospital Pharmacists.

Anderson KN et al, editors: *Mosby's medical, nursing, and allied health dictionary,* ed 5, St Louis, 1998, Mosby.

Carter BL, Furmaga EM, Murphy CM: Essential hypertension. In Young LY, Koda-Kimble MA, editors: *Applied therapeutics: the clinical use of drugs,* ed 6, Vancouver, Wash, 1995, Applied Therapeutics, Inc.

Desmond S et al.: Perceptions of hypertension in black and white adolescents, *Health Values* 16(2):3-10, 1992.

Levy RA: *Ethnic and racial differences in response to medicines: preserving individualized therapy in managed pharmaceutical programs,* Reston, Va, 1993, National Pharmaceutical Council.

Mosby: *Mosby's GenRx,* St Louis, 1998, Mosby.

Sagraves R, Letassy NA, Barton TL: Obstetrics. In Young LY, Koda-Kimble MA, editors: *Applied therapeutics: the clinical use of drugs,* ed 6, Vancouver, Wash, 1995, Applied Therapeutics, Inc.

Wolfe SM: Widely used calcium channel blocking drugs, *Worst Pills, Best Pills News* 1(9):1, 4, 1995.

CHAPTER 22

Calcium Channel Blockers

KEY DRUG

verapamil

KEY TERMS

automaticity, (p. 366)
calcium channel blockers, (p. 366)
peripheral vascular resistance, (p. 366)

CHAPTER FOCUS

The calcium channel blocking agents are used primarily for the treatment of angina, cardiac dysrhythmias, and hypertension. Nimodipine is only indicated for the treatment of subarachnoid hemorrhage. These drugs are frequently prescribed alone or in combination therapy, so it is important that healthcare professionals are knowledgeable about this drug category.

OBJECTIVES

After reading and studying this chapter, the student should be able to do the following:

1. *Define and discuss the key terms and key drug.*
2. *Relate the effects of the calcium channel blockers on cardiac muscle, the cardiac conduction system, and vascular smooth muscle.*
3. *Compare and contrast the effects and primary indications of the different calcium channel blocking medications.*
4. *Discuss the side effects and adverse reactions of this drug category.*
5. *Name and describe three potentially serious drug interactions reported with the calcium channel blockers.*

The **calcium channel blockers,** while having diverse chemical structures, all share a basic electrophysiologic property: they block the inward movement of calcium through the slow channels of the cell membranes of cardiac and smooth muscle cells. (See Chapter 18 for a discussion of the physiology of fast and slow channels of cardiovascular fibers.) This activity, however, varies according to the specific type of cardiovascular cells involved. The three types of tissues or cells are (1) cardiac muscle or myocardium, (2) cardiac conduction system (sinoatrial [SA] node and atrioventricular [AV] junction); and (3)vascular smooth muscle.

Action

Cardiac muscle or myocardium. Calcium channel blockers decrease the force of myocardial contraction by blocking the inward flow of calcium ions through the slow channels of the cell membrane during phase 2 (or plateau phase) of the action potential. (See Fig. 18-2 on p. 313.) The diminished entry of calcium ions into the cells thereby fails to trigger the release of large amounts of calcium from the sarcoplasmic reticulum within the cell. This free calcium is needed for excitation-contraction coupling, an event that activates contraction by allowing cross-bridges to form between the actin and myosin filaments of muscle. The force of the heart's contraction is determined by the number of actin and myosin cross-bridges formed within the sarcomere. Decreasing the amount of calcium ion released from the sarcoplasmic reticulum causes fewer actin and myosin cross-bridges to be formed, thus decreasing the force of contraction and resulting in a negative inotropic effect.

Cardiac conduction system (SA node and AV junction). In these tissues, calcium channel blockers decrease automaticity in the SA node and decrease conduction in the AV junction. **Automaticity** means that a cell depolarizes spontaneously and initiates an action potential without an external stimulus. Automaticity is a normal characteristic of the SA nodal cells. Depolarization (phase 0) of the action potential is normally generated by the inward calcium ion current through the slow channels. Thus, the agents that can block the inward calcium ion current across the cell membrane of SA junction tissue decrease the rate of depolarization and depress automaticity. The result is a decrease in heart rate (negative chronotropic effect). Similarly, an agent that decreases calcium ion influx across the cell membrane of the AV junction slows AV conduction (negative dromotropic effect) and prolongs AV refractory time. When AV conduction is prolonged, fewer atrial impulses reach the ventricles, thus slowing the rate of ventricular contractions. Diltiazem (Cardizem) depresses SA nodal automaticity, whereas verapamil (Calan, Isoptin) slows AV conduction. Therefore verapamil is preferred to treat supraventricular tachycardia.

Vascular smooth muscle. The smooth muscle of the coronary and peripheral vessels has a significant influence on the hemodynamics of circulation. Calcium channel blockers effectively inhibit calcium ion influx through the slow channels of the membrane of smooth muscle cells. The depressed interaction between actin and myosin results in a decreased force of smooth muscle contraction. As a consequence, coronary artery dilation occurs, which lowers coronary resistance and improves blood flow through collateral vessels, as well as oxygen delivery to ischemic areas of the heart. Hence drugs with these actions are useful in the treatment of angina pectoris.

Calcium channel blockers also inhibit the contraction of smooth muscle of the peripheral arterioles. This results in widespread reduction in **peripheral vascular resistance** (resistance to blood flow through the body determined by the tone of the vascular musculature and the diameter of the blood vessels) and blood pressure. The hemodynamic change reduces afterload, which also decreases oxygen demands of the heart. This indirectly provides a beneficial effect in the management of angina.

The calcium channel blockers include amlodipine (Norvasc), bepridil (Bepadin, Vascor), diltiazem (Cardizem), felodipine (Plendil), isradipine (DynaCirc), nicardipine (Cardene), nifedipine (Procardia), nisoldipine (Sular), nimodipine (Nimotop), and verapamil (Calan, Isoptin). Flunarizine (Sibelium), indicated for migraine prophylaxis, is only marketed in Canada. Verapamil was the first calcium channel blocker released and is the key drug for this category. It has direct effects on the heart and blood vessels resulting in reduced AV conduction, blocks the SA node resulting in a decrease in heart rate, increases coronary perfusion (coronary vasodilatation), and is considered a moderate peripheral vasodilator. Diltiazem has similar pharmacologic effects.

These agents dilate coronary arteries and arterioles, inhibit coronary artery spasm, and dilate peripheral arterioles and reduce total peripheral resistance (afterload), thus lowering arterial blood pressure at rest and during exercise. Table 22-1 shows a comparison of the effects of calcium channel blockers.

Therapeutically, the calcium antagonists have been used to treat chronic angina pectoris, supraventricular tachycardia, hypertension, Raynaud's syndrome, posthemorrhagic cerebral vasospasm, and vascular headache. Investigationally, verapamil is used to treat hypertrophic cardiomyopathy and vascular headaches. Because these agents differ in specificity and their individual effects on cardiac and peripheral tissues, they may have different indications. See Table 22-2 for Food and Drug Administration (FDA)-approved indications (Olin, 1998; USP DI, 1998).

Bepridil is only indicated for chronic stable angina. Its use is limited by its potentially serious adverse effects, serious ventricular dysrhythmia, and agranulocytosis. The action of diltiazem is largely restricted to dilating the coronary and peripheral blood vessels; the long-acting tablet is indicated for hypertension, regular tablets for angina, and parenteral dosage form for dysrhythmias. Felodipine, nicardip-

TABLE 22-1 Calcium Channel Blocking Agents: Comparison of Effects

Effects	*Amlodipine*	*Bepridil*	*Diltiazem*	*Felodipine*	*Nifedipine Nicardipine Isradipine*	*Verapamil*
Contractility	↑	↓	↓	↑	0/↓	↓↓
Vasodilation						
Coronary	↑	↑↑↑	↑↑↑	↑	↑↑↑	↑↑
Peripheral	↓↓↓	↓	↓	↓↓↓	↓↓↓	↓↓
Heart rate	+/−	↓	0/↓	↑	↑	↑↓
Cardiac output	↑	0	0/↑	↑	↑↑	↑↓

↑, slight increase; ↓, slight decrease; ↑↑, intermediate increase; ↓↓, intermediate decrease; ↑↑↑, significant increase; ↓↓↓, significant decrease; +/−, minimal effect; ↑↓, slight effect; 0, no effect.

TABLE 22-2 FDA-Approved Indications for Calcium Antagonists

Antianginal	amlodipine, bepridil, diltiazem, nicardipine, nifedipine, verapamil
Antiarrhythmic	diltiazem (parenteral), verapamil
Antihypertensive	amlodipine, diltiazem, felodipine, isradipine, nicadipine, nifedipine, nisoldipine, verapamil
Therapy for subarachnoid hemorrhage	nimodipine

ine, and nifedipine are used to treat hypertension and angina while isradipine is used to treat essential hypertension. Nicardipine is a very potent peripheral vasodilator that does not affect the SA node or AV junction. Because of its pronounced effect on the peripheral vascular bed, nifedipine causes the greatest hypotensive effect. However, it exerts minimal cardiac depressant action.

Nimodipine, which is highly lipophilic, crosses the blood-brain barrier and has a greater effect on the cerebral arteries than other arteries in the body. It is indicated for the treatment of cerebral arterial spasm after subarachnoid hemorrhage. It also inhibits platelet aggregation. The adult dose is 60 mg every 4 hours, starting within 96 hours after the subarachnoid hemorrhage and continuing for 3 weeks.

Pharmacokinetics

See Table 22-3 for pharmacokinetics of the calcium channel blocking agents. In addition, diltiazem is metabolized to a major metabolite, desacetyldiltiazem, which may be responsible for up to 50% of its coronary dilatation effect. Also, verapamil's active metabolite norverapamil accounts for about 20% of the antihypertensive effect of verapamil. Nifedipine has no known active metabolites while the other agents have metabolites, which may or may not have significant therapeutic effects.

Drug interactions

The following interactions may occur when calcium channel blocking agents are given with the drugs listed below:

Drug	**Possible effect and management**
Beta-adrenergic blocking agents, systemic and ophthalmic	Although advantageous in some patients, this combination should be closely monitored because adverse cardiac effects may occur (bradycardia, hypotension, and heart failure caused by prolonged AV conduction). In patients with impaired cardiac function, avoid concurrent use if possible.
Carbamazepine, cyclosporine, or quinidine	Diltiazem and verapamil may inhibit liver metabolism (cytochrome P450), resulting in increased serum levels drug toxicity. Nifedipine with quinidine may result in reduced serum levels of quinidine. Monitor such combinations closely because dosage adjustments may be necessary.
Digitalis glycosides	Increased serum levels of digoxin reported, especially when administered with verapamil (occurs to a lesser degree with other calcium antagonists); monitor digoxin serum levels closely whenever a calcium blocking agent is started or discontinued or when dosage is changed. Monitor for prolonged AV conduction, bradycardia, or AV blocks, especially during the initial week of therapy because digoxin dose may need to be changed.

TABLE 22-3 Calcium Channel Blocking Agents: Pharmacokinetics

Drug	Onset of Action (min)	Time to Peak Concentration (hr)	Duration of Action (hr)	Metabolism	Excretion	Usual Adult Daily Dose
amlodipine (Norvasc)	2-5 (IV)	6-12	N/A	Liver	Kidneys	PO: 5-10 mg; elderly start at 2.5 mg
bepridil (Vascor)	60	2-3	24	Liver	Kidneys	PO: 200-400 mg
diltiazem (Cardizem)	30	2-3	4-8	Liver	Kidneys and bile	PO: 120-360 mg Parenteral: 15-25 mg
Extended release	30-60	6-11	12	Same	Same	
felodipine (Plendil)	120-300	2.5-5	24	Liver	Kidneys	PO: 5-20 mg
isradipine (DynaCirc)	120	1.5	12	Liver	Kidneys	PO: 2.5-20 mg
nicardipine (Cardene)	N/A	½-2	8	Liver	Kidneys	PO: 60 mg
nifedipine (Procardia)	Oral: 20 (more rapid when given sublingually)	½-1	4-8	Liver	Kidneys	PO: 30-120 mg
nimodipine (Nimotrop)	N/A	1	Variable	Liver	Bile, feces	PO: 60 mg q4h
nisodipine (Sular)		N/A	24	Liver	Kidneys	PO: 20-40 mg
verapamil (Calan, Isoptin)	Oral: 60-120 IV: 1-5	1-2	IV: 2 Oral regular: 8-10 Oral extended release: 24	Liver	Kidneys and feces	PO: 240-480 mg Parenteral: 5-10 mg

N/A, not available.

disopyramide (Norpace)	Do not administer disopyramide within 48 hours before or 24 hours after verapamil because additive negative inotropic effects may result in serious reactions including death. If possible, avoid this combination. Caution is also necessary when flecainide is given concurrently with calcium antagonists.
Hypokalemia-producing drugs, such as corticosteroids and potassium-depleting diuretics	Increases the risk of bepridil-induced dysrhythmias.
procainamide, quinidine and any drugs that prolong Q-T interval	Both drug classifications have negative inotropic effects and when given concurrently, may result in serious adverse effects (such as hypotension, bradycardia, tachycardia, AV block, and pulmonary edema). Avoid such combinations if possible.

Color type indicates an unsafe drug combination.

Side effects and adverse reactions

These include headache, nausea, hypotension, dizziness, skin flushing or rash, edema of the ankles and feet, dry mouth, and tachycardia. See the boxes for geriatric implications of the use of the calcium channel blockers and for overdose treatment.

Warnings

Use with caution in patients with severe bradycardia, congestive heart failure (caution with felodipine, isradipine, nicardipine, nifedipine, and nimodipine as they have a slight negative inotropic effect), hypotension, acute myocardial infarction, and liver or kidney impairment.

Contraindications

Avoid use in persons with calcium blocking agent hypersensitivity, cardiac shock, hypokalemia (bepridil only), and severe bradycardia or congestive heart failure (use extreme caution with bepridil, diltiazem, and verapamil).

ADDITIONAL INFORMATION

Gingival hyperplasia is a rare side effect reported with amlodipine, diltiazem, felodipine, verapamil, and, most often, nifedipine. It starts as an inflammation of the gums, usually in the first 9 months of therapy. When the drug is discontinued, this effect usually improves within 1 to 4 weeks. Good dental hygiene, along with professional teeth cleaning, is necessary to reduce the potential for this adverse effect.

Proper dosing advice for these drugs includes the following:

- Bepridil or other calcium blocking agents produce nausea; the medication should be taken with food (meals) or at bedtime.

GERIATRIC IMPLICATIONS

Calcium Channel Blockers

The elderly are more susceptible to these agents and the side effects of increased weakness, dizziness, fainting episodes, and falls.

Although nitroglycerin (or other nitrates) may be taken concurrently with these agents, the patient should be advised to report any increase in frequency or intensity of angina attacks to his or her physician.

Nicotine may reduce the effectiveness of these agents; thus reduction or avoidance of tobacco smoking is advisable (Long, Rybacki, 1995).

Alcohol consumption may result in hypotensive episodes in some individuals. Whenever possible, the use of alcohol should be avoided.

Diltiazem, nimodipine, and verapamil half-lives may increase because of accumulation from decreased elimination in the elderly.

The risk of hypotension is increased with use of nimodipine.

These agents should not be discontinued abruptly, since severe rebound angina attacks may result (gradual drug withdrawal is recommended).

MANAGEMENT OF DRUG OVERDOSE

Calcium Blockers

- For symptomatic hypotension administer IV fluids plus IV dopamine or dobutamine, metaraminol, isoproterenol, calcium chloride, or norepinephrine. Use Trendelenburg (head lower than body and legs) position for parenteral verapamil-induced hypotension.
- Direct-current cardioversion, IV lidocaine, or IV procainamide is used for tachycardia, rapid ventricular rate in clients with antegrade conduction, in atrial flutter or fibrillation, and accessory pathway with Wolff-Parkinson-White syndrome.
- For bradycardia use IV atropine, isoproterenol, norepinephrine, or calcium chloride. In some instances an electronic cardiac pacemaker may be necessary.

- Diltiazem extended-release capsules should be swallowed whole; do not chew or crush. Use caution and do not switch brands, as Cardizem CD or Dilacor-XR are dosed once a day while Cardizem SR is dosed twice a day.
- Do not crush or chew extended dosage forms of nifedipine or verapamil or regular strength nifedipine. Procardia XL (nifedipine extended-release) tablet is formulated with a semipermeable membrane around the drug core. This system releases nifedipine at a regular rate over 24 hours, and afterward, the empty insoluble shell is excreted in the feces.
- The patient should also be advised to check with their prescriber or a healthcare professional before taking nonprescription or other medications.
- Caution the patient against smoking, because the effectiveness of the calcium channel blocking agents may be reduced in smokers (Jackson, 1993; Long, Rybacki, 1995).

SUMMARY

Calcium channel blocking agents block the inward movement of calcium through the slow channels of the cell membrane of cardiac and vascular smooth muscle cells. As a result, these agents decrease the force of myocardial contraction producing a negative inotropic effect, decrease automaticity in the SA node and decrease conduction in the AV junction (negative chronotropic and negative dromotropic effects), and inhibit calcium ion influx in smooth muscle cells (reduction in peripheral vascular resistance). These physiologic effects have resulted in the achievement of very effective medications for the treatment of angina, hypertension, and cardiac dysrhythmias.

Not all calcium channel blockers have equivalent therapeutic effects. For example, nicardipine and nifedipine are potent peripheral vasodilators with minimal cardiac effects; therefore, they are effective antihypertensive agents. Nimodipine is indicated for the treatment of subarachnoid hemorrhage while the other calcium channel blocking agents are used for their cardiovascular effects (antianginal, antidysrhythmic, and antihypertensive).

REVIEW QUESTIONS

1. Which calcium channel blocking agent causes the greatest antihypertensive effect?
2. Discuss the pharmacokinetic properties of nimodipine that limit its indication to the treatment of subarachnoid hemorrhage.
3. What advice would you give the elderly person with a prescription for a calcium channel blocking drug to reduce the potential for side effects and adverse reactions?

REFERENCES

Jackson G: The management of stable angina, *Hosp Pract* 28(1):59, 1993.

Long JW, Rybacki JJ: *The essential guide to prescription drugs,* New York, 1995, HarperCollins.

Olin BR: *Facts and comparisons,* Philadelphia, 1998, JB Lippincott.

United States Pharmacopeial Convention: *USP DI: drug information for the health care professional,* ed 18, Rockville, Md, 1998, The Convention.

ADDITIONAL REFERENCES

American Hospital Formulary Service: *AHFS drug information '98,* Bethesda, Md, 1996, American Society of Hospital Pharmacists.

Anderson KN et al, editors: *Mosby's medical, nursing, and allied health dictionary,* ed 5, St Louis, 1998, Mosby.

FDA News and Product Notes: New formulations/combinations—Tarka. *Formulary* 32 (1):24, 1997.

Foley JJ: Treatment of calcium-channel blocker overdose, *J Emerg Nurse* 20:314-315, 1994.
Kelly T: Medical management of calcium channel blocker overdoses, *Drug Newslett* 12(3)18, 1993.
Mosby: *Mosby's GenRx,* St Louis, 1998, Mosby.
Salerno SM et al: Calcium channel antagonists: what do the second-generation agents have to offer? *Postgrad Med* 95(1):181-188, 190, 201-202, 1994.
GD Searle: *Brief summary of Covera-HS,* Searle advertisement P96CV12022V, Chicago, 1996, The Company.
Talbert RL (1993). Ischemic heart disease. In DiPiro JT et al, editors: *Pharmacotherapy,* ed 2, Norwalk, Conn, 1993, Appleton & Lange.

CHAPTER 23

Vasodilators and Antihemorrheologic Agents

KEY DRUGS

nitroglycerin, (p. 372)
pentoxifylline, (p. 376)

KEY TERMS

angina pectoris (p. 372)
hemorrheology, (p. 376)
ischemic, (p. 372)
nitrates, (p. 372)

CHAPTER FOCUS

Nitroglycerin was discovered to be effective for the treatment of angina in 1879. While many other vasodilators were discovered and tested against nitroglycerin, none was found to be more effective for treatment of acute angina episodes (Katzung, Chatterjee, 1992). Recently, other agents such as the beta receptor blocking agents and the calcium channel blockers have also been found to be effective in preventing angina attacks. The antihemorrheologic agent pentoxifylline is used to improve microcirculatory flow.

OBJECTIVES

After reading and studying this chapter, the student should be able to do the following:

1. *Define and discuss the key terms and key drugs.*
2. *Describe the therapeutic effects of nitroglycerin in the treatment of angina pectoris.*
3. *Compare the effects of nitrates, beta blockers, and calcium blocking agents on ventricular volume, heart rate, coronary blood flow, and collateral blood flow.*
4. *Relate the mechanisms of action, side effects and adverse reactions, drug interactions, contraindications, and warnings for the nitrates.*
5. *Discuss the use of isoxsuprine for the treatment of cerebrovascular insufficiency and peripheral vascular disease.*
6. *Describe the mechanism of action, side effects and adverse reactions, contraindications, and dosage for pentoxifylline.*

Vasodilators are used for the treatment of vascular disorders, including peripheral vascular conditions. These agents produce peripheral vasodilation by relaxing smooth muscle in the blood vessel walls. Some drugs act primarily on veins or arterioles, while others dilate both types of blood vessels.

Vasodilators used to treat hypertension are reviewed in Chapter 21. This chapter addresses the use of vasodilators for angina and peripheral occlusive arterial disease and the use of antihemorrheologic agents for the treatment of peripheral vascular disease. The action for the antihemorrheologic drugs is to improve microcirculatory blood flow to **ischemic** (decrease in oxygenated blood supply to body organs or parts) tissues.

ANGINA

The term **angina pectoris** refers to temporary interference with the flow of blood, oxygen, and nutrients to heart muscle or intermittent myocardial ischemia. Angina is characterized by pain behind the sternum. The pain usually occurs with exercise or stress and is relieved by rest. Angina pectoris occurs when the workload on the heart is too great and oxygen delivery is inadequate. Coronary flow is very responsive to oxygen requirements of the heart. Inadequate oxygenation of the heart implies that coronary blood flow is less than the amount actually needed.

Therefore, angina pectoris is usually associated with myocardial ischemia. When coronary blood flow is inadequate, hypoxia causes an accumulation of pain-producing substances such as lactic acid (anaerobic metabolite) and other chemical irritants such as potassium ions, kinins, and prostaglandins. These products then stimulate the cardiac sensory nerve endings, which transmit impulses to the central nervous system to produce the typical anginal pain response.

Inadequate oxygenation may be caused by coronary atherosclerosis or vasomotor spasm of the coronary vessels. Other causes of anginal pain may be pulmonary hypertension and valvular heart disease. Individuals with severe anemia, even with minimal coronary artery disease, may suffer from anginal attacks because of inadequate oxygen supply. The presence of carbon monoxide hemoglobin (carboxyhemoglobin) in smokers, who have reduced amounts of available blood oxygen, is another factor in causing angina pectoris.

Drug therapy of angina pectoris is based on the belief that relaxation of coronary smooth muscle will bring about coronary vasodilation, which in turn will improve blood flow to the heart. However, coronary arteries narrowed by disorders such as sclerosis and calcification cannot respond to any coronary vasodilator. **Nitrates** are the primary drugs prescribed for the treatment of angina.

VASODILATORS

The nitrates, particularly nitroglycerin, are very effective drugs for the treatment of angina pectoris because of their dilating effect on the veins and arteries. The pooling of blood in the veins (capacitance blood vessels) decreases the amount of blood returned to the heart (preload), which reduces left ventricular end-diastolic volume. This decrease in blood return may help reduce the myocardial oxygen demand. Chest pain induced by angina pectoris largely results from an inadequate supply of oxygen to the heart (see Box 23-1 for types of angina pectoris).

BOX 23-1 Types of Angina Pectoris

Classic Angina (Stable or Effort)
Pain usually associated with coronary arteriosclerosis. The attack can be precipitated by exertion or stress (e.g., cold, fear, emotion) and by eating. The pain lasts about 15 minutes and disappears with rest or nitrates.

Unstable Angina (Crescendo or Preinfarction)
A progressive form of angina whereby pain occurs more frequently and becomes more severe in time. The attack may appear during rest and may last longer, with less relief from antianginal drugs. These individuals eventually show signs and symptoms of impending myocardial infarction or coronary failure.

Variant Angina (Prinzmetal's or Vasospastic)
Pain that may be associated with spasms of the coronary arteries and that usually occurs in the presence of coronary stenosis. The pain often happens during rest without any cause. Its occurrence follows a regular pattern (e.g., it appears at the same time during the night). Dysrhythmias often accompany the attack, and the electrocardiogram (ECG) shows an elevation in the S-T segment during the anginal episode. Nitroglycerin acts to increase the oxygen supply by relaxing or preventing spasms in the coronary arteries.

The ideal antianginal drug would (1) establish a balance between coronary blood flow and the metabolic demands of the heart, (2) have a local rather than a systemic effect (it would act directly on coronary vessels to promote coronary vasodilation with no effects on other organ systems), (3) promote oxygen extraction by the heart from arterial flow, (4) be effective when taken orally and have sustained action, and (5) have absence of tolerance.

Currently, no drug meets these criteria. Drugs presently available provide only temporary relief. Evidence is increasing that the nitrates exert their effect not so much by coronary vasodilation, but by lowering blood pressure and decreasing venous return and cardiac work. Box 23-2 gives a comparison of the effects of nitrates, beta blockers, and calcium blocking agents.

Nitrates

nitroglycerin (NTG)

Nitroglycerin is the key nitrate drug in this category. It is available as a sublingual tablet (Nitrostat), an extended-release buccal tablet (Nitrogard SR), a lingual aerosol (Ni-

BOX 23-2 Comparison of Effects of Nitrates, Beta Blockers, and Calcium Blocking Agents

	Nitrates	***Beta Blockers***	***Calcium Blocking Agents***
Systolic blood pressure	(−)	(−)	(−)
Ventricular volume	(−)	(+)	(−) or (0)
Heart rate	(+)	(−)	(−), (+), or (0)
Myocardial contractility	(0)	(−)	(−)
Coronary blood flow	(+)	(+) or (0)	(+)
Coronary vessel resistance	(−)	(+) or (0)	(−)
Coronary spasms	(−)	(+) or (0)	(−)
Collateral flow of blood	(+)	(0)	(−)

(−), decreased; (+), increased; (0), no change.

trolingual), extended-release capsules (Nitrocap), a parenteral injection (Nitro-Bid, Nitrol), an ointment (Nitro-Bid, Nitrostat), and transdermal topical systems (Nitrodisc, Transderm-Nitro, Nitro-Dur). The other drugs in the nitrate drug category include amyl nitrite inhalant, erythrityl tetranitrate (Cardilate), isosorbide dinitrate (Isordil, Sorbitrate), pentaerythritol tetranitrate tablet (Peritrate). pentaerythritol tetranitrate extended-release capsules (Duotrate), and others.

Mechanism of action

Nitrates dilate venous capacitance and arterial resistance vessels, which results in reduced myocardial oxygen demand and a more efficient distribution of blood in the myocardium. The antihypertensive effect of nitrates also is a result of peripheral vasodilation. The biochemical steps for the metabolism of nitrates to the active nitric oxide to the ultimate therapeutic effect of vasodilation are illustrated in Fig. 23-1.

Indications

Nitroglycerin and the other nitrates are used to reduce or prevent the pain of angina, to treat congestive heart failure associated or not associated with myocardial infarction, and as an antihypertensive agent (nitroglycerin injection).

Amyl nitrite has been used to treat acute angina attacks, but it has been replaced by the other, safer nitrate dosage forms. Although not approved by the Food and Drug Administration (FDA) for labeling in the United States, amyl nitrite has been used as an antidote for cyanide poisoning and in cardiac function tests to assess reserve cardiac function. This product has also been abused and used as a sexual stimulant or euphoric agent, but such applications are extremely dangerous and should be avoided.

Pharmacokinetics are detailed in Table 23-1.

Drug interactions

The concurrent use of nitrate with alcohol, antihypertensives, other hypotensive medications, and vasodilators may result in enhanced orthostatic hypotensive effects. Monitor closely as a dosage adjustment may be necessary.

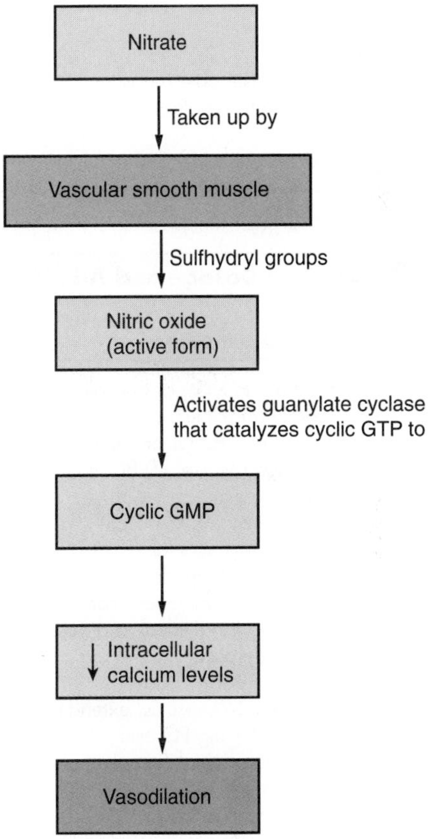

FIGURE 23-1
Biochemical steps of nitrates.

Side effects and adverse reactions

These include dizziness, headaches, nausea or vomiting, agitation, facial flushing, increased pulse rate, dry mouth, rash, prolonged headaches, and blurred vision.

Warnings

Use with caution in patients with cardiomyopathy, hypotension, and liver or kidney impairment.

TABLE 23-1 Nitrates: Pharmacokinetics

Drug	Onset of Action (min)	Duration of Action (hr)	Metabolism	Excretion
erythrityl tetranitrate				
Oral tablet	15-30	Up to 6	Liver	Kidneys
Sublingual tablet	5	2-3		
isosorbide dinitrate				
Oral tablet/capsule	15-40	4-6	Liver	Kidneys
Chewable tablet	2-5	1-2		
Extended-release	30	12		
Sublingual	2-5	1-2		
nitroglycerin				
Sublingual	1-3	½-1	Liver	Kidneys
Extended-release (buccal)	3	5		
Lingual aerosol	2-4	—		
IV infusion	Immediate	Several minutes		
Ointment	30	4-8		
Transdermal	30	8-24		
Extended-release tablet/capsule	—	8-12		
pentaerythritol tetranitrate				
Tablet	30	4-5	Liver	Kidneys
Extended-release tablet and capsule	Slow	12		

TABLE 23-2 Nitrates: Dosage and Administration

Drug	Usual Adult Dose
erythrityl tetranitrate	5-10 mg PO, SL, or buccally, 3 or 4 times daily (maximum of 100 mg/day)
isosorbide dinitrate	2.5-30 mg PO, SL or chewable every 6 hr Extended-release: 40-80 mg PO every 8-12 hr
nitroglycerin	0.15-0.6 mg SL or buccally, repeated at 5-min intervals for up to 3 doses (maximum dose is 10 mg/day) If relief is not obtained, contact prescriber or transport individual to a hospital. Lingual aerosol: 0.4-0.8 mg prn (maximum dose is 1.2 mg/day) Oral tablets/capsules, extended-release: 2.5, 6.5, or 9 mg PO every 12 hr IV infusion: initial 5 μg/min increased in increments of 5 μg/min at 3 or 5-min intervals as needed. Ointment: Apply 1-2 inches (15-30 mg) to skin every 6-8 hr (maximum is 5 inches [75 mg] per application) Transdermal topical system: apply one patch every 24 hr To reduce development of tolerance, it is recommended the patch be applied for 12-14 hr and removed for 10-12 hr.
pentaerythritol tetranitrate	10-20 mg PO 4 times daily (maximum of 160 mg/day) Extended-release: 30-80 mg PO every 12 hr (maximum of 160 mg/day)

SL, Sublingual.

Contraindications

Avoid use in persons with nitrate hypersensitivity, pericarditis, severe anemia, glaucoma, hyperthyroidism, and hypovolemia (for IV NTG only), and in those who have had recent myocardial infarction, head trauma, or cerebral hemorrhage.

Dosage and administration

See Table 23-2.

Dosage forms include the following:

- Sublingual, lingual aerosol, and extended-release buccal NTG tablets are prescribed to abort an acute attack of angina pectoris. Of these agents, the sublingual or lingual products are the preferred agents. The instructions are to place the sublingual tablet under the tongue or in the buccal pouch to allow it to dissolve fully or to spray the lingual aerosol on or under the tongue. Do not swallow, eat, drink, or smoke while the tablet is in the mouth. The dosage, if necessary, is repeated at 5-minute intervals for a total of three doses. If chest pain is not relieved within the 15-minute period, the prescriber should be contacted or the patient transported immediately to a hospital.
- After use of the sublingual preparations, the patient may experience a transient headache that lasts 5 to 20 minutes. If headaches persist, the prescriber should be notified. In some instances the headache may be relieved by aspirin or acetaminophen. If dizziness occurs, the patient should sit or lie down and move slowly when changing body positions. Flushing may also occur.
- The sublingual NTG tablets should be stored in a tightly closed dark container. Instruct the patient to date the bottle when it is opened. Inform the patient that he or she should not mix NTG with any medications or expose it to

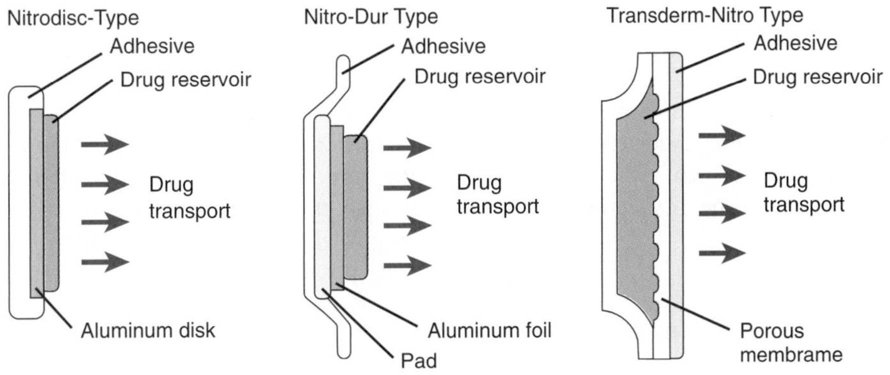

FIGURE 23-2

Transdermal systems. The Nitrodisc contains NTG mixed in a solid polymer similar to silicone and a cosolvent to enhance skin penetration. Nitro-Dur is a gel-like matrix surrounded by fluid. The NTG moves from the matrix to fluid to skin. Transderm-Nitro contains a semipermeable membrane between drug supply and skin. The membrane controls the drug delivery.

air, heat, and moisture. To maintain potency, many prescribers suggest the patient obtain a fresh supply of NTG every 6 months.

- Instruct the patient not to shake the lingual aerosol can and not to inhale the spray.
- Chewable NTG should be chewed well and held in the mouth for at least 2 minutes before swallowing.
- Oral sustained-release tablets/capsules need to be administered on an empty stomach (1 hour before or 2 hours after meals) with a full glass of water. The patient is advised not to chew or crush this medication.
- The use of nitroglycerin ointment requires careful patient instruction. Also advise the patient or caregiver to not get the ointment on the hands, as it may be absorbed and cause side effects such as headache.
- Transdermal nitroglycerin is a patch system that contains a drug reservoir from which the NTG is slowly released (passive diffusion). The NTG is absorbed through the skin and transported by blood to the site of action to produce its beneficial effects. This system is applied daily to a hairless skin area, usually on the chest (preferred site), shoulder, or inside upper arm. Avoid applying the patch to extremities, especially below the knee or elbow.

Transdermal systems are available in various strengths (releasing 0.1 mg/hr up to 0.8 mg/hr), and each has a different mechanism for drug delivery. Therefore, the systems should not be considered to be interchangeable. See Fig. 23-2 for an illustration of transdermal systems. As tolerance develops to this product, it is recommended that the patch be applied for 12 to 14 hours and removed for 10 to 12 hours each day. This drug-free interval will help to maintain the efficacy of the product.

Also advise the patient to use caution near microwave ovens while the system (with a metallic backing) is applied. Any leaking radiation from the oven could heat the backing and cause a burn.

Pregnancy safety for nitroglycerin has been established as FDA category C.

PERIPHERAL VASCULAR DISEASE

Peripheral vascular disease, which results in coolness or numbness of the extremities, intermittent claudication, and leg ulcers, is a common problem in the elderly. The primary pathophysiologic factor is atherosclerosis or hyperlipidemia. The use of various direct-acting vasodilators for peripheral occlusive arterial disease has generally been very disappointing. Because cyclandelate (Cyclospasmal) has been classified as ineffective by the FDA, it is not reviewed in this section. Papaverine (Cerebid, Pavabid) is an old drug that was exempted from the FDA's review on drug effectiveness. However, the advisory committee of the FDA, the Peripheral and Central Nervous System Drug Review Committee, concluded after reviewing studies and open hearings that papaverine has vasodilator effects but was not proved to be effective for its claimed indication, smooth muscle relaxation (USP DI, 1998).

The FDA requires substantial evidence of effectiveness to grade a drug "effective." The following drug lacks this information and is rated only "possibly effective" by the FDA.

isoxsuprine hydrochloride [eye sox′ syoo preen] (Vasodilan)

Isoxsuprine produces a direct relaxation effect on the smooth muscles of peripheral arterial walls located within skeletal muscle; it has little effect on cutaneous blood flow. It also causes an increase in heart rate, contractility, and cardiac output and uterine relaxation.

Isoxsuprine is considered "possibly effective" for the treatment of symptoms of cerebrovascular insufficiency and peripheral vascular disease and may relieve symptoms of Raynaud's syndrome, arteriosclerosis obliterans, and thromboangiitis obliterans (Buerger's disease).

Pharmacokinetics

Isoxsuprine has an onset of action of 10 minutes when given intravenously or 1 hour when administered orally. In adults, its half-life is 1.25 hours. It is partially metabolized in the blood and excreted via the kidneys. Side effects include nausea or vomiting, or, rarely, chest pain, rash, and respiratory difficulties. No significant drug interactions are reported with isoxsuprine.

Warnings

Use with caution in patients with bleeding disorders, glaucoma, and hypertension.

Contraindications

Avoid use in persons with isoxsuprine hypersensitivity, severe cerebrovascular disease, hypotension, severe coronary artery disease, tachycardia, and other cardiac arrhythmias.

Dosage and administration

The adult dose is 10 to 20 mg tablets PO three or four times a day. The dose to inhibit premature labor is 5 to 10 mg IM two to three times daily. Pregnancy safety has not been established although in near-term neonates the drug has a half-life of 1.5 to 3 hours.

HEMORRHEOLOGY

Hemorrheology is a science that deals with the deformation and flow properties of blood under physiologic and pathophysiologic conditions. Because arteriosclerosis reduces blood flow to tissues distal to the obstruction, blood viscosity is elevated, thereby diminishing the flow of blood still further. In addition, the impaired blood flow at the microcirculatory level affects the normal capacity of the red blood cells to flex as they enter the narrowed capillary lumen, which has a mean diameter smaller than the erythrocytes. A major function of red blood cells is to transport hemoglobin that carries oxygen, which during the metabolic process is converted to energy for muscle movement such as walking.

Accordingly, the decreased flexibility of the red blood cells and the elevated blood viscosity are responsible for diminishing tissue oxygenation. Hence, during exercise the demand for an increase in blood flow and tissue oxygenation may result in claudication, thereby limiting the distance a person can walk.

Intermittent claudication is a syndrome that results from an insufficient blood supply to skeletal muscles in the legs. Reduced microcirculatory blood flow causes ischemia and pain. This syndrome is a common complication of atherosclerosis and is characteristic of Buerger's disease. While walking, affected individuals experience first pain and then cramps and weakness in muscles.

ANTIHEMORRHEOLOGIC AGENT

pentoxifylline [pen tox i′ fi leen] (Trental)

Pentoxifylline represents an important concept in the therapy for peripheral vascular disorders, because the ability of vasodilators to improve blood flow by dilation of rigid, arteriosclerotic blood vessels is somewhat limited. Furthermore, because capillary walls lack smooth muscle, dilation by this group of drugs is often unlikely to occur.

Pentoxifylline improves hemorrheologic disorders in the microcirculation, which involves the flow of blood through the fine vessels (arterioles, capillaries, and venules). Although the mechanism of action of pentoxifylline is not completely understood, current evidence shows that the drug possesses several properties to improve microcirculatory blood flow to ischemic tissues. (1) It restores red blood cell flexibility, probably by its inhibition of phosphodiesterase, which results in an increase in cyclic adenosine monophosphate (AMP) in red blood cells. (2) It lowers blood viscosity by decreasing fibrinogen concentrations and inhibiting aggregation of red blood cells and platelets. The result is increased microcirculatory blood flow and oxygenation of tissues.

Indications

Pentoxifylline is indicated as an adjunct to surgery for the treatment of intermittent claudication caused by occlusive arterial disease of the limbs.

Pharmacokinetics

It is administered orally and on absorption binds to erythrocyte membranes. It has a half-life of 0.4 to 0.8 hours for the primary drug and 1 to 1.6 hours for the metabolites. The peak concentration in the blood occurs in 2 to 4 hours, and the onset of action with chronic dosing is between 2 and 4 weeks. It is metabolized by red blood cells and in the liver and is excreted primarily by the kidneys.

Drug interactions

Although no significant drug interactions are noted in the USP DI (1998), the professional should be aware that smoking may interfere with the effects of pentoxifylline. Concurrent use with antiplatelet and thrombolytic medications may increase prothrombin time and bleeding. Use with sympathomimetics and xanthines may result in an increase in central nervous system (CNS) stimulation. Monitor closely if these medications are used in combination.

Warnings

Use with caution in patients with bleeding problems or cerebrovascular or coronary artery disease.

Contraindications

Avoid use in persons with pentoxifylline hypersensitivity and liver or kidney impairment.

Side effects and adverse reactions

These include dizziness, headaches, abdominal distress, nausea, and vomiting. Rare adverse reactions are chest pain and an irregular heart rate. With an overdose the patient experiences increased sedation, flushing of skin, a feeling of faintness, increased excitability, or convulsions.

Dosage and administration

For adults the dose is 400 mg PO three times daily with meals. If undesirable side effects occur, such as gastrointestinal upset or CNS disturbances, the dosage should be decreased to 400 mg twice daily. Pregnancy safety for pentoxifylline has been established as FDA category C.

SUMMARY

The vasodilators and antihemorrheologic medications are both used to improve blood flow in the body. The vasodilators are used to treat vascular disorders by relaxing smooth muscle in the blood vessels, while the antihemorrheologic drug pentoxifylline improves microcirculatory blood flow by restoring red blood cell flexibility and lowering blood viscosity.

Nitroglycerin is a very effective drug for angina pectoris, although the continuous use of nitroglycerin products on a regular basis has resulted in the development of tolerance. To prolong the drug's therapeutic effect, drug-free time periods are recommended. The goal of therapy with the nitrates it to decrease pain duration and intensity, decrease the frequency of attacks, and improve the quality of life for the patient with angina.

REVIEW QUESTIONS

1. Name and describe the three types of angina pectoris.
2. Nitroglycerin sublingual tablets were prescribed for Mr. Jones with instructions to place one tablet under the tongue and repeat at 5-minute intervals if necessary, for a total of three doses. What additional instructions should be given to Mr. Jones about the use of this product?
3. What are the mechanism of action, onset of action, side effects and adverse reactions, and dose for pentoxifylline?

REFERENCES

Katzung BG, Chatterjee, K: Vasodilators and the treatment of angina pectoris. In Katzung BG: *Basic and clinical pharmacology,* ed 5, Norwalk, Conn, 1992, Appleton & Lange.

United States Pharmacopeial Convention: *USP DI: drug information for the health care professional,* ed 18, Rockville, Md, 1998, The Convention.

ADDITIONAL REFERENCES

American Hospital Formulary Service: *AHFS drug information '98,* Bethesda, Md, 1996, American Society of Hospital Pharmacists.

Anderson KN et al, editors: *Mosby's medical, nursing, and allied health dictionary,* ed 5, St Louis, 1998, Mosby.

Jackson G: The management of stable angina, *Hosp Pract* 28(1):59, 1993.

Mosby: *Mosby's GenRx,* St Louis, 1998, Mosby.

Olin BR: *Facts and comparisons,* Philadelphia, 1998, JB Lippincott.

UNIT VI

Drugs Affecting the Blood

CHAPTER 24

Overview of the Blood

CHAPTER FOCUS

Blood interacts with every system in the body to provide oxygen and nutrition and to remove body waste products. It is crucial for the maintenance of homeostasis, as a deficiency of any of its elements may result in illnesses such as anemia (deficiency in red blood cells), an increase in infection (decrease in leukocytes), or an increased tendency to bleed (decrease in platelets).

The study of hematology also includes knowledge of the hemostatic mechanism for coagulation and the different blood types.

OBJECTIVES

After reading and studying this chapter, the student should be able to do the following:

1. *Describe the composition and volume of blood.*
2. *Name and discuss the three types of blood cells.*
3. *Name and describe the five types of leukocytes found in the blood.*
4. *Discuss the intrinsic and extrinsic pathways for blood clotting.*
5. *Name and describe the functions of the three major proteins in blood.*

KEY TERMS

albumin, (p. 383)
anemia, (p. 382)
erythrocytes, (p. 382)
erythropoietin, (p. 382)
fibrinogen, (p. 384)
globulins, (p. 383)
hematocrit, (p. 382)
hemoglobin, (p. 382)
hemostasis, (p. 384)
leukocytes, (p. 382)
leukocytosis, (p. 383)
leukopenia, (p. 383)
phagocytosis, (p. 383)
plasma, (p. 382)
platelets, (p. 382)
thrombocytes, (p. 382)
thrombocytopenia, (p. 383)

Blood is the major transport system in the body. It is also vitally important for the proper functioning and regulation of the human body. Pumped by the heart, blood carries nutrients and oxygen from the digestive and respiratory systems to cells throughout the entire body. In addition, it picks up waste products from body cells and delivers them to the proper system for excretion, usually the liver, kidneys, and lungs. Hormones, enzymes, buffers, and many other biochemical substances are also transported by the blood from one site in the body to the receptors or target cells. Blood also helps to regulate body heat by absorbing and transporting heat from the body core where it can be more easily dispersed.

BLOOD VOLUME

Blood is composed of billions of cells and **plasma,** a fluid portion in which the cells are suspended. Although blood volume can vary from person to person, the average blood volume in a normal adult is approximately 5000 ml (5 L). Of this volume, 3000 ml is usually plasma and the remainder is primarily red blood cells. **Hematocrit** is the packed cell volume of the red blood cells expressed as a percentage of the total blood volume, or the blood viscosity. Hematocrit is measured by a laboratory test performed on a blood sample. The higher the hematocrit, the greater the blood viscosity. For example, persons with polycythemia may have a hematocrit of 60 or 70 because of an excessive number of red blood corpuscles. Increased blood viscosity can retard blood flow through blood vessels, resulting in headaches, fatigue, weakness, dyspnea, and perhaps an enlarged spleen and increased basal metabolism.

BLOOD COMPOSITION

Blood is composed of three types of blood cells: (1) red blood cells, or **erythrocytes,** which transport oxygen and carbon dioxide; (2) **leukocytes,** or white blood cells, which defend the body against bacteria and infections; and (3) **platelets,** or **thrombocytes,** which are necessary for blood coagulation. Proteins such as serum albumin, globulins, and fibrinogen are also present in the blood.

Plasma may contain thousands of other substances, such as glucose, electrolytes, vitamins, hormones, and waste products. However, this discussion on blood focuses on blood cells, blood proteins, and blood groups or types.

BLOOD CELLS

Red Blood Cells

Red blood cells are small and disk-shaped. They are the cells present in the largest quantities in the bloodstream. Their life span is approximately 120 days. The major function of red blood cells is to carry hemoglobin within the cell. Each **hemoglobin** molecule contains four iron atoms, which combine with four oxygen molecules to transport oxygen from the lungs to the tissues. Hemoglobin can also combine with carbon dioxide and carry it from the cells to the lungs for excretion. It also serves as an acid-base buffering system in whole blood.

After birth, red blood cells are produced by the bone marrow. They are manufactured by most bones in early life, but after 20 years of age most red blood cells are produced in the bone marrow of the vertebrae, sternum, ribs, and ilia.

Males have more hemoglobin in their blood than females do. Generally, most normal men have between 14 and 16 g/dl, while women have a range of 12 to 14 g/dl. **Anemia** is usually diagnosed if a person has a hemoglobin below 10. Anemias are classified according to both the size and the number of functional red blood cells in the blood.

Red blood cells are rapidly formed and destroyed in the body. It has been estimated that more than 100 million red blood cells are produced every minute during adulthood. The normal healthy adult has between 4.5 and 5.5 million cells/mm^3 of blood. The body balances production versus destruction of these cells to maintain a relatively constant body level of red blood cells. The exact body mechanism for this is unknown.

It is known that the rate of red blood cell production can be increased if a considerable decrease in red blood cells occurs or tissue hypoxia develops. Then the kidneys will be stimulated to increase secretion of **erythropoietin,** a hormone that acts to stimulate the production of red blood cells by the bone marrow. With maximum bone marrow stimulation, red blood cell production can be increased to nearly seven times over normal.

The bone marrow needs adequate supplies of vitamin B_{12}, iron, and other substances to make new red blood cells. A deficiency in absorption of vitamin B_{12} from the gastric tract, caused by a lack of intrinsic factor (see Chapter 60), can lead to pernicious anemia.

Anemias can also be induced by increased red cell destruction, which may occur with infections or cancer or from bone marrow suppression caused by radiation therapy and many cancer chemotherapeutic agents (Box 24-1).

Leukocytes

There are five types of leukocytes found in the blood. They are classified according to the presence or absence of granules in the cell cytoplasm. The granular leukocytes are neutrophils, eosinophils, and basophils; the nongranular leukocytes are lymphocytes and monocytes. The granular leukocytes have two or more nuclear lobes, so they are referred to as polymorphonuclear leukocytes or "polyps."

Blood in the normal person usually contains between 5000 and 9000 leukocytes/mm^3. A differential count may be ordered by the physician or healthcare provider to aid in diagnosis. For example, in acute appendicitis, the percentage of neutrophils increases, as does the total leukocyte count.

Leukocytes are produced primarily in the bone marrow. Lymphocytes are produced mainly in lymph tissues and organs such as the spleen, thymus, tonsils, and various other lymphoid tissue in the bone marrow, gastrointestinal

BOX 24-1 Drugs That Cause Bone Marrow Depression

amphotericin B, systemic (Fungizone)
antithyroid medications
azathioprine (Imuran)
busulfan (Myleran)
carmustine (BCNU; BiCNU)
chlorambucil (Leukeran)
chloramphenicol (Chloromycetin)
cisplatin (Platinol, Platinol-AQ ♣)
colchicine
cyclophosphamide (Cytoxan, Procytox ♣)
cytarabine (ara-C, Cytosar ♣)
dacarbazine (DTIC ♣, DTIC-Dome)
dactinomycin (Actinomycin D, Cosmegen)
daunorubicin (Cerubidine)
doxorubicin (Adriamycin RDF)
etoposide (VePesid, VP-16)
floxuridine (FUDR)
flucytosine (Ancobon, 5-FC, Ancotil ♣)
fluorouracil, systemic (5-FU, Adrucil)
hydroxyurea (Hydrea)
interferon (Roferon-A, Intron A)
lomustine (CCNU, CeeNU)
mechlorethamine, systemic (Mustargen, nitrogen mustard)
melphalan (Alkeran, L-PAM)
mercaptopurine (Purinethol)
methotrexate (Mexate)
mitomycin (Mutamycin)
pentamidine (Pentam)
plicamycin (Mithracin, mithramycin)
procarbazine (Matulane, Natulan ♣)
sodium iodide I 131 (Iodotope)
sodium phosphate P 32
streptozocin (Zanosar)
thioguanine (Lanvis ♣)
thiotepa
uracil mustard
vinblastine (Velban, Velbe ♣)
vincristine (Oncovin)
zidovudine (Retrovir)

tract, and elsewhere. Several terms are important to understand. **Leukopenia** refers to an abnormal decrease in the number of leukocytes to fewer than $5000/mm^3$; **leukocytosis** refers to an abnormal increase in the number of leukocytes.

Neutrophils, monocytes, lymphocytes, and basophils are very mobile. They can leave the capillaries and migrate to organisms or foreign particles that have entered the body. The neutrophils and monocytes ingest and destroy the invaders, a process known as **phagocytosis.** Lymphocytes defend the body against bacteria, fungus, and viruses by forming B lymphocytes or T lymphocytes. (See Chapter 54 for an overview of the immune system.)

BOX 24-2 Differential Normal Leukocyte Count

Neutrophils (polymorphonuclear)	62%
Eosinophils (polymorphonuclear)	2.3%
Basophils (polymorphonuclear)	0.4%
Monocytes	5.3%
Lymphocytes	30%

From Guyton, 1990.

Eosinophils are considered weak phagocytes and have limited mobility. An increased level is usually seen with allergic reactions or a cell injury caused by parasites (e.g., hookworm).

The life span of granulocytes is estimated to be 4 to 8 hours in the bloodstream and 3 to 5 days in body tissues. If involved in ingestion of invading organisms, this life span can be reduced to only a few hours, because during this process they are also destroyed. Monocytes also have a short life span in blood, but in the body tissues they can live for months or even years if not destroyed by phagocytosis. Monocytes in the tissues often increase in size to become tissue macrophages, so they often provide a first line of defense against tissue infections.

Platelets

Platelets or thrombocytes are small, round, or oval colorless cells produced by the bone marrow. They have a life span of 5 to 8 days. A normal platelet level in the blood is between 150,000 and $350,000/mm^3$.

Platelets are key substances for blood clotting in the body. If a blood vessel is injured and blood is escaping, platelets will quickly congregate at the site and clump together to form a plug to stop the bleeding. If the wound is large, platelets will set off a series of chemical reactions within the body to form a clot and seal the injury (Fig. 24-1).

Persons with a low quantity of platelets have thrombocytopenia. Such persons tend to bleed, and their skin usually displays small purple spots (hence the name thrombocytopenia purpura). Bleeding problems usually do not occur until the platelet level is below $50,000/mm^3$. **Thrombocytopenia** is often induced by irradiation injury to the bone marrow or from aplasia of the bone marrow induced by specific drugs.

Blood Proteins

The blood contains three major proteins: albumin, globulins, and fibrinogen. **Albumin** is responsible for the osmotic pressure gradient produced at the capillary membrane. This prevents plasma fluid from leaving the capillaries to enter the interstitial spaces.

Globulins are divided into alpha, beta, and gamma globulins. Gamma globulin and beta globulin (to a lesser extent) help to protect the body against infections. Gamma

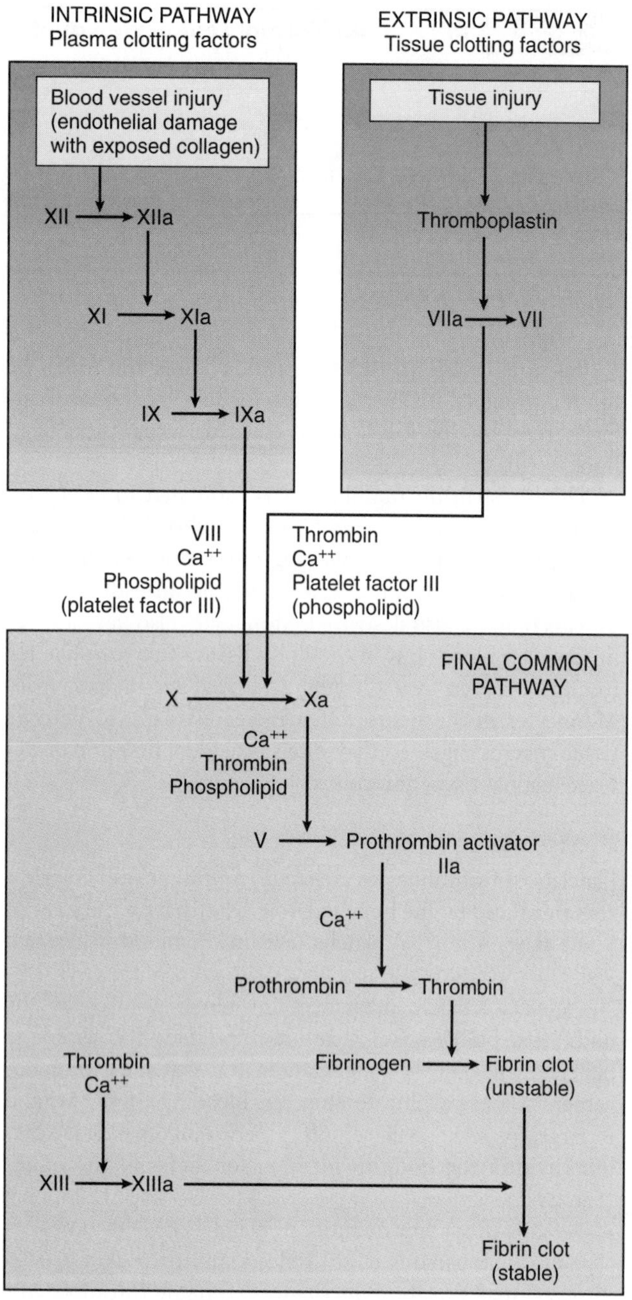

FIGURE 24-1
Coagulation mechanisms for intrinsic and extrinsic pathways for blood clotting. Final pathway (activation of factor X) is common to both the intrinsic and extrinsic coagulation systems.

globulin is involved with humoral immunity. Alpha and beta globulins are also believed to perform other functions, such as transportation of certain substances in the blood by reversibly combining with them. They may also be a substrate to form other substances.

Fibrinogen, a plasma protein that is converted to fibrin by thrombin in the presence of calcium ions, is necessary for coagulation.

COAGULATION

Hemostatic Mechanism

Hemostasis is a process that spontaneously stops bleeding from damaged blood vessels. Blood is normally fluid while circulating in the vessels, but with vessel injury, it rapidly clots at the site of injury.

After any injury to a blood vessel, hemostasis is achieved by three sequential steps: (1) blood vessels constrict to retard blood flow from the injured area; (2) platelet plugs form to temporarily seal the leaking small arteries and veins; and (3) blood coagulates to plug openings within the damaged vessels and wounds to prevent further bleeding.

Blood Vessel Constriction

Immediately after a blood vessel is injured, vascular constriction occurs as a reflex response. This response instantly slows the flow of blood from the ruptured vessel.

Platelet Plug Formation

After injury to a blood vessel, interruption of the continuity of its endothelial lining exposes the collagen (a fibrous protein) in the underlying connective tissue. Platelets immediately adhere to the exposed collagen to form a dense aggregate, a process known as platelet adhesion. This attachment triggers the release of adenosine diphosphate (ADP), which causes the outer surface of the platelets to become extremely sticky so that other adjacent platelets adhere to one another at the damaged site. This process eventually forms the platelet plug. Because this plug is relatively unstable, it can stop bleeding quickly as long as the damage to the vessel is minute. However, for long-term effectiveness the platelet plug must be reinforced with fibrin. This involves a chemical mechanism called blood coagulation.

Blood Coagulation

Blood coagulation is the final stage of a complex series of events in hemostasis. The process ultimately results in the formation of a stable fibrin clot, which is composed of a meshwork of fibrin threads that entraps platelets, blood cells, and plasma. Thus the physical formation of a blood clot or thrombus plays a key role in hemostasis by permanently closing the hole in the injured vessel to prevent further bleeding.

The chemical events in the blood coagulation mechanism involve two distinct pathways: the intrinsic pathway and the extrinsic pathway.

Intrinsic Pathway

Because all the chemical substances involved in coagulation are normally found in the circulating blood, this pathway is referred to as the intrinsic system of coagulation. In this pathway, activation of specific blood coagulation factors is initiated by injury to the endothelial lining of the blood vessel wall. When blood contacts the exposed underlying collagen, the Hageman factor (factor XII) is activated by enzy-

TABLE 24-1 Blood Coagulation Factors and Synonyms

Factor	Name or Synonym
I	Fibrinogen
II	Prothrombin
III	Tissue thromboplastin
IV	Calcium
V	Proaccelerin (labile factor, accelerator globulin)
VII	Proconvertin (stable factor, serum prothrombin conversion accelerator [SPCA])
VIII	Antihemophilic factor (AHF)
IX	Plasma thromboplastin component, Christmas factor
X	Stuart-Power factor
XI	Plasma thromboplastin antecedent (PTA)
XII	Hageman factor
XIII	Fibrin stabilizing factor

matically converting it to the active form (factor XIIa). The simultaneous damage of platelets also causes the release of platelet phospholipid (platelet factor III), which is required later in the coagulation process. Factor XIIa then activates factor XI to XIa. The reaction of factor XIa with factor IX requires calcium ions to form activated factor IX. In the presence of calcium ions and platelet phospholipid, factor IXa interacts with factor VIII and thrombin to form a complex. This combination then speeds up the activation of factor X. Factor Xa combines with factor V, calcium ions, and platelet phospholipid to form a complex known as the prothrombin activator (factor IIa). Factor IIa initiates the cleavage of prothrombin to form thrombin, which then enzymatically converts fibrinogen into fibrin, forming an unstable clot. The final step involves the action of factor XIII (a fibrin-stabilizing factor), thrombin, and calcium ions, which catalyze the formation of a stronger, stable fibrin clot. See Fig. 24-1 for a summary of the main events of the intrinsic pathway.

Extrinsic Pathway

The extrinsic pathway is activated by trauma to the vascular wall or to the tissues outside the blood vessels. In this pathway, clotting occurs when products of tissue damage gain access to the blood. The tissue factor thromboplastin is released and becomes part of a complex with factor VII and calcium ions. This combination of components activates factor X, which is the step at which the extrinsic pathway converges with the intrinsic pathway; coagulation then continues through a common route with the resultant formation of a final stable clot. See Fig. 24-1 for the extrinsic pathway; Table 24-1 lists blood coagulation factors.

The final pathway common to both the intrinsic and the extrinsic coagulation systems begins with the activation of factor X and ends in the formation of fibrin. Both systems function simultaneously in the body. The lack of a normal factor in either system will usually result in a blood disorder.

Blood Coagulation Abnormalities

Diseases associated with abnormal clotting vessels cause many deaths. It is estimated that over 1 million persons suffer from thrombosis or embolism in the United States each year. Diseases caused by intravascular clotting include some of the major causes of death from cardiovascular sources—coronary occlusion and cerebrovascular accidents. Therefore, drugs which inhibit clotting are important.

Local trauma, vascular stasis, and systemic alterations in the coagulability of blood are considered the main factors in the initiation of thrombosis. Basically, coagulation mechanisms are responsible for forming two kinds of thrombi: arterial thrombi and venous thrombi. Arterial thrombi are most frequently associated with atherosclerotic plaques, high blood pressure, and turbulent blood flow that damages the endothelial lining of the blood vessel and causes platelets to stick and aggregate in the arterial system. Arterial thrombi are mostly platelets, and their formation is associated with the intrinsic pathway of the coagulation mechanism.

Venous thrombi occur most often in areas where blood flow is reduced or static. This appears to initiate clotting and produces a thrombus in the venous system. Its formation involves the extrinsic pathway of the coagulation mechanism. Current anticoagulants are more effective in preventing venous rather than arterial thrombi.

BLOOD TYPES

Blood type refers to the type of antigen located on red blood cell membranes. Although many antigens have been identified, antigens A, B, and Rh are the most important blood antigens involved with blood transfusions and newborn survival. Every person belongs to one of the four blood groups and, in addition, is Rh positive or Rh negative. The ABO blood groups are as follows:

- Type A: A antigen on red blood cells (the plasma has antibody B)
- Type B: B antigen on red blood cells (the plasma has antibody A)
- Type AB: A antigen and B antigen on red blood cells (the plasma contains no antibodies)
- Type O: neither A nor B antigens on red blood cells (plasma contains A and B antibodies)

Persons with type A blood can safely receive blood from A and O donors. Persons with type B blood can safely receive blood from type B and O donors. People with AB blood are known as the universal recipients, because their blood is compatible with types AB, A, B, and O. Before transfusion, however, cross-matching of the blood is necessary because other agglutinins may be present. Type O persons can only receive type O blood, but they are called universal donors because they can donate blood to anyone. (See Chapter 31 for additional information on blood transfusion.)

A person who is Rh positive carries Rh antigen on the red blood cells. One who is Rh negative does not have any Rh antigens on the red blood cells. Approximately 85% of the population is Rh positive. Rh factor is particularly important when an Rh-negative woman is impregnated by an Rh-positive man. The mother may have antibodies against the Rh antigen, which can cross the placenta and attack the fetus should its blood be Rh positive. If this occurs, the infant may develop jaundice or be dead on delivery.

An Rh-negative woman could acquire Rh antibodies via blood transfusions. It is also possible for her to develop them if fetal blood enters her bloodstream during childbirth or miscarriage. Regardless, the first pregnancy usually has less risk associated with it than subsequent pregnancies.

Physicians can reduce this danger by administering an anti-Rh antibody (Gamulin Rh, RhoGAM, or HypRho-D) to Rh-negative women after each pregnancy. This will prevent their systems from making antibodies to Rh-positive blood. Rh-negative women who have a spontaneous or induced abortion or a termination of an ectopic pregnancy of up to and including 12 weeks' gestation are given a microdose of immune globulin (MICRhoGAM or Mini-Gamulin Rh) if the father is Rh positive.

SUMMARY

This chapter reviews the functions, volume, composition, and types of cells in blood. The proper composition and flow of blood are necessary for the continuous exchange of oxygen, nutrients, biochemicals, and waste products in the body. An understanding of the blood in maintaining homeostasis in the body is essential.

REVIEW QUESTIONS

1. What are the signs and symptoms of a patient with a red blood cell deficiency? A white blood cell deficiency? A platelet deficiency?
2. When a blood vessel is injured, how is hemostasis achieved? Outline the three steps.
3. What are the names and functions of the three globulins in blood?

REFERENCES

Guyton AC: *Textbook of medical physiology,* ed 8, Philadelphia, 1990, WB Saunders.

ADDITIONAL READINGS

Anderson KN et al, editors: *Mosby's medical, nursing, and allied health dictionary,* ed 5, St Louis, 1998, Mosby.

Guyton AC: *Human physiology and the mechanism of disease,* ed 4, Philadelphia, 1987, WB Saunders.

Olin BR: *Facts and comparisons.* Philadelphia, 1998, JB Lippincott.

Thibodeau GA, Patton KT: *Anatomy and physiology,* ed 4, St Louis, 1999, Mosby.

United States Pharmacopeial Convention: *USP DI: drug information for the health care professional,* ed 18, Rockville, Md, 1998, The Convention.

Van Wynsberghe D, Noback CR, Carola R: *Human anatomy and physiology,* ed 3, New York, 1995, McGraw-Hill.

CHAPTER 25

Anticoagulants, Thrombolytics, and Blood Components

CHAPTER FOCUS

Blood and its proper volume and composition are vital to the health of the individual. Injuries that lead to hemostasis or blood clotting require the use of anticoagulant medications. The formation of thrombi or acute thromboembolic disorders requires use of thrombolytic agents. Anticoagulants and thrombolytic agents are reviewed in this chapter. These are very potent and effective medications requiring a thorough pharmacologic knowledge for safe patient usage.

OBJECTIVES

After reading and studying this chapter, the student should be able to do the following:

1. *Define and discuss the key terms and key drugs.*
2. *Relate the different prophylactic uses for anticoagulant drug therapy.*
3. *Discuss the mechanisms of action, pharmacokinetics, onset of action, laboratory tests, and antidotes for parenteral and oral anticoagulants.*
4. *Describe the use of protamine and vitamin K as anticoagulant antagonists.*
5. *Differentiate between the therapeutic effects of thrombolytic and anticoagulant drugs on blood clots.*
6. *Name and discuss medications used to treat hemophilia.*
7. *Discuss use of systemic and topical hemostatic agents.*

KEY DRUGS

heparin sodium, (p. 388)
streptokinase, (p. 393)
warfarin, (p. 391)

KEY TERMS

antiplatelet drugs, (p. 397)
embolus, (p. 388)
fibrinolytic activity, (p. 388)
hemophilia, (p. 395)
hemostatic agents, (p. 398)
thrombolytic (fibrinolytic) drugs, (p. 393)
thrombus, (p. 388)

This chapter reviews drugs and substances that affect hemostasis or blood clotting, preformed thrombi, and blood administration. While normal blood clotting is a defense mechanism constantly available for protection against excessive hemorrhage, the development of a **thrombus** (an aggregation of platelets, fibrin, clotting factors, and the cellular elements of the blood that becomes attached to the inner wall of a blood vessel or blood clot) in a blood vessel can obstruct blood flow and cause an infarction with resultant tissue necrosis. An **embolus,** a mass of undissolved matter that breaks off from the thrombus, can travel in the blood vessel and lodge in areas of the body; this can cause death. By contrast, a defect in the blood clotting mechanism may lead to excessive bleeding or hemorrhage, even after a minor injury. Both thrombotic and hemorrhagic disorders can be treated with drugs. The following discussion describes the rationale for use of various groups of therapeutic agents.

PREGNANCY SAFETY

Category	Drug
B	aprotinin, dalteparin, dipyridamole, enoxaparin, ticlopidine, tranexamic acid, urokinase
C	abciximab, alteplase, aminocaproic acid, anistreplase, antiinhibitor coagulant complex, antithrombin III, factor IX, ardeparin, heparin, protamine, reteplase, streptokinase

Pregnancy safety is not established for warfarin and anisindione, but they both cross the placenta and should not be used during pregnancy.

ANTICOAGULANT DRUGS

Anticoagulant drug therapy is primarily prophylactic because these agents act by preventing (1) fibrin deposits, (2) extension of a thrombus, and (3) thromboembolic complications. Although long-term anticoagulant therapy remains controversial, there is evidence that anticoagulant therapy reduces the incidence of thrombosis and therefore prolongs life.

Anticoagulation therapy is focused on preventing intravascular thrombosis by decreasing blood coagulability. This therapy has no direct effect on a blood clot that has already formed or on ischemic tissue injured by an inadequate blood supply because of the clot. The two main groups of anticoagulant drugs are (1) parenteral anticoagulant drugs and (2) oral anticoagulant drugs. For effective anticoagulant therapy, the manner of use for both groups is important. They have been used to complement each other, and in some instances the administration of both a rapidly acting parenteral anticoagulant (heparin) and one of the synthetic oral anticoagulants is started simultaneously. Heparin is usually discontinued as soon as the prothrombin time has been sufficiently reduced and the oral compound is producing a full therapeutic effect. See the box for Food and Drug Administration (FDA) pregnancy safety classifications of the various anticoagulant agents.

PARENTERAL ANTICOAGULANT DRUGS

heparin sodium [hep′ a rin]
(Liquaemin, Hepalean)

Heparin is formed in especially large amounts in the mast cells of the liver, lungs, and intestinal mucosa. The source of heparin for injection is bovine (cattle) lung and the mucosal lining of pig intestines. It is a rapidly acting injectable anticoagulant.

Heparin produces its anticoagulant effect by combining with antithrombin III (heparin cofactor), a naturally occurring anticlotting factor in the plasma. This compound is unrelated to factor III (tissue thromboplastin), a factor in the process of blood coagulation. The binding of heparin with antithrombin III forms a complex that acts at multiple sites in the normal coagulation system, inactivating factors IXa, Xa, XIa, and XIIa. Inactivation of factor Xa of the intrinsic and extrinsic pathways prevents the conversion of prothrombin to thrombin, thereby inhibiting the formation of fibrin from fibrinogen. Furthermore, by preventing the activation of factor XIII (fibrin stabilizing factor), heparin also prevents the formation of a stable fibrin clot. As fibrin is associated with venous thrombi, heparin is useful in preventing venous thrombosis. The drug does not have **fibrinolytic activity.** This means that it will not dissolve existing clots but can prevent the extension of existing clots.

The normal function of antithrombin III is to maintain intravascular fluidity of the blood. Thromboembolism frequently occurs in individuals with acquired or congenital deficiency of this plasma protein. Therefore in the absence of antithrombin III, heparin is unable to perform its anticoagulating effect.

Indications

Heparin is used to prevent and treat all types of thromboses and emboli. It is used prophylactically to prevent blood clotting in surgery of the heart or blood vessels, during blood transfusion, in patients with disseminated intravascular coagulation (DIC), and in the hemodialysis process. It is considered the drug of choice for sudden arterial occlusion because its action is immediate and can be readily reversed if surgery is necessary.

Heparin is superior to the coumarin drugs in preventing pulmonary complications in cases of thrombophlebitis. It is also preferred for the treatment of thrombophlebitis during pregnancy, as it does not cross the placental barrier and is not excreted in breast milk. When rapid anticoagulation is necessary, it is used before the oral anticoagulants (Table 25-1).

TABLE 25-1 Anticoagulant Drugs: Comparison of Characteristics

	Heparin	*Coumarins/Indanediones*
Onset of action	Immediate	Slow (24-48 hr)
Route of administration	Parenteral	Oral
Duration of action	Short (less than 4 hr)	Long (approximately 2-5 days)
Laboratory test for dosage control	APTT, ACT	Prothrombin time
Antidote	Protamine sulfate	Vitamin K, whole blood, or plasma

APTT, activated partial thromboplastin time; ACT, activated clotting time.

Pharmacokinetics

It is administered parenterally because its large molecular size and polarity prevent any gastrointestinal absorption. By intravenous injection its onset of action is immediate. Subcutaneous injection usually results in an onset of action within 20 to 60 minutes. The half-life is dose dependent but averages 1.5 hours (range is 1 to 6 hours). It is highly protein bound, metabolized in the liver, and excreted via the kidneys.

Drug interactions

The following effects may occur when heparin is given with the drugs listed below:

Drug	Possible effect and management
aspirin, sulfinpyrazone (Anturane), nonsteroidal anti-inflammatory drugs (NSAIDs), or other platelet aggregation inhibitors	Increased risk of bleeding is present because of platelet inhibition by these drugs. Also, large doses of aspirin may produce hypoprothrombinemia. All drugs increase the risk of toxicity because of their potential to produce gastrointestinal ulceration and bleeding. Avoid or a potentially serious drug interaction may occur.
cefamandole (Mandol), cefoperazone (Cefobid), cefotetan (Cefotan), plicamycin (Mithracin), or valproic acid (Depakene)	Increased risk of bleeding and hemorrhage is possible with these drugs. These agents can cause hypoprothrombinemia and platelet inhibition. Avoid or a potentially serious drug interaction may occur.
methimazole (Tapazole) or propylthiouracil (PTU)	May produce a hypoprothrombinemic effect which can increase anticoagulant effect of heparin. Avoid or a potentially serious drug interaction may occur.
probenecid (Benemid)	May prolong and enhance heparin's anticoagulant effects. Avoid or a potentially serious drug interaction may occur. If necessary to give concurrently, monitor coagulation tests closely.
Thrombolytics, such as alteplase, (Activase) anistreplase (Eminase) reteplase (Retavase) streptokinase (Streptase) or urokinase (Abbokinase)	Increased risk of bleeding and hemorrhage is possible with this combination. Avoid or a potentially serious drug interaction may occur. Some studies indicate that heparin may be given with low doses of thrombolytic agents via the intracoronary route of administration. Also, heparin may be administered before or after thrombolytic therapy.

Color type indicates an unsafe drug combination.

Side effects and adverse reactions

Bleeding or hemorrhage is the most common adverse effect. Internal signs of bleeding include stomach pain, bloody or black stools, dizziness, persistent headaches, swollen, stiff or painful joints; vomiting, or coughing up of blood. Additional side effects include chest pain, chills, fever, respiratory difficulties, wheezing, rash, pruritus, hives, allergic reaction, anaphylaxis, paresthesia of hands or feet, blue tinge on arms or legs, and thrombocytopenia.

At the site of injection a hematoma or blood accumulation under the skin, pain, or a local skin reaction such as irritation, peeling, or sloughing may occur.

Early signs of heparin overdose includes increased bruising, nosebleeds, or excessive bleeding from minor cuts, wounds, brushing of teeth, or menstrual period.

Warnings

Use with caution in patients with asthma, a history of allergies, mild to moderate liver impairment, or hypertension.

Contraindications

Avoid use in persons with heparin hypersensitivity, cerebral aneurysm, cerebrovascular bleeding, hemorrhage, severe hypertension, hemophilia, peptic ulcer disease, severe liver or kidney disease, and blood dyscrasias, in women after recent childbirth, and in those who have recently had surgery or anesthesia.

Dosage and administration

Dosage is expressed in USP heparin units per milliliter in the United States. In Canada, dosage may be expressed in

USP units or in International Units (IU). USP heparin units are not equivalent to International Units. Because the potency may vary between USP units and International Units, the student should review the current package insert for dosage instructions whenever packages are labeled in International Units. The following recommended dosages will be given in USP units.

Heparin sodium adult dose is 10,000 to 20,000 USP units subcutaneously or 10,000 USP units intravenously initially or 5,000 to 10,000 units intravenously every 4 to 6 hours. Pediatric dose is usually 50 USP units/kg initially, followed by 50 to 100 units/kg every 4 hours.

Heparin dosage is closely monitored with coagulation tests such as the activated partial thromboplastin time (APTT), the activated clotting time (ACT), or other tests as ordered. For consistency it is recommended that a single laboratory be used to monitor a patient receiving heparin therapy.

LOW MOLECULAR WEIGHT (LMW) HEPARINS

The low molecular weight heparins are new antithrombin agents with the potential of being more effective than heparin. They have a longer half-life, require less laboratory monitoring, and are safe and effective for the management of thromboembolic disease (Turpie, 1995). Currently there are three drugs on the market: ardeparin, dalteparin, and enoxaparin.

ardeparin [arde′ pear in] (Normiflo)
dalteparin [dalt′ ta pear in] (Fragmin)
enoxaparin [en ox′ uh pear in] (Lovenox)

Enoxaparin was the first LMW heparin released in the United States for the prevention of postsurgical deep vein thrombosis after hip and knee replacement surgery. The LMW heparins appear to have the advantage of having slightly fewer hemorrhagic complications than standard heparin.

LMW heparins are made by chemically processing regular heparin into fragments that are based on molecular weight. These LMW heparins have a mean molecular weight between 4,000 to 6,000 daltons, while heparin's mean molecular weight ranges between 12,000 to 15,000 daltons. This difference in molecular weight produces an anticoagulant with considerably different properties than heparin. Both types of heparin can inactivate factor Xa, but to inactivate factor IIa (thrombin) requires the larger molecular weight heparin. See Table 25-2 for a comparison of heparin and LMW heparin.

Pharmacokinetics

The LMW heparins are administered subcutaneously and have a very low protein binding ratio; therefore their anticoagulant effect is more predictable. The time to peak serum level is reached in 2 to 4 hours with ardeparin, 4 hours with dalteparin, and 3 to 5 hours with enoxaparin. The elimination half-life for dalteparin is 3 to 5 hours and for enoxaparin is 3-6 hours (half-life not available for ardeparin).

These agents are primarily excreted by the kidney.

Drug interactions with enoxaparin are the same as those for heparin with the exception of methimazole (Tapazole), propylthiouracil, and probenecid (Benemid). Problems with these agents have not been reported. In addition, if enoxaparin is given concurrently with ticlopidine (Ticlid), inhibition of platelets resulting in an increased risk of bleeding may result. Monitor patient closely. Ardeparin and dalteparin drug interactions include using caution when these agents are prescribed with anticoagulants or platelet inhibitors, as the risk of bleeding episodes is increased.

Side effects and adverse reactions

These include local irritation effects such as erythema, hematomas, urticaria, and pain at injection site. Less frequently, thrombocytopenia and bleeding episodes may also occur.

Warnings

Use with caution in patients undergoing any medical procedure that increases the potential of bleeding.

Contraindications

Avoid use in persons with LMW heparin or heparin hypersensitivity, bleeding disorders, severe hypertension,

TABLE 25-2 Comparison of Regular Heparin and Low Molecular Weight Heparin (LMWH)

Properties	*Regular Heparin*	*LMWH*
Molecular weight range	3,000-30,000	1,000-10,000
Mean molecular weight	12,000-15,000	4,000-6,000
Mechanism of action	Inactivates factor Xa and IIa (thrombin)	Inactivates factor Xa
APTT monitoring required	Yes	No
Inhibits platelet function	++++ (high)	++ (medium)
Route of administration	IV, SC	SC only
Protein binding	++++ (high)	+ (low)
Vascular permeability increased	Yes	No
Treatment of drug overdose	Protamine	Protamine

stroke, thrombocytopenia, severe liver or kidney disease, endocarditis, and retinopathy and in those who have recently had surgery.

Dosage and administration

The usual ardeparin dose is 50 anti-Xa units/kg SC every 12 hours for up to 2 weeks or until the patient is mobile. The usual dalteparin dose is 25,000 IU SC 1 to 2 hours before abdominal surgery and then repeated daily for 5 to 10 days afterward, until the patient is mobile. For hip surgery, the dose is 5,000 IU SC the night before surgery and then repeated each evening for 5 to 10 days or until the patient is mobile. The usual enoxaparin dose is 30 mg SC twice a day for 7 to 10 days with first dose administered within 24 hours after surgery. Treatment is continued throughout the postoperative period until the risk for deep vein thrombosis declines.

PARENTERAL ANTICOAGULANT ANTAGONIST

protamine sulfate [proe′ ta meen] (heparin antidote)

Protamine sulfate, a protein-like substance derived from the sperm and mature testes of salmon and other fish, is an antidote for a heparin overdose. Protamine is a very weak anticoagulant alone, but when given in conjunction with heparin a combination is formed that dissociates the heparin–antithrombin III complex, thus reducing the anticoagulant action of heparin. Because protamine is a basic protein (many free amino groups), it is able to combine with the sulfuric acids of heparin and inactivate them.

Indications

Protamine is indicated for the treatment of a severe heparin overdose that has resulted in hemorrhaging. Blood transfusions may also be necessary. It is also used to neutralize the effects of heparin administered during dialysis or cardiac or arterial surgery.

Pharmacokinetics

It is administered intravenously and has an onset of action within 1 minute. Its duration of action is approximately 2 hours.

Side effects and adverse reactions

These include bradycardia, a sudden drop in blood pressure, shock, and dyspnea—all related to the too-rapid administration of protamine. Less often reported are bleeding (caused by protamine overdose or a rebound of heparin activity), hypertension, anaphylaxis, back pain, a feeling of warmth and/or tiredness, flushing, nausea, and vomiting.

Warnings

Use with caution in patients who have been exposed to protamine in the past, including protamine insulin. Protamine antibodies may have developed, which increases the risk of an allergic reaction.

Contraindications

Avoid use in persons with protamine hypersensivitiy.

Dosage and administration

Protamine is administered by slow intravenous injection at a rate of 1 mg/min. One milligram of protamine is necessary to neutralize approximately 100 USP units of heparin. It is recommended that not more than 50 mg of protamine be given in any 10 minute period and no more than 100 mg be administered over a 2 hour period. Close monitoring with blood coagulation tests is required.

ORAL ANTICOAGULANT DRUGS

There are two major types of oral anticoagulant drugs: coumarins and indanediones.

Coumarins

dicumarol [dye koo′ ma role]
warfarin [war′ far in] (Coumadin)

Indanediones

anisindione [an iss in dye′ one] (Miradon)

Both the coumarin and the indanedione derivatives interfere with liver synthesis of the vitamin K-dependent clotting factors. Thus they depress the synthesis of factors X, IX, VII, and II (prothrombin). Factor VII is depleted quickly; the sequential depletion of factors IX, X, and II follows. These agents do not affect established clots but do prevent further extension of formed clots, thereby diminishing the potential for secondary thromboembolic complications.

Indications

The oral anticoagulant drugs are used for the prophylaxis and treatment of deep venous thrombosis and pulmonary thromboembolism. They are also used for the prophylaxis of thromboembolism associated with chronic atrial fibrillation or myocardial infarction. The major advantages of these drugs are that they are effective orally and that they need to be given only once daily after the maintenance dose has been established.

Pharmacokinetics

With the exception of dicumarol, all the oral anticoagulants are well absorbed from the gastrointestinal tract. The absorption of dicumarol from the gastrointestinal tract is slow, incomplete, and erratic. Oral anticoagulants are highly protein bound (99%), metabolized in the liver, and excreted via the kidneys. For additional pharmacokinetics and dosage and administration, see Table 25-3. The elderly are more susceptible to anticoagulant effects; see the Geriatric Implications box for more information on anticoagulants.

Drug interactions

Many drugs interact with the oral anticoagulant drugs. See Box 25-1 for the significant drug interactions.

TABLE 25-3 Oral Anticoagulants: Pharmacokinetics and Dosage and Administration

Generic/Trade Name	Onset of Action (Days)	Duration of Action (Days)	Half-Life (Days)	Dosage and Administration
Coumarins				
dicumarol*	1-5	2-10	1-4 (dose dependent)	Adult: 25-200 mg daily orally as indicated by prothrombin time
warfarin (Coumadin)	.5-3	2-5	1.5-2.5	Adult: 10-15 mg orally for 2-4 days; then 2-10 mg daily as indicated by prothrombin time
Indanediones				
anisindione (Miradon)	2-3	1-3	3-5	Adult: 25-250 mg orally daily as indicated by prothrombin time

*Dicumarol activity is variable.

Side effects and adverse reactions

These may include alopecia, anorexia, abdominal cramps or distress, leukopenia, nausea, vomiting, diarrhea, purple toes syndrome (rare), and kidney damage (rare). Fetal abnormalities and facial anomalies have been reported. If an anticoagulant is necessary during pregnancy, heparin is usually the drug of choice because it does not cross the placenta.

Warnings

Use with caution in patients with a history of severe allergic or anaphylactic reactions, edema, elevated cholesterol or lipid levels, and hypothyroidism, in the elderly, and in unsupervised individuals who are alcoholics, psychotic, senile, or mentally unstable.

Contraindications

Avoid use in persons with known anticoagulant drug hypersensitivity, any medical or surgical condition associated with bleeding (aneurysm, cerebrovascular bleeding, surgery, and severe trauma), blood disorders, severe uncontrolled hypertension, pericarditis, severe diabetics, ulcers, visceral cancer, vitamin C or vitamin K deficiencies, endocarditis, and severe liver or kidney impairment.

ORAL ANTICOAGULANT ANTAGONISTS

Vitamin K

menadiol sodium diphosphate
[men a dye′ ole] (Synkayvite)
phytonadione [fye toe na dye′ one]
(Mephyton, AquaMEPHYTON)

Vitamin K is essential to the hepatic synthesis of prothrombin (factor II) and factors VII, IX, and X. It contributes to the activation of an enzyme necessary to the formation of prothrombin. A deficiency of vitamin K leads to hypoprothrombinemia and hemorrhage.

Indications

Vitamin K is used to prevent and treat hypoprothrombinemia. Prothrombin deficiency may occur because of inadequate absorption of vitamin K from the intestine (usually caused by biliary disease in which bile fails to enter the intestine) or because of destruction of intestinal organisms, which may occur with antibiotic therapy. It is also seen in the newborn, in which case it is probably caused by the fact that the intestinal organisms have not yet become established. It may result from therapy with certain medications such as salicylates, sulfonamides, quinine, quinidine, or broad-spectrum antibiotics.

Vitamin K is useful only in conditions in which the prolonged bleeding time is caused by a low concentration of prothrombin in the blood and not by damaged liver cells. Vitamin K is routinely administered to newborns to help prevent hemorrhage. Although prothrombin levels may be normal at birth, they decline until about the sixth to the eighth day, when the liver is able to form prothrombin. Phytonadione is usually the preferred agent.

Vitamin K is also indicated in the preoperative preparation of individuals with deficient prothrombin, particularly those with obstructive jaundice. In addition, it is given as an antidote for overdosage of oral anticoagulants.

It is important to measure prothrombin activity of the blood frequently when the patient is receiving a preparation of vitamin K. Parenteral preparations should be administered if intestinal absorption is impaired. Natural vitamin K is normally synthesized by the intestinal flora. When synthetic forms of vitamin K are administered, the absorption is good, but phytonadione requires the presence of bile salts.

Pharmacokinetics

The onset of action for menadiol sodium diphosphate injection is 8 to 24 hours, for oral phytonadione it is 6 to 12 hours, and for the injectable form it is 1 to 2 hours. Vitamin K is metabolized in the liver and excreted via the kidneys and in the bile.

Drug interactions

When vitamin K is given concurrently with the oral anticoagulants, a decrease in the anticoagulation effect is reported. If other hemolytics are used concurrently with vita-

GERIATRIC IMPLICATIONS

Anticoagulants

The elderly may be more susceptible to the effects of anticoagulants, such as warfarin (Coumadin) and dicumarol; thus a lower maintenance dose is usually recommended for the geriatric patient along with very close supervision and monitoring.

The primary adverse effects of excessive drug usage are prolonged bleeding from gums when brushing teeth or from small shaving cuts, excessive or easy skin bruising, blood in urine or stools, and unexplained nosebleeds. These may be early signs of overdose that indicate the need for medical intervention.

Caution patients to carry an identification card indicating the use of an anticoagulant. Also, remind patients to always consult their prescriber before starting any new drug, including OTC medications and vitamins, or if changing a medication dose or when any drug product is discontinued. Many medications can change the effects of an anticoagulant in the body.

Be aware that administration of concurrent drug therapy that may induce gastric irritation increases the risk for gastrointestinal bleeding. Drugs such as the nonsteroidal antiinflammatory agents (NSAIDs such as ibuprofin, indomethacin) that are commonly prescribed for the elderly person often cause gastrointestinal effects.

Alcohol consumption can alter the effect of this medication in the body. Individuals should be instructed to avoid alcohol or at the least limit their daily alcohol intake to one alcoholic drink a day. Alcohol may cause liver damage, which increases the individual's sensitivity to anticoagulants (*USP DI*, 1998.)

The healthcare professional should be aware that diet can interfere with the anticoagulant effect. In a previously stabilized person, vitamin C deficiency, chronic malnutrition, diarrhea, or other illnesses may result in an increased anticoagulant effect, while increased intake of green leafy vegetables (such as broccoli, cabbage, collard greens, lettuce, spinach, and others) or the consumption of a nutritional supplement or multiple vitamin containing vitamin K can result in decreased anticoagulant effectiveness.

min K, especially menadiol, the potential for toxic side effects may increase

Side effects and adverse reactions

Those reported are facial flushing, taste alterations, and redness or pain at the injection site.

Warnings

Use with caution in patients with glucose-6-phosphate dehydrogenase (G6PD) deficiency as menadiol may increase the potential for erythrocyte hemolysis.

Contraindications

Avoid use in persons with vitamin K analog hypersensivitiy and liver function impairment.

Dosage and administration

The dose of menadiol (vitamin K) as a nutritional supplement for hypoprothrombinemia is 5 mg/day orally or 5 to 15 mg IM or SC once or twice daily. As an antidote for drug-induced hypoprothrombinemia, the oral dose is 5 to 10 mg daily; the intramuscular or subcutaneous dose is 5 to 15 mg PO or IM daily.

THROMBOLYTIC AGENTS

Thrombolytic (fibrinolytic) drugs are used to treat acute thromboembolic disorders. Unlike anticoagulants, they dissolve clots and are used in a hospital setting only by healthcare providers who are experienced in the management of diseases caused by thrombosis. These agents alter the hemostatic capability of the patient more profoundly than does anticoagulant therapy. Consequently, when bleeding occurs, it is more severe and very difficult to control.

alteplase [al ti plase′] (Activase)
anistreplase [an eye′ strep lase] (Eminase)
reteplase [re ti plase′] (Retavase)
streptokinase [strep toe kye′ nase] (Streptase)
urokinase [yoor oh kin′ ase] (Abbokinase)

These agents dissolve clots via the endogenous fibrinolytic system. All five drugs have similar biochemical mechanisms of action on the fibrinolytic system: converting plasminogen in the blood to plasmin. Plasmin, a fibrinolytic enzyme, digests or dissolves fibrin clots wherever they exist and can be reached by plasmin. Streptokinase is a key drug because it was the first thrombolytic agent released. Alteplase, streptokinase, and urokinase are indicated for the treatment of acute pulmonary thromboembolism; currently only streptokinase is indicated for the treatment of an acute, deep venous thrombosis (USP DI, 1998). All five drugs can be used to treat an acute coronary arterial thrombosis associated with an acute myocardial infarction.

Pharmacokinetics

These agents are administered intravenously and/or intraarterially. Alteplase has an elimination half-life of 35 minutes; streptokinase and urokinase half-lives are 23 minutes and up to 20 minutes, respectively. Anistreplase, which is an acylated complex of streptokinase and human plasminogen, has a long half-life of approximately 90 minutes. The peak effect after IV injection is from 20 minutes to 2 hours. Duration of the thrombolysis effect is approximately 4 hours for alteplase, streptokinase, and urokinase; anistreplase thrombolysis effect occurs in 6 hours. Reteplase has an elimination half-life of 13 to 16 minutes and usually reaches a peak effect (fibrinogen levels decreased to less than 100 mg/dl) within 2 hours; mean fibrinogen levels return to

BOX 25-1 Significant Drug Interactions of Oral Anticoagulants

The oral anticoagulants have a great potential for causing drug interactions; therefore patients must be cautioned against taking any drug and/or making significant dietary changes without prior consultation with their prescriber. Check a current USP-DI for major drug interactions.

Agents That May Increase the Anticoagulant Effect, Often Necessitating a Dosage Reduction

allopurinol	clofibrate	indomethacin	propylthiouracil
amiodarone	danazol	mefenamic acid	quinidine
anabolic steroids	dextran	meperidine	salicylates
androgens	dextrothyroxine	methimazole	streptokinase
aspirin	diflunisal	metronidazole	sulfinpyrazone
azlocillin	dipyridamole†	mezlocillin	sulfonamides
cefamandole	disulfiram	nalidixic acid	sulindac
cefoperazone	erythromycins	phenytoin‡	thyroid hormone
chloral hydrate*	fenoprofen	piperacillin	ticarcillin
chloramphenicol	gemfibrozil	plicamycin	urokinase
cimetidine			

Agents That May Decrease the Anticoagulant Effect, Often Necessitating an Increase in Anticoagulant Dosage

oral antidiabetic agents§	colestipol	ethchlorvynol	primidone
barbiturates	contraceptives, oral	glutethimide	rifampin
carbamazepine	estramustine	griseofulvin	vitamin K
cholestyramine	estrogens		

*Usually occurs during first 2 weeks of therapy. With chronic concurrent therapy, the anticoagulant effect may return to normal or be decreased.
†With doses of dipyridamole >400 mg/day.
‡Increased anticoagulant effect occurs initially. With chronic concurrent therapy decreased activity may occur. May also see a decrease in metabolism of phenytoin, possibly leading to increased serum levels and toxicity.
§May initially increase anticoagulant effects, but with long-term concurrent therapy, such effects may decrease. Also, the decrease in metabolism of the antidiabetic agent may increase serum levels and cause prolonged half-life, hypoglycemia, and toxicity.

previous levels within 48 hours. It is metabolized in the liver and excreted by the kidneys.

Drug interactions

The following effects may occur when a thrombolytic agent is given with the drugs listed below:

Drugs	Possible effect and management
Anticoagulants, oral, enoxaparin (Lovenox),or heparin	Concurrent use increases hemorrhage risk, but the combination of heparin and thrombolytic therapy is often prescribed for treatment of an acute coronary arterial occlusion. Monitor closely if concurrent therapies are administered.
Antifibrinolytic drugs such as aminocaproic acid (Amicar), aprotinin (Trasylol), and tranexamic acid (Cyklokapron)	These agents may antagonize the action of the thrombolytic agents. Avoid concurrent drug administration.
cefoperazone (Cefobid), cefotetan (Cefotan), plicamycin (Mithracin), and valproic acid (Depakene)	Concurrent use with these medications which cause hypoprothrombinemia plus, plicamycin, and valproic acid may also inhibit platelet aggregation, which may result in an increased potential for severe bleeding. Avoid or a potentially serious drug interactions may occur.
NSAIDs, sulfinpyrazone (Anturane), ticlopidine (Ticlid)	Concurrent use may increase the risk of bleeding episodes. This therapy is not recommended with the exception of aspirin when indicated for an acute myocardial infarction.

Color type indicates an unsafe drug combination.

Side effects and adverse reactions

These include bleeding episodes, fever, headache, nausea, vomiting, hypotension, dysrhythmias, allergic reaction, facial flushing, arthralgia, and, perhaps, respiratory difficulties. With streptokinase and urokinase these include stomach pain or swelling, backache, bloody urine and stools, constipation, severe headaches, dizziness, swollen, stiff or painful joints and/or muscles, bleeding, tachycardia, bradycardia, and fever, which are seen more frequently with streptokinase than with urokinase.

Warnings

Use with caution in patients with a history of cerebrovascular disease, ulcers, recent bleeding episodes, uncontrolled hypertension, recent trauma, and acute pericarditis. In addition, for anistreplase and streptokinase allergic reactions have been reported. Also, use caution if the patient has received either of these drugs within the past year or has had a recent streptococcal infection, as both of these drugs are made from a streptococcal culture.

Contraindications

Avoid use in persons with bleeding disorders and in persons who have had an organ biopsy, severe gastrointestinal or other bleeding, or major surgery or had a child within the past 10 days. Avoid use in persons with bacterial endocarditis or mitral stenosis with atrial fibrillation, or who had a neurosurgical procedure performed more than 2 months earlier. In addition, for alteplase, avoid use if major signs of an cranial infarct or a severe neurological deficit are present.

Dosage and administration

In an acute coronary artery thrombosis evolving into a transmural myocardial infarction, thrombolytic therapy is most effective when started within 3 to 4 hours after the onset of symptoms. Usually alteplase is given at 1.25 mg/kg IV in divided doses over 3 hours for patients weighing less than 65 kg, or 100 mg intravenously for patients 65 kg or over (in divided doses over 3 hours). See current literature for recommended dosages over each of the 3 hours.

For reteplase, the usual adult dose is 10 units given IV over 2 minutes, repeated in 30 minutes. The dose of anistreplase is 30 units in solution administered by IV injection over 2 to 5 minutes.

For streptokinase, the dose is 1,500,000 IU IV administered within an hour. Smaller doses of 20,000 IU initially followed by an additional 2000 IU/min are used for intraarterial administration. Urokinase 6000 IU/min is administered intraarterially until the artery is opened. For other indications, refer to a current package insert or USP DI for dosing information.

antithrombin III (human) [an′ tee throm bin] (ATnativ)

Antithrombin III is prepared from pooled human plasma of healthy donors. It is indicated for the treatment or prevention of thromboembolism associated with a hereditary antithrombin III deficiency. Heparin and antithrombin III will enhance each other's effects; thus they have been administered concurrently, depending on the situation.

Drug interactions

No significant interactions are reported.

Side effects and adverse reactions

These include diuresis, hypotension, chest pain, fever, hives, and shortness of breath in some persons.

Dosage and administration

The usual adult dose is 50 to 100 IU/min IV, titrated to desired effect.

ANTIHEMOPHILIC AGENTS

Hemophilia is a hereditary disorder caused by a deficiency of one or more plasma protein clotting factors. This condition usually leads to persistent and uncontrollable hemorrhage after even minor injury. The symptoms include excessive bleeding from wounds and hemorrhage into joints, the urinary tract, and, on occasion, the central nervous system. There are two types of hemophilia: hemophilia A, the classic type in which factor VIII activity is deficient, and hemophilia B, or Christmas disease, in which factor IX complex activity is deficient. In recent years, a correct diagnosis of the coagulation disorder has led to specific factor replacement therapy, and this medical advance has resulted in effective management of the patient at home.

factor VIII (Koate-HP, Recombinate)

Factor VIII, or the antihemophilic factor, is a glycoprotein necessary for hemostasis and blood clotting. In the intrinsic pathway of the coagulation mechanism, the antihemophilic factor is required for the transformation of prothrombin to thrombin. In the treatment or prevention of hemophilia A, factor VIII administration is based on replacing the missing plasma clotting factor to control and prevent bleeding.

Pharmacokinetics

When administered intravenously, factor VIII has a distribution half-life of 2.4 to 8 hours and an elimination half-life of 8.4 to 19.3 hours. The time to peak effect is between 1 to 2 hours after IV administration.

Drug interactions

No significant drug interactions are reported with factor VIII.

Side effects and adverse reactions

Mild to severe allergic reactions have been reported, such as bronchospasm, elevated temperature, chills, or rash. Other side effects and adverse reactions, which may be related to the rate of infusion, include headache, increased heart rate, tingling of fingers, fainting, lethargy, sedation, hypotension, back pain, nausea or vomiting, visual disturbances, and chest constriction.

Warnings

Use caution in patients with sensitivity to mouse, hamster, or bovine proteins.

Contraindications

Avoid use in persons with antihemophilic factor hypersensitivity.

Dosage and administration

Dosage of factor VIII must be individualized according to the person's weight, severity of the deficiency, and the amount of blood loss. During hemorrhage, the dosage is adjusted so that a level of 25% of normal levels of factor VIII can produce hemostasis. Patients who develop inhibitors to factor VIII may not respond to factor VIII therapy. After careful evaluation of the individual, the administration of antiinhibitor coagulant complex, which reduces factor VIII inhibitors, may be indicated to correct this condition.

antiinhibitor coagulant complex

(Autoplex, Feiba VH Immuno)

Antiinhibitor coagulant complex is made from pooled human plasma. It contains variable quantities of clotting factors and kinin system factors and has been standardized to help correct clotting time in factor VIII-deficient individuals or to treat factor VIII-deficient individuals who have plasma-containing inhibitors to factor VIII.

Indications

Antiinhibitor coagulant complex is indicated for patients with factor VIII inhibitors who are bleeding or being prepared for surgery. Approximately 10% of factor VIII-deficient individuals have inhibitors to factor VIII present. Patients with factor VIII inhibitor levels greater than 10 Bethesda units are usually treated with this product.

Drug interactions

Concurrent administration with epsilon-aminocaproic acid or tranexamic acid is not recommended.

Side effects and adverse reactions

Allergic reactions and hypersensitivity (fever, chills, rash, and hypotension) reactions have been reported. If antiinhibitor coagulant complex is administered too rapidly, the recipient may experience flushing, headache, and changes in blood pressure and heart rate. These are indications to slow the rate of flow or stop the infusion until the symptoms disappear.

Dosage and administration

Antiinhibitor coagulant complex is administered only by intravenous infusion. The recommended dose varies from 25 to 100 units/kg depending on the site and severity of the hemorrhage. Check a current package insert or USP DI for specific recommendations.

factor IX complex (Konÿne 80, Proplex T)

Factor IX complex is a purified plasma fraction prepared from pooled units of plasma. It contains factors II, VII, IX, and X, which are known as the vitamin K coagulation factors.

Indications

This agent is used for therapy in individuals with a deficiency of these factors during hemorrhage or before surgery. It is also indicated for patients with hemophilia B in whom factor IX (Christmas disease) is deficient. Factor IX complex is used to prevent or control bleeding in individuals with factor IX deficiency. It is also used to treat patients with bleeding problems who have inhibitors to factor VIII and will reverse hemorrhage induced by coumarin anticoagulants.

Pharmacokinetics

Factor IX has an elimination half-life of 18 to 32 hours; its time to peak effect after IV administration is 10 to 30 minutes.

Drug interactions

No significant drug interactions are reported.

Side effects and adverse reactions

These include chills and fever, especially when large doses are given. Also, if the intravenous infusion is given too rapidly, headache, flushing, rash, nausea, vomiting, sedation, lethargy, elevated temperature, and tingling have been reported. The infusion should be stopped; in most persons it can be resumed at a much slower rate.

Thrombosis and DIC have occurred as a result of the administration of factor IX. Myocardial infarction, pulmonary embolism, and anaphylaxis have also been reported. It should not be used in individuals undergoing elective surgery, since they are at a greater risk for thrombosis.

Warnings

Use caution in patients with trauma injuries and severe liver impairment, and in those who have recently had surgery.

Contraindications

Avoid use in persons with factor IX, hamster protein or mouse protein hypersensitivity, DIC, and hyperfibrinoytic conditions and those with a history of thromboembolism.

Dosage and administration

Factor IX should be administered slowly by intravenous injection or by intravenous infusion. The dosage is individualized according to the patient's coagulation assay, which is performed before treatment. Check current references for specific dosing recommendations.

Antiplatelet Agents

The **antiplatelet drugs** or drugs that inhibit platelet aggregation include aspirin, dipyridamole (Persantine), ticlopidine (Ticlid), and abciximab (ReoPro). Aspirin inhibits cyclooxygenase, an enzyme necessary for thromboxane A_2 synthesis. As mentioned previously, thromboxane A_2 promotes platelet aggregation and vasoconstriction, and thus aspirin suppresses these actions (see Chapter 8). The other three drugs are discussed in this chapter.

The composition of arterial thrombi is primarily platelet aggregates; venous thrombi are usually composed of fibrin and red blood cells. Therefore the anticoagulant drugs are used to reduce the risks or complications of venous thrombi, whereas the antiplatelet agents are used for arterial thrombi.

dipyridamole [dye peer id′ a mole] (Persantine)

The mechanism of action for dipyridamole has been postulated to be inhibition of (1)thromboxane A_2 formation, a potent platelet activator; (2) phosphodiesterase, which results in an increase in cyclic-3′, 5′ monophosphate in the platelets; and (3) red blood cell uptake of adenosine, a platelet aggregation inhibitor.

Indications

Dipyridamole is used in combination with coumarin anticoagulants for the prevention of postsurgical thromboembolic complications after cardiac valve replacement.

Pharmacokinetics

After an oral dose, dipyridamole reaches peak serum levels in about 75 minutes. It is highly protein bound, metabolized in the liver, and excreted in bile.

Drug interactions

The following effects may occur when dipyridamole is given with the drugs listed below:

Drug	Possible effect and management
Oral anticoagulants, heparin	Concurrent use may increase risk of bleeding. While the combination of dipyridamole (up to 400 mg/day) and oral anticoagulants have been used together without affecting bleeding time, careful monitoring of prothrombin time is recommended.
aspirin and other salicylates and platelet inhibitors	Combined use increases the potential for bleeding episodes. Avoid or a potentially serious drug interaction may occur. Although the combination of aspirin and dipyridamole has been used commonly for additional therapeutic effects, studies have not proven the combination to more effective than aspirin alone (USP DI, 1998).
cefoperazone (Cefobid), cefotetan (Cefotan), plicamycin (Mithracin), or valproic acid (Depakene)	Concurrent use increases the risk of bleeding and hemorrhage. These agents can cause hypoprothrombinemia while plicamycin and valproic acid may also inhibit platelet aggregation. Avoid or a potentially serious drug interaction may occur.
Thrombolytic agents	Concurrent use increases risk of severe bleeding and hemorrhage. Avoid or a potentially serious drug interaction may occur.

Color type indicates an unsafe drug combination.

Side effects and adverse reactions

These include headache, dizziness, abdominal upset, rash, allergic reaction, angina pectoris, blood pressure lability (hypertension, hypotension), and tachycardia.

Warnings

Use caution in patients with unstable angina and hypotension.

Contraindications

Avoid use in persons with dipyridamole hypersensitivity and asthma.

Dosage and administration

The usual adult (adjunctive) dose is 75 to 100 mg PO four times daily.

ticlopidine [tye kloe′ pih deen] (Ticlid)

Ticlopidine is believed to produce an irreversible, adenosine diphosphate-induced inhibition of platelet-fibrinogen binding.

Indications

Ticlopidine is indicated to decrease the risk of stroke in patients who have had warnings of a thrombotic stroke or those who have had a thrombotic stroke.

Pharmacokinetics

Administered orally, it reaches peak serum levels in about 2 hours and peak effect with repeated dosing in 8 to 11 days. It is metabolized by the liver and excreted by the kidneys.

Drug interactions

With the exception of the cefamandole group of drugs, all other drug interactions are the same as those for dipyridamole above.

Side effects and adverse reactions

These include nausea, stomach cramps, bloating or gas, dizziness, skin rash, diarrhea, tinnitus, bleeding, pruritus, neutropenia, agranulocytosis, thrombocytopenia, purpura, hepatitis, and Stevens-Johnson syndrome.

Warnings

Use caution in patients planning dental or elective surgery (discontinue drug 10-14 days prior to elective surgery).

Contraindications

Avoid use in persons with ticlopidine hypersensitivity, hemophilia, bleeding disorders, current bleeding, and severe liver function impairment.

Dosage and administration

The recommended adult dose is 250 mg PO twice daily with food.

abciximab [ab six' i mab] (ReoPro)

Abciximab, a monoclonal antibody fragment, inhibits platelet aggregation by binding or blocking the glycoprotein (GPIIb/IIIa) receptor involved in the pathway for platelet aggregation.

Indications

Abciximab is indicated as adjunct therapy (to aspirin and heparin) for prevention of acute cardiac vessel ischemic complications in persons undergoing percutaneous transluminal coronary angioplasty or atherectomy.

Pharmacokinetics

Abciximab has a half-life of 30 minutes and a duration of action of 48 hours. It appears that this drug is catabolized like other natural proteins and excreted via the kidneys.

Drug interactions

The following effects may occur when abciximab is given with the drugs listed below:

Drug	Possible effect and management
Anticoagulants, oral	Administering abciximab within a week of the oral anticoagulants is not recommended, because of the increased risk of bleeding (exception, if the prothrombin time is < 1.2 the control).
dipyridamole (Persantine), platelet inhibitors, ticlopidine (Ticlid)	Monitor closely if administered concurrently as the risk of bleeding is increased.
dextran	Concurrent usage results in increased risk of bleeding and hemorrhage. Avoid or a potentially serious drug interactions may occur.
Thrombolytic medications	Combined use may result in increased risk of bleeding. Monitor closely if combination or sequential drug therapy is used.

Color type indicates an unsafe drug combination.

Side effects and adverse reactions

These include visual changes, confusion, hypesthesia, nausea, vomiting, major bleeding episodes, and hypotension.

Warnings

Use caution in pregnant patients and in the elderly.

Contraindications

Avoid use in persons with abciximab hypersensitivity,

Dosage and administration

The recommended adult dose is 0.25 mg/kg administered 10 to 60 minutes before the procedure. The maintenance dose by IV infusion is 0.01 mg/min for up to 12 hours.

HEMOSTATIC AGENTS

Hemostatic agents are compounds used to hasten clot formation to reduce bleeding. The purpose of these agents is to control rapid loss of blood.

Systemic Hemostatics

aminocaproic acid [a mee noe ka proe' ik] (Amicar)

Aminocaproic acid is a synthetic compound that inhibits fibrinolysis when excessive bleeding occurs. This drug acts as a competitive antagonist of plasminogen, therefore reducing the conversion of plasminogen to plasmin or fibrinolysin. To a lesser degree, it directly inhibits plasmin (fibrinolysin) by noncompetitive mechanisms.

Indications

Aminocaproic acid is used in the treatment of hyperfibrinolysis-induced hemorrhage such as fibrinolytic bleeding after heart surgery, prostatectomy, and nephrectomy and for hematologic disorders such as aplastic anemia, hepatic cirrhosis, and neoplastic disease states. Although not an approved indication, it has also been used as a specific antidote for an overdose of thrombolytic drugs.

Pharmacokinetics

Aminocaproic acid is absorbed orally and reaches a peak concentration within 2 hours. The therapeutic serum concentration is 130 μg/ml to inhibit systemic hyperfibrinolysis, or 150 to 300 μg/ml to prevent recurrent subarachnoid hemorrhage. It is excreted mainly by the kidneys.

Drug interactions

No significant drug interactions are reported although the healthcare professional should be aware that estrogens and oral estrogen-containing contraceptives increase the possibility for thrombus formation and that thrombolytic agents and aminocaproic acid are antagonistic to each other.

Side effects and adverse reactions

These include nausea, diarrhea, menstrual difficulties, increased weakness, weakness in muscles or severe muscle pain, a decrease in urination, edema of face, feet, or lower legs, unusual weight gain, slow or irregular heart rate, abdominal pain, rash, stuffy nose, tinnitus, bloodshot eyes, and thrombosis.

Warnings

Use with caution in patients with cardiac disease, hematuria, a history of thrombosis, and liver or kidney impairment.

Contraindications

Avoid use in persons with aminocaproic acid hypersensitivity and current problems with intravascular clotting.

Dosage and administration

The adult recommended dose is 5 g orally or parenterally (IV infusion) initially, followed by 1 g/hr for up to 8 hours or until the desired response is achieved. Maximum dose is 30 g/24 hr. The pediatric dose (oral or parenteral) is 100 mg/kg of body weight the first hour, followed by 33.3 mg/kg/hr up to 18 g/m^2/24 hr.

tranexamic acid [tran ex am′ ik] (Cyklokapron)

Tranexamic acid is a competitive inhibitor of plasminogen activation; at high doses, it is a noncompetitive inhibitor of plasmin. Its effects are similar to those of aminocaproic acid, but it is approximately 5 to 10 times more potent in vitro.

Indications

Tranexamic acid is used after dental surgery in patients with hemophilia to reduce or prevent bleeding episodes.

Pharmacokinetics

The peak plasma level (8 μg/ml after a 1 g dose) is reached 3 hours after oral administration. The duration of action in serum is 7 to 8 hours, and excretion is by the kidneys.

Drug interactions

No significant drug interactions have been reported although the same interactions mentioned for aminocaproic acid are possible with tranexamic acid.

Side effects and adverse reactions

These include nausea, vomiting, diarrhea, visual disturbance, thrombosis, hypotension, thrombosis, thromboembolism, and menstrual discomfort.

Warnings

Use with caution in women who are breastfeeding.

Contraindications

Avoid use in persons with tranexamic acid hypersensitivity, color vision defects, hematuria, subarachnoid hemorrhage, a history of thrombosis, and kidney function impairment.

Dosage and administration

The adolescent and adult dose before dental surgery in persons with hemophilia is 25 mg/kg PO three or four times daily, starting a day before the planned dental procedure. Clotting factors VIII or IX should also be given before surgery. Postsurgically the dose is 25 mg/kg PO three or four times daily for 2 to 8 days. By injection the dose is 10 mg/kg IV before surgery and 10 mg/kg postsurgically three or four times daily for 2 to 8 days. The parenteral postsurgical dose is usually reserved for persons unable to take the oral product.

aprotinin [aye pro′ tin in] (Trasylol)

Aprotinin is a proteinase inhibitor obtained from bovine lung that directly prevents fibrinolysis by inhibiting plasmin and kallikrein, an enzyme of the renal cortex.

Indications

It is used in cardiopulmonary bypass surgery to reduce blood loss and the need for blood transfusions.

Pharmacokinetics

Aprotinin is administered intravenously and is rapidly distributed in extracellular space with a terminal half-life between 5 and 10 hours. It is slowly metabolized by lysosomes in the kidneys and excreted primarily in urine.

Drug interactions

Concurrent administration of aprotinin with a thrombolytic agent may result in antagonistic effects.

Side effects and adverse reactions

These are rare but include allergic type reactions (skin rash, respiratory difficulties, nausea, tachycardia, hypotension, and bronchospasms) and anaphylaxis.

Warnings

Use with caution in patients with a history of allergies.

Contraindications

Avoid use in persons who had previous aprotinin therapy as reexposure increases the risk for allergic reactions. Also avoid in patients undergoing surgery of the aortic arch, especially if the person is older than 65 years of age as instances of renal failure and fatalities have been reported.

Dosage and administration

The recommended adult dose is 10,000 kallekrein inhibiting units (KIU) (1 ml) as a test IV dose first, administered at least 10 minutes before the loading dose. If no allergic type reaction occurs, all other dosages should be administered via a central venous line, and no other medications should be given in this line. See a current package insert or USP DI for dosing recommendations.

Topical Hemostatics

Absorbable Gelatin Sponge (Gelfoam)

Absorbable gelatin sponge is specially prepared nonantigenic gelatin capable of holding many times its weight in whole blood. It is used in thin strips to control capillary bleeding and may be left in place in a surgical wound because it is completely absorbed in 4 to 6 weeks. It should be well moistened with isotonic saline solution or thrombin solution before it is applied to a bleeding surface. Its presence does not induce excessive scar formation. Sterile technique must be used to avoid infection.

When inserted into cavities or tissue spaces, the gelatin sponge reduces bleeding by acting as a tampon. The contact with the sponge damages platelets, liberating the thromboplastin needed for clot formation. This product completely dissolves within 2 to 5 days when applied to bleeding areas on skin or in the nose, rectum, or vagina.

It is indicated in surgical procedures as an adjunct to hemostasis when bleeding is not controlled by ligature or when such methods are impractical. It is also used by dentists to aid in hemostasis.

Insertion of the gelatin sponge in the prostatic cavity promotes hemostasis in open prostatic surgery. The gelatin sponge may provide a site for infection. Monitor the surgical incision and implantation site closely for redness, swelling, or discomfort, as well as for signs of recurrent bleeding.

No significant drug interactions have been reported. This product is available in different sizes and diameters. Application instructions and size depend on the area to be treated.

Absorbable Gelatin Film (Gelfilm)

A sterile absorbable gelatin film (Gelfilm) is also available for specific indications, as in neurosurgery or thoracic or ocular surgery. When it is implanted in tissues, the rate of absorption could range from 2 to 5 months, depending on the site of implantation and the size of the film implanted. This product is useful as a dural substitute (neurosurgery) or to repair pleural defects during thoracic surgery.

Absorbable Gelatin Powder (Gelfoam)

A sterile absorbable gelatin powder (Gelfoam) is also available to promote hemostasis. This powder can be made into a paste to control bleeding from bone areas when standard procedures such as ligatures are ineffective or not practical. It is also used to treat chronic leg ulcers and decubitus ulcers.

Oxidized Cellulose (Oxycel, Surgicel)

Oxidized cellulose is a specially treated form of surgical gauze or cotton that exerts a hemostatic effect but is absorbable when buried in the tissues. The hemostatic action is caused by the formation of an artificial clot by cellulosic acid. Absorption of oxidized cellulose occurs between the second and the seventh days after implantation, although absorption of large amounts of blood-soaked material may take 6 weeks or longer. Oxidized cellulose is valuable in controlling bleeding for surgery of organs such as the liver, pancreas, spleen, kidney, thyroid, and prostate. Its hemostatic action is not increased by the addition of other hemostatic agents. It should not be used as a surface dressing except for the control of bleeding, because cellulosic acid inhibits the growth of epithelial tissue. It also interferes with bone regeneration, so it should not be implanted in fractures.

No significant drug interactions are reported. Do not moisten it, and use sterile techniques in applying or inserting the cellulose. Serious adverse reactions are related to site of application, amount used, and pressure applied to blood vessel or specific area. Careful application and monitoring are necessary to reduce complications such as obstruction, necrosis, and stenosis. When used after nasal polyp removal or hemorrhoidectomy, a burning sensation has been reported. Headache, stinging, and sneezing may also occur.

Microfibrillar Collagen Hemostat (Avitene)

This is an absorbable topical hemostatic substance that, when placed on a bleeding surface, will attract platelets and platelet aggregation in the area, forming thrombi. It is used as an adjunct to hemostasis during surgery when ligature or standard procedures are ineffective or impractical.

Adhesions, allergic or foreign body reactions, hematomas, or infections such as abscesses may occur. Monitor the patient closely because these conditions may cause serious problems. No significant drug interactions have been reported.

Generally, Avitene is applied directly on the source of bleeding in a dry form. Do not moisten or wet this substance and do not resterilize it. Apply pressure over the area with a dry sponge for a minute or more. Use dry forceps to handle it because it will adhere to wet gloves or instruments. Do not use gloved fingers to apply the necessary pressure.

Thrombin (Thrombinar, Thrombostat)

Thrombin is a hemostatic agent prepared as a sterile powder obtained from bovine prothrombin that has been treated with thromboplastin in the presence of calcium. Thrombin catalyzes the conversion of fibrinogen to fibrin. It has several additional mechanisms, which may include stimulating the release, reaction, and aggregation of platelets. It is used topically to treat capillary bleeding. It has also been used during various surgeries with absorbable gelatin sponge for hemostasis.

Fever and an allergic type of reaction have been reported

when thrombin was used for epistaxis. No significant drug interactions are reported.

Thrombin may be applied topically as a powder or solution. Concentration of the preparation varies with its use; see the package insert.

BLOOD AND BLOOD COMPONENTS

The bloodstream is the main mode of transport and distribution in the body. As such, it functions to deliver vital nutrients, water, and oxygen from the digestive and respiratory systems to all body parts. Wastes are retrieved for excretion by the bloodstream. In the kidneys, the bloodstream provides the hydrostatic pressure necessary to create urine as an excretory vehicle for those waste products. It conveys hormones from endocrine glands and enzymes, vitamins, buffers, and other biochemical substances to target areas. The bloodstream buffers and regulates the body's heat exchange processes by absorbing and transferring core body heat to the surface for dissipation, and it buffers the body's acid-base balance. The bloodstream also carries components such as platelets, blood cells, and antibodies to sites where a sudden need for these exists, as in hemorrhage, inflammation, or infection.

It creates oncotic or colloid osmotic pressure to regulate the volume of interstitial fluids. It also transports therapeutic additives such as medications, fluids, electrolytes, and nutrients to their respective sites of action.

Abnormal States of Blood Components

Normally, a thrifty bodily balance is maintained between the production and loss, attrition, or excretion of all components that comprise the bloodstream. Pathologic conditions result from a disturbance in production or an excessive loss or excretion of one or more components. Hemorrhage results in a generally impoverished bloodstream and may significantly alter many body functions. Impaired production or increased destruction of any one component may impinge on one or more functions. All this is a matter of degree. If the impairment is minor or is detected early, correction of the cause and replenishment by natural or therapeutic means may restore functioning.

Naturally harmful or foreign substances also may build up in the bloodstream when excretory systems fail (e.g., renal failure) or when metabolizing capabilities fail (e.g., liver failure). Some examples of abnormal states of blood components follow.

Depending on the individual's size and preexisting blood integrity, acute whole blood loss of more than 500 ml is manifested by signs of anemia. Chronic, gradual, unnoticed blood loss from gastrointestinal tract malignancy, ulcers, or hemorrhoids may be compensated for naturally, or iron deficiency anemia may develop. Signs of anemia usually reflect the true importance of red blood cell loss. Deficiencies in intake or functioning of certain essential nutritional elements may result in iron deficiency anemia or one of the megaloblastic anemias, which usually are caused by deficiencies in vitamin B_{12} or folic acid. A pathologic overabundance of erythrocytes can be compensation for long-standing hypoxia from pulmonary or cardiac disease, certain tumors, or polycythemia vera. Delayed or disordered production of erythrocytes (aplastic anemia) may result from disorders of the reticuloendothelial system, primarily the bone marrow, which is responsible for their systematic production. The bone marrow is particularly vulnerable to certain drugs, poisons, and antineoplastic agents. On the other hand, too-rapid destruction of erythrocytes can lead to hemolytic anemia.

Leukocytes also are lost in hemorrhage, but reductions in their numbers most often are associated with certain specific conditions. Each of the five types of white blood cells—neutrophils, eosinophils, basophils, lymphocytes, and monocytes—is associated with different disorders. For example, abnormally low neutrophil counts are associated with certain aplastic diseases, as well as with acute reactions to drugs such as sulfonamides, propylthiouracil, and chloramphenicol. Excessively high neutrophil counts are found primarily with bacterial infections, as well as with some inflammatory disorders, leukemia, and hyperplastic disorders.

Thrombocytes also may be present in inadequate numbers because of their rapid destruction, typically caused by idiopathic thrombocytopenia purpura. Conversely, excessive platelet counts are associated most often with hyperplastic disorders, iron deficiency anemia, splenectomy, and chronic inflammatory conditions such as tuberculosis. Other factors crucial to the clotting process may be absent in hemophilia and similar disorders.

Losses of the liquid portion of the blood can create dehydration problems, impede metabolic processes that function only through use of hydrogen or oxygen molecules, or subvert hydrodynamic and hydraulic processes.

In addition to hemorrhage, plasma proteins may be lost through burn wounds or wound drainage or may be insufficient because adequate available substrates such as amino acids are lacking. The results vary depending on the type of plasma protein and may include deficiencies in immune status, blood viscosity, or colloid osmotic pressure (oncotic pressure).

Replacement Therapies

Therapy to replace all or certain components of the bloodstream is a common practice in most health facilities. Since blood is considered a tissue, transfusions are technically tissue transplants. The usual treatment of choice is replacement of the sole blood component that is deficient rather than whole blood, since the body is better able to replace intravascular fluids than formed elements of the blood. Transfusing only the depleted blood fraction serves two other purposes: (1) it prevents fluid overload in high-risk individuals such as the elderly and those with cardiovascular or renal disease, and (2) it more efficiently uses the remaining blood fractions for other patients' needs. Table 25-4 outlines indications for this therapy.

TABLE 25-4 Indications for Common Blood Component Therapies

Component	Indications
Whole blood	Hemorrhage, hypovolemic shock
Fresh whole blood	Multiple transfusions, exchange transfusions; priming agent for hemodialysis machines (normal saline also may be used)
Packed red blood cells	Transfused when whole blood could result in circulatory overload
Deglycerolized or washed red cells	Transfused when hypersensitivity reactions are likely; as in immunosuppressed patients and those with a history of reactions or extreme hypersensitivity
Fresh-frozen plasma (FFP)	Clotting deficiencies, especially factors V and VII; blood volume expansion in burns, shock, or protein deficiencies (believed to be overused for these deficiencies)
Plasma exchange (plasmapheresis): blood drawn off, cleansed, and components returned	Immune-related disorders: multiple myeloma, glomerulonephritis, systemic lupus erythematosus, rheumatoid arthritis, myasthenia gravis
Plasma expanders (Dextran: large polysaccharide polymer)	Temporary volume expansion in hemorrhagic shock states (sole use for Dextran 70 or 75); not a substitute for blood or plasma
Granulocytes	Granulocyte counts <500
Platelets	Platelet counts $\leq 20,000/mm^3$
Cryoprecipitate (fresh-frozen plasma precipitate; contains factors I and VIII)	Hemophilia, fibrinogen deficiency, and von Willebrand's disease
Antihemophilic factor (AHF) concentrate	Treatment of hemophilia; preferred over FFP
Factor VII	
Factor IX complex	Hemophilia B; deficiencies of clotting factors II, VII, and X; coumarin overdose
Plasma protein fraction (PPF)	Hypovolemic shock; protein replacement; burns; adult respiratory distress syndrome, dehydration, and hypoalbuminemia; as additive to complement packed cells when necessary
Fibrinogen	When fibrinogen levels insufficient for adequate control of bleeding
Albumin	Blood volume expansion by oncotic pressure; prevention and treatment of cerebral edema
Gamma globulins	Exposure to hepatitis; to prevent complications of mumps

Healthcare professionals should be aware of transfusion hazards in certain blood-type combinations. Careful typing and cross-matching help to prevent serious complications. ABO antigen-antibody reactions result from the following and must be avoided:

RECIPIENT'S BLOOD TYPE	SHOULD NOT RECEIVE
A	Type B or AB
B	Type A or AB
O	Any except type O

Hypersensitivity is also common, as most of these products are essentially foreign proteins. Exceptions include autologous transfusions collected previously from the patient's own blood or transfusions of inert, synthetic products. Diphenhydramine (Benadryl) 25 mg, taken orally or injected into blood transfusion tubing before the transfusion, is recommended to prevent mild allergic reactions.

SUMMARY

This chapter reviews blood, blood types, anticoagulant therapy, thrombolytic therapy, antihemophilic agents, antiplatelet agents and hemostatic agents, systemic and topical. Anticoagulant therapy is primarily prophylactic while thrombolytic drugs are used to dissolve already formed clots in the treatment of acute thromboembolic disease states. The low molecular weight heparins are the new antithrombins with a longer half-life than heparin. They are considered safe and effective for the management of thromboembolic disease.

The hemostatic agents are used to promote clot formation to reduce blood loss whereas the antihemophilic drugs are specific factors from the clotting process used as replacement substances in persons with a factor deficiency. Selected antiplatelet drugs inhibit platelet aggregation and thus may be used to reduce the risk of stroke. Blood and its vital components are primarily used in replacement therapy.

REVIEW QUESTIONS

1. Compare the mechanisms of action and indications of the anticoagulant drugs (heparin and warfarin) with the thrombolytic agents.
2. What are the antidotes for heparin and warfarin overdosage toxicities? Describe how the antidotes are used.
3. Compare the low molecular weight heparins to regular heparin in chemical composition, mechanism of action, indications, route of administration, and side/adverse effects.

REFERENCES

Turpie AGG: Management of deep vein thrombosis: prevention and treatment, *P&T J* 20(6S):7S-15S, 1995.

United States Pharmacopeial Convention: *USP DI: drug information for the health care professional,* ed 18, Rockville, Md, 1998, the Convention.

ADDITIONAL REFERENCES

Abramowicz M, editor: Recombinant antihemophilic factor, *Med Lett* 35(898):51, 1993a.

Abramowicz M, editor: Enoxaparin: a low-molecular-weight heparin, *Med Lett* 35(903):75, 1993b.

Abramowicz M, editor: Ticlopidine for prevention of stroke, *Med Lett* 34(874):65, 1993c.

Agnelli G: Anticoagulation in the prevention and treatment of pulmonary embolism, *Chest* 107(1 suppl):39S-44S, 1995.

American Hospital Formulary Service: *AHFS drug information '98,* Bethesda, Md, 1996, American Society of Hospital Pharmacists.

Anderson KN et al, editors: *Mosby's medical, nursing, and allied health dictionary,* ed 5, St Louis, 1998, Mosby.

Bick RL, Strauss J: Thrombolytic therapy and its uses, *Lab Med* 26(5):330-337, 1995.

Majerus, P, Broze GJ Jr et al: Anticoagulant, thrombolytic, and antiplatelet drugs. In Hardman JG, Limbird LE, editors: *Goodman & Gilman's the pharmacological basis of therapeutics,* ed 9, New York, 1996, McGraw-Hill.

Mosby: *Mosby's GenRx,* St Louis, 1998, Mosby.

Olin BR: *Facts and comparisons.* Philadelphia, 1998, JB Lippincott.

Pagana KD, Pagana TJ: *Mosby's diagnostic and laboratory test reference,* ed 3, St Louis, 1997, Mosby.

Peterson FY, Kirshoff KT: Analysis of the research about heparinized versus nonheparinized intravascular lines, *Heart Lung* 20(6):631, 1991.

Wittkowdky AK: Thrombosis. In Young LY, Koda-Kimble MA, editors: *Applied therapeutics: the clinical use of drugs,* ed 6, Vancouver, Wash, 1995, Applied Therapeutics, Inc.

CHAPTER 26

Antihyperlipidemic Drugs

KEY DRUGS

cholestyramine (p. 409)
lovastatin, (p. 412)

KEY TERMS

atherosclerosis, (p. 405)
chylomicrons, (p. 405)
high-density lipoproteins (HDLs), (p. 405)
hyperlipidemia, (p. 405)
lipoprotein, (p. 405)
low-density lipoproteins (LDLs), (p. 405)
very-low-density lipoproteins (VLDLs), (p. 405)

CHAPTER FOCUS

Hyperlipidemia, or increased serum concentrations of cholesterol and triglycerides in the body, has been clinically associated with atherosclerosis. Atherosclerosis is a disorder of the arteries that is characterized by lipid deposits in the lining of the blood vessels, which obstruct blood flow, leading to coronary artery disease. Coronary artery disease may result in cardiovascular disease that may be health threatening and even fatal. Intensive research is ongoing for new and more effective antihyperlipidemic agents.

OBJECTIVES

After reading and studying this chapter, the student should be able to do the following:

1. *Define and discuss the key terms and key drugs.*
2. *Describe the four types of lipoprotein and differentiate them according to their lipid content.*
3. *Discuss the four primary goals of hyperlipidemia therapy.*
4. *Present the mechanisms of action, time for therapeutic response, and side/adverse effects for the reductase inhibitors.*

Hyperlipidemia is a metabolic disorder characterized by increased concentrations of cholesterol and triglycerides, two of the major serum lipids in the body. Antihyperlipidemic or antilipidemic drugs are used along with dietary modifications to treat hyperlipidemia. Clinical and experimental studies offer evidence that an important relationship exists between high levels of circulating triglycerides and cholesterol and atherosclerosis. **Atherosclerosis,** a disorder that involves large- and medium-sized arteries, is characterized by lipid deposits in the lining of the blood vessels, eventually producing degenerative changes and obstructing blood flow.

Atherosclerosis is a causative factor in coronary artery disease (CAD), which may result in angina, heart failure, and myocardial infarction; cerebral arterial disease that results in senility or cerebrovascular accidents; peripheral arterial occlusive disease (which may cause gangrene and loss of limb), and renal arterial insufficiency. It is also a factor in hypertension. Intensive research to develop more effective and safer antihyperlipidemic drugs is ongoing. If serum lipid or blood lipid levels could be controlled within normal limits, the development and progression of atherosclerosis might be inhibited or prevented.

HYPERLIPIDEMIC DISORDERS

Lipid compounds do not circulate freely in the bloodstream, but instead are bound to plasma proteins (albumin and globulin), which act as carriers. These complexes are called **lipoproteins.** The lipoprotein has a protein shell and interior composed of a core lipid (cholesterol and triglycerides) (Table 26-1). Hyperlipoproteinemia is always associated with an increased concentration of one or more lipoproteins, particularly cholesterol.

Classification of Lipoprotein

Lipoprotein complexes are classified according to their densities and electrophoretic mobilities. The three primary lipoproteins found in the blood of fasting individuals are **very-low-density lipoproteins (VLDLs), low-density lipoproteins (LDLs),** and **high-density lipoproteins (HDLs).**

The VLDLs contain a large amount of triglycerides (50% to 65%) and 20% to 30% cholesterol, which are formed in the liver from endogenous fat sources. These lipoproteins contain 15% to 20% of the total blood cholesterol and most of the triglyceride found in the body (McKenney, 1995). Because these particles are quite large, they are not believed to be involved in atherosclerosis.

After secretion from the liver, the VLDL particles will in time become smaller particles as the triglyceride content is removed. Two enzymes, lipoprotein lipase and hepatic lipase, are involved with triglyceride removal. The VLDL is eventually broken down into intermediate-density lipoprotein (IDL), which contains 50% each of cholesterol and triglycerides. About 50% of this substance is converted to the cholesterol-rich lipoprotein, or LDL. Therefore medications that increase the action of lipoprotein lipase will lower triglyceride levels.

The triglyceride-depleted lipoprotein now is smaller and contains a higher quantity of cholesterol. The smaller remnant VLDL particles now include VLDL, IDL, and LDL. These lipoproteins can now be involved in the development of atherosclerosis.

The LDLs contain the major portion of cholesterol in the blood and are considered to be the most harmful. They carry 60% to 70% of total blood cholesterol, and elevated LDL levels suggest that an individual has a greater potential for developing atherosclerosis.

The HDLs are the smallest and most dense lipoproteins. Their function is to transport cholesterol from peripheral cells to the liver where it is metabolized and excreted. Thus high levels of HDL are considered beneficial. The higher the HDL levels, the lower the potential risk for development of cardiovascular disease. This transport mechanism prevents the accumulation of lipids in the arterial walls, thereby providing protection against the development of coronary artery disease.

Chylomicrons are large particles that transport cholesterol and fatty acids from diet and the gastrointestinal (GI) tract to the liver. This is known as the exogenous system of transport. The lipoproteins transporting cholesterol to and from the liver to peripheral cells are part of the endogenous system. Chylomicrons consist mainly of triglycerides (85% to 95%). In a normal person, they are produced in the small intestine during absorption of a fatty meal and are cleared from the bloodstream by the enzyme lipoprotein lipase after 12 to 14 hours. A deficiency of the enzyme is rare; however, when present, it results in increased levels of chylomicrons, causing a disease called exogenous hyperlipoproteinemia. This condition is usually found in children, but it may also be induced by alcoholism. Therapy is focused on keeping the diet low in fat.

TABLE 26-1 Lipoproteins: Core Lipids and Transport/Function

Lipoproteins	*Core Lipid*	*Transports/Function*
Chylomicrons	Dietary triglycerides	Dietary triglyceride
Chylomicron remnants	Dietary cholesterol	Dietary cholesterol
VLDL	Endogenous cholesterol	Endogenous triglyceride
IDL	Endogenous cholesterol and triglycerides	Endogenous cholesterol
LDL	Endogenous cholesterol	Endogenous cholesterol
HDL	Endogenous cholesterol	Removes cholesterol

Apolipoproteins

Lipoproteins contain proteins on their surface called apolipoproteins. These proteins have a number of functions, which include helping the lipoprotein bind with cell receptors, activating the enzyme system, and providing structure for the lipoprotein. If apolipoprotein metabolism is impaired, an increased risk for atherosclerosis exists. Thus blood levels of apolipoproteins are important in evaluating lipid disorders. The clinically important apolipoproteins are A-I, A-II, B-100, C-II, and E. For example, a deficiency of the C-II apolipoprotein in VLDL particles results in impaired triglyceride metabolism and hypertriglyceridemia. The quantity of apoliproprotein B present is used to determine the number of VLDL and LDL substances in circulation. High levels of apolipoprotein A-I in HDL correlate with a lower risk for coronary heart disease than HDL particles that have both A-I and A-II (McKenney, 1995).

Fig. 26-1 reviews the normal lipid transport system. Dietary fats and cholesterol are consumed orally and transported into the system by bile acids; in endogenous transport, the liver converts excess calories from carbohydrates and fatty acids into triglycerides. The liver ultimately produces both HDL and LDL. The function of HDL is to carry about 25% of blood cholesterol to the liver, where it is processed into bile acids. Because the cholesterol it carries is for ultimate excretion, it is known as "good" cholesterol. LDL carries more than 50% by weight of cholesterol. This LDL-cholesterol combination can penetrate arterial walls, result-

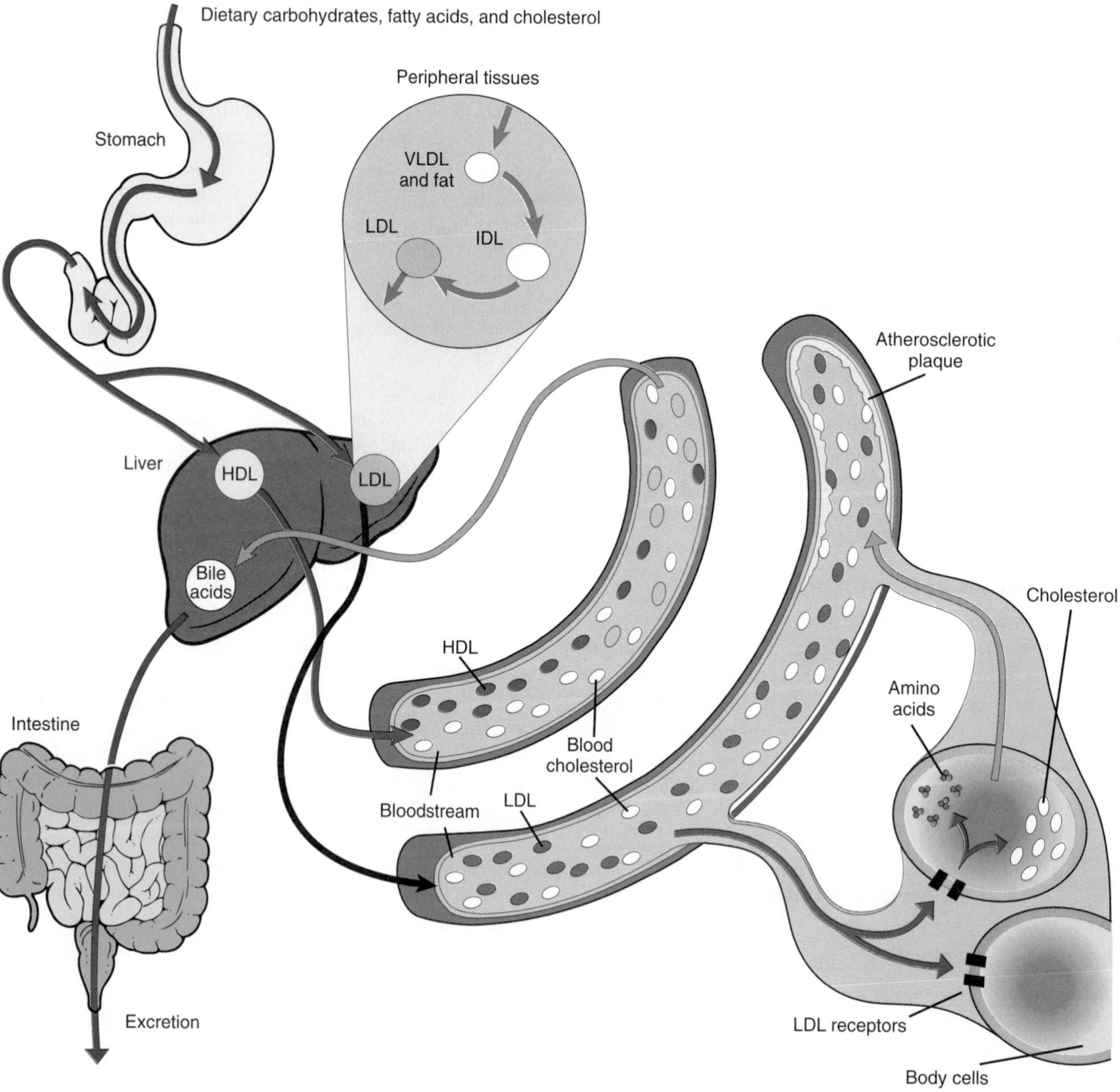

FIGURE 26-1
Dietary carbohydrates, fatty acids, and cholesterol: conversion sites and processes.

ing in atherosclerotic plaques; thus an excess of this combination is referred to as "bad" cholesterol.

Usually plasma lipoproteins are in a state of dynamic equilibrium because the LDL needed to transport fats such as fatty acids and cholesterol is present throughout the body. When cells outside the liver need cholesterol, they produce LDL receptors on their surfaces (Fig. 26-1). These receptors are necessary for LDL to enter the cell, where it is broken down into amino acids and free cholesterol. When the cellular need for cholesterol is met, the production of LDL receptors stops, and the excess cholesterol is discarded into the plasma. LDL receptors are also located in the liver where they function to monitor the plasma levels of LDL. When the appropriate level of LDL is present in the plasma, the liver will suppress its production. This is essentially a feedback system that functions like a thermostat in the home; it maintains adequate plasma levels of LDL to provide cholesterol to body cells on demand.

Table 26-2 describes the approach for drug treatment of lipid disorders, as recommended by the Adult Treatment Panel II (Expert Panel, 1994). Dietary modifications are important in the treatment of high LDL-cholesterol levels.

Dietary management consists of a two-step plan. The step I diet limits (1) saturated fat to 8% to 10% of total calories, (2) up to 30% of total calories obtained from fat, and (3) intake of less than 300 mg of cholesterol per day. If adherence to the step I diet does not meet the goal of lowering cholesterol, the step II diet plan is instituted. The step II diet limits saturated fat to 7% or less of total calories and cholesterol to 200 mg/day. Persons with coronary heart disease (CHD) are usually started on the step II diet. Dietary evaluation and consultation are highly recommended for the patient. If dietary changes fail to decrease hyperlipidemia, there may be a genetic cause, which usually requires drug treatment. Noncompliance with dietary restrictions may indicate a need for pharmacologic intervention.

Many drugs may affect serum levels of LDL-cholesterol, HDL-cholesterol, and triglycerides. Table 26-3 contains examples of effects of drugs on serum lipids.

TABLE 26-2 Drug Treatment for Lipid Disorders

Lipid Disorder	*Test Results*	*Drug Therapy Recommendations*
Hypercholesterolemia	↑ LDL, TG <200 mg/dL	Bile acid sequestering agent, niacin, or reductase inhibitor
Hypertriglyceridemia		Niacin, gemfibrozil, or reductase inhibitor
Combined hyperlipidemia	↑ LDL, TG 200-400 mg/dL	Niacin, reductase inhibitor, or gemfibrozil
Low HDL (<35 mg/dL)	LDL increased	Niacin, reductase inhibitor, or gemfibrozil
	TG increased	Niacin, gemfibrozil, or reductase inhibitor
	Alone, with CAD	Niacin, reductase inhibitor

From Expert Panel, 1994.
TG, Triglycerides.

TABLE 26-3 Effects of Drugs on Serum Lipids

	*Effect on Lipids**		
Drug	*LDL-Cholesterol*	*Triglycerides*	*HDL-Cholesterol*
Beta Blockers			
nonselective	N/C	I	D
selective	N/C	I	D
Corticosteroids	I	I	—
Diuretics			
thiazides	I	I	I
loop	N/C	N/C	D
Ethyl Alcohol	N/C	I	—
Oral Contraceptives			
monophasics	I	I	I/D
triphasics	I	I	I

From McKenney, 1995; USP DI, 1998.
I, Increased, D, decreased; N/C, no change; —, unknown.

Treatment Guidelines

Treatment recommendations are based on the patient's cholesterol level and the presence of CAD or two other risk factors, such as current cigarette smoking; hypertension; a family history of premature CAD (i.e., myocardial infarction or sudden death before age 55 in father or other male first-degree relatives or before age 65 in mother or other female first-degree relatives); male and age 45 or older, female and age 55 or older, or postmenopausal woman not receiving estrogen replacement; low HDL-cholesterol level (<35 mg/dl); and diabetes mellitus. A negative risk factor was added to the list: patients with an HDL-cholesterol level >60 mg/dl would reduce their total risk factors by one.

Total serum cholesterol and HDL-cholesterol should be evaluated in a nonfasting state at least every 5 years in adults 20 years of age and older. As noted in Table 26-4, an LDL–cholesterol level of 130 to 159 mg/dl is classified as borderline/high risk, whereas 160 mg/dl and over is considered a high-risk level. Assessment by a prescriber includes a clinical evaluation to determine if high LDL-cholesterol levels are secondary to other risk factors or causes and also to ascertain the presence of familial disorders.

The primary goals are as follows:

- Individuals without CAD and with fewer than two risk factors and LDL-cholesterol levels >160 mg/dl should receive dietary instructions and be reevaluated in 1 year. If such a person has a LDL-cholesterol level >190 mg/dl, drug therapy should be initiated.
- Individuals with no CHD but with two or more risk factors and an LDL-cholesterol level >130 mg/dl should receive a complete clinical evaluation plus dietary instructions. Further treatment will be based on findings of the clinical evaluation. If the LDL-cholesterol level is >160 mg/dl, drug therapy is indicated.
- Individuals with CHD and a LDL-cholesterol level of >100 mg/dl receive dietary instructions; if the LDL-cholesterol is ≥130 mg/dl, drug therapy should be instituted.
- If a negative response to dietary alterations is noted, then drug therapy may be indicated.

Hormone replacement therapy with estrogen in postmenopausal women to reduce menopause symptoms and osteoporosis may have the benefit also of reducing the risk of CHD by up to 50%. Doses of estrogen (e.g., 0.625 mg of conjugated estrogen or 2 mg of micronized estradiol per day) may reduce LDL-cholesterol by 25% and increase HDL-cholesterol by approximately 15%. Clinical studies have not been performed to evaluate the risk/benefit ratio of estrogen. Thus if it is used for its primary indications of treatment for menopausal symptoms or prevention of osteoporosis in women with hypercholesterolemia, the lipoprotein-cholesterol levels should also be monitored to evaluate the potential additional effect of estrogen (McKenney, 1993).

The references by McKenney (1995) and the Expert Panel (1994) contain detailed reviews of drug application and management.

Antihyperlipidemic agents offer the healthcare professional a pharmacologic method for reducing serum lipid levels and ideally reducing the risk of atherosclerosis with its many complications. Use of antihyperlipidemic agents is reserved for individuals who have specifically been identified to be at significantly increased risk and are unable to lower their serum lipid levels satisfactorily through exercise, diet, and other nondrug methods. Drug therapy for these patients augments the therapy aimed at lowering serum lipids and cardiovascular risk. See the Geriatric Implications box for more information.

TABLE 26-4 Guidelines for Cholesterol Levels

Risk	*Total Cholesterol (mg/dL)*	*LDL Cholesterol (mg/dL)*
Desirable	<200	<130
Borderline/high risk	200-239	130-159
High risk	≥240	≥160

From Expert Panel, 1994.

GERIATRIC IMPLICATIONS

Antihyperlipidemic Drugs

Dietary modifications and recommendations are vital to a successful lipid reduction program. When goals are not obtainable by diet alone, drug therapy should be considered.

The elderly often take multiple medications for their illnesses in addition to antihyperlipidemia medications. Therefore the healthcare professional should take a thorough drug history to determine if the person is taking medications that can increase lipid levels. For example, thiazides can increase triglycerides by 30% to 50%, nonselective beta blockers by 20% to 50%, ethanol by up to 50%, and so on (McKenney, 1995).

A common side effect, constipation (sometimes severe), has been reported in geriatric patients taking cholestyramine and colestipol. Encourage the patient to increase daily fluid intake to help reduce the constipating effects of this drug.

Be aware that long-term use of cholestyramine or colestipol may lead to deficiencies of vitamins A, D, E, and K, folic acid, and calcium. Additional nutritional supplementation may be necessary (Long, 1990).

Administer the antihyperlipidemic drugs before or with meals (follow manufacturer's instructions) because the drugs are generally not effective if not administered with food. Lovastatin is often given with supper to obtain its maximum beneficial effects, because the highest rate of cholesterol production occurs from midnight to 5 AM (Long, 1990).

BILE ACID SEQUESTERING AGENTS

cholestyramine [koe less' tir a meen] (Questran)

colestipol [koe les' ti pole] (Colestid)

Cholestyramine and colestipol are nonabsorbable anion-exchange resins, which are also called bile acid sequestrants. These drugs are used for their cholesterol-lowering effects. Cholesterol is the major precursor of bile acids that normally are secreted from the gallbladder and liver into the small intestine. Here the bile acids perform two functions: (1) they emulsify fat present in food to facilitate chemical digestion, and (2) they are required for absorption of lipids (including fat-soluble vitamins, A, D, E, and K). After their physiologic performance, the major portion of the bile acids is returned to the liver.

The anion-exchange resins bind bile acids in the intestine, thus preventing their absorption and producing an insoluble complex that is excreted in the feces. To compensate for the loss of bile acids removed by the drugs, the liver increases the rate of oxidation of cholesterol by converting more sterol to bile acids. Subsequently, the long-term fecal loss of bile acids causes a reduction of serum cholesterol levels and LDL-cholesterol.

Indications

Both cholestyramine and colestipol are used in treatment of the hyperlipidemia of primary hypercholesterolemia. Cholestyramine is also used to treat pruritus induced by bile acid deposits in dermal tissues (from partial biliary obstruction). While not approved indications, cholestyramine is also used as an antidiarrheal agent for diarrhea caused by bile acids (not for common diarrhea), and as an antidote for negatively charged drugs and other medications (e.g., digoxin, oral penicillin, tetracyclines, and thyroid medications).

Plasma cholesterol levels usually decrease within 1 to 2 weeks after initiation of therapy. With cholestyramine, plasma cholesterol levels may continue to fall for up to 1 year. After the initial decrease, plasma cholesterol levels in some individuals may increase to previous levels or even exceed these levels with continued therapy. Close monitoring for effectiveness is necessary. Diarrhea induced by increased bile acids will respond to cholestyramine within 24 hours, whereas it usually takes 1 to 3 weeks of therapy before a response is noted in patients with pruritus caused by cholestasis.

Pharmacokinetics

Colestipol's peak effect is noted within 1 month. After the initial decrease in cholesterol, some patients may exhibit an increased cholesterol level that equals or surpasses the previous level.

After withdrawal of colestipol and cholestyramine, plasma cholesterol levels will increase in about 2 to 4 weeks. Pruritus will return in about 1 to 2 weeks after discontinuance of the medication.

Drug interactions

The following effects may occur when the bile sequestering agents are given with the drugs listed below:

Drug	Possible effect and management
Oral anticoagulants, warfarin, or indanediones	Concurrent use significantly decreases absorption of oral anticoagulants and vitamin K; thus the anticoagulant effect may be increased or decreased. It is suggested that oral anticoagulants be given 6 hours before these drugs. Also, monitor prothrombin times closely because dosage adjustments may be necessary.
Digitalis glycosides, especially digitoxin	The half-life of digitalis glycosides, as well as GI absorption, may be reduced. It is recommended that cholestyramine or colestipol be administered at least 8 hours after digoxin to reduce the potential for interactions. Also, if cholestyramine or colestipol is discontinued in a patient also taking a digitalis product, the individual should be closely monitored for digitalis toxicity.
Thiazide diuretics (oral), phenylbutazone, oral propranolol, oral penicillin G, oral tetracyclines, or oral vancomycin	Decreased absorption of these medications has been reported. Give such medications several hours before or after cholestyramine or colestipol. Whenever possible, give these medications before cholestyramine or colestipol.
Thyroid hormones	Decreased absorption of thyroid products is reported. Give thyroid first and then give cholestyramine or colestipol several hours later.

Side effects and adverse reactions

These include constipation, indigestion, abdominal pain, nausea, vomiting, gas, dizziness, headache and, rarely, gallstones, pancreatitis, bleeding ulcers, and malabsorption syndrome.

Warnings

Use with caution in patients with gallstones, hypothyroidism, malabsorption problems, peptic ulcers, coronary heart disease, hemorrhoids, kidney disease, and bleeding disorders.

Contraindications

Avoid use in persons with cholestyramine or colestipol hypersensitivity, biliary obstruction, constipation, and phenylketonuria.

Dosage and administration

Cholestyramine is available as Questran and Questran Light (sugar free) powders for oral suspension. The adult dose is 4 g once or twice daily before meals; the maintenance dose is 8 to 24 g in two to six divided doses daily as necessary. The pediatric dose is 4 g/day in two divided doses initially, then 8 to 24 g in two or more divided doses as necessary.

The colestipol adult dose is 15 to 30 g orally before meals in two to four divided doses. The pediatric dosage has not been established.

ADDITIONAL ANTIHYPERLIPIDEMIC AGENTS

clofibrate [kloe fye′ brate] (Atromid-S, Claripex ✤)

The results of several large studies raise specific warnings concerning the use of clofibrate. First, there is the possibility of an increased risk of inducing malignancy and cholelithiasis in humans with the use of this product. Individuals taking clofibrate had twice the risk for cholelithiasis and cholecystitis that required surgery than nonusers. Second, there is no evidence of reduced cardiovascular mortality with its use. In fact, studies reported an increase in cardiac dysrhythmias, angina, and thromboembolic episodes (Olin, 1998). As a result, the clinical use of clofibrate has declined tremendously.

Clofibrate is more effective in reducing VLDLs rich in triglycerides than in lowering LDLs high in cholesterol. The exact mode of action of the drug is unknown although VLDL breakdown may contribute to its effect.

Indications

Clofibrate is indicated for the treatment of hyperlipidemia.

Pharmacokinetics

Clofibrate is slowly but completely absorbed from the intestines, is highly protein bound (96%), and reaches peak plasma levels in 2 to 6 hours after a dose. The peak effect with continued therapy is seen in approximately 3 weeks. A reduction in plasma VLDL concentrations is seen within 2 to 5 days. The half-life of this drug ranges from 6 to 25 hours for a single dose or 54 hours at steady state in normal healthy individuals. It is metabolized in the liver and gastrointestinal tract and excreted by the kidneys.

Drug interactions

When the oral anticoagulants are given concurrently with clofibrate, an increase in anticoagulant effect may result. Monitor closely as a decrease in the oral anticoagulant dose may be necessary.

Side effects and adverse reactions

These include diarrhea, nausea, muscle pain or cramps, fatigue, headache, weight gain, abdominal pain, gas, nausea, vomiting, flu-syndrome, and, rarely, anemia, leukopenia, angina, gallstones or pancreatitis, cardiac dysrhythmias, and kidney disease.

Warnings

Use with caution in patients with hypothydroidism, cardiovascular problems, gallstones, and peptic ulcers. See the box for Food and Drug Administration (FDA) pregnancy safety categories.

Contraindications

Avoid use in persons with liver or kidney function impairment.

Dosage and administration

The adult dose is 1.5 to 2 g orally daily in two to four divided doses. A pediatric dose has not been established.

gemfibrozil [jem fi′ broe zil] (Lopid)

Gemfibrozil is an agent that primarily decreases serum triglycerides found in VLDL and increases HDL. The mechanism of this action has not been established but it may involve an inhibition of peripheral lipolysis and a decrease in hepatic extraction of free fatty acids, which result in reduction of triglyceride production. In addition, the drug may accelerate turnover and removal of cholesterol from the liver, which is ultimately excreted in the feces.

Indications

Gemfibrozil is indicated for the treatment of hyperlipidemia.

Pharmacokinetics

Taken orally, gemfibrozil is well absorbed from the gastrointestinal tract and reaches peak levels in 1 to 2 hours. Its onset of action in reducing serum VLDL levels is within 2 to 5 days with the peak effect seen in 4 weeks. It is metabolized in the liver and excreted by the kidneys and in the feces.

Drug interactions

When gemfibrozil is given with oral anticoagulants, coumarin, or indanedione-type drugs, an increased anticoagulant effect is reported. Monitor prothrombin times closely

PREGNANCY SAFETY

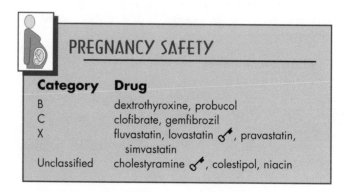

Category	Drug
B	dextrothyroxine, probucol
C	clofibrate, gemfibrozil
X	fluvastatin, lovastatin, pravastatin, simvastatin
Unclassified	cholestyramine, colestipol, niacin

because the anticoagulant dose may need to be decreased significantly. If administered with lovastatin, an increased risk of rhabdomyolysis and myoglobinuria may result in acute renal failure. This has been reported within 3 weeks to several months of combined drug therapy. If possible, avoid concurrent drug administration.

Side effects and adverse reactions

These include muscle aches and cramps, nausea, vomiting, rash diarrhea, gas, and abdominal distress.

Warnings

Use with caution in patients with gallstones or gallbladder disease.

Contraindications

Avoid use in persons with gemfibrozil hypersensitivity, liver or kidney disease, and especially primary biliary cirrhosis.

Dosage and administration

The adult dose is 1.2 g daily in two divided doses, preferably before breakfast and supper. The pediatric dosages have not been established.

dextrothyroxine [dex tro thy rox′ seen] (Choloxin)

Dextrothyroxine's mechanism of action as an antihyperlipidemic agent is not fully understood. Dextrothyroxine appears to act in the liver to increase formation of LDL and, to a greater extent, to increase the breakdown of LDL. The result is increased excretion of cholesterol and bile acids via bile into the feces, which causes a decrease in serum cholesterol and LDLs.

A definite relationship exists between thyroid function and serum cholesterol levels. Hypothyroidism is associated with high serum cholesterol levels, and administration of thyroid hormones lowers serum cholesterol. Dextrothyroxine apparently stimulates the liver to increase the rate of oxidation of cholesterol, and it promotes biliary excretion of cholesterol and its byproducts.

Indications

Dextrothyroxine is used as an adjunct to diet and other measures to reduce elevated serum cholesterol (LDL) levels in persons with no evidence of heart disease. Other antihyperlipidemic agents have replaced this drug because significant cardiac side effects are associated with its use.

Pharmacokinetics

Dextrothyroxine is approximately 25% absorbed from the gastrointestinal tract, is highly protein bound with a half-life of 18 hours, and reaches its peak effect as an antihyperlipidemic agent in 1 to 2 months. The duration of action after the drug is withdrawn is 6 weeks to 3 months. It is metabolized in the liver and excreted by the kidneys and in feces.

Drug interactions

When dextrothyroxine is administered concurrently with the oral anticoagulants, the anticoagulant effects may be increased or decreased depending on the patient's thyroid status. Monitor prothrombin times closely because the anticoagulant dose may need to be adjusted. If administered with cholestyramine or colestipol, dextrothyroxine absorption will be reduced. Separate these medications by approximately 4 to 5 hours.

Side effects and adverse reactions

These are rare and include nausea, vomiting, chest pain, abdominal pain, irregular heart rate, skin rash, and gallstones.

Warnings

Use with caution in patients with hypothyroidism.

Contraindications

Avoid use in persons with dextrothyroxine hypersensitivity, cardiac disease, diabetes mellitus, hyperthyroidism, and liver or kidney function impairment.

Dosage and administration

The adult dose for antihyperlipidemic effect is 1 to 2 mg PO daily, increased monthly if necessary, to achieve the desired effect. The maximum recommended dose is 8 mg/day. For children 2 years of age and older, the dose is 0.05 mg/kg daily, titrated monthly as necessary to achieve the desired effect. Maximum recommended dose is 4 mg/day.

niacin [nye′ a sin] (nicotinic acid, Nicobid)

Niacin is a water-soluble vitamin that can lower total cholesterol and triglyceride levels by inhibiting VLDL synthesis; it also increases the HDL-cholesterol serum level. It is used as an adjunct to other therapies because its vasodilating and other side effects limit its usefulness. Because nicotinic acid inhibits lipolysis in adipose tissue, it lowers the plasma concentration of free fatty acids, which usually is the main source of synthesis of triglycerides in the liver.

Indications

Niacin is used as an adjunct therapy in the treatment of both hypertriglyceridemias and hypercholesterolemia (types IIa, IIb, III, IV, or V). It is also used to prevent and treat niacin (vitamin B_3) deficiency.

Pharmacokinetics

It is well absorbed orally and has a half-life of approximately 45 minutes. It reduces cholesterol levels several days after therapy is started; a reduction in triglyceride levels occurs within several hours after oral doses are begun. Metabolism occurs in the liver, and the drug is excreted via the kidneys.

Drug interactions

No significant drug interactions have been reported to date.

Side effects and adverse reactions

These include increased feelings of warmth, flushing or red skin on the face and neck, headache, pruritus, skin rash, and rarely, anaphylactic reactions. With high dosages, dysrhythmias, dry skin or eyes, hyperglycemia, dizziness, diarrhea, hyperuricemia, myalgia, pruritus, and aggravation of peptic ulcers has been reported. Liver toxicity has been reported with chronic use with extended-release niacin.

Warnings

Use caution in patients with gout, glaucoma, and hypotension.

Contraindications

Avoid use in persons with niacin or niacinamide hypersensitivity, diabetes mellitus, peptic ulcer, liver disease, and bleeding disorders.

Dosage and administration

The adult dose for antihyperlipidemic effect is 1 g PO three times daily. The dosage may be increased to 500 mg/day every 2 to 4 weeks as necessary. The maximum dose is 6 g/day.

probucol [proe byoo′ kole] (Lorelco)

Probucol is an antihyperlipidemic agent for persons with primary hypercholesterolemia who have not responded to other measures. It lowers both LDL-cholesterol and the desired HDL-cholesterol levels, which limits its usefulness. In addition to lowering cholesterol levels, however, probucol also induces regression of xanthomas in persons with homozygous familial hypercholesterolemia and inhibits atherosclerosis as result of its antioxidant properties (Witztum, 1996).

Pharmacokinetics

Probucol is administered orally, and it has a variable absorption pattern. It tends to accumulate in fatty tissues with chronic therapy. Peak serum levels increase slowly and reach steady state after 3 or 4 months of treatment, whereas the peak effect usually occurs in 20 to 50 days after initiation of the drug. Its half-life ranges from 12 to 500 hours. Probucol is excreted as bile in the feces.

Drug interactions

No significant drug interactions are reported, although monitor closely if probucol is administered with antidysrhythmic drugs, tricyclic antidepressants, or phenothiazines as these agents increase the risk for ventricular tachycardia.

Side effects and adverse reactions

These include gas, diarrhea, nausea, vomiting, abdominal distress, ventricular dysrhythmias, and, rarely, anemia, angioneurotic edema, and thrombocytopenia.

Warnings

Use with caution in patients with severe bradycardia, gallstones, hypokalemia, hypomagnesemia, and liver function impairment.

Contraindications

Avoid use in persons with probucol hypersensitivity, biliary cirrhosis, congestive heart failure, and cardiac dysrhythmias.

Dosage and administration

The adult dose is 500 mg PO twice daily with breakfast and supper. A pediatric dose has not been established.

REDUCTASE INHIBITORS

atorvastatin [ator′ a sta tin] (Lipitor)
cerivastatin [seri′ va sta tin] (Baycol)
fluvastatin [floo′ va sta tin] (Lescol)
lovastatin [loe′ va sta tin] (Mevacor)
pravastatin [pra′ va sta tin] (Pravachol)
simvastatin [sim va stat′ in] (Zocor)

These agents are the most effective drugs to lower LDL-cholesterol levels. Reductase inhibitors are competitive inhibitors of hydroxymethylglutaryl coenzyme A (HMG-CoA) reductase, an enzyme necessary for cholesterol biosynthesis. The decrease in cholesterol production in the liver leads to an increase in the synthesis of cholesterol and also stimulates hepatocytes to produce more LDL receptors. The result is that more LDL-cholesterol is removed from the blood. In summary, these drugs convert HMG-CoA reductase to mevalonate, which results in an increase in HDL-cholesterol and a decrease in LDL-cholesterol, VLDL-cholesterol, and plasma triglycerides.

Indications

These agents are indicated as adjuncts for the treatment of primary hypercholesterolemia (types IIa and IIb) caused by an elevated LDL-cholesterol level that is not controlled by diet or other treatment measures.

Pharmacokinetics

On absorption they all have extensive first-pass hepatic extraction; all but pravastatin are highly protein bound. Peak serum levels are reached in 0.5 to 0.7 hour for fluvastatin, 1 to 2 hours for atorvastatin, 2.5 hours for cerivastatin, 2 to 4 hours for lovastatin, 1 hour for pravastatin, and 1.3 to 2.4 hours for simvastatin.

Cerivastatin, lovastatin, and simvastatin are converted by the liver to several active metabolites. The initial response is seen within 1 to 2 weeks, with the maximum therapeutic re-

TABLE 26-5 Summary of Comparison of Antihyperlipidemic Effects

	*Effect on Lipids**		*Effect on Lipoproteins*			
Drug	***Cholesterol***	***Triglycerides***	***VLDL***	***LDL***	***HDL***	***Typical Response***
cholestyramine	↓	0 or slight ↑	0 or ↑	↓	0 or ↑	Decreases cholesterol 20%-40%
colestipol	↓	0 or slight ↑	↑	↓	0 or ↑	Decreases cholesterol 20%-40%
clofibrate	↓	↓ (greatest effect)	↓	0 or ↓	0 or ↑	Lowers triglycerides; only slight decrease in cholesterol
dextrothyroxine	↓	0	0 or ↓	↓	0	
gemfibrozil	↓	↓	↓	0 or ↓	↑	Decreases triglycerides; only slight decrease in cholesterol; increases HDL
niacin	↓	↓	↓	↓	↑	Decreases triglycerides and cholesterol 10%-20%
probucol	↓	0 or ↑	↑ or ↓	↓	↓	Decreases cholesterol 12%-25%; also decreases HDL
lovastatin	↓	↓	↓	↓	↑	LDL cholesterol levels reduced 19%-39%, total cholesterol levels reduced 18%-34%

*↑, Increased; ↓, decreased; 0 no change. Typical response was approximated with individual taking drug while concurrently on specified diet.

sponse occurring within 4 to 6 weeks of chronic drug administration. Excretion is primarily fecal.

Drug interactions

A significant drug interaction may occur if the drugs are administered with cyclosporine (Sandimmune), gemfibrozil (Lopid), or niacin (B_3). An increased risk of rhabdomyolysis (necrosis of skeletal muscle with the release of myoglobulin, which may result in myopathy and acute renal failure) may occur. At the present time, such effects have only been reported with lovastatin, but the potential of inducing these effects exists with all six agents. Monitor closely if concurrent administration is necessary.

Side effects and adverse reactions

These include gas, stomach cramps or pain, rash, constipation or diarrhea, nausea, headaches, myalgia, myositis, rhabdomyolysis, and, rarely, impotency and insomnia.

Warnings

Use caution in patients alcoholics and history of liver disease

Contraindications

Avoid use in persons with hypersensitivity to any HMG-CoA reductase inhibitor, patients who have had an organ transplant and are receiving immunosuppressant drugs, and patients with any disease state or condition that may predispose them to renal failure.

Dosage and administration

The recommended adult dose for atorvastatin is 10 mg daily, titrated monthly as needed (the range is 10 to 80 mg/day), for cerivastatin is 0.3 mg daily in the evening, and for fluvastatin is 20 mg PO daily at bedtime, titrated monthly as necessary. The lovastatin adult dose is 20 mg daily with the evening meal, increased monthly as necessary, up to a maximum of 80 mg/day. The pravastatin adult dose is 10 to 20 mg at bedtime, with dosage adjustments at monthly intervals as needed. The simvastatin adult dose is 5 to 10 mg in the evening, titrated monthly as necessary and tolerated. The maximum dose is 40 mg/day. All of these drugs may be taken with or without food with the exception of lovastatin, which should be taken with the evening meal to increase bioavailability.

SUMMARY

The antihyperlipidemic medications are used to treat hyperlipidemia, a disorder characterized by increased levels of cholesterol and triglycerides in the body. High circulating levels of these lipids have been associated with atherosclerosis, a disorder in which lipids are deposited in the linings of medium- and large-sized arteries, which eventually produces degenerative changes and obstruction of blood flow.

Atherosclerosis is a causative factor in coronary artery disease which, in turn, may result in angina, heart failure, myocardial infarction, cerebral artery disease, peripheral artery occlusive disease, and renal arterial insufficiency. Although there are many contributing causes to and risk factors for atherosclerosis, it is believed that if serum lipid levels can be controlled, the progression of atherosclerosis may also be controlled.

Currently the medications available to treat hyperlipidemia include the bile acid sequestering agents, cholestyramine and colestipol, clofibrate, dextrothyroxine, probucol, gemfibrozil, niacin, and the reductase inhibitors. Each agent is indicated for specific types of hyperlipidemia. See Tables 26-2 and 26-5 for drug treatment approaches and a comparison of antihyperlipidemic effects.

REVIEW QUESTIONS

1. What is the best way to manage the drug interactions between digitoxin, oral anticoagulants (warfarin), and thyroid hormones with cholestyramine?
2. Name five major concerns for the administration of antihyperlipidemic drugs to geriatric patients.
3. What effects do thiazide diuretics, corticosteroids, and ethyl alcohol have on serum lipids?
4. Select one reductase inhibitor and present its pharmacokinetics, time for initial and maximum response, drug interactions, and usual adult dosage.

REFERENCES

Expert Panel on Detection, Evaluation, and Treatment of High Blood Cholesterol in Adults, National Cholesterol Education Program: Second report of the Expert Panel on Detection, Evaluation and Treatment of High Blood Cholesterol in Adults (Adult Treatment Panel II). *Circulation* 89:1329-1445, 1994.

Long JW: *The essential guide to prescription drugs,* New York, 1990, HarperCollins.

McKenney JM: Dyslipidemias. In Young LY, Koda-Kimble MA, editors: *Applied therapeutics: the clinical use of drugs,* ed 6, Vancouver, Wash, 1995, Applied Therapeutics, Inc.

Olin BR: *Facts and comparisons.* Philadelphia, 1998, JB Lippincott.

United States Pharmacopeial Convention: *USP DI: drug information for the health care professional,* ed 18, Rockville, Md, 1998, The Convention.

Witztum JL: Drugs used in the treatment of hyperlipoproteinemias. In: Hardman JG, Limbird LE, editors: *Goodman & Gilman's the pharmacological basis of therapeutics,* ed 9, New York, 1996, McGraw-Hill.

ADDITIONAL REFERENCES

American Hospital Formulary Service: *AHFS drug information '98,* Bethesda, Md, 1996, American Society of Hospital Pharmacists.

American Medical Association: *AMA drug evaluations 1995,* Chicago, 1995, the Association.

Anderson KN et al, editors: *Mosby's medical, nursing, and allied health dictionary,* ed 5, St Louis, 1998, Mosby.

Hardman JG, Limbird LE, editors: *Goodman & Gilman's the pharmacological basis of therapeutics,* ed 9, New York, 1996, McGraw-Hill.

Mishkel M: Dyslipidemia: practical goals and guidelines, *Med Clin North Am* 4(36):4476-4477, 1992.

Mosby: *Mosby's GenRx,* St Louis, 1998, Mosby.

Smith DA: Hypercholesterolemia: a guide to primary and secondary prevention, *Consultant* 34(6):844-850, 852, 1994.

Unit VII

Drugs Affecting the Urinary System

CHAPTER 27

Overview of the Urinary System

CHAPTER FOCUS

The urinary system affects all other body systems because of its important functions, which include regulating the volume and composition of fluid within the body, helping to retain essential materials, and excreting waste. Thus a healthy functioning urinary system plays a major role in the patient's general health. Many drug effects are increased or decreased by the activity of the urinary system; therefore the healthcare professional must be knowledgeable of its anatomy and physiology.

OBJECTIVES

After reading and studying this chapter, the student should be able to do the following:

1. *Define and discuss the key terms.*
2. *Present the anatomy and physiology of the urinary system.*
3. *Relate the functions of the different segments of the nephron.*
4. *Discuss the major functions of the kidneys.*
5. *Describe the sites of action and major effects of antidiuretic hormone, vasopressin, and aldosterone on the nephrons.*

KEY TERMS

electromagnetic gradient, (p. 418)
glomerular filtration, (p. 418)
glomerulus, (p. 418)
hypertonic, (p. 420)
hypotonic, (p. 420)
isotonic, (p. 419)
osmotic gradient, (p. 418)
threshold concentration, (p. 419)
tubular transport maximum, (p. 418)

The urinary system is composed of organs that manufacture and excrete urine from the body: two kidneys, two ureters, bladder, and urethra (Fig. 27-1). Urine formed in the kidneys flows through the ureters to the bladder, where it is stored.

When approximately 250 ml of urine is collected, the bladder expansion will result in a feeling of distention and a desire to void. The urine flows from the bladder into the urethra to be expelled from the body.

In males, the urethra is surrounded by the prostate gland; it then passes through fibrous tissue connected to the pubic bones and terminates at the urinary meatus, or tip of the penis (Fig. 27-2). The male urethra serves a dual purpose: the elimination of urine from the body and semen transport. In the female, the urethra is the final vehicle for urination (Fig. 27-3).

The kidneys regulate homeostasis in the body; they are responsible for the maintenance of body fluids, electrolytes, and acid-base balance in addition to elimination of body waste, urea, and urine. The primary focus of this chapter is the kidneys.

ANATOMY AND PHYSIOLOGY OF THE KIDNEY

The kidney is composed of millions of individual units called nephrons. Each nephron consists of a glomerulus and a tubular system. The volume and composition of urine as a result of concentration and dilution depend on three major processes in the kidney: glomerular filtration, tubular reabsorption, and tubular secretion.

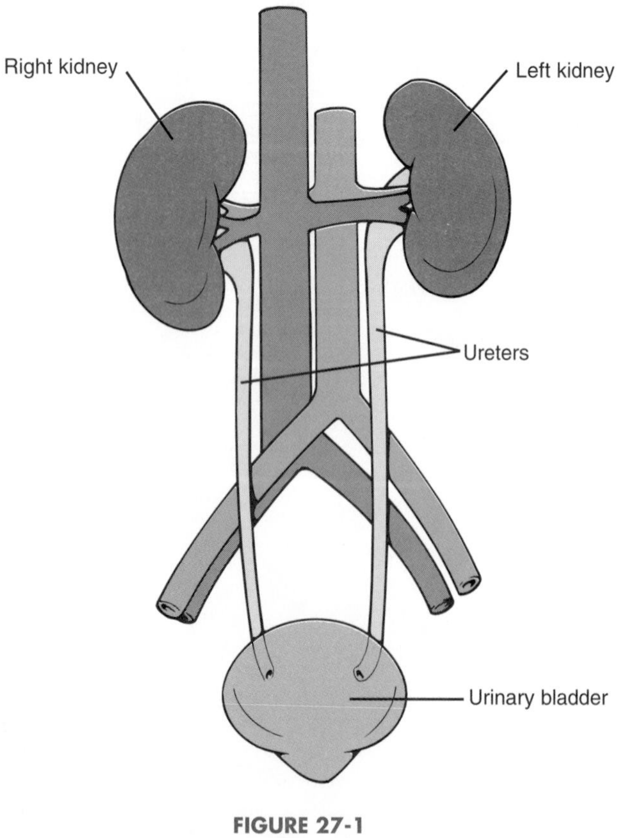

FIGURE 27-1
Urinary system.

Glomerular Filtration

Glomerular filtration occurs as a result of plasma flowing across a cluster of capillary blood vessels and into the urinary space of the Bowman's capsule. This capillary cluster is enveloped within a thin wall, giving off uriniferous tubules, and is called the **glomerulus.** The heart works to create pressure in the blood vessels, which in turn provides the force necessary to accomplish glomerular filtration. Blood flow to the kidney is 1200 ml/min, which is 20% to 25% of cardiac output. The blood pressure within the glomerular capillaries is about 60% of arterial pressure. Systemic blood pressure has to be significantly reduced before glomerular filtration is greatly altered. Usually some degree of filtration will exist if the mean blood pressure remains above 50 mm Hg. Maintenance of glomerular hydrostatic pressure is aided by the ability of the afferent and efferent arterioles to alter vessel resistance effectively. In the absence of disease, the glomerular membrane does not filter plasma proteins greater than 100 Å, such as hemoglobin and albumin and the small amount of protein-bound substances. The glomerular filtrate is otherwise almost identical to plasma. The rate of filtration in an average adult is approximately 125 ml/min; 99% of this tubular filtrate is ultimately reabsorbed throughout the tubule.

Tubular Reabsorption

Tubular reabsorption involves both active and passive transport of substances into the tubular epithelial cell and into the extracellular fluid compartment. Passive transport, or diffusion, through the tubular membrane occurs because of a difference in concentration of particles (**osmotic gradient**) or electrical charge (**electromagnetic gradient**).

In the proximal tubule, sodium is actively transported across the tubular cell membrane from tubule filtrate. Chloride follows passively because of an electromagnetic gradient. Water, in turn, follows passively in response to an osmotic gradient established by sodium chloride solute. Then diffusion of 60% of urea content occurs to maintain a chemical gradient. Depending on the amount of a drug in ionized or nonionized form and the pH of the tubular fluid, weak acids and weak bases may be reabsorbed by diffusion.

For almost every substance that is actively transported across the membrane, there is a maximum rate at which the transport mechanism can function, after which the excess substance will not be reabsorbed, and the substance will appear in the urine. This is called the **tubular transport maximum.** For example, the tubular transport maximum for glucose averages 320 mg/min for most adults. If the tubular load becomes greater than 320 mg/min, then the excess will not be reabsorbed but will appear in the urine. Every substance that has a tubular transport maximum also has a

threshold concentration, the plasma concentration below which none of the substance appears in the urine and above which progressively larger quantities appear.

Tubular Secretion

Tubular secretion affects the composition of urine by allowing compounds such as penicillin, histamine, probenecid, methotrexate, and thiazides to enter into tubular fluid from peritubular or interstitial capillaries. This is accomplished via specific transport mechanisms for secretion of organic compounds. Other important examples of tubular secretion include hydrogen ions, ammonia, and potassium ions.

Proximal Tubule

Most of the glomerular filtrate is reabsorbed in the proximal tubule and returned to the bloodstream. Approximately 70% of salt and water is reabsorbed rapidly, maintaining nearly the same osmolality between tubular fluid and interstitial fluid at the end of the proximal tubule (**isotonic**). The general mechanism for sodium, chloride, water, and urea reabsorption is under tubular reabsorption with respect to gradient transport. There are no dilutional or concentration changes of these ions in the proximal tubule.

Other substances reabsorbed in the proximal tubule include glucose, amino acids, phosphate, uric acid, and a major portion of potassium. Nearly 90% of bicarbonate in tu-

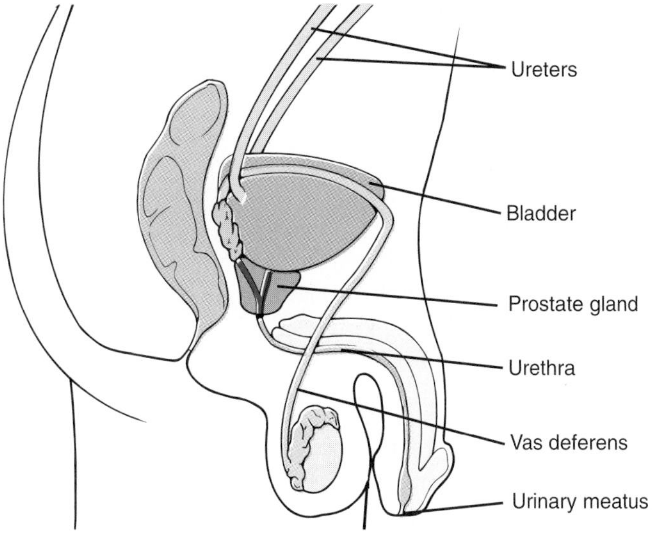

FIGURE 27-2
Sagittal section of male pelvis.

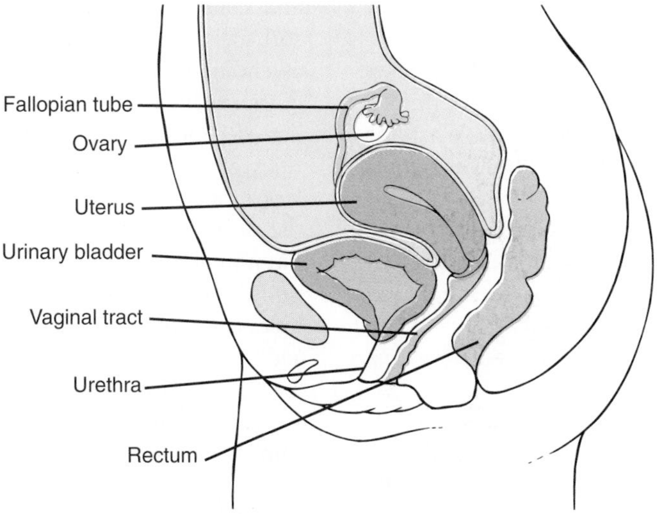

FIGURE 27-3
Sagittal section of female pelvis.

bular filtrate is reabsorbed as carbon dioxide if hydrogen ion is secreted in the tubular lumen. Plasma carbon dioxide is hydrolyzed in the tubular cell to form carbonic acid, which dissociates to give bicarbonate and hydrogen ion. This reversible reaction is catalyzed by carbonic anhydrase. The hydrogen ion secreted into the lumen combines with bicarbonate of the glomerular filtrate to form carbonic acid in the lumen. This again dissociates to give water and carbon dioxide, which are reabsorbed. This reaction is catalyzed at both steps by carbonic anhydrase. Proximal tubule reabsorption is usually constant in spite of moderate changes in the glomerular filtration rate.

Descending Loop of Henle

This portion of the nephron is permeable to water; water is passively taken up to equilibrate medullary interstitial osmolality. This produces a **hypertonic** (more concentrated) filtrate at the tip of the loop of Henle, the papilla. There is very low sodium and urea permeability in this segment.

Ascending Loop of Henle

Water permeability is almost nil in the ascending limb of the loop of Henle, whereas sodium and chloride permeability is high. Approximately 20% to 25% of sodium load in glomerular filtrate is reabsorbed and chloride follows passively. Consequently, two very important situations occur. The concentration of tubular filtrates becomes very dilute, or **hypotonic;** this is often termed "free water production." Meanwhile, the medullary interstitium becomes hypertonic, which is necessary to the concentration capacity of the countercurrent multiplier. The concentration gradient established across the tubular epithelium becomes multiplied in a longitudinal direction, resulting in a large osmotic gradient between the isosmotic renal cortex and the hyperosmotic medulla and papilla. The ascending limb of the loop of Henle is not responsive to any hormones as are other segments.

Distal Convoluted Tubule

Between 5% and 10% of sodium reabsorption actively takes place in the distal tubule. This uptake is largely determined by the presence of a hormone called aldosterone. When the extracellular fluid volume is decreased, the renin-angiotensin system is involved, stimulating the release of aldosterone. Increased levels of aldosterone act to increase the active reabsorption of sodium. Although an increase in potassium secretion is seen, a simple sodium-potassium exchange pump is no longer recognized.

Collecting Duct

The hypotonic fluid entering the collecting duct may be altered in the medullary portion by the presence of antidiuretic hormone (ADH), or vasopressin. The released ADH will act at the distal tubule and collecting duct to reabsorb water to increase plasma volume, thus lowering plasma osmolality. Urinary output is more concentrated, or fluid is lost because of the osmotic gradient set up by hypertonic medullary interstitium. Thus the collecting duct is responsible for urine concentration.

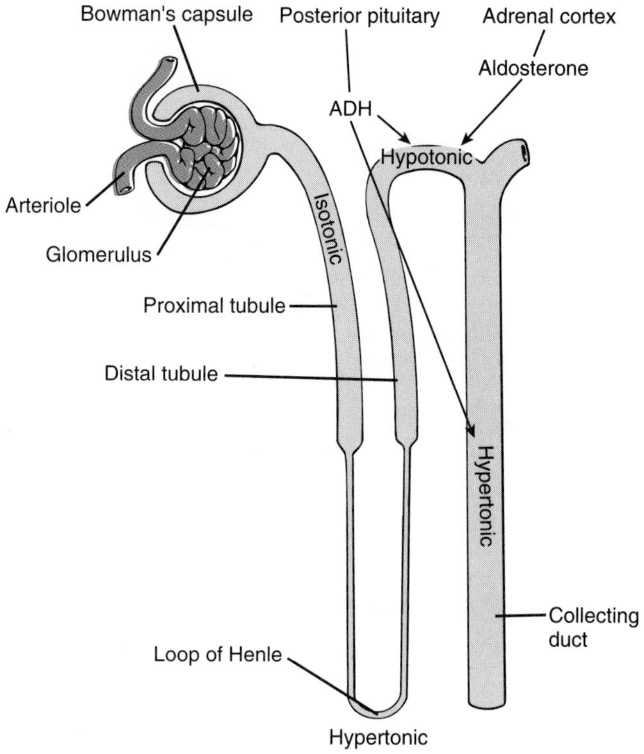

FIGURE 27-4
Components of a nephron.

PHYSIOLOGIC REGULATION BY THE KIDNEY

The kidneys excrete metabolic byproducts of the body, especially nitrogenous-type substances such as urea. They maintain electrolyte homeostasis (e.g., sodium, potassium, and chloride) and body fluids. Sodium is actively reabsorbed in the proximal tubules (approximately 65%) and ascending loop of Henle (27%). Approximately 8% of sodium reaches the distal tubules, and the rate of reabsorption here depends on the presence of aldosterone. If large quantities of aldosterone are present, sodium is reabsorbed. A lack of aldosterone will result in elimination of sodium in the urine. Generally, healthy kidneys excrete the daily sodium intake. Fig. 27-4 and Box 27-1 explain nephron functions. Potassium is also reabsorbed from the proximal tubules and loop of Henle in percentages equivalent to that of sodium. Thus approximately 8% of the filtered potassium reaches the distal tubules. Aldosterone controls potassium secretion; in its presence, sodium is reabsorbed and potassium is secreted in the distal tubules. The daily potassium intake is generally excreted daily in the kidneys.

ADH is a water-conserving hormone synthesized in the hypothalamus and stored in the posterior pituitary gland. When plasma osmolarity increases as a result of dehydra-

BOX 27-1 Nephron Functions

Site	*Major Functions*
Glomerulus	Filtration
Proximal tubule	Reabsorption of glucose, potassium, sodium, amino acids, water, and nutrients; remaining fluid isotonic
Loop of Henle	Sodium and chloride reabsorbed in ascending loop. Countercurrent mechanism produces decrease in osmolality of filtrate in ascending loop of Henle; i.e., sodium chloride is transported into the body but not water. Filtrate leaves loop of Henle as hypotonic urine.
Distal tubule	Sodium and bicarbonate reabsorbed. Potassium, hydrogen, and ammonia may be secreted. ADH necessary to reabsorb water at this site. Filtrate leaves distal tubule as hypotonic urine.
Collecting duct	ADH, if present, will reabsorb water at this site. Urine may be hypertonic. If ADH is unavailable or not functioning, dilute urine (hypotonic) may be excreted.

tion or water deprivation, osmoreceptors in the supraoptic area of the hypothalamus will stimulate the release of ADH. The released ADH will act at the distal tubule and collecting duct to reabsorb water to increase plasma volume, thus lowering plasma osmolality. Urine output is decreased and more concentrated.

Acid-base balance is partially controlled in the kidneys. The kidneys are one of three pH control mechanisms in the body; the others are the blood buffering and the respiratory adjustment mechanisms. As the blood pH becomes more acidic, the kidneys will respond by increasing the renal tubule excretion of hydrogen and ammonia, which results in an increase in blood bicarbonate and an increase in pH (toward normal). This is an effective method of adjusting hydrogen ions within the system.

The hormone erythropoietin is synthesized in the kidneys. A decrease in red blood cells below normal, or tissue hypoxia, will stimulate increased release of erythropoietin from the kidneys. The increased serum concentration of erythropoietin will stimulate the bone marrow to increase its production of red blood cells so that the red blood cell average is restored to normal.

SUMMARY

The kidneys control and regulate blood volume and red blood production, and they remove waste products from the blood. They are an important factor in controlling the concentration of ions in the blood and the pH of the blood. This system is vital for the maintenance of a normal environment for the body cells.

REVIEW QUESTIONS

1. Describe the processes of glomerular filtration, tubular reabsorption, and tubular secretion.
2. How would an elevated sodium level be processed by the proximal tubule, descending loop of Henle, ascending loop of Henle, distal convoluted tubule, and the collecting duct? What effect would large amounts of aldosterone have on the sodium?
3. Name the three body control mechanisms that regulate acid-base balance.
4. Discuss the function of the hormone erythropoietin in the body.

REFERENCES

Anderson KN et al, editors: *Mosby's medical, nursing, and allied health dictionary,* ed 5, St Louis, 1998, Mosby.

Martini F et al: *Fundamentals of anatomy and physiology,* ed 2, Englewood Cliffs, NJ, 1992, Prentice Hall.

Seeley RR, Stephens TD, Tate P: *Anatomy and physiology,* ed 3, New York, 1995, McGraw-Hill.

Thibodeau GA, Patton KT: *Anatomy and physiology,* ed 4, St Louis, 1999, Mosby.

Van Wynsberghe D, Noback CR, Carola R: *Human anatomy and physiology,* ed 3, New York, 1995, McGraw-Hill.

Wingard LB et al: *Human pharmacology,* St Louis, 1991, Mosby.

CHAPTER 28

Diuretics

KEY DRUGS

furosemide, (p. 427)
hydrochlorothiazide, (p. 424)
spironolactone, (p. 429)

KEY TERMS

diuretics, (p. 423)
loop diuretics, (p. 427)
osmotic diuretics, (p. 430)
potassium-sparing diuretics, (p. 429)
proximal tubule diuretics, (p. 423)
thiazide-type diuretics, (p. 424)

CHAPTER FOCUS

Diuretics increase the output of urine; thus they are often used as primary therapies in conditions such as congestive heart failure and hypertension. These drugs may also cause electrolyte imbalance and other side effects and adverse reactions; therefore the student needs a thorough understanding of this drug classification.

OBJECTIVES

After reading and studying this chapter, the student should be able to do the following:

1. *Define and describe the key terms and key drugs.*
2. *Describe the body's adaptation mechanisms to extracellular volume depletion.*
3. *Name one drug from each of the five classifications of diuretics and identify their primary sites of action in the nephron.*
4. *Name at least five concerns with the use of diuretics in the elderly.*
5. *Compare the efficacy and primary side effects and adverse reactions associated with each of the five diuretic classifications.*

Diuretics modify renal function to induce diuresis, or the loss of body water by urination. In addition to water, diuretics increase the excretion of electrolytes, primarily sodium chloride. Understanding their action requires knowledge of the events that take place along each of the tubular segments (see Chapter 27). Diuretics are among the most commonly used medications. They represent the mainstay in the treatment of hypertension (see also Chapter 21) and are an integral part of drug therapies in edematous conditions such as cirrhosis, nephrotic syndrome, chronic renal failure, and acute and chronic congestive heart failure.

Therapeutically, drug selection is best understood if each diuretic is presented according to its major site of action. This approach does not preclude drug effect at other sites in the nephron. Fig. 28-1 shows the various sites of action of diuretic drug groups by means of water and electrolyte transport system in a kidney nephron.

PROXIMAL TUBULE DIURETICS

Carbonic Anhydrase Inhibitors

acetazolamide [a set a zole′ a mide]
(Diamox, Acetazolam ♣)

Acetazolamide, a sulfonamide, is the prototype of the **proximal tubule diuretics** and will be discussed in this section. Other carbonic anhydrase inhibitors include dichlorphenamide (Daranide) and methazolamide (Neptazane). These drugs act primarily to reduce the volume of sequestered fluids, especially of the aqueous humor. They inhibit the action of the enzyme carbonic anhydrase, which in turn prevents the reabsorption of bicarbonate ions from the proximal tubules. These bicarbonate ions then act to increase tubular osmotic pressure, causing osmotic diuresis. With long-term use, however, the diuretic effect of these drugs is lost.

Acetazolamide is widely used as an antiglaucoma agent because it lowers intraocular pressure by decreasing the production of aqueous humor by more than 50%; this is discussed in Chapter 36.

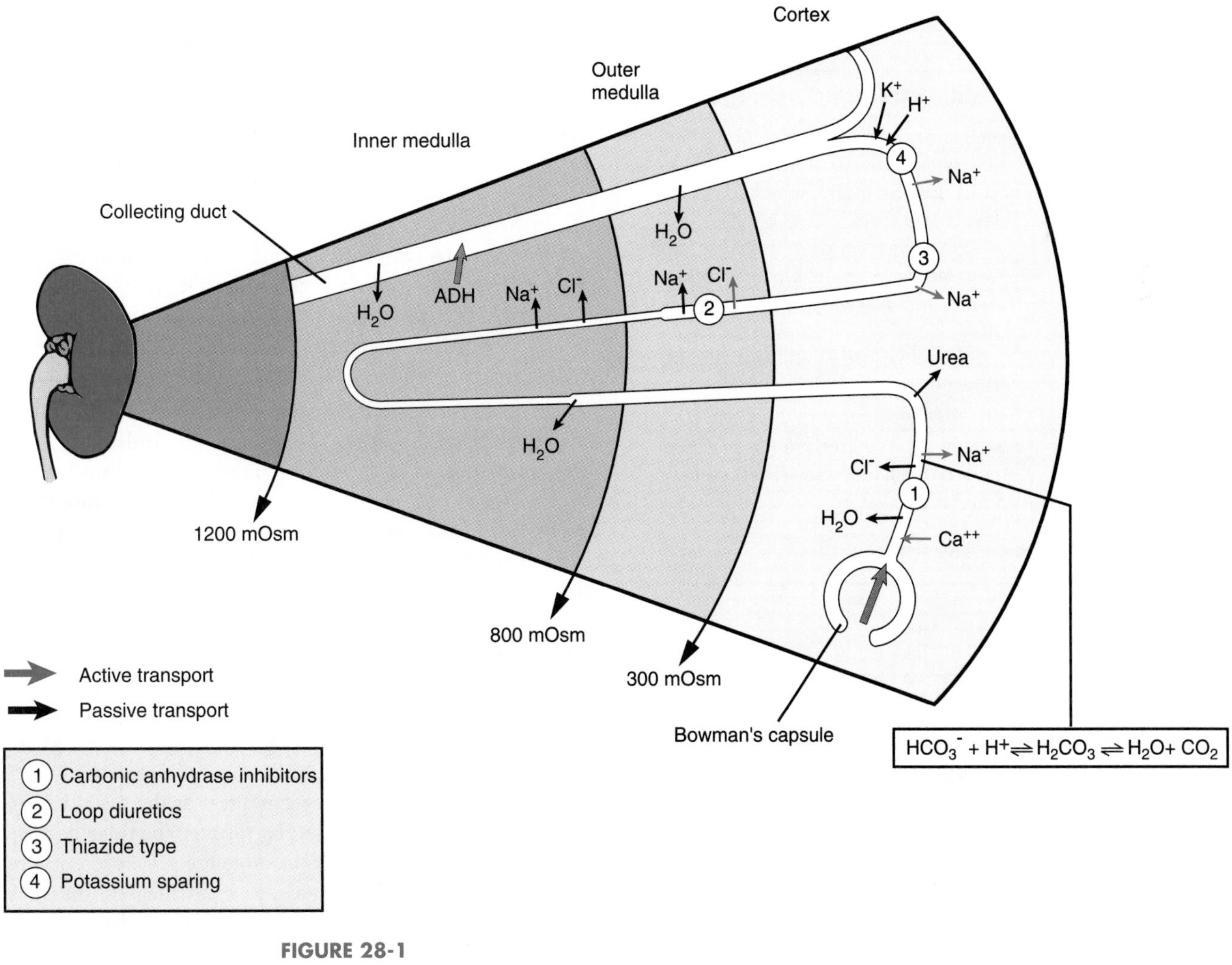

FIGURE 28-1
Site of action of diuretics by means of water and electrolyte transport.

Indications

Acetazolamide is indicated for the treatment of open-angle glaucoma and is also used as adjunct treatment with anticonvulsants to manage absence seizures (petit mal), generalized tonic-clonic seizures (grand mal), mixed seizure patterns, and myoclonic seizures. It has been found especially useful for women who experience an increase in seizures during their menstrual periods. When acetazolamide is taken orally, it has been found to decrease the incidence and severity of symptoms of altitude sickness in mountain climbers. In addition, acetazolamide produces an alkaline urine, which may help increase excretion of weakly acidic drugs in cases of drug overdose.

Pharmacokinetics

Acetazolamide is well absorbed orally and reaches a peak level in 2 to 4 hours after a 500 mg dose or 8 to 12 hours after a 500 mg extended-release capsule. Its half-life is 10 to 15 hours, and excretion is mainly by the kidneys.

Drug interactions

The following interactions may occur when acetazolamide is given with the drugs listed below:

Drug	Possible effect and management
Amphetamines, mecamylamine (Inversine), or quinidine	Because of alkalinization of urine, the excretion of these drugs is decreased. Therefore increased serum levels and toxicity may be seen. Avoid concurrent drug administration with mecamylamine. Dosage adjustments may be necessary with the other two drugs whenever a carbonic anhydrase inhibitor is started, dosage is changed, or medication is discontinued.
methenamine mandelate (Mandelamine)	Alkaline urine will reduce the effectiveness of methenamine. Avoid concurrent use.

Color type indicates an unsafe drug combination.

Side effects and adverse reactions

These include headaches, increased nervousness, anorexia, nausea or vomiting, depression, tremors, rash, alopecia, ataxia, chest, groin, or leg pain, weakness, increased frequency of urination, crystalluria, and, rarely, blood disorders; Stevens-Johnson syndrome; and metabolic acidosis.

Warnings

Use caution in patients with diabetes mellitus, gout, and pulmonary disease.

Contraindications

Avoid use in persons with carbonic anyhydrase inhibitor hypersensitivity, Addison's disease, hypokalemia, hyponatremia, liver or kidney disease or impairment, hyperchloremic acidosis, and a history of renal calcium calculi.

Dosage and administration

The adult dose for glaucoma is 250 mg PO one to four times daily. The anticonvulsant dose is 4 to 30 mg/kg orally divided into four doses per day. For altitude sickness the dose is 250 mg orally two to four times daily. The pediatric dose for glaucoma is 8 to 30 mg/kg orally per day in divided doses. Acetazolamide is also available parenterally for intravenous or intramuscular use. See a current package insert for dosing instructions.

DILUTING SEGMENT DIURETICS

Thiazide and Thiazide-Type Drugs

bendroflumethiazide
[ben droe floo me thy' a zide] (Naturetin)
benzthiazide [benz thy' a zide] (Exna, Hydrex)
chlorothiazide [klor oh thy' a zide] (Diuril)
chlorthalidone [klor' tha li done] (Hygroton)
cyclothiazide [sye kloe thy' a zide] (Anhydron)
hydrochlorothiazide [hydro klor oh thy' a zide] (HydroDIURIL, Esidrix)
hydroflumethiazide [hye droe meth' a zide] (Diucardin, Saluron)
methyclothiazide [met y clo thy' a zide] (Enduron)
metolazone [me toe' la zone] (Zaroxolyn)
polythiazide [pol ee thy' a zide] (Renese)
quinethazone [kwinth' a zone] (Hydromox)
trichlormethiazide [try klor me thy' a zide] (Metahydrin, Naqua)

Thiazide diuretics are the major diuretics active in the diluting segments of the kidney. They are synthetic drugs that are chemically related to the sulfonamides. Hydrochlorothiazide is one of the most commonly used thiazides. Because these agents are similar, all the diluting segment diuretics will be described collectively as the **thiazide-type diuretics** with important differences mentioned later. These agents are well absorbed orally and are usually excreted unchanged by the kidneys. For pharmacokinetics and dosages, see Table 28-1.

The primary action and site of action appear to be inhibition of sodium reabsorption in the early distal tubules in the nephron, the cortical diluting segment. These drugs are less potent than the loop diuretics, since the maximum portion of the sodium load they can affect at the distal tubule is less than 10% of the glomerular filtrate. The thiazide-type diuretics therefore primarily promote the renal excretion of water, sodium, chloride, potassium, and magnesium; they also may increase serum levels of calcium, glucose, and uric acid.

An especially important feature of the thiazides is their

TABLE 28-1 **Selected Diuretic Pharmacokinetics and Dosages***

Category/Generic (Trade Name)	Onset of Action (hr)	Peak Effect (hr)	Duration of Action (hr)	Initial Dose	
				Adults	Children
Thiazide Diuretics					
chlorothiazide (Diuril)	PO 2	4	6-12	250 mg q6-12h	6 months & older, 10-20 mg/kg/day
chlorthalidone (Hygroton)	PO 2	2	48-72	25-100 mg/day	2 mg/kg/day
hydrochlorothiazide (Esidrix)	PO 2	4	6-12	25-100 mg/day	1-2 mg/kg/day
metolazone (Zaroxolyn)	PO 1	2	12-24	5-20 mg/day	Not established
Loop Diuretics					
bumetanide (Bumex)	PO 0.5-1	1-2	4-6	0.5-2 mg/day	Not established
	IV min	0.25-0.5	0.5-1		
ethacrynic acid (Edecrin)	PO 0.5	2	6-8	50-100 mg/day	25 mg/day
	IV within 5 min	0.25-0.5	2		
furosemide (Lasix)	PO ⅓-1	1-2	6-8	20-80 mg/day	2 mg/kg/day
	IV within 5 min	0.5	2		
torsemide (Demadex)	PO 0.5-1	1-2	6-8	10-20 mg/day	Not established
	IV within 10 min	0.5-1	6-8		
Potassium-Sparing Diuretics					
amiloride (Midamor)	PO 1-2	6-10	24	5-10 mg/day	Not established
spironolactone (Aldactone)	PO 24-48	48-72	48-72	25-200 mg/day	1-3 mg/kg/day
triamterene (Dyrenium)	PO 2-4	24-72	7-9	25-100 mg/day	2-4 mg/kg/day
Osmotic Diuretics					
glycerin (Osmoglyn)	PO 20 min	1-1.5	5	1-1.5 g/kg initially, then 0.5 g q6h	Same initial dose; may repeat in 4-8 hr
isosorbide (Ismotic)	PO 10-30 min	1-1.5	5-6	1.5 g/kg 2-4 times/day	Not established
mannitol (Osmitrol)	IV 0.5-1	1	6-8	50-100 g as 5%-25% IV infusion	0.25-2 g/kg as 15%-20% IV infusion
urea (Ureaphil)	IV 20 min	1-2	3-10	0.5-1.5 g/kg as 30% IV infusion	2 years and older, see adult dose

*Doses are titrated as needed and tolerated (Olin, 1998; *USP DI,* 1998).

ability to impair free water clearance with no effect on concentration ability. The initial natriuretic effect lasts for about 1 week and then resets at a lower level. This diuretic tolerance occurs because of increased aldosterone levels and a decreased sodium load at the distal tubule. The mechanisms of antihypertensive action are believed to be initially due to the reduction in plasma and extracellular fluid volume, which results in a decrease in cardiac output. In time, the cardiac output returns to normal. The thiazides also decrease peripheral resistance by a direct action on the peripheral blood vessels.

When an increased sodium load is presented to the distal tubule, there is a corresponding increase in potassium secretion. In addition, as the extracellular fluid volume decreases, plasma renin activity and aldosterone levels increase, with resulting potassium loss (Fig. 28-2). Potassium is one of the most common electrolytes lost, with loss occurring in 14% to 60% of ambulatory hypertensive patients. This loss is dose related, occurring early in treatment (first month) and more frequently with the larger diuretic doses or with the long-acting type of diuretics (e.g., chlorthalidone) and in individuals with a high sodium intake (Tang, Lau, 1995). However, in many cases the loss is intermittent and neither harmful nor clinically observable. Potassium loss may be a serious threat in those who are taking digitalis preparations, since it can precipitate serious dysrhythmias as a result of digitalis toxicity. Hypokalemia may predispose the patient with cirrhosis to hepatic encephalopathy and coma.

Healthcare providers should caution patients for whom thiazide therapy is prescribed to increase their dietary intake of potassium (Box 28-1). If hypokalemia occurs, the prescriber may order oral potassium preparations; if urgent replacement is necessary, intravenous potassium chloride administration may be performed. Potassium loss may also be reversed by the addition of a potassium-sparing diuretic

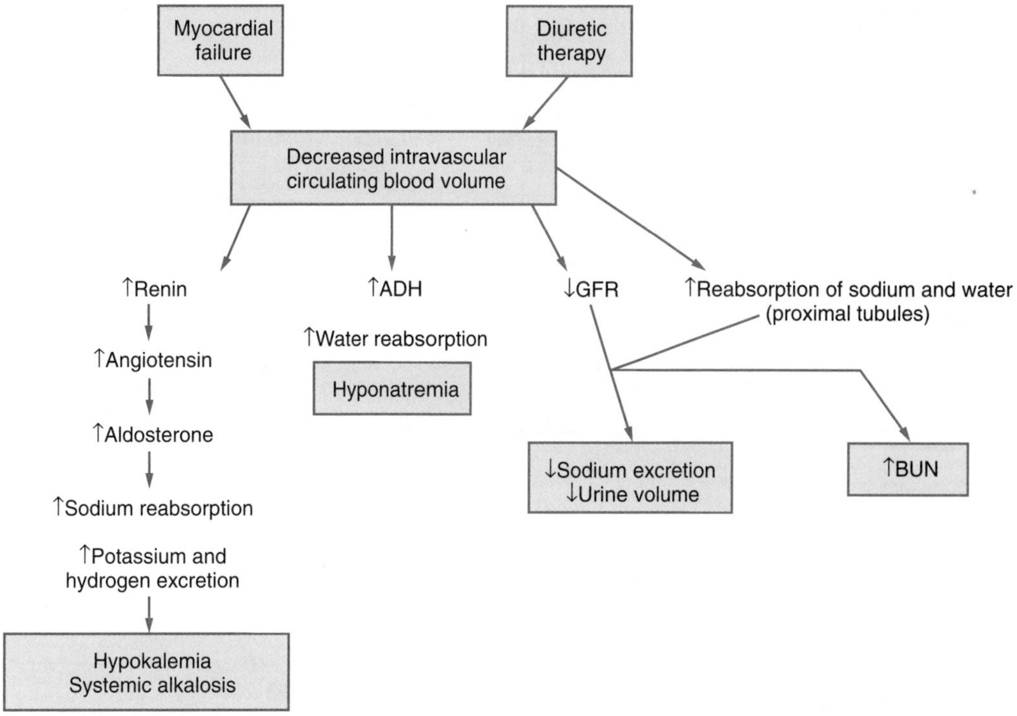

FIGURE 28-2
Body adaptation to extracellular volume depletion.

that acts to inhibit potassium loss at the distal tubule. However, potassium replacement is usually not necessary in 80% to 90% of individuals taking the thiazide diuretics, particularly for the treatment of nonedematous states. Potassium replacement may be dangerous in the elderly, in those with renal dysfunction, or when used in combination with potassium-sparing diuretics, since dangerously high serum potassium levels may occur.

Patients receiving the thiazide-type diuretics may have an increase in serum uric acid. The 1 to 2 mg/dl increase in serum uric acid level is persistent and probably results from inhibition of tubular secretion of uric acid. However, this effect is reversible when the drugs are discontinued. In the absence of gout or a genetic predisposition, the hyperuricemia is usually asymptomatic and requires no treatment. However, in a person with a history of gout the use of allopurinol or probenecid is suggested to counteract any elevation of serum uric acid.

Hyperglycemia or impaired glucose tolerance has also been reported with the thiazide-type and loop diuretics. This effect is reported most often in the elderly. The thiazides can precipitate diabetes in individuals with overt or subclinical disease patterns. Thiazide diuretics are not contraindicated for use in diabetic patients because if hyperglycemia is noted, it can usually be controlled by diet alterations or by increasing the insulin dose. When hyperglycemia does occur in the nondiabetic patient, many prescribers may try another type of diuretic such as furosemide to see if the problem can be reduced or alleviated.

The thiazide diuretics and perhaps furosemide have been associated with increasing serum levels of cholesterol and triglycerides. Because elevated serum lipid levels are associated with an increase in coronary heart disease, it is important that serum lipid levels be monitored and perhaps a specific dietary approach or weight loss program be implemented if necessary.

Indications

The indications for the thiazide diuretics include treating hypertension, edema associated with congestive heart failure, cirrhosis with ascites, and some types of renal impairment such as nephrotic syndrome, acute glomerulonephritis, and chronic renal failure.

Drug interactions

The following interactions may occur when thiazide or thiazide-type diuretics are given with the drugs listed below:

Drug	Possible effect and management
cholestyramine (Questran) or colestipol (Colestid)	Concurrent administration may reduce gastrointestinal (GI) absorption of thiazide diuretics. Schedule administration of diuretics 1 hour before or 4 hours after administration of these drugs.

BOX 28-1 **Foods Rich in Potassium**

Food	Amount	Potassium (mg)
Apricots		
Fresh	1	105
Canned in water	1 cup	409
Dried, uncooked	1 cup	1791
Avocado	1	1097
Banana	1	451
Figs		
Fresh	1	116
Canned in heavy syrup	1 cup	258
Dried, uncooked	1 cup	1418
Grapefruit		
Canned in water	1 cup	322
Fresh	½	312
Juice, canned, unsweetened	1 cup	378
Melon, fresh cantaloupe	1 cup	494
Orange		
Fresh	1	237
Juice, frozen, diluted	1 cup	474
Peaches		
Fresh	1	171
Canned in water	1 cup	241
Dried	1 cup	1594
Pears		
Fresh	1	208
Canned in juice	1 cup	238
Dried	1 cup	959
Prunes		
Juice, canned or bottled	1 cup	706
Dried	1 cup	1200
Raisins	1 cup	1089
Lima beans, frozen, cooked	1 cup	694
Beets, sliced, cooked	1 cup	532
Brussels sprouts, cooked	1 cup	494
Peanuts roasted in oil	1 ounce	200
Potato		
Baked	1	610
Boiled	1	515
Spinach		
Cooked, fresh	1 cup	838
Canned	1 cup	709
From frozen	1 cup	566
Squash		
Acorn, baked	1 cup	896
Hubbard, mashed	1 cup	504
Winter, mashed	1 cup	895
Zucchini, canned	1 cup	622
Sweet potato, baked	1	397
Tomato	1	297
Tomato juice, canned	1 cup	535

From Wardlaw et al, 1994.

Digitalis glycosides	Increases risk of digitalis toxicity in presence of hypokalemia. Monitor pulse and electrocardiogram (ECG) closely.
lithium	Increased risk of lithium toxicity is possible because of decreased lithium excretion. Also, lithium has the potential for nephrotoxic side effects. Avoid this combination.

Color type indicates an unsafe drug combination.

Side effects and adverse reactions

In addition to the previously mentioned electrolyte imbalance, these include anorexia, impotency, diarrhea, hypotension, photosensitivity, abdominal upset and, rarely, agranulocytosis, cholecystitis, liver function impairment, and thrombocytopenia.

Warnings

Use with caution in patients with diabetes mellitus, gout, liver function impairment, electrolyte imbalance (see Box 28-2 for signs and symptoms of fluid and electrolyte imbalances), hyperlipidemia, history of lupus erythematosus, pancreatitis, and sympathectomy. See the Geriatric Implications and Pregnancy Safety boxes for more information.

Contraindications

Avoid use in persons with thiazide or sulfonamide hypersensitivity and severe kidney impairment and in jaundiced infants.

LOOP DIURETICS

bumetanide [byoo met′ a nide] (Bumex)
ethacrynic acid [eth a krin′ ik] (Edecrin)
furosemide [fur os′ e myd] (Lasix, Furoside)
torsemide [tore′ seh mide] (Demadex)

These agents are **loop diuretics,** so called because they inhibit reabsorption of sodium and water in the ascending loop of Henle. Agents that work here at the Na^+-K^+-$2Cl^-$ cotransport (or carrier transfer site) in the ascending limb are most effective because the diuretic effect is greater than that reported with the other diuretic sites (Jackson, 1996). These drugs, for the most part, are very similar to the thiazide-type diuretics in pharmacology and in the side effects they produce. Hyperglycemia, hyperuricemia, and in-

BOX 28-2 Signs and Symptoms of Fluid and Electrolyte Imbalances Associated with Diuretic Therapy

Hypovolemia	Hypotension, weak pulse, tachycardia, clammy skin, rapid respirations, and reduced urinary output
Hyponatremia	Low serum sodium levels (normal range 135 to 145 mEq/L), lethargy, disorientation, muscle tenseness, seizures, and coma
Hypokalemia	Low serum potassium levels (normal range 3.5 to 5.0 mEq/L), weakness, abnormal ECG, postural hypotension, and flaccid paralysis
Hypocalcemia	Low serum calcium levels (normal range 8.4 to 10.2 mg/dL), irritability, vomiting, diarrhea, twitching, hyperactive reflexes, cardiac dysrhythmias, tetany, and seizures
Hypochloremia	Low blood chloride levels (normal range 100 to 110 mEq/L)
Hypomagnesemia	Low serum magnesium levels (normal range 1.3 to 2.1 mEq/L), nausea and vomiting, lethargy, muscle weakness, tremors, and tetany
With potassium-sparing diuretics, be alert for:	
Hyperkalemia	Above-normal values for potassium serum levels, nausea, diarrhea, muscle weakness, postural hypotension, and ECG changes

creases in low-density lipoprotein (LDL) cholesterol and triglycerides with a decrease in high-density lipoprotein (HDL) cholesterol plasma levels are reported. The loop diuretics also increase excretion of magnesium and calcium, which may result in hypomagnesemia and hypocalcemia; thus they are administered with a normal saline infusion to treat hypercalcemia (Jackson, 1996).

Bumetanide inhibits sodium reabsorption in the ascending limb of the loop of Henle, as shown by marked reduction of free water clearance during hydration and tubular free water reabsorption during dehydration. Reabsorption of chloride in the ascending loop is also blocked by bumetanide, which may have an additional action in the proximal tubule. Because phosphate reabsorption takes place largely in the proximal tubule, phosphaturia during bumetanide-induced diuresis indicates this additional reaction. Bumetanide does not appear to have a noticeable action on the distal tubule.

Indications

The indications for loop diuretics include treatment of edema associated with congestive heart failure, cirrhosis, and renal disease. Furosemide is also used to treat hypertension. In addition. these agents are used as adjunct therapy in patients with acute pulmonary edema and in persons whose conditions are refractory to the other diuretics.

GERIATRIC IMPLICATIONS

Diuretics

- The elderly may be more sensitive to diuretic-induced hypotension and electrolyte disturbances than the average adult.
- Pharmacologically, therapy for the elderly patient is started with the lowest dose possible, generally one-half the recommended adult dose and titrated slowly to effect (Menscer, 1992).
- Advise patients to drink sufficient fluids. Diuretics are often referred to as "water pills" with many persons believing fluid intake is restricted with this drug category. This erroneous belief should be discussed with the individual.
- Avoid or use *extreme* caution and close monitoring if concurrent potassium supplementation or a potassium chloride salt substitute is ordered for persons receiving a potassium-sparing diuretic. Hyperkalemia and death have been reported with this combination.
- Be aware that all diuretics will increase urinary incontinence.
- Report any signs and symptoms of diuretic toxicity to the prescriber, such as anorexia, nausea, vomiting, confusion, increased weakness, and paresthesia of the extremities.
- When a diuretic is to be discontinued, reduce the drug gradually to avoid the possibility of the development of fluid retention and edema.

PREGNANCY SAFETY

Category	Drug
B	amiloride, chlorothiazide, chlorthalidone, ethacrynic acid, hydrochlorothiazide, isosorbide, mannitol, methyclorthiazide, metolazone, torsemide, triamterene
C	acetazolamide, bendroflume-thiazide, benzthiazide, bumetanide, cyclothiazide, furosemide, glycerin, hydroflume-thiazide, trichlormethiazide, urea
Not established	spironolactone

Pharmacokinetics

The loop diuretics have fair-to-good absorption orally, are highly protein bound, are metabolized in the liver, and are excreted by the kidneys and in bile. For pharmacokinetics and dosage information, see Table 28-1.

Drug interactions

The following interactions may occur when loop diuretics are given with the drugs listed below:

Drug	Possible effect and management
amphotericin B injectable	Increases risk for ototoxicity, nephrotoxicity, and electrolyte imbalance (especially hypokalemia). Avoid or a potentially serious drug interaction may occur.
Anticoagulants; coumarin (Coumadin), indanedione-type, or heparin	Anticoagulant effects may be decreased with concurrent therapy. With ethacrynic acid the anticoagulant effects may be enhanced because of displacement of the anticoagulant from its protein binding sites. GI ulcers or bleeding is a possible adverse reaction to ethacrynic acid, which may increase the risk for hemorrhage. When possible, avoid giving ethacrynic acid to patients receiving anticoagulants. If loop diuretics are given concurrently, monitor patients closely for increased or decreased anticoagulant effectiveness.
Hypokalemia-causing drugs, lithium	Increased risk of hypokalemia when loop diuretics are administered concurrently. Monitor serum potassium levels and ECGs closely, as potassium supplements may be required. Increased risk of lithium toxicity because of reduced renal clearance. Monitor closely.
Nephrotoxic medications or other ototoxic medications	Increased risks for ototoxicity and nephrotoxicity, especially in patients with renal impairment. Avoid or a potentially serious interaction may occur.

Color type indicates an unsafe drug combination.

Side effects and adverse reactions

These include postural hypotension, blurred vision, headaches, abdominal distress, diarrhea, anorexia, anxiety, confusion, and ototoxicity. Photosensitivity has been reported with furosemide.

Warnings

Use with caution in patients with diabetes mellitus, gout, hearing impairment, liver function impairment, acute myocardial infarction, and pancreatitis and in patients at increased risk if hypokalemia is induced, such as persons taking digitalis glycosides or those with congestive heart failure, liver cirrhosis.

Contraindications

Avoid use in persons with loop diuretic hypersensitivity, anuria, or severe kidney disease or impairment.

DISTAL TUBULE DIURETICS/ POTASSIUM-SPARING DIURETICS

amiloride [a mill′ oh ride] (Midamor)
spironolactone [speer on oh lak′ tone] (Aldactone)
triamterene [trye am′ ter een] (Dyrenium)

The **potassium-sparing diuretics** are similar in action to other diuretics and are generally considered to be weak diuretics that act at the distal renal tubules. They block sodium reabsorption in the distal tubule, thus increasing sodium and water excretion while conserving potassium. Generally, they are primarily considered useful when combined with other potassium-losing diuretics.

Amiloride and triamterene directly inhibit reabsorption of sodium and water, while spironolactone is an aldosterone antagonist. Any of the three agents may be used when it is necessary to restore or preserve the normal serum potassium level if other concurrent diuretic therapy challenges it and when potassium supplementation by medication or diet is inappropriate. These agents are highly effective for this purpose. If prescribed singly, however, their efficacy may actually result in an undesirable and rapidly developing hyperkalemia.

Spironolactone, a synthetic steroidal compound, antagonizes aldosterone effect by binding competitively to the protein that permits potassium secretion at the distal tubule. This response is directly related to the amount of circulating aldosterone in the serum. Spironolactone produces a very mild diuresis of sodium and water at the distal tubule by means of this mechanism. It does not interfere with renal tubule transport of sodium and chloride and does not inhibit carbonic anhydrase. Triamterene directly depresses the renal tubular transport of sodium in the distal tubule independent of the presence of aldosterone.

Indications

The potassium-sparing diuretics are indicated for the prevention and treatment of hypokalemia. They are also used as adjunct therapy in the treatment of edema and hypertension, and spironolactone is indicated in the diagnosis and treatment of primary hyperaldosteronism.

Pharmacokinetics

These agents have low (amiloride), moderate (triamterene), or good (spironolactone) absorption from the gastrointestinal tract. Spironolactone and triamterene are metabolized in the liver, and amiloride and spironolactone are excreted mainly by the kidneys. Triamterene is excreted primarily in bile. For pharmacokinetics and dosages, see Table 28-1.

Drug interactions

The following interactions may occur when potassium-sparing diuretics are given with the drugs listed below:

Drug	Possible effect and management
Anticoagulants	Anticoagulant effects may be decreased when used concurrently with potassium-sparing diuretics as a result of plasma volume reduction concentrating procoagulant factors in the blood. Dosage adjustment of anticoagulants may be necessary.
lithium	Concurrent use increases the risk of lithium toxicity by reducing renal clearance.
Blood from bank, angiotensin-converting enzyme (ACE) inhibitors, cyclosporine, other potassium-sparing diuretics, low-salt milk, potassium-containing medications, or potassium supplements	May increase potassium levels and result in hyperkalemia. Monitor serum electrolytes closely.

Side effects and adverse reactions

These include abdominal cramps, diarrhea, nausea, vomiting, dry mouth, sedation, headache, and hyperkalemia. Photosensitivity is reported with triamterene.

Warnings

Use with caution in patients with diabetes mellitus, hyponatremia, and metabolic or respiratory acidosis.

Contraindications

Avoid use in persons with a potassium-sparing diuretic hypersensitivity, anuria, and liver or kidney function impairment and in seriously ill patients producing small urine volumes.

OSMOTIC DIURETICS

glycerin [gli′ ser in] (Osmoglyn)
isosorbide [eye sew sore′ bide] (Ismotic)
mannitol [man′ i tole] (Osmitrol)
urea [yoor ee′ a] (Ureaphil)

Osmotic diuretics include the parenteral agents, mannitol and urea, and the oral agents, glycerin and isosorbide. The two parenteral agents cause diuresis by adding to the solutes already present in the tubular fluid; they are particularly effective in increasing osmotic pressure because they are not reabsorbed by the tubules. Thus more water is pulled into tubular fluid, and less sodium, chloride, and water are reabsorbed by the kidneys in an effort to equalize the higher solute content. These excesses are then excreted in the urine.

Indications

The oral agents are primarily used to reduce intraocular pressure before and after intraocular surgery and to interrupt an acute attack of glaucoma. Parenteral agents (mannitol and urea) are used to treat cerebral edema and secondary glaucoma when other methods have been unsuccessful. Mannitol has also been used to increase urinary excretion of toxic substances (salicylates, barbiturates, lithium, and bromides), as an irrigating preparation to prevent hemolysis and hemoglobin accumulation during transurethral prostatic resection, and as an adjunct to other therapies in the treatment of edema in acute renal failure.

Drug interactions

When mannitol is given concurrently with a digitalis glycoside, the resulting hypokalemia may result in digitalis toxicity. Monitor closely.

Pharmacokinetics

Very little if any mannitol is metabolized in the liver. Urea is partially metabolized in the gastrointestinal tract to ammonia and carbon dioxide, which may be resynthesized into urea. Both mannitol and urea are excreted by the kidneys. Glycerin is metabolized in the liver and excreted by the kidneys. See Table 28-1 for pharmacokinetics and dosing.

Side effects and adverse reactions

For the parenteral agents (mannitol, urea) these include nausea, vomiting, dry mouth, headache, increased urination, and weakness. Mannitol may also cause visual disturbances, dizziness, and rash. Glycerin and isosorbide may induce nausea, vomiting, headache, increased thirst, dry mouth, diarrhea, and confusion.

Warnings

Use with caution in patients with hypovolemia, hyperkalemia, and hyponatremia. In addition, for urea use caution in patients with liver function impairment.

Contraindications

Avoid use in persons with drug hypersensitivity, severe cardiopulmonary function impairment , and severe kidney function impairment. In addition, for urea avoid use in persons with fructose intolerance (hereditary), severe dehydration, severe liver function impairment, and intracranial bleeding.

DIURETIC COMBINATIONS

As mentioned previously, a thiazide diuretic may be combined with a potassium-sparing diuretic. Fixed-dose combi-

BOX 28-3 Examples of Fixed-Dose Diuretic Combinations

Trade Name	*Contents*
Aldactazide 25/25	spironolactone, 25 mg; hydrochlorothiazide, 25 mg
Aldactazide 50/50	spironolactone, 50 mg; hydrochlorothiazide, 50 mg
Capozide 50/15, 25/25, & 50/25	captopril 25 or 50 mg with hctz* 15 or 25 mg
Dyazide	triamterene, 50 mg; hydrochlorothiazide, 25 mg
Hydropres-50	reserpine 0.125 mg with hctz* 50 mg
Hyzaar	losartan 50 mg with hctz* 12.5 mg
Inderide LA 80/50, 120/50, or 160/50	propranolol 80, 120, or 160 mg with hctz* 50 mg
Lopressor HCT 50/25, 100/25, or 100/50	metroprolol 50 or 100 mg with hctz* 25 or 50 mg
Maxzide	triamterene, 75 mg; hydrochlorothiazide, 50 mg
Timolide 10-25	timolol 10 mg with hctz* 25 mg
Ziac	bisoprolol fumarate 2.5, 5, or 10 mg with hctz* 6.25 mg

*hctz, hydrochlorothiazide.

nations, which are commercially available, may provide additional diuretic activity and decrease the potassium depletion characteristic of the thiazide diuretics. Additionally, diuretics are combined with antihypertensive agents to simplify medication regimens for patients whose hypertensive status has stabilized somewhat (Box 28-3).

SUMMARY

Diuretics are important therapeutic agents for the treatment of hypertension and for other conditions in which fluid volume excess is a problem, such as congestive heart failure, cirrhosis, and nephrotic syndrome. Diuretics are classified by the major site of their action along the tubule: proximal tubule diuretics, diluting segment diuretics, loop diuretics, and distal tubule diuretics. The osmotic diuretics enhance the flow of water from body tissues, and since they are not reabsorbed, they induce diuresis.

REVIEW QUESTIONS

1. Describe the use of acetazolamide in the treatment of glaucoma.
2. Describe the mechanisms and sites of action of the thiazide diuretics. Why are they less potent than the loop diuretics? What effect do they have on glucose, potassium, uric acid, serum levels of cholesterol, and triglycerides?
3. Compare the sites and mechanisms of action of the thiazide diuretics with the loop diuretics. Name a primary adverse reaction of concern and at least three serious drug interactions.
4. What are the advantages of combining a thiazide diuretic with a potassium-sparring diuretic or an antihypertensive drug with a diuretic?

REFERENCES

Jackson EK: Diuretics. In Hardman JG, Limbird LE, editors: *Goodman & Gilman's the pharmacological basis of therapeutics,* ed 9, New York, 1996, McGraw-Hill.

Menscer D: Hypertension. In Ham RJ, Sloane PD, editors: *Primary care geriatrics: a case-based approach,* ed 2, St Louis, 1992, Mosby.

Olin BR: *Facts and comparisons.* Philadelphia, 1998, JB Lippincott.

Tang I, Lau AH: Fluid and electrolyte disorders. In Young LY, Koda-Kimble MA, editors: *Applied therapeutics: the clinical use of drugs,* ed 6, Vancouver, Wash, 1995, Applied Therapeutics, Inc.

United States Pharmacopeial Convention: *USP DI: drug information for the health care professional,* ed 18, Rockville, Md, 1998, The Convention.

Wardlaw GM et al: *Contemporary nutrition: issues and insights,* ed 2, St Louis, 1994, Mosby.

ADDITIONAL REFERENCES

American Hospital Formulary Service: *AHFS drug information '98,* Bethesda, Md, 1996, American Society of Hospital Pharmacists.

American Medical Association: *AMA drug evaluations 1995,* Chicago, 1995, the Association.

Anderson KN et al, editors: *Mosby's medical, nursing, and allied health dictionary,* ed 5, St Louis, 1998, Mosby.

FDA: Regulatory actions, Demadex, *Hosp Formul* 29(4):226, 1994.

Mosby: *Mosby's GenRx,* St Louis, 1998, Mosby.

Williams SR: *Nutrition and diet therapy,* ed 8, St Louis, 1997, Mosby.

CHAPTER 29

Uricosuric Drugs

KEY DRUGS

allopurinol, (p. 434)
colchicine, (p. 433)

KEY TERMS

gout, (p. 433)
hyperuricemia, (p. 433)
urate neuropathy, (p. 434)

CHAPTER FOCUS

Gout is a disorder of uric acid metabolism that predominantly affects males in American society today. The onset of gout is usually during middle age, and it appears that less then 5% of all diagnosed cases are in postmenopausal women (probably because estrogen promotes excretion of uric acid [McCance, Huether, 1998]). This chapter reviews the primary drugs used in treatment and prevention of gout.

OBJECTIVES

After reading and studying this chapter, the student should be able to do the following:

1. *Define and discuss the key terms and key drugs.*
2. *Describe the cause and manifestation of gout in the body.*
3. *List the four treatment goals for gout.*
4. *Name three other disease states and four drugs that may cause hyperuricemia.*
5. *Discuss the mechanisms of action, indications, and significant drug interactions for colchicine, allopurinol, and probenecid.*

Hyperuricemia and gout occur in persons with an abnormality in uric acid production and/or excretion. Some of the risk factors for gout include obesity, hypertension, alcohol consumption, and lead exposure (Brooks, 1997). Recurrent gouty arthritis is painful and can cause crystal deposits throughout the body that results in an inflammatory response and in some instances, kidney stones.

GOUT

Gout is a disease associated with an inborn error of uric acid metabolism, which increases production or inhibits the excretion of uric acid. The hallmark of gout is **hyperuricemia,** or high levels of uric acid in the blood.

Gout is characterized by a defective purine metabolism and manifests itself by attacks of acute pain, swelling, and tenderness of joints, such as those of the big toe, ankle, instep, knee, and elbow. The amount of uric acid in the blood becomes elevated, and tophi, which are deposits of uric acid or urates, form in the cartilage of various parts of the body. These deposits tend to increase in size. They are seen most often along the edge of the ear. Chronic arthritis, nephritis, and premature sclerosis of blood vessels may develop if gout is uncontrolled.

Treatment goals for gout include the following: (1) end the acute gouty attack as soon as possible, (2) prevent a recurrence of acute gouty arthritis, (3) prevent the formation of uric acid stones in the kidneys, and (4) reduce or prevent disease complications that result from sodium urate deposits in joints and kidneys.

The drugs used to treat an acute gout attack include colchicine, nonsteroidal antiinflammatory drugs (NSAIDs), and corticosteroids. The NSAIDs are primarily used to treat the acute inflammation and have no effect on the underlying metabolic problem. They are often prescribed to relieve an acute gout attack while colchicine, because of its potentially toxic effects, is reserved for persons who are not responsive to these agents or individuals who cannot tolerate them (USP DI, 1998). The NSAIDs are discussed in Chapter 8. Colchicine, specifically used to treat gout, is reviewed in this chapter. To treat chronic gouty arthritis or to prevent gout attacks, allopurinol, probenecid, sulfinpyrazone, and salicylates have all been used. Salicylates require very high daily dosages (4 to 6 g/day). Because few individuals can tolerate such high dosages on a long-term basis, these agents are not commonly prescribed for gout.

The healthcare professional should be aware that low doses of aspirin can interfere with uric acid excretion, resulting in exacerbation of gout, and that a secondary hyperuricemia may occur from neoplastic diseases or cancer, psoriasis, Paget's disease, and other common and rare disease states. Many drugs have also been reported to cause an increase or a decrease in uric acid levels (Table 29-1). It is preferable for the prescriber to identify the cause of the hyperuricemia and then to decide whether or not to treat it. Asymptomatic hyperuricemia in an elderly person may or may not be drug induced and often is not treated by the prescriber because of the potential adverse drug reactions and the cost of the medications (Fig. 29-1). However, if symptoms are present or a treatable disease state is identified, then specific treatments would be indicated.

TABLE 29-1 Medications Affecting Serum Uric Acid Levels

Increase Levels	*Decrease Levels*
alcohol	acetohexamide
aminoglycosides	adrenocortitrophic hormone
cancer chemotherapeutic agents	allopurinol
diuretics (thiazides, furosemide)	chloramphenicol
ethambutol	probenecid
levodopa	radiopaque dyes
methyldopa	salicylates (more than 3 g/day)
pancrelipase	streptomycin
salicylates (less than 2 g/day)	tetracycline (outdated)

From Pagana, Pagana, 1997; USP DI, 1998; Young, Comagna, 1995.

Patients with gout should be instructed to avoid alcoholic beverages, because alcohol increases serum uric acid levels.

colchicine [kol' chi seen]

Colchicine's mechanism of action for gout is unknown, although it is reported to have antiinflammatory effects in gout. It also decreases phagocytosis, leukocyte motility, lactic acid production, and the release of a glycoprotein produced during urate crystal phagocytosis. These actions result in a decrease in urate deposits and inflammation even though the drug does not affect levels of uric acid in the circulatory system.

Indications

Colchicine is used in the treatment and prophylaxis of acute gouty arthritis and in the treatment of chronic gouty arthritis.

Pharmacokinetics

In acute gouty arthritis, colchicine has an onset of action within 12 hours after oral administration and intravenous injection. The peak effect for relief of pain and inflammation is reached in 1 to 2 days, but reduction of swelling may require 3 days or more. Colchicine is metabolized in the liver and excreted mainly in bile.

Drug interactions

When colchicine is given concurrently with radiation therapy or drugs that induce blood dyscrasia or bone marrow depression (such as phenylbutazone [Alka Butazolidine], chloramphenicol [Chloromycetin], antineoplastics, and others), the risk of bone marrow depression or other serious toxic hematologic effects are increased.

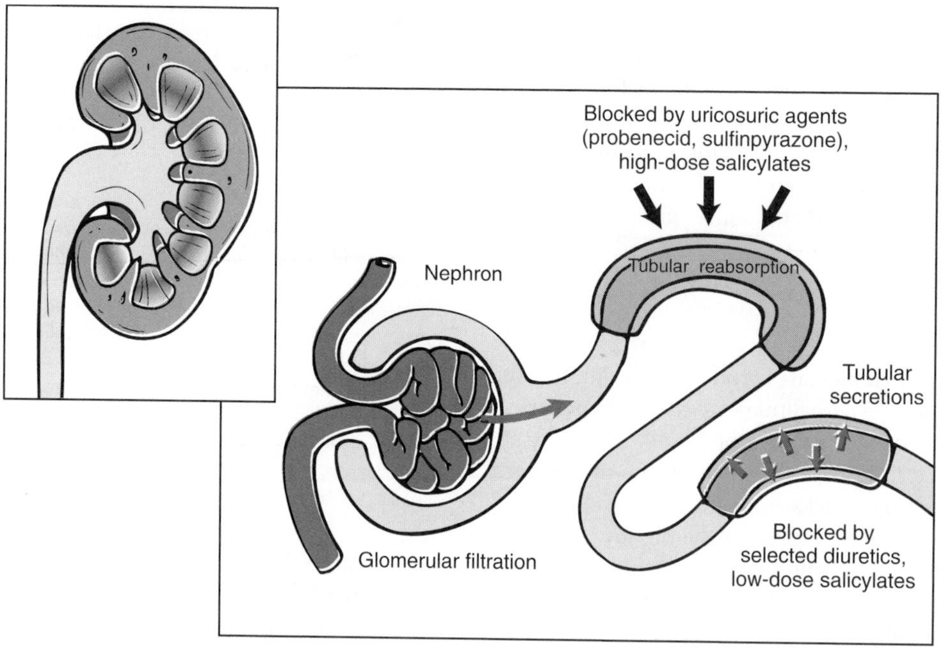

FIGURE 29-1
Drug effects on uric acid excretion in the kidney.

Side effects and adverse reactions

These include diarrhea, nausea, vomiting, abdominal pain, anorexia, and, with chronic therapy, alopecia. Rare adverse effects include hypersensitivity reactions, blood dyscrasias, neuropathy, myopathy, and bone marrow suppression.

Warnings

Use with caution in alcoholic patients. See the box for Food and Drug Administration (FDA) pregnancy safety categories.

Contraindications

Avoid use in persons with colchicine hypersensitivity, moderate to severe liver and kidney function impairment, leukopenia, blood dyscrasias, and cardiac and gastrointestinal (GI) disorders.

Dosage and administration

The adult antigout dosage for prophylaxis is 0.5 to 0.6 mg PO daily, increased if necessary to twice daily. The dose for acute gouty attacks is 0.5 to 1.2 mg (one to two tablets) initially, followed by one tablet every 1 to 2 hours until pain is relieved or the side effects of nausea, vomiting, or diarrhea have occurred or until the maximum dose of 6 mg has been reached. The pediatric dosage has not been established. The adult IV dose for prophylaxis is 0.5 to 1 mg once or twice daily. For use in acute gouty attacks, the dosage is 2 mg IV initially followed by 0.5 mg every 6 to 12 hours until the desired effect is achieved.

PREGNANCY SAFETY

Category	Drug
C	allopurinol
D	colchicine
Unclassified	probenecid, sulfinpyrazone

allopurinol [al oh pure′ i nole]
(Zyloprim, Purinol)

Allopurinol decreases the production of uric acid by inhibiting xanthine oxidase, the enzyme necessary to convert hypoxanthine to xanthine and xanthine to uric acid (Fig. 29-2). It also increases the reutilization of both hypoxanthine and xanthine for nucleic acid synthesis, thus resulting in a feedback inhibition of purine synthesis. The result is a decrease of uric acid in both the serum and urine.

This decrease of uric acid will prevent or decrease urate deposits, thus preventing or reducing both gouty arthritis and **urate nephropathy.** The reduction in urinary urate levels prevents the formation of uric acid or calcium oxalate calculi in the kidneys.

Indications

Allopurinol is indicated for the treatment of chronic gouty arthritis and for the prophylaxis and treatment

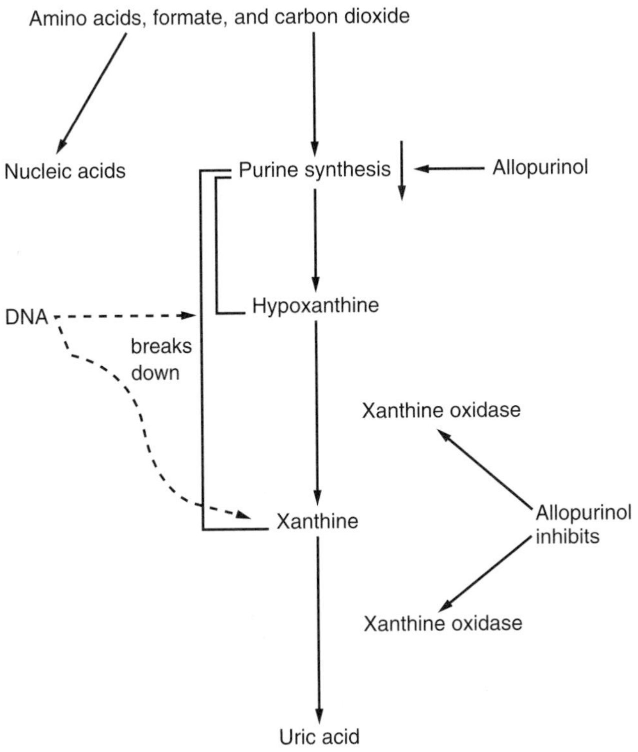

FIGURE 29-2
Uric acid production and allopurinol effects in the body.

of hyperuricemia, uric acid nephropathy, and renal calculi.

Pharmacokinetics

Allopurinol is well absorbed orally; the onset of action in reducing serum uric acid is 2 to 3 days. Approximately 70% of a dose is metabolized in the liver to an active metabolite, oxipurinol. Reduction of uric acid to a normal range occurs in 1 to 3 weeks, whereas a decrease in frequency of acute gout attacks may require several months of drug therapy. Excretion is via the kidneys.

Drug interactions

The following effects may occur when allopurinol is given with drugs listed below:

Drug	Possible effect and management
Anticoagulants, oral (coumarin or indanedione)	Allopurinol may inhibit metabolism of the oral anticoagulants, resulting in an increase in serum levels, activity, and perhaps toxicity. Monitor prothrombin levels closely because dosage adjustment may be necessary.
azathioprine (Imuran) or mercaptopurine (Purinethol)	Allopurinol's effect of inhibiting xanthine oxidase may result in decreased metabolism of these medications, leading to an increased potential for therapeutic and toxic effects (especially bone marrow depression). Monitor closely because interventions or dosage adjustments may be necessary.

Side effects and adverse reactions

These include pruritus, allergic reaction, rash, hives, diarrhea, abdominal distress, nausea, vomiting, alopecia, dermatitis, and, rarely, bone marrow depression, liver toxicity, a hypersensitivity reaction, peripheral neuritis, renal failure, and nosebleeds.

Warnings

Avoid use in patients with kidney function disease and any conditions that may predispose to changes in kidney function such as heart failure, diabetes mellitus, and hypertension.

Contraindications

Avoid use in persons with allopurinol hypersensitivity.

Dosage and administration

The adult antihyperuricemic dose is 100 mg daily initially, increased by 100 mg/day at 7-day intervals if necessary (the maximum dosage is 800 mg/day). The maintenance dosage is 100 to 200 mg two to three times daily or 300 mg once daily. For treatment of hyperuricemia (from antineoplastic therapy), initially administer 600 to 800 mg PO daily, beginning 2 to 3 days before chemotherapy or radiation therapy. For maintenance therapy, adjust the dosage according to serum uric acid levels, which are analyzed about 2 days after the initiation of allopurinol and periodically thereafter. Discontinue allopurinol during the period of tumor regression.

For treatment of uric acid calculi, the dosage is 100 to 200 mg PO one to four times daily or 300 mg daily as a single dose. For the pediatric dosage as an antihyperuricemic agent in antineoplastic therapy, see a current package insert or USP DI.

Patients should also be advised to increase their fluid intake, if not contraindicated, to 2.5 to 3 L/day, to reduce their risk of forming kidney stones. In addition, a neutral or slightly alkaline urine is also recommended, which can be accomplished by dietary means, such as consumption of milk, fruits (exception of plums, prunes or cranberries), and vegetables (exception of corn and lentils) and other dietary alterations as recommended by the prescriber or a dietitian.

probenecid [proe ben′ e sid] (Benemid, Benuryl)

Probenecid is indicated for the treatment of hyperuricemia and chronic gouty arthritis and as an adjunct to antibiotic therapy. It lowers serum levels of uric acid by competitively inhibiting the reabsorption of urate at the proximal renal tubule, thus increasing the urinary excretion of uric acid. It has no antiinflammatory action or analgesic effects.

As an adjunct to antibiotic therapy, probenecid competitively inhibits the secretion of weak organic acids, such as penicillin and some of the cephalosporins, at both the proximal and distal renal tubules in the kidneys. The result is an increase in blood concentrations and duration of action of these antibiotics. This combination is used to treat sexually transmitted diseases (e.g., gonorrhea, acute pelvic inflammatory disease, and neurosyphilis).

Pharmacokinetics

Probenecid is well absorbed orally and is highly bound to plasma proteins, especially to albumin. The therapeutic serum level for uricosuric effect is 100 to 200 μg/ml; for suppression of penicillin excretion it is 40 to 60 μg/ml. The peak uricosuric effect is reached within 30 minutes, whereas peak suppression of penicillin excretion is noted in 2 hours and lasts nearly 8 hours. Probenecid is metabolized in the liver and excreted by the kidneys.

Drug interactions

The following effects may occur when probenecid is given concurrently with the drugs listed below:

Drug	Possible effect and management
indomethacin (Indocin), ketoprofen (Orudis), and other NSAIDs	Probenecid decreases the renal excretion of ketoprofen by 66%, protein binding by 28%, and the formation of ketoprofen conjugates. This leads to an increase in ketoprofen serum levels and possibly toxicity. Avoid or a potentially serious drug interaction may occur. Probenecid may also decrease excretion of indomethacin and possibly other NSAIDs from the body, thus leading to increased serum levels, extended half-life, and increased potential for NSAID toxicity. Monitor closely because the prescriber may need to lower the daily dose of NSAID if adverse effects are reported.
Antineoplastic cytolytic drugs	Increased potential toxicity of uric acid nephropathy. Also, the rapidly acting antineoplastic drugs may increase plasma uric acid levels and interfere with any control of the previous hyperuricemia and gout. Avoid or a potentially serious drug interaction may occur.
aspirin or salicylates	Not recommended because salicylates in moderate to high doses given chronically will inhibit the effectiveness of probenecid. Also, if high doses of salicylates are being given for their uricosuric effects, probenecid may lower the excretion of salicylates, which may result in elevated serum salicylate levels and toxicity. Avoid or a potentially serious drug interaction may occur.
Cephalosporins, penicillins	Probenecid decreases the renal tubular secretion of penicillin and selected cephalosporins, which may result in an increased serum level and prolonged duration of action of the antibiotic. An increased risk of toxicity may also be present. Monitor serum levels closely if given concurrently. Cephalosporins not affected by probenecid include cefoperazone (Cefobid), ceforanide, ceftazidime (Fortaz), and ceftriaxone (Rocephin).
heparin	The anticoagulant effects of heparin may be enhanced and prolonged. Avoid or a potentially serious drug interaction may occur.
methotrexate (Folex, Mexate)	Probenecid may decrease the renal excretion of methotrexate, which may increase the risk of serious toxicity with methotrexate. If used concurrently, administer a lower dose of methotrexate and monitor closely for toxicity or monitor methotrexate serum levels.
nitrofurantoin (Furadantin)	Probenecid may decrease the renal tubular secretion of nitrofurantoin, resulting in an increase in serum levels and possibly toxicity. This may reduce the urinary levels and effectiveness of nitrofurantoin. A reduction in probenecid dosage may be necessary to use nitrofurantoin in urinary tract infections. Monitor effectiveness closely.
zidovudine (AZT)	Concurrent drug administration may lead to inhibition of zidovudine metabolism and secretion, resulting in elevated serum levels and an increased risk of zidovudine toxicity. The administration of probenecid may permit a reduced daily dose schedule for zidovudine. In one trial, a high incidence of skin rash was reported.

Color type indicates an unsafe drug combination.

Side effects and adverse reactions

These include headaches, anorexia, mild nausea or vomiting, sore gums, pain and/or blood on urination, lower back pain, frequent urge to urinate, renal stones, dermatitis, and, rarely, anaphylaxis, anemia, leukopenia, and nephrotic syndrome.

Warnings

Use with caution in patients with a history of peptic ulcer disease.

Contraindications

Avoid use in persons with probenecid hypersensitivity, in patients with any conditions that may increase uric acid formation such as a history of renal stones and moderate to severe kidney function impairment, or any patients undergoing treatment that may increase uric acid formation such as cancer chemotherapy, radiation therapy for cancer. Also avoid use in patients with blood disorders and kidney disease.

Dosage and administration

The adult dose is 250 mg twice daily for 7 days, increased to 500 mg twice a day. As an adjunct to penicillin/cephalosporin drug therapy the dose is 500 mg four times daily. The pediatric dosage as an antihyperuricemic agent is not established. As an antibiotic adjunct, check a current drug reference for recommended dosing schedules.

In addition, the patient should be instructed to maintain a high fluid intake and to take the medication with food or an antacid to reduce its potential for gastric irritation. If the prescriber suggests a diet for alkalinization of the urine the patient should be cautioned to closely follow the diet.

sulfinpyrazone [sul fin peer′ a zone] (Anturane)

The mechanism of action is similar to that of probenecid; it inhibits reabsorption of urate at the proximal renal tubule, thus increasing urinary uric acid excretion.

Indications

Sulfinpyrazone is indicated for the treatment of chronic gouty arthritis and hyperuricemia. Sulfinpyrazone is well absorbed orally and is highly bound to plasma proteins.

Pharmacokinetics

Sulfinpyrazone is metabolized in the liver into four active metabolites; the *p*-hydroxysulfinpyrazone metabolite produced contributes between 33% to 50% of the uricosuric effect of sulfinpyrazone. The duration of effect for the uricosuric effect is usually 4 to 6 hours. It is excreted by the kidneys.

Drug interactions

The following effects may occur when sulfinpyrazone is given concurrently with the drugs listed below:

Drug	Possible effect and management
Anticoagulants (coumarin or indanedione, heparin) or thrombolytics (streptokinase or urokinase)	Sulfinpyrazone may increase the anticoagulant effect by displacing coumarin or indanedione from its protein-binding site and by inhibiting metabolism. Monitor prothrombin time closely because dosage adjustments may be necessary. An increase in bleeding episodes or hemorrhage may result from concurrent administration of sulfinpyrazone and anticoagulant or thrombolytic therapy. The potential for this reaction is caused by the inhibitory effect of sulfinpyrazone on platelet aggregation and its possibility of causing gastrointestinal ulceration or hemorrhage. Avoid or a potentially serious drug interaction may occur.
alprostadil (Prostin VR), anagrelide, aspirin, dextran, carbenicillin (parenteral), dipyridamole (Persantin), divalproex (Depakote), moxalactam, NSAIDs, plicamycin (Mithracin), ticarcillin (Ticar), ticlopidine (Ticlid), or valproic acid (Depakene)	These drugs inhibit platelet aggregation; therefore concurrent drug administration may increase the potential of bleeding episodes. Monitor closely for early signs of bleeding.
Antineoplastic agents, rapidly cytolytic	Increased risk of inducing uric acid nephropathy or losing control of uric acid serum levels (preexisting levels) and gout is possible. Avoid or a potentially serious drug interaction may occur.
aspirin or salicylates	When salicylates are given long term in moderate to high doses, the uricosuric effect of sulfinpyrazone may be inhibited. See comments about probenecid. Avoid or a potentially serious drug interaction may occur.
cefotetan (Cefotan), cefamandole (Mandole), cefoperazone (Cefobid), or plicamycin (Mithracin)	These drugs can cause platelet function inhibition and hypoprothrombinemia (Moxalactam can cause irreversible platelet damage.) Monitor closely for bleeding tendencies. Avoid or a potentially serious drug interaction may occur.

nitrofurantoin (Furadantoin)	Sulfinpyrazone may decrease kidney excretion of nitrofurantoin, which may increase the risk of nitrofurantoin toxicity and reduce the effectiveness of nitrofurantoin as a urinary tract antiinfective agent. Avoid or a potentially serious drug interaction may occur.

Color type indicates an unsafe drug combination.

Side effects and adverse reactions

These include nausea, vomiting, abdominal pain, and rash or allergic reaction.

Dosage and administration

The adult antigout dosage is 100 to 200 mg PO twice daily initially, increased gradually at 2-day intervals as necessary (usually 400 to 800 mg/day). The maintenance dosage is 200 to 400 mg daily. The pediatric dosage has not been established.

Instruct the patient to take the medication with food to reduce the potential for gastric irritation. Also, a high fluid intake is recommended; if the prescriber suggests a alkaline urine, instruct the patient to closely follow dietary instructions.

The NSAIDs indomethacin (Indocin), naproxen (Naprosyn), phenylbutazone (Butazolidin), and sulindac (Clinoril) are also used in the treatment of acute gouty arthritis. Only the immediate-release dosage forms are used for the treatment of an acute attack. For information on these drugs, see Chapter 8.

SUMMARY

Gout is a metabolic disorder of uric acid metabolism that is characterized by hyperuricemia. The primary goals of therapy are to end the acute attack as soon as possible, to prevent a recurrence, to prevent the formation of uric acid stones in the kidneys, and to prevent or minimize the complications of sodium urate deposits in the joints. The primary medications used for these purposes are colchicine, allopurinol, probenecid, and sulfinpyrazone.

REVIEW QUESTIONS

1. Describe the effects of low-dose and high-dose aspirin on uric acid in gout.
2. Why does the prescriber often choose not to treat asymptomatic hyperuricemia, especially in the elderly patient?
3. Why is probenecid combined or given with antibiotic therapy, such as penicillin and some cephalosporins? Describe the site of action and ultimate effects.
4. What are the usual dietary and fluid, and alcohol intake recommendations suggested to the patient with gout?

REFERENCES

Brooks PM: Rheumatic disorders. In Speight TM, Holford NHG, editors: *Avery's Drug Treatment,* ed 4, Auckland, New Zealand, 1997 Adis International.

McCance KL, Huether SE: *Pathophysiology: the biologic basis for disease in adults and children,* ed 3, St Louis, 1998, Mosby.

Pagana KD, Pagana TJ: *Mosby's diagnostic and laboratory test reference,* ed. 3, St Louis, 1997, Mosby.

United States Pharmacopeial Convention: *USP DI: drug information for the health care professional,* ed 18, Rockville, Md, 1998, The Convention.

Young LY, Campagna KD: Gout and hyperuricemia. In Young LY, Koda-Kimble MA, editors: *Applied therapeutics: the clinical use of drugs,* ed 6, Vancouver, Wash, 1995, Applied Therapeutics, Inc.

ADDITIONAL REFERENCES

American Hospital Formulary Service: *AHFS drug information '98,* Bethesda, Md, 1996, American Society of Hospital Pharmacists.

American Medical Association: *AMA drug evaluations 1995,* Chicago, 1995, the Association.

Anderson KN et al, editors: *Mosby's medical, nursing, and allied health dictionary,* ed 5, St Louis, 1998, Mosby.

Abrams WB, Berkow R: *The Merck manual of geriatrics,* Rahway, NJ, 1990, Merck Sharp & Dohme Research Laboratories.

Mosby: *Mosby's GenRx,* St Louis, 1998, Mosby.

Olin BR: *Facts and comparisons.* Philadelphia, 1998, JB Lippincott.

Physicians' desk reference, ed 52, Montvale, NJ, 1998, Medical Economics Co.

Seeley RR, Stephens TD, Tate P: *Anatomy and physiology,* ed 3, New York, 1995, McGraw-Hill.

Thibodeau GA, Patton KT: *Anatomy and physiology,* ed 4, St Louis, 1999, Mosby.

CHAPTER 30

Drug Therapy for Renal System Dysfunction

CHAPTER FOCUS

Renal impairment or failure can alter the distribution and protein binding of drugs by modifying systemic pH, altering albumin, and drug renal excretion. This can be a significant problem when drug therapy is needed, as renal dysfunction may cause the parent drug or its toxic metabolites to accumulate. In addition, medications can cause drug-induced nephrotoxicity. Management of drug therapy in such patients is important for the healthcare professional.

OBJECTIVES

After reading and studying this chapter, the student should be able to do the following:

1. *Define and describe the key terms.*
2. *Discuss the differences between acute renal failure and chronic renal failure.*
3. *Describe and compare the uses of epoetin and erythropoietin. Review the pharmacokinetics of epoetin.*
4. *Discuss the serum creatinine and creatinine clearance tests and their relationship to renal function*
5. *Discuss several parameters for monitoring the patient with renal system dysfunction.*

KEY TERMS

acute renal failure, (p. 440)
azotemic, (p. 440)
chronic renal failure, (p. 440)
end-stage renal disease, (p. 440)
hemodialysis, (p. 440)
peritoneal dialysis, (p. 440)

The person with impaired renal function receiving standard drug dosages on a regular schedule may experience drug accumulation and toxicity. Therefore it is important for the healthcare provider to monitor persons with impaired renal function because drug dosages or time intervals frequently need to be adjusted.

ACUTE VERSUS CHRONIC RENAL FAILURE

Acute renal failure, a condition characterized by oliguria, by the rapid accumulation of nitrogenous wastes in the blood, and by a rapid decline in renal function, occurs in 2% to 5% of all hospitalized individuals and up to 1% of persons admitted to the hospital from the community (Bailie, 1995). Primary causes include trauma, pregnancy, renal ischemia as a result of surgery, severe hemorrhage, severe volume depletion, and shock. In some instances, nephrotoxic agents such as heavy metals and aminoglycosides may also induce acute renal failure. If recognized early and treated promptly, acute renal failure may be reversed before acute tubular necrosis or permanent damage occurs.

Chronic renal failure (CRF) is a progressive disease usually caused by an irreversible kidney injury that results in permanent nephron or renal mass loss. It is a major health concern in North America. In 1991, nearly 215,000 persons in the U.S. Medicare program had end-stage renal disease (Ateshkadi, Johnson, 1995). The most common causes of CRF are glomerulonephritis, diabetes mellitus, hypertension, polycystic kidney disease, and other diseases that may lead to destruction or impaired functioning of the kidneys. Individuals with CRF may be treated conservatively initially, but in **end-stage renal disease** (ESRD), hemodialysis, peritoneal dialysis, or organ transplantation may be necessary. **Hemodialysis** is a procedure in which impurities or wastes are removed from the blood, shunting the blood from the body through a machine for diffusion and ultrafiltration, then returning it to the patient's circulation. **Peritoneal dialysis** is another form of dialysis, but one in which the peritoneum is used as the diffusible membrane. A solution known as dialysate is placed via a catheter into the peritoneal cavity and retained for a specified time while osmosis, diffusion, and filtration pass needed electrolytes into the bloodstream and remove wastes into the dialysate, which is then drained by gravity from the abdominal cavity.

As the focus of this book is pharmacology, this chapter concentrates on the therapeutic regimen and recommendations for drug dosage adjustments in patients with impaired renal function.

SIGNS AND SYMPTOMS OF RENAL FAILURE OR INSUFFICIENCY

One of the more common signs of acute renal failure is a marked alteration in the expected urine output, which is usually significant (<400 ml/day). Thus the first phase is the oliguric phase. Phase two is the diuretic phase; in this phase the individual has an increase in urine volume for a few days but he or she is still **azotemic,** retaining excessive amounts of nitrogenous compounds (blood urea nitrogen and creatinine) in the blood. Phase three is considered the recovery phase as azotemia decreases and renal function is recovering. The recovery phase may occur over weeks to months, depending on the damage caused by the original insult to the kidneys (Bailie, 1995). Signs of acute renal failure, in the presence of reduced urine production are usually the result of fluid overload: edema, weight gain, weakness, hypertension, and tachycardia.

The most common complaints with CRF are increasing weakness, fatigue, and lethargy. Gastrointestinal signs include anorexia, gastrointestinal distress, nausea, vomiting, thirst, and weight loss. Paresthesias, peripheral neuropathy, convulsions, and neuromuscular irritability may also occur. On examination, the patient may appear pale and dehydrated and have an increased respiratory rate and uremic breath. Hypertension with retinopathy, cardiac hypertrophy, pulmonary edema, or pericarditis may often be present.

A detailed patient history, thorough physical examination, urinalysis, and measurement of blood chemistry levels are important for assessment, diagnosis, and determination of an appropriate treatment plan. The degree of renal impairment is usually estimated by reviewing the serum creatinine and blood urea nitrogen (BUN) levels. Elevated levels indicate a decrease in renal clearance, which, of course, predisposes the individual to drug toxicity.

MEASUREMENT OF RENAL FUNCTION

Many formulas and nomograms are available to determine the individual's approximate creatinine clearance and the appropriate drug dosage adjustment necessary to minimize the possibility of toxicity. Normal values may vary from laboratory to laboratory, but, in general, a normal BUN level ranges between 5 and 20 mg/dl, while the level of serum creatinine, which varies with age, usually ranges between 0.5 and 1.2 mg/dl. The most reliable test is the creatinine clearance test, but since accurate collection of all urine excreted for a 24 hour period is difficult, many clinicians use a formula to estimate creatinine clearance and others prefer to use a nomogram. The formulas most commonly used are noted in Box 30-1. The mean endogenous creatinine clearance in an adult is usually between 90 and 130 ml/min/1.73 m^2 body surface per 24 hours. Therefore reductions in this quantity signify impairment of renal function (Box 30-2).

Another important factor in evaluating drug blood levels in patients with renal failure or renal impairment is an assessment of serum albumin and total protein for the patient. Serum protein is decreased in individuals with renal insufficiency, which can alter the interpretation of serum levels of drugs that are protein bound (90% or more) in the normal person. Individuals with a lower albumin or protein value may have a drug concentration in the low range that appears to be therapeutic. This is possible if the laboratory does not differentiate between the bound and unbound drug in the testing. Lower protein levels may lead to a higher

BOX 30-1 Formulas for Estimating Creatinine Clearance

Adult male =

$$\frac{(140 - \text{age}) \times (\text{ideal body weight in kg})}{72 \times \text{serum creatinine (mg per dL)}}$$

Adult female =

$$\frac{(140 - \text{age}) \times (\text{ideal body weight in kg})}{72 \times \text{serum creatinine (mg per dL)}} \times 0.85$$

Ideal Body Weight (IBW) Calculations

IBW (males) = 50 kg + (2.3 kg × inches over 5 feet)

IBW (females) = 45 kg + (2.3 kg × inches over 5 feet)

From *USP DI,* 1998.

BOX 30-2 Typical Grading for Renal Impairment Using Creatinine Clearance

Degree of Renal Failure	*Creatinine Clearance*
Normal	Men: 90-139 mL/min Women: 80-125 mL/min
Mild impairment	50-80 mL/min
Moderate impairment	10-50 mL/min
Severe impairment	<10 mL/min

Data from Bennett WM et al, 1983.

unbound concentration of the drug (the active form), thus producing an adequate therapeutic response.

SPECIAL NEEDS OF THE CRF PATIENT

The individual in CRF has special dietary, electrolyte, and fluid requirements. In general, dietary protein is usually restricted to 0.5 to 1 g/kg of lean body weight daily. This limitation will reduce the incidence of azotemia, hyperkalemia, and acidosis. Fluid intake is based on daily losses and metabolic needs. Dietary sodium is restricted to approximately 2 g or 90 mEq/day. Potassium, magnesium, and phosphorus are also restricted. Often an aluminum hydroxide gel is prescribed to decrease phosphate absorption from the gastrointestinal tract. The reduced excretion of phosphates, magnesium, and potassium from the kidneys with CRF can lead to elevated serum levels or hypermagnesemia, hyperkalemia, and hyperphosphatemia, which in turn lead to hypocalcemia and osteodystrophy.

Thus dietary restrictions are absolutely necessary. Calcium supplements and vitamin D are often prescribed for these patients to reduce or prevent hyperparathyroidism and bone disease. Magnesium levels are kept somewhat in check by the patient's avoidance of magnesium-containing antacids and laxatives.

Production of red blood cells (erythropoiesis), which is usually decreased in CRF, leads to anemia, weakness, and fatigue. Iron therapy may be prescribed for those patients with iron deficiency anemia resulting from chronic blood loss; folic acid, vitamin C, and soluble B complex vitamins are often given to replace substances usually lost during dialysis. Therefore it is not unusual to care for CRF patients to have many dietary and fluid restrictions, as well as prescriptions for vitamins, calcium, specific antacids, and additional drugs as necessary. A drug specifically used to stimulate erythropoiesis in CRF is epoetin.

epoetin [eh poh′ ee tin] (Epogen)

Epoetin is a glycoprotein chemically identical to human erythropoietin. It is produced by recombinant DNA technology and contains the same 165 amino acids in the same sequence as human erythropoietin. Therefore epoetin stimulates bone marrow erythropoiesis and also induces the release of reticulocytes from the marrow so they can then mature into erythrocytes. Human erythropoietin is produced mainly in the kidneys.

Indications

Epoetin is indicated for the treatment of anemia associated with renal failure and severe anemia associated with acquired immunodeficiency syndrome (AIDS) but should not be considered a substitute for blood or blood transfusions.

Epoetin has the same biologic action as the endogenous hormone; it stimulates erythropoiesis in the bone marrow and also induces the release of reticulocytes from bone marrow. Because endogenous erythropoietin is manufactured mainly in the kidneys, anemia resulting from CRF is caused by inadequate production of the hormone.

Pharmacokinetics

With the use of epoetin, the initial increase in reticulocytes is seen within 7 to 10 days while an increase in red cell count, hematocrit, and hemoglobin occurs within 2 to 6 weeks. This product reaches its peak serum level within 15 minutes after intravenous administration and within 5 to 24 hours after a subcutaneous dose. The half-life is between 4 and 13 hours after intravenous or subcutaneous administration. When therapy is discontinued, the hematocrit decreases in approximately 2 weeks (duration of action).

Drug interactions

No significant drug interactions have been reported.

Side effects and adverse reactions

The most frequent side effects include arthralgias or bone pain, asthenia (severe muscle weakness), nausea and vomiting, increased weakness, diarrhea, chest pain, edema of extremities or face, weight gain, tachycardia, headache, and hypertension. The most common adverse reactions include clotting of the arteriovenous shunt and/or dialyzer, hypertension, and polycythemia

TABLE 30-1 Selected Medication Dosing for Adults in Renal Insufficiency

	Creatinine Clearance (mL/min)*			
		Renal Failure		
Medication	**Normal Dose >50**	**10-50**	**<10**	**t½ (hr)**
acyclovir (Zovirax)	5 mg/kg q8h	5 mg/kg q12-24h	2.5 mg/kg q24h	N: 2.5 A: 20
ampicillin (Omnipen-N)	1-2 g q4-6h	1-1.5 g q6h	1 g q8-12h	N: 0.8-1.5 A-20
cefazolin (Ancef)	1-2 g q8h	0.5-1.5 g q12h	0.5-1 g q24h	N: 1.8-2.6 A: 12-40
ciprofloxacin (Cipro)	250-750 mg PO q12h	250-500 mg q12h	250-750 mg q24h	N: 4 A: 8.5
fluconazole (Diflucan)	100-200 mg q24h	50-200 mg q24h	50-100 mg q24h	N: 20-50 A: 98
gentamicin (Garamycin)	1 mg/kg q8h	0.25-0.5 mg/kg q8h	0.1 mg/kg q8h	N: 1.5-3 A: 20-54
meperidine (Demerol)	50-100 mg IV/IM q3-4h	75%-100% of dose q6h	50% of dose q6-8h	N: 3-7 A: ?
vancomycin (Vancocin)	500 mg q6h	1 g q3-7 days	1 g q1-2 wk	N: 4-9 A: 129-190

From Aweeka, 1995; *USP DI*, 1998; *PDR*, 1998.
t½, half-life; *N*, normal; *A*, anuric.
*Creatinine clearance or glomerular filtration rate.

Warnings

Use with caution in patients with blood disorders including sickle cell anemia, vascular disease, history of convulsions, folic acid or vitamin B_{12} deficiency, infections, inflammation, and aluminum toxicity.

Contraindications

Avoid use in persons with hypertension.

Dosage and administration

The initial adult dose (IV and SC) is 50 to 100 units/kg three times a week. If hematocrit has not increased after 2 months of therapy by at least 5 to 6 points and the patient's level is still below the desired range of 30% to 33%, then dosage increments of 25 units/kg may be instituted. For maintenance, decrease the dose gradually by 25 units/kg monthly to the lowest dose that maintains hematocrit at the desired level. The dosage for children younger than 12 years of age has not been determined. Pregnancy safety has been established by the Food and Drug Administration (FDA) as category C.

TABLE 30-2 Medications Associated with Renal Toxicity or Dysfunction

Possible Toxicity or Dysfunction	**Medications**
Acute tubular necrosis	aminoglycoside antibiotics, cephalothin, vancomycin, amphotericin B, cyclosporine, anticancer medications (cisplatin, nitrosoureas)
Obstructive nephropathy	sulfonamides, cytotoxic agents such as methotrexate, acyclovir, ciprofloxacin, excessive amounts of vitamin D and calcium
Analgesic nephropathy	phenacetin, aspirin, NSAIDs
Chronic interstitial nephritis	cyclosporine, lithium, cisplatin, aminoglycosides
Membranes glomerulonephritis	gold salts, penicillamine

From Critchley, et al., 1997.

SELECTED DRUG MODIFICATIONS IN RENAL FAILURE

As previously mentioned, BUN and serum creatinine are waste products to be excreted by the kidneys. Serum levels of these substances are used to measure renal function. Unfortunately, neither test is useful in discovering early renal impairment because abnormal levels do not appear until 50% or more of renal function is impaired. Fortunately, human kidneys are functional even if 90% of the glomerular filtration rate is lost. However, the continuing progressive loss may result in end-stage renal disease, renal loss necessitating hemodialysis, peritoneal dialysis, kidney transplantation, and other interventions discussed in this chapter.

In individuals with renal insufficiency or impairment, the drug dosage may be decreased (dosage reduction method) while maintaining the usual interval, or if the dose is the usually prescribed one, the interval between doses is lengthened (interval extension method). Usually the dosage reduction method is preferred for drugs that require a constant blood therapeutic level. For most patients receiving a loading dose, the dose is similar to the dose given to a person without renal impairment. This permits a therapeutically desirable blood level that is then maintained by one of the above dosing methods. Table 30-1 gives typical dosing recommendations for selected medications, along with a list of drugs that may or may not be removed by hemodialysis or peritoneal dialysis. See Table 30-2 for the medications that have been associated with renal toxicity or dysfunction. The reader is referred to current package inserts or renal failure dosing guides for specific data.

SUMMARY

Renal system dysfunction may be a source of tremendous stress for the patient and family, and it also presents a challenge for the healthcare professional. Treatment is complicated by multiple drug therapy and altered pharmacokinetics. Drug interactions or adverse reactions may appear at any time, and make close monitoring of drug effects and renal function by the healthcare professional essential. In addition, nondrug therapy, such as diet modification and fluid restriction, and involvement of other body systems present additional areas for intervention.

REFERENCES

Ateshkadi A, Johnson CA: Chronic renal failure.In Young LY, Koda-Kimble MA, editors: *Applied therapeutics: the clinical use of drugs,* ed 6, Vancouver, Wash, 1995, Applied Therapeutics, Inc.

Aweeka FT: Dosing of drugs in renal failure. In Young LY, Koda-Kimble MA, editors: *Applied therapeutics: the clinical use of drugs,* ed 6, Vancouver, Wash, 1995, Applied Therapeutics, Inc.

Bailie GR: Acute renal failure. In Young LY, Koda-Kimble MA, editors: *Applied therapeutics: the clinical use of drugs,* ed 6, Vancouver, Wash, 1995, Applied Therapeutics, Inc.

Bennett WM et al: Drug prescribing in enal failure: dosing guidelines for adults. *Am J Kidney Dis* 3(3):155, 1983.

Critchley JAJH, Chan TYK, Cumming AD: Renal disease. In Speight TM, Holford HG, editors: *Avery drug treatment,* ed 4, Auckland, New Zealand, 1997, Adis International.

Physicians' desk reference, ed 52, Montvale, NJ, 1998, Medical Economics Co.

United States Pharmacopeial Convention: *USP DI: drug information for the health care professional,* ed 18, Rockville, Md, 1998, The Convention.

ADDITIONAL REFERENCES

Anderson KN et al, editors: *Mosby's medical, nursing, and allied health dictionary,* ed 5, St Louis, 1998, Mosby.

Baer C, Lancaster LE: Acute renal failure, CCNQ 14(4):1, 1992.

Brundage DJ: *Renal disorders,* St Louis, 1992, Mosby.

Mosby: *Mosby's GenRx,* St Louis, 1998, Mosby.

Pagana KD, Pagana TJ: *Mosby's diagnostic and laboratory test reference,* ed. 3, St Louis, 1997, Mosby.

Thibodeau GA, Patton KT: *Anatomy and physiology,* ed 4, St Louis, 1999, Mosby.

UNIT VIII

Drugs Affecting the Respiratory System

CHAPTER 31

Overview of the Respiratory System

CHAPTER FOCUS

The respiratory system maintains the exchange of oxygen and carbon dioxide in the lungs and cells and also regulates the pH of body fluids. Thus, any changes within the respiratory system affect other body systems. Disorders of other body systems (such as fever) may increase the body's oxygen requirement and therefore increase the work of respiration. Many patients in clinical settings have respiratory problems that require care and interventions by healthcare professionals. This chapter provides an anatomy and physiology review to prepare the student for understanding the drugs affecting the respiratory system in the following chapters.

OBJECTIVES

After reading and studying this chapter, the student should be able to do the following:

1. *Define and describe the key terms.*
2. *Describe the three interrelated respiration processes.*
3. *Name five factors that determine airway efficiency.*
4. *Name and describe the two sources of respiratory secretions.*
5. *Describe the beta$_2$ receptor theory of bronchodilation.*
6. *Discuss the central and peripheral regulation of respiration.*

KEY TERMS

bronchial glands, (p. 448)
bronchoconstriction, (p. 448)
bronchodilation, (p. 449)
cellular respiration, (p. 448)
gas transport, (p. 448)
goblet cells, (p. 448)
mucokinesis, (p. 448)
pulmonary ventilation, (p. 448)

The respiratory system includes all structures involved in the exchange of oxygen and carbon dioxide, such as the airway passages, lungs, nasal cavities, pharynx, larynx, trachea, bronchi, bronchioles, pulmonary lobules with their alveoli, diaphragm, and all muscles concerned with respiration itself.

The most urgent and critical need for maintaining life is a continued, uninterrupted supply of oxygen. Oxygen is supplied to the body through the process of respiration. Respiration is a term loosely used to describe three distinct but interrelated processes:

- **Pulmonary ventilation,** which involves the movement of air into and out of the lungs
- **Gas transport,** which involves the exchange of gases between the air in the lungs, the blood, and the cell
- **Cellular respiration,** which involves the utilization of oxygen in the catabolism of energy-yielding substances for the production of energy

Respiration, one of the body's regulating systems, helps maintain physiologic dynamic equilibrium. It also compensates for rapid adjustment to changes in metabolic states.

The air passages permit air to flow from the external environment to pulmonary blood and modify the air taken in by warming and moistening it and removing noxious substances. Airway efficiency is determined by the following factors:

- Shape and size of each portion of the respiratory tract (nasal cavity, pharynx, larynx, trachea, bronchi, bronchioles, and alveolar sacs)
- Presence of a ciliated, mucus-secreting, epithelial lining throughout most of the respiratory tract
- Character and thickness of respiratory tract secretions
- Compliance of the cartilaginous and bony supports
- Pressure gradients
- Traction on airway walls
- Absence of foreign substances in the lumen of the respiratory tract

Any alteration of any of these factors will affect the ease with which air flows through the air passages, or effective airway clearance. Congenital anomalies, injuries, allergies, or disease will cause air flow resistance if these factors are abnormally affected. For example, resistance occurs if there is stenosis or narrowing of any portion of the respiratory tract, a loss of cilia that ordinarily sweep out foreign substances, any thick or tenacious secretions, loss of elasticity, or the presence of foreign objects.

RESPIRATORY TRACT SECRETIONS

The tracheobronchial tree, made up of repeated branching tubes, is a tubular airway that serves as a conduit for passage of air from the external environment to the alveolar-capillary exchange unit. The inner surface of the tracheobronchial tree is lined with ciliated columnar epithelium interspersed with **goblet cells.** The gelatinous mucus (gel layer) produced by goblet cells is normally discharged into the tubular lumen. In some obstructive pulmonary diseases, mucus secretion is greatly increased, thus making it difficult for the cilia to transport secretions along the airway (Fig. 31-1).

The **bronchial glands,** which are located in the submucosa of the tracheobronchial tree, secrete a relatively watery fluid (sol layer) through ducts leading to the surface of the ciliated epithelium. Under vagal (parasympathetic) control, the glands can be stimulated by irritant agents or aerosol drugs to release their contents into the lumen of the airway (Fig. 31-1, *B*).

The products of these two sources—goblet cells and bronchial glands—form the sol-gel film that makes up the mucociliary blanket. This protective blanket of fluid bathes the ciliated epithelium of the tracheobronchial tree. In addition, the cilia continuously propel the sol gel film up toward the larynx along the respiratory tree. The normal adult produces approximately 100 ml of respiratory secretions per day and swallows this material without being aware of it. The process of moving mucus along the tracheobronchial tree is called **mucokinesis.** The mucociliary blanket is a basic concern in most chronic obstructive pulmonary disease. The cilia must sustain appropriate function; a dry atmosphere causes the respiratory secretions to become thick and tenacious, which tends to interfere with ciliary movements. Thus adequate humidity should be maintained to prevent the change in the normal consistency of the respiratory secretions.

BRONCHIAL SMOOTH MUSCLE

Smooth Muscle Arrangement

An important structure of the tracheobronchial tree is the smooth muscle. The mass of muscle fibers along the bronchi progressively increases as it extends down toward the distal bronchioles. Isolated muscle fibers may be found as far down as the alveolar ducts. The smooth muscle fibers are arranged along the length of the tubular tree in a double helical or spiral pattern, and this formation profoundly influences the diameter or the lumen of the airways. Because of this structural feature, the effect of muscle contraction reduces both the diameter and the length of the bronchus (Fig. 32-1, *C*).

Nerve Supply

The airway or tracheobronchial tree is innervated by the autonomic nervous system. The bronchial smooth muscle tone is influenced by the balance maintained between parasympathetic and sympathetic stimuli during rest. Activation of the parasympathetic fiber (vagus nerve) releases acetylcholine, which results in **bronchoconstriction,** a narrowing of the lumen of the bronchial airway. By contrast, the stimulation of the sympathetic fiber and the sympathoadrenal system releases epinephrine and norepinephrine from the adrenal medulla into circulation. Their action on the $beta_2$ receptor sites in the bronchial smooth muscle produces bronchodilation by means of smooth muscle relaxation, which improves ventilation to the lungs.

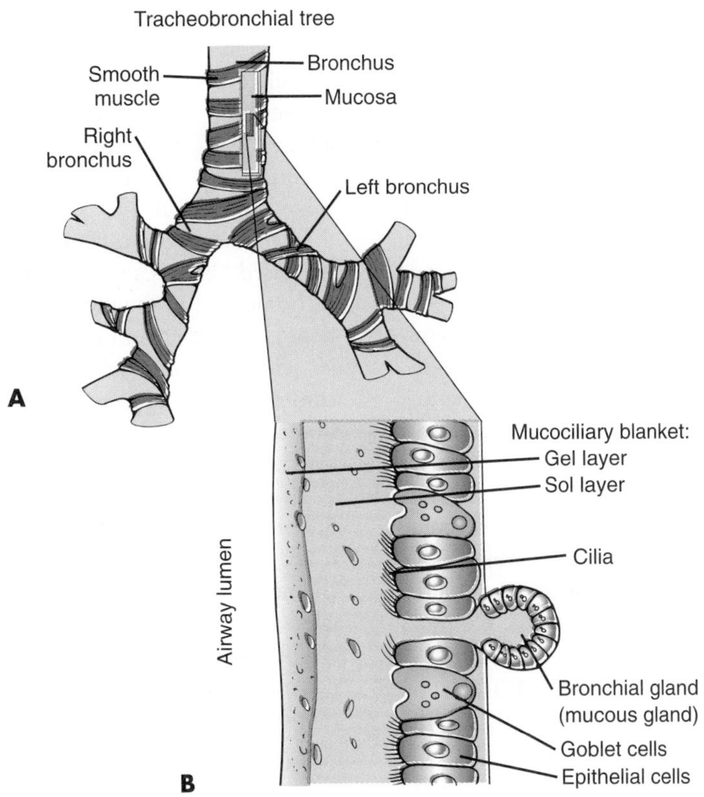

FIGURE 31-1

Tracheobronchial tree and bronchial smooth muscle. **A,** Diagram of tracheobronchial tree. **B,** Cut-out section of inner lining of bronchus.

Receptors

Several kinds of receptors are found along the bronchial airway. The release of acetylcholine activates muscarinic receptors during stimulation of the parasympathetic system, whereas the sympathetic system affects adrenergic receptors. Most of the adrenergic receptors present in the bronchial smooth muscle are $beta_2$ receptors that are stimulated mainly by epinephrine released from the adrenal medulla. $Beta_1$ receptors are also found, although the ratio of $beta_2$ to $beta_1$ receptors is approximately 3:1. Thus bronchial smooth muscle is supplied primarily by $beta_2$ receptors. The sympathomimetic drugs used principally as bronchodilators stimulate the $beta_2$ receptors. Because many of these agents are not purely selective in their pharmacologic effect, they also stimulate the $beta_1$ receptors in the heart, as well as alpha receptors in the lungs and peripheral arterioles. The side effects on the heart are increased cardiac output, tachycardia, and dysrhythmia. Few alpha receptors are present on the bronchial smooth muscle, and their stimulation results in only mild bronchoconstriction.

Bronchodilation

The $beta_2$-adrenergic receptors mediate **bronchodilation.** This mechanism presumably is initiated by epinephrine released from the adrenal medulla and norepinephrine released from the peripheral sympathetic nerves. Also located in the cell membrane is an enzyme system known as adenylate cyclase. In the presence of magnesium ions, adenylate cyclase catalyzes the action of adenosine triphosphate (ATP) in the cytoplasm of the cell to produce cyclic 3′,5′-adenosine-monophosphate (cyclic AMP or cAMP). Cyclic AMP then performs its important function, inducing relaxation of bronchial smooth muscle or bronchodilation. The hormone epinephrine is designated as the "first messenger" and cyclic AMP as the "second messenger." As a final action, cyclic AMP is inactivated by an enzyme, phosphodiesterase, which catalyzes it to the inactive 5′-AMP. This results in a fall in the cyclic AMP level. The action of phosphodiesterase may be inhibited by a xanthine drug such as theophylline. As a consequence, the cyclic AMP level remains elevated, thereby affecting smooth muscle dilation (see Fig. 32-4).

Circulating catecholamines can exert their effects on $beta_1$, $beta_2$, and alpha receptors. Persons with asthma may have a normal reaction to both alpha and beta stimulation through a reduced cyclic AMP response, by an abnormally sensitive response to alpha stimulation, and by an exaggerated response to the muscarinic agonists via the vagal pathways. This exaggerated bronchoconstrictive airway response may result from the effects of a decrease in cyclic AMP, histamine effects on smooth muscle, the vagal reflex pathway, an increase in cyclic guanylic acid secondary to calcium influx, and histamine-induced release of the contents of mast cells. Bronchodilation is induced by circulating catecholamines or administration of a sympathomimetic agent.

Circulating catecholamines reach the lung via circulation and interact with the beta$_2$-adrenergic receptors in the cell membrane of the bronchial smooth muscle cell.

Bronchoconstriction

The bronchial smooth muscle is innervated by the parasympathetic fibers from the vagus nerve. Acetylcholine released from the terminal interacts with the muscarinic receptors on the membrane of the cell. Stimulation of the muscarinic receptor increases the activity of the enzyme guanylate cyclase in the membrane, thereby promoting the rate of formation of cyclic 3′,5′-guanosine monophosphase (cyclic GMP) from guanosine triphosphate (GTP) (see Fig. 32-4). The cyclic GMP level affects the bronchial muscle by producing bronchoconstriction. In addition, alpha receptors found on the bronchial smooth muscle have a similar involvement with this mechanism. On activation, the alpha receptors also increase the cyclic GMP level. Further, cyclic GMP stimulates the release of chemical mediators from the mast cell during an asthmatic attack, and these mediators are responsible for causing bronchoconstriction.

CONTROL OF RESPIRATION

Central Control

The basic rhythm for respiration is initiated and maintained in the medullary rhythmicity area located beneath the lower part of the floor of the fourth ventricle in the medial half of the medulla. Neurons that control inspiration and expiration intermingle and discharge or fire impulses alternately. However, signals from the spinal cord, the cerebral cortex and midbrain, the apneustic area of the pons, and the pneumotaxic area of the upper pons can enter the medullary rhythmicity area, modify the rhythm of respiration, and contribute to the normal pattern of respiration.

Normally, the human organism is unaware of the respiratory process. However, voluntary influence and control of breathing are possible. This is important when a patient must learn to voluntarily control breathing patterns.

Peripheral Control

The medullary rhythmicity area is also influenced by various sensory and peripheral stimuli, the vasomotor center, reflex mechanisms (e.g., the Hering-Breuer reflex), the chemoreceptors in the carotid and aortic bodies, and the baroreceptors in the carotid sinus and aortic arch. Fear, pain, stress, blood pressure, body temperature, and blood levels of oxygen and carbon dioxide can all modify the activity of the respiratory centers.

Humoral regulation of respiration is achieved primarily through changes in the concentrations of oxygen, carbon dioxide, or hydrogen ions in body fluids. In a healthy individual, carbon dioxide is the chief respiratory stimulant. An increase in the carbon dioxide tension of the blood directly stimulates the inspiratory and expiratory centers, which increases both the rate and depth of breathing. This results in a blowing off of carbon dioxide to keep the carbon dioxide tension of the blood constant. The pH of the blood is determined by the ratio of bicarbonate ion (HCO_3^-) to carbon dioxide. When the carbon dioxide content of the blood is increased, there is a subsequent increase in the formation of carbonic acid in the blood. This alters the bicarbonate/carbonic acid ratio from the normal value of 20:1 and results in acidosis. Conversely, a decrease in the carbon dioxide content of the blood results in alkalosis. Therefore respiration is important for regulating the pH of the blood by controlling the carbon dioxide tension of the blood.

Basically, changes in arterial oxygen concentration have little if any direct effect on the respiratory center. However, if the arterial oxygen concentration falls below normal, the chemoreceptors in the carotid and aortic bodies are stimulated and in turn stimulate the respiratory center to increase alveolar ventilation. This mechanism operates primarily under abnormal conditions such as chronic obstructive pulmonary disease.

SUMMARY

The proper functioning of the respiratory system is necessary for the survival of the human organism. Through the processes of pulmonary ventilation, gas transport, and cellular respiration, oxygen is provided to various body tissues, organs, and cells. Generally, the rhythm and depth of pulmonary ventilation are initiated and maintained centrally in the medulla and are influenced peripherally by reflex mechanisms, chemoreceptors, and baroreceptors.

REVIEW QUESTIONS

1. What are the effects of the parasympathetic and sympathetic nervous system on the respiratory system?
2. Discuss the effect of arterial oxygen concentration on the respiratory system.

REFERENCES

Anderson KN et al, editors: *Mosby's medical, nursing, and allied health dictionary,* ed 5, St Louis, 1998, Mosby.

Guyton AC: *Textbook of medical physiology,* ed 8, Philadelphia, 1990, WB Saunders.

Martini F et al: *Fundamentals of anatomy and physiology,* ed 2, Englewood Cliffs, NJ, 1992, Prentice Hall.

McCance KL, Huether SE: *Pathophysiology: the biologic basis for disease in adults and children,* ed 3, St Louis, 1998, Mosby.

Seeley RR, Stephens TD, Tate P: *Anatomy and physiology,* ed 3, New York, 1995, McGraw-Hill.

Thibodeau GA, Patton KT: *Anatomy and physiology,* ed 4, St Louis, 1999, Mosby.

Van Wynsberghe D, Noback CR, Carola R: *Human anatomy and physiology,* ed 3, New York, 1995, McGraw-Hill.

Wingard LB et al: *Human pharmacology,* St Louis, 1991, Mosby.

CHAPTER 32

Mucokinetic and Bronchodilator Drugs

KEY DRUGS

KEY TERMS

CHAPTER FOCUS

This chapter reviews the various mucokinetic and bronchodilator drugs used in the treatment of asthma. Also discussed are the prophylactic medications (cromolyn and nedocromil), leukotriene antagonists, xanthine derivatives, and corticosteroids.

OBJECTIVES

After reading and studying this chapter, the student should be able to do the following:

1. *Define and describe the key terms and key drugs.*
2. *Describe the effects and advantages and disadvantages of water and saline solutions on respiratory secretions.*
3. *Name four objectives of aerosol therapy and explain the relationship of droplet sizes to aerosol effectiveness.*
4. *Discuss the three classifications of asthmatic patients.*
5. *Name one drug from each of the sympathomimetic bronchodilator drug category (i.e., nonselective adrenergic drugs, nonselective beta-adrenergic drugs, and selective beta$_2$ receptor drugs) and compare their mechanisms of action and effectiveness.*
6. *Describe the action of the leukotriene antagonists in asthma.*
7. *Discuss the drugs and mechanisms of action in the xanthine drug group and xanthine derivatives.*
8. *Review the actions of the prophylactic asthmatic drugs (cromolyn and nedocromil) and the corticosteroid drugs in the treatment of asthma.*

Mucokinetic and bronchodilator drugs, which help to maintain patency of the respiratory tract, are the two main groups of drugs discussed in this chapter.

MUCOKINETIC DRUGS

Mucokinetic agents promote the removal of abnormal or excessive respiratory tract secretions by thinning hyperviscous mucus, which allows for more effective ciliary action. These agents prevent sputum retention, which may result from abnormal ciliary activity, defects in airflow, or modification in cough effectiveness. **Sputum** (or phlegm) may be defined as an abnormal, viscous secretion that is an excretory product of the lower respiratory tree. It consists mainly of **mucus,** a proteinaceous material having a mucopolysaccharide as its major component. In addition, sputum contains deoxyribonucleic acid (DNA) molecules, which are derived from the breakdown of mucosal cells, leukocytes, and bacteria. These products are responsible for the characteristic heavy quality and yellow color of the sputum. The terms "sputum" and "mucus" should not be used interchangeably. Sputum is an abnormal secretion originating in the lower respiratory tract, whereas mucus is a normal secretion produced by the surface cells in the mucous membrane.

Individuals with respiratory disorders such as chronic bronchitis develop disturbances of the mucociliary blanket, resulting in a significant impairment of the mucus clearance process (Fig. 32-1). Consequently, mucus plugging and pathogenic colonization of microorganisms occur in the lower respiratory tract. These changes lead to overproduction of thick, tenacious sputum. Thus the advantage provided by the mucokinetic drugs is that they alter the consistency of the sputum, thereby promoting the eventual expectoration, or expulsion, of these secretions.

DILUENTS

Water

The most commonly used agent to dilute respiratory secretions is water. Persons with chronic obstructive pulmonary disease (COPD) frequently suffer from dehydration; thus respiratory secretions are retained. These secretions then become highly viscous in consistency and lead to widespread

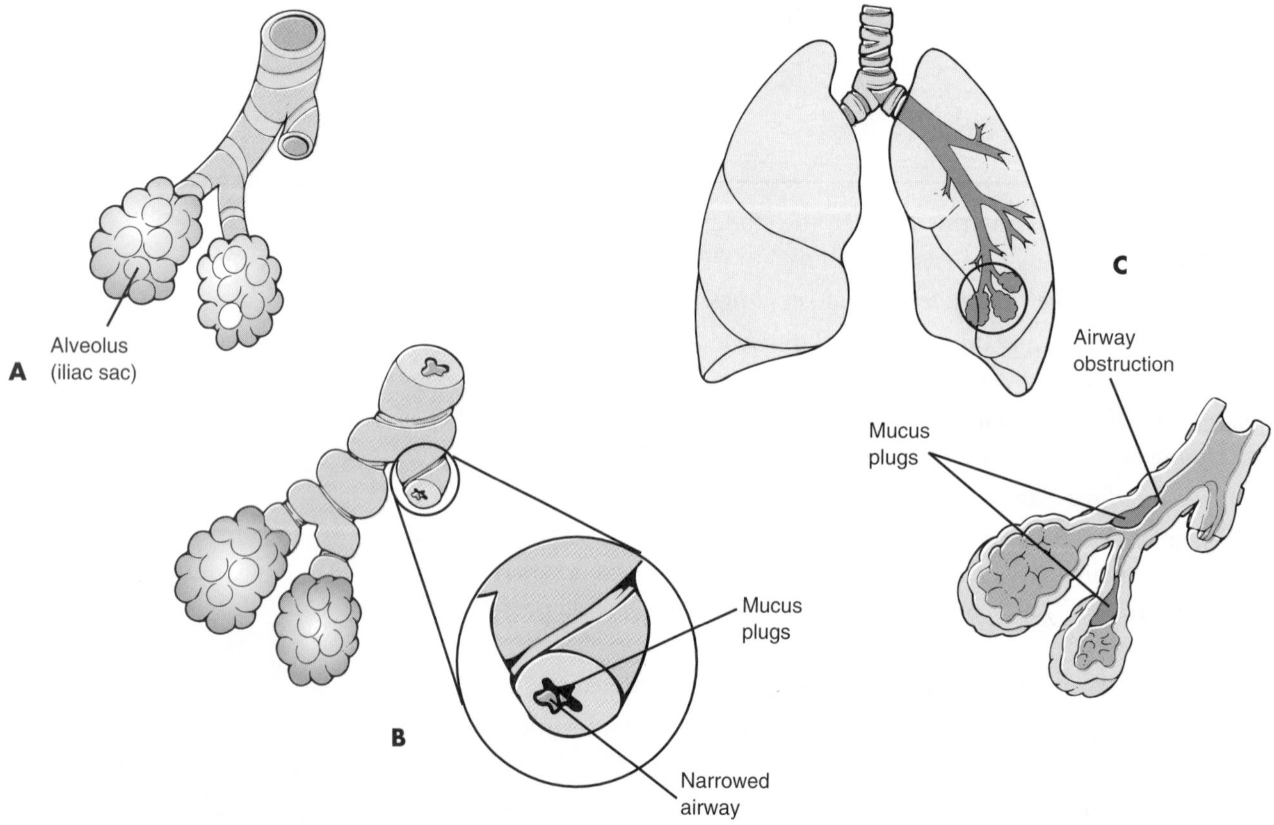

FIGURE 32-1
Bronchiole in normal state **(A)** and during an asthma attack **(B).** An asthmatic attack is illustrated by bronchial muscle spasms, inflammation, and excessive mucus, resulting in mucus plugs, edema, and trapped air in the air sacs (alveoli), which causes airway obstruction **(C).** Total amount of air inhaled and exhaled is decreased because of air trapped in the lungs after expiration.

plug formation in the respiratory tree. Water may be administered by ultrasonic nebulizer. Small amounts of water deposited on the gel layer of the respiratory tree appear to reduce the adhesive characteristics and general viscosity of the gelatinous substances found in this layer. Care is needed with persons receiving restricted fluid intake, since water can be absorbed through the inhalation route. If fluid intake is being measured, water added to the nebulizer and absorbed through the inhalation route must be added to the patient's intake record. Usually large amounts of water are needed to liquefy the respiratory secretions.

Saline Solutions

Normal saline (0.9% sodium chloride) is physiologic (isotonic) salt solution that exerts the same osmotic pressure as plasma fluids. Therapy by nebulization is well tolerated, resulting in hydration of respiratory secretions. Hypotonic solution (0.45% sodium chloride) is thought to provide deeper penetration into the more distal airways or in the alveoli via the inhalation route, whereas inhalation of hypertonic solution (1.8% sodium chloride) stimulates a productive cough since the particles deposited on the respiratory mucosa are irritating. Hypertonic solution osmotically attracts fluid out of the mucosa and into the respiratory secretions, thereby promoting their excretion.

AEROSOL THERAPY

Aerosol therapy is a form of inhaled, topical pulmonary treatment. An aerosol is a suspension of fine liquid or solid particles dispersed in a gas or in solution that is deposited in the respiratory tract. Dry powder inhalers are also available. Liquid or solid particles range in size from about 0.005 to 50 μm in diameter. **Nebulizers** are designed to deliver a maximum number of particles of a desired size. Thus aerosol therapy is delivered through nebulization. The terms "aerosol therapy" and "nebulization therapy" are often used interchangeably. Aerosol therapy promotes the following: bronchodilation and pulmonary decongestion; loosening of secretions; topical application of corticosteroids and other drugs; and moistening, cooling, or heating of inspired air

The effectiveness of nebulization therapy depends on the number of droplets that can be suspended in an inhaled aerosol. This number is directly related to the size of the droplets. Smaller droplets can be suspended in greater numbers than large droplets. Small droplets (about 2 to 4 μm in diameter) are more likely to reach the periphery of the lungs—the alveolar ducts and sacs. Larger droplets (8 to 15 μm in diameter) will be deposited primarily in the bronchioles and bronchi. Droplets of more than 40 μm will be deposited primarily in the upper airway (mouth, pharynx, trachea, and main bronchi).

Rate and depth of breathing are other factors that determine the effectiveness of nebulization therapy. Rapid or shallow breathing decreases the number, as well as the retention, of droplets reaching the periphery of the lungs. Rapid breathing permits escape of significant amounts of fine droplets during expirations, although few droplets will escape if the breath is held long enough after deep inspiration to permit droplet deposit in the lung periphery. Small droplets are more effective for absorption of bronchodilators.

Almost all large droplets will be retained somewhere in the larger air passages. Large droplets are used for keeping large airways (nose and trachea) moist and for loosening secretions. Slow and deep breathing is required for proper lung aeration and penetration of the mist into peripheral lung areas. The breath should be held for a few seconds after a full inspiration.

Droplet size can be controlled by the amount of pressure used to force oxygen or room air through the solution to produce a mist. The nebulizer tubing diameter, its length, and its number of bends affect turbulent flow and mist temperature. With most nebulizers the maximum density of the inhaled mist is achieved by making the flow of mist as smooth and direct as possible. Nebulizers commonly used in hospitals produce similar mists. Be aware, though, that drug reconcentration can occur with both jet and ultrasonic nebulizers if a humidity deficit occurs. That is, evaporation of water molecules causes a gradual increase in drug concentration in the droplets, thus increasing the risk of drug toxicity. Control of temperature and humidity can prevent this toxicity.

The main groups of drugs conventionally administered by aerosol include bronchodilators, cromolyn (Intal), nedocromil (Tilade), and steroid preparations. It is important to remember that the lung is an absorptive organ and thus is a route of access for drugs to enter the systemic circulation. For example, after inhalation anesthetic agents enter the blood, they exert their main effect on the central nervous system. Aerosol therapy, when used as a method of administering drugs, is supposed to minimize systemic absorption and side effects. Yet certain bronchodilator aerosols do produce cardiovascular effects simply because the drug may possess a property that adversely influences cardiac action after absorption into the bloodstream.

When combination inhalation aerosols are prescribed without specific prescriber instructions about the sequence of drug administration, the healthcare professional should be aware of the proper recommendations for drug administration. For example, if a corticosteroid (beclomethasone [Beclovent, Vanceril]) or cromolyn (Intal) or nedocromil (Tilade) is prescribed to be administered with ipratropium (Atrovent), the ipratropium should be administered 5 minutes before either of the other drugs to promote bronchodilation. Whenever a beta agonist (e.g., metaproterenol [Alupent] or albuterol [Proventil]) is prescribed with ipratropium (Atrovent), the beta agonist is always administered first with a 5-minute wait before administration of the second drug. Do not administer both aerosols in rapid sequence because of the possibility of inducing fluorocarbon toxicity; also, this rapid administration decreases drug effectiveness. Box 32-1 lists additional therapeutic tips.

BOX 32-1 | Therapeutic Tips

Selective $beta_2$ drugs such as albuterol, terbutaline, and others provide the most rapid relief of acute asthmatic symptoms. These drugs have no antiinflammatory effects, but they are very effective in the treatment of acute bronchospasm and asthma. Subcutaneous injection is not more effective than inhalation therapy, and it often causes more side effects and adverse reactions; therefore its use is usually reserved for persons with a very severe dyspnea that prevents them from responding to inhalation therapy.

Oral selective $beta_2$ drugs are considered less effective than the same agents administered by inhalation. They also have a longer onset of action time and frequently cause more tremor than inhaled preparations.

Corticosteroid inhalation products such as beclomethasone (Vanceril) and others are less toxic than oral preparations. Oral candidiasis can occur with use if proper preventive measures such as rinsing and gargling with water after each use are not performed. Other adverse effectives may occur with continuous, long-term use; check a current drug reference for information.

Theophylline is considered a less potent bronchodilator and potentially a more toxic agent than inhaled adrenergic drugs; thus it has limited usefulness in acute, intermittent asthma. Theophylline is more useful in chronic asthma.

Cromolyn decreases airway hyperreactivity. It has no bronchodilator effects and thus should not be used for the treatment of acute asthma.

Patients need to be taught about the proper techniques for use of a metered-dose inhaler (MDI) and other inhaling devices as ordered. Spacer units are often suggested for young children and, at times, other patients also benefit from their usage. Home use of peak flow meters is also often recommended for patients with moderate to severe asthma. With proper use, this device may help in the early detection of airflow obstruction, which then allows for a more timely intervention (NAEPP, 1998).

MUCOLYTIC DRUGS

Mucolytics are drugs that exert a disintegrating effect on mucus. These agents, also called **expectorants,** promote coughing or spitting and thereby the removal of mucus or other exudates from the lung, bronchi, or trachea. One of the more commonly used mucolytics is acetylcysteine.

acetylcysteine [a se teel sis′ tay een] (Mucomyst)

Acetylcysteine reduces the thickness and stickiness of purulent and nonpurulent pulmonary secretions by decreasing the viscosity of the respiratory mucoprotein molecules into smaller, more soluble, and less viscous strands. In addition, this drug also effects similar changes in the DNA molecule and cellular debris. The decrease in viscosity of bronchial secretions aids their removal by coughing, postural drainage, or suctioning.

Indications

Acetylcysteine is indicated as an adjunct treatment for thick or abnormal mucus in bronchopulmonary disease, cystic fibrosis, or atelectasis caused by a mucus obstruction. It is also used as a diagnostic aid in a variety of bronchial studies, such as bronchospirometry and bronchograms.

When administered systemically, it is a specific antidote for an acetaminophen overdose. Acetylcysteine reduces the extent of liver injury after acetaminophen overdose by altering hepatic metabolism; it maintains or restores glutathione concentrations. Glutathione is necessary for the inactivation of an intermediate metabolite of acetaminophen that on accumulation is believed to be hepatotoxic.

Pharmacokinetics

In inhalation therapy, some acetylcysteine is absorbed from the pulmonary epithelium, although its primary effects are local on the mucus in the lungs. When inhaled it produces an effect within 1 minute, although direct instillation via an intratracheal catheter produces an immediate effect. The peak response from inhalation occurs within 5 to 10 minutes. Acetylcysteine is metabolized in the liver.

Drug interactions

No significant drug interactions are reported.

Side effects and adverse reactions

These include fever, nausea, vomiting, runny nose, throat or lung irritation, unpleasant odor during drug administration, clammy skin, sore mouth, stomatitis, hemoptysis, rash, and respiratory difficulties.

Warnings

None are reported.

Contraindications

Avoid use in persons with acetylcysteine hypersensitivity and asthma and in patients who are unable to cough.

Dosage and administration

The usual adult and pediatric dose by nebulization using a face mask, mouthpiece, or tracheostomy is 3 to 5 ml of a 20% solution or 6 to 10 ml of a 10% solution inhaled three or four times daily. To treat an acetaminophen overdose, acetylcysteine is administered orally in a dose of 140 mg/kg initially, then 70 mg/kg every 4 hours for 17 additional doses.

Other Expectorants

Over the years, many other products have been used as expectorants in both prescription and over-the-counter (OTC) medications. Guaifenesin, the only expectorant listed by the Food and Drug Administration (FDA) in category I (safe and effective), is reviewed in Chapter 3. A prescribed respiratory inhalant product is recombinant human DNase or dornase alfa (Pulmozyme). This product is used to increase expectoration in cystic fibrosis.

dornase alfa (Pulmozyme)

Cystic fibrosis is a respiratory disease associated with thick secretions from an accumulation of DNA from degenerating neutrophils and inflammation. Dornase alfa is an enzyme that digests extracellular DNA, thus improving pulmonary function and reducing the risk of respiratory tract infections common with cystic fibrosis. The use of this product has resulted in a decrease in respiratory infections, hospitalizations, and medical costs (Franz et al, 1994).

Pharmacokinetics

Significant improvement in pulmonary function is seen within 3 to 7 days and a decrease in respiratory infections within weeks to several months.

Drug interactions

None are reported.

Side effects and adverse reactions

These include chest pain, sore throat, laryngitis, skin rash, conjunctivitis, hoarseness, upset stomach, dyspnea, fever, and rhinitis.

Warnings

None are reported.

Contraindications

Avoid use in persons with dornase alfa or Chinese hamster ovary cell product hypersensitivity.

Dosage and administration

The usual dose for children 5 years of age and older and adults is 2.5 mg daily inhaled via nebulization.

DRUGS THAT ANTAGONIZE BRONCHIAL SECRETIONS

Anticholinergic agents decrease secretions and also make them hard to expectorate. While not generally used for this purpose, atropine may be given cautiously to decrease secretions and excessive expectoration in certain forms of bronchitis. Many remedies used to treat colds contain atropine, an anticholinergic.

ipratropium [i pra troe′ pee um] (Atrovent)

Ipratropium is an anticholinergic drug that produces a local bronchodilation after inhalation. It is indicated for maintenance (not for acute episodes) therapy in persons with COPD (chronic bronchitis or emphysema).

Pharmacokinetics

After administration, onset of action is between 5 and 15 minutes, peak effect occurs in 1 to 2 hours, and duration of action is between 3 and 6 hours.

Drug interactions

No significant drug interactions are reported, although the student should be aware that concurrent administration of other anticholinergics (even eye drops) can increase the potential for side effects and toxicity. Also, avoid use of tacrine with ipratropium as the effects of either drug may be decreased.

Warnings

Use with caution in patients with urinary retention.

Contraindications

Avoid use in persons with ipratropium, belladonna alkaloid, soybean protein, or legume (e.g., peanut) hypersensitivity and in persons with narrow-angle glaucoma.

Side effects and adverse reactions

These include dry mouth or throat, coughing, headache, anxiety, gastrointestinal distress, and, rarely, eye pain, blurred vision, tremors, tachycardia, bronchospasms, glaucoma, hives, skin rash, or stomatitis.

Dosage and administration

The usual adolescent or adult dose is one or two inhalations three or four times daily, administered every 4 hours. Shake the unit well before using.

BRONCHODILATOR DRUGS

Bronchodilator drugs are primarily used to treat chronic pulmonary diseases such as asthma, chronic bronchitis, and emphysema. Major causes of ineffective airway clearance include (1) bronchial smooth muscle contraction (asthma), (2) mucus hypersecretion (chronic bronchitis), and (3) mucosal edema or inflammation (chronic bronchitis). Bronchial asthma may appear with some or all of these symptoms (Fig. 32-1).

In the past, asthma was classified on the basis of the stimuli that may induce an attack, such as intrinsic asthma caused by emotional factors or exercise and extrinsic asthma caused by pollens, molds, dust, or animal hair. Because many asthmatic patients have a combination type of asthma, this type of classification is not considered useful. The National Institutes of Health (NIH) defines asthma as a lung disease that has reversible airway obstruction, airway inflammation, and increased airway sensitivity to stimuli (Self, Kelly, 1995). Distinguishing between asthma and COPD is important, as asthma has a better prognosis with treatment. Asthmatic patients are classified according to the frequency and severity of their asthma attacks (mild, moderate, or severe) because this information is the most useful when considering pharmacologic interventions:

- *Mild:* intermittent attacks of less than one to two a week or nocturnal asthma less than one to two times monthly. Peak expiratory flow (PEF) >80%; normal after bronchodilator use; PEF variability <20%.
- *Moderate:* attacks more than twice weekly, nocturnal asthma symptoms more than twice a month and the use of a beta agonist inhaler nearly daily. PEF 60% to 80%; normal after bronchodilator use; PEF variability 20% to 30%.
- *Severe:* frequent and continuous asthmatic symptoms in-

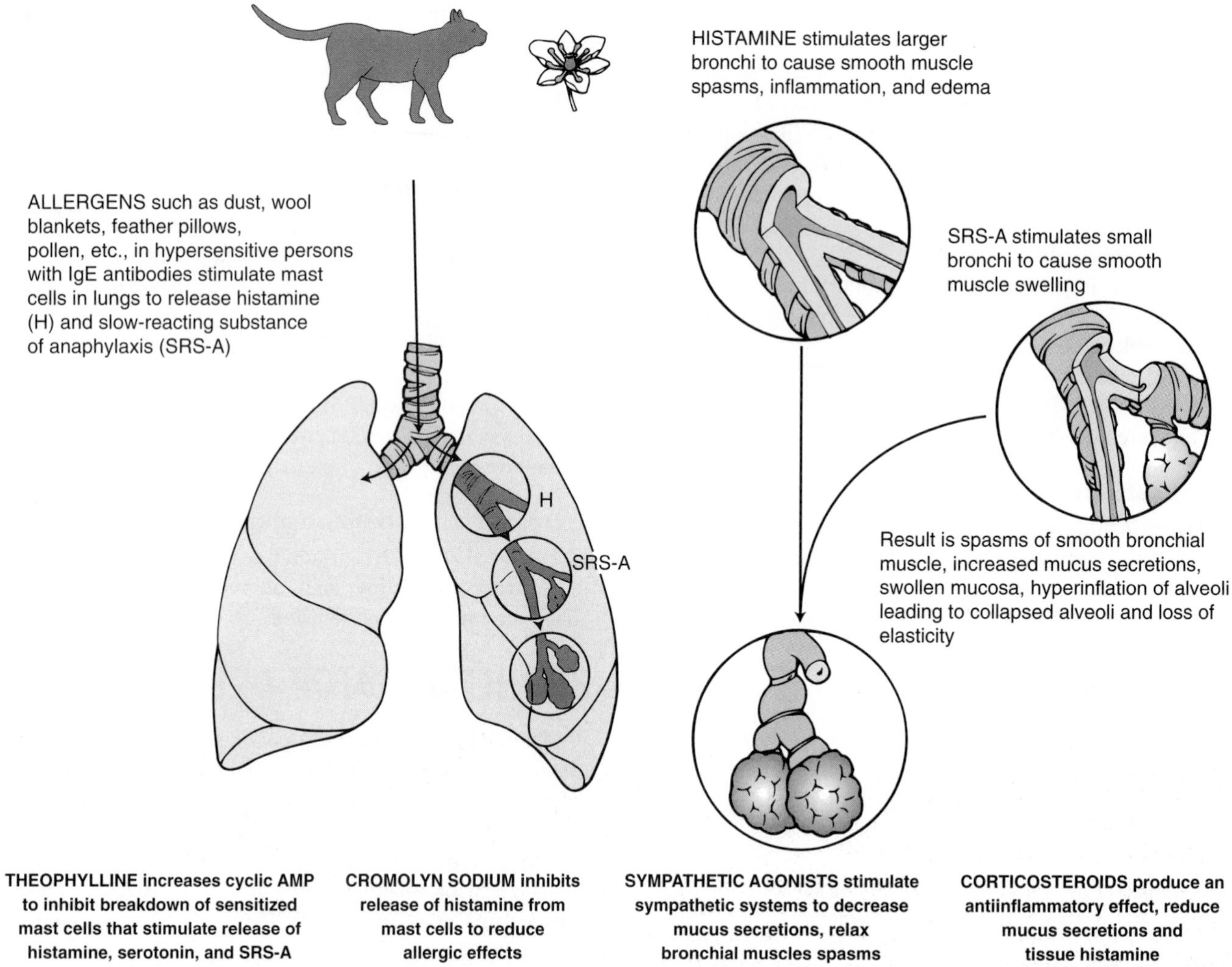

HISTAMINE stimulates larger bronchi to cause smooth muscle spasms, inflammation, and edema
ALLERGENS such as dust, wool blankets, feather pillows, pollen, etc., in hypersensitive persons with IgE antibodies stimulate mast cells in lungs to release histamine (H) and slow-reacting substance of anaphylaxis (SRS-A)
SRS-A stimulates small bronchi to cause smooth muscle swelling
H
SRS-A
Result is spasms of smooth bronchial muscle, increased mucus secretions, swollen mucosa, hyperinflation of alveoli leading to collapsed alveoli and loss of elasticity
THEOPHYLLINE increases cyclic AMP to inhibit breakdown of sensitized mast cells that stimulate release of histamine, serotonin, and SRS-A
CROMOLYN SODIUM inhibits release of histamine from mast cells to reduce allergic effects
SYMPATHETIC AGONISTS stimulate sympathetic systems to decrease mucus secretions, relax bronchial muscles spasms
CORTICOSTEROIDS produce an antiinflammatory effect, reduce mucus secretions and tissue histamine

FIGURE 32-2
Overview of the effects of various antiasthmatic medications.

cluding nocturnal asthma plus having been hospitalized for asthma in the previous year.

The major drugs used in treatment of asthma include sympathomimetic drugs, theophylline, cromolyn, nedocromil, and the corticosteroids. Fig. 32-2 gives an overview of the effects of antiasthmatic medications. Fig. 32-3 illustrates the primary action sites for these drugs. The principal agents used in the treatment of airway obstruction include sympathomimetic drugs and xanthine derivatives. Prophylactic antiasthmatic agents also prevent airway obstruction in individuals with certain types of asthma. Most of these drugs enhance the production of cyclic 3′,5′-adenosine monophosphate (cyclic AMP) in bronchial smooth muscle cells to effect bronchodilation (Fig. 32-4).

SYMPATHOMIMETIC DRUGS

Based on their receptor action, three types of sympathomimetic drugs are recognized: (1) nonselective adrenergic drugs which have alpha, $beta_1$ (cardiac), and $beta_2$ (respiratory) activities (e.g., epinephrine); (2) nonselective beta adrenergic drugs with $beta_1$ and $beta_2$ effects (e.g., isoproterenol); and (3) selective $beta_2$ agents (e.g., albuterol [Proventil], bitolterol [Tornalate], isoetharine [Bronkosol], metaproterenol [Alupent], pirbuterol [Maxair], salmeterol [Serevent], terbutaline [Brethine]) that act primarily on $beta_2$ receptors with minor activity at $beta_1$ receptors in the lungs (bronchial smooth muscle). Two additional bronchodilator drugs are available in Canada: fenoterol (Berotec 🍁) and procaterol (Pro-Air 🍁).

Nonselective Adrenergic Drugs

Nonselective adrenergic drugs such as epinephrine, ephedrine, and others possess both alpha- and beta receptor stimulating properties. Alpha activity appears to mediate vasoconstriction to reduce mucosal edema, while $beta_2$ stimulation produces bronchodilation and vasodilation. In contrast, $beta_1$ receptor action causes unwanted cardiac side effects such as increases in heart rate and force of myocardial contraction.

Undesirable effects on $beta_2$ receptors include skeletal

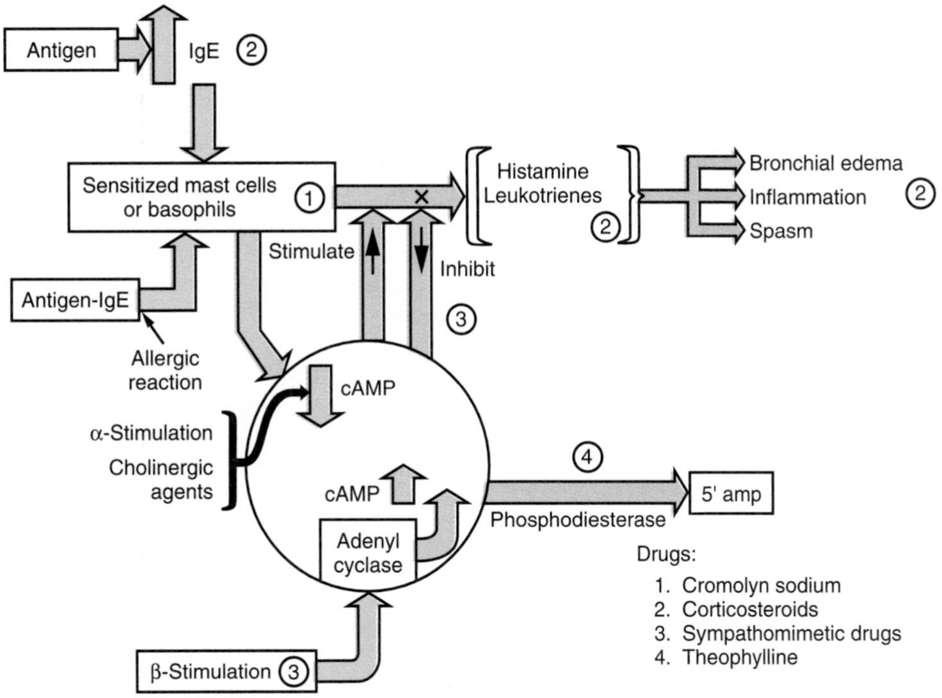

FIGURE 32-3
Major sites of action of drugs used to treat asthma.

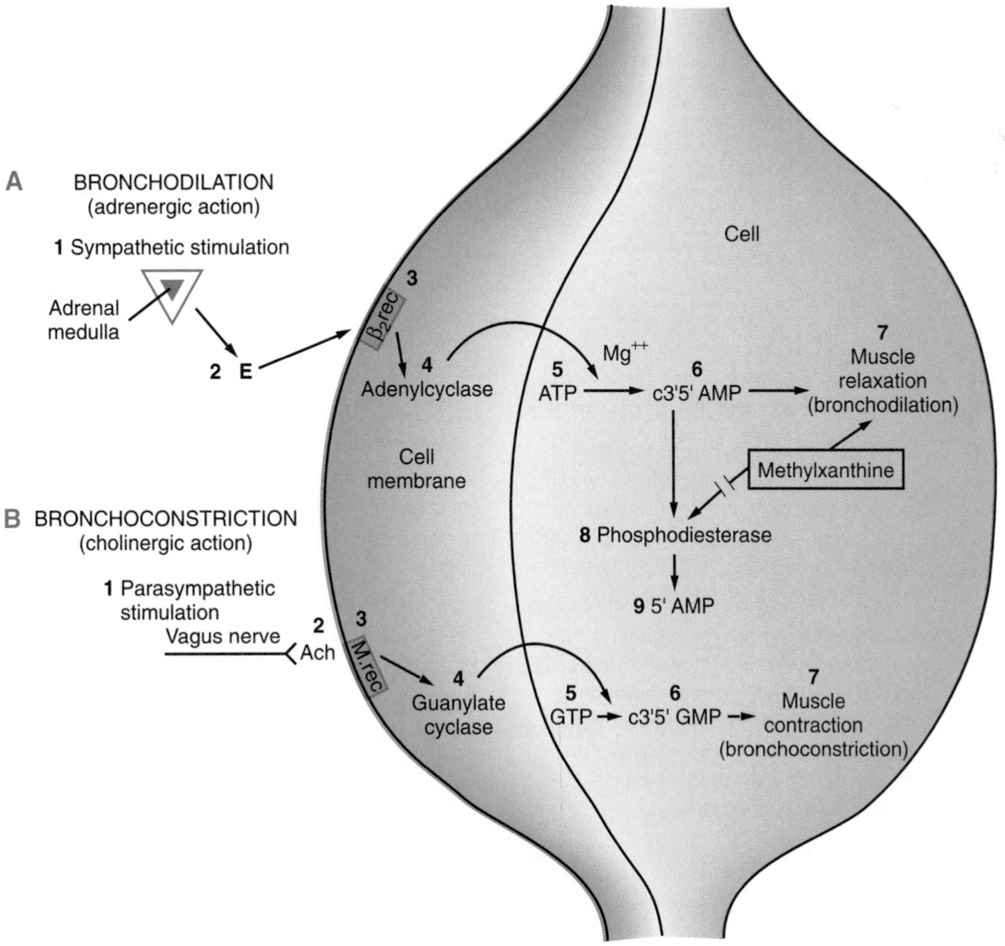

FIGURE 32-4
Mechanism of bronchial smooth muscle action. **A,** Bronchodilation pathway. **B,** Bronchoconstriction pathway. (*E,* Epinephrine; *Ach,* acetylcholine; β *rec,* β_2 receptor; *M. rec,* muscarinic receptor).

muscle tremors, tachycardia, palpitations, increased central nervous system (CNS) stimulation, hypokalemia (after large doses are administered), glycogenolysis, and gluconeogenesis.

epinephrine [ep i nef′ rin] (Adrenalin)

Epinephrine induces relaxation of bronchial smooth muscle (by stimulating $beta_2$ receptors in the lungs), thus relieving bronchospasm, increasing vital capacity, and reducing airway resistance. It also inhibits the bronchoconstriction induced by the release of histamine and substances released during anaphylaxis.

Indications

Epinephrine is indicated for the treatment of bronchial asthma, bronchitis, and other pulmonary disease states and the prevention of bronchospasm and bronchial asthma.

Pharmacokinetics

By inhalation, only slight absorption occurs, but if large doses of epinephrine are administered, systemic absorption increases. Systemic absorption is rapid by intramuscular or subcutaneous administration.

The onset of action is within 3 to 5 minutes by inhalation, between 6 and 15 minutes by subcutaneous injection, and variable by IM injection. The duration of action is between 1 and 3 hours by inhalation or 1 to 4 hours by the parenteral routes. It is metabolized at sympathetic nerve endings and other tissues with a small amount of excretion in the kidneys.

Drug interactions

The following effects may occur when epinephrine is given with the drugs listed below:

Drug	Possible effect and management
Inhalers that contain a fluorocarbon propellant	When epinephrine is given concurrently with other inhalers that contain a fluorocarbon propellant, fluorocarbon toxicity may result. Teach patient to allow at least a 5-minute interval between the use of such inhalants.
Alpha-adrenergic blocking agents (e.g., prazosin or tolazoline) or other medications with alpha blocking properties (e.g., phenothiazines or haloperidol) or the fast-acting vasodilators (nitrates)	Concurrent use of these drugs with epinephrine may result in severe hypotension and tachycardia. Monitor closely because medical interventions may be necessary. The vasodilator effects of nitrites may also be decreased with concurrent use.
Anesthetics, such as chloroform, cyclopropane, and halothane	Concurrent use with epinephrine increases the risk for severe dysrhythmias. Avoid if possible; if not, reduce dosages and monitor closely.
Tricyclic antidepressants, cocaine, and epinephrine	Concurrent use with epinephrine may increase the risk of cardiac dysrhythmias, tachycardia, hypertension, and hyperpyrexia. Such combinations should be avoided.
Beta-adrenergic blocking agents (oral, parenteral, and ophthalmic)	Concurrent use may decrease the therapeutic effects of both drugs. In addition, adverse cardiovascular side effects (e.g., hypertension, bradycardia, and heart block) may be enhanced. Whenever possible, avoid concurrent administration.
Digitalis glycosides (digoxin and digitoxin)	The combination of digitalis glycoside and epinephrine increases the risk for cardiac dysrhythmias. If concurrent therapy is necessary, monitor with an electrocardiogram.
ergotamine and ergoloid mesylates	This combination may result in peripheral vascular ischemia, gangrene, or with ergotamine, severe hypertension. This drug combination should be avoided.

Color type indicates an unsafe drug combination.

Side effects and adverse reactions

These include nervousness, insomnia, tachycardia, dizziness, headaches, hypotension, anorexia, nausea, a pounding tachycardia, sweating, vomiting, cold pale skin, trembling, increased anxiety or restlessness, blurred vision, mental alterations, severe muscle cramps, increased blood pressure, hallucinations, chills, fever, and difficulty in urination.

Warnings

Use with caution in patients with hypotension, hypertension, hyperthyroidism, angle-closure glaucoma, diabetes mellitus, Parkinson's disease, pheochromocytoma, prostatic hypertrophy, and a history of convulsions.

Contraindications

Avoid use in persons with sympathomimetic hypersensitivity, shock, organic brain damage, and cardiovascular disease.

Dosage and administration

Various forms of epinephrine are available: for example, epinephrine (Bronkaid Mist, Primatene Mist), epinephrine bitartrate (Asthmahaler, Medihaler-Epi), and racepinephrine (AsthmaNefrin, Vaponefrin). By inhalation, the adult dose is usually 10 drops of a 1% solution or a diluted racepinephrine solution (2.25%) in a nebulizer. Generally one inhalation of the former or two or three inhalations of the latter preparation is administered. Doses may be repeated at sufficient intervals as stated in the current package inserts or USP DI. With the aerosol preparations, one inhalation is administered, which if necessary may be repeated in 1 minute if needed. Subsequent doses are usually administered in 3 to 4 hours. Pediatric doses are individualized by the prescriber according to response.

Many other adrenergic bronchodilators are available. In choosing a beta receptor agonist, the $beta_2$ selectivity, potency, and duration of action of the drug are considered. The high incidence of undesirable cardiotoxic effects caused by the $beta_1$ property of sympathomimetic agents (nonselective agents) led to the search for a more specific $beta_2$ receptor agonist such as isoetharine and the noncatecholamine $beta_2$ receptor agonists, albuterol, metaproterenol, and terbutaline.

Nonselective Beta-Adrenergic Drugs

Nonselective beta-adrenergic drugs exhibit both $beta_1$ and $beta_2$ agonist activity. Their main action is on the bronchial smooth muscle as well as on the heart. Isoproterenol is the prototype example for this drug category.

isoproterenol solution [eye soe proe ter′ e nole] (Vapo-Iso, Isuprel)

Isoproterenol is indicated for the treatment of bronchial asthma, bronchitis, and other pulmonary disease states.

Pharmacokinetics

The onset of action by inhalation is within 2 to 5 minutes, sublingually (SL) within 15 to 30 minutes, and by intravenous injection, immediately. Its duration of action is 0.5 to 2 hours by inhalation, 1 to 2 hours SL, and less than 1 hour by IV injection. It is metabolized in the liver, lungs, and other body tissues and excreted by the kidneys.

Drug interactions

Significant drug interactions are similar to those of epinephrine, except for the interactions noted with parenteral local anesthetics, alpha blocking agents, and the ergoloid mesylates or ergotamine. These exceptions are due to the fact that isoproterenol does not have alpha effects.

Side effects and adverse reactions

These include restlessness, anxiety, insomnia, pink or red colored saliva, and a dry mouth or throat after inhalation usage. Dizziness, flushing of the skin, headache, tremors, palpitations, sweating, tachycardia, weakness, vomiting, and hypertension or hypotension have also been reported.

Warnings

Use with caution in patients with cardiac dysrhythmias, uncontrolled hypertension, uncontrolled hyperthyroidism, and pheochromocytoma.

Contraindications

Avoid use in persons with adrenergic bronchodilator or sulfite hypersensitivity and coronary insufficiency.

Dosage and administration

The adult bronchodilator inhalation dose is 6 to 12 inhalations of a 0.25% nebulized solution, which may be repeated at 15-minute intervals, if needed, for three doses. The maximum number of treatments recommended in a 24-hour period is 8. In an acute asthmatic attack, 5 to 15 deep inhalations of a 0.5% nebulized solution or 3 to 7 inhalations of 1% nebulized solution are administered. The sequence is repeated once after waiting 5 to 10 minutes if needed. Up to five subsequent doses per day may be administered, if necessary. For bronchospasm in COPD, a nebulizer of intermittent positive pressure breathing (IPPB) drug administration may be used. The pediatric dosage recommendations are similar to those for adults with the exception of using the 1% solution.

Isoproterenol injection is used IV as a bronchodilator for bronchospasm during anesthesia at a dose of 10 to 20 μg. If necessary, the dose may be repeated.

Selective $Beta_2$ Receptor Drugs

Catecholamine $Beta_2$ Agents

isoetharine inhalation [eye soe eth′ a reen] (Bronkosol)

Isoetharine is a direct-acting sympathomimetic catecholamine that selectively stimulates $beta_2$ receptors to relax bronchial smooth muscle. Because it possesses a weak $beta_1$ response, less risk of cardiotonic side effects exists than with epinephrine and isoproterenol. Its $beta_2$ adrenergic-receptor activity relieves bronchospasm, increasing vital capacity and decreasing resistance of bronchial airways. It may also inhibit antigen-induced release of histamine by stimulating the production of cyclic AMP, which stabilizes the mast cell.

Indications

Isoetharine has the same indications as epinephrine.

Pharmacokinetics

This drug has an onset of action of 1 to 6 minutes and a peak effect between 15 and 60 minutes. Its duration of action is 1 to 4 hours. It is metabolized in the liver, lungs, gastrointestinal tract, and other body tissues and is excreted by the kidneys.

Drug interactions

For significant drug interactions, see isoproterenol.

Side effects and adverse reactions

These include dizziness, headaches, dry mouth, and a foul taste in the mouth or throat after use of the inhalation product; nausea, anxiety, palpitations, tremors, insomnia, tachycardia, weakness, and vomiting have also been reported.

Warnings and contraindications

See discussion of isoproterenol.

Dosage and administration

The adult bronchodilator dose with a hand nebulizer is four inhalations of an undiluted 0.5% or 1% solution, usually administered every 4 hours. For IPPB or oxygen aerosolization dosage, see a current package insert or USP DI. The dosage in children has not been established.

Noncatecholamine Beta₂ Receptor Drugs

Noncatecholamine drugs have two advantages over the catecholamine-type agents: they are longer acting and have fewer cardiovascular side effects. Albuterol and metaproterenol will represent this category, although salmeterol (Serevent) is the first long-acting bronchodilator inhaler approved for twice daily dosing.

albuterol [al byoo′ ter ole] (Proventil, Ventolin)

Albuterol, a sympathomimetic bronchodilator, possesses a relatively selective specificity for $beta_2$-adrenergic receptors in the lungs and therefore is less likely to cause unwanted cardiovascular effects. Its interaction with the $beta_2$ receptor in the cell membrane of the bronchial smooth muscle stimulates the enzyme adenylate cyclase to produce cyclic AMP, which results in relaxation of the smooth muscle of the bronchi (Fig. 32-4), thus relieving bronchospasm and decreasing airway resistance. In addition, this mechanism causes relaxation of the smooth muscle of the uterus and blood vessels of skeletal muscle. However, it has been reported that high doses of the drug administered intravenously would be required to inhibit uterine contractions to delay premature labor (see the Pregnancy Safety box).

Indications

This drug is a bronchodilator and is also used as prophylaxis for exercise-induced bronchospasms.

Pharmacokinetics

By inhalation, albuterol has an onset of action between 5 and 15 minutes, a peak effect in 1 to 1½ hours after two inhalations, and a duration of action of 3 to 6 hours. Orally, its onset of action is between 15 and 30 minutes, peak effect is in 2 to 3 hours, and duration of action of 8 hours or more (12 hours for the sustained-release dosage form). The drug is metabolized in the liver and excreted by the kidneys and in feces.

PREGNANCY SAFETY

Category	Drug
B	cromolyn, ipratropium, terbutaline, zafirlukast
C	albuterol, beclomethasone, flunisolide, isoetharine, isoproterenol, metaproterenol, theophylline, zileuton
D	triamcinolone

Drug interactions

Significant drug interactions are similar to those of isoproterenol, with the exception of the interactions noted with alpha-adrenergic blocking agents, ergoloid mesylates, and ergotamine. Albuterol also has a significant drug interaction with monoamine oxidase inhibitors (MAO) inhibitors; that is, the effects of albuterol on the vascular system may be potentiated.

Side effects and adverse reactions

These include nausea, increased anxiety, palpitations, tremors, tachycardia, sedation, hypokalemia, difficulty in urination, flushing, anorexia, dizziness, headaches, heartburn, muscle cramping, insomnia, increased sweating, vomiting, increased weakness, hypotension or hypertension, and an unusual taste in the mouth.

Warnings

Use with caution in patients with diabetes mellitus, hyperthyroidism, ketoacidosis, and pheochromocytoma.

Contraindications

Avoid use in persons with sympathomimetic hypersensitivity and cardiovascular disease such as dysrhythmias, coronary insufficiency, hypertension, and ischemic heart disease.

Dosage and administration

The adult bronchodilator dosage for inhalation is 200 to 400 μg every 4 to 6 hours. The oral dosage is 2 to 6 mg orally, three or four times daily. This dose may be increased to a maximum of 8 mg four times daily if necessary. Extended-release tablets of 4 or 8 mg orally are administered every 12 hours. See a package insert for the pediatric dosage schedule.

metaproterenol [met a pro ter′ e nole] (Alupent, Metaprel)

The metaproterenol mechanism of action is the same as that for albuterol, while its indications are the same as those for epinephrine.

Pharmacokinetics

Metaproterenol inhalation has an onset of action within 1 minute, a peak effect in 1 hour, and a duration of action of 1 to 5 hours after a single dose. Orally its onset of action is within 15 to 30 minutes, its peak effect occurs in an hour, and its duration of action is up to 4 hours. It is metabolized in the liver and excreted in the kidneys.

Drug interactions

Significant drug interactions are similar to those for albuterol.

Side effects and adverse reactions

These include anxiety, restlessness, dizziness, headaches, hypertension, muscle cramps, nausea, vomiting, palpitations, tremors, sweating, tachycardia, and weakness. Respiratory difficulties are a rare adverse reaction seen with this drug.

Warnings

Use with caution in patients with diabetes mellitus, hyperthyroidism, seizure disorders, and pheochromocytoma.

Contraindications

Avoid use in persons with sympathomimetic hypersensitivity and cardiovascular disease such as dysrhythmias, coronary artery disease, and hypertension.

Dosage and administration

The adult bronchodilator inhalation dose is 1.3 to 2.25 mg (two or three inhalations) every 3 to 4 hours, not to exceed 9 mg (12 inhalations) in 24 hours. The oral dose is 20 mg three or four times daily. The dosage is not established for children younger than 6 years of age. For children 6 to 9 years of age who weigh up to 27 kg, the oral dosage is 10 mg three or four times daily. For children older than 9 years of age weighing at least 27 kg, apply the adult dosage scale.

terbutaline aerosol [ter byoo′ ta leen] (Brethaire) *terbutaline tablets and injection* (Brethine, Bricanyl)

The mechanism of action of terbutaline is similar to that for albuterol and indications are the same as those for epinephrine.

Pharmacokinetics

Terbutaline's onset of action by inhalation is within 5 to 30 minutes, peak effect within 1 to 2 hours, and duration of action within 3 to 6 hours. Orally its onset of action is within 1 to 2 hours, peak effect within 2 to 3 hours, and duration of action within 4 to 8 hours. Parenterally, its onset of action is within 15 minutes, peak effect within 0.5 to 1 hour, and duration of action within 1.5 to 4 hours. Terbutaline is metabolized in the liver and excreted in the kidneys.

Drug interactions

See discussion of albuterol.

Side effects and adverse reactions

These include tremors, increased anxiety, restlessness, dizziness, sedation, headaches, hypertension, muscle cramps, nausea, vomiting, palpitations, insomnia, sweating, tachycardia, weakness, dry mouth or throat, and an unusual taste in the mouth. Rare adverse reactions include chest pain and an increase in respiratory difficulties.

Dosage and administration

The adult bronchodilator dose is one to two inhalations (200 to 500 μg), with the second inhalation at least 1 minute after the first, then dosed every 4 to 6 hours. Orally a 2.5 to 5 mg tablet three times daily every 6 hours is recommended. For children 12 to 15 years of age, give 2.5 mg orally three times a day. Parenterally, a 250 μg subcutaneous dose is administered, which may be repeated in 15 to 30 minutes. A total dose of 500 μg is the maximum in a 4 hour period.

Leukotriene Antagonists

The first two drugs released in this category are zafirlukast and zileuton.

zafirlukast [za feer′ loo cast] (Accolate) *zileuton* [zye′ lu than] (Zyflo)

Zafirlukast blocks the **leukotriene receptors** (D_4 and E_4), which are components of slow-reacting substance of anaphylaxis while zileuton blocks leukotriene synthesis. Zileuton is the first lipoxygenase inhibitor approved in the United States. By blocking lipoxygenase, it interferes with the formation of substances that cause mucus plugs and constriction of bronchial airways. Therefore both drugs can reduce the inflammation, mucous secretion, and bronchoconstriction associated with asthma.

Indications

Zafirlukast and zileuton are indicated for the treatment and/or prophylaxis of chronic asthma.

Pharmacokinetics

Administered orally, both drugs are rapidly absorbed and bound to plasma proteins (mainly albumen): zafirlukast is 99% bound while zileuton is 93% bound. The onset of action for zileuton is 2 hours while it was approximately 1 week before improvement in asthma symptoms was noted with zafirlukast. These drugs are metabolized in the liver with zafirlukast excreted primarily in feces.

Drug interactions

The following effects may occur when either drug is given with the drugs listed below:

Drug	Possible effect and management
astemizole (Hismanal), cisapride (Propulsid), cyclosporine (Sandimmune), felodipine (Plendil), isradipine (DynaCirc), nicardipine (Cardene), nifedipine (Procardia), or nimodipine (Nimotop)	These drugs are metabolized by the cytochrome P450 isoenzyme CYP3A4; monitor if any of these drugs are given concurrently with zafirlukast or zileuton as both drugs are reported to inhibit CYP3A4 in vitro. Monitor closely if drugs are administered concurrently.

Beta receptor blocking agents	When zileuton and propranolol were administered concurrently, propranolol serum levels nearly doubled. Any beta receptor blocking agents administered concurrently with zileuton should be closely monitored.
carbamazepine (Tegretol), phenytoin (Dilantin), or tolbutamide (Orinase)	These agents are metabolized by cytochrome P450 2C9 isoenzyme. While information on combined use is unknown, it is known that zafirlukast inhibits cytochrome P4502C9 in vitro. If administered concurrently, monitor closely.
theophylline	Concurrent administration of theophylline and zileuton may result in doubling the serum level of theophylline. Management usually requires administering one half the theophylline dose and closely monitoring serum theophylline levels. When theophylline was administered with zafirlukast, the serum level of zafirlukast was reduced by approximately 30%. Monitor closely.
warfarin (Coumadin)	Concurrent use may increase prothrombin time. Monitor closely as warfarin dose may need to be reduced.

Side effects and adverse reactions

These include headache, nausea, increased incidence of infection, especially in the those older than 55 years of age, abdominal upset or pain, weakness, liver function impairment with zileuton (flu-like symptoms, fatigue, lethargy, pruritus, upper right abdominal pain, and jaundice), and perhaps Churg-Strauss syndrome with zafirlukast when corticosteroid therapy is reduced or discontinued. Churg-Strauss syndrome presents with flu-like syndrome, fever, muscle pain, weight loss, eosinophilia, vasculitic rash, cardiac problems, and neuropathy and, if untreated, major organ damage.

Warnings

Use either drug with caution in alcoholic (active) patients.

Contraindications

Avoid use in persons with zileuton or zafirlukast hypersensitivity, and liver disease or liver function impairment, and in pregnant or breastfeeding women.

Dosage and administration

The zileuton adult and adolescent dose is 600 mg PO four times daily. The zafirlukast adult and adolescent dose is 20 mg PO twice a day, 1 hour before or 2 hours after a meal.

XANTHINE DERIVATIVES

The xanthine group of drugs includes caffeine, theophylline, and theobromine. Beverages from the extracts of plants containing these alkaloids have been used by humans since ancient times. **Xanthine derivatives** relax smooth muscle (particularly bronchial muscle), stimulate cardiac muscle and the CNS, and also produce diuresis, probably through a combined action of increased renal perfusion and increased sodium and chloride ion excretion.

The drugs in this category are methylated forms of xanthines or methylxanthines. The effectiveness of these preparations as bronchodilators depends on their conversion to theophylline, which is the active constituent. Therefore, with the exception of dyphylline, the action of xanthine depends on the content of theophylline. Xanthines inhibit mast cell degranulation and the release of histamine and other mediators that are responsible for bronchoconstriction. Because the methylxanthines impede enzymatic action, they are also called phosphodiesterase inhibitors (Figs. 32-3 and 32-4).

The rate of absorption and therapeutic effects of theophylline products, especially slow-release products, can vary even if they have the same strength and active ingredient. It has been recommended that pharmacists not substitute for these drugs if the new product does not have proven bioequivalence (USP DI, 1998). Some states, such as Florida, do not permit generic substitution for theophylline slow-release products.

Although theophylline toxicity may occur in some persons at 15 μg/ml, the upper therapeutic level is 20 μg/ml. Dosage adjustment with theophylline is also necessary under certain conditions especially when concurrent factors affecting therapeutic effects are present. See Box 32-2 for factors affecting theophylline's therapeutic effects.

BOX 32-2 Factors Affecting Theophylline's Therapeutic Effects

May be Increased by:
Age: elderly and newborn
Drugs: erythromycin, cimetidine, ciprofloxacin
Disease states: cirrhosis, pulmonary edema, congestive heart failure, and severe COPD
Diet: high carbohydrate

May be Decreased by:
Substances: tobacco, marijuana
Drugs: phenobarbital, phenytoin
Diet: high protein
Age: adolescence

aminophylline [am in off′ i lin]
(Aminophylline, Palaron 🍁)
oxtriphylline [ox trye′ fi lin]
(Choledyl, Apo-Oxtriphylline 🍁)
theophylline [thee off′ i lin]
(Bronkodyl, Elixophyllin, and others)

Theophylline is the prototype of the xanthine derivatives. It competitively inhibits the action of phosphodiesterase, the enzyme that degrades cyclic AMP, which results in bronchodilation, as discussed previously (Fig. 32-4). These drugs are used for the prevention and treatment of bronchial asthma and treatment of bronchitis, pulmonary emphysema, and COPD.

Pharmacokinetics

Oral liquids and uncoated tablets of aminophylline, oxtriphylline, and theophylline are rapidly absorbed, whereas enteric-coated tablets have a delayed and at times an unreliable absorption pattern. Extended-release dosage forms are slowly absorbed and sometimes unreliable. The retention enema is rapidly absorbed, whereas rectal suppositories are slow and unreliable. Dyphylline has good oral absorption. The theophylline peak level is reached in 1 to 2 hours with the oral solution, immediate release capsules, or tablets, in approximately 4 hours with delayed release tablets, and in 4 to 13 hours for extended-release products. Theophylline's half-life varies by age and with concurrent illness. For example, in premature newborns, the half-life is approximately 30 hours during the first 15 days of life; for children 1 to 4 years of age, it is 3.4 hours; for the adult nonsmoker with uncomplicated asthma, it is 8.2 hours; and for the elderly, the half-life is nearly 10 hours. In patients with acute hepatitis the half-life is 19 hours, with cirrhosis 32 hours, and with hyperthyroidism 4.5 hours (USP DI, 1998). The theophylline half-life in an adult smoker is only 3 to 4 hours (Self, Kelly, 1995).

Drug interactions

The following effects may occur when xanthine products is give with the drugs listed below:

Drug	Possible effect and management
phenytoin (Dilantin)	Increased metabolism of xanthines occurs. Decreased absorption of phenytoin, leading to low serum levels, may be seen with concurrent administration. Serum levels of both drugs should be closely monitored, since dosage adjustments may be necessary.
Beta-adrenergic blocking agents, systemic or ophthalmic	Therapeutic effects of both drugs may be inhibited. Concurrent use may also decrease theophylline excretion. Monitor closely because dosage adjustments may be necessary.
cimetidine (Tagamet), erythromycin (Erythrocin), ranitidine (Zantac), or troleandomycin (Tao)	May decrease theophylline metabolism, resulting in elevated serum levels of theophylline and possible toxicity. Monitor closely because dosage adjustments may be necessary.
ciprofloxacin (Cipro), norfloxacin (Noroxin)	Concurrent drug administration may reduce theophylline excretion, resulting in an increase in theophylline half-life, serum level, and potential toxicity. Monitor serum levels closely because a dosage adjustment may be indicated.
Smokers of tobacco or marijuana	May result in increased metabolism of xanthines (except dyphylline), which may result in low serum theophylline levels. Dosage adjustments of 50% to 100% greater dosage has been required in smokers.
Nicotine chewing gum, or other smoking deterrents	Smoking cessation may increase the therapeutic effects of the xanthines (except dyphylline) by decreasing metabolism; however, nonsmoking normalization of xanthines levels may not occur for 3 months to 2 years after smoking cessation.

Aminophylline, oxtriphylline, and theophylline salts all release free theophylline in vivo. Theophylline is metabolized by the liver to caffeine. Caffeine concentrations may average about 30% of the theophylline concentration in adults, but in neonates it may be much more. Caffeine does not accumulate in adults.

Serum levels

The therapeutic serum levels for bronchodilator effects with theophylline are usually stated to be between 10 and 20 μg/ml. Some studies, however, have indicated that therapeutic response may be seen at the 5 to 15 μg serum level while some patients have minimal gain, and some experience toxicity in the 15 to 20 μg/ml range (Kelly, Hill, 1993).

Therefore, close supervision with dosage adjustments according to the patient's therapeutic response or the presence of toxic effects is necessary. As a respiratory stimulant, the theophylline serum level is between 5 and 10 μg/ml. Theophylline is metabolized in the liver and excreted by the kidneys.

Side effects and adverse reactions

These include nausea, increased anxiety, restlessness, gastric upset, vomiting, gastroesophageal reflux, headache, increase in urination, insomnia, trembling, increase nervousness, tachycardia and, with aminophylline, dermatitis.

Warnings

Use with caution in patients with fever, active gastritis or peptic ulcer disease, gastroesophageal reflux, tachycardia, and other tachydysrhythmias.

Contraindications

Avoid use in persons with theophylline or ethylenediamine hypersensitivity, heart failure, liver disease, hypothyroidism (uncontrolled), sepsis, pulmonary edema (acute), and convulsive disorders.

Dosage and administration

The dosage of theophylline preparations must be tailored to the medical circumstances in each case. The usual efficacy of a theophylline preparation depends on the attainment of a serum concentration of 10 to 20 μg/ml (see previous comments on serum levels). The rapid intravenous administration of theophylline and its derivatives has caused severe and even fatal acute circulatory failure; therefore the drug should be administered slowly over 20 to 30 minutes. Since theophylline has a low therapeutic index, using caution when determining the dosage is essential. See the box below right for management of xanthine overdose.

The various xanthine preparations contain the following:

DRUG	PERCENT ANHYDROUS THEOPHYLLINE PRESENT
aminophylline anhydrous	86
aminophylline dihydrate	79
oxtriphylline	64
theophylline monohydrate	91

PROPHYLACTIC ASTHMATIC DRUGS

cromolyn [kroe′ moe lin]
(Intal, Novo-Cromolyn)
nedocromil [ned o kroe′ mill] (Tilade)

Cromolyn and nedocromil are antiinflammatory agents that inhibit the release of histamine, leukotrienes, and other mediators of inflammation from mast cells, macrophages, and other cells associated with asthma. Neither drug has any bronchodilator effect, nor do they have any effect on any inflammatory mediators already released in the body. Nedocromil appears to be more effective than cromolyn (Serafin, 1996), and in some stabilized persons, it is therapeutically effective in twice daily dosing (USP DI, 1998).

Indications

Both drugs are indicated for prevention of bronchospasms and bronchial asthmatic attacks.

Pharmacokinetics

Administered by oral inhalation, cromolyn is approximately 8% to 10% absorbed in the lungs. It has an onset of action within 4 weeks and is excreted in the kidneys and bile. Nedocromil has systemic absorption of 7% to 9% and a half-life of 1.5 to 3.3 hours. Its onset of action as maintenance therapy is between 2 and 4 weeks. It is excreted by the kidneys. It can also prevent bronchospasm if given up to ½ hour before exposure to allergens or exercise.

Drug interactions

No significant drug interactions reported.

Side effects and adverse reactions

These include cough, headache, hoarseness, dry mouth or throat, running nose or stuffy nasal congestion, diarrhea, myalgia, difficulty sleeping, stomach pain, rash, sneezing, bronchospasm, and bad taste in the mouth after use of the inhaler.

Warnings

With cromolyn, use with caution in patients with liver or kidney function impairment.

Contraindications

Avoid use in persons with cromolyn or nedocromil hypersensitivity

Dosage and administration

The adult and children dose (5 years of age and older) oral inhalation dose of cromolyn to prevent bronchial asthma is two inhalations (1.6 or 2 mg) four times daily at 4- or 6-hour intervals. To prevent exercise-induced or allergen-induced bronchospasms, the dose is two oral inhalations approximately 10 to 15 minutes before exercise or

MANAGEMENT OF DRUG OVERDOSE

Theophylline (Xanthine)

- Treatment is supportive and symptomatic because there is no known specific antidote.
- To decrease drug absorption, administer an activated charcoal preparation orally or via a nasogastric tube. Charcoal should be premixed with sorbitol, or a single dose of sorbitol should follow the charcoal dose. Sorbitol is considered to be more effective than magnesium-containing laxatives.
- Gastric lavage is instituted early (within 1 hour of ingestion) or whole bowel irrigation with a polyethylene glycol and electrolyte solution is useful for very large overdoses of theophylline.
- If the client has seizures, establish an airway and administer oxygen. Diazepam or phenobarbital IV may be administered to control the seizures.
- Charcoal hemoperfusion may be necessary when the theophylline serum concentration is very high (greater than 40 μg/mL in chronic overdose or if other risk factors are present, such as an elderly patient, concurrent illnesses, etc.). Hemodialysis and peritoneal dialysis are less or ineffective, respectively, for theophylline toxicity (USP DI, 1998).
- Monitor vital signs and provide supportive care as required.

exposure. A dose is not established for children younger that 5 years of age.

The usual adult and adolescent dose for nedocromil is initially two oral inhalations four times daily. Reduction of doses to three and then twice daily may be attempted in persons whose symptoms are under good control.

Corticosteroid Drugs

Corticosteroid drugs are used in chronic asthma to decrease airway obstruction. As antiinflammatory agents, they stabilize the membranes of lysosomes, thus preventing the release of hydrolytic enzymes that produce the inflammatory process in the tissues. The exact mechanism in asthma is still poorly understood, but it does involve suppression of antibody formation that is responsible for provoking the asthmatic attack. In addition, corticosteroids inhibit leukotriene synthesis, thus reducing bronchoconstriction and secretion of mucus.

Daily administration of systemic corticosteroid therapy provides great therapeutic benefits, but the high incidence of side effects has led to the use of the alternate-day schedule of treatment. This regimen provides the best benefit/risk ratio for prolonged therapy because it minimizes the likelihood of unwanted side effects. The corticosteroids generally used have an intermediate-acting duration of action. These corticosteroids include prednisone, prednisolone, and methylprednisolone (see Chapter 41 for more detailed information on these drugs).

Chronic use of the steroid aerosols has resulted in a decrease in bronchial hyperreactivity and symptom prevention. Inhaled corticosteroids have been reported to be more effective than alternate-day therapy with oral steroids (Self, Kelly, 1995). Topical corticosteroid therapy offers the possibility of limiting action at the site of application and thereby avoiding systemic effects. By chemically modifying the structural arrangement of the steroid molecule, compounds were developed to diminish systemic absorption from the respiratory tract. The products available are beclomethasone (Vanceril, Beclovent), budesonide (Pulmicort), flunisolide (AeroBid), and triamcinolone (Azmacort).

These products offer the advantage of producing few systemic adverse effects, including limited or no adrenal suppression. This category also includes dexamethasone (Decadron), but it is less often used today because of a higher incidence of side effects than the other agents. Box 32-3 explains the step approach to therapeutic management of asthma for the current recommendations for corticosteroids. The aerosols are rapidly absorbed from pulmonary tissues with limited gastrointestinal absorption. The maximum improvement in pulmonary function may take 1 to 4 weeks.

Side effects and adverse reactions

These include abdominal distress, anorexia, cough without infection, dizziness, headache, unpleasant taste in mouth, and, rarely, an increase in bronchospasms, and oral fungal infection or candidiasis.

The beclomethasone (Vanceril, Beclovent) adult dosage is two oral inhalations three or four times daily. For severe asthma, use 12 to 16 inhalations initially a day, then decrease dosage when appropriate. For children younger than 6 years of age, the dosage is not established; for children 6 to 12 years of age, administer one or two metered sprays three or four times daily.

In severe asthma, the initial adult budesonide dosage for the inhalation powder (Pulmicort) is 0.2 to 2.4 mg daily, divided in two to four doses. The maintenance dose is 0.2 to 0.4 mg twice daily, adjusting dosage as necessary. This product is not recommended for children younger than 6 years of age; for children 6 to 12 years of age with severe asthma, the dose is 0.1 to 0.2 mg twice daily.

For flunisolide (AeroBid), the dose is two oral inhalations twice daily, morning and night, for children 4 years of age and older and adults.

The triamcinolone (Azmacort) adult dosage is two inhalations three or four times daily. In very severe asthma, 12 to 16 inhalations per day may be used. For children 6 to 12 years of age, one or two inhalations three or four times a day is recommended. Do not exceed 12 inhalations per day in children.

BOX 32-3 Step Approach for Therapeutic Management of Asthma

Step 4, severe	For long-term prophylaxis control, a high-dose corticosteroid inhaler *plus* a long-acting $beta_2$ agonist tablet, or inhaler or a long-acting theophylline *plus* corticosteroid oral (2 mg/kg/day, not exceeding 60 mg/day) daily should be utilized. A short-acting $beta_2$ agonist inhaler is available for symptom control.
Step 3, moderate	Intermediate dose corticosteroid inhaler *plus* a long-acting $beta_2$ agonist inhaler, tablets or long-acting theophylline daily. A short-acting $beta_2$ agonist inhaler is available for symptom control.
Step 2, mild (persistent)	Low dose corticosteroid inhaler or nedocromil daily. Children may start with cromolyn or nedocromil. Zafirlukast, zileuton or a long-acting theophylline product are alternatives for patients 12 years old or older. A short-acting $beta_2$ agonist inhaler is available for symptom control.
Step 1, mild (intermittent)	Short-acting $beta_2$ agonist inhaler is available for symptom control. If inhaler is used more than twice weekly, consider step 2 therapy.

From NAEPP, 1997.

SUMMARY

Patients with abnormal or excessive respiratory tract secretions or bronchospasms often need mucokinetic and bronchodilator drugs. The mucokinetic agents promote the removal of respiratory tract secretions by thinning hyperviscous secretions; thereby they enhance the ciliary action of the respiratory tract. Bronchodilators induce bronchial smooth muscle relaxation. Xanthine derivatives are also used as bronchodilators although they are no longer first-line therapy. The prophylactic agents for asthma include cromolyn and nedocromil, while the leukotriene antagonists are indicated for the treatment and/or prophylaxis of chronic asthma. Corticosteroids are also used in chronic asthma to prevent or minimize inflammation.

REVIEW QUESTIONS

1. An asthmatic patient has the following medications prescribed:

   metaproterenol (Alupent), 2 inhalations qid
   cromolyn (Intal), 2 inhalations qid
   ipratropium (Atrovent), 2 inhalations four times a day

   To obtain the maximum effects from combination drug inhalers, what instructions would you share with this patient on order (first, second, and third) of the drugs? State additional therapeutic tips.
2. What are the indications, mechanism of action, pharmacokinetics, and side effects and adverse reactions with the use of acetylcysteine?
3. Name the only OTC expectorant that has been found to be safe and effective by the FDA.
4. Discuss the use of dornase alfa in the treatment of cystic fibrosis.

REFERENCES

Franz MN, Cohn RC: Management of children and adults with cystic fibrosis: one center's approach, *Hosp Formul* 29(9):364-378, 1994.

National Asthma Education and Prevention Program: Considerations for the diagnosing and managing asthma in the elderly, http://www.nhlbi.nih.gov/nhlbi/lung/asthma/prof/as_elder.txt (June 16, 1998).

National Asthma Education and Prevention Program Expert Panel 2: Guidelines for the diagnosis and management of asthma, http://www.nhlbi.nih.gov/nhlbi/lung/asthma/prof/asthmgdln.htm (1997).

Self TH, Kelly HW: Asthma. In Young LY, Koda-Kimble MA, editors: *Applied therapeutics: the clinical use of drugs,* ed 6, Vancouver, Wash, 1995, Applied Therapeutics, Inc.

Serafin WE: Drugs used in the treatment of asthma. In Hardman JG, Limbird LE, editors: *Goodman & Gilman's the pharmacological basis of therapeutics,* ed 9, New York, 1996, McGraw-Hill.

United States Pharmacopeial Convention: *USP DI: drug information for the health care professional,* ed 18, Rockville, Md, 1998, The Convention.

ADDITIONAL REFERENCES

American Hospital Formulary Service: *AHFS drug information '98,* Bethesda, Md, 1996, American Society of Hospital Pharmacists.

Anderson KN et al, editors: *Mosby's medical, nursing, and allied health dictionary,* ed 5, St Louis, 1998, Mosby.

Ip M, Lam K, Kung A, Ng M: Decreased bone mineral density in premenopausal asthma patients receiving long-term inhaled steroids, *Chest* 105(6):1722-1727, 1994.

Kelly HW: *The 1997 Expert Panel Report II: guidelines for the diagnosis and management of asthma,* Pharmacist's Letter, document 130417, 1997.

Kelly HW, Hill MR: Asthma. In DiPiro JT, Talber R et al, editors: *Pharmacotherapy, a pathophysiologic approach,* ed 2, Norwalk, Conn, 1993, Appleton & Lange.

Mathewson HS, Kovac AL: Update on inhaled steroids, *Respir Care* 39(8):837-840, 1994.

McFadden ER, Gilbert IA: Asthma, *N Engl J Med* 327(27):1928, 1992.

Mosby: *Mosby's GenRx,* St Louis, 1998, Mosby.

Olin BR: *Facts and comparisons,* Philadelphia, 1998, JB Lippincott.

Public Health Service, US Department of Health and Human Services: *Executive summary: Guidelines for the diagnosis and management of asthma,* NIH Pub No 91-3042A, Washington, DC, 1991, National Institutes of Health.

Wingard LB et al: *Human pharmacology,* St Louis, 1991, Mosby.

CHAPTER 33

Oxygen and Miscellaneous Respiratory Agents

KEY DRUGS

cyproheptadine, (p. 479)
diphenhydramine, (p. 473)

KEY TERMS

analeptics, (p. 471)
hypercapnia, (p. 470)
hypoxemia, (p. 468)
hypoxia, (p. 468)
pulse oximetry, (p. 470)

CHAPTER FOCUS

This chapter reviews the therapeutic gases oxygen and carbon dioxide. Cough suppressants, histamine, and antihistamines, H_1 receptor antagonists, and serotonin and antiserotonin agents are discussed in this chapter. These agents cover a wide range of therapeutic effects on the respiratory system.

OBJECTIVES

After reading and studying this chapter, the student should be able to do the following:

1. *Define and describe the key terms and key drugs.*
2. *Describe the effects of oxygen and oxygen deprivation on the body.*
3. *Explain the differences between a nasal catheter, nasal cannula, oxygen mask, and oxygen tent.*
4. *Discuss the use and effects of carbon dioxide as a pharmacologic agent.*
5. *Explain the various actions of histamine (H_1 and H_2) in the body.*
6. *Review serotonin's sites of action, pharmacokinetics, pharmacologic effects, and relationship to morphine and monoamine oxidase inhibitor drugs.*

DRUGS THAT AFFECT THE RESPIRATORY CENTER

Therapeutic Gases

Oxygen

Oxygen is a gas that is essential for life; it is colorless, odorless, and tasteless. It is not flammable, but it supports combustion much more vigorously than does air.

Inspired air normally contains 20.9% oxygen, which, at an atmospheric pressure of 760 mm Hg, exerts a partial pressure (PO_2) or tension of 159 mm Hg. However, as oxygen passes through the bronchial airway, the inspired air becomes saturated with water vapor, which then reduces the PO_2 in the alveoli to approximately 100 mm Hg. Finally, the oxygen appears in dissolved form in the arterial blood. The PO_2 of arterial blood is normally greater than 80 mm Hg.

Oxygen must be continuously supplied to tissue cells, as no fiber or cell can remain without oxygen, or hypoxic, for very long and survive. The adult human brain consumes from 40 to 50 ml of oxygen per minute. The cortex consumes more than the centers in the medulla or spinal cord. Cerebral oxygen consumption proceeds without pausing, and the replenishment of oxygen by the blood must be maintained continuously. Whenever any circulatory stress exists, cerebral blood flow tends to be preserved at the expense of other less vital organs. Of all the tissues affected by hypoxia (inadequate cellular oxygen), the brain is most susceptible to disruption of normal function and irreversible damage. An acute reduction of the PO_2 to 50 mm Hg decreases mental functioning, emotional stability, and finer muscular coordination. Further reduction of the PO_2 to 40 mm Hg produces impaired judgment, decreased pain perception, and impairment of muscular coordination. When the PO_2 is reduced to 32 mm Hg or less, unconsciousness and a progressive descending depression of the central nervous system (CNS) ensue.

The kidneys are vital organs in which there must be constancy of blood flow and oxygen supply. Oxygen consumption is greater in the renal cortex; renal medullary tissue has an oxygen consumption that is 15% less than that of the renal cortex. This difference is related to the variation in pressure gradient and to the fact that cortical flow is rapid while the medullary flow is slower. The renal cortex is highly dependent on oxygen, whereas the renal medulla can function relatively independently of the oxygen supply.

The rate of oxygen consumption by the kidneys is approximately 0.06 ml/g/min, more than most other tissues. For each 100 ml of blood entering the kidney, 1.4 ml of oxygen is consumed. The oxygen consumed by the kidneys is primarily used for sodium reabsorption.

When the renal arterial content falls to less than 55% of normal, renal vasoconstriction occurs. This response is believed to be mediated by chemoreceptors, which stimulate the vasomotor center to produce renal vasoconstriction. Renal vasoconstriction also occurs as a result of the action of ether, barbiturates, and other anesthetics. Renal blood flow is also decreased during periods of exercise. It is important to note that autoregulation of renal perfusion does occur.

In skeletal muscles, oxygen consumption is related to blood flow. Oxygen consumption and blood flow are decreased when muscle is at rest and significantly increased during exercise.

Reduction of oxygen supply to the intestinal tract is regarded by some investigators as a key factor for inadequate splanchnic vasoconstriction during hypotension. Inadequate oxygen supply impairs myocardial metabolism and function.

Arterial blood pressure determinations, when used alone, are unreliable indicators of the adequacy of tissue perfusion. Therefore arterial blood gas determinations should be obtained, since these results provide a more accurate and reliable indication of shifts in the partial pressures of oxygen and carbon dioxide. Severe hypoxia may produce changes in the ST segment and T wave of the electrocardiogram (ECG), dysrhythmias, ectopic beats, and myocardial infarction.

Indications

Oxygen is used chiefly to treat **hypoxia** (inadequate oxygen at cellular level) and **hypoxemia** (an abnormal oxygen deficiency in arterial blood). The four types of hypoxia are as follows:

1. Hypoxic hypoxia: produced by any condition causing a decrease in PO_2
2. Ischemic hypoxia: inadequate blood flow to an organ or tissue in the presence of a normal PO_2 and hemoglobin content
3. Anemic hypoxia: inadequate hemoglobin to carry O_2 in the presence of a normal PO_2
4. Histotoxic hypoxia: adequate PO_2 and hemoglobin but inability of tissues to use oxygen delivered because of a toxic agent

Clinically, hypoxic hypoxia is the most common form of hypoxia. A variety of pathologic conditions result in hypoxic hypoxia, which makes the use of oxygen treatment necessary. Some of these conditions are hypoventilation, increased airway resistance, pneumothorax, respiratory center depression, abnormal ventilation perfusion ratio, congenital cyanotic heart disease, decreased pulmonary compliance, and breathing oxygen-poor air. The use of oxygen is also indicated in cardiac failure or decompensation and coronary occlusion, and anesthesia administration (to increase the safety of general anesthesia).

Administration

Oxygen is administered by inhalation. Various methods are used, each having advantages and disadvantages (Fig. 33-1).

A nasal catheter made of soft plastic is passed through the nose until the tip is just above the epiglottis. The catheter should not be inserted so far that the patient swallows oxygen, since this will cause stomach distention and

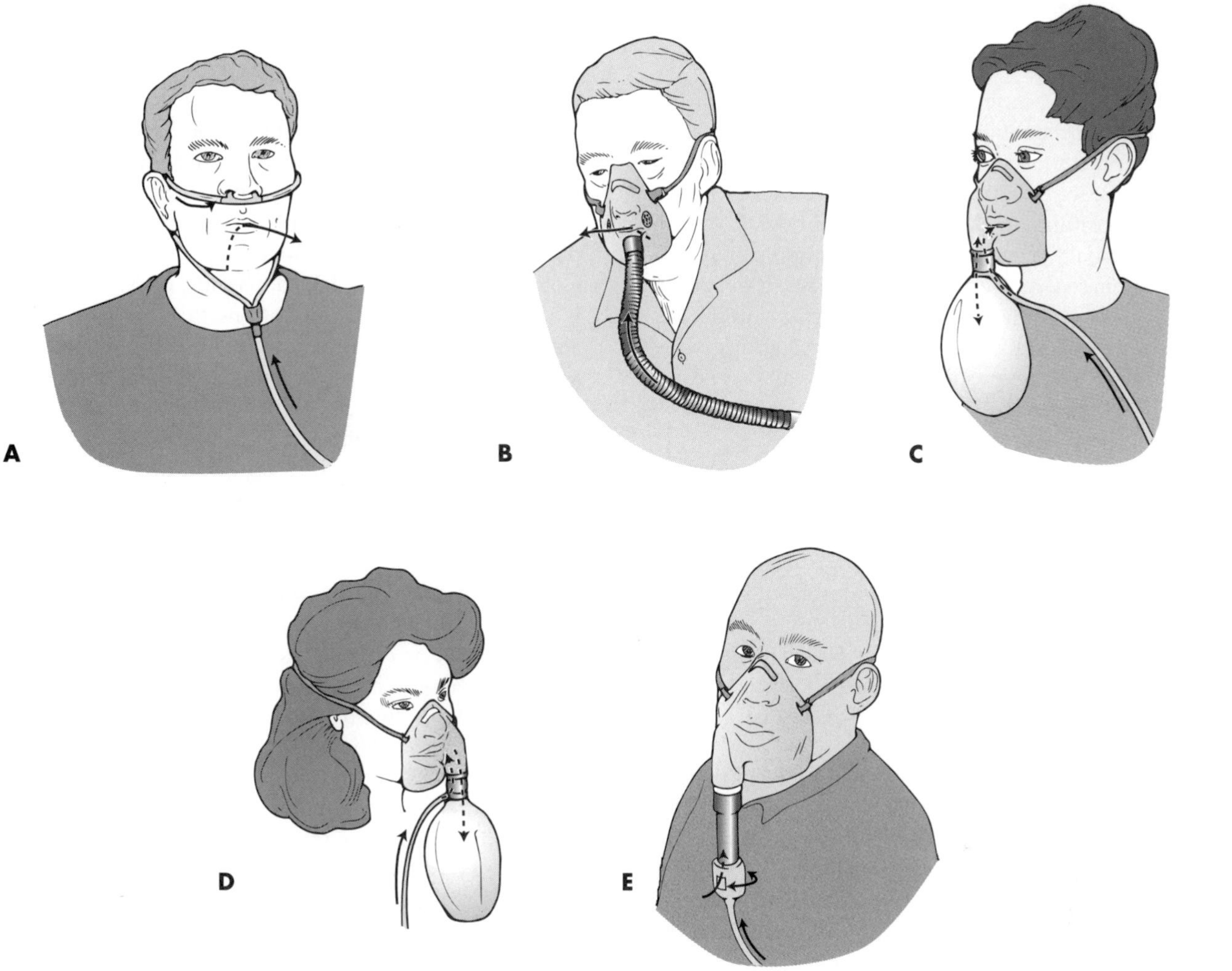

FIGURE 33-1
Various oxygen delivery systems. **A,** Nasal cannula. **B,** Simple face mask. **C,** Partial rebreathing mask. **D,** Nonbreathing mask. **E,** Venturi mask.

abdominal discomfort. The catheter is fastened with tape to the forehead and/or nose. The flow rate varies according to individual need, but 4 to 8 L/min of a 25% to 40% concentration of oxygen is commonly used. Because this form of therapy is very drying to the mucous membrane, the oxygen should be humidified. Most patients receiving oxygen therapy are mouth breathers, and frequent mouth care is required to prevent sores.

A nasal cannula is much more comfortable for the patient than is a catheter. Cannulas have either single or double short prongs that are inserted into the lower part of the nostrils. They are less likely to become obstructed with secretions. A flow of 1 to 6 L/min of a 23% to 40% concentration of oxygen is adequate for many patients.

An oxygen mask is the most effective means of delivering needed oxygen. Oxygen concentrations up to 90% can be administered by mask. To be effective, the mask must fit well over the nose and mouth. Masks are better tolerated when used intermittently or when disposable plastic masks are used. Only absolutely clean and uncontaminated rubber masks should be used, since they can be a source of nosocomial infection. There are two main types of oxygen masks: those that deliver low concentrations of oxygen and those that deliver high concentrations of oxygen.

A simple face mask, which is lightweight and disposable, is useful for short-term therapy of oxygen administration, such as in the early postoperative period or when intermittent oxygen therapy is required. The flow rate is only 6 to 10 L/min at a low oxygen concentration of 35% to 60%. Since the mask is loose fitting and can leak, simple face masks are suitable for individuals with carbon dioxide retention. It is also indicated for persons who cannot use a nasal cannula, for example, those who have a nasal obstruction.

A partial rebreathing mask is a disposable, light-weight plastic face mask consisting of a reservoir bag and a partial rebreathing valve. It is commonly used by individuals who require oxygen. On expiration, only a portion of the exhaled air enters the reservoir, so it conserves roughly one third of the patient's exhaled air. Because it comes from the trachea and bronchi and does not participate in gas exchange in the lungs, it is rich in oxygen.

Accordingly, to prevent the rebreathing of carbon dioxide, the reservoir bag should deflate only slightly on inhalation. By this method a concentration of 60% to 90% of oxygen can be delivered at a flow rate of 10 L/min.

A nonrebreathing mask is designed to fit tightly over the face and is usually made of rubber with a reservoir bag and a nonbreathing valve. On inhalation, oxygen flows into the bag and mask, and the one-way valve prevents exhaled air from flowing back into the bag. The expired air instead escapes through the one-way flap valve in the mask. The concentration of oxygen is 95%, which is high, and the flow is adjusted to keep the reservoir bag fully inflated.

This type of mask is used for short-term therapy such as counteracting smoke inhalation. The rubber can become hot and sticky so that prolonged use can cause discomfort.

An oxygen tent is of limited value, particularly when it is necessary to open the canopy for monitoring vital signs and administering care to the patient. The rate of flow is 20 L/min at an oxygen concentration of 60%. Obviously, the oxygen concentration falls, making the flow difficult to control each time the tent is opened. Consequently, oxygen tents are now used less frequently.

The Ventimask (Mix-O-Mask) originated from the Venturi mask, and it is used for patients with chronic alveolar hypoventilation and carbon dioxide retention. Exact low-flow concentrations of oxygen are delivered to the individual. The Ventimask provides an air-oxygen mixture at the desired oxygen concentration with the size of the orifice to the mask determining the concentration of oxygen: 24%, 28%, 35%, and 40% with flow rates of 4, 6, 8, and 10 L/min, respectively. A thin elastic band holds the Ventimask in position and tends to press into the skin behind the ears. A gauze padding under each side of the elastic band will alleviate this discomfort. The device must be removed when the person eats and may give the patient a feeling of being smothered.

Most of the oxygen administered in hospitals for therapy is provided from a central source where it is stored as a gas or liquid oxygen. The gas is piped into a patient's room at a standard pressure of 50 pounds per square inch (psi) at the gauge. Compressed oxygen is marketed in steel cylinders that are fitted with reducing valves for the delivery of the gas. The cylinders are usually color coded; green is used in the United States. Because the gas is under considerable pressure, the tanks must be handled carefully to prevent falling or jarring.

The effectiveness of oxygen administration depends on the carbon dioxide content of the blood. Individuals with chronic obstructive pulmonary disease (COPD) have difficulty with carbon dioxide and oxygen exchange and are subject to **hypercapnia** (high carbon dioxide content in the blood). Because of chronic hypercapnia, the medullary center of these individuals is relatively insensitive to stimulation of carbon dioxide; rather, a low partial arterial oxygen pressure (PaO_2) serves as a stimulant to respiration. Therefore oxygen flow rates are kept low (1 to 2 L/min) for patients with COPD.

The best method of measuring the need and effectiveness of oxygen is by arterial blood gas measurements or **pulse oximetry.** Pulse oximetry measures the wavelengths of light passing through living tissue and then analyzes the differences in absorption. For example, oxygenated hemoglobin will absorb the light differently, and this difference is used as the basis of calculations that compare oxygenated hemoglobin with nonoxygenated hemoglobin. The pulse oximeters have a small probe (the light source and detector) that is placed on the person's finger, toe, ear, bridge of nose, or temple. These devices are noninvasive and inexpensive and also safe and accurate with no calibration required. Pulse oximetry is frequently used to determine tissue oxygenation in any patients with respiratory problems.

Oxygen administration in the premature infant. Healthcare professionals caring for premature infants in incubators must be constantly aware of the danger of retrolental fibroplasia. This is a vascular proliferative disease of the retina that occurs in some premature infants who have had high concentrations of oxygen at birth.* The oxygen concentration should be kept between 30% and 40%. Higher concentrations can be administered to cyanotic infants without increasing the danger of retrolental fibroplasia because it is PaO_2, not inspired PO_2, that is implicated in this disease. Therefore careful monitoring of arterial blood gases is essential. Some incubators are equipped with a safety valve that automatically releases any excess oxygen outside the chamber.

Hyperbaric oxygen. Recently, hyperbaric oxygen has been used in the treatment of various conditions, such as infections caused by *Clostridium welchii,* the anaerobic bacillus producing gas gangrene. The intermittent use of hyperbaric oxygen has been valuable. It is believed that an increased oxygen pressure in the tissue may exert an inhibitory effect on enzyme systems of these bacteria. This same inhibitory effect may be implicated in the effect of hyperbaric oxygen on other anaerobic microorganisms.

Hyperbaric oxygen has also been used in certain circulatory disturbances such as air or gas embolism, decompression sickness, carbon monoxide and cyanide poisoning, and exceptional blood loss. It has also been used in certain local circulatory disturbances such as necrotizing soft tissue infections; acute traumatic ischemia, crush injury, and compartment syndrome; compromised (ischemic) grafts and flaps; radiation necrosis; refractory osteomyelitis; and enhancement of healing in selected problem wounds (Weaver, 1992).

*Excessive oxygen constricts the developing retinal vessels of the eye. Consequently, normal vascularization is suppressed. Because the endothelial cells become disorganized, they cause destruction of the immature retina. The result is blindness.

Helium-oxygen mixtures. Helium-oxygen mixtures have been used to treat obstructive types of dyspnea. Helium is an inert gas and so light that a mixture of 80% helium and 20% oxygen is only one third as heavy as air. Helium is only slightly soluble in body fluids and has a high rate of diffusion. Because of its low specific gravity, mixtures of this gas with oxygen can be breathed with less effort than either oxygen or air alone when air passages are obstructed.

These mixtures are recommended for individuals with status asthmaticus, bronchiectasis, and emphysema, as well as during anesthesia for a patient with respiratory tract obstruction.

Oxygen toxicity. Exposure to 100% oxygen for a period of 6 hours causes an inflammatory response with subsequent destruction of the alveolocapillary membrane of the respiratory tract. Toxicity is often difficult to recognize, but the most common symptoms are substernal distress (ache or burning sensation behind the sternum), an increase in respiratory distress, nausea, vomiting, restlessness, tremors, twitching, paresthesias, convulsions, and a dry, hacking cough.

Carbon Dioxide

Carbon dioxide is a colorless, odorless gas that is heavier than air. Carbon dioxide used as a pharmacologic agent affects respiration, circulation, and the CNS. Inhalation of carbon dioxide for a short period of time increases both rate and depth of respiration unless the respiratory center is depressed by narcotics or disease.

Carbon dioxide stimulates cells of the sympathetic nervous system, the respiratory center, and the peripheral chemoreceptors. Carbon dioxide also depresses the cerebral cortex, myocardium, and smooth muscle of the peripheral blood vessels. Carbon dioxide may also interfere with nerve conduction and transmission. When carbon dioxide increases the rate and force of respiration, venous return to the heart is usually enhanced as a result of decreased peripheral resistance; there is improved rate and force of myocardial contraction and less likelihood of myocardial irritability and dysrhythmias.

Too much carbon dioxide has a depressant effect and results in acidosis and unresponsiveness of the respiratory center to the gas. Therefore it is important that carbon dioxide be administered with caution.

Indications

The following are indications for use of carbon dioxide:

Carbon monoxide poisoning. A 5% to 7% concentration of carbon dioxide in oxygen is sometimes used in the treatment of carbon monoxide poisoning. Physiologically, carbon dioxide increases the rate of separation of carbon monoxide from carboxyhemoglobin.

General anesthesia. Most general anesthetics cause a reduction in response to carbon dioxide, which is reflected in CNS depression. The degree of depression is directly related to the depth of anesthesia. The more deeply the individual is anesthetized, the greater the depression of the CNS. Carbon dioxide initially speeds up anesthesia by increasing pulmonary ventilation. By lessening the sense of asphyxiation, it reduces struggling. In the postanesthesia period, it hastens the elimination of many anesthetics. Inhalation of 5% to 7% carbon dioxide increases cerebral blood flow by approximately 75%, primarily by dilation of cerebral vessels.

Respiratory depression. The use of carbon dioxide as a respiratory stimulant in the presence of depressed respiration is limited. When used, close monitoring by pulse oximetry and PaO_2 is important; if desired results are not obtained, it should be discontinued. Mechanical assistance to respiration and oxygen administration is the usual treatment in cases of respiratory depression.

Postoperative use. Occasionally, carbon dioxide is used postoperatively to increase ventilation and prevent atelectasis. Most investigators think that deep breathing exercises, coughing, frequent turning, tracheal suction, and intermittent positive pressure breathing produce better results.

Carbon dioxide administration has also been used in the treatment of postoperative hiccups. Relief of hiccups is apparently accomplished by stimulation of the respiratory center, causing large excursions of the diaphragm that suppress spasmodic contractions of that muscle, thereby promoting regular contractions.

Administration

Carbon dioxide is kept in metal cylinders and vaporizes as it is delivered from the cylinder. When carbon dioxide is used for medical purposes, it is administered in combination with oxygen. A 5% to 10% concentration of carbon dioxide delivered through a tight-fitting face mask is inhaled by the patient until the depth of respiration is definitely increased, which usually occurs within 3 minutes. For the postoperative individual, the procedure would be repeated every hour or two for the first 48 hours and then several times a day for several days.

Another way of administering carbon dioxide is to allow the patient to hyperventilate with a paper bag held over the face. Reinhaling expired air causes the carbon dioxide content to be continually increased.

Signs of carbon dioxide overdosage are dyspnea, breath holding, markedly increased chest and abdominal movements, nausea, and increased systolic blood pressure. Administration of the gas should be discontinued when these symptoms appear. The administration of 5% carbon dioxide may produce severe mental depression if given over 1 hour, and a 10% concentration can lead to loss of consciousness within 10 minutes. The administration should be stopped as soon as the desired effects on the patient's respiration have been obtained.

Direct Respiratory Stimulants

Direct respiratory stimulants come under a broader classification of CNS stimulants and are often referred to as **an-**

aleptics (see Chapter 12). These drugs act directly on the medullary center to increase respiratory rate and tidal exchange. Although these drugs are available for stimulating depth of respiration and rate of respiration, airway management and support of ventilation are more effective in the treatment of respiratory depression. The mechanical support of ventilation is often superior to the use of drugs, since respiratory stimulants in large doses can cause convulsions.

Respiratory stimulants (analeptics) have in the past been advocated in the treatment of drug-induced respiratory depression, but since these drugs are not specific antagonists to sedatives or narcotics, their use in drug-induced respiratory depression is now considered obsolete. Indeed, repeated doses of an analeptic may potentiate the depressant effects of CNS depressants. For information on the direct respiratory stimulant doxapram, see Chapter 12.

Reflex Respiratory Stimulants

Aromatic ammonia spirit is given by inhalation for its action as a reflex respiratory stimulant. In cases of fainting, it is administered by inhaling the vapor. Reflex stimulation of the medullary center occurs through peripheral irritation of sensory nerve receptors in the pharynx, esophagus, and stomach. The rate and depth of respiration are then increased through afferent messages to the respiratory control centers. Reflex stimulation of the vasomotor center results in a rise in blood pressure.

Respiratory Depressants

The most important respiratory depressants are opium and its derivatives and barbiturates. These agents depress the respiratory center, thereby making breathing slower and more shallow and lessening the irritability of the respiratory center. Respiratory depression, however, is seldom desirable or necessary, although it is sometimes unavoidable. It is a side/adverse effect of otherwise very useful drugs.

Occasionally, an opiate such as codeine is administered to inhibit the rate and depth of respiration for a painful or harmful cough. Concentrations of carbon dioxide that are too high in inhalation mixtures may paradoxically act to depress respiration.

COUGH SUPPRESSANTS

The over-the-counter (OTC) cough suppressants are reviewed in Chapter 3, and cough suppressants requiring prescriptions are discussed in this chapter. The prescribing of these agents is usually reserved for the nonproductive cough that is inadequately controlled or nonresponsive to the OTC medications.

Treatment of cough is secondary to treatment of the underlying disorder; that is, the therapeutic objective is to decrease the intensity and frequency of the cough yet permit adequate elimination of tracheobronchial secretions and exudates.

Opioid Antitussive Drugs

Opioids such as morphine and hydromorphone are potent suppressants of the cough reflex, but their clinical usefulness is limited by side effects. They inhibit the ciliary activity of the respiratory mucous membrane, depress respiration, and may cause bronchial constriction in allergic or asthmatic patients. In addition, they can cause drug dependence. Codeine and hydrocodone exhibit less pronounced antitussive effects, but they also have fewer side effects. They are widely used. (See Chapter 8 for opioid agents.)

Nonopioid Antitussive Drugs

The nonnarcotic drugs in this group have fewer gastrointestinal side effects than do codeine and related compounds.

benzonatate [ben zoe' na tate] (Tessalon)

Benzonatate, chemically related to the local anesthetic tetracaine, relieves coughing by peripherally anesthetizing the stretch or cough receptors in the lungs and respiratory passages. It may also have a central effect on the cough reflex.

Indications

Benzonatate is indicated for the symptomatic treatment of nonproductive cough.

Pharmacokinetics

After oral administration, the onset of action is within 15 to 20 minutes with duration of action up to 8 hours. It is metabolized, and the metabolites are excreted by the kidneys.

Drug interactions

No significant drug interactions are reported.

Side effects and adverse reactions

These include drowsiness, headaches, dizziness, tightness or numbness in chest, nausea, constipation, abdominal upset, skin eruptions, nasal congestion, and a vague sensation of chill.

Warnings

Use with caution in patients with persistent cough after medication was used for a week or with high fever, rash, or a persistent headache. See the box for Food and Drug Administration (FDA) pregnancy safety classifications.

Contraindications

Avoid use in persons with benzonatate or topical anesthetic hypersensitivity or if the patient has a productive cough.

Dosage and administration

The dosage for adults and children older than 10 years of age is 100 mg three times a day; the maximum daily dose is 600 mg.

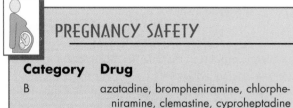

PREGNANCY SAFETY

Category	Drug
B	azatadine, brompheniramine, chlorpheniramine, clemastine, cyproheptadine, dexchlorpheniramine, dimenhydrinate, diphenhydramine, loratadine, triprolidine
C	astemizole, benzonatate, terfenadine
Unclassified	doxylamine, hydroxyzine, tripelennamine

diphenhydramine [dye fen hye′ dra meen] (Benylin, Benadryl, and others)

Diphenhydramine, available OTC and by prescription, depresses the cough center in the medulla of the brain (antitussive effect). It is reviewed in the antihistamine section of Chapter 3.

The adult dose for antitussive effect (syrup) is 25 mg orally every 4 to 6 hours, the antihistamine dose is 25 to 50 mg orally every 4 to 6 hours when necessary, and as a sedative-hypnotic, the dose is 50 mg given 20 to 30 minutes before bedtime. The antidyskinetic or antiparkinson effect dosage is 50 to 150 mg orally daily in divided doses. For antiemetic or antivertigo effects, the dose is 25 to 50 mg orally 30 minutes before traveling and before each meal as necessary. The elderly may be more sensitive to the effects of this drug; therefore lower adult doses should be prescribed with close monitoring for any adverse effects. The maximum daily dosage recommended is 300 mg in divided doses.

For children, the antihistamine dose is 1.25 mg/kg orally every 4 to 6 hours. The maximum daily dosage is 300 mg. Do not use diphenhydramine in premature or full-term neonates.

The adult dose of diphenhydramine injection used as an antihistamine or antidyskinetic is 10 to 50 mg IM or IV every 2 to 3 hours. As an antiemetic or antivertigo agent, the dose is 10 mg initially IM or IV, which may be increased to 20 to 50 mg every 2 or 3 hours. In children the antihistamine or antidyskinetic dose is 1.25 mg/kg IM four times daily. Do not use in premature or full-term neonates.

For information on dextromethorphan, another nonopioid antitussive drug, see Chapter 3.

HISTAMINE

Distribution

Histamine is a chemical mediator that occurs naturally in almost all body tissues. It is present in highest concentration in the skin, lung, and gastrointestinal tract. These structures are frequently exposed to environmental assaults and require protection against damage. When liberated from its cells, the free form of histamine plays an early transient role in the inflammatory process that defends the exposed tissues against injury.

TABLE 33-1 Histamine: Receptor-Mediating Effects

Structure	*Histamine Receptors*	*Pharmacologic Effects*
Vascular system		
Capillary (Microcirculation)	H_1 and H_2	Dilation Increased permeability
Arteriole (Smooth muscle)	H_1 and H_2	Dilation
Smooth muscle		
Bronchial, bronchiolar	H_1	Contraction
Gastrointestinal	H_1	Contraction
Exocrine glands		
Gastric	H_2	Gastric acid secretion (HCl)
Epidermis	H_1	Triple response (flush, flare, wheal)
Adrenal medulla	—	Epinephrine and norepinephrine release
Central nervous system	H_1	Motion sickness

In many tissues the chief site of production and storage of histamine is the cytoplasmic granules of the mast cell or, in the case of blood, the basophil that closely resembles the mast cell in function. The mast cells are small, ovoid structures widely distributed in the loose connective tissue. They are especially abundant along small blood vessels and along the bronchial smooth muscle cell, which appears to have the highest concentration of mast cells of any organ in the body. Both the mast cells and basophils make up the mast cell histamine pool. A second major site of histamine production is known as the non-mast cell pool, where the amine is stored in the cells of the epidermis, gastrointestinal mucosa, and the CNS. Although histamine is present in various foods and is synthesized by intestinal flora, the amount absorbed does not contribute to the body's stores of this amine.

Pharmacologic Actions

The reactions mediated by histamine are attributed to receptor activity, which involves two distinct populations of receptors called H_1 and H_2 receptors. The principal actions of histamine are listed in Table 33-1.

Vascular Effects

In the microcirculatory component of the cardiovascular system (arterioles, capillaries, and venules) the liberation of histamine has been shown to involve both the H_1 and H_2 receptors. Stimulation of these receptors dilates the capillaries and venules, producing an increased localized blood flow, increased capillary permeability, erythema, and edema. By activating the H_1 and H_2 receptors on the smooth muscles of the arterioles, histamine is also capable of eliciting a systemic response, that is, vasodilation of the arterioles, which can result in a profound fall in blood pressure.

Smooth Muscle Effects

Although histamine exerts a powerful relaxing effect on the smooth muscle of the arterioles, it produces a contractile action on the smooth muscles of many nonvascular organs, such as the bronchi and gastrointestinal tract. In sensitized individuals, activation of the H_1 receptors of the lungs can cause marked bronchial muscle contraction that often progresses to dyspnea and airway obstruction.

Exocrine Glandular Effects

While histamine stimulates the gastric, salivary, pancreatic, and lacrimal glands, the main effect is seen in the gastric glands. Stimulation of H_2 receptors in the exocrine glands of the stomach increases production of gastric acid secretions. Its high hydrochloric acid concentration is attributed to the activity of the parietal cells of the stomach and is implicated in the development of peptic ulcers.

Central Nervous System Effect

Histamine is also known to be present throughout the tissues of the brain. Its effects seem to involve both H_1 and H_2 receptor mediation. The activation of H_1 receptors of the semicircular canals is associated with motion sickness.

Pathologic Effects

Histamine as a chemical mediator is implicated in many pathologic disorders. Conditions for which drugs are used to counteract this compound are related to the hypersensitivity response known as the allergic reaction. Although four different types of hypersensitivity responses to immunologic injury exist, the type I anaphylactic reaction is the one associated with the disorders caused by histamine release.

Individuals with type I-mediated hypersensitivity develop allergies as a result of sensitization to a foreign agent that may be ingested, inhaled, or injected. An incalculable number of these agents acting as antigens exist. They vary widely in that different forms of allergic reactivity can develop in response to seasonal exposure to pollens, grasses, and weeds or nonseasonal agents such as house dust, feathers, molds, and other similar substances.

Hypersensitivity to a variety of foods such as shellfish or strawberries requires ingestion of the antigen. Insects such as bees or wasps and even drugs, particularly penicillin, also possess allergic properties that may induce a severe response in hypersensitive individuals.

Thus type I anaphylactic hypersensitivity accounts for a substantial number of allergic disorders, and it involves a complex series of anomalies that range from mild urticaria to anaphylactic shock. The mechanism of type I anaphylactic reaction involves the attachment of an antigen (Ag) to an antibody (Ab), specifically immunoglobulin E (IgE), and this complex in turn becomes fixed to the mast cell. The pathologic manifestations of Ag-IgE interaction are caused by mast cell degranulation, resulting in the release of histamine and other mediators responsible for producing the allergic symptoms. The type I anaphylactic reaction is responsible for various disorders, such as urticaria, atopy (allergic rhinitis, and hay fever), food allergies, bronchial asthma, and systemic anaphylaxis.

Urticaria

Urticaria is a vascular reaction of the skin characterized by immediate formation of a wheal and flare accompanied by severe itching. Contact with an external irritant such as drugs or foods produces the Ag-IgE–mediated response with resultant release of histamine from the mast cell into the skin. The local vasodilation produces the red flare, and the increased permeability of the capillaries leads to tissue swelling. These swellings are called "hives," and when giant hives occur, they are known as angioneurotic edema. Antihistaminic drugs administered before exposure to the antigen will prevent this response.

Atopy

Atopy occurs in genetically susceptible individuals and is usually caused by seasonal pollen. This condition is manifested as an upper respiratory tract disorder known as allergic rhinitis (hay fever) (Box 33-1). See Chapter 3 for additional information. After the interaction of Ag-IgE antibody on the surface of the bronchial mast cells, histamine is re-

BOX 33-1 Colds, Allergic Rhinitis, and Influenza: Signs or Symptoms

Signs or Symptoms	*Common Cold*	*Allergic Rhinitis*	*Influenza*
Fever	Rare	Absent	Common: sudden onset, 102-104° F
Aches and pains	Slight	Absent	May be severe
Sneezing	Usual	Common	Infrequent
Pruritus	Absent or rare	Common	Absent
Cough	Mild-moderate	Uncommon	Common
Headaches	Rare	Can occur	Prominent
Causative	Usually viruses	Usually allergens	Usually viruses
Occurrence	Anytime	Usually seasonal	Anytime
Complications	Sinus congestion, earache	Uncommon	Bronchitis, pneumonia

leased, producing local vascular dilation and increased capillary permeability. This change produces a rapid fluid leakage into the tissues of the nose, resulting in swelling of the nasal linings. In certain individuals antihistaminic therapy can prevent the edematous reaction if the drug is administered before antigenic exposure.

Food Allergies

Food allergies involve intestinal IgE-mast cell responses to ingested antigens. If the upper gastrointestinal tract is affected, vomiting results; if the lower gastrointestinal tract is invaded, cramps and diarrhea occur. This condition also has been known to produce systemic anaphylaxis after ingestion of a large amount of antigen.

Bronchial Asthma

When the inhaled antigen combines with the IgE antibody, stimulation of the mast cells triggers the release of mediators in the lower respiratory tract, usually in the bronchi and bronchioles. Histamine plays a minor role in this response because the slow-reacting substance of anaphylaxis (SRS-A) is a more potent mediator, causing long-term contraction of the bronchiolar smooth muscle. The difficulty in breathing may be relieved by a bronchodilator such as epinephrine. The administration of antihistaminic drugs actually does not help to relieve this condition, since more potent chemical mediators than histamine are responsible for causing the reaction.

Systemic Anaphylaxis

Systemic anaphylaxis is a generalized reaction manifested as a life-threatening systemic condition. The Ag-IgE mediator response involves the basophils of the blood and the mast cells in the connective tissue. The most common precipitating causes of this response are drugs, particularly penicillin, insect stings (wasps and bees), and occasionally certain foods. The release of massive amounts of histamine into the circulation causes widespread vasodilation, resulting in a profound fall in blood pressure. The excessive dilation also allows plasma to leave the capillaries, and a loss of circulatory volume ensues. When the reaction is fatal, death is usually caused not only by shock but also by laryngeal edema. The symptoms of the latter condition include smooth muscle contraction of the bronchi and pharyngeal edema, which usually leads to asphyxiation. Since the mediator, SRS-A, also is released from the cells, spasm of the smooth muscle of the bronchioles elicits the asthma-like attack.

Antihistaminic drugs are less effective against systemic anaphylaxis because these agents do not antagonize the SRS-A mediator that causes the severe bronchoconstriction. Accordingly, a drug such as epinephrine, a bronchodilator, is indicated for this life-threatening situation. The relief produced by this drug results from the beta_2 receptor action that relaxes bronchial smooth muscles.

Drug allergies frequently develop in susceptible individuals who show no adverse effects after the first dose of drug administration. However, a second or subsequent reexposure to even a minute amount of this same antigen may elicit an exaggerated IgE response either locally or systemically. Individuals who exhibit such reactions are said to be allergic to the drug. The IgE-mediated response, particularly with penicillin, may occur in either the skin, producing severe urticaria, or the respiratory tract, causing bronchial asthma.

On the other hand, even limited contact in certain sensitized individuals can produce a fatal systemic anaphylaxis. Some of the drugs that elicit an allergic response include penicillin, chloramphenicol, streptomycin, sulfonamides, aspirin, and phenacetin. Allergic reactions to penicillin account for nearly 100 deaths per year in the United States. Therefore if an individual exhibits even the mildest sign of an allergic response, such as a slight skin rash, this symptom should be reported immediately to the prescriber. In all probability the drug will be discontinued to avoid the possibility of an exaggerated type I hypersensitivity reaction.

Histamine Testing: Gastric Function

Histamine is used to test for gastric acid secretory functions. If achlorhydria is the response to histamine, then the person may have pernicious anemia, gastric polyps, gastric carcinoma, or atrophic gastritis. If gastric acid hypersecretion occurs after the histamine, then a duodenal ulcer or Zollinger-Ellison syndrome may be the problem.

This test is contraindicated in patients with a history of hypersensitivity to the drug, bronchial asthma, vasomotor instability, urticaria, or severe cardiac, pulmonary, or renal disease. Histamine should be used cautiously in individuals with pheochromocytoma. Histamine H_2 receptor antagonists, such as cimetidine and ranitidine, are not to be administered for the 24 hours before the test because they will antagonize the effects of the histamine. Antacids and anticholinergics are also withheld before the examination. The procedure and any anticipated effects of the histamine test should be explained to the patient.

The person should fast for a minimum of 12 hours and be at rest under basal conditions. Use a nasogastric tube to empty the stomach contents before the examination and to obtain specimens during the examination. The patient may swallow 300 ml of water; then the histamine dose of 0.01 mg/kg (equal to 0.0275 mg/kg of histamine phosphate) is given subcutaneously. If the side effects of flushing, headache, nasal stuffiness, dizziness, faintness, and nausea become too severe, epinephrine or ephedrine may be administered. These drugs antagonize the effects of histamine except for those on gastric secretion.

The pulse rate and blood pressure should be closely monitored. Prevent the patient from swallowing saliva; its alkalinity may interfere with test results. Obtain four samples for volume and acidity of gastric contents 15 minutes apart for analysis. The maximum effect from the histamine is usually seen in about 30 minutes. This test should be performed by or under the direction of a physician.

Other drugs are also used to induce gastric secretion. Besides histamine, pentagastrin (Peptavion), a synthetic compound, is also used as a diagnostic aid to evaluate gastric acid secretion.

ANTIHISTAMINES

Antihistamines are drugs that compete with histamine for its receptor sites. With the discovery of two histamine receptors, H_1 and H_2, the antihistamines should be divided into the H_1 receptor antagonists and the H_2 receptor antagonists. The H_2 receptor blocking agents, which include cimetidine (Tagamet), ranitidine (Zantac), and others, are discussed in Chapter 35, while the OTC antihistamines are reviewed in Chapter 3. This section reviews the prescription antihistamines.

H_1 Receptor Antagonists

Antihistamines prevent the physiologic action of histamine by preventing histamine from reaching its site of action; thus the H_1 antihistamines have the greatest therapeutic effect on nasal allergies. They do not inhibit histamine already attached to receptors; therefore these drugs are more effective if given before histamine is released. They relieve symptoms better at the beginning of the hay fever season than during its height but fail to relieve the asthma that frequently accompanies hay fever. These preparations are palliative and do not immunize the individual or protect him or her over time against allergic reactions. They do not replace other remedies such as epinephrine, ephedrine, and others.

In acute asthmatic reactions, the antihistamine drugs serve only as supplements to these remedies, and relief of various symptoms of allergy is obtained only while the drug is being taken. Dozens of antihistamine drugs are available; they generally differ from each other by potency, duration of action, and incidence of side effects, particularly sedation. It is often necessary to try different types of antihistamines to determine the appropriate one for an individual.

Antihistamines are indicated for the treatment of allergies, vertigo, motion sickness, antitussive effect (diphenhydramine), and sedative and local anesthetic effects in dentistry. Generally, their oral absorption pattern is good, and onset of action is within 15 to 60 minutes for most of them. With astemizole (Hismanal), the onset of action is 2 to 3 days. Dimenhydrinate (Dramamine) rectally has an onset of action within 30 to 45 minutes. The time to peak effect can vary with each individual preparation. For example, the peak effect of astemizole (Hismanal) occurs within 9 to 12 days while that for triprolidine (Myidil) is within 2 to 3 hours. Duration of action is also variable with dimenhydrinate between 3 and 6 hours, azatadine (Optimine) at 12 hours, and loratadine (Claritin) at least 24 hours. These agents are primarily metabolized in the liver and excreted in the kidneys with the exception of astemizole, which is mainly excreted fecally.

Drug interactions

The following effects may occur when antihistamines are given with the drugs listed below:

Drug	Possible effect and management
Alcohol, CNS depressants	Concurrent use may enhance CNS-depressant effects. If the CNS depressant also has anticholinergic side effects, enhanced effects may be seen. Monitor closely, as interventions may be necessary.
Anticholinergic medications, psychotropics, and others	Enhanced CNS-depressant and anticholinergic side effects may be noted. Monitor closely because intervention may be necessary.
erythromycin (Erythrocin)	If administered concurrently with astemizole, an increased risk of cardiotoxic effects has been reported. Avoid or a potentially serious drug interaction may occur.
ketoconazole(Nizoral)	If administered concurrently with astemizole and loratadine, increased levels of antihistamines may result, which increases the potential for cardiotoxicity. Avoid or a potentially serious drug interaction may occur.
Monoamine oxidase (MAO) inhibitors	Prolonged anticholinergic and CNS-depressant effects may result. Avoid or a potentially serious drug interaction may occur

Color type indicates an unsafe drug combination.

Side effects and adverse reactions

See discussion of diphenhydramine.

Warnings

Use with caution in patients with open-angle glaucoma.

Contraindications

Avoid use in persons with specific antihistamine hypersensitivity, hypokalemia, liver function impairment, prostatic hypertrophy, and urinary retention.

Dosage and administration

The antihistamine dosage varies with each drug's chemical classification and pharmacokinetic profile. The newer agents released generally are longer-acting drugs with fewer sedative side effects, such as loratadine (Claritin), which is taken once a day and has few, if any, sedative and anticholinergic side effects.

The older agents that usually exhibit these side effects carry warnings about the drug use in the elderly; the geri-

TABLE 33-2 Antihistamines: Recommended Dosages

Antihistamine	Adult Dosage	Children's Dosage
astemizole (Hismanal)	10 mg daily	6-12 yr, 5 mg/day
azatadine (Optimine)	1-2 mg q8-12h	12 yr and older, 0.5-1 mg twice daily
brompheniramine (Dimetane)	4 mg q4-6h (maximum of 24 mg/day)	0.5 mg/kg in 3 or 4 divided doses
	Extended release: 8 mg q8-12h or 12 mg q12h	6 yrs and older, 8 or 12 mg q12h
	Parenteral IM, IV, or SC: 10 mg q8-12h	12 yr and under, 0.125 mg/kg 3 or 4 times daily
cetirizine (Reactine)	5-10 mg daily	2-6 yr, 5 mg daily 6-11 yr, 10 mg daily
chlorpheniramine (Chlortrimeton)	4 mg q4-6h	6-12 yr, 2 mg 3 or 4 times a day
	Parenteral IM, IV, SC: 5-40 mg as single dose	SC: 87.5 μg/kg q6h
clemastine (Tavist)	1.34 mg twice daily or 2.68 mg 1 to 3 times a day	6-12 yr, 670 μg to 1.34 mg twice a day
cyproheptadine (Periactin)	4 mg q8h, increase as necessary (range 4 to 20 mg/day)	0.125 mg/kg q8-12h
dexchlorpheniramine (Polaramine)	2 mg q4-6h	150 μg/kg in 4 divided doses
	Extended release: 4 or 6 mg q8-12h	Not recommended
dimenhydrinate (Dramamine)	50-100 mg q4h	5 mg/kg in 4 divided doses
	Parenteral, IM, IV: 50 mg IM or 50 mg in 10 ml normal saline for IV q4h (administer IV slowly)	1.25 mg/kg IM or IV, q6h (maximum 300 mg/day)
diphenhydramine (Benadryl)	25-50 mg q4-6h	6-12 yr, 12.5-25 mg q4-6h
doxylamine (Unisom)	12.5-25 mg q4-6h	6-12 yr, 6.25-12.5 mg q4-6h
fexofenadine (Allegra)	60 mg PO twice daily	Not available
loratadine (Claritin)	10 yr old and adults: 10 mg daily, before eating	2-9 yr: 5 mg daily before eating
phenindamine (Nolahist)	25 mg q4-6h	6-12 yr, 12.5 mg q4-6h
tripelennamine (Pyribenzamine)	25-50 mg q4-6h	1.25 mg/kg q6h as needed (maximum 300 mg/day)
	Extended-release: 100 mg q8-12h	Not recommended
triprolidine (Myidil)	2.5 mg q4-6h	4 to 24 mo, 312 μg q6-8h; 2-4 yr, 625 μg q6-8h; 4 to 6 yr, 937 μg q6-8h; 6 to 12 yr, 1.25 mg q6-8h

atric patient is usually more sensitive to the effects of these drugs and may require a reduction in dosage. The adult and pediatric dosages are noted in Table 33-2.

Fexofenadine (Allegra), an antihistamine approved in 1996, is a metabolite of terfenadine (Seldane) that was chemically altered to eliminate the serious and potentially fatal cardiovascular drug interactions associated with terfenadine (Seldane). It is indicated for the treatment of seasonal allergic rhinitis (Rxtra Facts, 1996).

Many prescription antihistamine-decongestant formulations are also available, for example acrivastine-pseudoephedrine (Semprex-D), brompheniramine and pseudoephedrine (Bromfed), and others. The trend, however, is for more antihistamines and antihistamine combinations to be allowed OTC marketing status in the future. For a discussion on antihistamine combinations, see Chapter 3.

Inhibitor of Histamine Release

Cromolyn sodium provides a local protective effect in the mucosal airways by inhibiting the granulation of pulmonary mast cells and thereby preventing the release of histamine and SRS-A. See the section on cromolyn sodium in Chapter 32.

SEROTONIN

As with histamine, serotonin (5-hydroxytryptamine or 5-HT) has no therapeutic application; however, its importance is related to the action of other drugs and several disease states. Serotonin is widely distributed in nature, occurring in both plants (pineapples, bananas, strawberries, tomatoes, and nuts) and animals. In human beings, serotonin occurs in various body tissues, but primarily in three tissue types. (1) The largest fraction (90%) is synthesized and stored in the enterochromaffin cells of the gastrointestinal tract mucosa, particularly in the pylorus of the stomach and in the upper region of the small intestine. (2) A much smaller fraction is stored but not synthesized in platelets; on disintegration this fraction is released in serum and in the spleen. (3) In the CNS the greatest concentration occurs in the hypothalamus, midbrain, reticular formation, raphe (midline) regions of medulla and pons, and pineal gland. A neuron that releases serotonin is termed a serotoninergic or tryptaminergic fiber. Only a very low concentration of serotonin appears in cells.

Pharmacologic Actions

Serotonin appears to possess multiple pharmacologic actions, but because of discrepant experimental findings, this variability has caused much controversy. Despite the need for additional experimental analysis, it is now known that the primary function of serotonin is exerted on various smooth muscles and nerves. As previously stated, serotonin is not a therapeutic agent, but its more prominent effects are associated with its influence on other drugs and some disease states.

Gastrointestinal Tract

Serotonin is secreted from specialized cells of the stomach and intestine that are responsible for contraction of the gastrointestinal smooth muscle, thereby producing the peristaltic response.

Carcinoid syndrome is a condition elicited from carcinoid tumors that causes an overproduction of serotonin; bradykinin and histamine may also be released. Serotonin is responsible for causing this syndrome, which is characterized by paroxysmal flushing, hyperperistalsis, diarrhea, bronchoconstriction, and cardiac valvular lesions. The diagnosis of carcinoid syndrome is confirmed by the presence of excess 5-HT, which eventually is excreted in the urine.

Blood Platelets

Serotonin is released from platelets during their breakdown within the circulation. This compound then activates receptors on the surface of other blood platelets, thereby promoting platelet aggregation. It has been suggested that through this mechanism the discharge of serotonin from platelets may contribute to the formation of pulmonary embolism.

Central Nervous System

Serotonin is manufactured and stored in the neurons in the brain. The central action of the neuronal system appears to elicit primarily an inhibitory response from the specific nuclei of the brain. Researchers now postulate that altered function of serotoninergic pathways is a factor in various CNS dysfunctions.

Sleep

Serotonin-synthesizing cells are required for the induction of non-rapid eye movement (NREM) sleep (quiet brain and potentially excitable muscles) and the onset of rapid eye movement (REM) sleep (active brain, rapid eye movements, dreams, and atonic muscles). Normal sleep depends on serotonin along with the combined functions of norepinephrine and cholinergic systems. The basic sleep pattern consists of four to six cycles that alternate between NREM and REM sleep. Destruction of the raphe nuclei results in insomnia. Other disorders of sleep are quite common; for example, narcolepsy is characterized by a sudden change from wakefulness directly to REM sleep.

Sleep hypnotics such as barbiturates tend to decrease REM sleep, which is an essential component of restful sleep. Also, the drug *p*-chlorophenylalanine inhibits formation of serotonin, and this depletion can cause prolonged wakefulness when administered to animals.

Pain Perception

The serotoninergic neurons located in the raphe nuclei of the brainstem have axons that project to the spinal cord and forebrain. One important system related to the brain involves a substance called beta-endorphin, which is associated with neurons that interconnect various nuclei in the hypothalamus, limbic system, and thalamus. The beta-endorphin neurons mediate euphoric and emotional behavior. The thalamic nuclei mediates poorly localized deep pain, which is best influenced by opiates. The density of opiate receptors in the brain appears to be much greater in the medial and lateral thalamus. The extent of opiate addiction and withdrawal are influenced by the quantity of opiate receptors involved.

Serotonin also is implicated in the action of morphine. Studies suggest that as tolerance develops toward this narcotic, the synthesis but not the accumulation of serotonin doubles. In addition, a decrease in brain serotonin level increases a person's sensitivity to painful stimuli, thus decreasing the analgesic effect of morphine.

Mental Illness

CNS depression correlates with low levels of total brain serotonin. The enzyme MAO metabolizes serotonin, resulting in a lower level of the transmitter (Fig. 33-2). Accordingly, a MAO inhibitor blocks the degradation of serotonin and thereby increases the concentration level of the neurotransmitter in the brain. (The antidepressant effects of MAO inhibitor drugs are discussed in Chapter 13.) The tricyclic compounds also act as antidepressants, blocking the reuptake of serotonin and norepinephrine at the membrane of the neuron and thereby potentiating the action of the synapse.

ANTISEROTONINS

Antiserotonins, or serotonin antagonists, are considered complex compounds because they possess varying degrees of specificity, and thus the exact mechanism of action is unknown. In addition to performing serotonin-blocking activity, many other pharmacologic actions are involved in inhibiting responses to serotonin.

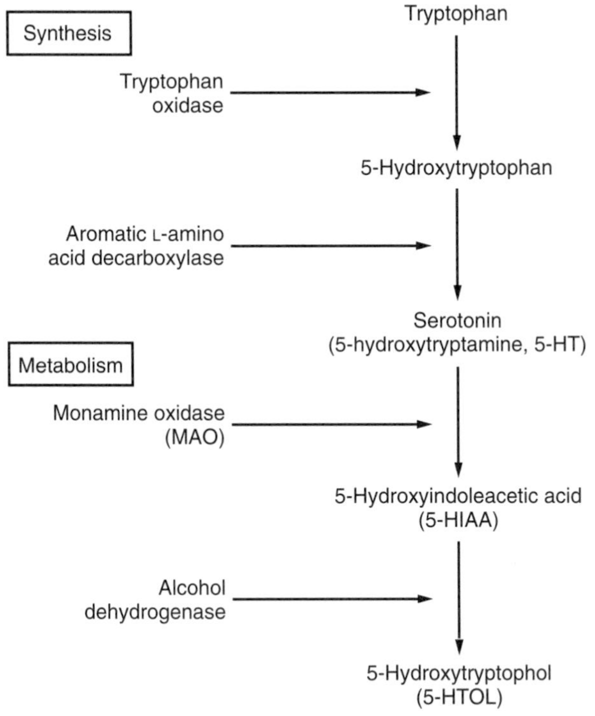

FIGURE 33-2
Synthesis and metabolism of serotonin.

cyproheptadine [si proe hep′ ta deen] (Periactin)

Cyproheptadine blocks serotonin activity in the smooth muscle of blood vessels and the intestine and also has antihistaminic and possibly anticholinergic properties. It may produce weight gain by blocking serotonin activity in the appetite center in the hypothalamus; in other words, cyproheptadine then stimulates appetite. Although not approved by the FDA, it has also been used to treat vascular headaches. It is administered primarily for allergic disorders. (See discussion of antihistamines.)

lysergic acid diethylamide (LSD)

The basic mechanism underlying LSD's hallucinogenic properties is not known. Experts agree, however, that its profound effects on behavior are mediated through the central neurotransmitter, serotonin. Studies in the 1970s suggested that the more powerful hallucinogenic drugs exert a dual function in the brain: they inhibit the action of serotonin and stimulate the norepinephrine system. See Chapter 6 for a discussion of LSD as a drug of abuse.

methysergide maleate [meth i ser′ jide] (Sansert)

Although its mechanism of action in preventing vascular headaches is unknown, methysergide is both a potent antiserotonin and a vasoconstrictor agent. These properties apparently help to relieve migraine and other vascular headaches (see Chapter 16).

SUMMARY

This chapter reviews a variety of pharmacologic agents used for the respiratory system. For example, oxygen is a therapeutic gas that is essential to sustain life, and it is used in many clinical situations. Carbon dioxide is another gas that is used as a pharmacologic agent affecting respiration, circulation, and the central nervous system.

Cough suppressants are used for nonproductive coughs as persistent coughing can be annoying, exhausting, and painful. (The opioid antitussive drugs are discussed in Chapter 8.) The healthcare professional should be aware, though, that the nonnarcotic antitussive drugs may be effective in many situations and generally have fewer gastrointestinal and other side effects.

Histamine is a natural chemical found in most body tissues and it has been implicated in a number of pathologic conditions such as urticaria, atopy, food allergies, bronchial asthma, and systemic anaphylaxis. Therefore antihistamines that compete at receptor sites with histamines to prevent their physiologic actions are extremely valuable medications. Serotonin is another naturally occurring substance that in itself, has no therapeutic application. However, it has been connected to the action of other drugs, such as the opioids, and CNS depression has been correlated with low levels of total brain serotonin. Methysergide maleate is an antiserotonin product used to relieve vascular headaches.

REVIEW QUESTIONS

1. What are the signs and/or symptoms of oxygen toxicity?
2. Discuss the action, indications, pharmacokinetics, side effects and adverse reactions, and advantages of a nonopioid antitussive medication.
3. Name four indications for the antihistamine, diphenhydramine.
4. Describe the relationship between histamine release and type I anaphylactic reaction.

REFERENCES

Rxtra Facts: Supplement to *Facts and Comparisons* 1(3):1, 1996.
Weaver LK: Hyperbaric treatment of respiratory emergencies, *Respir Care* 37(7):720-730, 1992.

ADDITIONAL REFERENCES

AARC Clinical Practice Guideline: Oxygen therapy in the home or extended care facility, *Respir Care* 37(3):918-920, 1992.
Abramowicz M: Acrivastine/pseudoephedrine (Semprex-D) for seasonal allergic rhinitis, *Med Lett* 36(930):78, 1994.
American Hospital Formulary Service: *AHFS drug information '98*, Bethesda, Md, 1998, American Society of Hospital Pharmacists.
Anderson KN et al, editors: *Mosby's medical, nursing, and allied health dictionary*, ed 5, St Louis, 1998, Mosby.
Branson RD: The nuts and bolts of increasing arterial oxygenation: devices and techniques, *Respir Care* 38(6):672-683, 1993.
Crocco JA, Francis PB: Acute oxygen therapy—when and how? *Patient Care* 25(14):69-74, 1991.

Feldman EG, Davidson DE: *Handbook of nonprescription drugs,* ed 9, Washington, DC, 1990, American Pharmaceutical Association and The National Professional Society of Pharmacists.

Mosby: *Mosby's GenRx,* St Louis, 1998, Mosby.

Olin BR: *Facts and comparisons.* Philadelphia, 1998, JB Lippincott.

Somerson SJ, Sicilia MR: Emergency oxygen administration and airway management, *Crit Care Nurse* 12(4):23-29, 1992.

United States Pharmacopeial Convention: *USP DI: drug information for the health care professional,* ed 18, Rockville, Md, 1998, The Convention.

Wilson SF, Thompson JM: *Respiratory disorders,* St Louis, 1990, Mosby.

UNIT IX

Drugs Affecting the Gastrointestinal System

CHAPTER 34

Overview of the Gastrointestinal Tract

CHAPTER FOCUS

The gastrointestinal (GI) system includes the neural, secretory, muscular, and glandular tissues from the mouth to anus. This chapter provides an overview of the anatomy and physiology of the GI tract, along with the disorders that affect each segment along the tract.

OBJECTIVES

After reading and studying this chapter, the student should be able to do the following:

1. *Define and describe the key terms.*
2. *Present and discuss the major parts of the GI tract.*
3. *Describe the functions of the various segments in the GI tract.*
4. *Present the usual functions and effects of the parasympathetic and sympathetic nervous systems on the GI tract.*

KEY TERMS

acute gastritis, (p. 485)
cholecystitis, (p. 486)
cholelithiasis, (p. 486)
chronic gastritis, (p. 485)
digestion, (p. 484)
peptic ulcer disease, (p. 485)
peristaltic process, (p. 485)

Disorders of the gastrointestinal (GI) tract such as indigestion, gastritis, constipation, and peptic ulcers are very common problems reported by large numbers of the population. Because the cause of many GI diseases remains unclear, pharmacologic management is often focused on relieving symptoms rather than on control or cure. In this chapter the anatomy and functions of the GI tract are reviewed.

The GI system itself is made up of the alimentary canal or digestive tract, the biliary system, and the pancreas (Fig. 34-1). The alimentary canal extends from the mouth to the anus. Food substances entering the canal undergo mechanical and chemical changes called **digestion.** These changes permit nutrients to be absorbed and undigestible materials to be excreted by the body. Absorbed nutrients may be used as an energy source or stored (glycogen for glucose or fat for carbohydrate). Movements by the smooth muscle fibers surrounding the canal (1) mix the contents by segmental contractions and (2) move the mass through the tract by peristalsis.

The secretory and muscular activities of the GI system are regulated by neural mechanisms. An interconnecting network of neurons is located in smooth muscle and secretory cells. This system is self-regulating; it is capable of controlling exocrine gland secretions and muscular contractions without any external influence.

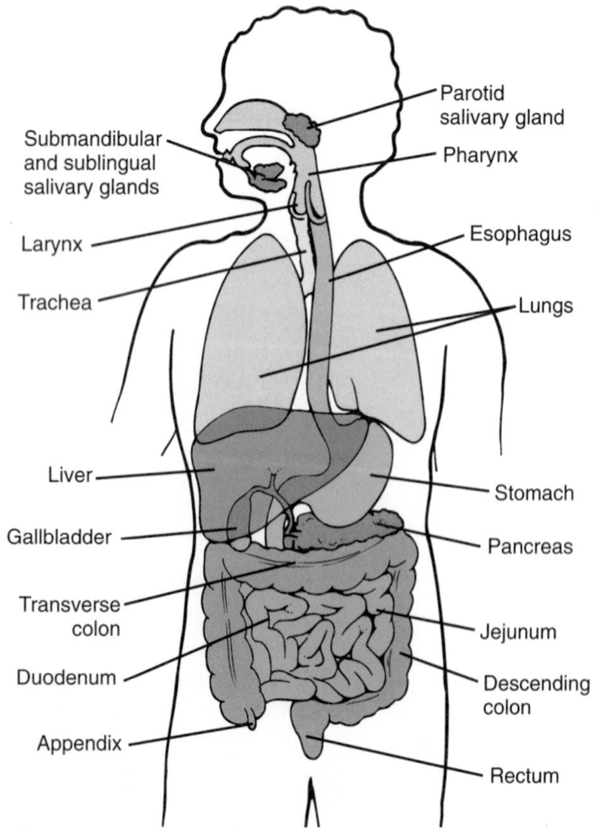

FIGURE 34-1
Gastrointestinal and respiratory systems.

By contrast, the external innervation of the GI system is supplied by the divisions of the autonomic nervous system. Their major function is to correlate activities between different regions of the GI system and also between this system and other parts of the body. The parasympathetic division, mediated by two branches of the vagus nerve, exerts an excitatory action, which increases digestive secretions and muscular activity. By contrast, the splanchnic nerves of the sympathetic division are primarily inhibitory, depressing digestive secretions and muscular activity. Under normal conditions, the two divisions of the autonomic nervous system maintain a delicate balance of control of functions.

Drugs affecting the GI tract exert their action mainly on muscular and glandular tissues. The action may be directly on the smooth muscle and gland cells or indirectly on the autonomic nervous system. Drugs also may cause increased or decreased function, tone, emptying time, or peristaltic action of the stomach or bowel. In addition, they may be used to relieve enzyme deficiency, to counteract excess acidity or gas formation, to produce or prevent vomiting, or to aid in diagnosis.

MOUTH (ORAL CAVITY)

The mouth, or oral cavity, functions as the starting point of the digestive process. Food is taken in, chewed, and mixed with saliva that contains the enzyme amylase (ptyalin), which begins the process of chemical digestion.

Three pairs of salivary glands secrete saliva into ducts emptying into the mouth. The sublingual and submandibular salivary glands are located beneath the tongue; the largest pair, the parotid glands, are found in front of and slightly below the ears. When the food bolus has been chewed and reduced in the mouth, it is swallowed. Swallowing (deglutition) is a complex process that begins as a voluntary movement but is continued as an involuntary muscular reflex as the food is propelled through the GI tract.

Disorders Affecting the Mouth

Systemic diseases, nutritional deficiencies, and mechanical trauma can cause irritation or inflammation of buccal structures. Dental disorders (e.g., caries, gingivitis, and pyorrhea) and bacterial, viral, or fungal infections (e.g., candidiasis or herpes simplex) can affect the structures of the oral cavity, causing symptoms such as mouth blistering or other lesions, swelling, pain, and inflammation.

Agents acting on the oral cavity are discussed in Chapter 35.

PHARYNX

The pharynx (throat), a tubelike passageway connecting the mouth and the esophagus, is important in swallowing. Food and fluid pass through the pharynx into the esophagus. During this passage the trachea is closed to prevent aspiration into the lungs.

Disorders Affecting the Pharynx

Like the mouth, the pharynx can be affected by various systemic diseases. It can become irritated and inflamed (e.g., from sinusitis or the "common cold") and treated symptomatically with an antiinflammatory agent. It can also become a locus of infection (e.g., with strep throat), requiring systemic antibiotic therapy.

ESOPHAGUS

The esophagus is a pliable muscular structure approximately 25 cm long that extends from the pharynx to the cardiac end of the stomach. It extends through the diaphragm as it drops from the thoracic cavity into the abdominal cavity.

The esophagus is considered the beginning of the digestive system proper, since the rest of the GI tract organs function only in digestion and/or excretion. The esophagus continues the process of swallowing and begins the **peristaltic process,** or the squeezing of the food bolus down the GI tract by band contraction. The peristaltic band wave stimulates the lower esophageal sphincter, which closes to prevent gastroesophageal reflux and then returns the esophagus to its normal resting state.

Disorders Affecting the Esophagus

Esophageal disorders are characterized by retrosternal pain (heartburn) and difficulty in swallowing (dysphagia). The sources of the pain are numerous; some potential causes include diffuse esophageal spasm, achalasia, pyloric or duodenal ulcers, scleroderma, postural changes (bending forward), excessive alcohol ingestion, and nonspecific dysmotility.

However, heartburn commonly results from reflux esophagitis, in which the incompetent lower esophageal sphincter permits gastric contents to flow back into the esophagus, or from hiatal hernia, in which a part of the stomach protrudes into the diaphragm. One type of hiatal hernia, paraesophageal hernia, may be associated with esophageal obstruction and strangulation. Difficulty in swallowing can be a symptom of esophageal obstruction, mechanical interference with or paralysis of the muscles of deglutition, neuromuscular incoordination, achalasia, carcinoma of the esophagus, anxiety states, hysteria, or schizophrenic hallucinations.

Inflammation of the esophagus can have many causes: reflux esophagitis associated with hiatal hernia, irritant ingestion, infection, peptic ulceration, prolonged gastric intubation, and uremia.

STOMACH

The stomach, a pouchlike structure lying below the diaphragm, has three divisions: the fundus, the body, and the pylorus. Two sphincter muscles, the cardiac sphincter and the pyloric sphincter, regulate the stomach opening. Gastric glands secrete mucus and gastric juice composed of enzymes and hydrochloric acid. They also produce intrinsic factor, a protein essential for absorption of vitamin B_{12}. Vitamin B_{12} in turn is needed for erythropoiesis (red blood cell formation).

The stomach functions as a temporary storage site for food as it is being digested. It also manufactures gastrin, a hormone that regulates enzyme production to facilitate digestion. The stomachs of men and women differ, both in food storage capacity and size. Females have smaller and more slender stomachs. The stomach is capable of holding 1500 to 2000 ml. It distends after eating and gradually collapses as the food bolus moves out into the small intestine. Its churning action further breaks down the food bolus and mixes it with gastric juice to continue chemical digestion. A limited amount of nutrient and drug absorption takes place in the stomach.

The time required for digestion in the stomach depends on the amount of food eaten. Normal emptying time is 2 to 6 hours. However, the gastric emptying time may be affected by drug administration, physical activity of the individual, and body position during digestion. Gastric emptying time is a factor to consider in the timing of drug administration, since the presence of food may block the absorption of some drugs.

Disorders Affecting the Stomach

Acute gastritis is an inflammatory response of the stomach lining to ingestion of irritants, such as ethanol or nonsteroidal antiinflammatory agents, including aspirin. Symptoms include epigastric discomfort, nausea, abdominal tenderness, and gastrointestinal hemorrhage. Treatment consists of lifestyle modifications and drugs such as antacids, antiemetic agents, anticholinergics, and antihistamines (see Chapter 35).

Chronic gastritis is a long-term inflammation of the stomach lining, generally with degeneration of the gastric mucosa, but its causes are not well established. It is more common in women, and the incidence increases with age, excessive smoking, and ethanol use. Symptoms are nonspecific but may include flatulence, epigastric fullness after meals, diarrhea, and bleeding. Treatment is the same as for acute gastritis. Iron deficiency anemia and pernicious anemia may result from chronic gastritis. Treatment of symptoms with antacids, anticholinergics, and sedatives, as well as vitamin B_{12} if pernicious anemia is present, and elimination of possible causative or aggravating factors (e.g., aspirin use) comprise the usual therapeutic regimen.

Peptic ulcer disease is a broad term encompassing both gastric and duodenal ulcers. Although both types of ulcers produce a "break" in the gastric mucosa, the causes differ. With gastric ulcers, the ability of the gastric mucosa to protect and repair itself seems to be defective; in duodenal ulcers hypersecretion of gastric acid is responsible for the erosion of the gastric mucosa. Gastric colonization with *Helicobacter pylori,* a gram-negative bacilli, has been identified as a causative agent in patients with peptic ulcer disease that was not caused by the nonsteroidal antiinflammatory drugs. Treatment with various antibacterial combinations has resulted in healing and a low peptic ulcer recurrence rate (Piper, de Carle et al, 1997). *H pylori* has been identified in approximately 90% of all persons with duodenal ulcer and also in nearly 70% of persons with gastric ulcers (Smith, 1995).

Duodenal ulcers are more common than gastric ulcers, accounting for nearly 80% of all peptic ulcers. Duodenal ulcers usually occur more frequently in younger persons. Overall, the reported incidence of peptic ulcers is much lower in females. In addition to antibacterial combination therapies, pharmacologic treatment of peptic ulcer disease may also include the use of antacids, H_2 receptor antagonists, and sucralfate. However, nondrug treatment (diet and lifestyle modifications) is equally important (see Chapter 35). Hereditary factors, use of some drugs (e.g., aspirin and corticosteroids), psychic factors, stress, and diet have been implicated in the development of peptic ulcer disease.

LIVER

Immediately under the diaphragm and above the stomach is the largest gland in the body, the liver. It weighs approximately 1.5 kg and is an extremely active and important organ that performs over 100 different functions.

The liver consists of two lobes composed of multitudes of lobules that function to remove toxins from the bloodstream, store nutrients such as iron and some vitamins, and secrete bile. Bile is transported via the hepatic ducts to the gallbladder for storage. In the intestine, bile aids in digestion, emulsification, and absorption of fat. Because it is normally alkaline, bile also functions to neutralize gastric acid in the duodenum.

Venous blood goes directly to the liver from the intestinal tract, so nutrients and absorbed drugs pass through the liver before reaching the systemic circulation. Thus the liver plays an active role in absorbing and metabolizing fats, carbohydrates, and proteins. It also stores vitamins A, B_{12}, and D and iron. Some drugs are taken up by the liver, released into the bile, and then excreted in the feces. Other drugs move from the bile into the small intestine, where they are reabsorbed and recirculated. Still other drugs are transformed by the liver and excreted in the urine. In all of these cases the liver metabolizes the drug to make it more water soluble. This biotransformation changes the parent compound to a metabolite that may have greater, lesser, or equal activity. Cytochrome P-450 in the liver is responsible for biotransformation. There are also drugs that pass through the body and are secreted unchanged in the urine.

Disorders Affecting the Liver

Viral hepatitis, Läennec's and postnecrotic cirrhosis, carcinoma, or chronic alcoholism causes damage to the liver and liver cell dysfunction.

GALLBLADDER

Lying on the undersurface of the liver is the gallbladder, a pear-shaped organ 7 to 10 cm long and 2.5 to 3.5 cm wide. The gallbladder can hold 30 to 50 ml of bile. It concentrates the bile and stores it until it is needed for digestion in the stomach and small intestine.

Disorders Affecting the Gallbladder

Cholecystitis, inflammation of the gallbladder, is often associated with the presence of gallstones (**cholelithiasis**). The stones lodge in the gallbladder neck or ducts, causing congestion and edema as bile builds up. This may be an acute or a chronic condition. Treatment of cholecystitis and cholelithiasis includes administration of analgesics, antispasmodics, and chenodeoxycholic acid. Malignant tumors of the gallbladder are infrequent.

PANCREAS

The pancreas is a gland about 15 to 20 cm long and 5 cm wide that weighs approximately 75 g. The gland has three major segments: the head (found in the curve of the duodenum), the body, and the tail (which touches or nearly touches the spleen). The role of the pancreas is twofold: the exocrine cells secrete the digestive enzymes found in pancreatic juice, and the endocrine cells help control carbohydrate metabolism with their production of glucagon and insulin.

Disorders Affecting the Pancreas

With the exception of diabetes mellitus, many pancreatic diseases have symptoms that are not readily diagnosed. Inflammation of the pancreas may be acute or chronic. Among the many causes are blockage of the pancreatic ducts, trauma to the pancreas, alcohol consumption, drug use, and tumors, cysts, or abscesses. Symptoms are nonspecific but ultimately include severe pain. Carcinoma of the pancreas is as difficult to diagnose as other pancreatic disorders.

SMALL INTESTINE

The small intestine is a coiled tube approximately 21 feet long. It consists of the duodenum, jejunum, and ileum. Within the small intestine the food bolus is thoroughly mixed with the digestive juices to complete the "breakdown" process. The intestinal mucosa then absorbs nutrients and drugs, which are filtered through the liver before entering the circulatory and lymphatic systems.

Disorders Affecting the Small Intestine

Two disorders affecting the entire lower gastrointestinal tract are diarrhea and constipation. These are discussed in Chapters 3 and 35 along with the drugs used in their treatment.

Other disorders affecting the small intestine include obstruction, malabsorption syndrome, and blind loop syndrome. Symptomatic treatment is customary while the underlying causative factors are investigated.

LARGE INTESTINE

The cecum, colon, and rectum make up the large intestine. The distal 2.5 cm of the rectum is known as the anal canal. The large intestine is approximately 5 feet long. It completes the digestive and absorptive processes. The large intestine is involved mainly with water absorption (from 1800 to 3000 ml/day) and synthesis of vitamin K. The lining of the large intestine secretes mucus to coat the undigested residue and protect the bowel lining. The undigestible residue is expelled through the reflex action known as defecation.

Disorders Affecting the Large Intestine

Diarrhea and constipation, discussed in Chapters 3 and 35, also affect the large intestine. Other disorders include diverticular disease, which has no specific therapy; ulcerative colitis, treated with lifestyle modifications, antidiarrheal agents, and steroids; carcinoma; and irritable bowel syndrome. Hemorrhoids (varicosities of the external or internal hemorrhoidal veins) are common.

SUMMARY

While food and water help to sustain life and to determine the individual's nutritional status, they also contribute to a person's state of health and development of resistance to and ability to handle disease. The primary function of the gastrointestinal tract, though, is to provide the body cells with nutrients, electrolytes, and water through the processes of ingestion, digestion, and food absorption, in addition to the excretion of waste products and residue. Many drugs may affect various areas of the gastrointestinal tract by acting primarily on muscular and glandular tissue. Such agents are reviewed in the next chapter.

REVIEW QUESTIONS

1. Name the functions of the oral cavity, pharynx, esophagus, stomach, liver, gallbladder, pancreas, and small and large intestines.
2. Name at least one disorder that is associated with each structure mentioned in the previous question.

REFERENCES

Piper DW, de Carle, DJ et al: Gastrointestinal and hepatic diseases. In Speight TM, Holford NHG, editors: *Avery's drug treatment,* ed 4, Auckland, New Zealand, 1997, Adis International.

Smith C: Upper gastrointestinal disorders. In Young LY, Koda-Kimble MA, editors: *Applied therapeutics: the clinical use of drugs,* ed 6, Vancouver, Wash, 1995, Applied Therapeutics, Inc.

ADDITIONAL REFERENCES

Anderson KN et al, editors: *Mosby's medical, nursing, and allied health dictionary,* ed 5, St Louis, 1998, Mosby.

Feldman M et al: Treating ulcers and reflux: What's new? *Patient Care* 26(13):53, 1992.

McCance KL, Huether SE: *Pathophysiology: the biologic basis for disease in adults and children,* ed 3, St Louis, 1998, Mosby.

Melmon KL et al: *Clinical pharmacology: basic principles in therapeutics,* ed 3, New York, 1992, McGraw-Hill.

Richter JE: Gastroesophageal reflux: diagnosis and management, *Hosp Pract* 27(1):39, 1992.

Thibodeau GA, Patton KT: *Anatomy and physiology,* ed 4, St Louis, 1999, Mosby.

Van Wynsberghe D, Noback CR, Carola R: *Human anatomy and physiology,* ed 3, New York, 1995, McGraw-Hill.

Wingard LB et al: *Human pharmacology,* St Louis, 1991, Mosby.

CHAPTER 35

Drugs Affecting the Gastrointestinal Tract

KEY DRUGS

cimetidine, (p. 501)
metoclopramide, (p. 494)
misoprostol, (p. 500)
omeprazole, (p. 500)
ondansetron, (p. 496)

CHAPTER FOCUS

This chapter reviews the various topical and systemic medications that are used to treat gastrointestinal (GI) illnesses or disorders affecting the upper and lower GI tract. These include agents that affect the mouth, stomach, vomiting reflex, gastrointestinal tract, and gallbladder. As many GI disorders, such as peptic ulcers, nausea, vomiting, constipation, and diarrhea, negatively affect the patient's quality of life, the healthcare professional needs to be informed on the proper treatment and management of GI tract disorders.

KEY TERMS

adsorbents, (p. 507)
antiemetics, (p. 493)
cathartics, (p. 504)
chemoreceptor trigger zone (CTZ), (p. 493)
constipation, (p. 503)
emetic center, (p. 493)
laxatives, (p. 504)

OBJECTIVES

After reading and studying this chapter, the student should be able to do the following:

1. *Define and describe the key terms and key drugs*
2. *Differentiate between various mouthwashes and gargles (i.e., alcoholic, antiseptic, oxygen-releasing, and fluoridated).*
3. *Discuss the mechanisms of action of the oral antifungal agents.*
4. *Review the use and side effects of antacids.*
5. *Name two digestant drugs used to promote the process of digestion.*
6. *Describe the vomiting reflex, chemoreceptor trigger zone, and other sites, along with the major pharmacologic antiemetic agents effective at these sites.*
7. *Name the emetic agents and describe their mechanisms of action and usage.*
8. *Discuss the effect of H_2 receptor antagonists metoclopramide, ondansetron, sucralfate, misoprostol, omeprazole, and ursodiol on the GI tract.*

DRUGS THAT AFFECT THE MOUTH

Medications generally have little effect on the mouth. Good oral hygiene, which includes brushing properly after meals and at bedtime, flossing, and gum stimulation, has more influence on the tissues of the mouth than most medicines. Many mouth and throat preparations that contain steroids, anesthetics, and antiseptics are available for various disorders of the oral cavity, including chapped lips, sun and fever blisters, inflammatory lesions, ulcerative lesions secondary to trauma, gingival lesions, teething pain, toothache, irritation caused by orthodontic appliances or dentures, and oral cavity abrasions. Most agents that affect the mouth may be purchased over the counter (OTC).

MOUTHWASHES AND GARGLES

Mouthwashes and gargles are dilute aromatic solutions that contain a sweetener and an artificial coloring agent. They may also contain an antiseptic (e.g., alcohol, cetylpyridinium chloride, or phenol), anesthetic (eugenol or clove oil), astringent (zinc chloride), and anticaries agent (sodium fluoride). Mouthwashes with a high alcohol content may be problematic in special populations (Box 35-1).

Although several products claim to contain ingredients that reduce plaque formation, clinical trials have demonstrated some success with volatile oils and cetylpyridinium chloride alone or in combination with domiphene bromide. Commercial products that contain at least one of these active ingredients include Cepacol (cetylpyridinium chloride), Listerine (volatile oils), and Scope (cetylpyridinium chloride and domiphene bromide). A detergent-type product to lessen plaque (Plax) is also available on the market. The patient should be informed that these products do not replace good oral hygiene but instead are recommended as an adjunct to proper brushing and flossing of the teeth (Flynn, 1996).

Mouthwashes are often used for halitosis, or "bad breath," or as gargles to treat colds or sore throats. They are generally not considered effective for such problems. Mouthwashes may improve mouth odor briefly, but if such a problem persists, the underlying cause needs to be identified and treated, such as poor dental hygiene, various gum diseases, and many other potential causes.

Sore throats are usually caused by infection, most often viral rather than bacterial. Gargling cannot reach the site of infection, which is usually deep in the throat tissues. Sodium chloride solution (½ teaspoon of salt to an 8 oz glass of warm water) has been recommended for use as a gargle and mouthwash and is probably as effective as some of the remedies sold today.

Oxygen-Releasing Agents

Hydrogen peroxide is a weak antibacterial agent used to clean wounds topically and orally. The antibacterial effect depends on the liberation of oxygen, which occurs when the peroxide comes in contact with the tissue enzyme catalase. The resulting effervescence (bubbling action) loosens pus and tissue debris, which helps reduce bacterial content. Hydrogen peroxide is usually used in a 1.5% to 3% solution for cleaning wounds or as a mouthwash. As a gargle, the 3% solution should be diluted with an equal amount of water before use.

A number of other oxygen-releasing products are commercially available. Perimax Perio Rinse (hydrogen peroxide) is used for treatment of canker sores, denture irritation, and irritation following orthodontic intervention. The solution is expectorated. Hydrogen peroxide gel (Peroxyl) is also available for minor mouth irritation and is applied and expectorated after use.

Fluoridated Mouthwash

A number of fluoride-containing preparations, including mouthwash (Fluorigard), toothpaste, tablets, and solutions, are available for use as anticaries agents. The exact mechanism of action of fluoride in preventing caries is not fully understood; however, fluoride ions appear to exchange for hydroxyl or citrate (anion) ions and then settle in the anionic space in the surface of the enamel (Marcus, 1996). This results in a harder outer layer of tooth enamel (a fluoridated hydroxyapatite) that is more resistant to demineralization. Fluoridated mouthwashes have been used in communities with both limited fluoridated and unfluoridated water supplies, and their use has been associated with a significant decrease (between 17% and 47%) in tooth decay (Flynn, 1996).

Mouthwashes are generally used once a day (rinsed for a minute and expectorated), preferably after brushing and flossing. The patient should be taught to avoid taking anything by mouth for approximately 30 minutes after usage (Box 35-2).

BOX 35-1 **Alcoholic Mouthwash Warnings**

Pediatric Alert
The leading mouthwashes usually contain from 14% to 27% alcohol. Because safety closures are not generally used with mouthwashes, parents of young children should be cautioned to store these products in a safe area, preferably a locked cabinet. The use of mouthwash in young children is not recommended since children often swallow the mouthwash rather than expectorate it.

Alcohol Abuse
Alcohol-containing products such as mouthwashes and cough-cold preparations may be substituted by alcoholics when beverage alcohol is not readily available. The healthcare professional should be alert for ingestion abuse of alcohol-containing products in persons with a history of alcohol abuse (Katzung, 1992).

BOX 35-2 Fluoride Toxicity

Fluoride is capable of producing an acute toxic reaction that may be fatal if not treated promptly. A chronic toxic state resulting in mottling or discoloration of the tooth enamel and possible osteosclerosis has been reported. This effect may occur when excessive fluoride is consumed during childhood. In severe cases, brown- to black-stained corroded areas appear on the teeth. Fluoridated water supplies usually contain 0.7 to 1 ppm (part per million) of fluoride, which is accepted as a safe level that is effective in reducing the incidence of caries in permanent teeth. Healthcare professionals, particularly in primary healthcare settings, need to be aware of the amount of fluoride in their water supplies and to recommend and/or closely supervise the use of additional fluoride products by their patients. Fluoride supplements are recommended when community drinking water contains less than 0.7 ppm of fluoride (Covington, 1996).

Antiseptic Mouthwash

Phenol penetrates plaque and is a local anesthetic and antimicrobial agent. Chloraseptic mouthwash contains phenol and sodium phenolate. Teething preparations that provide temporary relief of sore gums caused by teething often contain phenol or benzocaine. Phenol or phenol-type compounds are also present in several OTC lozenges, liquids, and sprays for the treatment of sore throat. The liquid is diluted with equal parts of water or may be sprayed full strength.

DENTIFRICES

A dentifrice is a substance used to aid in cleaning teeth. Ordinary dentifrice contains one or more mild abrasives, a foaming agent, and flavoring materials made into a powder or paste (toothpaste) to be used as an aid in the mechanical cleansing of accessible parts of the teeth. Fluoride dentifrices are effective anticaries agents. These products carry the American Dental Association Council on Dental Therapeutics seal to indicate its endorsement.

Dentifrices are also available for the treatment of hypersensitive teeth, which usually occur from exposed root areas at the cement-enamel junction. This exposed area allows pain stimuli access to the nerve fibers in the pulp area. Dentists often suggest desensitizing dentifrices that contain potassium nitrate, such as Promise, Mint Sensodyne, or Denquel.

ORAL ANTIFUNGAL AGENTS

clotrimazole [kloe trim′ a zole] (Mycelex)
ketoconazole [kee toe koe′ na zole] (Nizoral)
nystatin [nye stat′ in] (Mycostatin, Nilstat)

Clotrimazole, ketoconazole, and nystatin inhibit synthesis of sterols in the fungal wall, increasing permeability of the cell membrane, which results in the loss of important cellular contents. Ketoconazole and clotrimazole also inhibit oxidative enzyme activity, which may increase intracellular hydrogen peroxide to toxic levels and thus contribute to the destruction of the fungal cells and their contents. In addition, they inhibit fungal synthesis of triglycerides and phospholipids. These agents are indicated for the treatment of candidiasis or fungal infections caused by *Candida* species. Fluconazole (Diflucan) and itraconazole (Sporanox) are more potent drugs used to treat *Candida* infections. Only clotrimazole will be reviewed in this section; ketoconazole and nystatin are discussed in Chapter 52.

Pharmacokinetics

Clotrimazole is poorly absorbed and appears to bind to the oral mucosa from which it is slowly released. The duration of action is up to 3 hours. Any absorbed drug is metabolized in the liver and excreted in feces.

Side effects and adverse reactions

These include stomach pain or cramps, nausea, vomiting, and diarrhea.

Warnings

None are listed.

Contraindications

Avoid use in persons with clotrimazole hypersensitivity and in infants or children younger than 4 or 5 years of age.

Dosage and administration

The usual dosage for adults and children 5 years of age and older is one lozenge (10 mg) dissolved slowly in the mouth, five times a day for 2 weeks.

SALIVA SUBSTITUTES

Saliva substitutes (Orex, Xero-Lube, Moi-stir, and Salivart) are used for the relief of dry mouth and throat in xerostomia. They are available as solutions in squirt bottles and as pump or aerosol sprays. They contain electrolytes (potassium phosphate, magnesium chloride, potassium chloride, calcium, and sodium), sodium fluoride, sorbitol, and carboxymethylcellulose as the base.

DRUGS USED TO TREAT MOUTH BLISTERING

Acute and chronic diseases contribute to mouth blistering and erosions. Acute viral diseases such as herpes simplex, herpes zoster, and varicella have previously been treated only symptomatically. Acyclovir (Zovirax), an antiviral agent, is effective against herpes simplex virus and varicella zoster virus, the viruses associated with skin manifestations. It acts to reduce viral shedding, time to crusting, duration of local pain, and severity of symptoms (AHFS, 1998). Acyclovir is available in topical, oral, and parenteral dosage forms. It and other antiviral agents are covered in Chapter 52.

Mouth lesions or blistering (acute or chronic) may be caused by local irritation, medications, radiation, dental manipulations, or systemic disease. To properly treat, one must first identify the causative factor and then institute appropriate treatment.

DRUGS THAT AFFECT THE STOMACH

Conditions of the stomach requiring drug therapy include hyperacidity, hypoacidity, ulcer disease, nausea, vomiting, and hypermotility. Some of the drugs used for these conditions are not unique in their treatment of gastric dysfunction but are members of other major groups of drugs, such as anticholinergic preparations, antihistamines, and antidepressants.

DRUGS USED TO TREAT GASTRIC HYPERACIDITY

Antacids

Antacids are chemical compounds that buffer or neutralize hydrochloric acid in the stomach and thereby increase the gastric pH. The major ingredients in antacids include aluminum salts, calcium carbonate, magnesium salts, and sodium bicarbonate, alone or in combination. Most antacids may be purchased as OTC preparations.

Traditionally, the antacids have been termed "nonsystemic" or "systemic." Nonsystemic indicates the almost negligible amount of drug absorbed into the circulation; activity occurs only locally within the gastrointestinal tract. The nonsystemic metal ion, however, is absorbed to some degree. The aluminum ion is absorbed the most and magnesium the least; calcium is absorbed slightly more than magnesium. Long-term chronic use of antacids or their use in the presence of impaired renal function may result in increased adverse effects from metal ion absorption, especially of calcium carbonate or magnesium hydroxide.

Antacids are indicated for the relief of symptoms associated with hyperacidity related to the diagnosis of peptic ulcer, gastritis, gastroesophageal reflux disease (GERD), gastric hyperacidity, heartburn, or hiatal hernia. Antacids generally have a rapid onset of action. When administered in a fasting state, the antacid effect lasts from 20 to 40 minutes. If administered 1 hour after meals, though, the effects may be extended for up to 3 hours. A small amount of absorbable antacid is absorbed (15% to 30%), but the remainder is broken down via the digestive process and excreted via the feces.

Altered Drug Solubility, Stability, and Absorption

Many drugs are either weak acids or weak bases, and the pH of the stomach is an important factor in their absorption. Drugs that are weak acids are nonionized in the acidic environment of the stomach, are lipid soluble, and are absorbed by simple diffusion across the gastric mucosal cells. The administration of an antacid either with a weak acidic drug or shortly before or after will raise the pH of the stomach contents, causing the formation of a more ionized drug that will not be absorbed to the degree the nonionized, lipid-soluble form was absorbed. A weakly basic drug is absorbed in a more alkaline medium. Changes in pH modify drug solubility and stability, which also affect absorption. Consider then that antacids will affect the absorption of most drugs to some degree.

Drugs that are weak bases include morphine sulfate, quinine, pseudoephedrine, antihistamines, amphetamines, theophylline, tricyclic antidepressants, and quinidine. Examples of weak acids are isoniazid, barbiturates, nalidixic acid, nonsteroidal antiinflammatory agents, sulfonamides, salicylates, nitrofurantoin, and coumarins.

Additional Drug Interactions

Antacids have been reported to reduce the absorption of many drugs, such as quinolone antibiotics, tetracyclines, ketoconazole, sucralfate, and digoxin; therefore the healthcare professional should carefully watch how these medications are scheduled as the majority of medications need to be separated by hours from an antacid. Close monitoring for both therapeutic response and possible side effects is also recommended. For dosage and administration, see Chapter 3. The following effects may occur when antacids are given with the drugs listed below:

Drug	Possible effect and management
Fluoroquinolones	Aluminum- and magnesium-containing antacids may reduce absorption of these drugs. Advise taking of fluoroquinolones at least 2 hours before or 2 hours after antacid for norfloxacin (Noroxin) and ofloxacin (Floxin), 6 hours after antacid for ciprofloxacin (Cipro) and lomefloxacin (Maxaquin), and 8 hours after antacid for enoxacin (Penetrex).
Ion-exchange sodium polystyrene sulfonate resin (Kayexalate)	When calcium- or magnesium-containing antacids are given concurrently with resin, neutralization of gastric acid may be impaired. The binding of the calcium and magnesium may result in anion absorption and systemic alkalosis. Avoid oral administration of this combination.
isoniazid (INH)	Aluminum antacids interfere with the absorption of isoniazid. Separate the administration of these drugs by at least 1 hour or administer a non-aluminum-containing antacid to prevent this interaction.
ketoconazole (Nizoral)	Increased gastric pH may decrease absorption of ketoconazole. Advise patients to take antacids at least 3 hours after ketoconazole.

mecamylamine (Inversine)	Effects of mecamylamine may be prolonged because an alkaline urine decreases its excretion. Concurrent administration should be avoided.
methenamine (Mandelamine, Hiprex)	An alkaline urine may decrease methenamine's effectiveness by prohibiting its conversion to formaldehyde. Concurrent administration is not recommended. Because urine alkalinization may occur with antacids, monitor patient for increased risk of crystalluria and nephrotoxicity.
Tetracyclines, oral	Antacids may combine with tetracyclines, decreasing their absorption in the GI tract. Advise patients to take antacids at least 3 to 4 hours before or after tetracycline.

Color type indicates an unsafe drug combination.

Side effects and adverse reactions

See Table 3-2.

Warnings

Use with caution in patients with undiagnosed GI or rectal bleeding. For magnesium- and magaldrate-containing antacids, use caution in patients with colitis, diarrhea, diverticulitis, or a colostomy.

Contraindications

Avoid use in persons with hypersensitivity to antacid ingredients, intestinal obstruction, and appendicitis. For aluminum- and magaldrate-containing antacids, avoid use in persons with Alzheimer's disease and kidney function impairment.

Dosage and administration

See Chapter 3.

DIGESTANTS

Digestants are drugs that promote the process of digestion in the GI tract. Problems with digestion may be caused by a deficiency of hydrochloric acid, digestive substances, enzymes, or bile salts; organic disease states (stomach cancer, pernicious anemia, and cholecystectomy); or, possibly, a reaction to emotional situations or stress.

Digestive enzymes secreted by the mouth, stomach, small intestine, pancreas, and liver are necessary for the digestion of food. Pepsin is the stomach enzyme that reduces protein to smaller particles. It can be given alone or in combination with a hydrochloric acid source in hypochlorhydric or achlorhydric patients.

Hydrochloric acid keeps the gastric pH level below 4 and protects the proteolytic activity of pepsin. A pH level of 1.5 to 2.5 is usually the optimal range. Pepsin is not considered a critical enzyme because proteolytic enzymes released from the pancreas and intestine cause the same effects.

pancreatin [pan′ kree a tin] (Entozyme, Donnazyme)
pancrelipase [pan kre li′ pase] (Pancrease, Viokase)

The pancreas releases digestive enzymes and bicarbonate into the duodenum to help in the digestion of fats, carbohydrates, and proteins. Bicarbonate neutralizes acid and thus helps to protect the enzymes from both acid and pepsin. When acid chyme enters the duodenum, vagal stimulation regulates pancreatic secretion, so that enzyme replacement therapy may be necessary for patients who have had vagal fibers surgically severed or had surgical procedures that cause food to bypass the duodenum.

Both pancreatin and pancrelipase contain the enzymes amylase, trypsin, and lipase, but pancrelipase has greater enzyme activity in the neutral or alkaline media of the gastrointestinal tract. It has about 12 times the lipolytic and 4 times the proteolytic and amylolytic activities of pancreatin. These agents are not interchangeable because they are not bioequivalent.

Both pancreatin and pancrelipase aid in the digestion and absorption of fats, carbohydrates, and triglycerides. In addition, replacement therapy is usually necessary in exocrine pancreatic enzyme deficiency states, chronic pancreatitis, cystic fibrosis, pancreatic tumors, pancreatic obstruction, and pancreatectomy.

Both products are available in enteric-coated capsules to avoid destruction in the stomach. The enteric-coated microsphere formulation resists gastric inactivation, so enzymes reach the duodenum to hydrolyze fats into glycerol and fatty acids, proteins into proteases, and starch into dextrins and sugars.

Side effects and adverse reactions

These include nausea, abdominal cramps, hyperuricemia, intestinal obstruction, allergic reaction, and loose stool.

Avoid use of these agents in persons with pork protein, pancrelipase, or pancreatin hypersensitivity and acute pancreatitis. See the box for Food and Drug Administration

PREGNANCY SAFETY

Category	Drug
B	cimetidine, famotidine, granisetron, lansoprazole, metoclopramide, ondansetron, ranitidine, sucralfate, ursodiol
C	cisapride, difenoxin and atropine, diphenoxylate and atropine, dronabinol, ipecac, monoctanoin, nizatidine, omeprazole, pancreatin, pancrelipase, scopolamine
X	chenodiol, misoprostol
Not established	diphenidol, trimethobenzamide; thiethylperazine is not recommended for use during pregnancy

(FDA) pregnancy safety classifications. The usual adult pancreatin dose is one to two tablets with meals or snacks, while the dose for pancrelipase is one to three capsules or tablets or one or two packets before or with meals or snacks. Dosage should be adjusted as necessary. In extreme deficiency, the dosage interval may be changed to hourly if no nausea or diarrhea develops.

EMETIC (VOMITING) REFLEX

The vomiting or **emetic center** located in the medulla oblongata may be stimulated by smells, strong emotion, severe pain, increased intracranial pressure, labyrinthine disturbances (motion sickness), endocrine disturbances, toxic reactions to drugs, gastrointestinal disease, radiation treatments, and chemotherapy (Fig. 35-1). The stimuli may involve neurotransmitters and vagal and/or sympathetic afferent nerve transmission.

The **chemoreceptor trigger zone (CTZ)** is an area of sensory nerve cells activated by chemical stimuli that relays messages to the emetic center. It has various receptors (serotonin, dopamine, and opiate) that detect irritating drugs or toxins in the blood to stimulate or mediate emesis. The chemoreceptor trigger zone itself is not able to induce vomiting.

Because the CTZ is located close to the respiratory center in the brain, it is difficult to completely control vomiting initiated from this site without affecting respiration. The cerebral cortex area is involved in anticipatory nausea and vomiting, a conditioned response caused by a stimulus connected with a previous unpleasant experience. For example, unpleasant memories, such as receiving cancer chemotherapy that has resulted in vomiting, might make the patient vomit at the sight of the hospital, doctor, or nurse, even before treatment is given (Koda-Kimble, Young, 1995). See the discussion in Chapter 48.

If the emetic center is activated by stimuli, it sends impulses (via efferent nerves) to the diaphragm, stomach muscles, esophagus, and salivary glands, resulting in vomiting.

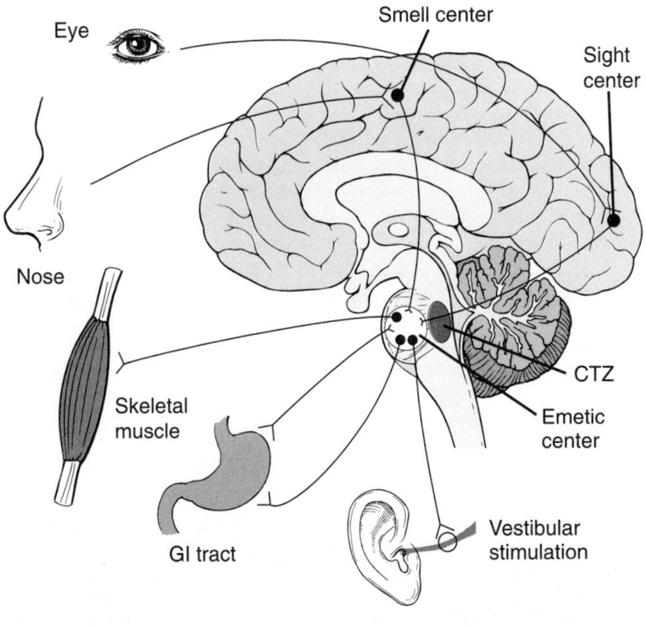

FIGURE 35-1
Chemoreceptor trigger zone (CTZ) and other sites activating the emetic center.

ANTIEMETICS

Antiemetics are drugs given to prevent or relieve nausea and vomiting. Control of vomiting is important and at times may be difficult. Numerous preparations have been used, but effective treatment usually depends on treating the cause. The primary pathways for the vomiting reflex are:

1. Higher CNS or cerebral cortex stimulation
   a. Emotional or anticipatory vomiting
2. Peripheral or central nerve transmission secondary to body tissue or organ alterations
   a. Irritation of GI tract
   b. Increased intracranial pressure
   c. Vestibular stimulation
3. Stimulation from the CTZ
   a. Toxins circulating in blood

Antiemetics may exert their effects on the vomiting center, the cerebral cortex, the CTZ, or the vestibular apparatus (Box 35-3).

The neurotransmitters and pharmacologic agents used to control and prevent nausea and vomiting include:

1. *Neurotransmitter:* Dopamine (D_2) receptors located in the GI tract and CTZ. *Pharmacologic agents:* Phenothiazines, such as chlorpromazine (Thorazine) and prometh-

BOX 35-3 Proposed Sites of Action for Antiemetic Drugs

Proposed Sites	***Drugs***
Emetic center	anticholinergics
	antihistamines
	thiethylperazine maleate*
Chemoreceptor trigger zone	benzquinamide hydrochloride
	butyrophenones
	dephenidol hydrochloride*
	metoclopramide 🔑*
	phenothiazine
	thiethylperazine maleate*
	trimethobenzamide HCl
Cerebral cortex	cannabinoids (THC, nabilone, dronabinol)
	diazepam
	lorazepam
	scopolamine*
	antihistamines
Peripheral	diphenidol hydrochloride*
	metoclopramide 🔑*
	scopolamine*
Unknown	corticosteroids

*Dual action.

azine (Phenergan), and metoclopramide (Reglan), are dopamine antagonists. They act on the CTZ, GI tract, and other dopamine neurotransmitter areas. These are the most effective antiemetics and often the drugs of choice.

2. *Neurotransmitter:* Acetylcholine (ACh) receptors in vestibular and vomiting center. Overstimulation of the labyrinth (inner ear) results in the nausea and vomiting of motion sickness. *Pharmacologic agents:* Anticholinergics, such as scopolamine, reduce the excitability of labyrinth receptors, depress conduction in the vestibular cerebellar pathways, or prevent impulses from stimulating the CTZ.
3. *Neurotransmitter:* Histamine (H_1) receptors in vestibular and vomiting centers. *Pharmacologic agents:* H_1 antihistamines affect neural labyrinth pathways; examples include cyclizine (Marezine), dimenhydrinate (Dramamine), and diphenhydramine (Benadryl). Many antihistamines have anticholinergic side effects (see 2 above).
4. *Neurotransmitter:* Serotonin (5-HT_3) receptors in the GI tract, CTZ, and vomiting centers (Lichter, 1993). *Pharmacologic agents:* Ondansetron (Zofran) and granisetron (Kytril) are selective serotonin receptor antagonists approved for prevention of nausea and vomiting induced by cancer chemotherapy.
5. *Miscellaneous agents:* Antacids relieve gastric irritation; diphenidol (Vontrol) acts on the vestibular apparatus, and benzquinamide (Emete-con) acts on the CTZ to reduce nausea and vomiting. Steroids (dexamethasone and methylprednisolone) and cannabinoids (nabilone and delta-9-tetrahydrocannabinol [THC]) are also used.

Cancer Chemotherapy–Induced Vomiting

Vomiting from cancer chemotherapy can be serious enough to limit the dosages of chemotherapeutic agents given to a patient. Because antiemetics are usually more effective in preventing vomiting than they are in treating it, they should be administered prophylactically before chemotherapy administration. Also, chemotherapy-induced vomiting may require several antiemetic agents with different sites of action for effectiveness, for example, metoclopramide (Reglan) and lorazepam (Ativan), metoclopramide and dexamethasone, or prochlorperazine (Compazine) and dexamethasone.

metoclopramide [met oh kloe′ pra mide] (Reglan, Maxeran)
cisapride [sis′ a pride] (Propulsid)

Metoclopramide has both central and peripheral actions in preventing or relieving nausea and emesis. Centrally it blocks dopamine receptors in the CTZ while peripherally it increases motility of the upper GI tract, increases peristalsis, and overcomes the immobility, dilation, and reverse motility that occurs with the vomiting reflex. Cisapride is chemically similar to metoclopramide although it lacks any dopamine receptor activity. Cisapride has been postulated to increase acetylcholine release from postganglionic nerves located in the myenteric plexus, which decreases esophageal reflux; it also enhances gastric and duodenal emptying by increased contractility. Therefore it increases transit in both the small and large intestine.

Metoclopramide is used for diabetic gastroparesis, gastroesophageal reflux, and parenterally for the prevention of nausea and vomiting secondary to emetogenic cancer chemotherapeutic agents, radiation, and opioid medications. It is also used as an adjunct for GI radiologic examinations because it hastens barium's transit through the upper GI tract by its stimulation of gastric emptying and acceleration of intestinal transit. Parenteral metoclopramide may be used to facilitate intestinal intubation. Cisapride is used to prevent or treat gastroesophageal reflux (USP DI, 1998).

Pharmacokinetics

Metoclopramide's onset of action is ½ to 1 hour after oral administration, 10 to 15 minutes after an intramuscular dose, and within 3 minutes after an intravenous dose. Its duration of action is 1 to 2 hours, and half-life is 4 to 6 hours. It is metabolized by the liver and excreted in the kidneys.

Cisapride's onset of action is ½ to 1 hour, its peak serum concentration is reached in 1 to 2 hours, and half-life is 7 to 10 hours. It is metabolized by the liver and excreted by the kidneys and in feces.

Side effects and adverse reactions

For metoclopramide these include diarrhea, sleepiness, restlessness, increased weakness, extrapyramidal (parkinsonian) effects, hypotension, hypertension, tachycardia, and, rarely, agranulocytosis.

Side effects and adverse effects for cisapride include stomach cramps, constipation or diarrhea, headache, nausea, drowsiness, and, rarely, convulsions.

Drug interactions

The following effects may occur when metoclopramide and cisapride are given with the drugs listed below:

Drug	Possible effect and management
Alcohol and CNS-depressant medications	Concurrent administration may increase the CNS-depressant effects of either or both drugs. It may also result in an increased rate of absorption of alcohol from the small intestine. Avoid or a potentially serious drug interaction may occur.
Anticholinergic agents and opioid analgesics	Concurrent administration of these agents may antagonize motility effects of metoclopramide and cisapride and increase the sedative effects of all the agents.

itraconazole (Sporanox), IV miconazole (Monistat IV), and troleandomycin (Tao)	Concurrent administration of these agents markedly increases cisapride plasma concentrations because of inhibition of the hepatic enzymes responsible for cisapride metabolism. Avoid or a potentially serious drug interaction may occur.
Oral ketoconazole (Nizoral)	Concurrent use may result in markedly elevated cisapride plasma concentrations and a prolonged Q-T interval associated with ventricular dysrhythmia. Avoid or a potentially serious drug interaction may occur.

Color type indicates an unsafe drug combination.

Warnings

Use cisapride with caution in patients with a history of seizures, liver or kidney function impairment, electrolyte imbalance, and cardiac (Q-T syndrome or prolongation) disease. Use metoclopramide cautiously in patients with asthma, hypertension, liver failure, and Parkinson's disease.

Contraindications

Avoid cisapride and metoclopramide in persons with drug hypersensitivity, or GI bleeding, obstruction, or ulceration. In addition, avoid the use of metoclopramide in persons with pheochromocytoma and severe chronic kidney failure.

Dosage and administration

To treat diabetic gastroparesis or gastroesophageal reflux in an adult, the oral dose of metoclopramide is 10 mg 30 minutes before each meal and at bedtime (up to four times daily). Check the package insert for further instructions. The IV dose is 10 mg as a single dose. The adult antiemetic dose (for chemotherapy-induced emesis) is 2 mg/kg by IV infusion 30 minutes before chemotherapy; the dose may be repeated every 2 to 3 hours as necessary.

The oral pediatric dose is 0.1 to 0.2 mg/kg per dose 30 minutes before meals and at bedtime to increase peristalsis. See current references for additional dosing recommendations.

The adult dose of cisapride to prevent gastroesophageal reflux is 10 mg PO twice a day, before breakfast and at bedtime. To treat reflux, the dose is 5 to 10 mg three to four times daily, 15 minutes before meals and at bedtime. The pediatric dose is 0.15 to 0.3 mg/kg body weight PO three or four times daily before meals.

diphenidol [di phen′ i dol] (Vontrol)

Diphenidol may decrease vestibular stimulation and have a potential effect on the medullary CTZ. It is used to prevent and control vertigo (Ménière's disease, labyrinthitis after middle or inner ear surgery, and motion sickness), nausea, and vomiting.

Pharmacokinetics

Diphenidol is well absorbed orally, reaches peak serum levels in 1.5 to 3 hours, has a half-life of 4 hours, and is excreted by the kidneys.

Drug interactions

When diphenidol is given with alcohol or other CNS depressants, the effects of either drug may be potentiated. Monitor closely for enhanced CNS-depressant effects.

Side effects and adverse reactions

These include drowsiness, dry mouth, headache, insomnia, weakness, rash, dizziness, indigestion and, rarely, disorientation, delusion, and hallucinations.

Warnings

Use with caution in patients with gastrointestinal or genitourinary tract obstruction and glaucoma.

Contraindications

Avoid use in persons with hypotension and kidney function impairment.

Dosage and administration

The adult dosage for antiemesis and antivertigo is 25 to 50 mg PO every 4 hours as needed.

thiethylperazine maleate

[thye eth il per′ a zeen] (Torecan)

Thiethylperazine is a phenothiazine derivative with antiemetic effects, probably by an inhibitory action on the CTZ and vomiting center. It is used to prevent nausea and vomiting caused by toxins, surgery, chemotherapy, and radiation therapy. For pharmacokinetics, see the discussion of phenothiazines in Chapter 13.

Drug interactions

The following effects may occur when thiethylperazine is given with the drugs listed below:

Drug	Possible effect and management
Alcohol and CNS depressants	Concurrent use may result in increased CNS and respiratory depression. Dosage reductions of either drug may be necessary.
epinephrine (Adrenalin)	Avoid use of epinephrine to treat severe hypotension induced by thiethylperazine or a potentially serious drug interaction may occur. Norepinephrine and phenylephrine are drugs of choice for this purpose.

levodopa (l-dopa)	Concurrent administration may cancel the therapeutic antiparkinson's effect of levodopa. Avoid concurrent drug administration.
metrizamide, intrathecal (Amipaque)	Concurrent drug administration may result in an increased risk of seizures because thiethylperazine lowers the seizure threshold. Avoid or a potentially serious drug interaction may occur. Thiethylperazine should be discontinued at least 48 hours before metrizamide is administered.
Phenothiazines, other extrapyramidal effect-causing medications	Monitor for increased potential and severity of extrapyramidal reactions.
quinidine	An increase in adverse cardiac effects may result with this combination. Avoid or a potentially serious drug interaction may occur.

Color type indicates an unsafe drug combination.

Side effects and adverse reactions

These include sleepiness, dizziness, dry mouth, skin rash, fever, ringing of the ears, headache, extrapyramidal effects (parkinsonism in the elderly and dystonia in younger persons), and also agranulocytosis and cholestatic jaundice. Confusion, seizures, and peripheral edema have also been noted.

Dosage and administration

The adult dose is 10 mg one to three times daily orally, intramuscularly, or rectally. Thiethylperazine is not recommended for children. For additional information including phenothiazine warnings and contraindications, see Chapter 13.

trimethobenzamide [trye meth oh ben′ za mide] (Tigan)

Trimethobenzamide may depress the CTZ in the medulla rather than the vomiting center directly. As an antiemetic, it is not as effective as metoclopramide (Brunton, 1996). Trimethobenzamide is metabolized in the liver and excreted in the urine.

Drug interactions

When trimethobenzamide is given concurrently with CNS drugs, enhanced CNS depression or other CNS effects may occur. Use with caution and monitor closely.

Side effects and adverse reactions

These include sleepiness, blurred vision, diarrhea, dizziness, headache, muscle cramps, and, rarely, allergic reactions, seizures, blood dyscrasias, impaired liver function, tremors, Reye's syndrome, and depression (USP DI, 1998).

Warnings

Use with caution in patients with electrolyte disturbances, encephalitis, high fever, or gastroenteritis and in dehydrated patients.

Dosage and administration

The oral adult dose of trimethobenzamide is 250 mg three or four times per day. Rectally or intramuscularly, 200 mg is given three or four times per day. For children 15 mg/kg/day is given orally, divided into three or four doses. See a current drug reference for additional recommendations.

scopolamine transdermal (Transderm-Scop)

Scopolamine is an anticholinergic agent used to prevent motion-induced nausea and vomiting by depressing conduction in the labyrinth of the inner ear. Overstimulation in this area is responsible for the nausea and vomiting of motion sickness. Scopolamine is metabolized in the liver and excreted by the kidneys. The side effects and adverse reactions of scopolamine are related to its anticholinergic effects; these include decreased sweating, sleepiness, and dry mouth, nose, throat, or skin. In the elderly, impaired memory and insomnia (paradoxical reaction) have been reported.

Scopolamine transdermal is recommended for use in adults only. In the United States, the product is a four-layered film that releases 0.5 mg of scopolamine over a 3-day period. It is applied on the skin behind the ear usually 4 hours before the antiemetic effect is desired. In Canada, it is formulated to release 1 mg of scopolamine over the 3-day period, and it should be applied 12 hours before the antiemetic effect is desired. See Chapter 15 for additional information.

ondansetron [on dan′ si tron] (Zofran)
granisetron [gran iz′ e tron] (Kytril)

Ondansetron was the first of a new class of serotonin receptor ($5\text{-}HT_3$) antagonists approved by the FDA for the prevention of nausea and vomiting associated with the use of antineoplastic agents. Granisetron, released in 1995, is also a selective serotonin antagonist. Serotonin receptors are located peripherally on the vagus nerve terminal and centrally in the CTZ. It is believed that antineoplastic agents cause the release of stored serotonin from the enterochromaffin cells of the GI tract (USP DI, 1998). The serotonin stimulates serotonin receptors located in the vagus nerve in the GI tract, which then stimulates serotonin receptors in the CTZ, inducing vomiting. When ondansetron or granisetron is administered before antineoplastic therapy, the serotonin receptors in the brain stem and GI tract are blocked. As a result, serotonin released in response to the administration of antineoplastic agents cannot bind with the serotonin receptors and so prevents vomiting.

Pharmacokinetics

Ondansetron administered orally peaks in 1 to 2 hours, its elimination half-life is 3 to 4 hours, and it is metabolized in the liver and excreted primarily by the kidneys. Pharmacokinetic information on granisetron is limited. Its elimination half-life after IV administration may range from 9 to 12 hours, and it is metabolized in the liver and excreted in the urine and feces.

Drug interactions

No significant drug interactions are reported.

Side effects and adverse reactions

For granisetron these include stomach pain, diarrhea or constipation, headache, increased weakness and, rarely, cardiac dysrhythmias, fainting, and hypersensitivity or allergic type reactions.

The side effects and adverse reactions for ondansetron include fever, headache, constipation, diarrhea and, rarely, anaphylaxis, chest pain, and bronchospasm.

Warnings

Use ondansetron with caution in patients with liver function impairment and those who have had abdominal surgery (may mask an ileus or gastric distention).

Contraindications

Avoid use in persons with granisetron or ondansetron hypersensitivity.

Dosage and administration

To prevent cancer chemotherapy-induced nausea and vomiting in adults and children 4 to 18 years of age the IV dosage of ondansetron is 0.15 mg/kg infused over 15 minutes beginning 30 minutes before the start of chemotherapy, followed by 0.15 mg/kg at 4 and 8 hours after the first dose of ondansetron. The oral adult dose is 8 mg 30 minutes before cancer chemotherapy, then 8 mg at 8 hours after the first dose, followed by 8 mg every 12 hours for several days.

The dosage of IV granisetron to prevent cancer chemotherapy–induced nausea and vomiting in children 2 years of age and older and adults is 10 μg/kg given over 5 minutes, 30 minutes before the chemotherapy or radiotherapy. The oral dosage is 1 mg twice a day with the first dose administered an hour before chemotherapy and the second dose 12 hours after the first dose (USP DI, 1998; Olin, 1998).

Cannabinoids

dronabinol [droe nab′ i nol] (Marinol)

Dronabinol, the synthetic derivative of THC, is indicated for the treatment of nausea and vomiting related to cancer chemotherapy. Dronabinol is used as a second line agent to prevent nausea and vomiting associated with chemotherapy when other antiemetics are ineffective. It is also used as an appetite stimulant to treat anorexia and weight loss in persons with acquired immunodeficiency syndrome (AIDS).

Pharmacokinetics

Dronabinol reaches peak serum levels in 2 to 4 hours. Its duration of action is 4 to 6 hours for psychic effects and 1 day or longer for appetite-stimulating effects. It is metabolized in the liver and excreted mainly in the feces.

Drug interactions

When administered with CNS-depressant drugs it may result in potentiated CNS-depressant effects. Monitor closely.

Side effects and adverse reactions

These include ataxia, lightheadedness, nausea, vomiting, blurred vision, dry mouth, restlessness, weakness, drowsiness, tachycardia, or bradycardia and CNS side effects, such as confusion, delusions, hallucinations, depression, mood alterations, restlessness, and anxiety. The elderly are particularly prone to the CNS adverse reactions.

Warnings

Use with caution in patients with hypertension, cardiac disease, a history of drug abuse, mania, depression, or schizophrenia.

Contraindications

Avoid use in persons with dronabinol or sesame oil hypersensitivity.

Dosage and administration

The adult oral dose is 5 mg/m^2 of body surface 1 to 3 hours before chemotherapy, then every 2 to 4 hours afterward for four to six doses daily. If the initial dose is ineffective, it may be increased in increments of 2.5 mg/m^2 (maximum dose is 15 mg/m^2). The appetite stimulant dose is 2.5 mg twice daily before lunch and supper, which may be increased if necessary up to a maximum of 20 mg/day. Pediatric dosage is similar to adult dose.

nabilone [na′ bi lone] (Cesamet 🍁)

Nabilone is a synthetic derivative of cannabinoid (not THC) approved for selected persons receiving emetogenic chemotherapy nonresponsive to other first-line antiemetic agents.

Pharmacokinetics

It has an onset of action within ½ to 1 hour and peak effect in 2 hours. It is metabolized in the liver and excreted primarily in feces.

Drug interactions

When administered concurrently with alcohol or other CNS-depressant drugs, it may result in enhanced CNS-depressant effects. Monitor closely.

Side effects and adverse reactions

These include ataxia, sedation, dry mouth, euphoria, mood disorders, hallucinations, hypotension, tachycardia, weakness, headache, and difficulty in concentration.

Warnings

Use with caution in patients with severe liver impairment, hypertension, hypotension, cardiac disease, and a history of drug abuse.

Contraindications

Avoid use in persons with schizophrenia, mania, or clinical depression.

Dosage and administration

The adult dose is 1 or 2 mg twice daily. The pediatric dose is not established.

Corticosteroids

Corticosteroids have been reported to be effective for chemotherapy-induced nausea and vomiting alone or when used in combination with other antiemetics (Koda-Kimble, Young, 1995). The mechanism of action is unknown, but it has been proposed that these drugs may inhibit prostaglandin synthesis, which may be involved in cancer chemotherapy–induced vomiting. Research has indicated that certain prostaglandins (especially the E series) can induce nausea and vomiting.

Many studies with corticosteroids have involved the use of dexamethasone and methylprednisolone, although corticotropin and hydrocortisone may also be used. Their effectiveness as antiemetics was a serendipitous discovery: patients receiving various chemotherapeutic regimens had less nausea and vomiting when prednisone was one of the agents administered. Thus the corticosteroids are used as antiemetics in cancer chemotherapy, especially for persons not responsive to other drug therapies. Discussion related to corticosteroids may be found in Chapter 41.

EMETIC AGENTS

Emetic drugs exert their effects on the same centers as antiemetic drugs but with the opposite effect. They are used to induce vomiting as part of the treatment for certain drug overdoses and poisonings.

ipecac syrup [ip′ e kak]

Ipecac syrup is an OTC drug for home emergency treatment; it is the emetic of choice. Its major alkaloids are emetine and cephaeline, which stimulate the CTZ and irritate the gastric mucosa to induce vomiting (Box 35-4).

Approximately 80% to 90% of patients vomit within ½ hour after oral drug administration; the average time for vomiting is 20 minutes. Although this product is generally given in the home, a poison control center or healthcare provider should be called for advice before administration. However, if medical help is not available, one could still use this product. Vomiting-induced gastrointestinal contents recovered may range up to 78% (mean 28%). Therefore patients need further monitoring and/or treatment, since not all the toxic substances are recovered from the gastrointestinal tract.

BOX 35-4 Ipecac Syrup Precaution

Ipecac syrup is the only product to be used as an emetic. *Do not use ipecac fluidextract,* because it is 14 times more concentrated than the syrup, and its use has resulted in serious injury and sometimes death. Although the fluidextract is no longer commercially produced in the United States, this product may still be on the shelves of some older pharmacies.

Ipecac syrup has the advantage of oral administration. The active alkaloid emetine is a cardiotoxic substance. Although administration of a single dose does not usually lead to major problems, serious complications including fatalities have resulted from chronic use of this product by persons with an eating disorder, such as anorexia or bulimia. Emetine is excreted very slowly, so with repeated doses, it will accumulate in the body. It may produce systemic effects for months, even after the drug is discontinued.

Myopathy, or muscle aching and weakness, especially in the muscles of the neck and extremities, hyporeflexia, slurred speech, and dysphagia have been reported. Cardiotoxicity has caused some fatalities. Cardiac and muscle effects are due to emetine toxicity and are usually symptoms associated with misuse or overdose of this drug.

The contraindications for ipecac include any condition that has an associated increased potential for vomiting aspiration such as unconsciousness, shock, a depressed gag reflex, decreased alertness, or a history of convulsions. Also, do not use if the patient ingested any corrosive substances such as strong acids or lye.

For adults and children older than 12 years of age, the dose is 15 to 30 ml (1 oz) orally. Children 1 to 12 years are given 15 ml orally. For adults, follow each dose of ipecac syrup with 8 oz (240 ml) of water; for children 4 to 8 oz of water is given. If vomiting does not occur in 20 to 30 minutes, a second dose may be given. If vomiting does not occur then, gastric lavage should be implemented.

DRUGS USED TO TREAT PEPTIC ULCERS

Treatment of peptic ulcer disease may include a variety of drugs: antimicrobials, antacids, anticholinergics, antidepressants, anxiolytics, H_2 receptor antagonists, and cytoprotective agents (substances that protect cells from damage) such as sucralfate. This section is limited to the more specific agents: the cytoprotective agents and the H_2 receptor antagonists. See the box for geriatric implications of the antiulcer therapies.

Helicobacter pylori has been found in persons with gastritis and gastric and duodenal peptic ulcers. It has been re-

GERIATRIC IMPLICATIONS

Antiulcer Therapies

Gastrointestinal symptoms are very common in elderly patients. Every symptom should be properly evaluated before instituting drug therapy.

Acid secretion reaches its peak during sleep, between the hours of 10 PM and the early morning hours (Covington, 1995). Therefore, H_2 receptor antagonists prescribed as a daily dose should be administered at bedtime.

Cigarette smoking, which increases the amount of acid produced in the stomach, may decrease the effect of H_2 blockers. Patients should be advised to stop smoking if possible, or at least not to smoke after the last daily dose of medication is taken (USP DI, 1998).

With the routine administration of H_2 blockers, confusion and dizziness are more commonly reported by the elderly than by younger adults (USP DI, 1998). With cimetidine, famotidine, and ranitidine, mental status changes have been reported, especially in elderly persons who have impaired liver or renal function or are severely ill. Acute mental changes in the elderly may indicate the need for lowering the drug dose or discontinuing the medication.

Antacids effectively neutralize gastric acid while food also serves as a buffer for gastric acid. Thus antacids are most beneficial if administered between meals and at bedtime.

When H_2 receptor antagonists are prescribed with antacids, schedule medications at least 1 hour apart, administering the antacid first.

ported that persons who have a colony of this bacteria in the stomach are more prone to gastritis and gastric and duodenal ulcers (Fedotin, 1993). It has been recommended that all persons with non-drug-induced peptic ulcer be treated with a combination of antibacterial agents to eradicate *H pylori.* Controlling or eradicating this bacteria vastly improves the chances of nonrecurrence of the ulcer. The drug regimen usually includes a bismuth preparation (Pepto-Bismol), tetracycline, and metronidazole (Flagyl) plus an H_2 blocking agent. Some resistance has been reported to metronidazole in addition to side effects with all three drugs, which has lead to the use of other combinations, such as bismuth and amoxicillin or amoxicillin and omeprazole (Abramowicz, 1994; Graham, 1993; Smith, 1995).

Several combination medications were also released in 1996. Ranitidine bismuth citrate (Tritec) is used in combination with clarithromycin while bismuth subsalicylate, metronidazole, and a tetracycline combination (Helidac) may also be used to treat active duodenal ulcers associated with *H pylori* infection (Olin, 1998). Combining individual agents in a single product helps to simplify a complicated drug schedule.

Cytoprotective Agents

sucralfate [soo kral′ fate] (Carafate, Sulcrate ✦)

Sucralfate is a local topical agent composed of sulfated sucrose and aluminum hydroxide that in the presence of albumin and fibrinogen forms a protective, acid-resistant shield in the ulcer crater. This barrier hastens the healing of the peptic ulcer by protecting the mucosa for up to 6 hours. It is administered orally with minimal systemic absorption (up to 5%). Excretion is primarily by the fecal route.

Indications

This product is indicated for short-term (up to 8 weeks) duodenal ulcer treatment.

Drug interactions

The following effects may occur when sucralfate is administered with the following drugs:

Drug	Possible effect and management
Antacids	Concurrent use may interfere with sucralfate binding, thus reducing its effect. Administer antacids either 30 minutes before or 1 hour after sucralfate administration.
ciprofloxacin (Cipro), norfloxacin (Noroxin). or ofloxacin (Floxin)	Sucralfate is reported to decrease absorption and serum levels of these antibiotics. Advise patients to take antibiotics 2 to 3 hours before sucralfate.
digoxin (Lanoxin) or theophylline (Elixophyllin)	Sucralfate interferes with absorption of digoxin and theophylline. Advise patients to take digoxin or theophylline two hours before or after sucralfate.
phenytoin (Dilantin)	Concurrent administration with sucralfate may decrease phenytoin serum levels, resulting in a loss of seizure control. Advise patients not to take sucralfate within 2 hours of phenytoin administration.

Side effects and adverse reactions

These are minimal; the most commonly one reported is constipation. Other possible effects include diarrhea, nausea, gastric discomfort, dry mouth, dizziness, drowsiness, back pain, rash, and itching.

Warnings

Use with caution in patients with dysphagia, GI obstruction, and kidney failure.

Contraindications

Avoid use in persons with sucralfate hypersensitivity.

Dosage and administration

The adult dose for treatment of a duodenal ulcer is 1 g four times daily 1 hour before each meal and at bedtime. The dose for prophylaxis of duodenal ulcer is 1 g twice daily on an empty stomach.

misoprostol [mye soe prost′ ole] (Cytotec)

Misoprostol, a gastric mucosa-protecting agent, is indicated for the prevention of gastric ulcers associated with the use of nonsteroidal antiinflammatory drugs (NSAIDs), especially in persons at increased risk of developing complications from gastric ulcers. Normally, prostaglandins protect the stomach by decreasing gastric acid secretion and increasing gastric cytoprotective mucus and bicarbonate. The NSAIDs inhibit prostaglandin synthesis, which reduces the protective mechanisms and may result in gastric ulcers. Misoprostol, a synthetic prostaglandin E_1 analog, suppresses gastric acid secretion and thus helps to heal gastric ulcers (Brunton, 1996).

Pharmacokinetics

Misoprostol is rapidly absorbed orally, reaching a peak serum level in approximately 15 minutes with a duration of action of 3 to 6 hours. It is metabolized to an active metabolite that is later metabolized to inactive metabolites in various body tissues. It is excreted primarily by the kidneys.

Drug interactions

No significant drug interactions are reported.

Side effects and adverse reactions

These include stomach distress and diarrhea, which are dose related. Less frequent side effects include constipation, gas, headache, nausea, and vomiting.

Warnings

Use with caution in patients with epilepsy and coronary artery and cerebral vascular disease.

Contraindications

Avoid use in persons with misoprostol and prostaglandin hypersensitivity.

Dosage and administration

The adult dose is 0.2 mg four times daily after meals and at bedtime or 0.4 mg twice daily, taking the last dose at bedtime. The pediatric dosage has not been established.

Proton Pump Inhibitors

Proton pump inhibitors suppress gastric acid secretion by inhibiting the hydrogen/potassium adenosine triphosphatase (ATPase) enzyme system at the secretory surface of the gastric parietal cells. Therefore they block the final step of acid production, inhibiting both basal and stimulated gastric acid secretion. Omeprazole binds irreversibly at this site while lansoprazole's effects are dose related.

lansoprazole [lan soe′ pra zole] (Prevacid)
omeprazole [oh me′ pray zol] (Prilosec)

Omeprazole, the prototype drug, and lansoprazole are indicated for the treatment of severe erosive esophagitis that occurs with gastroesophageal reflux, for treatment of duodenal ulcer, and for the long-term treatment of hypersecretory gastric conditions.

Pharmacokinetics

Administered orally, omeprazole's onset of action is within 1 hour, its peak effect is in 2 hours, and its duration of action is 3 to 4 days (time needed for production of new enzyme). It is metabolized in the liver and excreted by the kidneys. Lansoprazole's onset of action is within 1 to 3 hours (depending on dose), and it has a duration of action longer than 24 hours. It is metabolized in the liver and excreted primarily in bile and feces.

Drug interactions

Lansoprazole absorption will be decreased if administered with sucralfate. Administer lansoprazole 30 to 60 minutes before sucralfate. Concurrent administration of omeprazole with oral anticoagulants, diazepam (Valium), or phenytoin (Dilantin) may result in a decrease in metabolism of the latter medications causing increased serum levels and perhaps, toxicity. This effect is secondary to omeprazole's inhibition of the cytochrome P-450 enzyme systems.

Side effects and adverse reactions

These include stomach colic or pain for omeprazole and diarrhea for lansoprazole. Other potential side effects include abdominal distress, increased weakness, muscle aches, dizziness, headache, sedation, chest pain, heartburn, constipation or diarrhea, gas, nausea, vomiting, or skin rash. Rare adverse reactions reported with omeprazole include anemia, neutropenia, pancytopenia, thrombocytopenia, and urinary tract infections.

Warnings

Use lansoprazole with caution in patients with liver function impairment.

Contraindications

Avoid use in persons with lansoprazole or omeprazole hypersensitivity. Also avoid omeprazole in patients with acute or chronic liver disease or a history of liver disease.

Dosage and administration

The adult oral dose for omeprazole for gastroesophageal reflux is 20 mg (delayed-release capsule) daily for 1 to 2 months. For gastric hypersecretory conditions, the oral dose is 60 mg daily, adjusting as necessary. For elderly patients the dosage should not exceed 20 mg/day. The pediatric dosage has not been established.

The lansoprazole adult dose for duodenal ulcer is 15 mg orally before breakfast for up to 1 month, the dose for erosive esophagitis is 30 mg daily before breakfast for up to 2 months, and the dose for hypersecretory conditions is 60 mg before breakfast daily. The pediatric dose has not been established.

H_2 Receptor Antagonists

Histamine, found in the mucosal cells of the GI tract, activates H_2 receptors to increase gastric acid secretion. The major components of gastric secretion include hydrochloric acid (HCl) and intrinsic factor, produced by the parietal (acid-forming) cells; pepsinogen, synthesized by the chief cells; and mucus. The principal function of mucus is to protect the epithelial cells of the gastrointestinal tract from attack by pepsin and irritation by the HCl secreted by the stomach. Pepsinogen, an enzyme, is the precursor of pepsin; HCl catalyzes the cleavage of pepsinogen to active pepsin by providing a low pH environment in which pepsin can initiate the digestion of proteins.

Gastric secretion is regulated by a neural mechanism, parasympathetic (vagus) fibers, and a hormonal mechanism, gastrin. Activation of the vagus nerve causes secretion of vast quantities of pepsinogen and HCl. In contrast, the hormonal mechanism involves the actual presence of food, which distends the stomach and stimulates the antral mucosa to release gastrin. This hormone is then absorbed into the blood and carried to the parietal cells and chief cells secreting HCl and pepsinogen, respectively. Histamine is believed to activate the gastric mucosa much the same as gastrin does. In addition, caffeine and alcohol are potent stimuli for gastrin release. When the acidity of the gastric juice is increased to a pH of 2, a negative feedback mechanism helps to block production of gastric secretion from the parietal and chief cells. Thus inhibition of gastric gland secretion plays an essential role in protecting the stomach against excessively acidic secretions, which are responsible for causing peptic ulcerations.

Normally, the mucosal surface of the stomach and upper duodenum is protected from the irritation of gastric acid by a layer of mucus. If a circumscribed area of the mucosal surface is damaged and fails to repair rapidly, it may become eroded, forming an ulcer at one of these sites. When gastric acid comes in contact with this inflamed region, pain may result. Moreover, clinical studies have suggested that esophageal, gastric, and duodenal ulcers (peptic ulcers) are associated with the excessive production of gastric acid.

Clinical evidence has shown that histamine released by severe injuries, particularly burns, may lead to the formation of peptic ulcers.

The H_2 receptor blocking agents include cimetidine (Tagamet), ranitidine (Zantac), famotidine (Pepcid), and nizatidine (Axid). They act to prevent histamine from stimulating the H_2 receptors located on the gastric parietal cells, thus resulting in a reduction in the volume of gastric acid secretion (from stimuli such as food, pentagastrin, histamine, caffeine, and insulin) and the concentration (acid content) of the secretions. All four drugs are presently considered to be equally potent and effective, although pharmacokinetics, side effects and adverse reactions, and drug interactions may differ.

cimetidine [sye met′ i deen] (Tagamet) 🔑
ranitidine [ra nye′ te deen] (Zantac)
famotidine [fa moe′ ti deen] (Pepcid)
nizatidine [ni za′ ti deen] (Axid)

Indications

These agents are used to treat and prevent duodenal ulcer and to treat gastric ulcer, gastroesophageal reflux, and hypersecretory gastric states.

Pharmacokinetics

See Table 35-1.

Drug interactions

Since cimetidine, unlike the other H_2 receptor antagonists, inhibits the liver drug metabolism systems, the major drug interactions noted are with cimetidine. All of the H_2 receptor antagonists, though, may exhibit a similar effect with ketoconazole and antacids.

TABLE 35-1 H_2 Receptor Antagonists: Pharmacokinetics

Drug	Absorption	Time to Peak Plasma Level	Plasma Half-Life (hr)	Duration of Action (hr)	Metabolism/ Excretion
cimetidine 🔑 (Tagamet)	Very good orally, 60%-70%	45-90 min after oral dose	2	4-5 basal 6-8 nocturnal	Liver/kidneys
famotidine (Pepcid)	Fair orally, 40%-45%	1-3 hr after oral dose	2.5-3.5	10-12 basal and nocturnal	Liver/kidneys
nizatidine (Axid)	Very good orally, 90%	0.5-3 hr after oral dose	1-2	Up to 8 basal Up to 12 nocturnal	Liver (has active metabolite)/kidneys
ranitidine (Zantac)	Good orally, 50%	2-3 hr after oral dose	2-2.5	Up to 4 hr basal; up to 13 hr (nocturnal)	Liver/kidneys

Drug	Possible effect and management
Anticoagulants (coumarin, indanedione); antidepressants, tricyclic; metoprolol (Lopressor); phenytoin (Dilantin); propranolol (Inderal), or xanthines (exception: dyphylline)	When administered with cimetidine, a decrease in metabolism and excretion of these medications may occur. Because dosage adjustments may be necessary, blood concentration (for phenytoin and xanthines), prothrombin time (for anticoagulants), and blood pressure monitoring (for metoprolol and propranolol) are indicated.
Antacids	Concurrent use is often prescribed, but if the H_2 receptor antagonist (all four agents) is given concurrently with an antacid, absorption of the antagonist may be decreased. Antacids should not be administered within 1 hour of administration of the H_2 receptor antagonist.
ketoconazole (Nizoral)	An increase in GI pH induced by the H_2 receptor antagonist (all four agents) may result in a reduced absorption of ketoconazole. Advise patients to take the H_2 receptor antagonist at least 2 hours after ketoconazole.

Side effects and adverse reactions

For H_2 receptor blockers these include diarrhea, constipation, headache, stomach cramps or pain, dizziness, rash, and breast swelling or pain in males and females. Famotidine may also cause dry mouth or skin, anorexia, and tinnitus. The less common and rare adverse effects include confusion, neutropenia, bradycardia, tachycardia, and agranulocytosis.

Warnings

Use with caution in patients with cirrhosis or liver impairment and in immunocompromised persons (the decrease in gastric acids may increase the possibility of strongyloidiasis).

Contraindications

Avoid use in persons with hypersensitivity to any histamine H_2 receptor antagonists.

Dosage and administration

For treatment of duodenal and benign active gastric ulcer, the adult dosage is as follows:

- cimetidine: 300 mg orally 4 times daily with meals and at bedtime, or 600 mg twice a day, or 800 mg at bedtime. Adult dose by IM, IV, or IV infusion is 300 mg every 6 to 8 hours
- famotidine: 40 mg at bedtime. Parenteral adult dose is 20 mg IV or IV infusion every 12 hours
- nizatidine: 300 mg at bedtime
- ranitidine: 150 mg twice a day or 300 mg at bedtime. The parenteral dose is 50 mg IM, IV, or IV infusion every 6 to 8 hours

See a current reference for additional dosing recommendations.

DRUGS THAT AFFECT THE GALLBLADDER

chenodiol [kee noe dye′ ole] (Chenix, Chendol ♣)

Chenodiol (chenodeoxycholic acid) is a normal bile acid synthesized in the liver. Cholesterol is broken down by bile acids and lecithin, so when the amount of cholesterol exceeds the capacity of bile acids and lecithin to perform this effect, crystallization and gallstones may result. Chenodiol blocks liver synthesis of cholesterol, thus reducing biliary cholesterol levels, leading to gradual dissolving of floating, radiolucent cholesterol gallstones.

Indications

Chenodiol is indicated for the patient with radiolucent stones who has a well-opacified, functioning gallbladder, but who is at increased risk with elective surgery because of systemic disease, age, or cardiovascular, renal, or respiratory disease.

Pharmacokinetics

Chenodiol is absorbed in the small intestine, metabolized by the liver, and excreted in feces.

Drug interactions

No significant drug interactions are reported.

Side effects and adverse reactions

These include dose-related diarrhea, which may occur with initial therapy or any time during the treatment period. Most cases of diarrhea are mild and tolerated, so they do not interfere with therapy. In some persons, a dosage decrease and/or an antidiarrheal agent may be required. Other side effects include fecal urgency, cramps, heartburn, constipation, nausea, vomiting, anorexia, flatulence, and nonspecific abdominal pain.

Warnings

Use with caution in patients with atherosclerosis.

Contraindications

Avoid use in persons with any bile duct abnormality or gallstone complications.

Dosage and administration

The adult oral dose is 13 to 16 mg/kg/day in two divided doses taken with milk or food in the morning and at night. The initial dose is 250 mg twice daily for 2 weeks and increased by 250 mg/day each week thereafter until either the maximum tolerated dose or the recommended dose is attained.

monoctanoin [mon oh ock′ ta noyn] (Moctanin)

Monoctanoin is a solubilizing agent (dissolves cholesterol stones) indicated for the treatment of cholesterol gallstones in the bile duct or after a unsuccessful cholecystectomy. It is more effective for a single radiolucent stone than for multiple gallstones. Monoctanoin is administered directly into the common bile duct.

This product is absorbed by the portal vein and metabolized by pancreatic lipases to fatty acids and glycerol. The most common side effect reported is abdominal irritation and pain. Less frequently reported side effects include diarrhea, anorexia, nausea, or vomiting.

The adult dose via catheter (continuous perfusion) is 3 to 5 ml/hr administered at a pressure of 10 cm of water for 1 to 3 weeks. Do not administer this drug by IM or IV administration.

ursodiol [yoos oh dye′ ole] (Actigall)

Ursodiol, an analog of chenodiol, is an oral product used to dissolve cholesterol gallstones in patients with uncomplicated gallstone disease. It is more effective against small, floatable stones and is not indicated for the treatment of calcified cholesterol stones, radiopaque (calcium-containing) stones, or radiolucent bile pigment type stones or when surgery is clearly necessary.

Although its exact mechanism of action is unknown, ursodiol inhibits intestinal absorption of cholesterol and also decreases cholesterol synthesis and secretion in the liver. It concentrates in bile. A decrease in cholesterol saturation allows for the gradual dissolution of cholesterol from the gallstones. Ursodiol also increases bile flow in the body. Be aware, however, that gallstone dissolution may necessitate 6 to 24 months of oral therapy, depending on the composition and size of the stone. This therapy is monitored by performing ultrasonograms at 6-month intervals during the first year. If partial effectiveness is not recorded after 1 year of treatment, then ursodiol is usually determined to be ineffective and drug therapy is discontinued. If successful, ursodiol is recommended for at least 3 months after complete dissolution of the stones to ensure the removal of small particles that are not visible via the ultrasonogram.

Pharmacokinetics

Administered orally, ursodiol is absorbed from the small intestine; reaches a peak concentration in 1 to 3 hours, and is metabolized by the liver to taurine and glycine conjugates that are secreted in bile. Excretion is mainly in the feces. An infrequent side effect reported with ursodiol is diarrhea. Ursodiol may cause hepatotoxicity, but to date liver injuries have not been reported.

Drug interactions

No significant drug interactions have been reported with ursodiol, but healthcare professionals should keep in mind that antacids (containing aluminum), cholestyramine, or colestipol may decrease the absorption and effectiveness of ursodiol when administered concurrently. Space such medications at least 2 hours apart from ursodiol.

Side effects and adverse reactions

These include diarrhea, back pain, hair loss, dizziness, heartburn, nausea, vomiting, and psoriasis.

Warnings

Use with caution in patients with chronic liver impairment.

Contraindications

Avoid use in persons with ursodiol or bile acid hypersensitivity and gallstone complications.

Dosage and administration

The oral dose is 8 to 10 mg/kg daily, divided into two or three doses taken with meals. A pediatric dose has not been established.

DRUGS THAT AFFECT THE LOWER GASTROINTESTINAL TRACT

Bowel elimination is often a major concern of patients, particularly constipation in the older patient and diarrhea in children and immunosuppressed patients. Most of the agents that affect the lower gastrointestinal tract may be purchased OTC and therefore are discussed in Chapter 3.

Constipation is defined as difficult fecal evacuation as a result of degree of hardness and perhaps infrequent movements. Each person has regular bowel movements that may range from three per day to three per week. Chronic constipation is sometimes caused by organic disease, such as tumors; bowel obstruction; megacolon; metabolic abnormalities, such as diabetes mellitus or hypercalcemia; rectal disorders; diseases of the liver, gallbladder, or muscles; neurologic abnormalities, such as multiple sclerosis and Parkinson's disease; and pregnancy. Persons who suffer from disorders of the gastrointestinal tract frequently complain of constipation. On the other hand, many persons complain of constipation when no organic disease or lesion can be found.

When not a result of organic factors, constipation is generally attributable to faulty eating habits, a failure to respond to defecation impulses, insufficient fluid intake or exercise, or hospitalization, that is, off the usual routine and in a strange place. For example, a diet that provides inadequate bulk and residue will contribute to the development of constipation. The GI tract should function normally if fluids and residue are supplied in sufficient quantities to keep the stool formed but soft.

Another common cause of constipation is a failure to respond to the normal defecation impulses and insufficient time to permit the bowel to produce an evacuation. In addition, sedentary habits and insufficient exercise may be factors. Patients with impaired physical mobility may be constipated because of inactivity or an unnatural position for defecation, such as using a bedpan.

Another causative factor is the effect of drugs. The use of antacids, diuretics, morphine, tricyclic antidepressants, codeine, aluminum hydroxide, and anticholinergics often leads to constipation as a side effect. Constipation can also be a symptom of both functional and organic disorders, such as febrile states, psychosomatic disorders, anemias, and tension headaches. In addition, a less frequent cause of constipation may be atonic and hypotonic conditions of the musculature of the colon. These may result from habitual use of **cathartics,** substances that produce a liquid or fluid evacuation of the bowel.

LAXATIVES

Laxatives are drugs given to induce defecation. Laxatives may be classified according to their source, site of action, degree of action, or mechanism of action (see Chapter 3). Box 35-5 summarizes the types of laxatives discussed in Chapter 3. Only the monographs for the prescription laxatives Lactulose and GoLYTELY are in this section (Table 35-2).

BOX 35-5 | Selected Types of Laxatives

Saline laxatives retain and increase water content of feces by virtue of osmotic qualities.
Stimulant laxatives increase peristalsis in the colon by irritating intramural sensory nerve plexi endings in the mucosa.
Bulk laxatives absorb water and increase the volume, bulk, and moisture of nonabsorbable intestinal contents, thereby distending the bowel and initiating reflex bowel activity.
Intestinal lubricants mechanically lubricate feces to facilitate defecation.
Emollients, or fecal softening agents act as dispersing wetting agents, facilitating mixture of water and fatty substances within the fecal mass; when a homogenous mixture is produced, the feces become soft.
Hyperosmotic agents increase the intraluminal osmotic pressure in the bowel; because they are not absorbed, they draw water into the intestine, resulting in an increased volume that stimulates peristalsis.

lactulose [lak′ tyoo lose] (Chronulac, Duphalac ♣)

Lactulose is composed of galactose, fructose, and other sugars, and in the GI tract, the normal colonic bacteria *(Lactobacillus* and *Bacteroides, Escherichia coli,* and *Streptococcus faecalis)* metabolize lactulose syrup to organic acids, primarily lactic, acetic, and formic acids. These acids produce an osmotic effect, an increase in fluid accumulation, distention, peristalsis, and bowel movement within 24 to 72 hours. Lactulose is also used to decrease blood ammonia levels in persons with hepatic encephalopathy secondary to chronic liver disease.

Pharmacokinetics

After oral administration absorption is minimal; it is excreted via the kidneys. Lactulose syrup is used in patients with a history of chronic constipation that generally does not respond sufficiently to the bulk laxatives. It increases the number of bowel movements daily and the number of days on which bowel movements occur.

Drug interactions

The effectiveness of lactulose may be reduced if it is used concomitantly with an antibiotic that destroys the normal colonic bacteria. A nonabsorbed antibiotic such as neomycin destroys enough luminal colonic bacteria to interfere with lactulose. Most systemic, highly absorbable antibiotics do not affect the colonic bacteria in the lumen.

Side effects and adverse reactions

These include dose-related flatulence and intestinal cramps, increased thirst, diarrhea, and belching. Excessive doses may produce some diarrhea (hypokalemic) and nausea (caused by the sweet taste).

Contraindications

Avoid use in persons with a sensitivity to the laxative class, appendicitis, heart failure, hypertension, diabetes mellitus, intestinal obstruction, and undiagnosed rectal bleeding.

Dosage and administration

The adult dose is 1 to 2 tablespoons (15 to 30 ml) daily, increased in 5 and 10 ml increments to 60 ml daily after breakfast. Teach the patient to take a full glass of water with each dose, plus additional fluids during the day. If taste is a problem, suggest fruit juice or a citrus flavored carbonated beverage after taking a dose of medication. Lactulose produces its effects in 24 to 48 hours after a dose.

polyethylene glycol (PEG) and electrolytes (GoLYTELY)

This powder consists of a mixture of polyethlylene glycol (nonabsorbable osmotic substance) with sodium salts (sulfate, bicarbonate, and chloride) and potassium chloride that is isotonic with body fluids. Because it is isotonic, fluids and electrolytes will be neither absorbed nor secreted in the GI tract, thus it can be used in dehydrated persons and in individuals with renal impairment or cardiac disease.

The drug acts as an osmotic agent.

Indications

GoLYTELY is used for bowel cleansing before colonoscopy and before administration of a barium enema for radiologic examination.

Drug interactions

Do not administer this product with other oral medications or within an hour of its administration, as the other medications may be excreted without absorption.

Side effects and adverse reactions

These include a low incidence of nausea, vomiting, bloating, cramps, and abdominal fullness with GoLYTELY.

Warnings

Use with caution in patients with severe colitis, an impaired gag reflex, or a predisposition to aspiration or regurgitation or unconscious or semiconscious persons.

Contraindications

Avoid use in persons with a toxic megacolon or toxic colitis, paralytic ileus, perforated bowel, or a GI obstruction.

Dosage and administration

After reconstitution of the powder, refrigerating the solution improves palatability. The reconstituted solution must be used within 48 hours. GoLYTELY is given orally, 4 L at a rate of 240 ml every 10 minutes (rapidly swallowed). Fasting for 3 to 4 hours before use is necessary. Generally, a midmorning examination permits 3 hours for consumption, followed by a 1 hour period for bowel movement. Less stool is retained after its use, but the water or electrolyte balance does not change. Only clear liquids are permitted after its administration and before examination.

ANTIDIARRHEALS

This section focuses on the prescription drugs with a direct pharmacologic effect on the gastrointestinal tract. The antidiarrheal preparations that may be purchased OTC were discussed in Chapter 3. OTC antidiarrheals may contain the following ingredients: limited amounts of opiates; adsorbents such as bismuth salts, aluminum salts, attapulgite, kaolin, pectin, activated charcoal, and belladonna alkaloids (hyoscyamine, hyoscine, scopolamine, and atropine); and calcium salts. Inactive ingredients vary, but the healthcare professional should be aware of the variation in alcohol content (1.5% to 18%).

While antidiarrheal products have a warning stating that they are not to be used for longer than 2 days, not to be used if a fever is present, and not to be used in infants or children younger than 3 years of age, the physician may modify these instructions.

The intractable diarrhea of infancy is traditionally treated with clear liquids and gradual reintroduction of milk or formula, with the addition of oral elemental diets or total parenteral nutrition. The infant syndrome is described as loose stools, resulting in dehydration and a failure to thrive. Because a newborn's total body weight is usually 75% water, a 10% or greater weight loss may occur if the infant has severe diarrhea. If an infant has 8 to 10 bowel movements in a 24-hour period, the fluid loss may cause circulatory collapse and renal impairment. Diarrhea in infants should be considered serious enough to warrant referring the patient to a prescriber for evaluation.

Persistent diarrhea in the elderly can result in fluid and electrolyte loss, dehydration, and perhaps more serious medical complications. Such patients should be referred to their prescriber.

TABLE 35-2 Prescription Laxative Overview

	Lactulose Syrup/PEG 3350*
Disadvantages with repeated frequent (long-term) administration	Early, transient flatulence and cramps; nausea reported
Increases rate of transit in small bowel	Possibly
Causes net secretion of water and electrolytes in small bowel	No
Inhibits absorption in small bowel	Not reported
Increases mucosal permeability in small bowel	No
Causes mucosal damage in small bowel	No
Acts only in colon (not small bowel)	Yes
Indicated for long-term treatment	Yes: lactulose No: PEG
Examples of type	Chronulac (lactulose) CoLyte GoLYTELY (PEG 3350)
Physical or chemical property responsible for action	Colon-specific increase in stool water content and stool softening by increase in osmotic pressure (hyperosmotic) and colon acidification

*PEG 3350, Polyethylene glycol electrolyte solution.

Prescription Antidiarrheal Agents

Opioids

The opioids (codeine and paregoric) act by virtue of their constipative and sedative action. They lower the propulsive motility of the bowel, reduce pain, and relieve tenesmus (rectal spasms). The delay in transit time of food permits contact time of intestinal contents with the absorptive surface of the bowel, which increases the reabsorption of water and electrolytes and reduces stool frequency and net volume.

The anticholinergics and opium derivatives decrease the motility of the bowel. They should not be used when the cause of diarrhea is an invading organism (toxigenic bacteria or pseudomembranous enterocolitis) because these drugs decrease intestinal motility and subsequently lower excretion of the organisms and their toxins, resulting in epithelial penetration and multiplication of the organisms.

Codeine and paregoric cause depression and sedation. This factor must be considered if the patient is taking other CNS-depressant drugs because of the additive effects. The opiates are short acting; frequent administration (4- to 6-hour intervals) is needed to control the gastrointestinal smooth muscle function. The opiates are discussed in greater detail in Chapter 8.

opium tincture, deodorized

Tincture of opium, a hydroalcoholic (19% alcohol) solution, contains 10% opium, with an average dosage of 0.6 ml four times daily. This is a class II prescription under the Controlled Substances Act.

paregoric

Paregoric (camphorated opium tincture, although camphor is no longer required in the United States in this formulation) requires a prescription. It is a class III drug that is equivalent to 2 mg of morphine per 5 ml. It is important that the healthcare professional does not confuse opium tincture, deodorized (10 mg of morphine equivalent per 1 ml), and camphorated opium tincture (0.4 mg of morphine equivalent per 1 ml), because opium tincture, deodorized, has 25 times more morphine equivalent than camphorated opium tincture. Addiction liability has been reported with these preparations. When paregoric is combined with another drug, it becomes a class V product if the combination contains no more than 100 mg of opium or 25 ml of paregoric per 100 ml of the mixture. The adult antidiarrheal dose is 5 to 10 ml one to four times daily. The pediatric dosage is 0.25 to 0.5 ml/kg one to four times daily.

Synthetic Opioids

The synthetic opioids used to treat diarrhea include diphenoxylate and difenoxin.

diphenoxylate and atropine [dye fen ox′ i late] (Lomotil)

Diphenoxylate, a class V product, inhibits intestinal propulsive motility by acting directly on intestinal smooth muscles and thus decreases transit time.

Indications

It is indicated as an adjunct to fluid and electrolyte replacement for the treatment of acute and chronic diarrhea in adults. It is not recommended for use in children.

Pharmacokinetics

The onset of diphenoxylate effect is between 45 and 60 minutes, the half-life is 2.5 hours, and the duration of action is 3 to 4 hours. It is metabolized in the liver and excreted primarily by the kidneys.

Drug interactions

The following effects may occur when diphenoxylate and atropine is given with the drugs listed below:

Drug	Possible effect and management
Alcohol, CNS depressants	Concurrent use may result in increased CNS-depressant effects; if tricyclic antidepressants are used with atropine, potentiated anticholinergic effects may result.
Anticholinergics or other drugs with anticholinergic effects	An increase in anticholinergic effects may result. A dosage adjustment may be required.
Monoamine oxidase inhibitors (MAO inhibitor)	Concurrent use with diphenoxylate may result in a hypertensive crisis, while this combination with atropine may potentiate atropine's effects. Avoid or a potentially serious drug interaction may occur.
naltrexone (ReVia)	If naltrexone is administered to a person dependent on an opioid such as diphenoxylate, withdrawal symptoms may occur within 5 minutes and persists for up to 2 days. In addition, naltrexone will block the antidiarrheal effects of diphenoxylate; therefore combined drug usage is not recommended.

Color type indicates an unsafe drug combination.

Side effects and adverse reactions

These include drowsiness, dizziness, tachycardia, dry mouth, hyperthermia, abdominal distress, rash, agitation, numbness of hands or feet, gum swelling, trembling, and, infrequently, a toxic megacolon or paralytic ileus.

Warnings and contraindications

See the discussion of morphine in Chapter 8.

Dosage and administration

For adults and children 12 years of age and older, the dosage is one to two tablets orally three or four times daily.

difenoxin and atropine [dye fen ox′ in] (Motofen)

A third product in this category is difenoxin with atropine (Motofen). Difenoxin is the active metabolite derived from diphenoxylate, therefore it is effective at one fifth the dose of diphenoxylate.

Indications

It is indicated for the treatment of acute nonspecific diarrhea and acute exacerbations of chronic diarrhea.

Pharmacokinetics

Peak serum levels are reached between 40 to 60 minutes. It is metabolized in the liver and excreted primarily by the kidneys and in feces.

Drug interactions

See diphenoxylate.

Side effects and adverse reactions

These include dry mouth, difficult urination, blurred vision, dizziness, sedation, headache, insomnia, weakness, confusion, and, less frequently or rarely, toxic megacolon or paralytic ileus.

Warnings and contraindications

See morphine in Chapter 8.

Dosage and administration

The adult oral dose is two tablets initially, then one tablet after each loose stool or one tablet every 3 to 4 hours as needed. The maximum daily dose is eight tablets.

Adsorbents

Adsorbents are substances that take up or attach to (adsorb) another substance. They act by coating the wall of the GI tract, absorbing the bacteria or toxins causing the diarrhea, and passing them out with the stools. Examples of drugs in this class requiring a prescription are the anion exchange resins, colestipol, and cholestyramine.

cholestyramine [koe less′ tir a meen] (Questran)

Cholestyramine has a direct adsorbent affinity for acidic materials (e.g., bile acids). It is indicated as adjunctive therapy to diet in the treatment of hypercholesterolemia. Although not an FDA-approved indication, cholestyramine has been used to treat diarrhea. For additional information, see cholestyramine in Chapter 26.

SUMMARY

Numerous medications that affect the upper and lower gastrointestinal tract are reviewed in this chapter. Drugs affecting the stomach include antacids, antiflatulents, digestants, antiemetics, emetics, and agents used to treat peptic ulcers. Antacids are used to neutralize hydrochloric acid in the stomach, while digestants are used to enhance the process of digestion in instances of specific deficiencies. Antiemetics are given for the relief of nausea and vomiting, while emetics are used to induce vomiting, usually for drug overdoses or poisonings. The drugs used in the treatment of peptic ulcer include the cytoprotective agents to promote healing and the H_2 receptor antagonists to reduce gastric acid secretion. Several medications, chenodiol and ursodiol, are used to dissolve radiolucent cholesterol gallstones in high-risk patients.

Drugs affecting the lower gastrointestinal tract are primarily laxative or antidiarrheal medications. The primary goal in using these agents is to return the patient to a normal bowel pattern.

REVIEW QUESTIONS

1. Name and describe the three significant antacid drug interactions that should be avoided in clinical practice.
2. In some patients, two or three antiemetics may be necessary to prevent nausea and vomiting. Present a case or situation where this might be necessary.
3. Describe the mechanism of action and effects of metoclopramide in nausea and vomiting. Explain why some patients may experience extrapyramidal reactions with this medication.
4. Explain the use of ipecac syrup in a home emergency. When can it be used? When should it be avoided?

REFERENCES

Abramowicz M: Drugs for treatment of peptic ulcers, *Med Lett* 36(927):65-67, 1994.

American Hospital Formulary Service: *AHFS drug information ’98,* Bethesda, Md, 1998, American Society of Hospital Pharmacists.

Brunton LL: Agents affecting gastrointestinal water flux and motility; emesis and antiemetics; bile acids and pancreatic enzymes. In Hardman JG, Limbird LE, editors: *Goodman & Gilman’s the pharmacological basis of therapeutics,* ed 9, New York, 1996, McGraw-Hill.

Covington TR, editor: *Handbook of nonprescription drugs,* ed 11, Washington, DC, 1996, American Pharmaceutical Association.

Fedotin MS: *Helicobacter pylori*-associated ulcer disease: current treatment options, *Hosp Formul* 28(7):632-634, 636, 639-640, 1993.

Flynn AA: Oral health products. In Covington TR, editor: *Handbook of nonprescription drugs,* ed 11, Washington, DC, 1996, American Pharmaceutical Association.

Graham DY: Treatment of peptic ulcers caused by *Helicobacter pylori, N Engl J Med* 328(5):349-350, 1993.

Katzung BG: *Basic and clinical pharmacology,* ed 5, Norwalk, Conn, 1992, Appleton & Lange.

Koda-Kimble MA, Young LY: Nausea and vomiting. In Young LY, Koda-Kimble MA, editors: *Applied therapeutics: the clinical use of drugs,* ed 6, Vancouver, Wash, 1995, Applied Therapeutics, Inc.

Lichter I: Forum: which antiemetic? *J Palliat Care* 9(1):42, 1993.

Marcus R: Agents affecting calcification and bone turnover. In Young LY, Koda-Kimble MA, editors: *Applied therapeutics: the clinical use of drugs,* ed 6, Vancouver, Wash, 1995, Applied Therapeutics, Inc.

Olin BR: *Facts and comparisons.* Philadelphia, 1998, JB Lippincott.

Smith C: Upper gastrointestinal disorders. In In Young LY, Koda-Kimble MA, editors: *Applied therapeutics: the clinical use of drugs,* ed 6, Vancouver, Wash, 1995, Applied Therapeutics, Inc.

United States Pharmacopeial Convention: *USP DI: drug information for the health care professional,* ed 18, Rockville, Md, 1998, The Convention.

ADDITIONAL REFERENCES

Ahronheim JC: *Handbook of prescribing medications for geriatric patients,* Boston, 1992, Little, Brown.

Anderson KN et al, editors: *Mosby's medical, nursing, and allied health dictionary,* ed 5, St Louis, 1998, Mosby.

Cerda JJ et al: A revolution in peptic ulcer disease, *Patient Care* 28(9):18-22, 24, 25-28, 1994.

Hamacher DR: Mouthwash, *NARD J* 115(6):57, 1993.

Mosby: *Mosby's GenRx,* St Louis, 1998, Mosby.

Ofman J et al: Peptic ulcer disease dealing with H. pylori-induced ulceration, *Consultant* 34(7):987-990, 992-994, 1994.

Plezia PM et al: Randomized crossover comparison of high-dose intravenous metoclopramide versus a five-drug antiemetic regimen, *J Pain Sympt Manage* 5(2):101, 1990.

UNIT X

Drugs Affecting the Visual and Auditory Systems

CHAPTER 36

Overview of the Eye and Ophthalmic Drugs

CHAPTER FOCUS

The eye, the organ for sight, is a structure that captures light and transforms it into images. Any impairment of sight may result in visual disorders that reduce the individual's ability to function fully and/or independently in a complex environment. The early detection and treatment of many ophthalmic disorders may help to decrease visual impairment. The ophthalmic medications available have made a significant contribution to the treatment of eye disorders and the preservation of vision.

OBJECTIVES

After reading and studying this chapter, the student should be able to do the following:

1. *Define the key terms.*
2. *Describe the anatomy and physiology of the eye.*
3. *Name the four physiologic functions that protect the eye.*
4. *Contrast the functions and muscles involved with miosis and mydriasis.*
5. *Name and describe the mechanisms of action for the three primary medication groups used to treat glaucoma.*
6. *Discuss the systemic side effects and adverse reactions induced by ophthalmic drugs.*
7. *Review the indications and mechanisms of action for the ophthalmic anticholinergics, adrenergic agonists, and antiviral preparations.*

KEY TERMS

accommodation, (p. 512)
cataract, (p. 512)
cornea, (p. 512)
cycloplegia, (p. 513)
glaucoma, (p. 513)
miosis, (p. 512)
miotics, (p. 512)
mydriasis, (p. 512)

OVERVIEW OF THE EYE

The eye is the receptor organ for one of the most delicate and valuable senses—vision. Fig. 36-1 shows the parts of the eye. The eyeball has three layers or coats: the protective external layer (cornea and sclera), the middle layer (which contains the choroid, iris, and ciliary body), and the light-sensitive retina.

The eyeball is protected in a deep depression of the skull called the orbit. It is moved in the orbit by six small extraocular muscles.

The anterior covering of the eye is the **cornea.** The cornea is normally transparent, so it allows light to enter the eye. The cornea has no blood vessels and receives its nutrition from the aqueous humor and its oxygen supply by diffusion from the air and surrounding structures. The corneal surface consists of a thin layer of epithelial cells, which are quite resistant to infection. However, an abraded cornea is very susceptible to infection. The cornea is also supplied with 60 to 80 sensory fibers that elicit pain whenever the corneal epithelium is damaged. Seriously injured corneal tissue is replaced by scar tissue, which is usually not transparent. Increased intraocular pressure results in loss of transparency.

The sclera, which is continuous with the cornea, is nontransparent; it is the white fibrous envelope of the eye. The conjunctiva is the mucous membrane lining the anterior part of the sclera and the inner surfaces of each eyelid.

The iris gives the eye its brown, blue, gray, green, or hazel color. It surrounds the pupil; the sphincter and dilator muscles in the iris alter pupil size. The sphincter muscle, which encircles the pupil, is parasympathetically innervated; the dilator muscle, which runs radially from the pupil to the periphery of the iris, is sympathetically innervated. Contraction of the sphincter muscle, either alone or with relaxation of the dilator muscle, causes constriction of the pupil, or **miosis.** Contraction of the dilator muscle and relaxation of the sphincter muscle causes dilation of the pupil, or **mydriasis** (Fig. 36-2). Drugs producing miosis (**miotics**) act by (1) interfering with cholinesterase activity or (2) acting like acetylcholine at receptor sites in the sphincter muscle. Drugs producing mydriasis (mydriatics) act by (1) interfering with the action of acetylcholine or (2) stimulating sympathetic or adrenergic receptors. Pupil constriction normally occurs in bright light or when the eye is focusing on nearby objects. Pupil dilation normally occurs in dim light or when the eye is focusing on distant objects.

The lens is situated behind the iris. It is a transparent mass of uniformly arranged fibers encased in a thin elastic capsule. Its protein concentration is higher than that of any other tissue of the body. The function of the lens is to ensure that the image on the retina is in sharp focus. The lens does this by changing shape (**accommodation**) to adjust to variations in distance. This occurs readily in young persons, but with age the lens becomes more rigid. The ability to focus on close objects is then lost, and the near point (the closest point that can be seen clearly) recedes.

With age, the lens may also lose its transparency and become opaque; this is known as a **cataract.** Unless it can be treated or removed surgically, blindness can occur. However, if the opaque (cataract) portion is located peripherally in the lens, vision is not compromised.

The lens has suspensory ligaments called zonular fibers around its edge, which connect with the ciliary body. Their

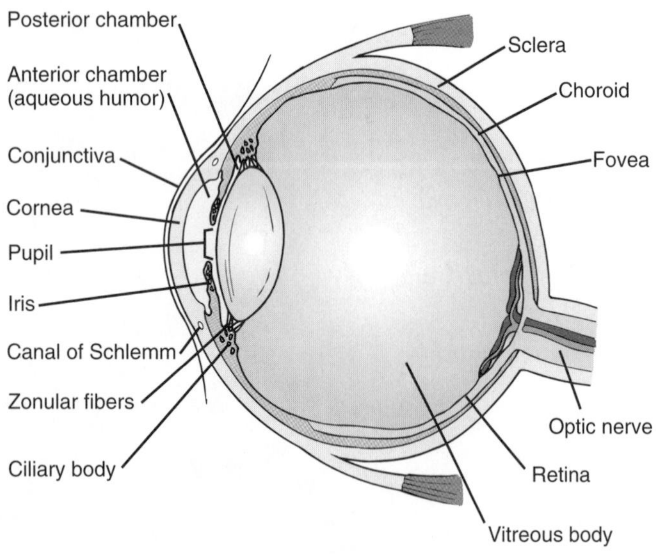

FIGURE 36-1
Parts of the eye.

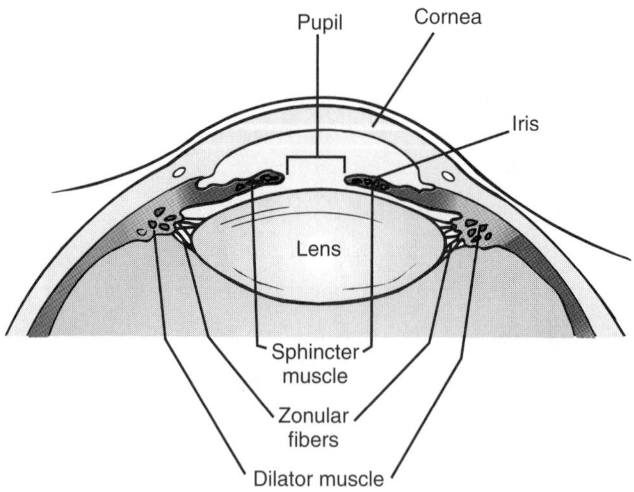

FIGURE 36-2
Accommodation and pupillary alterations. When zonular fibers contract, the pupil dilates, resulting in sharp distant vision and blurred near vision (unaccommodated eye). Parasympathetic stimulation accommodates the eye for near vision; the pupil constricts in response to contraction of the sphincter muscle. The zonular fibers are relaxed. Pupillary diameter: Constriction (miosis): contraction of sphincter muscle (parasympathetic stimulation) alone or with relaxation of dilator muscle. Dilation (mydriasis): contraction of dilator muscle (sympathetic stimulation) alone or with relaxation of dilator muscle.

tension helps to change the shape of the lens. In the unaccommodated eye the ciliary muscle is relaxed and the zonular fibers are taut. When zonular fibers contract, the pupil dilates, resulting in sharp distant vision and blurred near vision (unaccommodated eye). Parasympathetic stimulation accommodates the eye for near vision; the pupil constricts in response to contraction of the sphincter muscle. The zonular fibers are relaxed.

Accommodation depends on two factors: (1) ciliary muscle contraction and (2) the ability of the lens to assume a more biconvex shape when tension on the ligaments is relaxed. The ciliary muscle is innervated by parasympathetic fibers. Paralysis of the ciliary muscle is termed **cycloplegia.**

Aqueous humor is formed by the ciliary body. It bathes and feeds the lens, iris, and posterior surface of the cornea. After it is formed, it flows forward between the lens and the iris into the anterior chamber. It drains out of the eye through drainage channels located near the junction of the cornea and sclera. A trabecular meshwork called the canals of Schlemm drains the aqueous humor into the venous system of the eye (see Fig. 36-1).

The retina contains nerve endings plus the rods and cones that function as visual sensory receptors. It is connected to the brain by the optic nerve, which leaves the orbit through a bony canal in the posterior wall.

Eyelashes, eyelids, blinking, and tears all serve to protect the eye. Each eye has about 200 eyelashes. A blink reflex occurs whenever a foreign body touches the eyelashes. The lids close quickly to prevent the foreign substance from entering the eye. Blinking, which is bilateral, occurs every few seconds during waking hours. It keeps the corneal surface free of mucus and spreads the lacrimal fluid evenly over the cornea. Tears are secreted by lacrimal glands and contain lysozyme, a mucolytic enzyme with bactericidal action. Tears provide lubrication for lid movements. They wash away noxious agents. By forming a thin film over the cornea, tears provide it with a good optical surface. Tear fluid is lost by evaporation and by draining into two small ducts (the lacrimal canaliculi) at the inner corners of the upper and lower eyelids.

OPHTHALMIC DRUGS

Drugs used to treat eye disorders can be divided into three major groups: the antiglaucoma agents, the mydriatics and cycloplegics, and the antiinfective/antiinflammatory agents. There are many eye preparations available, including ophthalmic diagnostic products, enzymes, irrigating solutions, eye washes, and hyperosmolar preparations. This chapter discusses the major groups and selected other eye preparations, along with their major dosage and administration considerations and side effects and adverse reactions.

ANTIGLAUCOMA AGENTS

Glaucoma is an eye disease characterized chiefly by abnormally elevated intraocular pressure (IOP) that may result from excessive production of aqueous humor or diminished ocular fluid outflow. Increased pressure, if sufficiently high and persistent, may lead to irreversible blindness. Although it is primarily a disease of middle age, occurring in approximately 2% of all persons 40 years of age and older, it has also been diagnosed in younger adults and children. There are three major types of glaucoma: primary, secondary, and congenital.

Primary glaucoma includes angle-closure (acute congestive) glaucoma and open-angle (chronic simple) glaucoma (Fig. 36-3). Persons with angle-closure glaucoma have closure of the angle of the anterior chamber, possibly because of a physiologic or anatomic predisposition. Drugs are needed to control the acute attack associated with angle-closure glaucoma, followed usually by surgery, such as iridectomy or laser surgery. Open or wide-angle glaucoma is more common, occurring in approximately 90% of the individuals with primary glaucoma. The increased IOP is secondary to an increased production of aqueous humor or a decreased outflow caused by degenerative changes in the outflow system. It has a gradual insidious onset, and its control depends on drug therapy or perhaps a peripheral iridectomy. Secondary glaucoma may result from previous eye disease or may follow cataract extraction (Abel, 1995). Therapy for secondary glaucoma usually involves drugs, while congenital glaucoma requires surgical treatment. See the box for Food and Drug Administration (FDA) pregnancy safety classifications.

Primary medications used to treat glaucoma include beta-adrenergic blocking agents, cholinergics, and sympathomimetics; selection of a drug is determined largely by the requirements and individual response of the person.

Beta-Adrenergic Blocking Agents

The beta-adrenergic blocking agents include betaxolol (Betoptic), carteolol (Ocupress), levobunolol (Betagan C Cap), metipranolol (OptiPranol), and timolol (Timoptic). Betaxolol is a cardioselective ($beta_1$) blocking agent, whereas all the other beta blockers are noncardioselective (i.e., they block both $beta_1$ and $beta_2$ adrenergic receptors). These agents work alone or in combination with other drugs to decrease the production of aqueous humor, thus reducing IOP in open-angle glaucoma. The exact mechanism of action for these agents, though, is unknown.

Timolol is also used to treat secondary glaucoma in selected patients. Betaxolol is indicated for the treatment of open-angle glaucoma and ocular hypertension and may be a drug of choice for patients with pulmonary disease because of its selective $beta_1$ blocking effects, although the patient should be monitored for possible respiratory difficulties.

Side effects and adverse reactions

These are primarily local reactions, such as burning, stinging, or eye irritation. Rare effects include eye inflammation, visual disturbance, pruritus, or allergic reaction.

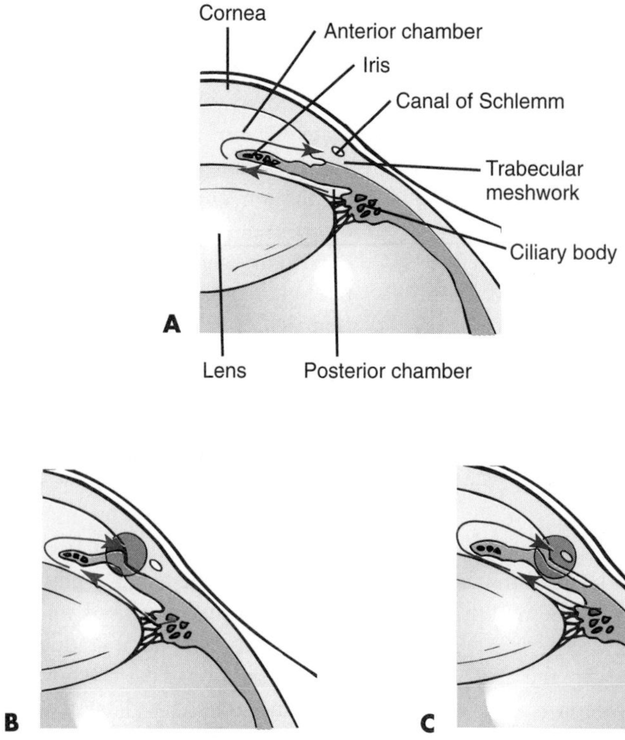

FIGURE 36-3
Main structures of the eye and enlargement of the canal of Schlemm showing aqueous flow in normal **(A)**, angle-closure **(B)**, and open-angle glaucoma **(C)**.

PREGNANCY SAFETY

Category	Drug
B	cromolyn, dipivefrin, erythromycin, lodoxamide, tobramycin
C	acetazolamide, atropine, betaxolol, carbachol, carteolol, cyclopentolate, dichlorphenamide, dorzolamide, echothiophate, epinephrine, homatropine, idoxuridine, lantanoprost, levocabastine, levobunolol, methazolamide, metipranolol, naphazoline, natamycin, norfloxacin, phenylephrine, pilocarpine, polymyxin B, proparacaine, sulfonamides, tetracaine, timolol, trifluridine, vidarabine
X	demecarium, isoflurophate
Unclassified	chymotrypsin, gentamycin, hydroxyamphetamine, oxymetazoline, scopolamine, tetrahydrozoline, tropicamide

These agents can be systemically absorbed to cause bradycardia or tachycardia, confusion, insomnia, weakness, wheezing, respiratory difficulties, depression, ataxia, edema of lower extremities, nausea, and vomiting. Hallucinations have been reported with timolol only. Table 36-1 lists beta-adrenergic blocking agents, pharmacokinetics, and dosing information.

Cholinergic Agents

Cholinergic medications or miotics, so called because they cause pupillary constriction, are topically applied agents useful in treating open-angle and angle-closure glaucoma. Cholinergic miotics (direct acting) are chemically related to acetylcholine, the neurotransmitter that mediates nerve impulse transmission at all cholinergic or parasympathetic nerve sites. Applied topically to the eye, cholinergic drugs cause contraction of the sphincter muscle of the iris, resulting in pupil constriction (miosis), and contraction of the ciliary muscle attached to the trabecular meshwork, thus opening the spaces in the meshwork and increasing the outflow of aqueous humor. The ciliary muscle effect leaves the eye in accommodation of near vision.

Anticholinesterase drugs (indirect acting) such as carbachol (Carboptic) and pilocarpine (Isopto Carpine) inhibit the enzymatic destruction of acetylcholine by inactivating cholinesterase. This permits acetylcholine to act on the iris sphincter and ciliary muscles, producing pupil constriction (miosis) and ciliary muscle contraction (accommodation).

The irreversible anticholinesterase drugs, (echothiophate [Phospholine Iodide] and isoflurophate [Floropryl]), form stable complexes with cholinesterase and thus irreversibly impair the destructive function of the enzyme. Destruction of acetylcholine then depends on synthesis of new enzymes.

TABLE 36-1 Beta-Adrenergic Blocking Agents: Pharmacokinetics and Dosing

Drug	Onset of Action (hr)	Peak Effect (hr)	Duration of Action (hr)	Usual Adult Dosage
betaxolol (Betoptic)	0.5	2	12	0.25%, 0.5%: instill 1 drop twice daily
carteolol (Ocupress)	N/A	2	6-8	1%: instill 1 drop twice daily
levobunolol (Betagan C Cap B.I.D.)	1	2-6	Up to 24	0.25%: instill 1 drop 1-2 times daily; 0.5%: instill 1 drop daily
metipranolol (OptiPranolol)	0.5	2	24	0.3%: instill 1 drop twice daily
timolol (Timoptic)	0.5	1-2	Up to 24	0.25%, 0.5%: instill 1 drop 1-2 times daily

N/A, not available.

TABLE 36-2 Cholinergic Agents: Pharmacokinetics and Dosing

Drug	Onset of Action (hr)	Peak Effect (hr)	Duration of Action (hr)	Usual Adult Dosage
Miotics—Direct Acting				
carbachol (Carboptic)	0.25	Miosis: 2-5 min IOP: within 4	24	0.75%-3%: 1 drop topically 3 times daily
pilocarpine (Isopto Carpine)	Up to 0.5	1-1.25	4-8	0.25%-4%: 1 drop topically up to 4 times daily
Miotics—Cholinesterase Inhibitors				
demecarium (Humorsol)	Miosis: <1 IOP: 4	2 Within 24	24-48	0.125%-0.25%: 1 drop topically once or twice daily
echothiophate (Phospholine Iodide)	Same as demecarium			0.03%-0.25%: 1 drop topically once or twice daily
isoflurophate (Floropryl)	Same as demecarium			0.025% ointment: thin strip topically once every 3 days to 3 times daily

Demecarium (Humorsol) is more toxic than the other agents in this category, so it is not as commonly used. Although it is a reversible inhibitor, its prolonged action has results similar to that of the irreversible inhibitors.

The cholinesterase inhibitors, though, are usually reserved for persons that have an inadequate response to the first-line agents such as beta blockers, cholinergics (pilocarpine), and sympathomimetics (epinephrine).

Side effects and adverse reactions of cholinergic agents include visual blurring, irritation, myopia, ciliary spasm, brow pain, and headache resulting from stimulation of accommodative ancillary muscles. Miosis also makes it difficult to adjust quickly to changes in illumination. This may be serious in elderly persons, since their light adaptation and visual acuity are often reduced. Nighttime is particularly hazardous for these individuals.

Cysts of the iris, synechiae, retinal detachments, obstruction of tear drainage, and even cataracts may develop with prolonged use, especially with the long-acting anticholinesterases. Generally side effects of direct-acting cholinergic agents are less severe and occur less frequently than those caused by anticholinesterase agents. Systemic side effects include salivation, nausea, vomiting, diarrhea, precipitation of asthmatic attacks, a fall in blood pressure, and other symptoms of parasympathetic stimulation. Table 36-2 lists the pharmacokinetics and dosing of cholinergic agents.

Sympathomimetic Agents

The primary sympathomimetic agents are dipivefrin (Pro-Pine), which is converted to epinephrine by enzyme hydrolysis in the eye, and epinephrine, a direct acting sympathomimetic agent. Dipivefrin's chemical modification results in a more lipophilic compound that facilitates absorption and penetration through the cornea into the anterior chamber of the eye. The penetration and absorption of dipivefrin is greater than that of epinephrine. The mechanism of action is unknown, although it appears that they lower IOP by decreasing aqueous humor production and increasing its outflow. They are indicated for the treatment of open-angle glaucoma.

Side effects and adverse reactions are rarely troublesome; they include burning, stinging or eye irritation, headache, brow pain, and watering of the eyes. The signs and symptoms of systemic absorption include tachycardia, palpitations, hypertension, increased sweating, tremors, and lightheadedness.

Epinephrine's onset of action is within 1 hour, the peak effect is reached in 4 to 8 hours, and the duration of action is up to 24 hours. Available in 0.1% to 2% strengths, the usual adult dose is 1 drop topically, once or twice daily. Dipivefrin has an onset of action within 30 minutes and reaches its peak effect in 1 hour. The pediatric and adult dose is 1 drop (0.1%) topically every 12 hours.

TABLE 36-3 Antiglaucoma Agents: Pharmacokinetics and Dosing

Drug	Onset of Action (hr)	Peak Effect (hr)	Duration of Action (hr)	Usual Adult Dosage
Carbonic Anhydrase Inhibitors				
Oral				
acetazolamide (Diamox)				
capsules	2	8-12	18-24	500 mg PO twice daily, morning and evening
tablets	1-1.5	2-4	8-12	250 mg PO 1-4 times daily
IV	2 min	15 min	4-5	500 mg IV
dichlorphenamide (Daranide)	0.5-1	2-4	6-12	100-200 mg initially, then 100 mg every 12 hr; maintenance dose 25-50 mg 1-3 times daily
methazolamide (Neptazane)	2-4	6-8	10-18	50-100 mg 2 or 3 times daily
Eyedrops				
dorzolamide (Trusopt)	N/A	N/A	N/A	2% solution: 1 drop 3 times daily
Prostaglandin Agonist				
latanoprost (Xalatan)	N/A	2	N/A	1 drop in affected eye(s) in the evening

N/A, not available.

Carbonic Anhydrase Inhibitor Agents

The oral carbonic anhydrase inhibitors include acetazolamide (Diamox), dichlorphenamide (Daranide), and methazolamide (Neptazane). Acetazolamide, the most widely used drug of this class, is the focus of this discussion. The carbonic anhydrase inhibitors are sulfonamides (nonbacteriostatic) with an undetermined mechanism of action, but they appear to lower IOP by decreasing the aqueous production to about half of its baseline measurement. The topical sulfonamide dorsolamide, a carbonic anhydrase inhibitor, is systemically absorbed to produce its antiglaucoma effects. The 2% eyedrop solution three times a day is approximately equivalent in effect to an oral 2 mg dose twice a day.

Drug interactions

The following effects may occur when the carbonic anhydrase inhibitor agents are given with the drugs listed below:

Drug	Possible effect and management
Amphetamines, quinidine, and mecamylamine (Inversine)	Carbonic anhydrase inhibitors decrease excretion of these drugs because of alkalinization of the urine, which may result in a prolonged duration of drug action and, possibly, increased side effects. Avoid concurrent use of mecamylamine. Monitor other agents closely because dosage adjustments are usually necessary.
methenamine (Mandelamine)	Alkalinization of the urine prevents conversion of methenamine to formaldehyde, thus reducing the effectiveness of methenamine. Concurrent drug administration is not recommended.

The oral drugs are used for the treatment of open-angle, secondary, and angle-closure glaucoma while the eyedrop is indicated for open-angle glaucoma and ocular hypertension. Side effects with the oral agents include diarrhea, discomfort, diuresis, anorexia, metallic taste in the mouth, nausea, vomiting, tingling or numbness (paresthesia) of fingers, hands, and toes, and weight loss. Prescriber intervention is necessary if the patient has the signs and symptoms of acidosis, blood dyscrasias, or hypokalemia. Eyedrop side effects include topical allergic reaction of the eye, bitter taste in the mouth, photosensitivity, and superficial punctate keratitis. Table 36-3 lists the pharmacokinetics and dosing of antiglaucoma agents.

Prostaglandin Agonist

Latanoprost (Xalatan) is the first prostaglandin agonist approved to treat open-angle glaucoma and ocular hypertension. It reduces IOP by increasing aqueous humor outflow.

Side effects and adverse reactions include blurred vision, burning and stinging, itching, photophobia, and conjunctival hyperemia. Systemic effects include upper respiratory tract type infection, muscle, joint, back or chest pain, angina, and rash. Patients should be informed that this drug can cause an increase in iris pigmentation (brown).

Osmotic Agents

Osmotic agents are given intravenously or orally to reduce IOP. These agents generally do not cross the blood aqueous barrier into the anterior chamber of the eye and are rarely found in ocular humor. The osmotic agents are discussed in Chapter 28.

MYDRIATIC AND CYCLOPLEGIC AGENTS

Adrenergic agonists cause pupil dilation (mydriasis), while cycloplegic agents paralyze ciliary muscle (accommodation). These agents are primarily used for diagnosis of oph-

TABLE 36-4 Anticholinergic Agents: Pharmacokinetics and Dosing

Drug	Time to Maximal Mydriasis (min)	Recovery (days)	Time to Maximal Cycloplegia (min)	Recovery (days)	Usual Adult Dose
atropine	30-40	7-10	60-180	6-12	1%: 1 drop
cyclopentolate	30-60	1	25-75	6-24 hr	0.5%-2%: 1 drop
homatropine	40-60	1-3	30-60	1-3	2%-5%: 1 drop
scopolamine	20-130	3-7	30-60	3-7	0.25%: 1 drop
tropicamide	20-40	6 hr	30	6 hr	1%: 1 drop

	Indication	Usual Adult Dosage
Combination Eyedrops		
cyclopentolate and phenylephrine (Cyclomydril)	Mydriasis	1 drop in each eye every 5-10 min as necessary; do not exceed 3 doses
scopolamine and phenylephrine (Murocoll 2)	Mydriasis, cycloplegia, and posterior synechiae in iritis	Mydriasis: 1-2 drops in eye, repeated in 5 min if necessary
tropicamide and hydroxyamphetamine (Paremyd)	Mydriasis with partial cycloplegia	1-2 drops in conjunctival sac

From Moroi, Lichter, 1996; Olin, 1998; USP DI, 1998.

thalmic disorders. The effects of these agents depend on the patient's age, race, and color of iris. For example, mydriatic agents evoke less of a response in persons with heavily pigmented (dark) irides than in those with lighter-pigmented (blue) irides. Thus blacks tend to respond less to the agents than whites. Anticholinergic agents produce both mydriasis and cycloplegia via blockade of muscarinic receptors. Contraction of the iris sphincter leads to relaxation and possibly, an increase in IOP. This discussion focuses on anticholinergic agents and adrenergic agonists.

Anticholinergic Agents

Anticholinergic agents are indicated for the treatment of inflammations such as uveitis and keratitis to relieve ocular pain by relaxing inflamed intraocular muscles. They are also used for relaxation of ciliary muscle for accurate measurement of refractive errors, which permits proper lens determination for eyeglasses, and for preoperative and postoperative use in intraocular surgery.

Local side effects and adverse reactions include stinging or an increase in IOP. With chronic use, allergic lid reactions, red eye, and various eye irritation injuries may be induced. If absorbed systemically, mild to serious adverse reactions may result, such as dryness of the mouth, inhibition of sweating, flushing, tachycardia, ataxia, hallucinations, psychiatric and behavioral problems, fever, delirium, convulsions, respiratory depression, and coma. Deaths have been recorded in children after systemic absorption.

Pupillary dilation from either local or systemic administration can precipitate acute glaucoma in predisposed persons. If unrecognized or untreated, this can result in blindness. Table 36-4 lists the pharmacokinetics and dosing of anticholinergic agents.

Combination eyedrops include Cyclomydril, Murocoll 2, and Paremyd. These agents in combination produce a greater mydriasis than either drug alone. Table 36-4 gives indications and dosage.

Adrenergic Agonist Agents

Topical adrenergic agents mimic (direct acting) or potentiate (indirect acting) the action of epinephrine on the dilator muscle of the iris resulting in mydriasis and decreased congestion of conjunctival blood vessels. The primary adrenergic drugs used in ophthalmology include epinephrine (Epifrin, Glaucon), phenylephrine (Ak-Nefrin, Prefrin, Neo-Synephrine), oxymetazoline (Ocuclear), hydroxyamphetamine (Paredrine), naphazoline (Allerest, VasoClear), and tetrahydrozoline (Murine Plus, Visine).

Adrenergic drugs applied topically to the eye elicit the following sympathetic responses: vasoconstriction, pupil dilation, an increase in outflow of aqueous humor plus a decrease in aqueous humor formation, and relaxation of the ciliary muscle. Exactly how these effects are produced remains uncertain, but there is some evidence that alpha-adrenergic receptors are present in the outflow mechanism of the eye. When stimulated, they increase outflow of aqueous humor. It has also been shown experimentally that vasoconstriction decreases the rate of aqueous humor formation (Abel, 1995).

Adrenergic drugs are used to treat wide-angle glaucoma and glaucoma secondary to uveitis, to produce mydriasis for ocular examination, and to relieve congestion and hyperemia. Adrenergic drugs are contraindicated in the treatment of narrow-angle glaucoma or abraded cornea because dilation of the pupil will further restrict ocular fluid outflow, which may cause an acute attack of glaucoma. See the discussion of pharmacokinetics of adrenergic agents in Chapter 16.

Serious systemic side effects from these drugs are unusual and include local pain and brow ache. Systemic absorption, though, is a concern, especially in patients with cardiovascular disease because tachycardia and elevated blood pressure can occur with these agents. Sweating, tremors, and confusion may also occur. As with other ophthal-

TABLE 36-5 Adrenergic Ophthalmic Agents

Drug	Duration of Action (hr)	Market Availability	Usual Adult Dosage
epinephrine (Epifrin, Glaucon)	V+ <1 IPO 12-24	Rx	0.5%-2%: 1 drop once or twice daily
hydroxyamphetamine (Paredrine)	1-3	Rx	1%: 1 or 2 drops for dilation of pupil
naphazoline			
(Allerest, VasoClear)	3-4	OTC	0.012%-0.03%: 1 drop up to 4 times daily
(Albalon, Vasocon)	3-4	Rx	0.1%: 1 drop every 3-4 hr as necessary
oxymetazoline (OcuClear)	4-6	OTC	0.025%: 1 drop every 6 hr as necessary
phenylephrine			
(Ak-Nefrin, Prefrin)	0.5-1.5	OTC	0.12%: 1 or 2 drops up to 4 times daily as necessary
(Neo-Synephrine)	1-7	Rx	2.5%, 10%: 1 drop as necessary
tetrahydrozoline (Murine Plus, Visine)	1-4	OTC	0.05%: 1 or 2 drops up to 4 times daily

From Olin, 1998; USP DI, 1998.
V+, vasoconstriction; IOP, reduction in intraocular pressure; Rx, prescription.

mic drugs, the potential for systemic drug interactions exists if significant absorption occurs.

Apraclonidine (Iopidine) reduces IOP in patients with glaucoma and also after laser trabeculoplasty or iridotomy. This drug is a selective alpha agonist that does not have any local anesthetic action.

The onset of action is usually within 60 minutes; maximum IOP reduction occurs within 3 to 5 hours. After topical application, apraclonidine is absorbed and may induce systemic side effects and adverse reactions such as stomach pain, diarrhea, vomiting, and dry mouth. Ophthalmic side effects include burning, pruritus, dryness, blurred vision, conjunctival blanching, and mydriasis. Table 36-5 lists adrenergic ophthalmic drugs, duration of action, market availability, and usual adult dosage.

ANTIINFECTIVE/ANTIINFLAMMATORY AGENTS

To treat ocular infections, the drug of choice and the dose required should be determined by laboratory isolation of the offending organism. The initial culture from the infected area is obtained before any ophthalmic agent is applied. However, treatment is not withheld if the time required to make these determinations may cause increased severity of infection and if the type of infection (e.g., most cases of conjunctivitis, which tend to be self-limiting) does not warrant the expense of laboratory analysis.

Prophylactic use of antiinfective/antiinflammatory agents in general is useless, wasteful, and potentially dangerous because a large proportion of the inflammatory diseases seen in ophthalmology are caused by viruses or other agents that are not susceptible to any currently available antiinfective agents. Systemic medications that can induce ocular side effects need to be considered before an antiinfective or antiinflammatory agent is introduced. See Table 36-6 for drugs that induce ocular side effects.

Most antiinfective agents do not readily penetrate the eye when applied. However, some drugs will penetrate the inflamed eye when the blood-aqueous barrier is decreased by injury or inflammation. Topically applied antiinfective agents can cause sensitivity reactions (stinging, itching, angioneurotic edema, urticaria, and dermatitis). Individuals sensitized to one drug may show cross reactions to chemically related drugs. Topical application of antiinfective agents may also interfere with the normal flora of the eye, which may encourage growth of other organisms.

Eye infections require prompt treatment to help prevent spread of infection because severe infections may damage the eye and impair vision. Solutions are preferred for treatment of eye infections, since ointment bases often tend to interfere with healing.

Antibacterials

Antibiotics

To avoid possible sensitization to systemic antiinfective drugs and to discourage development of resistant strains of offending organisms, the antibiotic of choice is not given systemically. Rather, these agents are administered topically, subconjunctivally, or intrauveally. Selection of an antibiotic for ocular infection is based on (1) clinical experience, (2) the nature and sensitivity of the organisms most commonly causing the condition, (3) the disease itself, (4) the sensitivity and response of the patient, and (5) laboratory results.

Some of the common ocular infections treated with antibiotics include the following:

- *Conjunctivitis.* Acute inflammation of the conjunctiva resulting from bacterial invasion or viral infection. It is a common sign in severe colds. "Pink eye" is the acute contagious epidemic form of conjunctivitis usually caused by *Haemophilus* organisms. Symptoms include redness and burning of the eye, lacrimation, itching, and, at times photophobia. Conjunctivitis is usually self-limiting. The eye should be protected from light.
- *Hordeolum (sty).* An acute localized infection of the eyelash follicles and the glands of the anterior lid margin, resulting in the formation of a small abscess or cyst.
- *Chalazion.* Infection of the meibomian (sebaceous)

TABLE 36-6 **Ocular Side Effects Induced by Systemic Medications**

Drug	*Possible Ocular Side Effect Induced*
allopurinol	Retinal hemorrhage, exudative lesions
aspirin	Allergic dermatitis including keratitis and conjunctivitis
barbiturates	Nystagmus
busulfan	Cataracts
cannabis, marijuana	Nystagmus, conjunctivitis, double vision
chloral hydrate	Eyelid edema, conjunctivitis, miosis
chloroquine	Lenticular and corneal opacity, retinopathy
clomiphene citrate	Blurred vision, light flashes
clonidine	Miosis
corticosteroids	Cataracts, increased intraocular pressure, papilledema
diazoxide	Oculogyric crisis
digitalis glycosides	Scotomas, optic neuritis
ethyl alcohol	Nystagmus
guanethidine	Miosis, ptosis, blurred vision
hydralazine	Lacrimation, blurred vision
ibuprofen	Altered color vision, blurred vision
indomethacin	Mydriasis, retinopathy
isoniazid	Optic neuritis
lithium carbonate	Exophthalmos
nitroglycerin	Transient elevation in intraocular pressure
opiates	Miosis, nystagmus
phenothiazines	Corneal and conjunctival deposits, cataracts, retinopathy, oculogyric crisis
phenytoin	Nystagmus
quinine	Blurring of vision, optic neuritis, blindness (reversible)
thiazide diuretics	Acute transient myopia, yellow coloring of vision
vincristine	Ptosis, paresis of extraocular muscles
vitamin A overdose or toxicity	Papilledema, increased intraocular pressure
vitamin D toxicity	Calcium deposits in cornea

glands of the eyelids. A hard cyst may form from blockage of the ducts.

- *Blepharitis.* Inflammation of the margins of the eyelid resulting from bacterial infection or allergy. Symptoms are crusting, irritation of the eye, and red and edematous lid margins.
- *Keratitis.* Corneal inflammation caused by bacterial infection; herpes simplex keratitis is caused by viral infection.
- *Uveitis.* Infection of the uveal tract, or the vascular layer of the eye, which includes the iris, ciliary body, and choroid.
- *Endophthalmitis.* Inner eye structure inflammation caused by bacteria.

Antibiotic ophthalmic preparations include bacitracin, chloramphenicol, ciprofloxacin, erythromycin, gentamicin, norfloxacin, ofloxacin, polymyxin B, and tobramycin. Combination preparations usually contain various combinations of these ingredients and/or neomycin, gramicidin, oxytetracycline, or trimethoprim. The following are examples of selected antibiotic ophthalmic products.

triple antibiotic ophthalmic ointment

(neomycin, polymyxin B sulfate, and bacitracin ophthalmic ointment) [nee oh mye′ sin, pol i mix′ in, bass i tray′ sin] (Mycitracin, Neosporin)

Bacitracin is rarely used systemically because of its nephrotoxic effects. It is particularly useful in treating surface superficial infections caused by gram-positive bacteria (it inhibits protein synthesis). Bacitracin does penetrate the conjunctiva or the cornea slightly, but in therapeutic amounts it is nonirritating to the eye, is excreted in the nasolacrimal system, and produces no systemic effects.

A broader spectrum of antimicrobial activity is produced when bacitracin is used in combination with other antibiotics than when it is used alone. Although all three of these agents have been or are available as single ophthalmic drugs, reports of sensitization to the individual drug have somewhat limited their usefulness. The combination dosage form provides a bactericidal effect against many gram-positive and gram-negative organisms. It is indicated for the treatment of superficial ocular infections caused by susceptible organisms. A small amount (1 cm) of ointment is usually applied to the conjunctiva every 3 to 4 hours.

chloramphenicol [klor am fen′ i kole] (Chloroptic)

A bacteriostatic agent, chloramphenicol prevents peptide bond formation and protein synthesis in a wide variety of gram-positive and gram-negative organisms. Thus it is an extremely useful drug for superficial intraocular infections.

Side effects are rare. Burning and stinging on instillation have been reported. Irreversible aplastic anemia has not been reported with this form of chloramphenicol, although it would be prudent to monitor for blood dyscrasias.

When treating adults, apply a thin strip of ointment (1% solution) to the conjunctiva every 3 hours or more often if necessary. The solution dosage for adults is 1 drop into the conjunctiva every 3 hours for several days. Prolonged use is not recommended with this drug as it has been implicated in the development of aplastic anemia after continuous usage. See Table 36-7 for systemic effects from a variety of ophthalmic agents.

erythromycin [er ith roe mye′ sin] (Ilotycin)

Erythromycin ophthalmic ointment is a bacteriostatic agent, but in high concentrations against very susceptible organisms it may be bactericidal. It is indicated for the treatment of neonatal conjunctivitis caused by *Chlamydia trachomatis* and for the prevention of ophthalmia neonatorum (against *Neisseria gonorrhoeae* or *C trachomatis*) and other ocular infections caused by susceptible organisms.

Eye irritation not present before therapy is rarely reported with this drug. For adults and children with ocular

TABLE 36-7 Ophthalmic Drugs: Adverse Systemic Effects

Ophthalmic Drug	Reported Adverse Effect
Antimicrobial Agents	
chloramphenicol eyedrops	Aplastic anemia
sulfacetamide eyedrops	Stevens-Johnson syndrome, systemic lupus erythematosus
Anticholinergic Drugs	
atropine eyedrops	Tachycardia, elevated temperature, fever, delirium
cyclopentolate	Convulsions, hallucinations
scopolamine eyedrops	Acute psychosis
Antiglaucoma Medications	
beta blocking agents (timolol)	Bradycardia, syncope, low blood pressure, asthmatic attack, congestive heart failure, hallucinations, loss of appetite, headaches, nausea, weakness, depression
anticholinesterase (echothiophate)	Asthmatic attack, systemic cholinergic effects
parasympathomimetic (pilocarpine)	Nausea, stomach pain, increased sweating, salivation, tremors, bradycardia, lightheadedness
Adrenergic Medications	
phenylephrine (10%)	Severe hypertension, cerebral hemorrhage, dysrhythmias, myocardial infarction
epinephrine eyedrops	Tremors, increased sweating, headaches, hypertension

infections apply a thin ointment strip to the conjunctiva daily or more often (up to 6 times daily) if necessary.

Aminoglycosides

gentamicin [jen ta mye′ sin] (Garamycin, Genoptic)
Gentamicin is effective against a wide variety of gram-negative and gram-positive organisms. It is particularly useful against *Pseudomonas, Proteus,* and *Klebsiella* organisms and *Escherichia coli,* as well as staphylococci and streptococci that have developed resistance to other antibiotics. It is applied as an ointment two or three times daily, or 1 drop of solution every 4 hours.

tobramycin [toe bra mye′ sin] (Tobrex)
This water-soluble aminoglycoside is used topically for a wide variety of gram-positive and gram-negative external ophthalmic pathogens and is particularly valuable for treating gentamicin-resistant infections. Adverse reactions include ocular toxicity and hypersensitivity, including lid itching, swelling, and conjunctival erythema. When topical aminoglycosides are used concurrently with systemic aminoglycosides, the total serum concentration will be affected and should be monitored. Systemic toxicity from absorption may occur from excessive use.

The dose for mild to moderate infection is 1 drop in the affected eye every 4 hours.

Sulfonamides

sulfacetamide [sul fa see′ ta mide] (Bleph-10, Sulamyd)
sulfisoxazole [sul fi sox′ a zole] (Gantrisin)
Ophthalmic bacteriostatic antiinfective agents block the synthesis of folic acid in susceptible bacterial organisms. The action of sulfonamides, though, is reduced by the presence of *p*-aminobenzoic acid (PABA) or its derivatives, procaine and tetracaine, and also by the presence of purulent drainage or exudate (purulent matter contains PABA). Therefore lid exudate should be removed before the drugs are instilled.

Because the activity of sulfacetamide may be inhibited by concurrent administration of ophthalmic anesthetics, such drugs are applied 30 to 60 minutes apart. Sulfonamides are physically incompatible with thimerosal and silver preparations.

Before administration the patient should check to see that the solution has not darkened in color; if so, discard it. Solutions are instilled at a rate of 1 drop every 1 to 3 hours during the day, with increased time intervals during the night. Instillation of the drops may cause some mild pain and discomfort.

Antifungal Agents

natamycin [na ta mye′ sin] (Natacyn)
Natamycin ophthalmic suspension is used to treat fungal blepharitis, conjunctivitis, and keratitis. By binding to steroids in the cell membrane of the fungus, natamycin produces an altered membrane permeability causing a loss of the cellular constituents. Because it is mainly retained in the conjunctival area, significant drug levels in the ocular fluids are not achieved. It is not systemically absorbed. Natamycin may cause irritation of the eye. For fungal keratitis, 1 drop of the 5% solution is instilled into the conjunctiva at 1- to 2-hour intervals initially for 3 or 4 days followed by six to eight times daily dosing afterward. For fungal blepharitis and conjunctivitis, 1 drop four to six times daily is usually adequate.

Antiviral Agents

Antiviral ophthalmic preparations include idoxuridine, trifluridine, and vidarabine.

idoxuridine [eye dox yoor′ i deen] (Stoxil, Herplex)

Idoxuridine resembles thymidine, a substance necessary for viral deoxyribonucleic acid (DNA); thus it replaces it and inhibits the replication of the viral DNA. It is indicated for the treatment of herpes simplex virus keratitis. Less frequent side effects and adverse reactions include hypersensitivity (eye redness, pruritus, and irritation), visual disturbance, and photosensitivity that were not present before therapy.

The adult dosage of idoxuridine solution for treatment of herpes simplex virus keratitis is 1 drop hourly during waking hours and every 2 hours during the night. For ointment, apply a thin strip every 4 hours (five times daily) during waking hours.

trifluridine [trye flure′ i deen] (Viroptic)

For mechanism of action and indications, see idoxuridine. In addition, trifluridine is used to treat herpes simplex virus keratoconjunctivitis. A frequent side effect reported is burning or stinging on application. Rare side effects and adverse reactions include increased IOP, blurred vision, and hypersensitivity reaction, evidenced by redness, swelling, or eye irritation not present before therapy.

The usual adult dose is 1 drop (1% solution) into the conjunctiva every 2 hours during waking hours. The maximum daily dose is 9 drops. Continue therapy until the cornea has recovered then reduce dosage to 1 drop every 4 hours during waking hours (minimum of 5 drops/day) for 1 week.

vidarabine [vye dare′ a been] (Vira-A)

The antiviral mechanism of action is due to vidarabine's conversion to substances intracellularly that inhibit viral DNA polymerase or other virus DNA specific enzymes. It is indicated for the treatment of herpes simplex virus keratitis and keratoconjunctivitis. Systemic absorption is not expected after ocular administration.

The side effects and adverse reactions of vidarabine include increased tear flow and a sensation of something being in the eye. The prescriber should be contacted if photosensitivity, redness, eye swelling, or increased eye irritation not present before treatment occurs.

The usual adult dose is application of a thin strip of ointment to the conjunctiva every 3 hours five times daily. Therapy is continued until cornea is completely reepithelialized, then the dose is decreased to twice daily for 7 to 10 days.

Antiseptics

Many antiseptics that were used to treat surface infections of the eye before the advent of antibiotics are now obsolete. Inorganic mercuric salts such as yellow mercuric oxide ophthalmic ointment (1% to 2%), thimerosal (Merthiolate), and ammoniated mercury formerly served as bacteriostatic agents. They are seldom used today because they do not completely sterilize, spores are resistant to them, and they are irritating to the eye.

silver nitrate

Two drops of a solution of 1% silver nitrate is routinely instilled in each eye immediately after birth as a prophylaxis against gonorrheal ophthalmia neonatorum. In many states this is required by law. The gonococci are particularly susceptible to silver salts. Liberated silver ions precipitate bacterial proteins. Silver nitrate is preferred over effective antibiotic agents, since these may sensitize the patient, and silver nitrate has stood the test of time.

Silver nitrate ophthalmic solution is available in collapsible capsules containing about 5 drops of a 1% solution. The solution should be in contact with the conjunctival sac for not less than 30 seconds to produce a mild chemical conjunctivitis. Irrigation after use is not recommended.

Corticosteroids

Many corticosteroids are available for ophthalmic use as topical solutions, suspensions, or ointments. They include betamethasone (Betnesol), dexamethasone (Maxidex, Decadron), fluorometholone (FML S.O.P., FML), hydrocortisone (Cortamed), medrysone (HMS Liquifilm), and prednisolone (Pred Forte, Predair-A). These are available in varying strengths and in combination with various antibiotics or mydriatics. They are indicated for the treatment of allergic and inflammatory ophthalmic disorders of the conjunctiva, cornea, and anterior segment of the eye.

Side effects and adverse reactions

These include burning or lacrimation, blurred vision or visual disturbances, eye pain, headaches, ptosis, or enlarged pupils. These should be reported to the prescriber. For dosage and administration, see USP DI or current package inserts.

TOPICAL ANESTHETIC AGENTS

Local anesthetics stabilize neuronal membranes so that they become less permeable to ions; this prevents initiation and transmission of nerve impulses. It is theorized that sodium ion permeability is limited by these agents.

Local anesthetics are used to prevent pain (deep anesthesia) during surgical procedures (removal of sutures and foreign bodies) and tonometry examinations. The local anesthetics have rapid onset (within 20 seconds) and last for 15 to 20 minutes.

proparacaine [proe par′ a kane] (Ophthaine, Ophthetic)

Proparacaine is similar to tetracaine. A 0.5% solution is administered by topical instillation. Anesthesia is produced within 20 seconds and lasts for 15 minutes. Proparacaine is relatively free from the burning and discomfort of other anesthetics, but it is highly toxic if it enters the systemic circulation. Side effects and adverse reactions include allergic contact dermatitis, softening and erosion of corneal epithelium, pupillary dilation, cycloplegia, conjunctival congestion and hemorrhage, and stromal edema.

tetracaine [tet′ ra kane] (Pontocaine)

Tetracaine is widely used topically for rapid, brief, superficial anesthesia. One to 2 drops of a 0.5% solution of tetracaine will produce anesthesia within 30 seconds; the patient may feel a burning or stinging sensation. The anesthetic effect lasts for 10 to 15 minutes. Tetracaine can cause epithelial damage and systemic toxicity; therefore it is not recommended for prolonged home use by patients. It is physically incompatible with the mercury or silver salts often found in ophthalmic products.

OTHER OPHTHALMIC PREPARATIONS

Artificial Tear Solutions and Lubricants

Lubricants or artificial tears are used to provide moisture and lubrication in diseases in which tear production is deficient, to lubricate artificial eyes and moisten contact lenses, to remove debris, and to protect the cornea during procedures on the eye. These agents are also incorporated in ophthalmic preparations to prolong the contact time of topically applied drugs.

Such products have a balanced salt solution (equivalent to 0.9% sodium chloride), buffers to adjust pH, highly viscous agents (methylcellulose, propylene glycol, and others) to extend eye contact time, and preservatives to maintain sterility. These products are usually administered three or four times a day.

An artificial tear insert (Lacrisert) was devised to extend the effect of the preparation. It is usually inserted daily or at most twice a day for selected patients.

Ointment preparations are also used as ocular lubricants. They will help to protect the eye (such as during and after eye surgery) and to lubricate the eye. They are particularly valuable for patients who have an impaired blink reflex and for nighttime use. Examples include Lacri-Lube, Duratears, and Hypo Tears.

Antiallergic Agents

Three antiallergic ophthalmic agents are available: cromolyn, levocabastine, and lodoxamide tromethamine.

cromolyn sodium (Opticrom)

Cromolyn sodium inhibits degranulation of sensitized mast cells occurring after exposure to a specific antigen. This mast cell release inhibition prevents the mediators of inflammation (histamine and slow-releasing substance of anaphylaxis [SRS-A]) from producing their characteristic effects. The drug is used for allergic eye disorders (vernal and allergic keratoconjunctivitis, papillary conjunctivitis, and keratitis) that have symptoms of itching, tearing, redness, and discharge.

Side effects and adverse reactions

These include stinging and burning sensation in the eyes. Concomitant use of corticosteroids may be necessary. For adults and children (older than 4 years of age), instill 1 drop in each affected eye four to six times a day at regular intervals.

levocabastine (Livostin)

Levocabastine is a topical antihistamine indicated for allergic conjunctivitis. The side effects are mild and include burning, stinging, visual alterations, eye pain, red eyes, and headaches. The usual adult dose is 1 drop in the eyes four times a day.

lodoxamide [loe dox′ a mid] (Alomide)

Lodoxamide ophthalmic, an antiallergic and mast cell stabilizer, is used for the treatment of vernal conjunctivitis, vernal keratitis, and several other eye disorders. Lodoxamide inhibits type I immediate hypersensitivity reactions by interfering with histamine release and inhibits the release of SRS-A and eosinophil chemotaxis.

Side effects and adverse reactions

These include a transient burning of the eye, blurred vision, pruritus of the eye, tearing, or eye irritation. The usual dose for children 2 years of age and older and adults is 1 to 2 drops to the conjunctiva four times daily for up to 3 months.

Diagnostic Aids

fluorescein [flure′ e sceen] (Fluorescite, Fluor-I-Strip)

Fluorescein is a nontoxic water-soluble dye that is used as a diagnostic aid. When applied to the cornea, it stains corneal lesions or ulcers a bright green; foreign bodies appear to be surrounded by a green ring. These effects permit detection of corneal epithelial defects caused by injury or infection and location of foreign bodies in the eye. The dye is also used in fitting hard contact lenses. Areas that lack fluorescein-stained tears will appear black under ultraviolet light, indicating that the contact lens is touching the cornea at those areas. Fluorescein is used in retinal photography to determine retinal vascular status and to identify defects in the retinal pigment epithelium. In addition, it may be used to test lacrimal apparatus patency; if after the dye is instilled into the eye it appears in the nasal secretions, the nasolacrimal drainage system is open.

Injection is used in ophthalmic angiography to examine the fundus, vasculature of the iris, and aqueous flow, to make differential diagnosis of cancerous and noncancerous tumors, and to determine time for circulation in the eye. Side effects and adverse reactions after injection include nausea, headache, abdominal distress, vomiting, hypotension, hypersensitivity reactions, and anaphylaxis.

A topical solution is used to detect foreign bodies and corneal abrasions (1 or 2 drops of 2% solution). For strip application and injection, check a current drug reference for instructions.

Enzyme Preparation

chymotrypsin [kye' moe trip sin] (Catarase)

Chymotrypsin, a proteolytic enzyme, is used in selected patients to facilitate cataract extraction. Injected behind the iris into the posterior chamber, it dissolves the filaments or zonules that hold the lens, thereby facilitating intracapsular lens extraction. This effect is usually obtained in 5 to 15 minutes with total lysis of the entire zonular membrane reported within 30 minutes. Side effects and adverse reactions include a transient postoperative glaucoma lasting about 1 week, which can be relieved by the use of pilocarpine.

Hyperosmolar Preparation

sodium chloride ointment (Muro 128)
sodium chloride solution (Adsorbonac)

This 5% ointment and 2% or 5% solution are used to reduce the corneal edema that occurs in certain corneal dystrophies and after cataract extraction. The dose is 1 to 2 drops or a small amount of ointment in the affected eye(s) every 3 to 4 hours as directed.

Nonsteroidal Antiinflammatory Agents

Flurbiprofen, suprofen, diclofenac, and ketorolac tromethamine are available topically for ophthalmic use. These agents are nonsteroidal antiinflammatory drugs (NSAIDs). They have the following indications:

- Flurbiprofen [flure bee proe' fen] (Ocufen) and suprofen [sue' proe fen] (Profenal) are used to inhibit intraoperative miosis.
- Diclofenac [dye kloe' fen ak] (Voltaren) is used to treat postoperative inflammation after a cataract extraction.
- Ketorolac [kee' toe role ak] (Acular) is used to treat conjunctivitis and seasonal allergic ophthalmic pruritus.

These agents, if absorbed, may produce a systemic effect. Because they have the potential to cause increased bleeding, monitor their use closely in patients who are known to have bleeding tendencies. The most common side effect reported is transient burning or stinging on application. Other minor symptoms of ocular irritation have also been reported, such as itching, redness, discomfort, and allergic reaction. For dosing recommendations, see a current package insert or drug reference.

Irrigating Solutions

The sterile isotonic external irrigating solutions are used in tonometry, fluorescein procedures, and removal of foreign material, and to cleanse and soothe the eyes of patients wearing hard contact lenses. These external products do not require a prescription and are available as drops, irrigations, and eyewashes. Examples of irrigating solutions include BSS Plus, Surgisol, and Lavoptik Eye Wash.

SUMMARY

Although there are many ophthalmic preparations available, the drugs to treat eye disorders can be divided into the following major headings: antiglaucoma agents, carbonic anhydrase inhibitor agents, mydriatics and cycloplegics, antiinfective/antiinflammatory agents, antifungal/antiviral agents, anesthetic agents, antiallergic agents, diagnostic aids, enzyme preparations, nonsteroidal antiinflammatory agents, irrigating solutions, and artificial tear solutions and lubricants. The indications, mechanisms of action, side effects and adverse reactions topically and systemically and drug dosages were discussed in this chapter.

REVIEW QUESTIONS

1. Explain the theories on how timolol (Timoptic), pilocarpine, and epinephrine lower the intraocular pressure of glaucoma.
2. What are the indications for the use of anticholinergic and adrenergic agonist ophthalmic medications? Describe their mechanisms of action.
3. Name the ocular side effects induced by aspirin, marijuana, digitalis glycosides, ethyl alcohol, and ibuprofen.
4. Name the serious adverse systemic effects that may be induced by the following ophthalmic drugs: chloramphenicol, atropine, scopolamine, beta blocking agents, and epinephrine.

REFERENCES

Abel SR: Eye disorders. In *Applied therapeutics,* ed 6, Vancouver, 1995, Applied Therapeutics.

Moroi SE, Lichter PR: Ocular pharmacology. In Hardman JG, Limbird LE, editors: *Goodman & Gilman's the pharmacological basis of therapeutics,* ed 9, New York, 1996, McGraw-Hill.

Olin BR: *Facts and comparisons.* Philadelphia, 1998, JB Lippincott.

United States Pharmacopeial Convention: *USP DI: drug information for the health care professional,* ed 18, Rockville, Md, 1998, The Convention.

ADDITIONAL REFERENCES

American Hospital Formulary Service: *AHFS drug information '98,* Bethesda, Md, 1998, American Society of Hospital Pharmacists.

Anderson KN et al, editors: *Mosby's medical, nursing, and allied health dictionary,* ed 5, St Louis, 1998, Mosby.

DiPiro JT, Talber R et al, editors: *Pharmacotherapy, a pathophysiologic approach,* ed 2, Norwalk, Conn, 1993, Appleton & Lange.

Eye drops and infection: The solution may be the problem, *Emerg Med* 24(4):142, 1992

Mosby: *Mosby's GenRx,* St Louis, 1998, Mosby.

Schein OD et al: Eye drops and infection, *Arch Ophthamol* 110:82, 1992.

Seeley RR, Stephens TD, Tate P: *Anatomy and physiology,* ed 3, New York, 1995, McGraw-Hill.

Thibodeau GA, Patton KT: *Anatomy and physiology,* ed 4, St Louis, 1999, Mosby.

Van Wynsberghe D, Noback CR, Carola R: *Human anatomy and physiology,* ed 3, New York, 1995, McGraw-Hill.

Wingard LB et al: *Human pharmacology,* St Louis, 1991, Mosby.

CHAPTER 37

Overview of the Ear and Auditory Drugs

CHAPTER FOCUS

Knowledge of the anatomy and physiology of the ear is necessary to understand the medications used to treat ear disorders. Individuals with ear disorders may have pain, vertigo, and difficulty with balance and communication. The pharmacologic agents used to treat ear disorders are limited, but the healthcare professional should be aware that many systemic agents can affect the ear therapeutically and adversely (e.g., causing ototoxicity). This chapter reviews these agents.

OBJECTIVES

After reading and studying this chapter, the student should be able to do the following:

1. *Describe the external, middle, and inner ear and name the three bones of the inner ear.*
2. *Review the eustachian tube functions.*
3. *Name two of the most common ear disorders.*
4. *List several drugs that are commonly used to treat ear infections.*
5. *Discuss the two types of drug-induced ototoxicity.*
6. *List four drugs reported to cause ototoxicity.*

KEY TERMS

auditory ossicles, (p. 525)
cerumen, (p. 526)
cochlea, (p. 525)
eustachian (auditory) tube, (p. 525)
external ear, (p. 525)
inner ear, (p. 525)
middle ear, (p. 525)
otitis media, (p. 525)
ototoxicity, (p. 527)
tinnitus, (p. 527)
tympanic membrane, (p. 525)
vertigo, (p. 527)

OVERVIEW OF THE EAR

ANATOMY AND PHYSIOLOGY

The ear consists of three sections or parts: external ear, middle ear, and inner ear (Fig. 37-1). The **external ear** has two divisions: the outer ear, or pinna, and the external auditory canal. The external auditory canal leads to the eardrum, or tympanic membrane, a thin, transparent partition of tissue between the canal and the middle ear. The function of the external ear is to receive and transmit auditory sounds to the eardrum. The **tympanic membrane** protects the middle ear from foreign substances and transmits sound to the bones of the middle ear.

The **middle ear** is an air-filled cavity in the temporal bone that contains three small bones called the **auditory ossicles.** The ossicles are the malleus (hammer), incus (anvil), and stapes (stirrup). The tip of the malleus is attached to the surface of the tympanic membrane. Its head is attached to the incus, which in turn is attached to the stapes. The ossicles amplify and transmit sound waves to the inner ear. The middle ear is also directly connected to the nasopharynx by the **eustachian (auditory) tube.** The eustachian tube is usually collapsed except when the individual swallows, chews, yawns, or moves the jaw. This tube joins the nasopharynx, and the tympanic cavity, which allows for the equalization of the air pressure in the inner ear with atmospheric pressure to prevent the tympanic membrane from rupturing. On airline flights pressure changes are relieved by action of the eustachian tube when the individual chews gum, yawns, or deliberately swallows.

The **inner ear** is the complex structure of the ear that communicates directly with the acoustic nerve, which transmits sound vibrations from the middle ear. The inner ear, also referred to as the labyrinth because of its series of canals, has two main divisions. The bony labyrinth consists of the vestibule, cochlea, and semicircular canals, and the membranous labyrinth consists of a series of sacs and tubes within the bony labyrinth. The **cochlea,** through which passes fibers of the cochlear division of the acoustic nerve, is the primary organ of hearing, and the vestibular apparatus is necessary to maintain equilibrium and balance (Fig. 37-1).

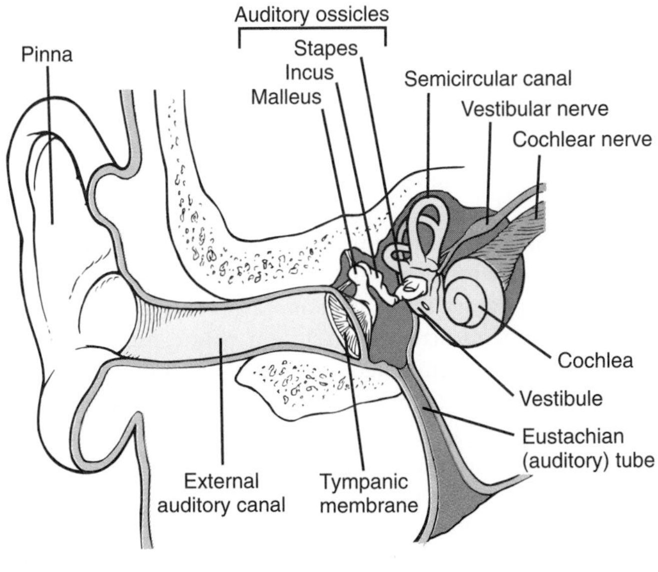

FIGURE 37-1
Anatomy of the ear.

COMMON EAR DISORDERS

The most common ear disorders include infections of the ear (bacterial or fungal), earwax accumulation, and various other painful or distressing conditions. Many ear disorders are minor and easily treated or are self-limiting. Persistent pain or ear problems should be professionally evaluated because some untreated disorders can lead to hearing loss.

External ear disorders usually include trauma, such as lacerations or scrapes to the skin. These are often minor and heal with time. If the injury results in bleeding and perhaps a hematoma, referral to a primary healthcare provider is necessary. Localized infections of the hair follicles resulting in boils may occur. Patients with recurring boils and small boils who do not respond to good hygiene and topical compresses should be referred to a provider for evaluation and, possibly, systemic antibiotics.

Dermatitis of the ear, itching, local redness, weeping, and drainage are also reported. Such conditions must be evaluated individually, since the causes can vary from inflammation induced by seborrhea, psoriasis, or contact dermatitis to head trauma producing ear discharge. Self-medication should be discouraged when infection is suspected or in the presence of known injuries of the ear or whenever drainage, pain, and dizziness are present.

Middle ear disorders are not to be treated with over-the-counter (OTC) medications. The most commonly reported problem is middle ear inflammation, **otitis media.** This occurs most often in children, although chronic otitis media may be caused in adults by a nasopharyngeal tumor. Pain, fever, malaise, pressure, a sensation of fullness in the ear, and hearing loss are common symptoms. Individuals with such conditions should be treated promptly by a prescriber. Acute tympanic membrane perforation from foreign objects or from water sports (such as diving or water skiing) will result in a multitude of symptoms, if untreated. Pain at the time of injury which subsides, diminished hearing acuity, tinnitus, nausea, vertigo, and otitis media or mastoiditis may be noted. A physician's examination is vital when a perforated tympanic membrane is suspected.

Loss of hearing, especially unilateral hearing loss, may result from viral infection of the inner ear. Hearing deficits may be caused by genetic diseases or slowly progressive diseases such as otosclerosis or Ménière's disease. Untreated external and middle ear infections may also affect hearing and the functioning of the inner ear.

Healthcare professionals should be aware of drugs that have ototoxicity as an adverse effect, which results in impaired hearing for the patient. These will be identified later in this chapter.

AUDITORY DRUGS

Disorders and infections of the external ear canal are treated with antibiotic solutions, corticosteroids, and miscellaneous preparations such as wax emulsifiers, antibacterials, antifungals, local anesthetics, antiinflammatory agents, and local analgesic-type preparations. The potent systemic medications that may adversely affect the patient's hearing and balance will also be reviewed.

ANTIBIOTIC EAR PREPARATIONS

Antibiotic ear preparations are used to treat infections of the external auditory canal surface as a topical agent. For serious inner ear infections, systemic antibiotics are indicated.

chloramphenicol [klor am fen′ a kole] (Chloromycetin Otic)

Chloramphenicol, a broad-spectrum antibiotic (bacteriostatic) solution, is used to treat external ear infections caused by *Staphylococcus aureus, Escherichia coli, Pseudomonas aeruginosa, Enterobacter aerogenes, Haemophilus influenzae,* and other susceptible organisms.

Potential side effects include burning, redness, rash, swelling, or other signs of topical irritation that were not present before the start of therapy. The medication should be discontinued if this hypersensitivity reaction occurs. The usual dosage for adults and children is two or three drops inserted in the ear canal every 6 to 8 hours.

gentamicin sulfate otic solution [jen ta mye′ sin] (Garamycin)

Gentamicin, a bactericidal antibiotic, is another antibiotic that is not presently available in the otic preparation in the United States but is available in Canada. Although it is not Food and Drug Administration (FDA) approved, prescribers sometimes use the ophthalmic preparation marketed in the United States for otic infections.

Side effects are similar to those of chloramphenicol. The dose is three or four drops inserted in the ear canal three times daily.

CORTICOSTEROID EAR PREPARATIONS

Corticosteroid otic solutions include betamethasone and hydrocortisone, only available in Canada (Betnesol 🍁 and Cortamed 🍁), and dexamethasone (Decadron) available in both countries. Hydrocortisone combinations with acetic acid (VōSoL HC, Acetasol HC), with alcohol (EarSoL-HC), or with acetic acid and benzethonium (AA-HC Otic) are also available. Acetic acid, boric acid, benzalkonium chloride, benzethonium, and aluminum acetate (Burow's solution) are used for their antibacterial or antifungal effects. Hydrocortisone is included for its antiinflammatory, antipruritic, and antiallergic effects (USP DI, 1998).

TABLE 37-1 Selected Examples of OTC Otic Solutions

Ingredients (Trade Names)	*Use/Indications*
carbamide peroxide (Auro Ear Drops)	Ear wax
isopropyl alcohol (Auro-Dri Ear Drops)	Swimmer's ear
boric acid and isopropyl alcohol (Aurocaine 2)	Swimmer's ear
isopropyl alcohol in glycerin (Swim-Ear Drops)	Swimmer's ear
carbamide peroxide and glycerin (Dent's Ear Wax Drops, E.R.O. Ear Drops, Ear Wax Removal System)	Ear wax
hydrocortisone, propylene glycol, alcohol, benzyl benzoate (EarSoL-DC Drops)	Antiinflammatory, antipruritic

Modified from American Pharmaceutical Association, 1997.

Corticosteroid may be combined with the antibiotics neomycin and polymyxin B to treat external ear canal infections and mastoidectomy cavity infections. Many such products are available that may also include other ingredients, such as those included in the OTC otic preparations. These are prescription otic solutions such as AK-spore HC, Cort-Biotic, Cortisporin, Cortomycin, and others (USP DI, 1998).

OTHER OTIC PREPARATIONS

OTC otic preparations often contain acidified (acetic acid) solutions of alcohol, glycerin, or propylene glycol to help restore the normal acid pH to the ear canal, especially after the person swims or bathes. Glycerin, mineral oil, and olive oil (sweet oil) are used as emollients to help relieve itching and burning in the ear, while propylene glycol enhances the antibacterial effect and acidity of acetic acid. Carbamide peroxide (urea hydrogen peroxide) is an antibacterial agent that releases oxygen to help remove **cerumen** (ear wax) accumulations. Thus combinations of these ingredients are often included in OTC otic solutions (Covington, 1996).

A wide variety of both single and combination products is used to treat impacted cerumen, inflammation, bacterial or fungal infections, ear pain, and other minor or superficial problems associated primarily with the external ear canal. More serious problems such as an earache secondary to an upper respiratory tract infection, ear discharge or drainage, persistent or recurrent otitis, or ear pain caused by recent injury or head trauma require a healthcare provider's thorough evaluation and intervention to prevent complications. In such cases, systemic medications with or without ear preparations are usually necessary.

Although most OTC otic preparations are considered safe and effective, patients should be advised to see a provider if symptoms do not improve within several days of using these preparations or if an adverse reaction occurs. See Table 37-1 for selected examples of OTC otic solutions.

TABLE 37-2 Selected Drugs Reported to Cause Ototoxicity

Drug	*Comments*
Analgesics	
aspirin and nonsteroidal antiinflammatory drugs (NSAIDs)	Salicylates, especially in high doses, can cause tinnitus, vertigo, and hearing loss. It is generally reversible if drug use is reduced or discontinued, although some cases of irreversible hearing loss are documented. With NSAIDs, hearing disturbances and loss are reported.
Antibiotics	
aminoglycosides	Incidence of ototoxicity is 1%-5% and may be irreversible.
clarithromycin	Hearing loss has been reported (usually reversible). It occurs more often in elderly women.
erythromycin	Reversible hearing loss has been reported in persons with liver and/or kidney impairment, in persons 50 years of age and older, and in individuals who received high doses (>4 g/day). IV erythromycin has resulted in irreversible ototoxicity.
vancomycin	Hearing loss has been reported, especially in persons with kidney impairment or those receiving another ototoxic medication concurrently.
Antineoplastic Agents	
cisplatin	Ototoxicity with tinnitus, hearing loss, and possible deafness has been reported. This effect is especially severe in children (younger than 12 years of age). This effect is accumulative; therefore audiometric testing is recommended.
mechlorethamine	Tinnitus and, less frequently, hearing loss have been reported.
Loop Diuretics	
bumetanide, ethacrynic acid, furosemide	Reversible and irreversible hearing loss has been reported, usually with too rapid IV injection, high diuretic dosages, and concurrent use with other ototoxic medications, and in persons with renal impairment.

DRUG-INDUCED OTOTOXICITY

Many medications have reportedly caused **ototoxicity** in humans. The ototoxicity may affect the person's hearing (auditory or cochlear function), balance (vestibular function), or both. The most common symptom reported is **tinnitus,** a ringing or buzzing sound in the ears.

Cochlear ototoxicity causes a progressive or continuing hearing loss. High-pitched tinnitus, or the loss of the highest tones, occurs first, then progresses to affect the lowest tones. Because of this slow progression, most patients are not aware that it is occurring. Vestibular toxicity may start with a severe headache of 1 to 2 days duration, followed by nausea, vomiting, dizziness, ataxia, and difficulty with equilibrium. The person may feel as though the room is in motion (**vertigo**). Ototoxicity is usually bilateral and may be reversible, but it can become irreversible if not recognized early enough to stop the offending medications. Most drug-induced ototoxicity is associated with the use of aminoglycosides, such as streptomycin, gentamicin, tobramycin, and others. Table 37-2 lists selected drugs reported to induce ototoxicity.

SUMMARY

Although therapeutic agents for the treatment of ear disorders are limited, knowledge of the anatomy and physiology of the ear is necessary. Drugs are available to treat ear infections and inflammation and to remove cerumen, or ear wax. In addition, an awareness of the systemic medications that can cause ototoxicity is important as a lack of this recognition can cause irreversible hearing loss.

REVIEW QUESTIONS

1. Describe the function of the eustachian tube on airline flights. What advice can you offer the traveler to reduce the problem with air pressure changes?
2. What part of the ear is the primary organ of hearing? For equilibrium and balance?
3. Name three causes of pain in the ear.

REFERENCES

American Pharmaceutical Association: *Nonprescription products: formulations and reatures '97-'98,* Washington, DC, 1997, The Association.

Covington TR, editor: *Handbook of nonprescription drugs,* ed 11, Washington, DC, 1996, American Pharmaceutical Association.

United States Pharmacopeial Convention: *USP DI: drug information for the health care professional,* ed 18, Rockville, Md, 1998, The Convention.

ADDITIONAL REFERENCES

Anderson KN et al, editors: *Mosby's medical, nursing, and allied health dictionary,* ed 5, St Louis, 1998, Mosby.

Covington TR: *Product update, handbook of nonprescription drugs,* ed 10, Washington, DC, 1995, American Pharmaceutical Association.

Mosby: *Mosby's GenRx,* St Louis, 1998, Mosby.

Olin BR: *Facts and comparisons.* Philadelphia, 1998, JB Lippincott.

Semia TP et al: *American Pharmaceutical Association geriatric dosage handbook,* Hudson, OH, 1993, Lexi-Comp.

Thibodeau GA, Patton KT: *Anatomy and physiology,* ed 4, St Louis, 1999, Mosby.

UNIT XI

Drugs Affecting the Endocrine System

CHAPTER 38

Overview of the Endocrine System

CHAPTER FOCUS

The endocrine system comprises glands that produce hormones necessary for a variety of vital functions in the body. The endocrine glands are also called the ductless glands because they secrete their hormones directly into the bloodstream, where they are then carried to other organs or tissues in the body that they affect, control, or regulate. This chapter reviews the anatomy and physiology of the endocrine system.

OBJECTIVES

After reading and studying this chapter, the student should be able to do the following:

1. *Define and describe the key terms.*
2. *Identify the major hormones and explain their functions in the body.*
3. *Name and describe the three hormones released from the adrenal glands.*
4. *Discuss the contrasting effects of insulin and glucagon on blood glucose levels.*

KEY TERMS

glucagon, (p. 539)
glucocorticoids, (p. 538)
goiter, (p. 536)
hormones, (p. 532)
insulin, (p. 539)
mineralocorticoids, (p. 538)
myxedema, (p. 537)
negative feedback, (p. 532)
oxytocin, (p. 534)
thyrotoxicosis, (p. 537)
vasopressin (antidiuretic hormone), (p. 534)

HORMONES

Hormones are active, natural chemical substances secreted into the bloodstream from the endocrine glands that initiate or regulate the activity of an organ or group of cells in another part of the body. They have specific, well-defined physiologic effects on metabolism. The list of major hormones includes the products of the secretions from the anterior and posterior pituitary glands, the thyroid hormones, parathyroid hormone, pancreatic insulin and glucagon, epinephrine and norepinephrine from the adrenal medulla, several potent steroids from the adrenal cortex, and the gonadal hormones of both sexes (Fig. 38-1).

The major types of hormones are the steroid hormones and the amino acid-derived hormones. Steroid hormones are those substances secreted by the adrenal gland and the sex glands. They transport proteins in the plasma; their physiologic effect begins when the steroid enters the cell, with subsequent binding to the specific cytosol or nuclear protein receptor.

Hormones from the various endocrine glands work together to regulate vital processes, including the following: (1) secretory and motor activities of the digestive tract; (2) energy production; (3) composition and volume of extracellular fluid; (4) adaptation, such as acclimatization and immunity; (5) growth and development; and (6) reproduction and lactation.

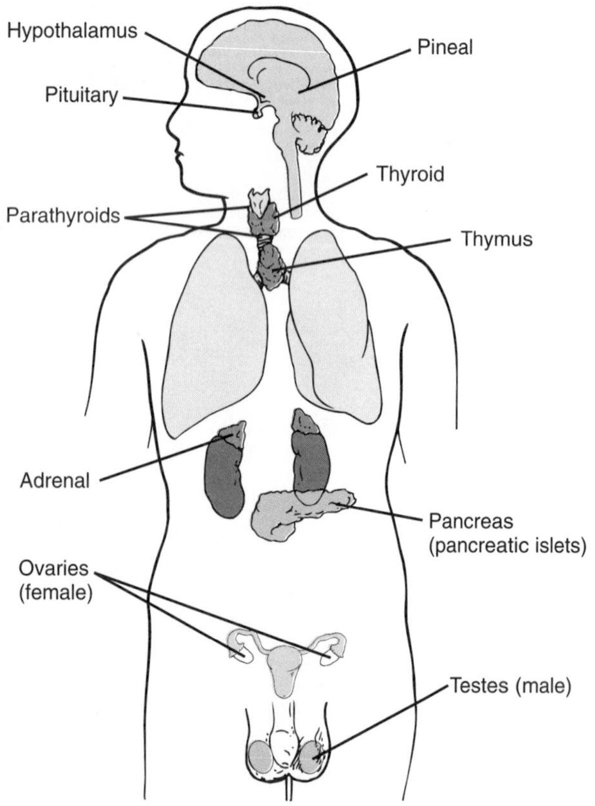

FIGURE 38-1
Locations of the major endocrine glands.

Hormones may exert their effects by controlling the formation or destruction of an intracellular regulator cyclic 3′,5′-adenosine monophosphate (cyclic AMP), controlling protein synthesis, or controlling membrane permeability and the movement of ions and other substances. The effect of a hormone depends on its interaction with a receptor and is determined by the level of the circulating active hormone.

To maintain the internal environment, hormone secretion must be controlled. This is achieved by a self-regulating series of events known as **negative feedback;** that is, a hormone produces a physiologic effect that. when strong enough, inhibits further secretion of that hormone, thereby inhibiting the physiologic effect. Increased hormonal secretions may be evoked in response to stimuli from the external environment; cessation of external stimuli ends the internal secretion response (Fig. 38-2).

Hormones are not "used up" in exerting their physiologic effects but must be inactivated or excreted if the internal environment is to remain stable. Inactivation occurs enzymatically in the blood or intercellular spaces, liver or kidney, or target tissues. Excretion of hormones is primarily via the urine and, to a lesser extent, the bile. Most hormones are destroyed rapidly, having a half-life in blood of 10 to 30 minutes. However, some such as the catecholamines have a half-life of seconds, and thyroid hormones have a half-life measured in days. Some hormones exert their physiologic effects immediately, while others require minutes or hours

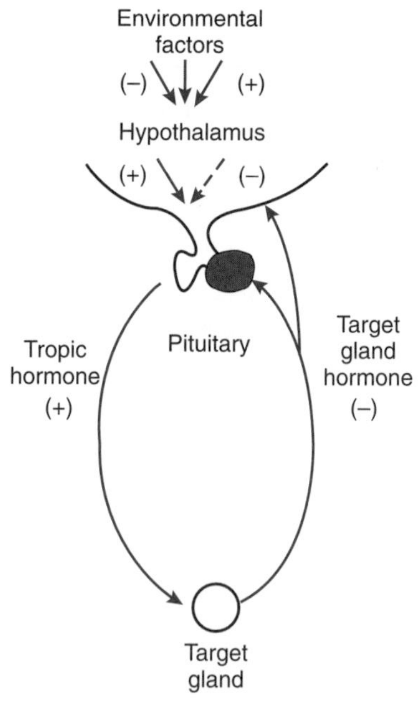

FIGURE 38-2
Various internal and external factors may inhibit or stimulate the hypothalamus to secrete inhibitory (–) or releasing (+) factors to control output of hormones from the anterior pituitary gland and ultimate hormone release from target glands.

before their effects occur. In addition, some effects end immediately when the hormone disappears from the circulation. Other responses may persist for hours after hormone concentrations have returned to basal levels. The exposure of a tissue to an active hormone also is controlled by that hormone's pathway for metabolism, including molecular alterations, consumption at the site of action, and hepatorenal excretion. This wide range of onset and duration of hormonal activity contributes to the flexibility of the endocrine system.

One of the major developments of this century in the fields of biology and medicine has been the recognition, isolation, purification, and chemical and cellular understanding of most known hormones. In addition, once their chemical structure is known, duplicating hormones by chemical synthesis becomes theoretically possible. This has been accomplished for some but not all hormones.

In medicine, hormones generally are used in three ways: (1) for replacement therapy, exemplified by the use of insulin in diabetes or of adrenal steroids in Addison's disease; (2) for pharmacologic effects beyond replacement, as in the use of larger-than-endogenous doses of adrenal steroids for their antiinflammatory effects; and (3) for endocrine diagnostic testing.

Research in endocrinology has advanced the concept of specific receptors within or on the surface of cells. This has led to knowledge of hormone specificity and the essential cellular mechanisms involved in the hormone-receptor complex. The recognition and activation properties found in the hormone-receptor complex come from different receptor molecular sites. Only specific receptor material binds a hormone and begins its activity; the hormone has no effect on other tissues that do not carry specific receptors.

Alterations in either hormone secretion or hormone receptor responses may culminate in endocrine disease states. Certain cell surface receptors may become antigenic and develop antibodies that accelerate receptor destruction, block receptor function, or mimic the action of the target tissue. Among the receptor-like disorders, referred to as antireceptor autoimmune diseases, are myasthenia gravis, Graves' disease, insulin-resistant diabetes mellitus, and bronchial asthma.

PITUITARY GLAND

The hormones of the pituitary gland exert an important effect in regulating the secretion of other hormones. The pituitary body is about the size of a pea and occupies a niche in the sella turcica of the sphenoid bone. It consists of an anterior lobe (adenohypophysis), a posterior lobe (neurohypophysis), and a smaller pars intermedia composed of secreting cells. The anterior lobe is particularly important in sustaining life. The function of the pars intermedia is not well understood. Fig. 38-3 shows the major pituitary hormones and their principal target organs.

Regulation of Anterior Pituitary Function

The pituitary and target glands have a negative feedback relationship. A trophic hormone from the pituitary stimulates the target gland to secrete a hormone that inhibits further secretion of the trophic hormone by the pituitary. When the serum concentration of the target gland hormone falls below a certain level, the pituitary again secretes the trophic hormone until the target gland produces enough hormone to inhibit the pituitary secretion. However, the negative feedback concept alone is not enough to account for changes in serum levels of target gland hormones, especially those caused by changes in the external environment. Thus the central nervous system is believed to play a decisive role in regulating pituitary function to meet environmental demands.

The discovery of various hypothalamic-releasing factors is of great research interest. These factors cause the release of inhibition of the various hormones from the anterior pituitary. Among these releasing factors are thyroid-stimulating hormone releasing factor, corticotropin releasing factor, growth hormone-releasing hormone, growth hormone-inhibiting hormone (somatostatin), luteinizing hormone-releasing hormone, and prolactin inhibitory factor.

Anterior Pituitary Hormones

The number of hormones secreted by the anterior pituitary gland is unknown, but at least seven extracts have been prepared in a relatively pure state, and they have definite specific action.

1. A growth factor influences the development of the body. It promotes skeletal, visceral, and general growth. Acromegaly, gigantism, and dwarfism are associated with pathologic conditions of the anterior lobe of the pituitary gland.

   Growth hormone (GH) (somatotropin, somatropin, somatotropic hormone, STH) has been obtained as a small crystalline protein, but thus far no established place in medicine has been found for GH except in documented clinical and laboratory evidence of GH deficiency associated with chronic renal insufficiency (Olin, 1998). Its use in various clinical conditions is largely experimental. See Chapter 39 for further discussion on growth hormone.
2. Follicle-stimulating hormone (FSH) stimulates the growth and maturation of the ovarian follicle, which in turn brings on the characteristic changes of estrus (menstruation in women). This hormone also stimulates spermatogenesis in the male. FSH appears to be a protein or is associated with a protein, but this human pituitary gonadotropin has not yet been obtained in a highly purified form.
3. Luteinizing hormone (LH), also known as the interstitial cell-stimulating hormone (ICSH), together with FSH

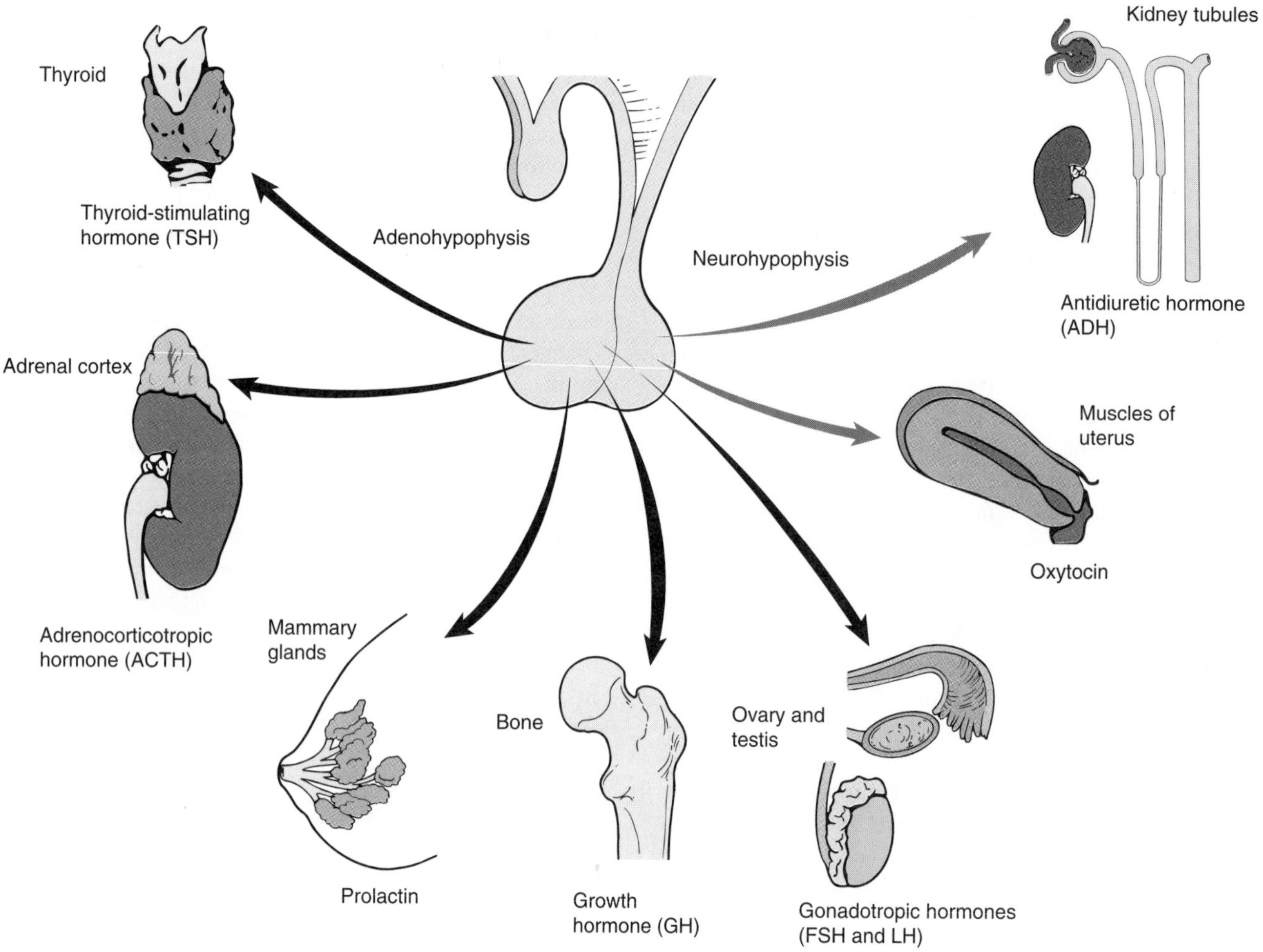

FIGURE 38-3
Pituitary hormones. Some of the major hormones of the adenohypophysis and neurohypophysis and their principal target organs.

(Pergonal) causes maturation of the graafian follicles, ovulation, and the secretion of estrogen in the female. It causes spermatogenesis, androgen formation, and growth of interstitial tissue in the male. LH also promotes the formation of the corpus luteum in the female.

4. Thyroid-stimulating hormone (TSH, thyrotropic hormone, thyrotropin) is necessary for normal development and function of the thyroid gland. If too much is present, it is known to produce hyperthyroidism and increase the size of the gland in laboratory animals.
5. A lactogenic factor (prolactin or mammotropin) plays a part in the proliferation and secretion of the mammary glands of mammals. This may be identical to the hormone responsible for the development of the corpus luteum. In its absence the corpus luteum fails to produce progesterone.
6. Adrenocorticotropic hormone (ACTH, corticotropin) stimulates the cortex of the adrenal gland.
7. Melanocyte-stimulating hormone (MSH, intermedin) is probably produced in the intermediate lobe. Its physiologic role is unknown, but when injected in human beings it darkens the skin.

The hormones produced by the anterior lobe of the pituitary gland are important physiologically, and recently purified preparations became available, at least for clinical study. Such preparations are both expensive and limited in supply. They may become useful in combating certain disorders in the future; however, as chemically defined preparations become available.

Posterior Pituitary Hormones

Two hormones obtained from the posterior lobe of the pituitary gland have been identified and chemically analyzed. These compounds, **oxytocin** (a hormone that stimulates the smooth muscle of the uterus to contract) and **vasopressin (antidiuretic hormone)**, are both peptides, and each contains eight amino acids. It has proven possible to synthesize them chemically. Availability of these hormones in pure form has clarified their mechanism of action and has allowed better control of their therapeutic use. For example, a certain overlap of pharmacologic action exists even in the pure preparation: pure oxytocin has some vasopressor activity and vice versa. The antidiuretic potency of vasopressin is much greater than its pressor potency.

Although vasopressin is available in a natural state, synthetic formulations such as lypressin and desmopressin, have been developed, and they act primarily as ADH. They have very little, if any, pressor or oxytocic activity.

Oxytocin is discussed in Chapter 45.

THYROID GLAND

The thyroid gland, one of the most richly vascularized tissues of the body, secretes three hormones essential for proper regulation of metabolism: thyroxine (T_4), triiodothyronine (T_3), and calcitonin. Because of its role in calcium metabolism, calcitonin is discussed in greater detail in the section on parathyroid gland hormones (see Chapter 40).

The thyroid gland is composed of at least two types of cells: follicular, which produce T_3 and T_4; and parafollicular, the source of calcitonin.

Thyroid Hormones

The large amount of iodine in thyroid hormones and the availability of radioactive iodine have led to detailed knowledge about thyroid physiology and its role in metabolism. Iodine is essential for thyroid hormone synthesis. About 1 mg of iodine is required per week, most of which is ingested in food, water, and iodized table salt. About two thirds of this iodine is reduced in the gastrointestinal tract, enters the circulation as iodide, and is excreted into the urine. The remaining third is taken up by the thyroid gland for hormone synthesis. This process is aided by the "iodide pump," which takes up the iodide from the extracellular fluid, traps it, and concentrates it to many times that found in plasma. The ratio of iodide in the thyroid gland to that in the serum is expressed as the T/S ratio; normally this ratio is 20:1. In hypoactivity the ratio may be 10:1; in hyperactivity it may be as great as 250:1.

Thyroglobulin is synthesized first. It contains tyrosine, an amino acid that reacts with iodine to form thyroid hormones. The thyroglobulin-thyroid hormone complex is stored in the follicles of the thyroid gland and is called "colloid." About 30% of the thyroid mass is stored thyroglobulin, which contains enough thyroid hormone to meet normal requirements for 2 to 3 months without any further synthesis.

Normally, thyroglobulin is not released into the circulation but undergoes proteolytic digestion (a coupling reaction), which releases the active thyroid hormones T_3 and T_4. Hormone synthesis—iodine trapping, iodination and proteolysis of thyroglobulin, and hormone release—is controlled by THS from the beta cells of the anterior pituitary gland. Thyroid secretion is maintained by this TSH secretion. Decreased serum levels of T_3 and T_4 stimulate thyrotropin-releasing hormone (TRH) from the hypothalamus, which stimulates the pituitary gland to secrete TSH; this in turn stimulates release of thyroxin from thyroglobulin.

TSH secretion is negatively regulated by T_3 and T_4, which directly inhibit the pituitary gland's thyrotropic cells. An increase in free, unbound thyroid hormone causes a decrease in TSH secretion and inhibits TRH production, and a decrease in the free unbound hormone causes an increase in TSH secretion and stimulates TRH production—a negative feedback mechanism.

Physiologic Effects of Thyroid Hormones

The precise physiologic role of the thyroid hormones is not yet known, although several hormonal actions have been identified and studied. Three generalizations can be made about thyroid hormones.

1. They have a diffuse effect and do not seem to have any specific target organ effect; no special cells or tissues appear to be particularly affected by the thyroid hormones.
2. Their long delay in onset of action and their prolonged action rule them out as minute-to-minute regulators of physiologic function. Instead, their role is more likely to be that of establishing and maintaining long-term functions such as growth, maturation, and adaptation.
3. They are not necessary for survival, although reduced levels can affect quality of life.

T_3 and T_4 appear to have the same physiologic actions, although T_3 is far more potent than T_4.

Growth and maturation

A normal, functioning thyroid is essential for normal growth. Thyroid hormones stimulate production of messenger ribonucleic acid (RNA) molecules, which are involved in the synthesis of various proteins, thus facilitating growth and development. The hormones must be present in the right amounts for growth to occur at the normal rate. In children who are hypothyroid the rate of growth is retarded, which may lead to shortness of stature. Conversely, children who are hyperthyroid may have excessive skeletal growth and become taller than they otherwise would. If there is premature closing of the epiphyses because of accelerated bone maturation, however, stunting of growth results. In the adult, excess thyroid hormone causes increased demineralization of bone and increased loss of calcium and phosphate.

Cells in the interstitial tissue between follicles of the thyroid gland produce calcitonin; the effect of this hormone is to reduce the blood calcium ion concentration, an effect that is the exact opposite of that of parathyroid hormone. Calcitonin is essential for bone formation in children because it promotes deposition of calcium. In the adult, calcitonin has a very weak effect on plasma concentration because absorption and deposition of calcium are slow in the adult and calcitonin effects are rapidly overridden by parathyroid hormone.

Central nervous system function

From the time of birth through the first year of life, thyroid hormone must be present for normal development of the cerebrum; if the hormone is not present, irreversible mental retardation occurs. In the adult, hypothyroidism causes listlessness, a general dulling of mental capacity, decreased sensory capacity, slow speech, impaired memory, and somnolence. Hyperthyroidism in the adult results in hyperexcitability, irritability, restlessness, exaggerated responses to environmental stimuli, and emotional instability. Psychosis can occur in either hypothyroidism or hyperthyroidism.

Basal metabolic rate

Thyroid hormones increase oxygen consumption in most cells of the body with the exception of the lungs, spleen, gastric smooth muscle, gonads, and accessory sex organs. In hypothyroidism the basal metabolic rate is subnormal; in hyperthyroidism it may be 40% to 60% above normal.

Carbohydrate and lipid metabolism

Thyroid hormones accelerate glucose catabolism, increase cholesterol synthesis, and enhance the liver's ability to excrete cholesterol in the bile. Because the effect on cholesterol excretion is greater than that on cholesterol synthesis, the result is a decrease in plasma cholesterol level. The hormones also stimulate the mobilization of fatty acids from adipose tissue. The hypothyroid individual will have an elevated serum cholesterol level and increased blood levels of phospholipids and triglycerides.

Protein metabolism

Thyroid hormones are essential for the development of protein mass. In hypothyroidism both the synthesis and the breakdown of protein are diminished, but the effect on protein synthesis is more profound. In addition, deposition of mucoproteins occurs in subcutaneous spaces, which osmotically attract water, causing "puffiness." In hyperthyroidism increased catabolism of protein, or breakdown of muscle mass, and increased nitrogen excretion occur.

Gastrointestinal function

Thyroid hormones increase gastrointestinal motility, absorption of food, and secretion of digestive juices. Hypothyroidism decreases both intestinal absorption and secretion of pancreatic enzymes. Constipation also may occur.

Water and electrolyte balance

In thyroid hormone deficiency, water and electrolytes accumulate in subcutaneous spaces; administering thyroid hormone results in diuresis and a loss of fluid and electrolytes from the subcutaneous spaces.

Cardiovascular function

Because the thyroid hormones increase metabolism, the tissues have an increased need for oxygen and nutrients, which in turn demands increased blood flow. In hyperthyroidism these effects cause increased cardiac output, increased pulse pressure, and tachycardia. If these effects are prolonged, cardiac hypertrophy and even high-output myocardial failure may occur. The opposite effects occur in hypothyroidism.

Muscle function

Moderate increases in thyroid hormone make muscles react with vigor; large increases result in muscle weakness because of excess protein catabolism. A characteristic sign of hyperthyroidism is a fine muscle tremor. Hypothyroidism causes the muscles to be sluggish.

Temperature regulation

Thyroid hormones must be present for an increase in heat production or a decrease in heat loss to occur. Although the hormones do not initiate the physiologic response to cold, they appear to magnify the body's response to catecholamine effects, which innervate the sympathetic system during cold exposure. Hypothyroidism causes decreased tolerance to cold.

Lactation

Thyroid hormone is necessary for normal milk production; without thyroid hormone, the fat content of milk and total milk production are greatly reduced.

Reproduction

Thyroid hormone is required for normal rhythmicity in the reproductive cycle.

Thyroid Gland Disorders

Goiter

The synthesis of the thyroid hormones and their maintenance in the blood in adequate amounts depend largely on an adequate intake of iodine. Iodine ingested by way of food or water is changed into iodide and is stored in the thyroid gland before reaching the circulation. Prolonged iodine deficiency in the diet results in enlargement of the thyroid gland, known as a simple **goiter.** When thyroid hormones fail to be synthesized because of a lack of iodine, the anterior lobe of the pituitary is stimulated to increase the secretion of thyrotropic hormone, which in turn causes hypertrophy and hyperplasia of the gland. The enlarged thyroid then removes residual traces of iodine from the blood. This type of goiter (simple or nontoxic) can be prevented by providing an adequate supply of iodine for young persons. Iodine is not abundant in most foods except fish and seafood, and iodized salt is frequently the primary source of iodine in areas where seafood is expensive or not readily available.

Hypothyroidism

Patients with primary hypothyroidism have decreased T_3 and T_4 levels and an elevated TSH level. Those with pituitary (secondary) hypothyroidism and hypothalamic (tertiary) hypothyroidism have decreased levels of T_3, T_4, and TSH.

The TSH test, the most sensitive index of hypothyroidism, is elevated in primary hypothyroidism and depressed in secondary hypothyroidism. The free thyroxine index (FTI) is depressed in patients with both primary and secondary hypothyroidism but elevated in patients with hyperthyroidism. T_3 resin uptake (T_3RU) is depressed in pregnant patients and in patients with primary and secondary hypothyroidism but elevated in patients with hyperthyroidism. The serum T_3 level is depressed in both secondary and primary hypothyroidism but elevated in hyperthyroid states and T_3 thyrotoxicosis. The T_4 (measured by the Murphy-Pattee technique) level is elevated in pregnancy and hyperthyroidism but depressed in both primary and secondary hypothyroidism. The free T_4 (unbound) level is depressed in both primary and secondary hypothyroid states but is elevated in hyperthyroid states.

Hypothyroidism in the young child is known as cretinism and is characterized by cessation of physical and mental development, which leads to dwarfism and mental retardation. Individuals with cretinism usually have thick, coarse skin; a thick tongue; gaping mouth; protruding abdomen; thick, short legs; poorly developed hands and feet; and weak musculature. This condition may result from faulty development or atrophy of the thyroid gland during fetal life. Failure of development of the gland may be caused by lack of iodine in the mother.

In children, normal skeletal growth is evidence of adequate therapy; an increase in serum alkaline phosphatase indicates that growth will occur. In cretinism, thyroid hormone levels equal to or above those required for the adult must be established immediately after birth to prevent permanent mental and physical retardation. Treatment of the older cretin will not reverse the mental retardation that has already occurred. Persons with hypothyroidism need to be informed of their lifelong need for replacement therapy.

Severe hypothyroidism in the adult is called **myxedema** (acid mucopolysaccharide accumulation). When it is the last stage of long-standing, inadequately treated, or untreated hypothyroidism, coma sets in accompanied by hypotension, hypoventilation, hypothermia, bradycardia, hyponatremia, and hypoglycemia. The development of myxedema is usually insidious and causes gradual retardation of physical and mental functions. There is gradual infiltration of the skin and loss of facial lines and facial expression (resulting in a puffy, expressionless face). The formation of subcutaneous connective tissue causes the hands and face to appear puffy and swollen. The basal metabolic rate becomes subnormal, the skin is cold and dry, the hair becomes scant and coarse, movements become sluggish, cardiac output is reduced, and the patient becomes hypersensitive to cold.

Hyperthyroidism (Thyrotoxicosis)

Excessive formation of the thyroid hormones and their escape into the circulation result in a toxic state called **thyrotoxicosis.** This occurs in the condition known as diffuse toxic goiter, or exophthalmic goiter (Graves' disease) or in some forms of adenomatous goiters.

Primary hyperthyroidism is characterized by elevated levels of T_3 and T_4 and decreased level of TSH. In pituitary (secondary) hyperthyroidism levels of T_3, T_4, and TSH increase. Hyperthyroidism leads to symptoms quite different from those seen in myxedema. The metabolic rate is increased, sometimes as much as 60% or more. The body temperature frequently is above normal, the pulse rate is fast, and the patient complains of feeling too warm. Other symptoms include restlessness, anxiety, emotional instability, muscle tremor and weakness, sweating, and exophthalmos. The increased T_4 levels may cause cardiomegaly, tachycardia, congestive heart failure, hepatic alterations (necrosis, dysfunction, and fatty changes), lymphoid hyperplasia, osteoporosis, pretibial myxedema, and neurologic irritability. In thyroid storm, a sudden onset of hyperthyroid symptoms occurs, especially those affecting the nervous and cardiovascular systems, because of elevated T_4 levels. Before the advent of antithyroid drugs, treatment was limited to a subtotal resection of the hyperactive gland. Propylthiouracil is the most commonly used antithyroid medication. However, antithyroid drugs provide less rapid control of hyperthyroidism than do surgical measures. Radioactive therapy is used primarily in treatment of middle-aged and elderly patients.

PARATHYROID GLANDS

Lying just above and behind the thyroid gland are bean-shaped glands known as the parathyroids. Humans have two pairs. The adult glands consist of encapsulated masses of cells, between which are abundant adipocytes and vascular channels. The primary function of the parathyroids is to maintain adequate levels of calcium in the extracellular fluid. Parathyroid hormone has multiple effects, ultimately culminating in mobilization of calcium from bone. It also reduces phosphate concentration, permitting more calcium to be mobilized.

Parathyroid Hormones

Parathyroid hormone (PTH) is a polypeptide. The active component has a half-life of 30 minutes and the inactive component of 7 to 10 days. PTH circulates in elevated concentrations in patients with hyperplastic parathyroid glands as a result of diminished calcium levels, as found in persons with impaired renal function or intestinal malabsorption. These elevated PTH levels may cause metabolic bone disease, including osteoporosis and osteomalacia.

The mechanism of PTH action in the bone or kidney is incompletely understood. Some researchers suggest that PTH receptor-binding and adenylate cyclase activity are coupled events subject to down-regulation of the receptors. Patients with hyperparathyroidism may be resistant to PTH action on kidney and bone. The decreased number of these receptors, not their altered affinity, produces a reduction in PTH-stimulated adenylate cyclase activity.

Cholesterol-derived provitamin D is converted to vitamin D_3 by the action of sunlight on the skin. The vitamin is also present as a milk additive. Along with PTH, vitamin D_3 is converted to its active form in the kidney. It is involved in calcium, phosphate, and magnesium metabolism in bone and the gastrointestinal tract. Primary hyperparathyroidism is the most common parathyroid disorder. Generally it is caused by adenomas, chief cell hyperplasia, or hypertrophy. PTH elevations produce altered function of renal tubular cells, bone cells, and gastrointestinal tract mucosa. Elevated levels of calcium and increased bone resorption with the development of renal calculi occur generally in hyperparathyroidism. In secondary hyperparathyroidism, an overactive parathyroid gland causes increased calcium excretion and possibly kidney stones, but serum calcium levels generally remain stable because of an effective feedback mechanism.

Hypoparathyroidism leads to manifestations of hypocalcemia and tetany, the symptoms of which include muscle spasms, convulsions, gradual paralysis with dyspnea, and death from exhaustion. Before death, gastrointestinal hemorrhages and hematemesis frequently occur. At death the intestinal mucosa is congested, and the calcium content of the heart, kidney, and other tissues is increased.

The symptoms of tetany are relieved by administration of calcium salts. Large doses of vitamin D also help to relieve tetany and to restore the normal calcium level in the blood. The patient is hospitalized because frequent assessment of blood calcium and phosphate levels is essential.

ADRENAL GLANDS

The adrenal glands are located just above the kidneys. They consist of two parts: the inner medulla and the outer cortex. The adrenal cortex synthesizes three important classes of hormones: the glucocorticoids (cortisol), mineralocorticoids (primarily aldosterone), and androgens (primarily dehydroepiandrosterone). The **glucocorticoids,** adrenocortical steroid hormones that increase glyconeogenesis, exert an antiinflammatory effect, and influence many body functions, are synthesized primarily in the zona fasciculata and are under the control of ACTH from the pituitary gland.

Although the basal production rate averages 30 mg every 24 hours, under stressful conditions (trauma, major surgery, and infection) there is a reserve capacity production of up to 300 mg daily. Increases in glucocorticoid production may be related to proportional increases in the release of ACTH by the pituitary. For more information, see the discussion of steroid abuse in Chapter 6.

The **mineralocorticoids** are synthesized specifically in the zona glomerulosa of the adrenal cortex. Production is primarily under the control of both the renin-angiotensin axis system (discussed later) and the blood potassium level. The production of aldosterone is stimulated by salt depletion and causes sodium retention in the kidney at the distal convoluted tubule to preserve the extracellular fluid volume. Mineralocorticoids also increase the urinary excretion of potassium and hydrogen ions and maintain normal blood volume.

The androgens are synthesized in the zona fasciculata and the zona reticularis and essentially enhance male characteristics and control growth of the hair follicles in the skin.

Normally a reaction to serious stress causes a prompt and noticeable increase in cortisol and aldosterone production; these hormones operate together to maintain the cardiovascular tone essential for survival. A person under stress who has impaired ability to produce these hormones incurs the risk of developing acute adrenal crisis. The production of cortisol is under the control of a continuous feedback mechanism involving the pituitary and ACTH production, which is in turn inhibited by the circulating cortisol levels. Stress is a stimulus to override this inhibition and initiates secretion of corticotropin-releasing factor, which culminates in ACTH release and activation of the adrenal cortex, leading to an increased production of cortisol.

Mineralocorticoids: Aldosterone

Aldosterone is the primary mineralocorticoid to regulate sodium and potassium balance in the blood. It is synthesized in the adrenal zona glomerulosa, which is the outer edge of the adrenocortical tissue below the adrenal capsule. Aldosterone production is maintained primarily by the renin-angiotensin system and the concentration of circulating serum potassium. A drop in the circulating arterial volume stimulates volume receptors in the juxtaglomerular apparatus. As a result, renin (a proteolytic enzyme) is produced and acts on angiotensinogen, which is synthesized by the liver to form angiotensin I. When the angiotensin I passes through the pulmonary circulation, two amino acids are cleared from it to form angiotensin II. Angiotensin II stimulates the adrenal zona glomerulosa to produce aldosterone. Aldosterone promotes sodium reabsorption in the kidney at the distal convoluted tubule to preserve extracellular fluid volume. In the normal patient, aldosterone secretion is stimulated by a decrease in circulating volume (e.g., loss of blood, excessive diuresis, and low salt intake) and increased potassium levels. Aldosterone secretion is suppressed by an elevation of sodium levels in the blood (e.g., by excessive dietary salt intake). It restricts the loss of sodium and its accompanying anions, chloride and bicarbonate, and thereby helps to maintain extracellular fluid volume. It also maintains acid-base and potassium balance.

In adrenal insufficiency, aldosterone deficit occurs, sodium reabsorption is inhibited, and potassium excretion decreases. Hyperkalemia and mild acidosis occur. With adrenalectomy the loss of aldosterone leads to an overall reduction of sodium reabsorption and a powerful and uncontrolled loss of extracellular fluid. Plasma volume drops, and a state of hypovolemic shock may ensue. This may cause death unless a mineralocorticoid, salt, and water are administered. In excessive doses aldosterone increases potassium excretion, and unless dietary intake compensates for the loss, hypokalemia results. Acidification of the urine then occurs, leading to metabolic alkalosis.

Aldosterone has much more potent electrolyte effects than desoxycorticosterone, although it a therapeutic status comparable to that of desoxycorticosterone has not yet been established. Its use has been limited because of its cost and relative unavailability and because it must be administered intramuscularly.

The amount of aldosterone secreted by the adrenal cortex apparently is affected by the concentration of sodium in body fluids rather than by the stimulation of the adrenal cortex by ACTH.

PANCREAS

The pancreas is a gland that lies transversely across the posterior wall of the abdomen. It secretes a limpid, colorless fluid that digests proteins, fats, and carbohydrates. It also produces internal secretions, insulin and glucagon, that affect blood glucose levels.

Insulin is a hormone secreted by the beta cells of the islets of Langerhans in the pancreas in response to increased levels of glucose in the blood. On hydrolysis, this hormone yields several amino acids. In its crystalline state it appears to be chemically linked with certain metals (zinc, nickel, cadmium, or cobalt). Normal pancreatic tissue is rich in zinc, which may be significant to the natural storage of the hormone. Insulin consists of two polypeptide chains and contains 48 amino acids, the exact sequence of which is known. Insulin is stored in the beta cells as a larger protein known as proinsulin. Because relatively small amounts of insulin are necessary in the body tissues, it is thought that insulin acts as a catalyst in cellular metabolism.

Carbohydrate metabolism is controlled by a finely balanced interaction of several endocrine factors (adrenal, anterior pituitary, thyroid, and insulin), but the particular phase of carbohydrate metabolism that is affected by insulin is not entirely known. When insulin is injected subcutaneously, however, it produces a rapid lowering of the blood glucose. This effect is produced in both diabetic and nondiabetic persons. Moderate amounts of insulin in the diabetic animal promote the storage of carbohydrate in the liver and also in the muscle cells, particularly after the feeding of carbohydrate. In the normal animal the deposit of muscle glycogen also increases, but apparently the level of liver glycogen does not. In both diabetic and nondiabetic persons the oxygen consumption increases and the respiratory quotient rises.

Glucagon, like insulin, is a pancreatic extract and is thought to oppose the action of insulin. Glucagon is a product of the alpha cells of the islets of Langerhans. Glucagon acts primarily by mobilizing hepatic glycogen and converting it to glucose, which produces an elevation in the concentration of glucose in the blood.

Diabetes Mellitus

Diabetes mellitus is a heterogeneous complex disorder of carbohydrate, fat, and protein metabolism that is primarily a result of a relative or complete lack of insulin or defects of the insulin receptors. Insulin action is ineffective at the tissue site, or not enough insulin is available. Obesity, certain drugs, viruses, autoimmune phenomena, genetic predisposition, and age may have roles in its development. The blood glucose becomes elevated, and when it exceeds a certain amount, the excess is secreted by the kidney (glycosuria). Symptoms include increased appetite (polyphagia), thirst (polydipsia), weight loss, increased urine output (polyuria), weakness (fatigue), and itching such as pruritus vulvae.

In diabetes mellitus, glycogen fails to store in the liver, although the conversion of glycogen back to glucose or the formation of glucose from other substances (gluconeogenesis) is not necessarily impaired. As a result, the level of blood glucose level rises rapidly. This derangement of carbohydrate metabolism results in an abnormally high metabolism of proteins and fats. The ketone bodies, which result from oxidation of fatty acids, accumulate faster than the muscle cells can oxidize them, resulting in ketosis and acidosis.

The course of untreated diabetes mellitus is progressive. The symptoms of diabetic coma and acidosis are directly or indirectly the result of the accumulation of acetone, beta-hydroxybutyric acid, and diacetic acid. Respirations become rapid and deep, the breath has an odor of acetone, the blood glucose level is elevated, the patient becomes dehydrated, and stupor and coma develop unless treatment is started promptly.

The long-term complications of diabetes mellitus can lead to an increase in morbidity and mortality. Some of the most commonly associated problems are peripheral atherosclerosis, which may result in coronary artery disease, infections, gangrene, or strokes, and diabetic retinopathy, which can include vitreal hemorrhage, retinal detachment, and blindness. Renal disease, peripheral sensory neuropathy, and cardiomyopathy leading to heart failure are also reported.

Diabetes mellitus usually is treated with exogenous insulin, diet, and exercise. Glucose and insulin promote the formation and retention of glycogen in the liver, and the oxidation of fat in the liver is arrested. Therefore the rate of formation of acetone bodies is slowed, and the acidosis is checked. Other supportive measures, such as restoring the fluid and electrolyte balance of the body, are very important in its treatment.

Recent advances in diabetic therapy include (1) the synthesis of human insulin by bacteria genetically altered by recombinant DNA technology, (2) islet cell and/or pancreas transplantation, and (3) external and implanted continuous insulin infusion pumps.

SUMMARY

The endocrine system is involved with integrating and regulating body function with the use of hormones. This system is composed of specialized glands and their hormones that act on specific target cells to produce various responses. Pathologic conditions in this system usually involve the overproduction or underproduction of hormones. For hormonal underproduction, replacement hormone therapy is usually prescribed as discussed in the following chapters.

REVIEW QUESTIONS

1. Name six vital processes produced by hormones from different endocrine glands.
2. Maintenance of the internal environment is similar to the functioning of a thermostat. Explain the negative feedback mechanism.
3. Describe the effect of thyroid hormones on growth, central nervous system function, basal metabolic rate, food metabolism, temperature regulation, and cardiovascular function.
4. Explain the effects of the mineralocorticoids produced by the adrenal glands.

REFERENCES

Olin BR: *Facts and comparisons.* Philadelphia, 1998, JB Lippincott.

ADDITIONAL REFERENCES

Anderson KN et al, editors: *Mosby's medical, nursing, and allied health dictionary,* ed 5, St Louis, 1998, Mosby.

Hershman JM et al: A savvy approach to thyroid testing, *Patient Care* 26(3):134, 1992.

Melmon KL et al: *Clinical pharmacology: Basic principles in therapeutics,* ed 3, New York, 1992, McGraw-Hill.

Seeley RR, Stephens TD, Tate P: *Anatomy and physiology,* ed 3, New York, 1995, McGraw-Hill.

Thibodeau GA, Patton KT: *Anatomy and physiology,* ed 4, St Louis, 1999, Mosby.

Wingard LB et al: *Human pharmacology,* St Louis, 1991, Mosby.

CHAPTER 39

Drugs Affecting the Pituitary Gland

CHAPTER FOCUS

Although the pituitary gland secretes many hormones, this chapter is limited only to growth hormone and antidiuretic hormone, vasopressin. The other hormones will be discussed in the appropriate chapters more directly involved with the endocrine glands affected.

OBJECTIVES

After reading and studying this chapter, the student should be able to do the following:

1. *Define and describe the key terms and key drugs.*
2. *Name and discuss the primary functions of the anterior and posterior pituitary hormones.*
3. *Describe the indications and mechanisms of action for somatrem, somatropin, octreotide, and vasopressin.*
4. *Discuss the primary effects of lypressin nasal spray.*

KEY DRUGS

somatrem, (p. 542)
vasopressin, (p. 543)

KEY TERMS

diabetes insipidus, (p. 544)
dwarfism, (p. 542)
gigantism, (p. 542)
growth hormone-inhibiting hormone (somatostatin), (p. 542)
growth hormone-releasing hormone (GHRH), (p. 542)

The variety of preparations available that affect the pituitary gland are generally used as replacement therapy for hormone deficiency or drug therapy for specific disorders using such preparations to produce a therapeutic hormonal response and as diagnostic aids to determine hypofunctional or hyperfunctional hormone states.

A number of hormones have been identified, and many have been synthesized, including the following: growth hormone-releasing hormone (GHRH), growth hormone-inhibiting hormone (somatostatin), thyrotropin-releasing hormone (TRH), corticotropin-releasing hormone (CRH), gonadotropin-releasing hormone (GnRH, gonadorelin), and prolactin-inhibiting hormone (PIH, dopamine). Six anterior pituitary hormones and two posterior pituitary hormones have also been identified. The anterior pituitary hormones include growth hormone (GH), thyrotropin (TSH), adrenocorticotropin (ACTH), follicle-stimulating hormone (FSH), luteinizing hormone (LH), and prolactin. The posterior pituitary hormones are vasopressin and oxytocin. This chapter covers specific agents affecting the pituitary gland.

Of the previously mentioned hormones, GnRH is discussed in Chapter 44, and TRH and CRH are discussed in Chapters 40 and 41, respectively. While a true hormone with prolactin-inhibiting effects has not been identified, the substance is believed to be dopamine. Bromocriptine, a drug with dopamine-agonist properties, is reviewed in Chapters 17 and 45.

Of the remaining substances, **growth hormone-releasing hormone (GHRH)** has been identified in vivo but is still under investigation. This substance has been found to stimulate the release of growth hormone after intranasal application. It is currently listed as an orphan drug manufactured by Fujisawa. Information on orphan drug availability may be obtained from the Office of Orphan Products Development (HF-35), 5600 Fishers Lane, Rockville, Md 20857 (Olin, 1998).

Growth hormone-inhibiting hormone (somatostatin) was obtained from human cadaver pituitaries, but its distribution in the United States was stopped in 1985. Creutzfeldt-Jakob disease (a neurotropic virus), which is rare in young people, was diagnosed in some patients and resulted in the death of several persons 5 to 7 years after receiving this product. Several biosynthetic hormones grown through recombinant deoxyribonucleic acid (DNA) technology are available in the United States. Growth hormone preparations include somatrem and somatropin while octreotide is used to inhibit the release of growth hormone.

ANTERIOR PITUITARY HORMONES

somatrem [soe' ma trem] (Protropin)

Somatrem contains the identical sequence as the pituitary-derived human growth hormone plus one additional amino acid, methionine. In tests it has been demonstrated to be therapeutically equivalent to somatropin, the pituitary human growth hormone.

Mechanism of action

Somatrem's anabolic effects are due to the indirect effect of another hormone, known as somatomedin C or insulin-like growth factor 1 (IGF-1). IGF-1 is directly responsible for skeletal and soft tissue growth, and it also increases cell numbers in the body rather than cell size. Therefore a major pharmacologic consequence of somatrem use is an increase in longitudinal growth, whereas a deficiency in growth hormone usually results in **dwarfism.**

Somatrem also has metabolic effects: it decreases insulin sensitivity and may also affect glucose transport; it increases lipolysis; it promotes cellular growth by retaining phosphorus, sodium, and potassium; and it enhances protein synthesis by increased nitrogen retention.

Indications

Somatrem is indicated for the treatment of growth failure in children caused by a pituitary growth hormone deficiency. It is sometimes abused by athletes seeking increased size and strength. For the major effects and adverse effects associated with the use of anabolic steroids, see Chapter 6.

Pharmacokinetics

The half-life of parenteral (IV) somatrem is 20 to 30 minutes (IM and SC, 3 to 5 hours), and the duration of action is 12 to 48 hours. It is metabolized in the liver and excreted by the kidneys.

Drug interactions

When somatrem is given concurrently with adrenocorticoids, glucocorticoids, or ACTH, the growth response effects of somatrem may be impaired. ACTH should not be given concurrently, and if it is necessary to treat with an adrenocorticoid agent, the daily dosages should be limited. For example, the total daily dose per square meter of body area should not be greater than the following: cortisone (12.5 to 18.8 mg), hydrocortisone (10 to 15 mg), methylprednisolone (2 to 3 mg), prednisone or prednisolone (2.5 to 3.75 mg), betamethasone (300 to 450 µg), and dexamethasone (250 to 500 µg).

Side effects and adverse reactions

Antibodies to somatrem have been reported in 30% to 40% of treated patients during the first 3 to 6 months of therapy, but only 5% of the patients develop neutralizing antibodies. It is rare for a patient not to respond to therapy. However, pain and edema have been reported at the site of injection and, rarely, an allergic type reaction (rash and itching). Excessive doses may produce **gigantism,** an abnormal condition characterized by excessive size and stature, in children. Therefore before the drug is used, growth failure must be carefully documented, and dosages and individual responses closely monitored. Hypothyroidism has been rarely reported.

Warnings

Use with caution in patients with hypothyroidism and cancer.

Contraindications

Avoid use in persons with somatrem hypersensitivity.

Dosage and administration

The dosage of somatrem (Protropin) for children is up to 0.1 mg/kg injected IM or SC (preferred) three times weekly. Monitor the growth rate response in 3 to 6 months to determine if dosage adjustment is necessary. Therapy is usually continued until epiphyseal closure occurs, or there is no further response. If therapy is unsuccessful (growth of <2 cm per year), the treatment should be discontinued and the child reevaluated (Olin, 1998; USP DI, 1998).

somatropin, recombinant [soe ma troe′ pin] (Humatrope)

Somatropin is a DNA recombinant product that is identical to the amino acid sequence of human growth hormone. It is used to stimulate linear growth in patients who lack sufficient endogenous growth hormone, thus resulting in increased skeletal growth (an increased length of the epiphyseal plates of long bones reported). The number and size of muscle cells, organs, and red cell mass are also increased. An increase in cellular protein synthesis and lipid mobilization resulting in a decrease in body fat stores is also reported.

The mechanism of action, indications, warnings, and other properties of somatropin are similar to those of somatrem.

The recommended pediatric dosage is individualized up to 0.06 mg/kg SC or IM three times weekly (Olin, 1998).

octreotide [ok tree′ oh tide] (Sandostatin)

Octreotide is a long acting agent with an effect similar to that of somatostatin, the growth hormone-inhibiting hormone, although it is a more potent inhibitor of growth hormone, glucagon, and insulin (Olin, 1998).

Indications

Octreotide is indicated to lower blood levels of growth hormone and IGF-1 to normal in persons with acromegaly who are unable to have or have not responded to other therapies, such as surgery, radiation, and bromocriptine. It is also used to treat the symptoms associated with carcinoid tumors, such as flushing and severe diarrhea. It also has many unapproved uses, including the treatment of acquired immunodeficiency syndrome (AIDS)-associated diarrhea. See a current reference for additional indications, approved and unapproved.

Pharmacokinetics

It is rapidly absorbed after SC injection, reaching a peak serum concentration in about 25 minutes with a half-life of 1.7 hours. Its duration of action is variable but depending on the tumor can be up to 12 hours. The IV and SC doses of octreotide are considered equivalent in effect.

Drug interactions

Concurrent use of octreotide with the sulfonylurea antidiabetic agents, glucagon, growth hormone, or insulin may result in hypoglycemia or hyperglycemia. Closely monitor as dosage adjustments may be needed.

Side effects and adverse reactions

These include pain, swelling, and pruritus at the injection site; sinus bradycardia, diarrhea, and stomach distress (30% to 58% in acromegalic patients, but only 5% to 10% in other disorders); headache; dysrhythmias; and cold-like symptoms. Hyperglycemia, hypoglycemia, and hypothyroidism are also reported, primarily in acromegalic patients. Check a current reference for list of other potential side effects and adverse reactions.

Warnings

Use with caution in patients with diabetes mellitus and severe kidney impairment.

Contraindications

Avoid use in persons with octreotide hypersensitivity and gallbladder disease.

Dosage and administration

The dose in acromegaly is 50 μg three times a day, SC or IV, adjusted according to the patient's response and the presence of side effects and adverse reactions.

POSTERIOR PITUITARY HORMONES

The posterior pituitary gland hormones are oxytocin and vasopressin (antidiuretic hormone [ADH]). Oxytocin is discussed in Chapter 45 with the drugs related to labor and delivery. Vasopressin is obtained from natural sources whereas lypressin and desmopressin are synthetic derivatives of vasopressin. Desmopressin has a longer duration of activity than the other agents.

vasopressin [vay soe press′ in]) (Pitressin)
desmopressin [des moe press′ in] (DDAVP, Stimate)
lypressin [lye press′ in] (Diapid)

The ADH effect is the result of increasing water reabsorption in the collecting ducts of the nephron, resulting in a decreased urine volume with a higher osmolarity. At higher than physiologic dosages, vasopressin stimulates peristalsis through a direct effect on gastrointestinal motility, increases secretion of corticotropin, growth hormone, and FSH and may increase blood pressure secondary to a vasoconstriction effect.

TABLE 39-1 Posterior Pituitary Hormones: Side/Adverse Effects

Drug	Side Effects*	Adverse Reactions†
desmopressin (DDAVP, Stimate)	Less frequent: headache, nausea, mild stomach cramps, vulval pain Injection: local redness, burning or swelling, facial flush, slight increase or decrease in blood pressure	Rare: severe allergic reaction including anaphylaxis with parenteral administration
lypressin (Diapid)	Less frequent: abdominal distress, headache, heartburn, eye pain, nasal irritation or itching, runny nose, increase in bowel movements	Rare: continuous coughing, chest pain, shortness of breath, difficult breathing
vasopressin (Pitressin)	Less frequent: abdominal distress, gas, sweating, nausea, vomiting, tremors, increased pressure for bowel evacuation, headache	Rare: chest pain due to angina or myocardial infarction, allergic reaction, increased or continuing headaches, confusion, coma, convulsions, weight gain, drowsiness, urinary difficulties (usually the result of water retention or intoxication)

*If side effects continue, increase, or disturb the patient, inform the prescriber.
†If adverse reactions occur, contact the prescriber because medical intervention may be necessary.

Indications

Vasopressin (Pitressin) is used to treat **diabetes insipidus,** a metabolic disorder characterized by extreme polyuria and polydipsia caused by the deficient production or secretion of the antidiuretic hormone centrally. It is not effective for polyuria induced by renal impairment, nephrogenic diabetes insipidus, psychogenic diabetes insipidus, or drug-induced (lithium or demeclocycline) diabetes insipidus.

The synthetic formulations (desmopressin [DDAVP] and lypressin [Diapid]) act as ADH with little vasopressor activity. Lypressin is used to treat persons who are either nonresponsive to or unable to tolerate other interventions. This product prevents or controls the polydipsia, polyuria, and dehydration caused by diabetes insipidus (insufficient ADH). Vasopressin, desmopressin, and lypressin are not effective for polyuria induced by renal impairment, nephrogenic diabetes insipidus, psychogenic diabetes insipidus, hypokalemia, hypercalcemia, or drug-induced diabetes insipidus (e.g., by lithium or demeclocycline).

Desmopressin intranasal is used for primary nocturnal enuresis. The oral, intranasal, and parenteral dosage forms are used to treat central diabetes insipidus, while only the parenteral dosage form of desmopressin is used for hemostasis in hemophilia A and von Willebrand's disease patients.

Pharmacokinetics

Vasopressin administered IM or SC has a half-life of 10 to 20 minutes; the duration of effect is 2 to 8 hours. It is metabolized in the liver and kidneys and excreted by the kidneys.

Lypressin nasal spray has an immediate onset of antidiuretic activity, peaks in ½ to 1½ hours, and has a duration of action of 3 to 8 hours. Desmopressin nasal has a half-life of approximately 3.5 hours, and the peak serum concentration is reached in 40 to 45 minutes. For the oral and intranasal dosage forms the peak serum level is reached in 1 to 1½ hours. The onset of antidiuretic effects the tablets is within 1 hour while the maximum effect is reached between 4 and 7 hours.

Drug interactions

No significant drug interactions are reported.

Side effects and adverse reactions

See Table 39-1.

Dosage and administration

The adult dosage of aqueous vasopressin injection (Pitressin) is 5 to 10 units IM or SC two or three times a day when needed to treat central diabetes insipidus. In children the dosage for treatment of central diabetes insipidus is 2.5 to 10 units three or four times daily.

The adult lypressin nasal spray dose is 1 or 2 sprays to one or both nostrils when urination frequency increases or a significant thirst sensation occurs. The usual pediatric and adult dose is 1 or 2 sprays in each nostril four times a day.

For children 6 years of age and older and adults, the desmopressin intranasal dose for primary nocturnal enuresis is 10 μg (0.2 ml) intranasal at bedtime, adjusted as necessary. The central diabetes insipidus adult dose is 0.1 to 0.4 mg daily as a single dose or in divided doses. The parenteral dose is 0.5 to 1 ml SC or IV daily in two divided doses. The oral adult dose starts with 0.05 mg twice daily and is adjusted according to response.

SUMMARY

The drugs in this chapter are usually used for replacement therapy, that is, hormone deficiency, such as drug therapy for a specific disorder. Somatrem is used for growth failure in children; desmopressin, lypressin, and vasopressin are used for central diabetes insipidus or to control excess blood levels of growth hormone, such as octreotide. In addition, desmopressin is also used to treat primary nocturnal enuresis and hemophilia A or von Willebrand's disease. The parenteral form of desmopressin is used to maintain hemostasis before surgery or can help to stop bleeding in patients with IM hematomas or mucosal bleeding.

Somatrem is equivalent to somatropin (or the human growth hormone from the anterior pituitary) and is used to treat growth failure in children caused by a hormone deficiency while octreotide is similar to somatostatin, the growth-hormone-inhibiting agent, so it is used in acromegaly. It also has additional uses as discussed in this chapter.

REVIEW QUESTIONS

1. Describe the mechanism of action for somatrem's anabolic effects. What metabolic effects does it have? What side effects and adverse reactions?
2. What effects does octreotide have in the body? What are its indications, pharmacokinetics, and side effects and adverse reactions?
3. Compare the effects, indications, and dosage and administration of vasopressin, desmopressin, and lypressin.

REFERENCES

Olin BR: *Facts and comparisons.* Philadelphia, 1998, JB Lippincott.

United States Pharmacopeial Convention: *USP DI: drug information for the health care professional,* ed 18, Rockville, Md, 1998, The Convention.

ADDITIONAL REFERENCES

American Hospital Formulary Service: *AHFS drug information '98,* Bethesda, Md, 1998, American Society of Hospital Pharmacists.

Anderson KN et al, editors: *Mosby's medical, nursing, and allied health dictionary,* ed 5, St Louis, 1998, Mosby.

Ascoli M, Segaloff DL: Adenohypophyseal hormones and their hypothalamic releasing factors. In Hardman JG, Limbird LE, editors: *Goodman & Gilman's the pharmacological basis of therapeutics,* ed 9, New York, 1996, McGraw-Hill.

Jaffe CA, Barkan AL: Acromegaly: recognition and treatment, *Drugs* 47(3):425-445, 1994.

Mosby: *Mosby's GenRx,* St Louis, 1998, Mosby.

CHAPTER 40

Drugs Affecting the Parathyroid and Thyroid Glands

KEY DRUGS

propylthiouracil, (p. 553)
thyroid (p. 549)

CHAPTER FOCUS

Thyroid and parathyroid disorders have a large influence on the endocrine system. They affect growth and development, metabolic rate, energy level, and reproductive systems. Healthcare professionals need to be knowledgeable about these preparations to ensure safe and effective management of their patients.

KEY TERMS

iodine, (p. 551)
myxedema, (p. 549)
primary hyperparathyroidism, (p. 547)

OBJECTIVES

After reading and studying this chapter, the student should be able to do the following:

1. *Define and describe the key terms and key drugs.*
2. *Describe the signs and symptoms associated with hypothyroidism, hyperthyroidism, hypoparathyroidism, and hyperparathyroidism.*
3. *Describe the need for and dosage of calcium and vitamin D products in the treatment of hypoparathyroidism.*
4. *Name the primary agents used to treat hypothyroidism.*
5. *Discuss the two diagnostic agents used to assess thyroid function.*
6. *Present the effects of iodine (iodide ion), radioactive iodine, and thioamide drugs in treating hyperthyroidism.*

This chapter reviews the wide variety of medications available to treat the various conditions of the thyroid and parathyroid glands.

PARATHYROID GLANDS

In idiopathic hypoparathyroidism, serum calcium levels are decreased while serum phosphate levels are increased. Usually vitamin D levels are low. The administration of vitamin D and calcium supplements usually will restore the calcium and phosphorus levels to normal (Box 40-1). Calcitriol (Rocaltrol) is an active metabolite form of vitamin D that is also used to elevate serum calcium levels. Table 40-1 lists drugs used to treat hypocalcemia.

Primary hyperparathyroidism is a hyperactivity of the parathyroid glands with excessive secretion of parathyroid hormone that results in increased resorption of calcium from the skeletal system and increased absorption of calcium by the kidneys and the gastrointestinal (GI) system. The urine phosphate level is high (serum level is low to normal), which can lead to renal stones, bone pain with skeletal lesions, and possibly pathologic fractures. Because adenomas or tumors may cause this syndrome, surgery is usually the primary treatment. In patients with mild hypercalcemia or mild hyperparathyroidism, a thorough examination by a physician determines whether or not surgery is indicated. High serum levels of calcium may require immediate treatment. Table 40-2 describes typical recommendations for treatment of hypercalcemia.

Calcitonin and other synthetic drugs are used to treat hypercalcemia, osteoporosis, and Paget's disease. Two calcitonin products are available: salmon calcitonin (Calcimar) and human calcitonin (Cibacalcin), and both products produce the same effect although the salmon calcitonin has a slightly longer half-life (70 to 90 minutes versus 60 minutes).

Indications

Both calcitonins are indicated for the treatment of Paget's bone disease; in addition, calcitonin-salmon is also indicated for hypercalcemia and postmenopausal osteoporosis.

Pharmacokinetics

Onset of the therapeutic effect with either calcitonin in Paget's disease may range from 6 to 24 months of regular treatment although some improvement (a decrease in serum alkaline phosphatase levels) may occur within the first few months. The peak effect of calcitonin-salmon in hypercalcemia is 2 hours and duration of action is 6 to 8 hours. Excretion is via the kidneys.

Drug interactions

No significant drug interactions are reported.

TABLE 40-1 Hypocalcemia Treatment

Drug	*Usual Adult Dose*
calcium gluconate	IV: 970 mg given slowly at rate not exceeding 5 mL (47.5 mg) per min
Vitamin D Analogs	
calcifediol (Calderol)	Oral: 50 μg daily per week; adjust dose monthly if necessary
calcitriol (Rocaltrol)	Oral: 0.25 μg daily, increased every 2-4 weeks if necessary IV: 0.5 μg three times a week, increased every 2-4 weeks if necessary
dihydrotachysterol (Hytakerol)	Oral: 0.12-2 mg daily
ergocalciferol (Calciferol)	Oral: individualized dosing; prophylaxis dose is 5-10 μg daily

BOX 40-1 Calcium Supplements

The activity of calcium depends on calcium ion (elemental) content. The following calcium salts are listed by milligrams per gram, milliequivalents per gram, and percent of calcium in the preparation.

Preparation	*Calcium (mg/g)*	*Calcium (mEq/g)*	*Percent of Calcium*	*Calcium/Salt in Tablet (mg)**	*Tablets Needed to Provide 1000 mg of Calcium*
calcium carbonate	400	20.0	40	250/625 500/1250	4 2
calcium chloride	272	13.6	27.2		
calcium citrate	211	10.5	21.1	200/950	5
calcium gluceptate	82	4.1	8.2		
calcium gluconate	90	4.5	9	45/500	22
calcium lactate	130	6.5	13	42/325	24
calcium phosphate				115/500	9
dibasic	230	11.5	23		
tribasic	400	20	38		

TABLE 40-2 Hypercalcemia: Treatment Recommendations

Increase Calcium Excretion	
saline diuresis	Infuse normal saline (100-200 mL/hr) to increase calcium excretion. Monitor fluid intake, output, and electrolytes. Watch closely for evidence of fluid overload.
furosemide (Lasix)	Often used with the administration of normal saline as above. Usual dose is 20-40 mg IV bid to qid.
Inhibit Bone Resorption	
calcitonin-salmon (Calcimar)	IM or SC: 4-8 IU/kg every 6-12 hours. Tolerance can develop in 24-72 hours; therefore corticosteroids may be prescribed concurrently.
etidronate (Didronel)	IV infusion: 7.5 mg/kg in 250 mL of normal saline, administered over 2 hr daily until calcium level is normal or for a maximum of 1 week.
pamidronate (Aredia)	IV infusion: 60-90 mg in 1 L of normal saline infused over 24 hr. The advantage of this product is that it is effective in a single dose.
plicamycin (Mithracin)	More toxic than other agents. Reserve for individuals who do not respond to other therapies. Usual dose is 25 μg/kg in 500 mL of dextrose in water administered IV over 4-60 hr.

From Tang, Lau, 1995; Woodley, Whelan, 1992.

Side effects and adverse reactions

For the parenteral dosage form these may include flushing or a tingling sensation of the face, ears, hands and feet, gastric distress, anorexia, diarrhea, abdominal pain, increased urinary frequency, respiratory difficulties, nausea, vomiting, and pain or swelling at the injection site. For the nasal spray (Miacalcin) effects include rhinitis, nasal irritation and redness, muscle and back pain, epistaxis, and headache.

Contraindications

Avoid use in persons with a history of protein allergy or calcitonin hypersensitivity.

Dosage and administration

The usual salmon-calcitonin adult dose for Paget's disease is 100 IU (IM or SC) daily, decreasing to 50 IU daily, every other day and then three times weekly. For postmenopausal osteoporosis, the parenteral dose is 100 IU (IM or SC) daily; the nasal dose is 200 IU intranasally daily, alternating nostrils each day.

To reduce the occurrence of nausea or flushing, bedtime administration is suggested or, if necessary, a reduction in dosage may be required. It is also recommended that patients take 1.5 g of a calcium carbonate supplement and 400 units of vitamin D daily. For the treatment of hypercalcemia, see Table 40-2.

Bisphosphonates

Alendronate (Fosamax), etidronate (Didronel), pamidronate (Aredia), and tiludronate (Skelid) are bisphosphonates that are incorporated into bone to inhibit normal and abnormal resorption, primarily by decreasing activity of osteoclasts. In addition, etidronate reduces bone formation while alendronate and pamidronate inhibit bone resorption without inhibiting bone formation.

Mechanism of action

Multiple mechanisms may be involved, but the action of these agents is believed to be due to binding to hydroxyapatite in bone, decreasing dissolution of mineral bone content, or their effect on bone resorbing cells. For example, alendronate incorporation in bone will decrease bone resorption by suppressing the number and action of osteoclasts. Tiludronate is the newest biphosphonate released and has an action similar to alendronate. It also decreases abnormal bone growth in Paget's disease because unlike etidronate it does not interfere with bone mineralization.

Indications

Alendronate is indicated for the treatment of postmenopausal osteoporosis and Paget's disease; etidronate and pamidronate are indicated for the treatment of Paget's disease and hypercalcemia associate with cancer. In addition, etidronate is used for heterotopic ossification while pamidronate is also used as a treatment adjunct for osteolytic metastases (bone metastases). Tiludronate is indicated for the treatment of Paget's disease.

Drug interactions

The following effects may occur when alendronate or tiludronate is given with the drugs listed below:

Drug	Possible effect and management
Oral medications including antacids, mineral supplements, food, or beverages	Food and other items may interfere with the absorption of alendronate, etidronate, and tiludronate. Separate medications by at least two hours.
Salicylates	Patients who take more than 10 mg/day of alendronate concurrently with salicylates will have an increased potential for upper GI tract adverse effects with alendronate. Salicylates will decrease tiludronate absorption by up to 50% if taken within 2 hours after tiludronate. Space medications at least 2 hours before or after tiludronate.

pamidronate	When pamidronate is administered concurrently with calcium preparations, vitamin D, calcifediol, or calcitriol, the effects of pamidronate may be antagonized when used for the treatment of hypercalcemia may be antagonized.

Side effects and adverse reactions

With alendronate these include gas production, acid regurgitation, esophageal ulcer, gastritis, dysphagia, constipation, diarrhea, muscle pain, and headaches; with etidronate, bone pain (and perhaps bone fractures and osteomalacia), nausea, diarrhea, metallic taste, and, rarely, hypersensitivity; and with pamidronate, fever, nausea, vomiting, anorexia, leukopenia, hypocalcemia (more common with dosages of 90 mg), and muscle stiffness. Tiludronate may cause upper respiratory or flu-like syndrome (fever, nasal congestion, and sore throat), back or body pain, abdominal distress, nausea, headache, diarrhea, arthralgia, conjunctivitis, pharyngitis, rash, nausea, vomiting, cataract, glaucoma, and chest pain.

Warnings

Use all bisphosphonates (with the exception of pamidronate) with caution in patients with hypocalcemia or vitamin D deficiency

Contraindications

Avoid use of alendronate and tiludronate in persons with GI diseases and kidney impairment, especially when creatinine clearance is <30 to 35 ml/min. Avoid use of etidronate in persons with hypercalcemia, heart failure, bone fractures, enterocolitis, and impaired kidney function (serum creatinine level is 2.5 to 4.9 mg/dl). For pamidronate, avoid use in persons in heart failure or with kidney function impairment (serum creatinine level is 5 mg/dl or more). Avoid use of any of these agents if the patient is reportedly hypersensitive to it.

Dosage and administration

The usual adult dose of alendronate for Paget's disease is 40 mg daily (at least 30 minutes before breakfast) for 6 months, for etidronate the dose is 5 mg/kg PO (at least 2 hours before or after food) daily for 6 months or 7.5 mg/kg by IV infusion daily for 3 consecutive days, and for pamidronate the dose is 30 mg/day on 3 consecutive days by IV infusion, up to 30 mg weekly for 6 weeks (90 to 180 mg total dose per treatment) given at a rate of 15 mg/hr. For other dosages, see a current reference. For treatment of hypercalcemia, see Table 40-2. The adult dose of tiludronate for Paget's disease is 400 mg at least 2 hours before or after food, beverages, or other medications. Take all oral dosage forms with 6 to 8 oz of water.

THYROID GLAND

Thyroid Preparations

Individuals with hypothyroidism require thyroid replacement therapy. For many years, natural or desiccated thyroid was used for replacement therapy, but the synthetic thyroids available today are more standardized and stable formulations and so are generally prescribed. Thyroid USP is derived mainly from hog thyroid glands, although cattle and sheep thyroid glands have also been used.

The thyroid gland produces two iodine-containing active hormones, thyroxine (T_4) and triiodothyronine (T_3), which are essential for human growth and development and also to maintain metabolic homeostasis. These hormones have been synthesized and are available as liothyronine (for T_3), levothyroxine (for T_4), and liotrix (both T_3 and T_4). See Chapter 38 for further information on the functioning of the thyroid gland. Table 40-3 illustrates equivalent dosages and the usual adult dose for thyroid products.

The goal of treatment of patients with hypothyroidism or **myxedema** (adult hypothyroidism) is to eliminate their symptoms and to restore them to a normal emotional and physical state. Box 40-2 lists the clinical features of hyperthyroidism versus hypothyroidism. Clinical response is more important than blood hormone level; however, laboratory assessments of T_3, T_4, serum cholesterol, and thyrotropin levels are used as criteria for adequacy of therapy.

Thyroid hormone concentrations are regulated by the hypothalamic-anterior pituitary and thyroid body feedback mechanism (Box 40-3).

Indications

Thyroid supplements are indicated for the treatment of hypothyroidism, treatment and prevention of goiter, treatment and prevention of thyroid carcinoma, and thyroid function diagnostic tests.

Pharmacokinetics

Thyroid and levothyroxine are incompletely absorbed from the gastrointestinal tract (50% to 75%), whereas liothyronine is nearly completely absorbed (95%). They are highly protein bound with a peak effect in 3 to 4 weeks and duration of action of 1 to 3 weeks for thyroid, thyroglobulin, and levothyroxine after withdrawal of chronic therapy. Liothyronine peaks in 2 to 3 days and has a duration of action of up to 3 days after withdrawal. These agents are metabolized the same as endogenous thyroid hormone—some in peripheral tissues and smaller amounts in the liver—and excreted in bile.

Drug interactions

The following effects may occur when thyroid hormone preparations are given with the drugs listed below:

TABLE 40-3 Thyroid Preparations: Equivalent and Usual Adult Dose

Drug	Equivalent Dose	Usual Adult Dose
levothyroxine (Synthroid)	100 μg (0.1 mg)	Orally: 12.5-50 μg daily (geriatric patients or those with cardiovascular disease, dose range is 12.5-25 μg daily), adjusting dose every 2-3 weeks as necessary. Injection: 50-100 μg IM or IV daily. For myxedema, stupor, or coma, the dose is 200-500 μg IV initially, even in geriatric patients. If improvement is not noted by the second day, additional 100-200 μg (0.1 to 0.3 mg) may be given. Switch to oral dose form as soon as possible.
liothyronine (Cytomel)	25 μg (0.025 mg)	Orally: 25-50 μg daily, adjusting dose every 1-2 weeks as needed. For myxedema and simple, nontoxic goiter, dose is 2.5-5 μg daily (increasing at 5-10 μg increments every 7-14 days) as necessary. Maintenance myxedema dose is 25-50 μg/day; for simple goiter, it is 50-100 μg/daily.
liotrix (Thyrolar)	50-60 μg of levothyroxine and 12.5-15 μg of liothyronine	Orally: myxedema, 50-60 μg of levothyroxine and 12.5-15 μg of liothyronine daily; increase monthly if necessary. Geriatric dose is 25%-50% of the usual adult dose, adjusted as necessary at 6- to 8-week intervals.
thyroid	60 mg	Orally: 60-120 mg daily. For myxedema or hypothyroidism with cardiovascular disease, initial dose is 15 mg daily, increased as necessary every 2 weeks. Geriatric dose is 7.5-15 mg daily, doubled every 6-8 weeks if necessary.

Pregnancy safety for all thyroid products has been established as Food and Drug Administration (FDA) category A.

Drug	Possible effect and management
Anticoagulants, oral (coumarin or indanedione)	May alter the therapeutic effects of the oral anticoagulant. An increase in thyroid hormone may require a decrease in anticoagulant oral dosage. Monitor coagulation time closely using the prothrombin time (PT) test.
cholestyramine (Questran) or colestipol (Colestid)	May bind thyroid hormones, delaying or decreasing their absorption from the gastrointestinal tract. A 4- to 5-hour interval is recommended between administration of these drugs.
Sympathomimetics	The effects of one or both medications may be increased. An increased risk of coronary insufficiency may result if the individual has coronary artery disease. If a thyroid preparation is given with tricyclic antidepressants, an increase in cardiac dysrhythmias may result. Monitor closely, since dosage adjustments may be necessary.

Side effects and adverse reactions

Side effects are dose related and may occur more rapidly with liothyronine than with the other products mainly because it has a faster onset of action. The general signs of underdosage or hypothyroidism are dysmenorrhea, ataxia, coldness, dry skin, constipation, lethargy, headaches, drowsiness, tiredness, weight gain, and muscle aching. During the early period of treatment, hair loss may occur in children but with chronic therapy, normal hair growth will resume.

A rare adverse reaction is an allergic skin rash. Overdose with thyroid products results in hyperthyroidism: alterations in appetite and menstrual periods, elevated temperature, diarrhea, hand tremors, increased irritability, leg cramps, increased nervousness, tachycardia, irregular heart rate, increased sensitivity to heat, chest pain, respiratory difficulties, increased sweating, vomiting, weight loss, and insomnia.

Warnings

Use with caution in patients with diabetes mellitus and malabsorption problems.

Contraindications

Avoid use in persons with adrenocortical or pituitary insufficiency, cardiac disease, hyperthyroidism, thyrotoxicosis, and thyroid hypersensitivity.

Dosage and administration

See Table 40-3 and the Geriatric Implications box.

Diagnostic Testing for Hypothyroidism

Protirelin (Thypinone, Relefact TRH) and thyrotropin (thyroid-stimulating hormone, TSH) are diagnostic agents used to assess thyroid function. The TSH stimulation test is a very sensitive test used to diagnose hypothyroidism. Thyroid-releasing hormone (TRH) is administered to measure the pituitary's response to TRH. For example, in hypothalamic hypothyroidism, the pituitary responds slowly to

BOX 40-2 **Hyperthyroidism vs. Hypothyroidism: Clinical Features**

	Hyperthyroidism	*Hypothyroidism*
Eyes	Prominent	Eyelids edematous, ptosis
Hair	Thin, fine texture	Dry, brittle, thin
Temperature	Intolerance to heat	Intolerance to cold
Weight	Appetite increases, weight loss	Appetite decreases, weight gain
Emotional	Increased nervousness, irritability, insomnia	Lethargic, depressed, increase in sleeping needs
Gastrointestinal	Diarrhea	Constipation
Neuromuscular	Fast deep tendon reflexes	Slow or delayed deep tendon reflexes
Extremities	Hot, moist skin	Cold, dry skin

BOX 40-3 **Thyroid Feedback Mechanism**

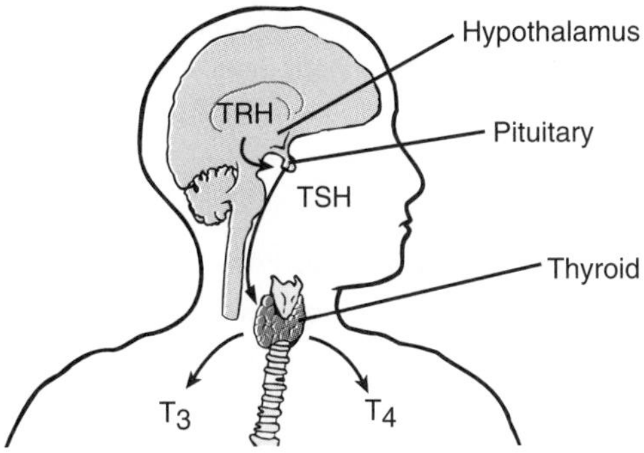

Physiology of Influences on the Thyroid

When serum levels of T_3 and T_4 are increased, the release of TRH from the hypothalamus and TSH from the anterior pituitary gland is reduced, thus inhibiting their effects on the thyroid gland.

When serum levels of T_3 and T_4 are decreased, TRH release triggers the release of TSH from the pituitary. TSH effects on the thyroid are an increase in the size and number of follicular cells in the thyroid, thus increasing their ability to absorb iodide, and an increase in thyroglobulin breakdown, which releases T_3 and T_4 hormones from the thyroid gland into the bloodstream, thus increasing blood levels of the thyroid hormones.

GERIATRIC IMPLICATIONS

Thyroid Hormones

Since the elderly are usually more sensitive to and experience more adverse reactions to thyroid hormones than other age groups, it is recommended that thyroid replacement doses be individualized. In some persons, the dose should be 25% lower than the usual adult dose.

Hypothyroidism, the second most common endocrine disease in the elderly, is often misdiagnosed. Only one third of the geriatric patients exhibit the typical signs and symptoms of cold intolerance and weight gain. Most often the symptoms are nonspecific, such as failing to thrive, stumbling and falling episodes, incontinence, and, if neurologic involvement has occurred, a misdiagnosis of dementia, depression, or a psychotic episode may be made (USP DI, 1998; Rizzolo, 1992).

Laboratory tests for serum T_4 and TSH are used to confirm hypothyroidism.

Levothyroxine (Synthroid, others) is usually the drug of choice for thyroid replacement.

exogenous TRH and produces a slow but rising TSH. In patients with primary hypothyroidism, TSH basal levels are increased, and the pituitary is hyperreactive to TRH stimulation. If the patient has hypothyroidism resulting from hypopituitarism, no response to TRH is expected. Therefore the TSH stimulation test can differentiate a primary from a secondary hypothyroidism and also differentiate hypopituitary from hypothalamic hypothyroidism. See Box 40-3 for an illustration of this thyroid feedback mechanism.

ANTITHYROID AGENTS

An antithyroid drug is a chemical agent that lowers the basal metabolic rate by interfering with the formation, release, or action of thyroid hormones. Antithyroid drugs that interfere with the synthesis of the thyroid hormones are known as goitrogens. A variety of compounds are included in this category of antithyroid drugs, but only iodine (iodide ion), radioactive iodine, and thioamide derivatives are discussed here.

Iodine and Iodides

Iodine, an essential micronutrient, almost 80% of which in the body is in the thyroid gland, is the oldest of the antithyroid drugs. Although a small amount of iodine is necessary for normal thyroid function and to synthesize thyroid hormones, the response of the patient with thyrotoxicosis to iodine administration is inhibition of thyroid hormone synthesis and thyroid release from the hyperfunctioning thyroid gland.

Thyroid-Iodide Pump

Iodide from the diet is rapidly absorbed into the bloodstream. Approximately one third of it is removed from the blood by the iodide pump in the thyroid. The initial iodide removed from the blood is usually sodium or potassium iodide. The enzyme peroxidase converts the iodides to iodine, which is then used to form monoiodotyrosine (MIT) and diiodotyrosine (DIT), which are the components of T_3 and T_4. The synthesized hormones (T_3 and T_4) are stored within thyroglobulin until they are released into the blood circulation. These activities involve a complex negative feedback mechanism between the thyroid gland and the hypothalamus-pituitary gland. Low levels of circulating thyroid hormone increase the release of TSH from the pituitary and appear to influence the secretion of thyrotropin-releasing factor (TRF) from the hypothalamus. Increased levels of TSH increase iodide trapping by the gland, which results in an increase in synthesis and circulating thyroid hormones. As thyroid hormone levels increase, the hypothalamic and pituitary centers stop the release of TRF and TSH. This process is repeated if thyroid hormone levels decrease again, in response to the declining levels of circulating thyroid hormones. For more information about the thyroid feedback mechanism, see Box 40-3.

The inhibition of thyroid hormone release for several weeks leads to an increase in TSH secretion that can overcome this blockade. Thus large doses of iodides are generally used for 7 to 14 days before thyroid surgery to decrease the thyroid's size and vascularity, resulting in diminished blood loss and a less complicated surgical procedure.

Radioactive iodine (RAI) is preferred for persons who are poor surgical risks, such as debilitated patients, those with advanced cardiac disease, and the elderly. It is also used for patients who have not responded adequately to drug therapy or who have had recurrent hyperthyroidism after surgery. The primary disadvantage of using surgery or RAI therapy, in addition to the risk involved with surgery and postsurgical complications, is the induction of hypothyroidism.

Iodine Products

strong iodine solution (Lugol's solution) *potassium iodide*

Iodine is indicated to protect the thyroid gland from radiation before and after the administration of radioactive isotopes of iodine or in radiation emergencies and may be used with an antithyroid drug in patients with hyperthyroidism in preparation for thyroidectomy. Therapeutic effects may be noted within 24 hours with maximum effects achieved within 10 to 14 days of continuous therapy.

Strong iodine solution is a combination of 5% iodine and 10% potassium iodide. The iodine is converted to iodide in the GI tract before systemic absorption.

Potassium iodide liquid or tablets are also commonly known as KI or SSKI.

Drug interactions

The following effects may occur when iodide products are given with the drugs listed below:

Drug	Possible effect and management
Antithyroid drugs	May increase the hypothyroid and goitrogenic effects of the drugs. Monitor closely for decreased metabolic activity.
Diuretics, potassium-conserving type	If these diuretics are used concurrently with potassium iodide, increased levels of potassium may result in hyperkalemia, cardiac dysrhythmias, or cardiac arrest. Monitor serum potassium levels closely.
lithium	The hypothyroid and goitrogenic effects of both drugs may be potentiated. Obtain and monitor baseline thyroid status periodically to plan appropriate interventions.

Side effects and adverse reactions

These include diarrhea, nausea, vomiting, stomach pain, rash, swelling of the salivary gland, and with prolonged usage, severe headaches, sore gums or teeth, increased salivation, burning sensation in the mouth or throat, and a metallic taste in the mouth.

Warnings

Use with caution in patients with tuberculosis, hyperthyroidism, and, for potassium iodide only, myotonia congenita.

Contraindications

Avoid use of strong iodine solution in persons with iodine or potassium iodide hypersensitivity, bronchitis, pulmonary edema, hyperkalemia, and kidney impairment. For potassium iodide, avoid use in persons with potassium iodide hypersensitivity, hyperkalemia, and kidney impairment.

Dosage and administration

The adult dose of strong iodine solution before thyroid surgery is 3 to 5 drops administered in a full glass of water, fruit juice, or milk three times daily.

The potassium iodide adult oral dose is 100 to 150 mg 24 hours before radiation, then daily for 3 to 10 days afterward. Children 1 year of age and older are given a 130 mg oral dose daily for 10 days after exposure to radioactive iodine. To reduce GI injury, it is recommended that potassium iodide be administered in a full glass of water, fruit juice, or milk. In addition, the tablet dosage form should be dissolved in ½ glass of water or milk before ingestion.

While unclassified regarding pregnancy safety, strong iodine solution and potassium iodide do cross the placenta and may produce abnormal thyroid function in infants.

sodium iodide (^{131}I, Iodotope)

Sodium iodide, a radioactive isotope of iodine, accumulates in thyroid tissue and selectively damages or destroys it.

Indications

It is indicated for the treatment of hyperthyroidism and thyroid carcinoma.

Pharmacokinetics

Administered orally, it has an onset of effect within 2 to 4 weeks; the peak therapeutic effect occurs between 2 and 4 months; and it is mainly excreted by the kidneys. Up to 20% of the dose may appear in breast milk within 24 hours. It has a radionuclide half-life of approximately 8 days; principal types of radiation are beta and gamma rays.

Drug interactions

Although no significant drug interactions are noted with this product, many drugs are capable of interfering with test results. See a current reference for possible drug interference and current dosage recommendations.

Side effects and adverse reactions

These include sore throat, neck swelling or pain, temporary loss of taste, nausea, vomiting, and painful salivary glands. After treatment for hyperthyroidism, the patient may experience increased or unusual irritability or tiredness. After treatment for thyroid carcinoma, the patient may experience fever, sore throat, chills (due to leukopenia), and increased bleeding episodes (thrombocytopenia).

If hypothyroidism occurs after treatment, monitor for changes in menstrual cycle, ataxia, cold feelings, sedation, dry puffy skin, headaches, muscle aches, dry or thin hair, weakness, and unusual weight gain.

Warnings

Use with caution in patients with diarrhea, vomiting, nephrosis, low serum chloride level, kidney function impairment, and severe thyrotoxic cardiac disease, especially the elderly.

Contraindications

Avoid use in persons with hypersensitivity to radiopharmaceutical preparations.

Dosage and administration

Pregnancy safety is classified as FDA category X.

Thioamide Derivatives

methimazole [meth im′ a zole] (Tapazole)
propylthiouracil [proe pill thye oh yoor′ a sill] (Propyl-Thyracil)

Thioamide derivatives, or antithyroid agents, inhibit thyroid hormone synthesis by inhibiting incorporation of iodide into tyrosine and the coupling of iodotyrosines. They do not affect exogenous thyroid hormones.

Propylthiouracil (not methimazole) also inhibits the conversion of T_4 to T_3, which may make it more effective for treatment of thyroid crisis or storm.

Indications

These agents are indicated for the treatment of hyperthyroidism, before surgery or radiotherapy, or as adjunct therapy for treatment of thyrotoxicosis or thyroid storm (propylthiouracil preferred for the latter indication).

Pharmacokinetics

The half-life of methimazole is 5 to 6 hours and of propylthiouracil us 1 to 2 hours. The peak effect occurs in 7 weeks with methimazole and 17 weeks with propylthiouracil. They are metabolized in the liver and excreted by the kidneys.

Drug interactions

The following drug interactions may occur when methimazole or propylthiouracil is administered with the drugs listed below:

Drug	Possible effect and management
amiodarone, iodinated glycerol, lithium, or potassium iodide	Amiodarone contains 37% iodine by weight. Increased or excess amounts of amiodarone, iodide, or iodine may result in a decreased response to the antithyroid drugs. Iodine deficiency, however, may result in an increased response to the antithyroid medications. Monitor closely.
Anticoagulants (coumarin or indanedione)	As thyroid status approaches normal, the response to anticoagulants may decrease, or, if the thioamide produces a drug-induced hypoprothrombinemia, the anticoagulant response may increase. Monitor closely because anticoagulant doses are adjusted based on prothrombin time test results.
Digitalis glycosides	As thyroid status approaches normal, serum levels of digoxin and digitoxin may increase. Monitor closely as dosage adjustments may be necessary.
sodium iodide ^{131}I	Thyroid uptake of ^{131}I may be decreased by the antithyroid agents. Monitor closely.

Side effects and adverse reactions

These include rash, pruritus, dizziness, loss of taste, nausea, vomiting, paresthesias, stomach pain, fever, chills, sore throat, weakness, jaundice of skin and eyes (due to cholestatic hepatitis) and, rarely, edema, backache, nephritis, joint pain, swollen lymph nodes, and increased bleeding tendencies or bruising.

Warnings

Use with caution in patients with a low leukocyte count.

Contraindications

Avoid use in persons with a history of methimazole or propylthiouracil hypersensitivity and liver impairment.

Dosage and administration

The methimazole oral adult dosage is 15 to 60 mg daily for hyperthyroidism. The maintenance dose is 5 to 30 mg daily in one or two divided doses. To treat thyrotoxic crisis, the dosage is 15 to 20 mg every 4 hours for 24 hours used as an adjunct to other therapies. The pediatric dose for hyperthyroidism is 0.4 mg/kg daily; the maintenance dose is 0.2 mg/kg daily.

The propylthiouracil oral adult dosage is 300 to 900 mg daily in divided doses. Children between 6 and 10 years of age receive 50 to 150 mg daily, while children older than 10 years of age receive 50 to 300 mg daily. For neonatal thyrotoxicosis, the dose is 10 mg/kg daily in divided doses.

Pregnancy safety has been established as FDA category D; both drugs cross the placenta and can cause fetal hypothyroidism and goiter.

SUMMARY

Improper functioning of the parathyroid or thyroid glands necessitates medical interventions. For example, if the patient has hypoparathyroidism, the use of vitamin D and calcium supplements will usually restore the calcium and phosphorus levels to normal. However, with hyperparathyroidism, the primary approach is usually surgery.

The patient with hypothyroidism has many undesired signs and symptoms, therefore the therapeutic goal is to eliminate the symptoms with thyroid replacement therapy.

Hyperthyroidism is managed by large doses of iodides to inhibit thyroid hormone release and reduce the size of the thyroid, a thioamide derivative that inhibits thyroid synthesis, radioactive iodine, or surgery.

Generally, these therapies provide hormone replacement or hormone inhibition; therefore close patient monitoring is necessary to avoid over- or undertreatment of the pathologic state.

REVIEW QUESTIONS

1. Describe the condition and treatment for idiopathic hypoparathyroidism and primary hyperparathyroidism.
2. Present the actions, indications, drug interactions, major side effects and adverse reactions, and dosage and administration for the bisphosphonates.
3. Name and describe the two active hormones in the thyroid. What are the names for the synthesized thyroid hormones? Discuss the indications, pharmacokinetics, and drug interactions of the thyroid hormones.
4. Discuss the use of iodine products and the thioamide derivatives on the thyroid gland.

REFERENCES

Rizzolo P: Thyroid. In Ham RJ, Sloane PD, editors: *Primary care geriatrics: a case-based approach,* ed 2, St Louis, 1992, Mosby.

Tang I, Lau AH: Fluid and electrolyte disorders. In Young LY, Koda-Kimble MA, editors: *Applied therapeutics: the clinical use of drugs,* ed 6, Vancouver, Wash, 1995, Applied Therapeutics, Inc.

United States Pharmacopeial Convention: *USP DI: drug information for the health care professional,* ed 18, Rockville, Md, 1998, The Convention.

Woodley M, Whelan A: *Manual of medical therapeutics,* ed 27, Boston, 1992, Little, Brown.

ADDITIONAL REFERENCES

American Hospital Formulary Service: *AHFS drug information '98,* Bethesda, Md, 1998, American Society of Hospital Pharmacists.

American Medical Association: *AMA drug evaluations 1995,* Chicago, 1995, the Association.

Anderson KN et al, editors: *Mosby's medical, nursing, and allied health dictionary,* ed 5, St Louis, 1998, Mosby.

Katzung BG: *Basic and clinical pharmacology,* ed 5, Norwalk, Conn, 1992, Appleton & Lange.

Kovacs CS, MacDonald SM, Chik CL, Bruera E: Hypercalcemia of malignancy in the palliative care patient: a treatment strategy, *J Pain Sympt Manag* 10(3):224-232, 1995.

McCance KL, Huether SE: *Pathophysiology: the biologic basis for disease in adults and children,* ed 3, St Louis, 1998, Mosby.

Melmon KL et al: *Clinical pharmacology: basic principles in therapeutics,* ed 3, New York, 1992, McGraw-Hill.

Mosby: *Mosby's GenRx,* St Louis, 1998, Mosby.

Olin BR: *Facts and comparisons.* Philadelphia, 1998, JB Lippincott.

Toft AD: Thyroxine therapy, *N Engl J Med* 331(3):174-180, 1994.

CHAPTER 41

Drugs Affecting the Adrenal Cortex

KEY DRUGS

cortisone (p. 556)
fludrocortisone, (p. 561)

CHAPTER FOCUS

This chapter discusses the medical approach to management of hyposecretion or hypersecretion of the adrenal cortex and reviews the rhythms that appear to influence glucocorticoid function (circadian and ultradian). The glucocorticoids affect numerous normal and pathologic conditions in the body; therefore the healthcare professional must have knowledge about the drugs that affect the adrenal cortex.

OBJECTIVES

After reading and studying this chapter, the student should be able to do the following:

1. *Define and describe the key terms and key drugs.*
2. *Describe the major effects of the glucocorticoids in the human.*
3. *Name and discuss a potentially serious drug interaction with a corticosteroid.*
4. *Discuss the recommended method for discontinuing corticosteroid treatment.*
5. *Name five major adverse reactions reported with the use of the corticosteroids.*

KEY TERMS

circadian rhythm, (p. 556)
corticosteroid, (p. 556)
glucocorticoids, (p. 556)
mineralocorticoids, (p. 556)
septic shock, (p. 557)
ultradian rhythms, (p. 556)

The adrenal cortex produces three types of steroid hormones: **glucocorticoids, mineralocorticoids,** and androgens. This chapter discusses the glucocorticoids and mineralocorticoids, otherwise referred to as corticosteroids (or adrenocorticoids).

The term **corticosteroid** refers to the natural or synthetic hormones associated with the adrenal gland. The principal glucocorticoid is cortisone, and the principal mineralocorticoid produced in humans is aldosterone. Corticosteroids are divided into two classes: glucocorticoids (an adrenocortical hormone that has antiinflammatory effects, increases glyconeogenesis, and has many other effects in the body [see discussion below]) and mineralocorticoids (an adrenocortical hormone that helps maintain blood volume, promotes retention of sodium and water, and increases urinary excretion of potassium and hydrogen ions).

Cholesterol, which is used for the biosynthesis of corticosteroids, is synthesized and stored in the adrenal cortex. Corticosteroid synthesis depends on pituitary adrenocorticotropin (ACTH), which is governed by the corticotropin-releasing hormone (CRH) from the hypothalamus. Evidence suggests that increased levels of corticosteroids can inhibit the adrenal glucocorticoid system by inhibiting the release of CRH from the hypothalamus and by inhibiting the release of ACTH from the pituitary.

GLUCOCORTICOIDS

Two rhythms appear to influence glucocorticoid function: circadian (daily) rhythm and ultradian rhythm. **Circadian rhythm,** a pattern based on a 24-hour cycle, with the repetition of certain physiologic phenomena, is controlled by the dark/light and sleep/wakefulness cycles. Normal persons sleeping in the dark at night will have increased plasma cortisol levels in the early morning hours that reach a peak after they are awake. These levels then slowly fall to very low levels in the evening and during the early phase of sleep. The importance of this rhythm is emphasized by the finding that corticosteroid therapy is more potent when given at midnight than when given at noon.

Ultradian rhythms are periodic or intermittent functions with frequencies greater than once every 24 hours. In human beings, four to eight adrenal glucocorticoid bursts occur each 24 hours, which may follow bursts in CRH and ACTH releases. These bursts are clustered close together and are very pronounced during the circadian rise in plasma glucocorticoid levels in the early hours of the morning. At other times they may be so widely spaced that adrenal secretion is zero. Consequently the adrenal cortex secretes glucocorticoids only about 25% of the time in unstressed individuals.

Cortisone (Cortone) is considered the key or prototype drug for this classification, and it and its synthetic analogs have similar effects in the body. These include the following pharmacologic actions:

- *Antiinflammatory action.* Glucocorticoids and especially cortisol in larger than normal dosages can stabilize lysosomal membranes and prevent release of proteolytic enzymes during inflammation. They can also potentiate vasoconstrictor effects.
- *Maintenance of normal blood pressure.* Glucocorticoids potentiate the vasoconstrictor action of norepinephrine. When glucocorticoids are absent, the vasoconstricting action of the catecholamines is diminished and blood pressure falls.
- *Carbohydrate and protein metabolism.* Glucocorticoids help to maintain the blood sugar level and liver and muscle glycogen content. They facilitate breakdown of protein in muscle and extrahepatic tissues, which leads to increased plasma amino acid levels. Glucocorticoids increase the trapping of amino acids by the liver and stimulate the deamination of amino acids. They also increase the activity of enzymes important to gluconeogenesis and inhibit glycolytic enzymes. This can produce hyperglycemia and glycosuria. They are diabetogenic. These effects can aggravate diabetes, bring on latent diabetes, and cause insulin resistance. Inhibition of protein synthesis can delay wound healing and cause muscle wasting and osteoporosis. In young persons these effects can inhibit growth.
- *Fat metabolism.* Glucocorticoids promote mobilization of fatty acids from adipose tissue, increasing their concentration in the plasma and their use for energy. Despite this effect, individuals taking glucocorticoids may accumulate fat stores (rounded face, buffalo hump). The effect of glucocorticoids on fat metabolism is complex and little known.
- *Thymolytic, lympholytic, and eosinopenic actions.* Glucocorticoids can cause atrophy of the thymus and decrease the number of lymphocytes, plasma cells, and eosinophils in blood. By blocking the production and release of cytokines, corticosteroids interfere with the integrated role of T and B lymphocytes, macrophages, and monocytes in immune responses (Schimmer, Parker, 1996) and also ultimately interfere with allergic responses. This, along with their antiinflammatory action, makes them useful immunosuppressants for delaying rejection in patients with organ or tissue transplants as well as useful antiallergenics for the treatment of acute allergic reactions such as urticaria, bronchial asthma, and anaphylactic shock. However, steroids can also be a source of danger in infections by limiting useful protective inflammation. These hormones also inhibit activity of the lymphatic system, causing lymphopenia and reduction in size of enlarged lymph nodes.
- *Stress effects.* During stressful situations (e.g., injury and major surgery), corticosteroids are suddenly released or are necessary to help maintain homeostasis. This sudden release is believed to be a protective mechanism for the individual. Without steroid administration, hypotension and shock may occur (Fig. 41-1). During stress, epinephrine and norepinephrine also are released from the adrenal medulla, and these catecholamines have a synergistic action with the corticosteroids.

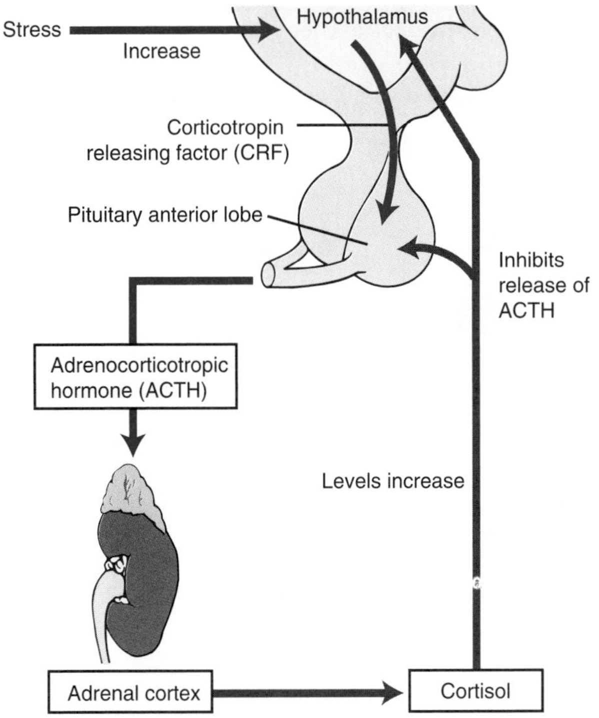

FIGURE 41-1
Glucocorticoid secretion.

BOX 41-1 Septic Shock

Septic shock usually results from a gram-negative bacteremia that leads to circulatory insufficiency. The inadequate tissue perfusion generally results in hypotension, oliguria, tachycardia, elevated temperature, and tachypnea.

Mechanism
Septic shock may be caused by bacterial substances that interact with body cell membranes and systems, especially coagulation and the complement system, resulting in injury to cells and alterations in blood flow in the body.

Treatment
Treatment may consist of volume replacement, antibiotics, surgery (if the client has an abscessed or necrotic bowel or organs/tissues), vasoconstricting agents (dopamine, norepinephrine, or levarterenol), diuretics, and glucocorticoids (steroids). Use of steroids is somewhat controversial, but several published studies have reported a benefit if they are used early in the treatment of shock.

Steroid Beneficial Effects
Beneficial effects of steroids include protecting cellular membranes from injury, decreasing platelet aggregation, reducing extracellular release of leukocyte enzymes, and preventing the formation of vasoactive substances in the body.

- *Central nervous system.* Corticosteroids effect mood and behavior and possibly cause neuronal or brain excitability. Some persons report euphoria, insomnia, anxiety, depression, and increased motor activity or may become psychotic.

Indications

Glucocorticoids are used as replacement therapy for adrenocortical insufficiency, to treat severe allergic reactions, anaphylactic reactions not responsive to other therapies, collagen disorders such as systemic lupus erythematosus, dermatologic conditions, hematologic disorders, ophthalmic disorders, respiratory disorders, rheumatic disorders, shock, and other conditions, and as adjunct treatment for neoplastic disease (Box 41-1).

Pharmacokinetics

The glucocorticoids are well absorbed orally; parenterally (IM) the soluble esters (sodium phosphate and sodium succinate) are rapidly absorbed while the poorly soluble agents (acetate, acetonide, diacetate, hexacetonide, and tebutate) are slowly but completely absorbed. Topically, the soluble esters are less rapidly absorbed while the poorly soluble agents are slowly but completely absorbed. Rectally about 20% of the drug is absorbed normally, but if the rectum is inflamed, absorption may increase up to 50%.

These agents are mainly metabolized in the liver and excreted by the kidneys. Cortisone and prednisone are inactive until metabolized to hydrocortisone and prednisolone, respectively. The fluorinated adrenocorticoids are more slowly metabolized than the other drugs.

For onset of action, peak effect, and duration of action, see Table 41-1. For the relative potency of the major short-acting, intermediate-acting, and long-acting adrenocorticoids, see Table 41-2.

Drug interactions

The following effects may occur when a corticosteroid is given with the drugs listed below:

Drug	Possible effect and management
aminoglutethimide (Cytadren)	Suppresses adrenal function; therefore do not administer corticotropin concurrently. When aminoglutethimide is given, glucocorticoid supplements are often prescribed. Be aware that aminoglutethimide can increase the metabolism of dexamethasone, reducing its half-life significantly. Hydrocortisone is recommended, however, because its metabolism does not appear to be affected by aminoglutethimide.

TABLE 41-1 Adrenocorticoids/Corticotropin: Pharmacology and Pharmacokinetics

Drug (Route)	*Onset of Action*	*Peak Effect*	*Duration of Action*
betamethasone (PO)	—	1-2 hr	3.25 days
(IM, IV)	Rapid	—	—
acetate/sodium phosphate (IM)	1-3 hr	—	7 days
corticotropin repository (IM)	—	—	12-24 hr
cortisone acetate (PO)	Rapid	2 hr	30-36 hr
(IM)	Slower	20-48 hr	—
dexamethasone (PO)	—	1-2 hr	66 hr
(IM)	—	8 hr	6 days
(IV)	Rapid	—	—
hydrocortisone (PO)	—	1 hr	30-36 hr
(IM)	—	4-8 hr	—
rectal enema (retention)	3-5 days	—	—
rectal foam	5-7 days	—	—
cypionate (PO)	Slow	1-2 hr	
(IM)	Rapid	1 hr	Varies
methylprednisolone (PO)	—	1-2 hr	30-36 hr
(IM)	6-48 hr	4-8 days	1-4 wk
(IA) (IL) (ST)	Very slow	7 days	1-5 wk
sodium succinate (IV, IM)	Rapid	—	—
prednisolone (PO)	—	1-2 hr	30-36 hr
acetate/sodium phosphate (IM)	—	—	Up to 4 wk
(IB, IS, IA, ST)	—	—	3-28 days
sodium phosphate (IV, IM)	Rapid	1 hr	—
prednisone (PO)	—	1-2 hr	30-36 hr
triamcinolone (PO)	—	1-2 hr	52 hr
(IM)	1-2 days	—	1-6 wk

From USP DI, 1998.
—, Not available; PO, orally; IM, intramuscularly; IV, intravenously, IA, intraarticularly; IL, intralesion; ST, in soft tissue; IB, intrabusal; IS, intrasynovial.

TABLE 41-2 Major Adrenocorticoids: Relative Potency and Half-Life

Adrenocorticoids	*Equivalent Glucocorticoid Dose (mg)**	*Relative Glucocorticoid Potency†*	*Relative Mineralocorticoid Potency‡*	*Half-Life (hr)*	
				Serum	*Tissue*
Short-acting					
cortisone	25	0.8	2	0.5	8-12
hydrocortisone	20	1	2	1.5-2	8-12
Intermediate					
methylprednisolone	4	5	0§	>3.5	18-36
prednisolone	5	4	1	2.1-3.5	18-36
prednisone	5	4	1	3.4-3.8	18-36
triamcinolone	4	5	0§	2->5	18-36
Long-acting					
betamethasone	0.6	20-30	0§	3-5	36-54
dexamethasone	0.5-0.75	20-30	0§	3-4.5	36-54

*Approximate dosages, applies to PO and IV only.
†Refers to antiinflammatory, immunosuppressant, and metabolic-type effects.
‡Potassium excretion and sodium and water retention.
§Some hypokalemia and/or sodium and water retention may occur, depending on dose and individual response.

amphotericin B parenteral (Fungizone)	May result in severe hypokalemia. If given concurrently, monitor serum potassium levels closely. May also decrease the adrenal gland response to corticotropin.
Antacids	When given concurrently with prednisone or dexamethasone, a decrease in steroid absorption may result. Monitor closely, as steroid dosage adjustments may be necessary.
Antidiabetic drugs (oral) or insulin	Glucocorticoids may elevate serum glucose levels (both during therapy and after, if the glucocorticoid is stopped); therefore a dosage adjustment of one or both drugs may be necessary.
Digitalis glycosides	May result in increased potential for toxicity (dysrhythmias) associated with hypokalemia.
Diuretics	The sodium- and fluid-retaining effects of the adrenocorticoids may reduce the effectiveness of the diuretic agents. Monitor closely for edema and fluid retention. Potassium-depleting diuretics given with adrenocorticoids may result in severe hypokalemia. Monitor potassium serum levels. The effects of potassium-sparing diuretics may be decreased. Monitor serum potassium levels and patient response closely.
Hepatic enzyme-inducing agents	Barbiturates, carbamazepine, phenytoin, and others may decrease the adrenocorticoid effect because of increased metabolism. Dosage adjustment may be necessary. Monitor serum cortisol levels closely.
mitotane (Lysodren)	Mitotane will decrease the adrenal gland's response to corticotropin. Avoid concurrent use. Adrenocorticoids are usually necessary during mitotane administration because mitotane suppresses adrenocortical function. Usually, higher than normal doses of glucocorticoids are needed.
Potassium supplements	These reduce the effect of either one or both medications on serum potassium levels. Monitor serum levels if given concurrently.
ritodrine (Yutopar)	When ritodrine is given to inhibit premature labor in the pregnant woman and the long-acting glucocorticoids are given to enhance fetal lung maturity, the result may be pulmonary edema in the mother. Monitor pregnant women closely for the first signs of pulmonary edema (shallow, rapid, difficult breathing; anxiety; restlessness; increased heart rate and blood pressure; enlarged peripheral and neck veins; edema of extremities; lung rales; and diaphoresis); early detection and treatment are necessary to prevent a potentially serious adverse effect or fatality.
Sodium-containing foods or medications	Concurrent usage may result in edema and hypertension. Monitor weight, intake and output, and blood pressure closely.
somatrem or somatropin	The growth response to somatrem or somatropin may be inhibited with concurrent chronic therapy with corticotropin or with daily doses of glucocorticoids above certain levels, such as daily doses of prednisone or prednisolone above 2.5 to 3.75 mg/m^2 of body surface. For dosages for other glucocorticoids, refer to a current USP DI.
vaccines, live virus, and other immunizations	Generally, immunizations are not recommended for patients receiving pharmacologic or immunosuppressant doses of glucocorticoids. Because corticosteroids inhibit antibody response, the immunization effect will be reduced or ineffective and the patient may develop neurologic complications. Avoid or a potentially serious drug interaction may occur. If live virus vaccines are given to individuals receiving immunosuppressant glucocorticoid therapy, the patient may develop the viral disease or at least have a reduced response to the vaccine. Avoid or a potentially serious drug interaction may occur. Also, do not administer the oral polio vaccine to persons in close contact with a person receiving immunosuppressant glucocorticoid therapy.

Color type indicates an unsafe drug combination.

Side effects and adverse reactions

These include euphoria, an increase in appetite (anorexia with triamcinolone), insomnia, restlessness, anxiety, gas, hyperpigmentation, hypotension, headache, increased hair growth, lowered resistance to infections, visual disturbances (cataracts), increased urination or thirst, and decreased growth in children. Parenterally at the injection site, redness, swelling, rash, pain, tingling, or numbness may occur. Chronic use may result in abdominal pain, acne, gastrointestinal (GI) bleeding, peptic ulcers, round face (Cushing's syndrome), hypertension, edema, weight gain, muscle cramps, weakness, irregular heart rate, nausea, vomiting, bone pain, increased bruising, and difficulty in wound healing.

Warnings

Use with caution in patients with hypertension, colitis, diverticulitis, open angle glaucoma, liver or kidney disease, oral herpes lesions, hyperlipidemia, hyperthyroidism, hypoalbuminemia, hypothyroidism, osteoporosis, systemic lupus erythematosus, and uncontrolled infections. See the box for Food and Drug Administration (FDA) pregnancy safety classifications.

Contraindications

Avoid use in persons with corticosteroid hypersensitivity, acquired immunodeficiency syndrome (AIDS) or human immunodeficiency virus (HIV) infection, heart disease, heart failure, severe kidney disease, chickenpox, measles, peptic ulcer, esophagitis, systemic fungal infection, diabetes mellitus, herpes simplex (eye), myasthenia gravis, and tuberculosis.

Dosage and administration

The betamethasone (Celestone) adult dose is 0.6 to 7.2 mg/day; the pediatric dose for adrenocortical insufficiency is 17.5 μg/kg in three divided doses. The parenteral adult drug dosage (IM, IV, intraarticular, intralesional, or soft tissue injections) is up to 9 mg/day. The dose of corticotropin (Acthar) as an adult diagnostic aid is 10 to 25 units in 500 ml of 5% dextrose in water (D_5W); the therapeutic dose (IM or SC) is 40 to 80 units/day. The pediatric dose (IV, IM, or SC) is 1.6 units/kg/24 hr in divided doses. The cortisone (Cortone) adult oral dose is 25 to 300 mg daily. The pediatric oral dose for adrenocortical insufficiency is 0.7 mg/kg daily in divided doses. For additional corticosteroid drug dosing, see Table 41-3.

PREGNANCY SAFETY

Category	Drug
C	corticotropin, fludrocortisone
D	aminoglutethimide
X	trilostane
Not established	other glucocorticoids

Additional comments

When cortisone or hydrocortisone is used as replacement therapy, the drug should be scheduled according to the normal endogenous corticosteroid secretion in the body; that is, give two thirds of the dose in the morning and one third in the evening. Other corticosteroids have a longer duration of action; therefore once daily dosing is usually sufficient.

To reduce the potential of suppressing the hypothalamic-pituitary-adrenal axis and producing undesirable side effects with chronic corticosteroid therapy, an alternate day schedule may be used. A drug is selected from the short-or intermediate-acting corticosteroids, and when the patient's condition is stabilized on a dose, a taper-down schedule on 1 day and increased dose on the next is used until the patient is taking approximately two to three times the daily dose every other day (Small, Cooksey, 1995).

The oral dosage form should be taken with food to reduce gastric distress. Avoid alcohol consumption as concurrent use will increase the potential for peptic ulcers. To discontinue these drugs, a gradual dose reduction is recommended.

MINERALOCORTICOIDS

Mineralocorticoids such as aldosterone are secreted by the adrenal cortex to increase the rate of sodium reabsorption by the kidneys, thereby increasing blood levels of sodium. This results in increased water reabsorption by the kidneys

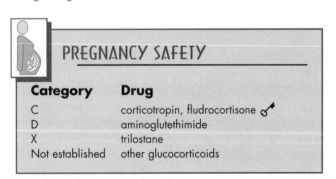

TABLE 41-3 Corticosteroid Preparations and Dosing

	Usual Dosage	
Drug	***Adult***	***Child***
dexamethasone (Decadron and others)	PO: 0.5-9 mg daily	Adrenocortical insufficiency: 23.3 μg/kg daily in three divided doses
hydrocortisone (Cortef and others)	PO/IM: 15-20 mg up to 240 mg daily	Oral: 0.56 mg/kg/day IM: 0.56 to 4 mg/kg/day
enema (Cortenema)	Rectal: 100 mg retention enema nightly for 3 wk	Not established
methylprednisolone (Medrol)	PO: 4-48 mg daily	Adrenocortical insufficiency: 117 μg/kg daily in three divided doses
prednisolone (Delta-Cortef and others)	PO: 5-60 mg daily (maximum 250 mg/day)	Adrenocortical insufficiency: 140 μg/kg daily in three divided doses
prednisone (Deltasone and others)	PO: 5-60 mg daily	Dosage varies, see current references
triamcinolone (Aristocort, Kenacort)	PO: 4-48 mg daily	Adrenocortical insufficiency: 117 μg/kg daily

Dexamethasone, methylprednisolone, prednisolone, and triamcinolone are also available in short-acting and long-acting preparations; see current references for dosing information.

and increased blood volume. They also increase potassium and hydrogen ion excretion into the urine, thereby decreasing blood levels of potassium and hydrogen ions. In adrenal cortex insufficiency, replacement of a glucocorticoid and in some individuals, a mineralocorticoid such as fludrocortisone is necessary.

fludrocortisone [floo droe kor′ ti sone] (Florinef)

Fludrocortisone has potent mineralocorticoid activity with some moderate glucocorticoid effects, although it is used primarily for its mineralocorticoid effects. It acts primarily on the renal distal tubule to reabsorb sodium and enhance excretion of potassium and hydrogen and is indicated for the treatment of Addison's disease (chronic primary adrenocortical insufficiency) and congenital adrenogenital syndrome.

Pharmacokinetics

Fludrocortisone has good oral absorption and a half-life of about 3.5 hours in the plasma with a biologic half-life of activity in the body of 18 to 36 hours. Its duration of action is 24 to 48 hours with metabolism in the liver and kidneys and excretion by the kidneys.

Drug interactions

The following effects may occur when fludrocortisone is given with the drugs listed below:

Drug	Possible effect and management
Digitalis glycosides	Hypokalemic effect may potentiate the risk for cardiac dysrhythmias or digitalis toxicity. Monitor closely with electrocardiogram (ECG) and pulse readings.
Diuretics	Effectiveness of diuretics may be decreased with these medications. Concurrent use of potassium-depleting diuretics or hypokalemic-inducing medications may produce severe hypokalemia. Monitor serum potassium levels closely.
Hepatic enzyme inducers	Increased metabolism of mineralocorticoids may result in a decrease in the effectiveness of these drugs.
Sodium in food or medications	In type IV renal tubular acidosis, concurrent use of sodium with fludrocortisone may result in hypertension, hypernatremia, and edema. Monitor sodium intake closely and advise patients on safe consumption of foods and medications to avoid hypernatremia. Instruct patients to read labels on both foods and medication.

Side effects and adverse reactions

These include severe or persistent headaches, hypertension, dizziness, edema of the lower extremities, joint pain, hypokalemia, increased weakness, tingling or numbness in the legs that may progress to arms, trunk, and face, congestive heart failure, and anaphylaxis. Such adverse reactions should be reported immediately to the prescriber.

Warnings

Use with caution in patients with peripheral edema, acute glomerulonephritis, liver impairment, hypothyroidism, hyperthyroidism, chronic nephritis, and osteoporosis.

Contraindications

Avoid use in persons with fludrocortisone hypersensitivity, congestive heart failure, heart disease, hypertension, and kidney function impairment.

Dosage and administration

The adolescent and adult oral dose is 0.1 mg daily. The usual pediatric dose is 50 to 100 μg daily.

ANTIADRENALS (ADRENAL STEROID INHIBITORS)

Aminoglutethimide, metyrapone, and trilostane are antiadrenals or adrenal steroid inhibitors. They inhibit or suppress adrenal cortex function.

aminoglutethimide [a mee noe gloo teth′ i mide] (Cytadren)

Aminoglutethimide inhibits the enzyme conversion of cholesterol or pregnenolone, thereby blocking the synthesis of adrenal steroids, and may have other suppression effects in the synthesis and metabolism of the steroids. It also inhibits estrogen production from androgens by blocking an enzyme in the peripheral tissues and may enhance estrone metabolism; thus it is used investigationally to treat breast cancer.

Indications

Aminoglutethimide is indicated for the treatment of Cushing's syndrome associated with adrenal carcinoma, ectopic adrenocorticotropic hormone tumors, or adrenal gland hyperplasia.

Pharmacokinetics

Aminoglutethimide is absorbed orally and has a half-life of 13 hours, which is reduced to 7 hours after chronic therapy. The time to peak concentration is 1.5 hours with adrenal function suppression occurring within 3 to 5 days of therapy. Aminoglutethimide is metabolized in the liver and excreted by the kidneys.

Drug interactions

The only significant drug interaction reported in the USP DI (1998) is with dexamethasone, i.e., aminoglutethimide increases the metabolism of dexamethasone, thus reducing its effectiveness. If a glucocorticoid is necessary for a patient receiving aminoglutethimide, hydrocortisone is usually the drug of choice.

Side effects and adverse reactions

These include ataxia, dizziness, sedation, loss of energy, and uncontrolled eye movements. Central nervous system (CNS) effects are usually dose related (effects may decline in 2 to 6 weeks of continuous therapy but, if severe, the drug may need to be stopped), anorexia, nausea, vomiting, a measles-like rash on the face and/or palms of hands, and, rarely, fever, chills, sore throat (caused by leukopenia or agranulocytosis), jaundice of eyes and skin, increased bleeding episodes, or unusual bruising (thrombocytopenia).

Warnings

Use with caution in patients with liver or kidney function impairment and hypothyroidism.

Contraindications

Avoid use in persons with aminoglutethimide or glutethimide hypersensitivity, chickenpox, herpes zoster, and infection.

Dosage and administration

The adult oral dosage is 250 mg two or three times daily for approximately 14 days; the maintenance dose is 250 mg every 6 hours four times daily. A pediatric dose has not been established.

trilostane [trye' loe stane] (Modrastane)

Trilostane suppresses synthesis of adrenal steroids by inhibiting specific enzymes in the adrenal cortex. It is indicated for the treatment of Cushing's syndrome.

Pharmacokinetics

Trilostane has a half-life of 8 hours and is metabolized by the liver.

Side effects and adverse reactions

These include diarrhea, stomach distress, muscle aches, headache, fever, flushing, increased salivation, nausea, dizziness, gas, burning sensation in the mouth or nose, watery eyes, and, rarely, darkening of the skin, sedation, anorexia, vomiting, rash, and depression.

Warnings

Use with caution in patients with liver or kidney function impairment.

Contraindications

Avoid use in persons with trilostane hypersensitivity, infection, and shock and in persons who have recently had surgery or severe trauma.

Dosage and administration

The oral adult dosage is 30 mg four times daily increased as necessary according to patient response. The maximum dose is 480 mg/day. The pediatric dosage has not been established.

SUMMARY

The corticosteroids, or glucocorticoids and mineralocorticoids that originated in the adrenal cortex, are discussed in this chapter. The many pharmacologic actions of the glucocorticoids such as antiinflammatory effect; fat, carbohydrate, and protein metabolism; thymolytic, lympholytic, and eosinopenic actions; and others were reviewed. In addition, the mineralocorticoids act in the kidneys to reabsorb sodium and enhance the excretion of potassium and hydrogen. The actions of these agents are vitally important in helping the body to maintain homeostasis. The adrenal steroid inhibitors, aminoglutethimide, and trilostane are used for the treatment of Cushing's syndrome.

REVIEW QUESTIONS

1. Name the three types of steroid hormones produced by the adrenal cortex. Review the primary functions of the glucocorticoids and mineralocorticoids.
2. Discuss the relationship of circadian and ultradian rhythms to plasma cortisol levels.
3. Explain the thymolytic, lympholytic, and eosinopenic effects of the glucocorticoids.
4. What effect does stress have on corticosteroids?
5. When cortisone or hydrocortisone is prescribed, what is the suggested schedule? Name three additional points to be discussed with the patient concerning the proper use of an oral corticosteroid.

REFERENCES

Schimmer BP, Parker KL: Adrenocorticotropic hormone: adrenocortical steroids and their synthetic analogs; inhibitors of the synthesis and actions of adrenocortical hormones. In Hardman JG, Limbird LE, editors: *Goodman & Gilman's the pharmacological basis of therapeutics,* ed 9, New York, 1996, McGraw-Hill.

Small, RE, Cooksey, LJ: Connective tissue disorders: the clinical use of corticosteroids. In Young LY, Koda-Kimble MA, editors: *Applied therapeutics: the clinical use of drugs,* ed 6, Vancouver, Wash, 1995, Applied Therapeutics, Inc.

United States Pharmacopeial Convention: *USP DI: drug information for the health care professional,* ed 18, Rockville, Md, 1998, The Convention.

ADDITIONAL REFERENCES

American Hospital Formulary Service: *AHFS drug information '98,* Bethesda, Md, 1996, American Society of Hospital Pharmacists.

Anderson KN et al, editors: *Mosby's medical, nursing, and allied health dictionary,* ed 5, St Louis, 1998, Mosby.

Epstein CD: Adrenocortical insufficiency in the critically ill patient, *AACN Clin Issues Crit Care Nurs* 3(3):705-713, 1992.

Greenberger PA: Corticosteroids in asthma: rationale, use, and problems, *Chest* 101(6):418S, 1992.

Hilton G, Frei J: High-dose methylprednisolone in the treatment of spinal cord injuries, *Heart Lung* 20(6):675, 1991.

Katzung BG: *Basic and clinical pharmacology,* ed 5, Norwalk, Conn, 1992, Appleton & Lange.

Melmon KL et al: *Clinical pharmacology,* ed 3, New York, 1992, McGraw-Hill.

Mosby: *Mosby's GenRx,* St Louis, 1998, Mosby.

Olin BR: *Facts and comparisons.* Philadelphia, 1998, JB Lippincott.

CHAPTER 42

Drugs Affecting the Pancreas

KEY DRUGS

acarbose, (p. 572)
glucagon, (p. 575)
insulin (p. 565)
tolbutamide (p. 570)

CHAPTER FOCUS

Diabetes mellitus is a common disorder that affects approximately 16 million Americans. Unfortunately, however, in about one half of these individuals the disorder has not been diagnosed. Diabetes mellitus is a disorder of carbohydrate metabolism resulting from a relative or absolute insulin deficiency. The frequency of diabetes increases with age and is equal in males and females. Uncontrolled diabetes is a devastating disease; it is the seventh leading cause of death in the United States and the major cause of new cases of blindness, end-stage renal disease, and lower limb amputations. Healthcare professionals should be well informed on the pathophysiology, management, and treatment of diabetes mellitus.

KEY TERMS

glucagon, (p. 565)
gluconeogenesis, (p. 570)
glycogenesis, (p. 565)
glycogenolysis, (p. 565)
insulin, (p. 566)
lipoatrophy, (p. 566)
type 1 diabetes, (p. 565)
type 2 diabetes, (p. 565)

OBJECTIVES

After reading and studying this chapter, the student should be able to do the following:

1. *Define and describe the key terms and key drugs.*
2. *Discuss the contrasting features of insulin-dependent (type 1) and non–insulin-dependent (type 2) diabetes mellitus.*
3. *Name and describe the different insulin preparations.*
4. *Discuss the mechanisms of action and differences between the first-generation, second-generation, and miscellaneous oral hypoglycemic agents.*
5. *Name the hyperglycemic medications, including their indications, mechanisms of action, and side effects and adverse reactions.*

The primary hormones released by the pancreas are insulin and glucagon. When serum blood glucose declines, **glucagon,** which is synthesized in the alpha cells of the pancreatic islets, facilitates the catabolism of stored glycogen in the liver. The result is **glycogenolysis,** or the conversion of glycogen to glucose, resulting in an increase in blood glucose (Fig. 42-1). The release of glucagon stimulates insulin secretion, which then inhibits the release of glucagon. Thus the feedback mechanism serves to keep glucose within a desired serum level.

On the other hand, when blood glucose increases, **glycogenesis,** or the conversion of excess glucose to glycogen for storage in skeletal muscle and the liver occurs. The most important disease involving the endocrine pancreas is diabetes mellitus, a disorder of carbohydrate metabolism that involves either an insulin deficiency, insulin resistance, or both. All causes of diabetes lead to hyperglycemia (see Chapter 38).

DIABETES MELLITUS

Diabetes mellitus affects approximately 16 million Americans and in nearly half of this population, the disorder has not been diagnosed (Beier, 1997). Uncontrolled diabetes is a devastating disease that is the leading cause of new cases of blindness, end-stage renal disease, and lower limb amputations and is the seventh leading cause of death in the United State (Baker, 1997). Diabetes affects males and females equally while the incidence of diabetes increases with age.

The two general classifications for diabetes mellitus are **type 1 diabetes,** or insulin-dependent diabetes mellitus (IDDM), and **type 2 diabetes,** or non–insulin-dependent diabetes mellitus (NIDDM). Patients with type 1 diabetes have very little or usually no endogenous insulin capacity. This type of diabetes usually occurs before the age of 30 and was previously called juvenile-onset diabetes. The patient

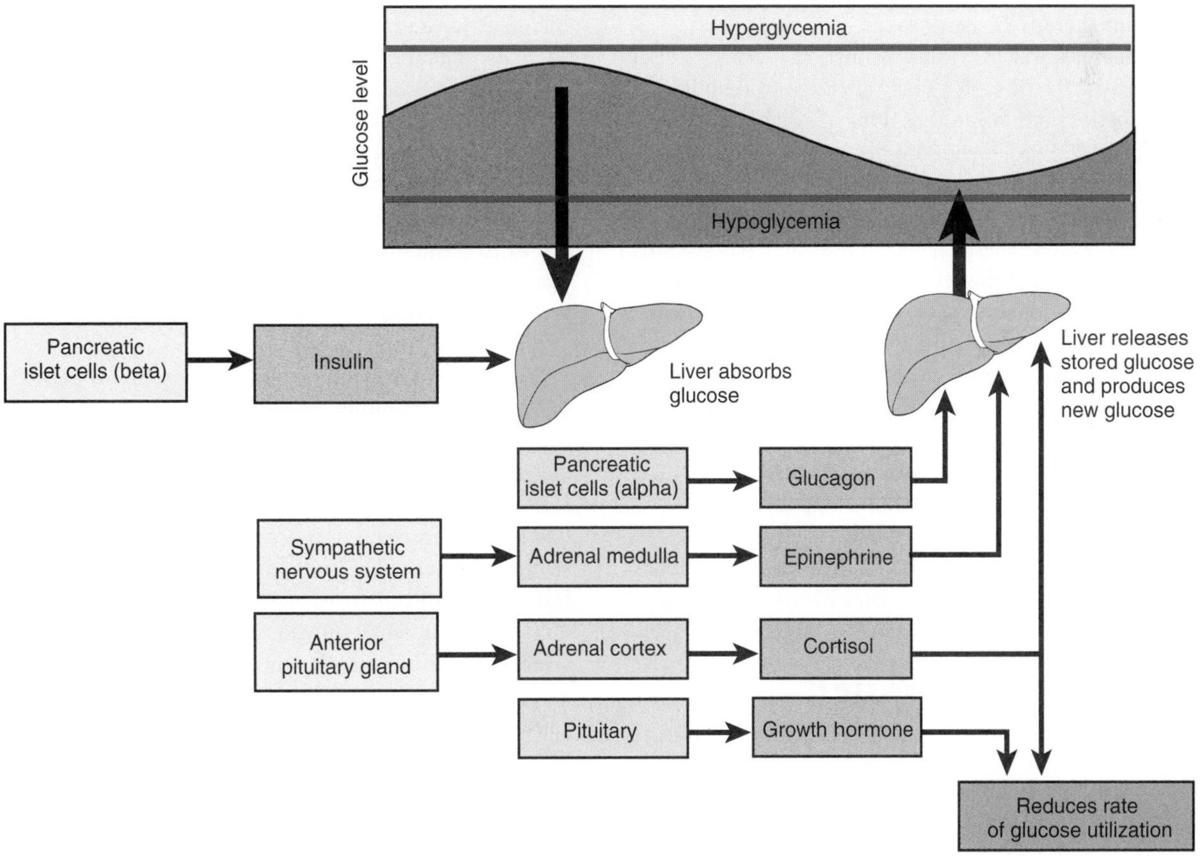

FIGURE 42-1

Insulin causes the liver to absorb excess blood glucose. When blood glucose levels are low, the alpha cells in the islets of Langerhans secrete glucagon, which stimulates liver glycogenolysis and gluconeogenesis. The sympathetic nervous system signals the adrenal medulla to secrete epinephrine while the anterior pituitary gland affects the adrenal cortex to release cortisol. Both substances enhance gluconeogenesis while epinephrine also increases glycogenolysis and cortisol slows down the rate of glucose utilization and also increases the plasma level of amino acids available for glucose production. The pituitary secretes growth hormone that decreases cellular glucose utilization and promotes glycogenolysis.

BOX 42-1 Features of Insulin-Dependent (IDDM) and Non–Insulin-Dependent (NIDDM) Diabetes

Feature	IDDM	NIDDM
Synonym	Type 1	Type 2
Age of onset	Usually <30 years	Usually >35 years
Onset of symptoms	Sudden (symptomatic)	Gradual (usually asymptomatic)
Body weight	Usually nonobese	Obese (80%)
Family history	Usually negative	Often positive
Incidence	10%	90%
Insulin levels	Low then absent	May be low, normal, or high (insulin resistance)
Insulin dependent	Yes	Usually not required
Insulin resistance	No	Yes
Receptors	Normal	Usually decreased or defective
Plasma insulin	Decreased	Normal or increased
Complications	Frequent	Frequent
Ketoacidosis	Prone to	Usually resistant
Dietary modifications	Mandatory	Mandatory

with type 1 diabetes is prone to ketosis and requires exogenous insulin therapy for survival.

Type 2 diabetes was previously known as maturity-onset diabetes because the onset is usually after age 40. About 90% of the diabetic population has type 2 diabetes (Koda-Kimble, Carlisle, 1995). Generally, persons with this type of diabetes have some insulin function, so they are not fully dependent on insulin for survival. Often weight reduction through dietary adjustments will help reduce hyperglycemia in patients with type 2 diabetes. The vast majority of individuals with type 2 diabetes are obese, and ketosis is rare. Although insulin resistance may occasionally occur with type 1 diabetes, it is believed to be more common in type 2 diabetes because of receptor and postreceptor defects. The risk factors for type 2 diabetes include age, obesity, family history, physical inactivity, and impaired glucose tolerance. See Box 42-1 for features of insulin-dependent and non-insulin-dependent diabetes.

The treatment plan for diabetes mellitus usually includes diet, exercise, and, if necessary, an oral hypoglycemic agent or insulin to help control blood glucose levels.

INSULIN PREPARATIONS

Insulin, which is normally synthesized and secreted by the beta cells of the pancreas, is composed of two amino acid chains: A (acidic) and B (basic), joined together by disulfide linkages. It is synthesized in the pancreatic beta cells, which are located in the islets of Langerhans and released when blood glucose levels are elevated.

Insulin preparations are derived from animals (extracted from beef or pork pancreas) or synthesized in the laboratory from either an alteration of pork insulin or recombinant DNA technology using strains of *Escherichia coli* to form human insulin (a biosynthetic human insulin). Beef insulin differs from human insulin by three amino acids, whereas the pork insulin differs from human insulin by only a single amino acid. The human (or recombinant) insulin is identical to the insulin produced by the pancreas.

Many diabetic patients do well when receiving the beef-pork combination insulins if they have not developed insulin resistance, insulin allergies, or **lipoatrophy** (a breakdown of subcutaneous fat occurring after repeated injections) at the same insulin injection sites. The beef-only insulins were indicated mainly for patients who are allergic to pork or for use in patients who must avoid the use of pork for religious reasons. There is a higher degree of immunogenicity reported with beef and beef-pork insulin than with pork insulin (Koda-Kimble, Carlisle, 1995).

Pork insulin has been found to be useful for patients who have local or systemic allergies, insulin resistance, or lipoatrophy, or for individuals who have a short-term need for insulin. The pure pork insulin is closer in composition to human insulin than beef insulin, and in many instances its use has resulted in reduction of the insulin dose (in insulin resistance) and in the improvement of local allergy (erythema, induration, and pruritus at injection site) in approximately 80% of the patients with insulin allergies.

Human insulin can be substituted for the same reasons as pork insulin, especially in persons allergic to pork, because it is much less antigenic than the animal-based insulin. Subcutaneously administered human insulin may also be absorbed faster and have a shorter duration of action than the animal insulins. It is standard practice now to prescribe human insulin whenever possible. Patients switched from an animal to human insulin should be closely monitored initially because a dosage adjustment may be necessary. As a result of the decreased allergenic effects, skin allergies, and resistance reported with human insulin, it is a commonly prescribed insulin for persons with newly diagnosed diabetes and pregnant women (Davis, Granner, 1996; Melmon et al, 1992).

A new, fast-acting insulin analog, insulin lispro (Humalog) was approved for release in 1996. This insulin uses

TABLE 42-1 Characteristics of Insulin Preparations After Subcutaneous Administration

Insulins *	Onset (hr)	Peak Effect (hr)	Duration of Action (hr)
Rapid Acting			
insulin lispro (Humalog)	0.25	1	4
insulin injection (Regular Insulin, Humalin R)†	½-1	2-4	5-7
Intermediate Acting			
isophane insulin suspension (NPH Insulin)	3-4	6-12	18-28
insulin zinc suspension (Lente Insulin)	1-3	8-12	18-28
Long Acting			
extended insulin zinc suspension (Ultralente Insulin)	4-6	18-24	36
Combinations			
isophane human insulin (50%) and human insulin (50%) (Humalin 50/50)	½	3	22-24
isophane human insulin (70%) and human insulin (30%) (Humalin 70/30, Novalin 70/30)	½	4-8	24

*Semilente Insulin is available in Canada but is no longer available in the United States. Onset of action of Semilente Insulin is 1-3 hr, peak effect is in 2-8 hr, and duration of action is 12-16 hr.
†These insulins may be administered intravenously. Intravenously, the onset of action is within ⅙ to ½ hr, peak effect within ¼ to ½, and duration of action within ½ to 1 hr.

regular human insulin and reverses the sequence of two amino acids in it. The primary advantage of the new insulin is it has a more rapid onset of action than regular insulin; therefore it can be administered 15 minutes before a meal. It also has an earlier peak effect and a shorter duration of action, so persons with type 1 diabetes will usually require concurrent use of a long-acting insulin product (Rodgers, 1996).

Mechanism of action

Insulin controls the storage and metabolism of carbohydrate, protein, and fat binding to receptor sites on cellular plasma membranes, especially in the liver, muscle, and adipose tissues. While insulin's exact molecular mechanism of action is still being investigated, it is known that insulin influences cell membrane transport, cell growth, enzyme activation and inhibition, and the metabolism of protein and fats.

Indications

Insulin is indicated for the treatment of type 1 diabetes and for treatment of type 2 diabetes during emergencies or in specific situations, such as supplementation in the patient with a low physiologic endogenous insulin level during high fevers, severe infection, ketoacidosis, severe burns, after major surgery and severe trauma, or during pregnancy.

Pharmacokinetics

The wide variety of insulins (including combination mixtures) available allow for sufficient blood glucose control to meet the diabetic patient's individual need and lifestyle. Table 42-1 notes the onset of action, peak effect and duration of action for the rapid-acting, intermediate-acting, long-acting and combination insulin preparations. Fig. 42-2 illustrates the duration of action of the insulins, and Box

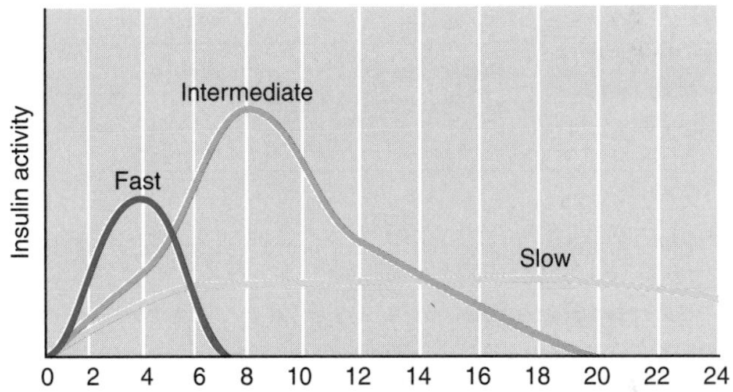

FIGURE 42-2
Insulin pharmacokinetics (see Table 42-1).

42-2 notes the symptoms of hypoglycemia and hyperglycemia. Maintaining glucose levels as close to normal as possible will help to improve the person's quality of life and also reduce the progression of complications associated with diabetes (Campbell, 1992).

Drug interactions

The following effects may occur when insulin is given with the drugs listed below. Many additional medications may also cause hyperglycemia or hypoglycemia; therefore the patient's medication regimen should always be closely monitored. For more information, see Box 42-3.

Drug	Possible effect and management
Adrenocorticoids, glucocorticoids	Adrenocorticoids and glucocorticoids may increase blood glucose levels. A dosage adjustment of insulin may be necessary. Monitor closely.

Alcohol	May increase the hypoglycemic effect of insulin. Monitor closely, as dosage adjustments may be necessary. If possible, avoid the concurrent use of alcohol.
Beta-adrenergic blocking agents (including eye preparations)	These agents may mask symptoms of hypoglycemia, such as increased pulse rate and decreased blood pressure. May also prolong hypoglycemia by blocking gluconeogenesis. Dosage adjustments of insulin may be necessary. Selective beta blockers in low dosages, such as metoprolol and atenolol, cause fewer problems than the other beta-adrenergic blocking agents. Propranolol may cause hyperglycemia or hypoglycemia when given concurrently with insulin. Periodic blood glucose tests are recommended to monitor the combined effects and allow for adjustment of insulin dose if necessary.

BOX 42-2 Symptoms of Hypoglycemia and Hyperglycemia

Persons administering insulin should be aware of the symptoms of hypoglycemia and hyperglycemia and know what action to take if they occur.

Hypoglycemia: Increased anxiety, blurred vision, chilly sensation, cold sweating, pallor, confusion, difficulty in concentrating, drowsiness, headache, nausea, increased pulse rate, shakiness, increased weakness, increased appetite

Hyperglycemia: Drowsiness; red, dry skin; fruity breath odor; anorexia; abdominal pain; nausea and vomiting; dry mouth; increased urination; rapid, deep breathing; unusual thirst; rapid weight loss.

BOX 42-3 Drugs Reported to Cause Hyperglycemia or Hypoglycemia

Hyperglycemia	***Hypoglycemia***
baclofen	anabolic steroids
corticosteroids	beta-adrenergic blocking agents
diuretics	disopyramide
estrogens (oral contraceptives)	ethanol
glucagon	monoamine oxidase inhibitors (MAOIs)
nonsteroidal antiinflammatory drugs (NSAIDs)	NSAIDs
pentamidine (toxic to pancreatic islet cells)	pentamidine (increases insulin release)
phenytoin	salicylates
sympathomimetics	sulfonamides
thyroid hormones	

From USP DI, 1998.

Many commonly abused drugs may also affect the management of diabetes (Box 42-4). In addition, many over-the-counter (OTC) medications may contain a sugar that can affect the diabetic's glucose control. See Box 42-5 for a list of sugar-free OTC medications.

Warnings

Use with caution in patients with liver or kidney disease, high fever, severe infection, hyperthyroidism, inadequately controlled adrenal or pituitary insufficiency, diarrhea, intestinal obstruction, vomiting, and gastroparesis and in patients who have had recent surgery or trauma.

Dosage and administration

There is no average dose of insulin for the diabetic person; each patient's needs must be determined individually

BOX 42-4 Effects of Commonly Abused Drugs on Diabetes Management

Many drugs can increase or decrease blood glucose levels, but rarely are the commonly abused drugs reviewed in relation to diabetes. Because substance abuse by the person with diabetes can be very problematic, the most commonly abused drugs are reviewed here.

Alcohol
Alcohol promotes hypoglycemia and blocks the formation, storage, and release of glycogen. It also may interact with many other drugs, including oral hypoglycemic agents such as chlorpropamide. In alcoholics who have decreased their food intake, alcohol can cause a serious drop in blood glucose levels, leading to a need for acute intervention.

Central Nervous System (CNS) Stimulants
Amphetamines, sympathomimetics, anorexics, cocaine, psychedelic drugs, and others may result in hyperglycemia and an increase in liver glycogen breakdown. Large amounts of caffeine in products such as coffee, tea, and cola drinks can also increase blood glucose levels.

Marijuana
Marijuana may increase appetite and food consumption. Heavy use may produce a glucose intolerance leading to hyperglycemia.

Cigarettes
Nicotine in cigarettes is a potent vasoconstrictor. It can decrease the absorption of subcutaneous insulin or increase the person's insulin requirements by 15% to 20%. Cigarette smoking can cause a drop of 1 to 2 degrees in skin temperature. It also is a risk factor for the development of diabetic nephropathy.

Abuse of CNS-Acting Drugs
CNS-acting drugs (such as stimulants, depressants, sedative-hypnotics, opiates, marijuana, and alcohol) can impair judgment and alter perceptions (time and place) and thus interfere with the individual's control of the diabetic state.

to attain euglycemia and to avoid hypoglycemia and hyperglycemia. Box 42-2 lists the symptoms of hypoglycemia and hyperglycemia.

Insulin dosage is expressed in units rather than in milliliters. Insulin injection is standardized so that each milliliter contains 100 USP units. Insulin is classified according to its duration of action (short- or rapid-acting, intermediate-acting, and long-acting) (Fig. 42-2). Generally, meals should occur at the same time that administered insulin reaches its peak effect. Insulin requirements can vary widely among individuals, so dosages must be adjusted to an individual's needs. During pregnancy, insulin is the drug of choice to control diabetes. Insulin requirements may drop for 24 to 72 hours after delivery and slowly return to prepregnancy levels in about 6 weeks.

Individuals with diabetes who become hyperglycemic, perhaps because of hospitalization or an infection, may need insulin coverage in addition to their regular insulin. The amount of insulin given will vary with the blood glucose values or (in some instances) with the glucose in the urine; this titration is known as "sliding-scale" administration of insulin. The latter method of testing urine may be used in some healthcare settings, but it is rarely used now to monitor blood glucose. If at all possible, urine glucose tests should not be used to determine insulin dosages. Because there may be variations between urine glucose tests, they should not be used interchangeably for urine glucose monitoring. The specific instructions for testing urine for glucose using a particular reagent is included with the testing kit.

Dietary intake, physical activity, ability to manage the therapeutic regimen, and the patient's glucose tolerance are all taken into consideration when insulin dosages are established. Insulin dosages should not be considered to be a fixed regimen; the dosage may need to be adjusted as a result of physical growth (child growing into adulthood), illness, stress, the development of antiinsulin antibodies, concomitant administration of certain medications, or changes in exercise and diet. Specific instructions should be obtained regarding insulin administration for the preoperative patient because of the alteration in the patient's dietary patterns and metabolic requirements as the result of the surgical procedure. Treatment programs need to be reviewed and adjusted as necessary with the prescriber, healthcare professional, and patient working closely to manage hypoglycemia and hyperglycemia and, if possible, avoid their complications.

Insulin is given subcutaneously (or intravenously, regular insulin only). It cannot be given by mouth because it is destroyed by digestive enzymes. Regular insulin is usually given about 15 to 30 minutes before meals.

Vials of insoluble preparations (all except regular insulin) should be rotated between the hands and inverted end-to-end several times before a dose is withdrawn. A vial should not be shaken vigorously or the suspension made to foam. Do not interchange human, beef, or pork insulins, since species differences may require a dosage change, or use insulin that has become clumped or granular in appearance.

Portable insulin pumps have improved the metabolic state of some type 1 patients who did not have adequate diabetic control after intensive dietary restrictions and multiple daily injections of insulin. The insulin pump is battery-operated and connected to a small computer that is programmed to release small amounts of insulin per hour. It does not analyze the blood glucose level; however, it is programmed based on the individual's daily insulin needs, diet, and physical exercise. The patient can also push a button that releases a bolus dose to cover each meal consumed.

Although the pumps are effective and useful in individuals who are properly trained, healthcare professionals need to be aware of several problems associated with them. Malfunction of the insulin infusion may occur because of battery failure, and defects in the tubing may cause leakage of insulin solution or may block the infusion tubing. Therefore it is vitally important to teach the person to change the infusion set and battery. Patients must be highly motivated and educated in the handling of insulin pumps. The patient should be capable of keeping records and following specific procedures and should be willing to perform blood tests daily or more often. Also, these pumps are very expensive.

BOX 42-5 Sugar-Free Over-The-Counter Medications

Advise clients to always read bottle labels or check with their pharmacists before purchasing medications. The sugar contents of OTC medications are changed often by the manufacturers, so the best advise is to check the list of contents every time a medication is purchased. The following is a select listing of medications that are currently sugar-free.

Antacids, Antiflatulents
Maalox Anti-Gas
Maalox Extra Strength
Mylanta
Riopan
Titralac Extra Strength Antacid
Titralac Plus Tablets/Liquids

Antipyretics
Acetaminophen Solution
Bayer Aspirin
Cama-In-Lay Tablets
Motrin IB
Panadol Children's Liquid
Tempra 3 chewable tablets
Tylenol Children's Fruit Flavor

Cough-Cold Preparations
Benadryl cold
Benylin Expectorant
Diabetic Tussin DM
Diabetic Tussin EX
Naldecon Senior DX and EX
Tussar-SF

From Covington, 1996.

Therefore insulin pumps currently are not recommended for every type 1 diabetic patient.

Needleless injectors, such as the Vitajet, Medi-jector, and Precijet 50, are also available. These devices are expensive and appear to have limited usefulness in practice. Many devices are also available for the visually impaired patient with diabetes. Information on injection aids for the blind may be obtained from state and national associations such as the American Foundation for the Blind and the American Diabetic Association.

Glucose Monitoring

To maintain euglycemia, blood glucose levels are frequently determined by blood glucose monitoring, which has been simplified by the availability of both visual test strips and strips used in blood glucose meters or instruments. Such devices allow patients to monitor their diabetes and make the necessary adjustments with medication, diet, and exercise, as instructed by their physician or healthcare provider. The visual glucose testing strips are less expensive than the testing instruments, but the meter readings are much more precise (if properly calibrated). Thus persons with visual problems or those who need a more accurate blood glucose reading will benefit from using a blood glucose meter instrument.

Another diabetic evaluation test is to determine the patient's glycosylated hemoglobin (hemoglobin A_{1c}) value. When patients have prolonged hyperglycemic serum levels, the level of hemoglobin A_{1c} will increase. Red blood cells have a life span of 4 months; therefore a measurement of the glycosylated hemoglobin will give the prescriber an evaluation of the individual's long-term diabetic control. In other words, diabetic patients may have undetected periods of hyperglycemia that alternate with a postinsulin time period of euglycemia or hypoglycemia. An elevated hemoglobin A_{1c} value indicates adequate or inadequate diabetic control for the previous 3 to 5 weeks (Watson, Jaffe, 1995). For diabetic patients, the usual target goal for hemoglobin A_{1c} is 7% or under.

ORAL HYPOGLYCEMIC AGENTS

Type 2 diabetic patients are treated with the oral hypoglycemics, diet, exercise, and, when necessary, insulin. Currently there are three classifications of oral agents: first- and second-generation sulfonylureas and a miscellaneous group that includes acarbose (Precose), metformin (Glucophage), miglitol (Glyset), repaglinide (Prandin), and troglitiazone (Rezulin). Although these drugs are sometimes called "oral insulins," this description is incorrect since chemically they are completely different from insulin. They also differ from insulin in mode of action. See Table 42-2 for pharmacokinetics and usual adult dose.

The first-generation sulfonylureas include acetohexamide (Dymelor), chlorpropamide (Diabinese), tolazamide (Tolinase), and tolbutamide (Orinase), which are considered to be equally effective although they may differ in pharmacokinetics and, perhaps, side effects and adverse reactions. The second-generation agents include glipizide (Glucotrol) and glyburide (DiaBeta, Micronase), which are much more potent than the previous generation but have not proven to be more therapeutically or clinically effective (Koda-Kimble, Carlisle, 1995).

The advantages in using the second-generation agents are that they have a long duration of action and have fewer side effects and adverse reactions. Of the first-generation agents, tolazamide also has similar advantages.

The sulfonylureas enhance the release of insulin from the beta cells in the pancreas, decrease liver glycogenolysis (the breakdown of glycogen stored in the liver to glycogen) and **gluconeogenesis** (the conversion of excess glucose to glycogen for storage in the skeletal muscle and liver), and increase the cellular sensitivity to insulin in body tissues. Therefore they reduce blood glucose concentration in persons with a functioning pancreas (Fig. 42-3). In addition, chlorpropamide has an antidiuretic effect; it increases the effect of low levels of antidiuretic hormone present in persons with central diabetes insipidus.

Indications

Oral hypoglycemic agents are indicated for the treatment of uncomplicated type 2 diabetes in persons whose diabetes cannot be controlled by diet only.

Pharmacokinetics

See Table 42-2.

Side effects and adverse reactions

These include hypoglycemia and nocturnal hypoglycemia symptoms of nausea, vomiting, headache, cold sweats, blurred vision, confusion, sedation, increased appetite, anxiety, troubled sleep patterns, tremors, weakness, nightmares, and tachycardia. The patient may also experience changes in taste sensation, dizziness, abdominal distress, polyuria, photosensitivity, and, rarely, anemia, blood disorders, and liver function impairment. With chlorpropamide and, very rarely, tolbutamide, monitor for the syndrome of inappropriate antidiuretic hormone (SIADH).

Warnings

Use with caution in patients with hypothyroidism.

Contraindications

Avoids use in persons with antidiabetic drug, sulfonamide or thiazide-type diuretic hypersensitivity, acidosis, severe burns, severe diarrhea, gastrointestinal (GI) obstruction, and other severe GI disorders, liver disease, and any conditions that may cause hyperglycemia (e.g., high fevers and severe infection), hyperthyroidism, hypoglycemia (e.g., adrenal insufficiency), and kidney function impairment. Avoid use also in patients in diabetic coma (or with ketoaci-

TABLE 42-2 Hypoglycemic Agents: Pharmacokinetics and Usual Adult Dose

Generic (Brand Name)	Onset of Action (hr)	Peak Effect (hr)	Duration of Action (hr)	Usual Adult Dose	Comments
Sulfonylureas					
First Generation					
acetohexamide (Dymelor, Dimelor 🍁)	1	1.5-6*	8-24	250-1000 mg/day	Use with caution in the elderly and patients with renal insufficiency
chlorpropamide (Diabinese)	1	2-4	24-72	250-500 mg/day	Is longest acting hypoglycemic with more reported side effects than other agents.
tolazamide (Tolinase)	4-6	3-4	10-20	100-500 mg with breakfast	Active metabolites may be increased in renal impairment.
tolbutamide 🔑 (Orinase, Mobenol 🍁)	1	3-4	6-12	250-2000 mg daily in divided doses	Is shortest acting agent and rapidly metabolized to inactive metabolites.
Second Generation					
glimepiride (Amaryl)	1	2-3	24	1-2 mg with breakfast	
glipizide (Glucotrol)	1-1.5	1-3	12-24	5-40 mg before meals in divided doses	Dose is 30 min before meals.
glipizide extended release (Glucotrol XL)	N/A	6-12	24	5-20 mg with breakfast	
glyburide nonmicronized (Diabeta, Micronase)	2-4	4	24	1.25-20 mg with breakfast, divide dosages >10 mg	Use with caution in elderly patients in renal failure.
glyburide micronized (Glynase Pres Tab)	1	3	24	0.75-12 mg/day; doses >6 mg divided and given with meals	Micronized formula has increased bioavailability; thus a lower dose is required.
Miscellaneous					
Alpha-glucosidase inhibitors					
acarbose 🔑 (Precose)	N/A	metabolites: 12-24	N/A	50-100 mg with meals	Most effective if given with high fiber diet
miglitol (Glyset)	N/A	2-3	N/A	25-100 mg tid	Reduces glycosylated hemoglobin in type 2 diabetes; take with first bite of food
Biguanide					
metformin (Glucophage, Novo-Metformin 🍁)	—	2-3	6-12	500 or 850 mg bid or tid	Take with food to reduce nausea and vomiting
Meglitinide					
repaglinide (Prandin)	N/A	1	N/A	0.5-2 mg before each meal	Take within 15 min of meal
Thiazolidinedione					
troglitazone (Rezulin)	N/A	2-3	24	200-400 mg daily	Food increases absorption; take with meals

From Davis, Granner, 1996; Koda-Kimble, Carlisle, 1995; Olin, 1998; Ponte, 1997; USP DI, 1998.
N/A, not available.
*Includes active metabolite, hydroxyhexamide.

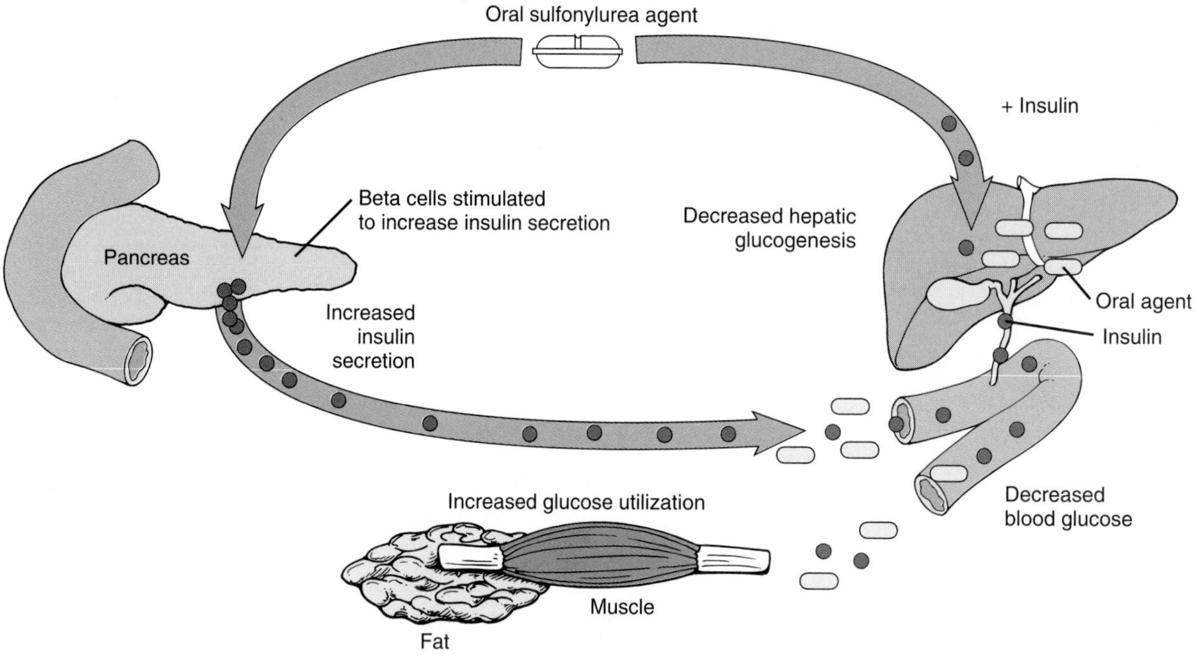

FIGURE 42-3
Mechanism of action of oral sulfonylurea agents. *(From Beare, Myers, 1998.)*

PREGNANCY SAFETY

Category	Drug
B	acarbose ♂, glucagon ♂, metformin, miglitol, troglitazone
C	acetohexamide, chlorpropamide, diazoxide, glipizide, glyburide, repaglinide, tolazamide, tolbutamide ♂

dosis) and in those who have had recently had major surgery or severe trauma.

Dosage and administration

See Table 42-2. Also see the box for Food and Drug Administration (FDA) pregnancy safety classifications.

MISCELLANEOUS HYPOGLYCEMICS

The miscellaneous hypoglycemics include the alpha-glucosidase inhibitors (acarbose and miglitol), a biguanide (metformin), a meglitinide (repaglinide), and a thiazolidinedione (troglitazone).

Alpha-Glucosidase Inhibitors

acarbose [ah car′ bohse] (Precose) ♂
miglitol [mig le′ tol] (Glyset)

Acarbose and miglitol are oral alpha-glucosidase inhibitors that delay digestion and absorption of carbohydrates in the small intestine; therefore after a meal, a smaller increase in blood glucose is noted.

Indications

They are indicated as an adjunct to diet for the treatment of type 2 diabetes. These drugs do not increase insulin secretion or cause hypoglycemia, lactic acidosis, or weight gain. They may be given alone or in combination with a sulfonylurea to lower blood glucose.

Pharmacokinetics

Acarbose absorption is minimal (approximately 2%) and later, metabolites (35%) may be absorbed from GI tract. For half-life, peak effect, and duration of action, see Table 42-2. Unabsorbed acarbose is primarily excreted in feces.

Drug interactions

The following effects may occur when acarbose or miglitol is given with the drugs listed below:

Drug	Possible effect and management
Adsorbents such as charcoal or digestive enzymes	Concurrent use is not recommended, as these drugs may decrease the effectiveness of acarbose.

Corticosteroids, diuretics (especially thiazides)	These drugs may cause hyperglycemia, which may require a antidiabetic drug dose adjustment. Monitor closely so proper adjustments may be instituted.
propranolol (Inderal), ranitidine (Zantac)	Studies indicate that miglitol decreases the availability of propranolol by 40% and ranitidine by 60%. Monitor closely as dosage adjustments may be necessary.

Side effects/adverse reactions

Because acarbose is poorly absorbed, it may cause dose-related side effects of malabsorption, abdominal gas, stomach pain, bloating (Davis, Granner, 1996, USP DI, 1998), and, rarely, jaundice. Miglitol side effects and adverse reactions include stomach pain, diarrhea, gas, and rash.

Warnings

Use acarbose with caution in patients with fever and infection and in patients who have recently had surgery or trauma.

Contraindications

Avoid use in persons with acarbose or miglitol hypersensitivity, diabetic ketoacidosis, intestinal disorders, and kidney function impairment. In addition, avoid use of acarbose in persons with cirrhosis.

Dosage and administration

See Table 42-2.

Biguanide

metformin [met fore′ man] (Glucophage)

Another nonsulfonylurea antihyperglycemic agent for the treatment of type 2 diabetes is metformin, classified as a biguanide. The first drug released in this chemical category was phenformin, but it was withdrawn from the market due to its association with lactic acidosis. Metformin has been associated only rarely with this complication (Davis, Granner, 1996).

Pharmacokinetics

Metformin decreases glucose absorption from the intestines and glucose production in the liver and also improves insulin sensitivity in peripheral tissues. It does not affect the pancreatic beta cells; therefore it does not increase insulin release nor cause hypoglycemia. For pharmacokinetics and dosing, see Table 42-2.

Drug interactions

The following effects may occur when metformin is given with the drugs listed below. In addition, see Box 42-3 for drugs that are reported to cause hyperglycemia or hypoglycemia.

Drug	Possible effect and management
Alcohol	May result in disulfiram (Antabuse)-type reaction, primarily with chlorpropamide (Diabinese). The reaction may include stomach pain, nausea, vomiting, facial flushing, lowered blood glucose levels, and headaches. Avoid or a potentially serious drug interaction may occur. This problem is reported less often with glipizide (Glucotrol) and glyburide (DiaBeta, Micronase).
Beta-adrenergic blocking agents (including ophthalmics)	Increased risk of hyperglycemia or hypoglycemia. See insulin for further information.
cimetidine (Tagamet) and other cationic medications excreted by renal tubular transport, such as amiloride, calcium blockers, digoxin, morphine, procainamide, quinidine, quinine, ranitidine, triamterene, trimethoprim, and vancomycin	Concurrent use with cimetidine may decrease metformin excretion (because cimetidine inhibits renal tubular secretion). Monitor closely as a dosage adjustment for metformin may be necessary. The cationic medications are also excreted by renal tubular transport, which may decrease metformin's excretion or interfere with metformin's plasma levels. Monitor blood glucose levels as drug dosage adjustment may be necessary.
furosemide (Lasix)	May increase metformin serum level; monitor closely.

Color type indicates an unsafe drug combination.

Side effects and adverse reactions

These include anorexia, abdominal gas or pain, headache, nausea, vomiting, weight loss, and, rarely, anemia, hypoglycemia, and lactic acidosis.

Warnings

Use with caution in patients with diarrhea and other GI tract problems, hyperglycemia-causing conditions (e.g., high fever), uncontrolled hyperthyroidism, and hypothyroidism- and hypoglycemia-causing conditions.

Contraindications

Avoid use in persons with metformin hypersensitivity, severe liver or kidney disease, lactic acidosis, cardiac disorders, severe burns, dehydration, and severe infections, in persons in diabetic coma or with ketoacidosis, and in those who have recently had major surgery or trauma.

Dosage and administration

See Table 42-2.

Meglitinide

repaglinide [re pagle′ nide] (Prandin)

Repaglinide is a nonsulfonylurea, hypoglycemic agent. It stimulates the beta cells of the pancreas to produce insulin, and it improves insulin secretion in response to increased glucose levels by regulating the ATP-sensitive K^+ channel at a different binding site than the sulfonylurea agents.

Pharmacokinetics

See Table 42-2. This drug is shorter acting and excreted faster than the oral sulfonylurea drugs, and it produces glucose control that is similar to that with glyburide therapy.

Drug interactions

The following effects may occur when repaglinide is given with the drugs listed below:

Drug	Possible effect and management
Antifungals such as ketoconazole (Nizoral) and miconazole (Monistat) or antibacterials such as erythromycin	These drugs may inhibit the metabolism of repaglinide, resulting in increased serum levels. Monitor closely.
troglitazone (Rezulin), rifampin, barbiturates, or carbamazepine (Tegretol)	These drugs induce the liver P450 enzyme system CYP3A4, which may increase the metabolism of repaglinide. Monitor closely as dosage adjustment may be necessary.

See Box 42-3 for other drugs that are reported to cause hyperglycemia or hypoglycemia.

Side effects and adverse reactions

These are the same as for the oral sulfonylurea agents, except the potential for adverse cardiovascular effects (e.g., hypertension, dysrhythmias, and myocardial infarction) may be at a higher level than with with glyburide (Baker, 1997).

Warnings

Use with caution in patients with liver impairment.

Contraindications

Avoid use in persons with repaglinide hypersensitivity and cardiac disorders.

Dosage and administration

See Table 42-2.

Thiazolidinedione

troglitazone [tro glit′ azone] (Rezulin)

Troglitiazone is the first agent in a new classification of drugs that lowers insulin resistance in patients with poorly controlled type 2 diabetes. This product appears to resensitize the body to its own insulin; thus it may reduce and, in some instances, eliminate the need for insulin.

Troglitiazone enters fat and muscle cells to stimulate the release of proteins that work with insulin to transfer sugar molecules from the bloodstream into body cells. In other words, it lowers blood glucose levels by improving the target cell response to insulin. This mechanism of action is totally different from that of all other hypoglycemic agents. Be aware, though, that this medication is not indicated for diabetic patients who cannot produce insulin (type 1 diabetes).

Pharmacokinetics

It is rapidly absorbed, especially in the presence of food, and is very highly protein bound (>99%) to serum albumin. It reaches a peak serum level in 2 to 3 hours and steady-state levels in 3 to 5 days and has a half-life of 16 to 34 hours. It is excreted primarily in feces.

Drug interactions

The following effects of troglitiazone may occur when it is given with the drugs listed below:

Drug	Possible effect and management
cholestyramine (Questran)	Concurrent administration reduces troglitiazone absorption by approximately 70%. Do not administer concurrently.
Oral contraceptives containing ethinyl estradiol and norethindrone and other drugs metabolized by the liver P450 CYP3A4 system (astemizole [Hismanal], calcium blockers, cisapride [Propulsid], corticosteroids, cyclosporine, hydroxymethylglucose-coenzyme A reductase inhibitors tacrolimus [Prograf], triazolam [Halcion], or terfenadine [Seldane])	Troglitiazone may induce drug metabolism of other drugs by the cytochrome P450 CYP3A4 system; therefore monitor concurrent drug therapy closely as dose adjustments may be necessary.

Side effects and adverse reactions

These include dizziness, headache, nausea, weakness, diarrhea, pharyngitis, rhinitis, jaundice, back pain, infection, peripheral edema, and urinary tract infection.

Contraindications

Avoid use in persons with troglitazone hypersensitivity, type 1 diabetes, diabetic ketoacidosis, heart failure, and liver function impairment.

Dosage and administration

The adult monotherapy dose is 400 to 600 mg daily, taken with a meal. If given in combination with insulin or a sulfonylurea, the starting oral dose is 200 mg daily with a meal, titrated as necessary (maximum dose is 600 mg/day).

Elderly patients. Elderly persons tend to be more sensitive to the effects of the oral hypoglycemic agents. Because hypoglycemia may be more difficult to recognize in these patients, they require lower dosages and closer monitoring.

HYPERGLYCEMIC AGENTS

glucagon [gloo′ ka gon]

Glucagon (for injection) is a natural polypeptide hormone secreted by pancreatic alpha cells in response to hypoglycemia. It is released to maintain plasma levels of glucose by stimulating hepatic glycogenolysis and gluconeogenesis (the conversion of glycerol and amino acids to glucose) and by inhibition of glycogen synthesis. Glucagon's effect is accelerated by stimulation of the synthesis of cyclic 3′,5′-adenosine monophosphate (cyclic AMP). Hepatic and adipose tissue lipolysis is enhanced by activation of adenylate cyclase, producing free fatty acids and glycerol, which stimulate ketogenesis and gluconeogenesis.

Indications

Glucagon is indicated for the treatment of severe hypoglycemia in persons with diabetes and as an adjunct for gastrointestinal radiography. It is useful in hypoglycemia only if liver glycogen is available; thus it is ineffective for chronic hypoglycemia, starvation, and adrenal insufficiency. As an adjunct to barium in gastrointestinal radiography, it produces relaxation of the esophagus, stomach, duodenum, small bowel, and colon (hypotonicity) and decreases peristalsis, thus improving outcome of the examination.

Pharmacokinetics

Parenterally administered (IM, IV, or SC), it has a half-life of 10 minutes and an onset of action (hyperglycemic) according to route of administration: IV, 5 to 20 minutes; IM, 15 minutes; and SC, 30 to 45 minutes. Its duration of action is 1.5 hours. It is metabolized in the liver and excreted by the kidneys.

Drug interactions

No significant drug interactions are reported.

Side effects and adverse reactions

For glucagon these are not usually severe and may include nausea or vomiting and an allergic reaction.

Contraindications

Avoid use in persons with glucagon hypersensitivity, diabetes mellitus, pheochromocytoma, or a history of insulinoma.

Dosage and administration

The adolescent and adult dose for hypoglycemia is 0.5 to 1 mg IM, IV, or SC, repeated in 20 minutes when necessary. The pediatric dose is 0.025 mg/kg up to a maximum dose of 1 mg (IM, IV, or SC).

diazoxide [dye az ox′ ide] (Proglycem)

Oral diazoxide produces a prompt, dose-related increase in blood glucose levels by inhibition of pancreatic insulin release. It may also have an extrapancreatic effect. It is indicated for the treatment of hypoglycemia caused by hyperinsulinism, secondary to an inoperable islet cell adenoma or carcinoma, an extrapancreatic malignancy, or an islet cell hyperplasia. It is not indicated for treatment of functional hypoglycemia. It is also available in parenteral dosage form to treat hypertensive emergencies.

Pharmacokinetics

Diazoxide is rapidly absorbed orally, has an onset of action within 1 hour, a duration of effect less than 8 hours, and a half-life between 20 and 36 hours in normal individuals. It is highly protein bound, metabolized in the liver, and excreted by the kidneys.

Drug interactions

The following effects may occur when diazoxide is given with the drugs listed below:

Drug	Possible effect and management
Anticonvulsants and hydantoin (phenytoin)	May decrease or nullify the action of both drugs. Monitor effects of both drugs and adjust doses accordingly.
Medications that induce hypotension (alcohol, diuretics, calcium channel blocking agents, and beta-adrenergic blocking drugs) and peripheral vasodilators	Concurrent use may cause an enhanced severe hypotensive effect. Monitor closely as dosage adjustments may be necessary.

Side effects and adverse reactions

These include taste alterations, constipation, anorexia, nausea, vomiting, abdominal pain, edema, tachycardia, allergic reaction, and, rarely, angina pectoris and myocardial infarction. With chronic drug administration, it may cause increased hair growth on arms, legs, back, and forehead (hypertrichosis). Hyperglycemia and ketoacidosis are typical symptoms reported with a diazoxide overdose.

Warnings

Use with caution in patients with gout or hyperuricemia, liver disease, and liver or kidney function impairment.

Contraindications

Avoid use in persons with diazoxide, sulfonamides or thiazide hypersensitivity, coronary or cerebral insufficiency, and acute aortic dissection and in patients who have an inadequate cardiac reserve or a compensatory hypertension.

Dosage and administration

The adult diazoxide dose is 1 mg/kg every 8 hours, adjusting the dosage as necessary. The maintenance dosage is 3 to 8 mg/kg orally daily, divided into two or three equal doses and administered every 12 or 8 hours. The maximum dose is usually 15 mg/kg/day.

glucose [gloo′ koes] (Glutose, Insta-Glucose)

Glucose is a monosaccharide that is absorbed from the intestine and then either used or stored by the body. It is indicated to treat or manage hypoglycemia. Glucose provides 4 calories/g.

The only side effects have been some reports of nausea. No significant drug interactions are reported.

In adults, approximately 10 to 20 g is administered orally and repeated in 10 minutes if necessary.

SUMMARY

The primary hormones of the pancreas are insulin and glucagon. Normally, when the blood glucose levels decrease, glucagon release is increased, which then facilitates the breakdown of glycogen stored in the liver to increase and restore blood glucose levels. In addition, the release of glucagon stimulates insulin secretion, inhibits the release of glucagon, and maintains the homeostasis of carbohydrate metabolism.

Diabetes mellitus is a disorder of carbohydrate metabolism that results from a relative or absolute insulin deficiency (in other words, an insulin deficiency or resistance or both). Diabetes mellitus is classified as type 1 (insulin-dependent diabetes mellitus) and type 2 (non-insulin-dependent diabetes mellitus or, formerly, maturity-onset diabetes). Persons with type 1 diabetes require insulin, while those with type 2 diabetes may require insulin at some time. Usually type 2 diabetes is managed by dietary treatment, weight reduction, and, if necessary, oral hypoglycemic agents.

The various insulin products and oral hypoglycemic agents are also reviewed in this chapter. In addition, hyperglycemic agents are available for the treatment of hypoglycemia

REVIEW QUESTIONS

1. What are the major complications of uncontrolled diabetes mellitus?
2. Why is human insulin preferred over use of animal-based insulins? In switching a patient to human insulin, what precautions should the healthcare professional take?
3. Name four drugs that may cause hyperglycemia and hypoglycemia.
4. What are the symptoms of hypoglycemia and hyperglycemia?
5. What is the longest-acting sulfonylurea agent that reportedly has more side effects than the other agents?
6. What are the mechanisms of action for the five miscellaneous oral hypoglycemic agents?

REFERENCES

Baker DE: Management of type 2 diabetes, *Clin Pharm Newswatch Parke-Davis* 4(4):1-6, 1997.

Beare PG, Myers JL: *Adult health nursing,* ed 3, St Louis, 1998, Mosby.

Beier MT: Incidence of NIDDM and impact of tight glucose control: implications for long-term care, *Consult Pharmacist Suppl A* 12:3-6, 1997.

Campbell RK: The clinical use of insulin, *US Pharmacist Diabetes Suppl,* Nov 1992.

Covington TR, editor: *Handbook of nonprescription drugs,* ed 11, Washington, DC, 1996, American Pharmaceutical Association.

Davis SN, Granner DK: Insulin, oral hypoglycemic agents, and the pharmacology of the endocrine pancreas. In Hardman JG, Limbird LE, editors: *Goodman & Gilman's the pharmacological basis of therapeutics,* ed 9, New York, 1996, McGraw-Hill.

Koda-Kimble MA, Carlisle BA: Diabetes mellitus. In Young LY, Koda-Kimble MA, editors: *Applied therapeutics: the clinical use of drugs,* ed 6, Vancouver, Wash, 1995, Applied Therapeutics, Inc.

Melmon KL et al: *Melmon and Morrelli's clinical pharmacology,* ed 3, New York, 1992, McGraw-Hill.

Olin BR: *Facts and comparisons.* Philadelphia, 1998, JB Lippincott.

Ponte CD, Chair: *New product bulletin: Rezulin (troglitazone),* American Pharmaceutical Association PD-168-Bk-2137-A1 (107) 709B59, 1997.

Rodgers K: New ammon: faster-acting insulin set to debut in August, *Drug Top* 140(13):59, 1996.

United States Pharmacopeial Convention: *USP DI: drug information for the health care professional,* ed 18, Rockville, Md, 1998, The Convention.

Watson J, Jaffe MS: *Nurse's manual of laboratory and diagnostic tests,* Philadelphia, 1995, FA Davis.

ADDITIONAL REFERENCES

American Diabetic Association: *Physician's guide to non–insulin-dependent (type 2) diabetes: diagnosis and treatment,* Alexandria, Va, 1990, The Association.

American Hospital Formulary Service: *AHFS drug information '98,* Bethesda, Md, 1996, American Society of Hospital Pharmacists.

Anderson KN et al, editors: *Mosby's medical, nursing, and allied health dictionary,* ed 5, St Louis, 1998, Mosby.

Betz JL: Pharmacy update: fast-acting human insulin analogues: a promising innovation in diabetes care, *Diabetes Educator* 21(3):195, 197-198, 200, 1995.

Katzung BG: *Basic and clinical pharmacology,* ed 5, Norwalk, Conn, 1992, Appleton & Lange.

Mosby: *Mosby's GenRx,* St Louis, 1998, Mosby.

UNIT XII

Drugs Affecting the Reproductive System

CHAPTER 43

Overview of the Female and Male Reproductive Systems

CHAPTER FOCUS

Because secrecy and cultural sensitivity often influence perceptions of reproductive disorders, care for patients with dysfunctions of the reproductive system is particularly challenging for the healthcare professional. The patient may experience disturbance of self-esteem, altered sexual patterns, and sexual dysfunction, thus requiring knowledge of reproductive anatomy and physiology and associated drugs for sensitive and appropriate teaching and counseling. This chapter reviews the anatomy and physiology of the female and male reproductive systems as groundwork for the next four chapters, which discuss the drugs affecting the reproductive system. The following objectives and key terms are important for a good understanding of this chapter.

OBJECTIVES

After reading and studying this chapter, the student should be able to do the following:

1. *Identify the anterior pituitary gland hormones that influence the female and male reproductive systems.*
2. *Describe hormonal influences on uterine function during the menstrual cycle.*
3. *Identify the primary male and female hormones.*
4. *Describe the effects of estrogen and progesterone during the proliferative stage.*
5. *Trace the transport of sperm in the male body from production to ejaculation.*

KEY TERMS

androgens, (p. 582)
estrogens, (p. 582)
follicle-stimulating hormone (FSH), (p. 582)
luteinizing hormone (LH), (p. 583)
ovulation, (p. 584)
progestogens, (p. 582)
testosterone, (p. 585)

Reproduction is the sum of genetic and hormonal influences originating from the sexes of a species to perpetuate the species. In human beings, the reproductive process in both sexes is highly complex, involving follicle-stimulating hormone (FSH), which stimulates the growth and maturation of graafian follicles in the ovary and spermatogenesis in the testes, and luteinizing hormone (LH), which stimulates the secretion of sex hormones by the ovary and the testes and is involved in the maturation of the spermatozoa and ova; both hormones are secreted from the anterior pituitary gland. The hormones from the reproductive systems of the male (**androgens**) and the female (**estrogens** and **progestogens**) are also involved in the reproductive process.

ENDOCRINE GLANDS

The reproductive system of the human female consists of the ovaries, fallopian tubes, uterus, and vagina. The male reproductive system consists of the testes, seminal vesicles, prostate gland, bulbourethral glands, and penis. The reproductive organs of both male and female are mainly under the control of the endocrine glands. The ovaries and testes, known as gonads, not only produce ova and sperm cells but also form endocrine secretions that initiate and maintain the secondary sexual characteristics in men and women. The structure and physiologic functions of the pituitary gland are reviewed in Chapter 39; the discussion of the pituitary gland in this chapter is limited to its effect on the female and male reproductive systems.

PITUITARY GONADOTROPIC HORMONES

The gonadotropins or pituitary hormones responsible for the development and maintenance of sexual gland functions are the following:

1. **Follicle-stimulating hormone (FSH)**, which stimulates the development of the ovarian (graafian) follicles up to the point of ovulation in the female; in the male, FSH stimulates the development of the seminiferous tubules and promotes spermatogenesis.
2. **Luteinizing hormone (LH)**, or interstitial cell-stimulating hormone (ICSH), which acts in the female to promote the growth of the interstitial cells in the follicle and the formation of the corpus luteum; in the male, ICSH stimulates the growth of interstitial cells in the testes and promotes the formation of the hormone androgen, testosterone.
3. Luteotropic hormone, or luteotropin, which is identical to the lactogenic hormone, or prolactin.

In the female, FSH initiates the cycle of events in the ovary. Under the influence of both FSH and LH the graafian follicle grows, matures, secretes estrogen, ovulates, and forms the corpus luteum. LH promotes the secretory activity of the corpus luteum and the formation of progesterone. In the absence of LH the corpus luteum undergoes regressive changes and fails to make progesterone.

FEMALE REPRODUCTIVE SYSTEM

Fig. 43-1 illustrates the effects of the pituitary hormones, ovarian hormones, and uterine functions during the menstrual cycle.

Day 1 of the menstrual cycle is the onset of menses, and day 5 usually signifies the end of menstruation. During this time, FSH is stimulating follicular growth in the ovary and also stimulating the ovary to produce estrogen, which is low at the beginning of the cycle. As estrogen levels increase, FSH levels decrease. The rising estrogen levels are preparing the uterus for a fertilized ovum, which is known as the proliferative stage of the uterus and results in the following: (1) the growth of glandular surface of the endometrium, or inner lining of the uterus; and (2) the production, by the endocervical glands, of a more plentiful, viscous mucus that contains nutrients that can be used by the sperm.

The increasing levels of estrogen also stimulate the pituitary gland to release LH. As FSH is decreasing, LH is increasing. At this time (day 14), **ovulation** occurs when the mature follicle ruptures and releases its ovum. The ovum travels through the fallopian tube to the uterus. Female pelvic organs are shown in Fig. 43-2.

The increasing levels of LH will affect the ruptured follicle by changing the follicle capsule into the corpus luteum. Under the influence of LH, the corpus luteum releases estrogen and progesterone. In the second phase, or secretory phase, both uterine hormones increase secretion of the glands of the endometrium. If the ovum is fertilized and reaches this area on approximately the 18th day of the cycle, it will be able to thrive on the nutrient secretions of the endometrium.

However, if fertilization does not occur, the pituitary will respond to the increased levels of estrogen and progesterone by shutting off the release of FSH and LH. Without the central stimulation, the corpus luteum cannot produce estrogen or progesterone, so the surface layer of the endometrium will slough off, resulting in menstruation. Fig. 43-3 depicts the feedback mechanism of FSH and LH and their main effects on the ovaries.

Most women demonstrate month-to-month variations in their menstrual cycles; therefore ovulation is not always predictable. The previous description of the menstrual cycle is based on a 28-day cycle, but ovulation varies and occurs on different days in different length cycles. Physiologically, this is the primary reason for the unreliability of the rhythm method of contraception, which depends on predicting the day of ovulation based on previous menstrual cycles.

Female Sexual Response

For both males and females, psychic stimulation and local sexual stimulation are necessary for a satisfactory sexual experience. Psychic stimulation may be aided by an individual's erotic thoughts, although sexual desire is also affected by increasing levels of estrogen secretion, especially during the preovulatory period.

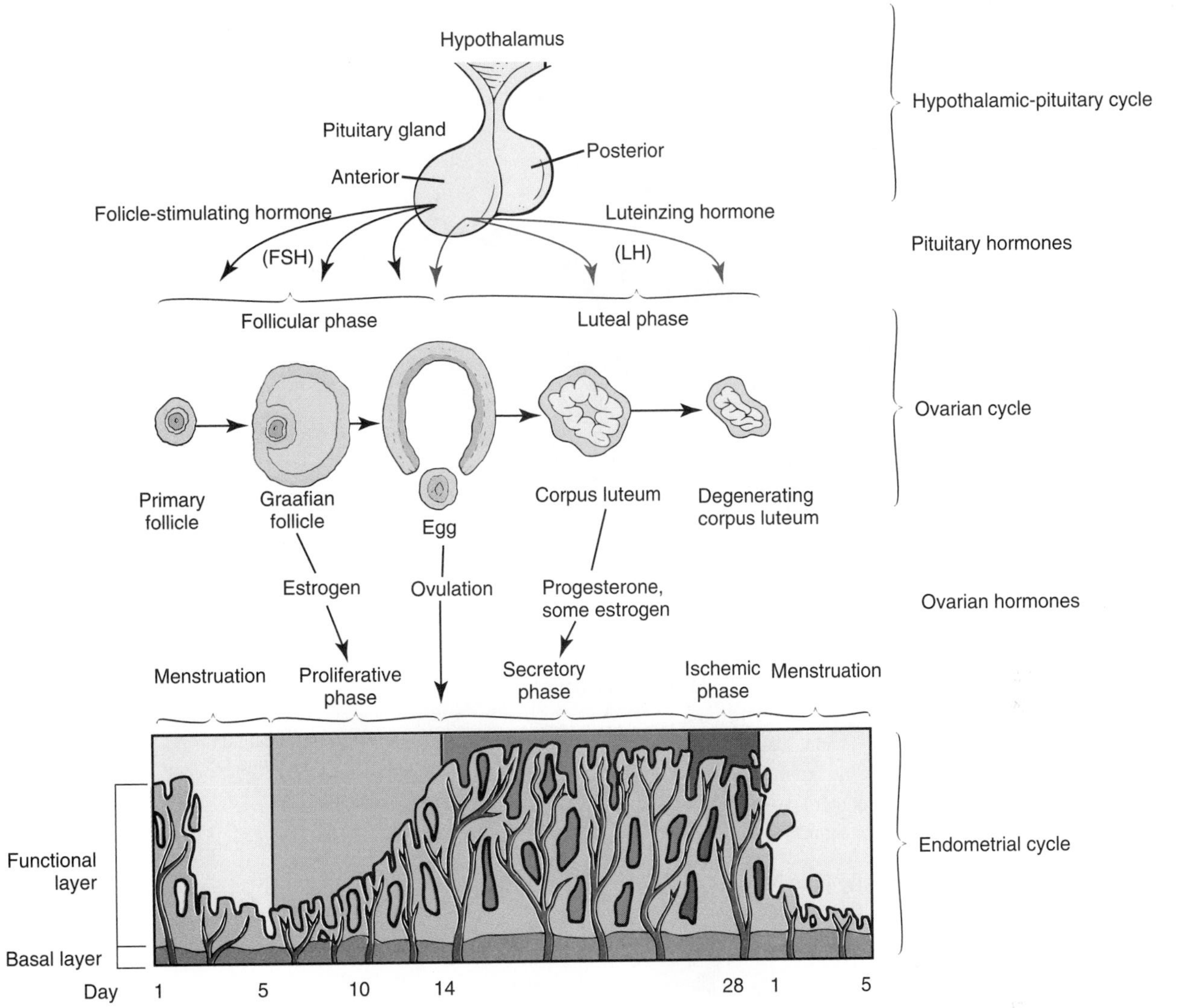

FIGURE 43-1
Menstrual cycle. *(Modified from Lowdermilk et al, 1997.)*

Local sexual stimulation causes similar responses in both sexes; that is, massage, increasing stimulation or irritation of the perineal region or sexual organs, can result in an enhancement of sexual sensations. In the female, the clitoris is very sensitive, and its stimulation can initiate a sexual sensation. Erectile tissue is located in the introitus (vaginal opening) and clitoris areas. This tissue is under parasympathetic nerve control; therefore in early stimulation, the parasympathetic nerves dilate the arteries located in the erectile tissues. Blood collects in the erectile tissue in the area so that the introitus will tighten around the penis, which aids male satisfaction for sexual stimulation, thus leading to ejaculation.

The parasympathetic nerves also signal the Bartholin's glands situated near the labia minora, which results in increased mucus secretion inside the introitus. This secretion, in addition to mucus from the vaginal epithelium, serves as a lubricant during sexual intercourse.

The female climax, or orgasm, is reached when the local sexual stimulation reaches the maximum sensation or intensity. It is considered similar to emission and ejaculation in the male and may also help to promote fertilization of the ovum. It has been theorized that orgasm produces a rhythm in the female tract from spinal cord reflexes that increase both uterine and fallopian tube motility and may result in cervical canal dilation for up to 30 minutes. This will allow for easy sperm transport in the female.

The intense sexual sensations that develop during orgasms also result in an increase in muscle tension throughout the body. After the sexual act, this tension subsides into relaxation or feelings of satisfaction, sometimes referred to as resolution.

MALE REPRODUCTIVE SYSTEM

The effects of FSH and LH or ICSH in the male were described in the section on pituitary gonadotropic hormones.

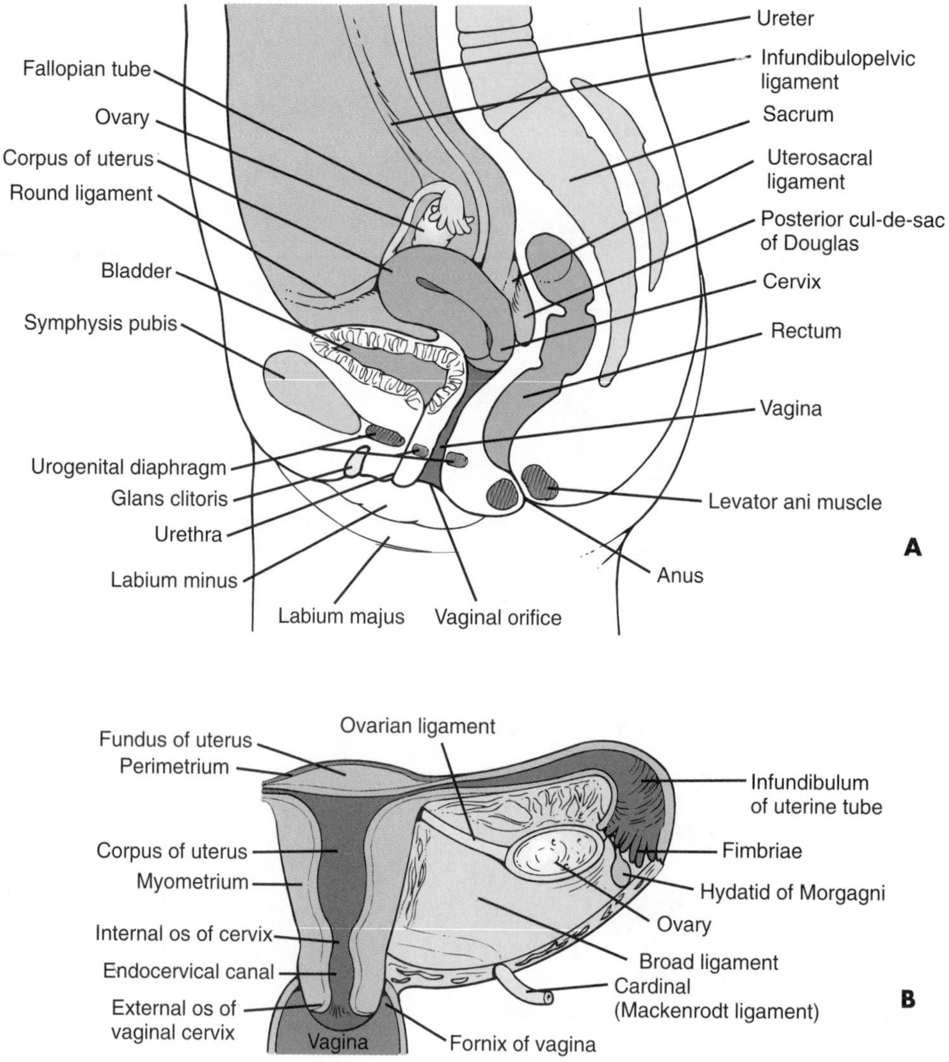

FIGURE 43-2
A, Female reproduction system. **B,** Cross-section of uterus, adnexa, and upper vagina. *(Modified from Beare, Myers, 1998.)*

The effects of ICSH on secretion of testosterone are seen in Fig. 43-4. **Testosterone,** an androgen, performs numerous functions, which are described below. FSH from the anterior pituitary gland stimulates the seminiferous tubules to increase production of spermatozoa, while ICSH stimulates the interstitial cells to increase secretion of testosterone. A high level of testosterone will inhibit the pituitary's release of FSH and ICSH.

Testosterone has many functions in the male. It aids in developing and maintaining the male secondary sex characteristics and male accessory organs, such as prostate, seminal vesicles, and bulbourethral glands. Testosterone promotes adult male sexual behavior, as well as regulating metabolism and protein anabolism, resulting in the growth of bone and skeletal muscles. This hormone affects fluid and electrolyte metabolism by reabsorbing sodium and water and increasing excretion of potassium. FSH and ICSH secretion are also inhibited from the anterior pituitary by testosterone.

Transport of Sperm in the Male

Sperm produced in the testes mature by spending 1 to 3 weeks in the epididymis of the male. The sperm, in seminal fluid, then travels through the epididymis (ducts that lie around the top of the testes) to the vas deferens. The vas deferens, a duct extension of the epididymis, extends over the bladder surface (posteriorly) to the ampulla to form the ejaculatory duct. Sperm can be stored in the vas deferens in excess of 1 month without loss of fertility depending on sexual activity. Thus a vasectomy, or severing of the vas deferens, will make a man sterile primarily because it interrupts the journey of spermto the ejaculatory duct and urethra.

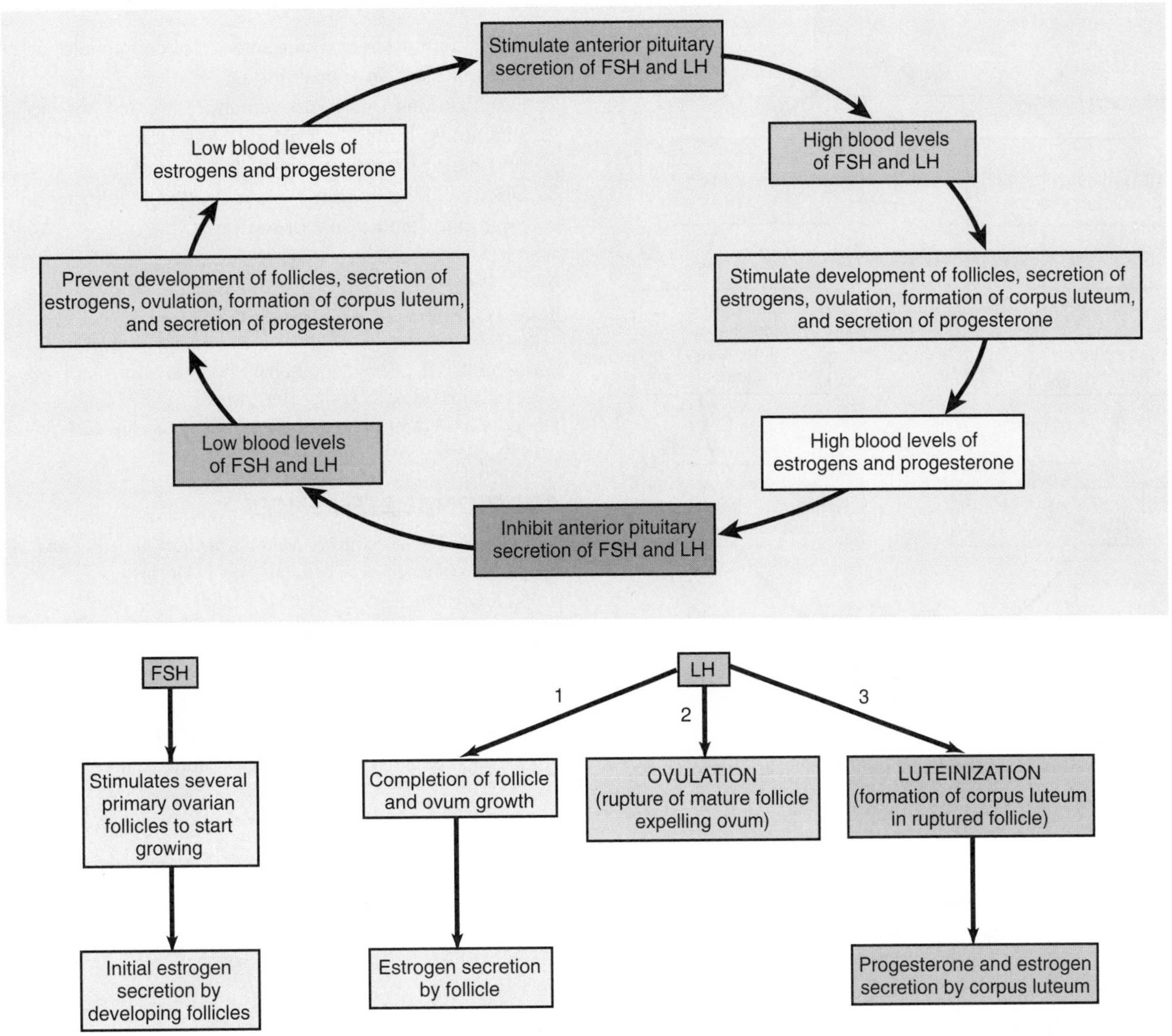

FIGURE 43-3
Feedback mechanism of FSH and LH and their main effects on the ovaries. *(Modified from Thibodeau, Patton, 1999.)*

Male pelvic organs and the anatomy of the ejaculatory ducts are shown in Fig. 43-5.

Male Sexual Response

Penile erection is a parasympathetic response that consists of dilation of the arteries and arterioles in the penis, which compresses the veins in this area. Thus more blood enters the penis than leaves, the penis becomes larger, and erection occurs. Emission and ejaculation of the sperm or semen is a reflex response. The stimulus that initiated erection will also help to move the sperm and secretions (semen) from the genital ducts to the prostatic urethra. Orgasm, the climax of the sexual act, moves the semen through the ejaculatory ducts. During coitus, the sperm can be transferred from male to female.

Later in life gonadal function ceases. Women undergo menopause or cessation of menses, and men have a decrease in sex hormone production, which is sometimes called the male climacteric.

SUMMARY

Disorders of the reproductive system of men and women result in acute and chronic physical and emotional stress. The healthcare professional requires a sound knowledge of the anatomy and physiology of the reproductive system to assess patients for health adaptations and alterations and to assist patients with complex health issues in this domain.

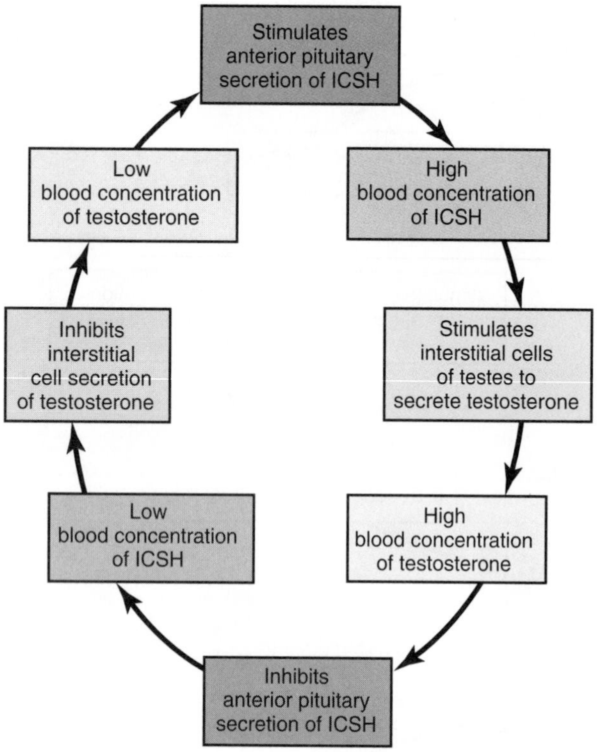

FIGURE 43-4

Effect of ICSH on testosterone. *(Modified from Thibodeau, Patton, 1999.)*

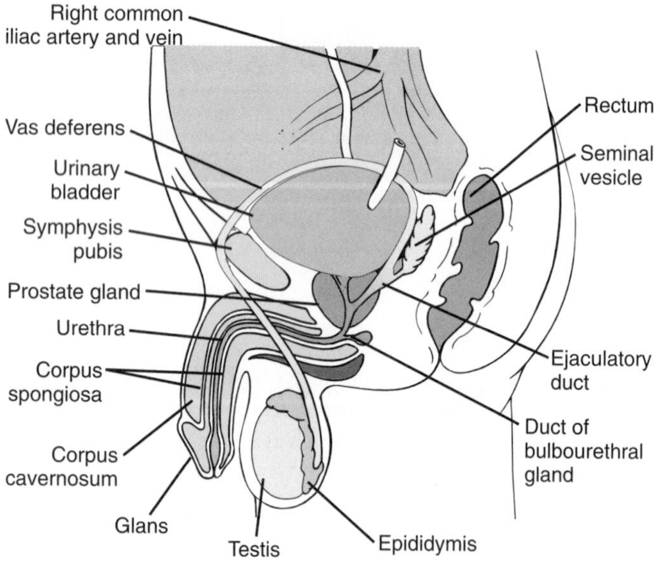

FIGURE 43-5

Male reproductive system. *(Modified from Thibodeau, Patton, 1999.)*

REVIEW QUESTIONS

1. Describe the effect of the interstitial cell-stimulating hormone (ICSH) on testosterone.
2. Describe the feedback mechanisms for the follicle-stimulating hormone (FSH) and luteinizing hormone (LH) and their primary effects on the ovaries.
3. Discuss the autonomic nervous system effects on the male and female sexual reponses.

REFERENCES

Beare PG, Myers JL: *Adult health nursing,* ed 3, St Louis, 1998, Mosby.

Lowdermilk DL, Perry SE, Bobak IM: *Maternity and women's health care,* ed 6, St Louis, 1997, Mosby.

Thibodeau GA, Patton KT: *Anatomy and physiology,* ed 4, St Louis, 1999, Mosby.

ADDITIONAL REFERENCES

Anderson KN et al, editors: *Mosby's medical, nursing, and allied health dictionary,* ed 5, St Louis, 1998, Mosby.

Gray M: *Genitourinary disorders,* St Louis, 1992, Mosby.

Guyton AC: *Textbook of medical physiology,* ed 8, Philadelphia, 1990, WB Saunders.

Seeley RR, Stephens TD, Tate P: *Anatomy and physiology,* ed 3, New York, 1995, McGraw-Hill.

Van Wynsberghe D, Noback CR, Carola R: *Human anatomy and physiology,* ed 3, New York, 1995, McGraw-Hill.

CHAPTER 44

Drugs Affecting the Female Reproductive System

KEY DRUGS

estrogen, (p. 590)
progestin, (p. 591)

KEY TERMS

anovulation, (p. 595)
biphasic oral contraception, (p. 594)
estrogens, (p. 590)
menotropin, (p. 589)
monophasic oral contraception, (p. 594)
oral contraception, (p. 592)
progestogens, (p. 590)
triphasic oral contraception, (p. 594)

CHAPTER FOCUS

Drugs that affect the female reproductive system therapeutically are synthetic or natural analogs of homogeneous hormones. They are administered to mimic the biologic effects of endogenous hormones, to supplement inadequate production (e.g., menopause), to correct hormonal balance (e.g., dysfunctional bleeding), to reverse an abnormal process (anovulation), and for contraception. Whatever the indication, the healthcare professional needs to be knowledgeable about these drugs to support the patient's need for intervention and instruction. The following objectives and key terms are important for a good understanding of this chapter.

OBJECTIVES

After reading and studying this chapter, the student should be able to do the following:

1. *Define and describe the key terms and key drugs.*
2. *List drugs affecting the female reproductive system.*
3. *Describe the source and action of chorionic gonadotropin.*
4. *Discuss the function of the primary female sex hormones.*
5. *Discuss the side effects and adverse reactions of estrogens and progestins.*
6. *Compare and contrast monophasic, biphasic, and triphasic oral contraceptives.*
7. *Implement care of patients receiving drug therapy affecting the female reproductive system.*

Synthetic and natural substances that affect the female reproductive system include gonadotropin-releasing hormones, nonpituitary chorionic gonadotropin, menotropins, female sex hormones, oral contraceptives, ovulatory stimulants, and drugs used for infertility.

GONADOTROPIN-RELEASING HORMONE (GnRH)

Five preparations of GnRH are available: leuprolide (Lupron) and goserelin (Zoladex), which are reviewed in Chapter 49, and gonadorelin, nafarelin, and histrelin, which are discussed in this chapter.

gonadorelin [goe nad oh rell′ in] (Factrel)

Gonadorelin is a synthetic GnRH used as an adjunct to other tests to diagnose hypogonadism in males and females. It is chemically identical to the natural GnRH; it stimulates the synthesis and release of luteinizing hormone (LH) and to a lesser extent follicle-stimulating hormone (FSH) from the anterior pituitary. In the diagnosing of hypogonadism, multiple dosing may be more valuable than a single dose test in differentiating between hypothalamic function impairment and pituitary function impairment.

Pharmacokinetics

Intravenously, it has an initial half-life of 2 to 10 minutes followed by a terminal half-life of 10 to 40 minutes. It is metabolized rapidly in the body and excreted by the kidneys.

Drug interactions

No significant drug interactions are reported with its use.

Side effects and adverse reactions

These include anaphylaxis, pain or inflammation at the injection site, and, rarely, stomach distress, flushing, headaches, nausea, and lightheadedness.

Contraindications

Avoid use in persons with gonadorelin hypersensitivity.

Dosage and administration

In children 12 years of age and older and adults, the dose to diagnose hypogonadism is 100 μg SC or IV. In females, the drug should be administered in the early follicular phase of the menstrual cycle, preferably within the first week.

GONADOTROPIN-RELEASING HORMONE AGONIST

nafarelin [naf′ a re lin] (Synarel)

Nafarelin is a potent agonist of GnRH that initially stimulates the release of LH and FSH but with continued dosing results in decreased secretion of the gonadotropins. The continuous stimulation of the GnRH receptors results in desensitization and ultimately decreased production of LH and FSH. It is indicated for the treatment or management of endometriosis.

Pharmacokinetics

This product is administered nasally with maximum serum levels reported in 10 to 40 minutes. It has a half-life of 3 hours with a maximum effect within 1 month.

Drug interactions

There are no recorded significant drug interactions with nafarelin usage.

Side effects and adverse reactions

These include breakthrough bleeding, spotting, amenorrhea, hypoestrogen (acne, hot flashes, decreased libido, vaginal dryness, and oily skin), headaches, mood swings, breast pain, rhinitis, weight changes, joint pain, and, rarely, galactorrhea, ovarian cysts, and immediate hypersensitivity.

Warnings

Use with caution in patients with low bone mineral content, as its usage increases the potential for osteoporosis.

Contraindications

Avoid use in persons with nafarelin hypersensitivity.

Dosage and administration

The dosage is one nasal spray of 200 μg in one nostril in the morning and one spray in the other nostril at night. It is usually administered for a period of 6 months.

histrelin [his′ tre lin] (Supprelin)

Histrelin is a synthetic GnRH agonist that is more potent than the natural hormone. It controls pituitary gonadotropin secretion, which results in a decrease in sex steroid levels and regression of secondary sexual characteristics in children with precocious puberty. It is used only in patients with centrally mediated precocious puberty before the age of 8 in girls and 9.5 in boys. In females, it decreases estradiol levels; in males it inhibits testosterone. Decreases in LH, FSH, and sex steroid serum levels are noted within 3 months of therapy.

Side effects and adverse reactions

These include vasodilation, vaginal dryness, breast edema and pain, gastric distress, urticaria, seizures, visual disturbances, hot flashes, mood alterations, headaches, fever, arthralgia, anxiety, and reactions at the site of injection. Vaginal bleeding usually occurs once in 1 to 3 weeks of therapy.

Contraindications

Avoid use in persons with histrelin hypersensitivity, in pregnant women or in women who may become pregnant, and in nursing mothers.

Dosage and administration

The usual dose for central precocious puberty is 10 μg/kg by daily SC injection.

NONPITUITARY CHORIONIC GONADOTROPIN

Certain gonadotropic substances formed by the placenta during pregnancy are extracted from the urine of pregnant women. The action of human chorionic gonadotropin is nearly equivalent to the pituitary's LH with little or no follicle-stimulating effects. A discussion of nonpituitary chorionic gonadotropin and menotropins is found later in this chapter.

gonadotropin, chorionic [goe nad′ oh troe pin] (A.P.L., Pregnyl)

This drug is administered to make up for a deficiency in LH. Chorionic gonadotropin is indicated for:

- Treatment of prepubertal cryptorchidism and hypogonadotropic hypogonadism. Stimulation of androgen production in the testes may enhance testes descent and increase development of the secondary male sex characteristics.
- Treatment of male and female infertility. In females it is combined with other drugs, such as menotropins. Men may receive it alone or in combination.
- Stimulation of multiple oocytes in ovulatory women in conjunction with other procedures.

Pharmacokinetics

Administered IM, the drug has a half-life of between 11 and 23 hours, and ovulation usually occurs within 32 to 36 hours of administration. It is excreted by the kidneys within 24 hours. It has no significant drug interactions.

Side effects and adverse reactions

These include increased irritation, headache, tiredness, edema, depression, precocious puberty, gynecomastia, aggression, ovarian hyperstimulation, and arterial thromboembolism.

Warnings

Use with caution in women who are lactating and in persons with epilepsy, migraine headaches, asthma, and heart and kidney disease.

Contraindications

Avoid use in persons with chorionic gonadotropin hypersensitivity, precocious puberty, and prostate cancer and in pregnant women

Dosage and administration

The adult dosage for male hypogonadotropic hypogonadism is 1000 to 4000 units IM two to three times a week for several weeks to months or in some cases indefinitely. For induction of ovulation, a dose of 5000 to 10,000 units IM is administered after the last dose of menotropins or from 5 to 9 days after the last dose of clomiphene.

For children with prepubertal cryptorchidism, the dose is 1000 to 5000 units IM two or three times a week for a maximum of 10 doses or the therapy is stopped when the desired response is achieved.

MENOTROPINS

Menotropin is a human pituitary gonadotropin, a purified preparation of FSH and LH obtained from the urine of postmenopausal women. It is sometimes called human menopausal gonadotropin (HMG).

menotropins [men oh troe′ pins] (Pergonal)

The mechanism of action is equivalent to effects produced by FSH and LH; menotropins stimulate the development of the ovarian follicle, causes ovulation, and may stimulate corpus luteum development. In males, it stimulates sperm production.

Menotropins are indicated in the treatment of the following conditions:

- Female infertility caused by ovulatory dysfunction, administered in combination with chorionic gonadotropin. Menotropins are considered the treatment of choice for individuals with hypothalamic hypogonadism or for those who did not respond to clomiphene.
- Male infertility, used in combination with chorionic gonadotropin to stimulate spermatogenesis in primary or secondary hypogonadotropic hypogonadism (male infertility).
- Stimulation of multiple oocyte development in ovulatory patients who are using other technologies to conceive, such as gamete intrafallopian transfer or in vitro fertilization, used in combination with chorionic gonadotropin.

Pharmacokinetics

Menotropins are administered IM with excretion via the kidneys.

Drug interactions

There are no reported significant drug interactions.

Side effects and adverse reactions

These include gastric distress, severe pelvic pain, weight gain, edema, shortness of breath, decreased urine output, abdominal bloating or pain, ovarian enlargement, or cysts (usually in females). For males these include breast enlargement and erythrocytosis.

Contraindications

Avoid use in women with vaginal bleeding (that is abnormal and undiagnosed) and ovarian cysts or enlargement.

Dosage and administration

The adult menotropin dosage for induction of ovulation is 1 ampule (75 units of FSH and LH activity) IM daily for a week or more, followed by 5000 to 10,000 units of chorionic gonadotropin, a day after the last menotropin dose. If necessary, the ampule dose may be increased every 4 to 5 days, up to a maximum of 6 ampules. For treatment of male infertility, administer 1 ampule IM three times weekly (in addition to chorionic gonadotropin twice a week) for a minimum of 4 months after pretreatment with chorionic gonadotropin for 4 to 6 months.

FEMALE SEX HORMONES

The ovaries, in addition to providing ova, manufacture and secrete female hormones that control secondary sex characteristics, the reproductive cycle, and the growth and development of the accessory reproductive organs in the female. Two main types of hormones are secreted by the ovary: (1) the follicular or estrogenic hormones (**estrogens**) produced by the cells of the developing graafian follicle and (2) the luteal or progestational hormones (**progestogens**) derived from the corpus luteum that is formed in the ovary from the ruptured follicle. The periodic cycling of the female sex hormones depends on an interaction between FSH and LH with the ovarian hormones estrogen and progesterone. This results in a menstrual cycle that normally continues throughout life, except during pregnancy, until menopause. Although estrogens are primarily secreted by the ovarian follicles, some may also be secreted by the adrenal glands, corpus luteum, placenta, and testes.

Estrogens

Estrogens are available from natural sources (the urine of pregnant mares) in conjugated dosage forms and have been synthetically formulated. Examples of natural steroidal estrogens include estradiol, estrone, esterified estrogens, and estrone; nonsteroidal estrogens include diethylstilbestrol (DES), dienestrol, and chlorotrianisene.

estrogen [ess′ troe jen] (various manufacturers)

Estrogen increases the synthesis of deoxyribonucleic acid (DNA), ribonucleic acid (RNA), and protein in estrogen-responsive tissues. Elevated estrogen serum levels inhibit secretion of FSH and LH from the pituitary, which results in inhibition of lactation and ovulation and the development of a proliferative endometrium.

Estrogen is indicated for the following conditions:

- Treatment of estrogen deficiency: atrophic vaginitis, female hypogonadism, insufficient primary ovarian function, abnormal uterine bleeding, severe vasomotor symptoms in menopause, and postmenopausal osteoporosis.
- Treatment of cancer: selected metastatic breast carcinomas in postmenopausal women with tumor estrogen-negative receptors, selected male breast carcinomas, and advanced prostatic carcinomas.

Menopause

The use of estrogen therapy in postmenopausal women has resulted in reports of a significant decrease in the risk of heart disease (Pharmacy Practice News, 1995), including a reduction in the death rate of women with coronary artery disease in America (Belchetz, 1994). Mosca et al (1998) report on an analysis of published studies in the United States indicating that use of postmenopausal estrogen reduces the incidence of coronary heart disease by 35% to 50%. Several studies also indicated an increase in life expectancy secondary to postmenopausal estrogen usage. Other studies reported a decreased in many diseases except for breast cancer and venous thromboembolism (Mosca et al, 1998). Investigational studies are ongoing to identify the unknown selection factors necessary to determine who can safely take estrogen. Until this is known, physicians are weighing risk versus benefit before prescribing estrogens during menopause. The student should be aware, though, that the estrogen dose for postmenopausal hormone replacement usage is considerably less than the dose used in oral contraceptives (Williams, Stancel, 1996).

Pharmacokinetics

Estrogen is protein bound, metabolized in the liver, and excreted by the kidneys.

Drug interactions

The following effects may occur when estrogen is given with the drugs listed below:

Drug	Possible effect and management
bromocriptine (Parlodel)	Concurrent use may result in amenorrhea and may also interfere with bromocriptine's therapeutic effect. Avoid or a potentially serious drug interaction may occur.
cyclosporine (Sandimmune)	Metabolism is inhibited, which may result in increased cyclosporine plasma levels and increased risk of hepatotoxicity and nephrotoxicity. Use concurrently only with very close monitoring of cyclosporine serum levels and liver and kidney function.
Hepatotoxic drugs, especially dantrolene	Estrogens increase the risk of inducing hepatotoxicity: females older than 35 years of age are at increased risk. Avoid or a potentially serious drug interaction may occur.
Tobacco (smoking)	Tobacco smoking increases the risk of serious cardiac adverse reactions, such as cerebrovascular accident, transient ischemic attacks, thrombophlebitis, and pulmonary embolism. The risk is higher in women older than 35 years of age who smoke. Avoid or a potentially serious drug interaction may occur.

Color type indicates an unsafe drug combination.

Side effects and adverse reactions

These include stomach cramps or gas, anorexia, nausea, chloasma, headaches, nausea, vomiting, a change in female libido and decrease in male sex drive, edema of the lower extremities, breast pain and enlargement, and changes in menstrual bleeding.

Warnings

Use with caution in patients with endometriosis, gallbladder disease, liver disease, pancreatitis, uterine leiomyoma, and hyperlipoproteinemia (familial).

Contraindications

Avoid use in persons with estrogen hypersensitivity, hypercalcemia, and estrogen-induced thrombophlebitis and thrombosis (except for the treatment of breast cancer or prostate cancer; for such usage, evaluate the risk versus benefit).

Dosage and administration

The lowest effective dose of estrogens should be administered for the shortest time period to reduce the possibility of serious adverse effects. When continuous therapy is required, the prescriber should reevaluate the patient at least annually.

To avoid overstimulation of estrogen-sensitive tissues, a cyclic dosing schedule of 3 weeks of estrogen administration and 1 week off or the addition of a progestin for the last 10 to 13 days of the cycle will most closely approximate the natural hormonal cycle. This is not the schedule for oophorectomized individuals or patients with cancer who are receiving hormonal therapy.

Estradiol and estrone are naturally occurring steroidal estrogens that are principal endogenous estrogens. Estradiol is available alone or synthetically as estradiol cypionate, estradiol valerate, ethinyl estradiol, and polyestradiol phosphate. The primary pharmacologic effects of all estrogens are similar.

Conjugated estrogens (Premarin), a mixture of estrogenic substances (especially estrone and equilin), are available in oral, parenteral, and vaginal cream dosage formulations. Dosage must be individualized according to diagnosis and therapeutic response, for example, vasomotor symptoms associated with menopause. The usual oral adult dose for esterified estrogens is 0.3 to 1.25 mg daily cyclically or continuously. Some women may require higher dosages.

DES is a synthetic nonsteroidal estrogen primarily used as an antineoplastic agent.

Transdermal estradiol (Estraderm) is used for women with estrogen deficiency. Applied topically to intact skin, 50 μg (0.05 mg) or 100 μg (0.1 mg) daily is released from the transdermal patch. It should be replaced twice weekly and is usually worn continuously.

The following precautions should be kept in mind when estrogen therapy is given:

1. The risk of endometrial cancer increases with prolonged use of estrogens in postmenopausal women. However, low-dose estrogen given cyclically or the use of a progestin (concurrently or sequentially) may reduce the risk of inducing endometrial cancer.

PREGNANCY SAFETY

Category	Drug
B	gonadorelin
C	chorionic gonadotropin, clomiphene
D	hydroxyprogesterone, progesterone
X	estrogens, histrelin, levonorgestrel, megestrol suspension, menotropins, nafarelin, norethindrone, norgestrel, oral contraceptives, urofollitropin

2. Estrogens, especially DES, should not be administered during pregnancy because of an increased risk of congenital malformations. See the box for Food and Drug Administration (FDA) pregnancy safety categories.
3. Estrogens are excreted in breast milk and will also inhibit lactation; therefore administration of estrogens to nursing women is not recommended.

Progesterone and Progestins

Progesterone produced by the ovaries is a naturally occurring progestin. The anterior pituitary LH stimulates the synthesizing and secretion of progesterone from the corpus luteum, mainly during the latter half of the menstrual cycle. Progesterone may also be formed from steroid precursors available in the ovaries, testes, adrenal cortex, and placenta.

Progesterone and synthetic progestins have similar pharmacologic effects in the body. Progestins were developed because progesterone was not always therapeutically satisfactory. The advantages with progestins are (1) greater potency that lowered the dose necessary to produce an response equivalent to that of progesterone; (2) a longer duration of action; and (3) an effective oral/sublingual dosage form that is available for some products.

progesterone [proe jess′ ter one]
progestin [proe jess′ tin]
(various manufacturers)

Progesterone and progestins (hydroxyprogesterone, norethindrone, and others) produce biochemical changes in the endometrium to prepare for the implantation and nourishment of the embryo. They also (1) supplement the action of estrogen in its effects on the uterus and mammary glands, (2) cause suppression of ovulation during pregnancy, (3) cause relaxation of the uterine smooth muscles, (4) increase the synthesis of DNA and RNA, and (5) inhibit, in large doses, the secretion of LH from the anterior pituitary.

Indications

Progesterone and progestins are indicated for the treatment of female hormonal imbalance of amenorrhea and dysmenorrhea, endometriosis, and specific carcinomas. They are also used to diagnose endogenous estrogen deficiency and to prevent pregnancy.

Pharmacokinetics

They are metabolized primarily in the liver and excreted by the kidneys.

Drug interactions

The following effects may occur when progestin is given with the drugs listed below:

Drug	Possible effect and management
aminoglutethimide	Concurrent use with oral and parenteral medroxyprogesterone has resulted in a decrease in serum levels of medroxyprogesterone. Monitor patients closely.
Liver enzyme-inducing drugs, such as carbamazepine (Tegretol), phenobarbital, phenytoin (Dilantin), rifabutin (Mycobutin), or rifampin (Rifadin)	Concurrent use may decrease the effectiveness of some progestins including levonorgestrel. Monitor patients closely.

Side effects and adverse reactions

These include weight gain, stomach pain and cramps, swelling of face and lower extremities, headache, mood alterations, anxiety, increased weakness, nervousness, ovarian enlargement or cyst formation, nausea, melasma, hot flashes, amenorrhea, breakthrough bleeding, hyperglycemia, menorrhagia, galactorrhea, rash, acne, insomnia, and breast pain.

Warnings

Use with caution in patients with asthma, cardiac insufficiency, epilepsy, hypertension, migraine, kidney or liver function impairment, central nervous system (CNS) disorders, diabetes mellitus, hyperlipidemia, pregnancy, thrombophlebitis and uterine, genital, or urinary tract bleeding (undiagnosed).

Contraindications

Avoid use in persons with progestin hypersensitivity, breast cancer, liver disorders, and thromboembolic disease.

Dosage and administration

Because dosage and method of administration for progestins can vary according to indications and current standards of practice, the student is referred to a current package insert or USP DI for the most recent recommendations. The following are examples of selected progestins and dosing regimens.

hydroxyprogesterone [hye drox ee proe jess′ ter one] (Hylutin and others)

For amenorrhea or dysfunctional bleeding of the uterus, administer 375 mg IM.

megestrol [me jess′ trole] (Megace)

For breast cancer, the dose is 40 mg PO four times daily or 160 mg as a single dose. To treat endometrial cancer, the dose is 40 to 320 mg daily in divided doses. Allow 2 months of therapy with megestrol before evaluating its effectiveness.

norethindrone [nor eth in′ drone′] (Micronor, Norlutate)

The contraceptive dose is 0.35 mg/day. For amenorrhea or dysfunctional uterine bleeding the dose is 2.5 to 10 mg PO from day 5 through day 25 of the menstrual cycle. For endometriosis, the dose is 5 mg initially, increased by 2.5 mg daily at 2-week intervals until 15 mg/day is reached. This dose is continued for 6 to 9 months.

progesterone [proe jess′ ter one] (Gesterol and others)

When used to treat amenorrhea caused by female hormone imbalance, the dose is 5 to 10 mg IM daily for 6 to 10 days. Bleeding will usually occur within 2 to 3 days after the last injection; normal menstrual cycles may then follow. Discontinue injections if menstrual bleeding occurs during the series of injections.

ORAL CONTRACEPTIVES

The most effective form of birth control presently available is **oral contraception.** Millions of women have used oral contraceptives, and through experience an enormous amount of information about effectiveness, estrogen-progestin combination, and relationship of risk factors to major side effects and mortality has been collected. For example, the newer, low-dose oral contraceptives have (1) a lower risk for adverse cardiovascular effects, (2) an increased risk for a myocardial infarction in smokers and women older than 35 years of age, (3) a lower risk for stroke or thromboembolic disease than with the older oral contraceptives although there is still a higher risk than for nonusers, (4) a decreased rate of ectopic pregnancies, (5) a decreased risk for ovarian cysts, epithelial ovarian cancer, and endometrial cancer, and (6) an increased risk for cervical cancer, liver cancer, and possibly an earlier onset of breast cancer after long-term use (Kenyon, 1995).

For safe oral contraceptive therapy, the prescriber should perform a thorough history and physical examination, including a complete drug history. Patient teaching and monitoring are also necessary.

estrogens and progestins (oral contraceptives) (various manufacturers)

The combination oral contraceptives inhibit ovulation by increasing serum levels of estrogens and progestins, which in turn inhibits secretion of FSH and LH from the pituitary.

In addition, changes in the endometrium impair ova implantation and an increase in cervical mucus impedes the passage of sperm.

Indications

Estrogens and progestins are indicated for the prevention of pregnancy and for treatment of hypermenorrhea.

Pharmacokinetics

The oral contraceptives are protein bound, metabolized mainly in the liver, and excreted primarily by the kidneys.

Drug interactions

The following effects may occur when an estrogen and progestin combination is given with drugs listed below:

Drug	Possible effect and management
Corticosteroids (glucocorticoid)	Concurrent use with estrogens may decrease glucocorticoid metabolism and decrease protein binding and also excretion of metabolites, which may result in an increased duration of action and glucocorticoid effects. Monitor closely as lower dosages of the glucocorticoid may be necessary.
cyclosporine (Sandimmune)	Concurrent use may result in an increased serum level of cyclosporine, which may increase its effects and potential for toxicity. Monitor closely as a lower dose of cyclosporine may be necessary.
Liver enzyme-inducing medications	See comments on progestins above.
Hepatotoxic drugs, especially troleandomycin	Concurrent use may increase the potential for hepatotoxicity. Monitor hepatic function closely.
ritonavir (Norvir)	Combined use may decrease the estrogen serum level by up to 40%. An increase in estrogen dosage or an alternate birth control method may need to be used.
Smoking (tobacco)	See comments on estrogens above.
theophylline	Concurrent use may increase both theophylline and ethinyl estradiol serum levels. Monitor closely as a dosage adjustment (lower) of theophylline may be necessary.
troglitazone (Rezulin)	Combined use may reduce serum levels of ethinyl estradiol and norethindrone by 40%, which can make the oral contraceptive ineffective. An alternate method of contraception may be necessary.

Side effects and adverse reactions

Hormone-related side effects are caused by an excess or a deficiency in estrogen or progestin or by an androgen excess. Androgen effects are more common with norgestrel and levonorgestrel than with the other progestins. Reporting side effects to the prescriber is useful because a more appropriate oral contraceptive for the individual may be chosen.

Excesses and deficiencies of estrogen and progestins elicit a variety of symptoms. Estrogen excess side effects include nausea, dizziness, abdominal bloating, leg pain, chloasma, hypertension, cyclic weight gain, hypertension, breast tenderness, and an increase in breast size. A deficiency in estrogen may produce an increase in anxiety, hot flashes, midcycle spotting, a decrease in menstrual flow, and a possible decrease in libido. An excess in progestins may result in alopecia, oily skin (acne) and scalp, increased fatigue, increased appetite and weight gain that is noncyclic, a decrease in the length of menstrual flow, breast tenderness, and increased breast size. A progestin deficiency may manifest itself as dysmenorrhea, heavy menstrual flow, weight loss, and a delayed onset of menses. An androgen excess may result in hirsutism, oily skin or skin rash, acne, pruritus, increased appetite and weight gain (noncyclic), and cholestatic jaundice.

Warnings

Use with caution in patients with a strong family history of breast cancer, benign breast disease, diabetes mellitus, epilepsy, gallbladder disease, hypertension, depression, migraine, obstructive jaundice, and chorea gravidarum, and in patients who have recently had major surgery or an extended period of immobilization.

Contraindications

Avoid use in persons with breast or endometrium cancer or any suspected estrogen-dependent tumor, coronary artery disease, cerebrovascular disease, cardiac insufficiency, liver disorders, tumors, or impairment, thrombophlebitis, thrombosis, and abnormal uterine bleeding (undiagnosed).

Dosage and administration

1. Although the use of exogenous estrogenic substances alone will inhibit ovulation, undesirable bleeding frequently occurs during the latter phase of the cycle. If estrogen levels are increased to prevent this, severe nausea and breast tenderness may occur. This is why estrogens are combined with progestins in oral contraceptives.
2. Because naturally occurring progesterone is inactivated or extremely weak in its effect when taken orally and must be given by injection to be effective, progestins (steroidal compounds related to progesterone) were developed. The majority of the oral contraceptives contain a synthetic progestin, usually norethynodrel, norethindrone, or norgestrel.
3. Norethynodrel is a basic progestin, norethindrone is a more androgenic progestin, and norgestrel is a synthetic progestogen similar to norethindrone. Norethindrone is

TABLE 44-1 Selected Oral Contraceptives

Brand Name	Estrogen (μg)	Progestin (mg)
Monophasic*		
Brevicon (21, 28†)	ethinyl estradiol 35	norethindrone 0.5
Ovcon-35 (21, 28†)	ethinyl estradiol 35	norethindrone 0.4
Demulen (21, 28†)	ethinyl estradiol 35	ethynodiol diacetate 1
Lo/Ovral (21, 28†)	ethinyl estradiol 30	norgestrel 0.3
Biphasic		
Ortho-Novum 10/11	Phase 1, ethinyl estradiol 35 (10 tabs)	norethindrone 0.5
	Phase 2, ethinyl estradiol 35	norethindrone 1
Triphasic		
Ortho-Novum 7/7/7	Phase 1, ethinyl estradiol 35	norethindrone 0.5
	Phase 2, ethinyl estradiol 35	norethindrone 0.75
	Phase 3, ethinyl estradiol 35	norethindrone 1
Triphasil	Phase 1, ethinyl estradiol 30	levonorgestrel 0.05
	Phase 2, ethinyl estradiol 40	levonorgestrel 0.075
	Phase 3, ethinyl estradiol 30	levonorgestrel 0.125

*Low-dose combination oral contraceptives.
†28s have 7 placebo tablets.

sometimes recommended for patients having excess side effects from estrogen, such as greater weight gain and amenorrhea. Norethynodrel is good for patients with oily skin, acne, hirsutism, and breakthrough bleeding.

4. Several methods of oral contraception are available: combination estrogen and progestin, low-dosage progestogens (minipill), and phasic (bi- and tri-) oral contraceptives with varying amounts of progestin (and sometimes estrogen) administered in two or three phases. The purpose of the phasic dosing was a belief that it might be less apt to interfere with women's normal metabolism. Clinically though, this has not been substantiated. Table 44-1 lists the composition, doses, and brand names of oral contraceptives used in these three methods.
5. Combination estrogen and progestin contraceptives are divided into three types:
   - **Monophasic oral contraception** is a fixed ratio of estrogen and progestin that is taken for 21 days of the normal menstrual cycle.
   - **Biphasic oral contraception** supplies two different amounts of progestin during the first and second phases of the menstrual cycle, that is, low levels of progestin in the follicular phase (first 7 to 10 days), which are increased during the next 11 to 14 days of the luteal phase of the menstrual cycle. The 28-day biphasic cycle has placebo tablets of a third color so that the proper sequence is clearly marked to reduce any possibility of confusion.
   - **Triphasic oral contraception** most closely simulates the normal estrogen and progesterone levels during the menstrual cycle. The dose of estrogen is kept at a low and constant level during the 21-day dosing period while the progestin is progressively increased (three times) to mimic the natural release of hormones in the female. Because the lowest dosages of hormones possible are used in this type of formulation, the incidence and severity of adverse reactions reported are considerably lower than with the monophasic or biphasic formulations.
6. Low-dosage progestogens (minipill) oral contraceptives do not contain estrogen. They are generally prescribed for 28 days of the menstrual cycle, are usually less effective than the combination products, and have a higher incidence of spotting and breakthrough bleeding. An advantage is that they generally do not cause the more serious adverse reactions associated with estrogen therapy.
7. Long-acting progestin-only contraceptives include levonorgestrel implants (Norplant), intrauterine progesterone (Progestasert), and medroxyprogesterone injection (Depo-Provera). Side effects and adverse reactions include vaginal bleeding, muscle pain, stomach distress, vaginitis, melasma, breast discharge, and weight gain. Rarely reported is thrombus formation or thromboembolism.

The levonorgestrel system is a set of six Silastic capsules that contain 36 mg each of levonorgestrel; it is implanted under the skin of the medial aspect of the upper arm (Fig. 44-1). The progestin is released at a constant rate for approximately 5 years. It is then removed and a new set is inserted if continuing contraceptive action is desired. Fertility will return after removal of the implants.

The intrauterine progesterone system is a unit containing 38 mg of progesterone that is inserted in the uterine cavity. It is indicated for women in a stable, monogamous relationship that have had at least one child and do not have any history of pelvic inflammatory disease. This system releases an average of 65 μg/day of progesterone for 1 year.

Medroxyprogesterone IM is administered to women every 3 months to inhibit gonadotropin secretion resulting in contraception.

Table 44-2 lists recommendations for selection of an oral contraceptive.

New Combination Oral Contraceptive

Estrostep is a graduated estrophasic dosage form of an oral contraceptive. It contains norethindrone acetate and ethinyl estradiol, 20 μg of estrogen/1 mg progestin for the first 5 days and then 30 μg/1 mg for days 6 through 12 and 35 μg/1 mg for days 13 through 21 of the cycle. A second formulation is a 28-day regimen that contains an additional 7 days of ferrous fumarate, taken on days 22 through 28. The

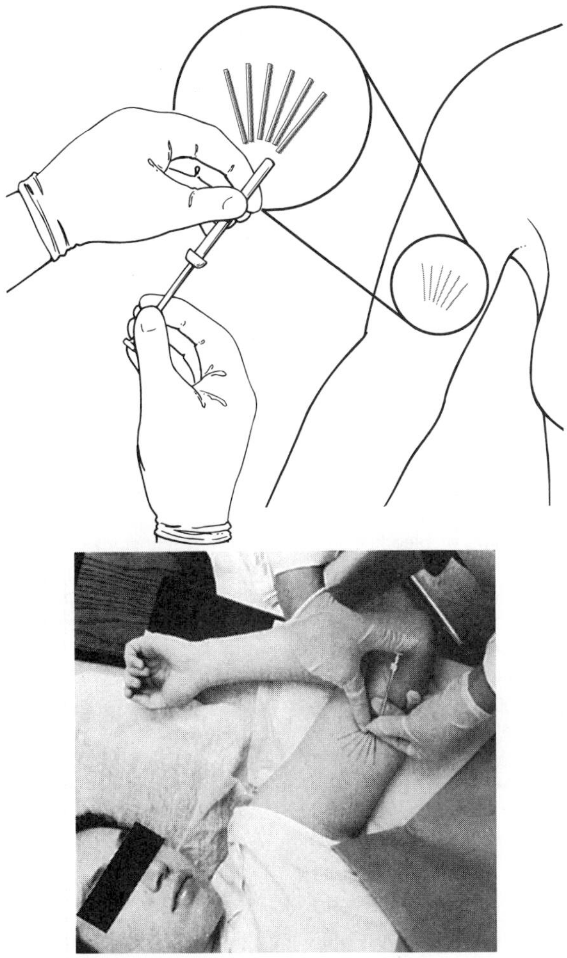

FIGURE 44-1
Norplant is another form of contraceptive therapy. Porous capsules containing progestin are placed just under the skin on the inside of the upper arm. *(From Haas, Haas, 1993.)*

manufacturer reports that clinical studies found this product was more effective (>99%) than other combination oral contraceptives (FDA News and Product Notes, 1997).

OVULATORY STIMULANTS AND DRUGS USED FOR INFERTILITY

Anovulation, the absence of ovulation, is physiologic in women who are pregnant, breastfeeding, or postmenopausal. It becomes a suspected pathologic condition in individuals with abnormal bleeding or infertility. The incidence of anovulation is unknown and cannot be ascertained, but diagnostic tests may determine its presence. Clomiphene and urofollitropin are ovulation stimulants used to treat infertility in the female.

clomiphene citrate [kloe′ mi feen] (Clomid, Serophene)

Clomiphene has antiestrogenic effects with some estrogen effects. Although its exact mechanism of action is unknown, it has been postulated that its competition with estrogen for receptor sites in the hypothalamus causes an increased secretion of FSH and LH. The result is ovarian stimulation, maturation of the ovarian follicle, and development of the corpus luteum.

Indications

Clomiphene is indicated to treat female infertility.

Pharmacokinetics

It is well absorbed orally and recirculated in the enterohepatic system, which may account for its prolonged duration of action in the body. It has a plasma half-life of 5 to 7 days with ovulation usually occurring between 4 to 10 days after the first day of treatment. Clomiphene is metabolized in the liver and excreted in the feces and bile.

Drug interactions

It has no known significant drug interactions.

Side effects and adverse reactions

These include hot flashes, abdominal pain or gas, visual disturbances, headache, nausea, vomiting, depression, anxiety, hot flashes, gynecomastia in males, breast discomfort in females, spotting, insomnia, weakness, ovarian enlargement or cyst formation, enlarged uterine fibroid tumors, hepatotoxicity, and photophobia.

Contraindications

Avoid use in persons with clomiphene hypersensitivity, liver function impairment, depression, ovarian cyst or enlargement that is not associated with polycystic ovary syndrome, thrombophlebitis, abnormal vaginal bleeding (undiagnosed), endometriosis, fibroid tumors in the uterus, and polycystic ovary syndrome.

Dosage and administration

The adult dose for female infertility is 50 mg PO daily for 5 days, starting on the fifth day of the menstrual period if bleeding occurs or at any time in women who have no recent uterine bleeding. This cycle is repeated until conception occurs, up to three or four cycles. If ovulation does not occur, the dose is increased to 75 to 100 mg/day for 5 days, which may be repeated if necessary.

urofollitropin [yur oh foe li′ troe pin] (Metrodin)

Urofollitropin, obtained from the urine of postmenopausal women, contains FSH. Human chorionic gonadotropin (action very similar to LH) is administered after urofollitropin to simulate natural ovulation. Urofollitropin is used to treat female infertility.

Side effects and adverse reactions

These include ovarian cysts or ovarian enlargement and pain and redness that may occur at the injection site. Other effects include severe stomach pain, bloating, a decrease in urination, severe nausea, vomiting or diarrhea, weight gain, swelling of the lower extremities, breathing difficulties, se-

TABLE 44-2 Recommendations for Selection of an Oral Contraceptive (OC)

Conditions	Contraceptive Management
Age	
Sexually active teenagers to 35 years of age	Low estrogen (30-35 μg)/low progestin Discourage smoking
Heavy smokers* and women >35 years of age and nonsmokers >40 years of age	Increased risk of serious cardiovascular side effects Use alternative methods of contraception
Concurrent disease states	
Cancer (breast, uterus, cervix, liver)	Oral contraceptives contraindicated
Cerebrovascular disease, coronary artery disease, and thromboembolic disorders	Oral contraceptives contraindicated
Liver impairment; smokers >35 years of age; history of CVA, uncontrolled hypertension, and migraine	Progestin only minipill
Management Side Effects	
Acne, oily skin, hirsutism, sebaceous cysts, weight gain	Trial with OCs with low progestin dose
Breakthrough bleeding	Early to mid-cycle bleeding or bleeding that never completely stops after menses is usually due to estrogen deficiency, while late breakthrough bleeding is due to progestin deficiency; prescribers often continue with same OC for 3 to 4 months because intermenstrual bleeding usually decreases with continued use; if bleeding continues, estrogen and/or progestin dosage may be adjusted to minimize effects
Withdrawal bleeding absent	First rule out pregnancy; if not pregnant, then an OC with a low progestin dose may be prescribed; some prescribers use ethinyl estradiol 20 μg for 3 months in addition to the OC (Ruggiero, 1995)

Data from Olin, 1998; Ruggiero, 1995; *USP DI*, 1998.
*>15 cigarettes/day.

vere pelvic pain as a result of the syndrome of severe ovarian hyperstimulation, skin rash, elevated temperature, and chills.

Contraindications

Avoid use in persons with urofollitropin or other gonadotropin hypersensitivity, abnormal vaginal bleeding (undiagnosed), and ovarian enlargement or cyst that is not caused by polycystic ovary syndrome.

Dosage and administration

The usual adult dose is 75 units daily for 1 week or more, followed by 5000 to 10,000 units of human chorionic gonadotropin 1 day after the last dose of urofollitropin.

SUMMARY

Drugs used for diagnostic purposes, to treat disorders, or to alter the normal functioning of the female reproductive system include many substances, such as gonadotropin-releasing hormone, nonpituitary chorionic gonadotropin, menotropins, female sex hormones, oral contraceptives, ovulatory stimulants, and drugs used for infertility. Gonadotropin-releasing hormone, or gonadorelin, is used for the diagnosis of hypogonadism in both males and females and, investigationally, for the treatment of primary hypothalamic amenorrhea. The gonadotropin-releasing hormone agonist, nafarelin, is used in the management of endometriosis. A deficiency in luteinizing hormone is the indication for chorionic gonadotropin. Menotropins are used in the treatment of both male and female infertility.

Estrogens, progesterone, and progestins are the more commonly used drugs in this group. Estrogen is used for hormonal replacement therapy, treatment of breast and prostatic carcinomas, and prevention of osteoporosis in postmenopausal women. Progesterone and progestins are indicated for hormonal replacement, the treatment of endometriosis and specific carcinomas, and the prevention of pregnancy.

Oral contraception with combinations of estrogen and progestin is the most effective form of birth control currently available. Because these drugs are primarily for self-administration, the emphasis for the healthcare professional is on patient education for accurate and safe administration and for early recognition of adverse reactions, particularly thromboembolism. Clomiphene and urofollitropin, on the other hand, are indicated for the treatment of infertility.

Because all of these drugs affect sexual identity, the healthcare professional must be sensitive to the patient's needs as a sexual being and alert to cues that reflect problems such as a disturbance of self-concept.

REVIEW QUESTIONS

1. Discuss the indications, advantages, disadvantages, and precautions with estrogen use during menopause.

2. Name the two naturally occurring endogenous estrogens, and discuss the typical approach for dosage and administration of estrogen products.
3. Name four progestins and their primary indications.
4. Discuss why estrogen is combined with progestin in oral contraceptives. Describe the three types of combination estrogen and progestin contraceptives.

REFERENCES

Belchetz PE: Hormonal treatment of postmenopausal women, *N Engl J Med* 330(15):1062-1071, 1994.

Haas K, Haas A: *Understanding sexuality,* ed 3, New York, 1993, McGraw-Hill.

Kenyon J, editor: Assessment of long-term risks and benefits of combined oral contraceptives, *Drugs Ther Perspect* 6(10):9-11, 1995.

Mosca L et al: Cardiovascular disease in women: a statement for healthcare professionals from the American Heart Association, http://www.americanheart.org/Scientific/statements/1997/109701.html (June 30, 1998).

Olin BR: *Facts and comparisons.* Philadelphia, 1998, JB Lippincott.

Pharmacy Practice News: Hormone replacement scores in landmark trial, *Pharm Pract News* 22(4):43, 1995.

Ruggiero R: Contraception. In Young LY, Koda-Kimble MA, editors: *Applied therapeutics: the clinical use of drugs,* ed 6, Vancouver, Wash, 1995, Applied Therapeutics, Inc.

United States Pharmacopeial Convention: *USP DI: drug information for the health care professional,* ed 18, Rockville, Md, 1998, The Convention.

Williams CL, Stancel GM: Estrogens and progestins. In Hardman JG, Limbird LE, editors: *Goodman & Gilman's the pharmacological basis of therapeutics,* ed 9, New York, 1996, McGraw-Hill.

ADDITIONAL REFERENCES

American College of Physicians: Guidelines for counseling postmenopausal women about preventive hormone therapy, *Ann Intern Med* 117(12):1038-1041, 1992.

American Hospital Formulary Service: *AHFS drug information '98,* Bethesda, Md, 1998, American Society of Hospital Pharmacists.

Anderson KN et al, editors: *Mosby's medical, nursing, and allied health dictionary,* ed 5, St Louis, 1998, Mosby.

FDA News and Product Notes: New formulations/combinations, *Formulary* 32(1):23, 1997.

Gordon L, editor: Cardiac benefits of ERT confirmed, *Med Trib Fam Physician* 36(1):17, 1995.

Henderson BE et al: Postmenopausal estrogen and prevention bias, *Arch Intern Med* 155:455-456, 1991.

Henrich JB: The postmenopausal estrogen/breast cancer controversy, *JAMA* 268(14):1900-1902, 1992.

Kritz-Silverstein D, Barrett-Connor E: Bone mineral density in postmenopausal women as determined by prior oral contraceptive use, *Am J Public Health* 83(1):100-102, 1993.

Melmon KL et al: *Melmon and Morelli's clinical pharmacology,* ed 3, New York, 1992, McGraw-Hill.

Mosby: *Mosby's GenRx,* St Louis, 1998, Mosby.

Sobel NR: Progestins in preventive hormone therapy, including pharmacology of the new progestins, desogestrel, norgestimate, and gestodene: are there advantages? *Obstet Gynecol Clin North Am* 21(2):299-319, 1994.

CHAPTER 45

Drugs for Labor and Delivery

KEY DRUGS

oxytocin, (p. 599)
ritodrine, (p. 601)

KEY TERMS

oxytocics, (p. 599)
tocolytics, (p. 599)

CHAPTER FOCUS

The drugs discussed in this chapter are limited to those that induce labor (oxytocics), inhibit premature labor (tocolytics), and suppress lactation. These are the typical medications used to treat labor and delivery in women.

OBJECTIVES

After reading and studying this chapter, the student should be able to do the following:

1. *Define and describe the key terms and key drugs.*
2. *Describe the effect of labor and delivery on drug pharmacokinetics.*
3. *Discuss oxytocic effects on the uterus.*
4. *Explain the source, mechanism of action, and three primary indications for the use of oxytocin.*
5. *Note the indications, side effects and adverse reactions, warnings, and contraindications of ergonovine and methylergonovine.*
6. *Discuss the mechanism of action and indications for ritodrine.*

As many drugs are available for use during labor and delivery, it is important to consider the benefit versus risk to the fetus. The pharmacokinetics of drugs may be altered during labor and delivery, for example, during labor, gastric emptying is delayed and vomiting may result, which would alter drug absorption. Vomiting may also be exacerbated by the use of opioid analgesics. Because oral drug absorption is unpredictable at this time, parenteral routes should be used. Drug metabolism and excretion may be altered and prolonged during labor, and although clinical data are currently sparse, the potential for inducing adverse or undesirable effects is always a concern. If a drug such as an opioid analgesic or sedative may be potentially harmful to the fetus, then the smallest possible dose should be used if alternate methods are not available.

Complications in pregnancy may also dictate the use of additional medications, such as those to treat diabetes, hypertension, preeclampsia, eclampsia, and systemic infections. These medications and their proper use are discussed in the appropriate pharmacologic sections of this textbook. For example, magnesium sulfate for toxemia of pregnancy is reviewed in Chapter 11. Discussion in this chapter is limited to the drugs used to induce labor (**oxytocics**), inhibit premature labor (**tocolytics**), and suppress lactation.

DRUGS AFFECTING THE UTERUS

The uterus is a highly muscular organ that exhibits a number of characteristic properties and activities. The smooth muscle fibers extend longitudinally, circularly, and obliquely in the organ. The uterus has a rich blood supply; however, when the uterine muscle contracts, blood flow is diminished. Profound changes occur in the uterus during pregnancy: it increases in weight from about 50 g to approximately 1000 g, its capacity increases 10-fold in length, and new muscle fibers may be formed. These changes are accompanied by changes in response to drugs.

Drugs that act on the uterus include oxytocics, those that increase uterine contractility, and tocolytics, those that decrease it.

Oxytocics

Agents that stimulate contraction of the smooth muscle of the uterus, resulting in contractions and spontaneous labor, are oxytocics. The most commonly used oxytocics are alkaloids of synthetic oxytocin and ergot, although many other drugs may have some effect on uterine contractility.

oxytocin [ox i toe′ sin] (Pitocin, Syntocinon) 🔑

Oxytocin is one of two hormones secreted by the posterior pituitary; the other hormone is vasopressin, or antidiuretic hormone (ADH). Oxytocin means "rapid birth," a term derived from its ability to contract the pregnant uterus. It also facilitates milk ejection during lactation.

The nonpregnant uterus is relatively insensitive to oxytocin, but during pregnancy uterine sensitivity to oxytocin gradually increases, with the uterus being most sensitive at term. Oxytocin secretion may precede and possibly trigger delivery of the fetus. Large amounts of oxytocin have been detected in the blood during the expulsive phase of delivery. A positive feedback mechanism may be operant; more forceful contractions of uterine muscle and greater stretching of the cervix and vagina result in more oxytocin release. Oxytocin acts directly on the myometrium, having a stronger effect on the fundus than on the cervix.

Oxytocin also transiently impedes uterine blood flow and stimulates the mammary gland to increase milk excretion from the breast, although it does not increase the production of milk.

Indications

This product is indicated for induction of labor, control of postpartum and postabortion hemorrhage, and stimulation of lactation.

Pharmacokinetics

This product is available parenterally and in a rapidly absorbed nasal dosage form (Syntocinon). Because the effect of the intranasal product may be erratic, it is primarily used before nursing or pumping of the breasts.

Oxytocin has a half-life of 1 to 6 minutes and an onset of action as follows: nasal, within a few minutes; IM, within 3 to 5 minutes; and IV, immediate, although uterine contractions increase gradually over 15 to 60 minutes before they stabilize. Duration of action is as follows: nasal, 20 minutes; IM, 30 to 60 minutes; and IV, within an hour after the infusion is stopped. Oxytocin is metabolized and excreted via the kidneys.

Drug interactions

When used concurrently with sodium chloride or urea for intraamniotic abortion or with other oxytocics, uterine rupture or severe cervical laceration may occur. Whenever such combinations are used, the patient should be very closely monitored

Side effects and adverse reactions

These include nausea, vomiting, tachycardia, and irregular heart rate with the parenteral drug. Oxytocin may occasionally cause fetal bradycardia, dysrhyhmias, neonatal jaundice, postpartum excessive bleeding, and, rarely, hematoma in the pelvic area. Prolonged therapy may result in water intoxication and possibly maternal death because of its slight antidiuretic effects. Monitor patients closely during prolonged use as hypertension or subarachnoid hemorrhage may occur.

Warnings

Use with caution in patients with hypertension and cardiac or kidney disease.

PREGNANCY SAFETY

Category	Drug
B	ritodrine
X	oxytocin

Ergot products are contraindicated during pregnancy.

Contraindications

Avoid use in persons with oxytocin hypersensitivity, hypertonic uterus, uterine inertia, and any other contraindications to a vaginal delivery.

Dosage and administration

The dose to induce labor is 0.5 to 2 mU/min by IV infusion, increased every 15 to 60 minutes by 1 to 2 mU/min until a contraction pattern is established that simulates normal labor (up to a maximum of 20 mU/min).

For control of postpartum uterine bleeding, the dose is 10 units at a rate of 20 to 40 mU infused intravenously after birth of the infant. The dose for the nasal solution is 1 spray in one or both nostrils 2 or 3 minutes before nursing or pumping of breasts.

See the box for Food and Drug Administration (FDA) pregnancy safety classifications.

ergonovine [er goe noe′ veen] (Ergotrate)

Ergonovine increases the force and frequency of uterine contractions by direct stimulation of the smooth muscle of the uterine wall. It is indicated to prevent and treat postpartum hemorrhage.

Pharmacokinetics

Administered orally or parenterally, ergonovine has an onset of action orally within 6 to 15 minutes, IM within 2 to 3 minutes, and IV within 1 minute. The duration of uterine contraction PO and IM is approximately 3 hours and IV about 45 minutes, but rhythmic contractions can persist for up to 3 hours. The drug is metabolized in the liver and excreted via the kidneys.

Drug interactions

Ergonovine has no significant drug interactions.

Side effects and adverse reactions

These include nausea, vomiting, diarrhea, dizziness, tinnitus, increased sweating, confusion, hypertension, chest pain and, rarely, respiratory difficulties, pruritus, pain in arms, legs or lower back, cold hands or feet, and leg weakness. A dose-related effect is abdominal cramping.

Warnings

Use with caution in patients with hypocalcemia.

Contraindications

Avoid use in persons with ergonovine or other ergot alkaloid hypersensitivity, unstable angina, a recent myocardial infarction, a history of cerebrovascular accident, transient ischemic attack, or hypertension, cardiac or coronary artery disease, eclampsia or preeclampsia, severe Raynaud's disease, sepsis, and liver or kidney function impairment.

Dosage and administration

Orally the dosage for ergonovine maleate tablets is 0.2 to 0.4 mg two to four times a day (on a schedule of every 6 to 12 hours). The usual treatment course is 48 hours. Parenterally, 0.2 mg is administered intramuscularly or intravenously and repeated in 2 to 4 hours if necessary for up to five doses. The intravenous route is usually only recommended in emergencies or in patients with excessive uterine bleeding.

methylergonovine [meth ill er goe noe′ veen] (Methergine)

The mechanism of action is direct stimulation of the smooth muscle of the uterine wall, which results in hemostasis.

Indications

Methylergonovine is indicated to prevent and treat postpartum hemorrhage.

Pharmacokinetics

It may be administered orally or parenterally, with a postpartum uterine contraction effect noted within 5 to 10 minutes (PO), 2 to 5 minutes (IM), or immediately (IV). The duration of action orally and intramuscularly is approximately 3 hours, while with intravenous administration the effect lasts about 45 minutes. The drug is metabolized in the liver and excreted by the kidneys.

Drug interactions

It has no reported significant drug interactions.

Side effects and adverse reactions, warnings, and contraindications

See ergonovine.

Dosage and administration

The oral dose is 200 to 400 μg orally two to four times daily (spaced every 6 to 12 hours) until uterine bleeding and atony are under control. Usually oral dosing follows the administration of an initial parenteral dose.

Premature Labor Inhibitors

Preterm labor, or labor that occurs before the 37th week of pregnancy, is a major problem in obstetrics. It occurs in approximately 10% to 15% of all pregnancies. Premature birth increases the possibility of neonatal morbidity and mortality. Ritodrine is currently the prototype for premature labor inhibitors, but terbutaline is being used investigationally (Box 45-1).

BOX 45-1 Update: Terbutaline in Premature Labor

Terbutaline, a $beta_2$-adrenergic stimulant (betamimetic) is used investigationally for the inhibition of premature labor. Studies indicate that parenterally terbutaline is as effective as ritodrine although the incidence of side effects and adverse reaction is significantly higher with terbutaline. The adverse effects with terbutaline, though, may be dose related. To prevent recurrent labor, oral terbutaline (30 mg/day) was more effective than oral ritodrine (120 mg/day) (Sagraves et al, 1995).

ritodrine [ri' toe dreen] (Yutopar)

Ritodrine, a $beta_2$-adrenergic stimulant that relaxes the uterine muscle by inhibiting uterine contractions, is indicated to prevent and treat premature labor (uncomplicated) in pregnancies of 20 or more weeks gestation.

Pharmacokinetics

It is available orally and parenterally. After oral administration the drug has an onset of action within ½ to 1 hour and intravenously within 5 minutes. The time to peak serum concentration by both routes is within 1 hour. Its half-life orally is biphasic: 1.3 and 12 hours (in male testing). Its half-life intravenously has three phases: 6 to 9 minutes, 1.7 to 2.6 hours, and 15 to 17 hours in nonpregnant females. The drug is metabolized in the liver and excreted by the kidneys.

Drug interactions

The following effects may occur when ritodrine is given with the drugs listed below:

Drug	Possible effect and management
Beta-adrenergic blocking agents (labetalol, nadolol, propranolol, and others)	Usage is not recommended because the two drugs are antagonistic toward each other. Drugs with greater $beta_1$ selectivity may be less antagonistic.
Corticosteroids, long-acting (betamethasone, dexamethasone, and paramethasone)	Concurrent drug use has resulted in pulmonary edema and death in pregnant women. Avoid or a potentially serious drug interaction may occur. If concurrent drug administration is absolutely necessary, monitor closely and discontinue both drugs at the first sign of pulmonary edema.

Color type indicates an unsafe drug combination.

Side effects and adverse reactions

With the IV dosage form these include increased maternal heart rate and increased systolic and decreased diastolic maternal blood pressure. The oral dosage forms may cause small increases in maternal heart rate but do not affect maternal blood pressure or fetal heart rate. With both dosage forms, trembling or tremors, anxiety, or restlessness may occur. With the IV form, nausea, vomiting, headaches, tachycardia, irregular heart rate are reported, and, rarely, chest pain and respiratory difficulties.

Warnings

Use with caution in patients with hypertension and migraine headaches.

Contraindications

Avoid use in persons with ritodrine or sulfite hypersensitivity, cardiac disease, uncontrolled hyperthyroidism or hypertension, pulmonary hypertension, hypovolemia, pheochromocytoma, chorioamnionitis, intrauterine fetal death, eclampsia, maternal complications (e.g., abruptio placentae and hemorrhage), and diabetes mellitus.

Dosage and administration

The adult oral dose is 10 mg initially ½ hour before the intravenous infusion is stopped and then 10 mg every 2 hours for 24 hours. The maintenance dose is 10 to 20 mg orally every 4 to 6 hours until birth or as directed by the prescriber. The maximum recommended daily dosage is 120 mg.

The adult dose is 50 to 100 μg/min intravenously increased every 10 minutes if necessary by increments of 50 μg to an effective dosage. The maintenance dose is 150 to 350 μg/min intravenously, which is continued for 12 to 24 hours after labor contractions have stopped. Oral therapy is then instituted.

LACTATION INHIBITORS

Estrogens such as chlorotrianisene (TACE) and bromocriptine (Parlodel) have been used to treat postpartum breast engorgement and to inhibit lactation, respectively. The use of estrogens for breast engorgement has declined over the years, mainly because the incidence of painful engorgement is considered low, and studies have indicated that analgesics or other supportive therapies are quite effective. The prescriber must also weigh the benefit of using estrogens for this purpose against the risk, particularly that of inducing a thromboembolism.

Bromocriptine directly inhibits the release of prolactin from the anterior pituitary gland, resulting in suppression of lactation. For further information on bromocriptine, see the drug monograph for dopamine agonists in Chapter 17.

SUMMARY

This chapter reviews the drugs that induce labor (oxytocics), inhibit premature labor (tocolytics), and suppress lactation. Any drugs given to the female at this time may have altered pharmacokinetics. Therefore before any medications are administered, the benefit versus risk to the fetus should be evaluated. If the drug is administered, the patient should be closely monitored by the healthcare professional.

The oxytocic drugs such as oxytocin, ergonovine, and methylergonovine are used to induce labor. These are drugs that affect or increase uterine contractility. Ritodrine is a medication used for preterm labor, that is, labor that occurs before the 37th week of pregnancy. It is a $beta_2$-adrenergic stimulant that relaxes uterine muscle and inhibits uterine contractions.

REVIEW QUESTIONS

1. Describe the effect of oxytocin on the pregnant and nonpregnant uterus.
2. What is the danger involved in the use of several oxytocics or an oxytocic with sodium chloride or urea for intraamniotic abortion?
3. Name and describe the most serious drug interaction with ritodrine.
4. Why has the use of lactation inhibitors declined over the years?

REFERENCES

Sagraves R, Letassy NA, Barton TL: Obstetrics. In Young LY, Koda-Kimble MA, editors: *Applied therapeutics: the clinical use of drugs,* ed 6, Vancouver, Wash, 1995, Applied Therapeutics, Inc.

ADDITIONAL REFERENCES

American Hospital Formulary Service: *AHFS drug information '98,* Bethesda, Md, 1998, American Society of Hospital Pharmacists.

Anderson KN et al, editors: *Mosby's medical, nursing, and allied health dictionary,* ed 5, St Louis, 1998, Mosby.

Faller HS: Among women: characteristics and birth outcomes, 1990, *Birth* 19(3):144-150, 1992.

Mosby: *Mosby's GenRx,* St Louis, 1998, Mosby.

United States Pharmacopeial Convention: *USP DI: drug information for the health care professional,* ed 18, Rockville, Md, 1998, The Convention.

CHAPTER 46

Drugs Affecting the Male Reproductive System

KEY DRUG

testosterone, (p. 604)

KEY TERMS

anabolic agents, (p. 604)
androgens, (p. 604)
hypogonadism, (p. 604)
testosterone, (p. 604)

CHAPTER FOCUS

Androgens, primarily testosterone, are male sex hormones used for replacement therapy (androgen deficiency), for treatment of advanced stages of breast cancer, and for anemia that is refractory to all other therapies (an unapproved Food and Drug Administration [FDA] use in United States). Benign prostatic hyperplasia is a very common disorder that occurs in aging men. The use of finasteride for this purpose is reviewed in this chapter.

OBJECTIVES

After reading and studying this chapter, the student should be able to do the following:

1. *Define and describe the key terms and key drug.*
2. *Compare the pharmacokinetics of oral, buccal, parenteral, and transdermal testosterone.*
3. *Discuss the three approved indications for testosterone therapy.*
4. *Name the side effects and adverse reactions of androgen therapy in males and females.*
5. *Discuss the mechanism of action, side effects and adverse effects, and dosage and administration of finasteride for benign prostatic hypertrophy.*

Androgens, primarily testosterone, are male sex hormones necessary for the normal development and maintenance of male sex characteristics. Testosterone, its derivatives and synthetic agents are commonly used as replacement therapy for males who lack the hormone. In individuals with **hypogonadism** or eunuchoidism (a deficiency of male hormone), the androgens produce marked changes in growth of the male sex organs, body contour, voice, and other secondary sex characteristics.

Hypertrophy of the glandular and connective tissue in the portions of the prostate that surround the urethra, benign prostatic hypertrophy (BPH), is considered a normal age-related change in men. Finasteride (Proscar) is a welcome addition to the treatment of BPH, which has been almost exclusively surgical.

TESTOSTERONE

Testosterone, a naturally occurring androgenic hormone produced primarily by the testes, regulates male development. It is available in combination with esters to prolong the medication's duration of action. For example, testosterone propionate is formulated in an oily solution that produces hormonal effects for 2 or 3 days, whereas testosterone cypionate and testosterone enanthate in oil are much longer acting. They are usually administered once every 2 to 4 weeks. Testosterone pellets are available for subcutaneous implantation. This form will also provide an extended duration of action; depending on the number of pellets used, it may extend from 2 to 6 months before replacement pellets are necessary.

In 1996, a transdermal testosterone system (Testoderm) was marketed. This is applied to scrotal skin where testosterone is highly absorbed at a rate at least five times greater than at other skin sites. A second transdermal testosterone system (Androderm) is also available and it is applied to nonscrotal skin. This system requires the application of two patches nightly (total dose of 5 mg/day), every 24 hours. Either system requires approximately 10 pm nightly application so that maximum serum concentrations are achieved in the morning, which simulates the normal circadian rhythm in healthy young males (Olin, 1998).

Oral testosterone is absorbed but is highly metabolized by the liver before it reaches systemic circulation. Administering methyltestosterone by the buccal route of administration increases its serum level and effectiveness. Fluoxymesterone is a synthetic androgen that is effective orally in tablet form.

Mechanism of action

As a natural hormone in normal males, androgens are responsible for the stimulation of spermatogenesis, the development of male sex characteristics (secondary), and, at puberty, sexual maturity. Testosterone also stimulates the synthesis and activity of ribonucleic acid (RNA), which results in increased protein production. Androgens are also potent **anabolic agents;** they stimulate the formation and maintenance of muscular and skeletal protein. They bring about retention of nitrogen (essential to the formation of protein in the body) and enhance storage of inorganic phosphorus, sulfate, sodium, and potassium. Athletes have used androgens to increase weight, musculature, and muscle strength. Weight gains may be caused by fluid retention, a side effect of androgen therapy. The potential risk of developing the major serious adverse reactions from androgens far outweighs the advantages to be gained in athletic events. Many major sporting events disqualify athletes whose use of such products is documented. Additional information on the abuse of androgens can be found in Chapter 6.

Indications

Testosterones are indicated for the following:

1. Treatment of androgen deficiency, such as testicular failure caused by cryptorchidism (failure of one or both testes to descend into the scrotum), orchitis (inflammation of the testes), orchidectomy (surgical removal of one or both testes), or pituitary-hypothalamic insufficiency.
2. Treatment of delayed male puberty when not induced by a pathologic condition.
3. Treatment of breast carcinoma: palliative or secondary treatment for inoperable metastatic breast cancer in postmenopausal women who have demonstrated a previous response to hormone therapy.
4. Treatment of anemia: stimulation of erythropoiesis, the production of erythrocytes, in certain types of anemia (refractory to other therapies primarily), although this is not an approved indication for these products in the United States.

Pharmacokinetics

The half-life of testosterone (IM) in plasma is 10 to 20 minutes, of fluoxymesterone is 9.2 hours, and of methyltestosterone is between 2.5 and 3.5 hours. The time to peak concentration for methyltestosterone, buccal tablet, is 1 hour and for the oral tablet is 2 hours. The duration of action depends on the dose and the ester formulation administered. The longest duration of action for testosterone preparations is with enanthate, then cypionate, and propionate; the base form has the shortest duration of action. Testosterone is metabolized in the liver and excreted by the kidneys.

Drug interactions

Significant drug interactions have been reported when testosterone was given concurrently with oral anticoagulants (coumarin or indanedione) or with other hepatotoxic medications. With the former, the anticoagulant effects are enhanced or increased; with the latter, the risk of inducing hepatotoxicity is increased.

Side effects and adverse reactions

In females, the most frequent adverse reactions are an increase in oily skin or acne, deepening of the voice, increased hair growth or alopecia, enlarged clitoris, and irregular menses. The deep voice or hoarseness may not be reversed, even when the medication is stopped. The adverse reactions reported in males are urinary urgency, breast swelling or tenderness (gynecomastia), and frequent or continuous erections. The less frequent side effects occurring in both sexes include abdominal pain, insomnia, diarrhea or constipation, dizziness, increased weakness, red skin or changes in skin color, redness at the site of injection, mouth soreness, frequent headaches, confusion, respiratory difficulties, depression, nausea, vomiting, pruritus, edema of the lower extremities, jaundice, an increase in bleeding episodes, and an unusual increase or decrease in libido.

Dosage and administration

The choice of dosage and length of therapy depend on the diagnosis, the patient's age and sex, and the intensity of the side effects/adverse reactions. See the box for FDA pregnancy safety categories.

Usually males with delayed puberty and hypogonadal (a decrease in androgen secretion from gonads) males, dosage regimens are started in the lower ranges and gradually increased according to the individual's needs and response. In delayed puberty, after 4 to 6 months of therapy, the androgens are discontinued for 1 to 3 months while x-ray examinations are performed to determine the drug's effect on bone growth. The hypogonadal male will receive the androgens through puberty with dosage adjustments as required. Usually lower maintenance dosages are used after puberty.

Androgen antineoplastic therapy usually requires a 3-month period to evaluate its effectiveness. Women with metastatic breast cancer should receive a shorter-acting androgen, especially during the initial therapies. It has been reported that androgens occasionally increase the extent of breast cancer.

Temporary withdrawal of the drug is required if the male experiences priapism (persistent, abnormal penis erection). This is an indication of excessive dosing of the androgen.

Dosage and administration

Sterile testosterone suspension. The usual adult dose is 25 to 50 mg IM two or three times a week. The dose for antineoplastic therapy for metastatic female breast cancer is 50 to 100 mg three times a week. The pediatric dosage for delayed puberty in males is 100 mg IM monthly for 4 to 6 months.

PREGNANCY SAFETY

Category	Drug
C	terazosin
X	androgens, finasteride

Testosterone enanthate injection. The usual adult dose is 50 to 400 mg IM every 2 to 4 weeks. For antineoplastic therapy for inoperable female breast cancer, the dose is 200 to 400 mg every 2 to 4 weeks. The pediatric dosage for delayed puberty in males is 100 mg monthly for approximately 4 to 6 months.

Methyltestosterone capsules (Metandren). The adult oral dosage for replacement therapy (hypogonadism, climacteric, or impotence) is 10 to 50 mg daily, for cryptorchidism is 10 mg three times a day; and for metastatic female breast carcinoma is 50 mg one to four times a day. The pediatric dose for delayed puberty in males is 5 to 25 mg/day for approximately 4 to 6 months.

Methyltestosterone buccal tablets (Metandren). The dose is one half the capsule dosage.

Fluoxymesterone tablets (Halotestin). The usual adult dose is 5 mg one to four times a day. For metastatic female breast carcinoma, it is 20 to 50 mg daily for 2 to 6 months. The pediatric dosage for treatment of delayed puberty in males is 2.5 to 10 mg daily for approximately 4 to 6 months.

BENIGN PROSTATIC HYPERPLASIA

BPH, the hypertrophy of the glandular and connective tissue in the portions of the prostate that surround the urethra, is considered a normal age-related change that begins around age 40 in men. By age 70, about 75% of men will develop BPH symptoms severe enough to require professional intervention (Thompson, 1995).

BPH obstructs the bladder neck and compresses the urethra, which results in urinary retention, increasing the risk of bacteriuria. If untreated, it may affect the ureters and kidneys and result in hydroureter, hydronephrosis, and renal impairment. The symptoms of BPH include hesitancy (difficulty starting the urinary stream), a decrease in the diameter and force of the stream, inability to terminate urination abruptly resulting in postvoid dribbling, and a sensation of incomplete bladder emptying resulting in frequency and nocturia.

Because the pathophysiology of BPH may also include impaired detrusor contractility, sensory abnormalities of the bladder wall, and contractility of the smooth muscle of the prostatic urethra with functionally important alpha$_1$-adrenergic receptors, pharmacologic treatment of BPH with nonselective adrenergic blockers was tried. Although prazocin (Minipress) is used investigationally for this purpose, terazocin (Hytrin) is approved for the treatment of BPH (USP DI, 1998). (See Chapter 16 for a discussion of adrenergic blockers.) Finasteride, a 5-alpha reductase inhibitor, is also available for the treatment of BPH.

finasteride [fin ass′ te ride] (Proscar)

Finasteride inhibits 5-alpha reductase, the enzyme that converts testosterone into the potent androgen 5-alpha-dihydrotestosterone (DHT), a substance responsible for prostate gland growth. Finasteride decreases serum DHT by nearly 70%, thus causing shrinkage of the enlarged prostate gland. It is the first of a new class of drugs approved by the FDA indicated for the treatment of symptomatic BPH. Gormley et al (1992) report that men treated with a daily dose of 5 mg of finasteride had a significant decrease in their urinary symptoms, an increase in their urinary flow rate, and a 19% decrease in prostate volume.

Pharmacokinetics

Finasteride is 90% protein bound to plasma proteins, with maximum plasma concentrations being reached in 1 to 2 hours after oral administration. No dosage adjustments are required for elderly patients.

Drug interactions

No significant drug interactions are reported.

Side effects and adverse reactions

These include gynecomastia, rash, stomach or back pain, diarrhea, headache, decreased libido, impotency, and a decreased amount of ejaculate.

Warnings

Avoid use in patients with liver disease and obstructive uropathy.

Contraindications

Avoid use in persons with finasteride hypersensitivity.

Dosage and administration

The drug is administered orally, 5 mg daily.

SUMMARY

This chapter reviews the androgen testosterone, the male sex hormone necessary for the normal development and maintenance of male sex characteristics. Testosterone is indicated for hormonal replacement therapy in males as well as for the treatment of breast carcinoma and anemia. The side effects and adverse reactions, such as gynecomastia in males and virilism in female patient, may be troubling to some individuals. The monitoring and support of healthcare professionals is important for such patients. In addition, finasteride, a drug indicated for the treatment of benign prostatic hypertrophy, is also reviewed.

REVIEW QUESTIONS

1. Discuss the similarities and differences between the use of the two transdermal testosterone systems (Testoderm and Androderm).
2. What are the mechanism of action, uses, and dosage and administration for testosterone?
3. Describe benign prostatic hyperplasia and the use of finasteride in treatment.

REFERENCES

Gormley GJ et al: The effect of finasteride in men with benign prostatic hyperplasia: the Finasteride Study Group, *N Engl J Med* 327(17):1185-1191, 1992.

Olin BR: *Facts and comparisons.* Philadelphia, 1998, JB Lippincott.

Thompson JF: Geriatric urological disorders. In Young LY, Koda-Kimble MA, editors: *Applied therapeutics: the clinical use of drugs,* ed 6, Vancouver, Wash, 1995, Applied Therapeutics, Inc.

ADDITIONAL REFERENCES

American Hospital Formulary Service: *AHFS drug information '98,* Bethesda, Md, 1998, American Society of Hospital Pharmacists.

Anderson KN et al, editors: *Mosby's medical, nursing, and allied health dictionary,* ed 5, St Louis, 1998, Mosby.

Hardman JG, Limbird LE, editors: *Goodman & Gilman's the pharmacological basis of therapeutics,* ed 9, New York, 1996, McGraw-Hill.

Mosby: *Mosby's GenRx,* St Louis, 1998, Mosby.

United States Pharmacopeial Convention: *USP DI: drug information for the health care professional,* ed 18, Rockville, Md, 1998, The Convention.

CHAPTER 47

Drugs Affecting Sexual Behavior

CHAPTER FOCUS

Sexual behavior and sexual function are an integral part of an individual's identity. Many medications can influence both sexuality and sexual function. Whenever possible, the healthcare professional should be aware of all medications (legal and illegal) their patients are taking so that viable information on the drug's side effects and adverse reactions can be provided.

KEY TERMS

impotence, (p. 608)
libido, (p. 608)
premenstrual syndrome (PMS), (p. 610)

OBJECTIVES

After reading and studying this chapter, the student should be able to do the following:

1. *Define and describe the key terms*
2. *Name commonly prescribed drugs, such as antihypertensives, diuretics, antihistamines, antianxiety, and psychotropic drugs, and describe their effects on sexual function.*
3. *Describe the effect of depression and antidepressants on sexual interest and activity.*
4. *Name and discuss drugs that may enhance libido or sexual gratification.*

Sexuality and sexual behavior have physiologic, psychologic, and social ramifications that reflect a higher level of complexity that a discussion of drugs that affect sexuality would imply. Many contributing factors are involved, such as self-esteem, general health, partner availability, appropriate environment, religious beliefs, society's standards, and others. Because drugs can affect sexual activities or sexual identity, healthcare professionals should be aware of patients' needs and problems in this area.

Various drugs can produce one or more side effects or adverse reactions such as decreased levels of testosterone, which is normally present in both sexes and enhances **libido** or sexual drive; increased or decreased levels of estrogen; clinical depression that may limit interest or response to sexual stimuli; or autonomic nervous system blockade, which may interfere with lubrication, erection, or ejaculation. The references at the end of this chapter and information in Chapter 43 provide a better understanding of the structure and function of the reproductive systems.

Many physiologic functions significant to sexual pleasure are controlled by the psyche and the autonomic nervous system (see also Chapter 14). This system comprises two parts—the sympathetic (adrenergic) and parasympathetic (cholinergic) systems—and its functional units are nerves, nerve plexuses, and ganglia. Although viewed as physiologic antagonists, the two systems often have synergistic effects on sexual functioning. The male and female sexual organs are composed of homologous tissues; although the shapes of the organs differ, they correspond, part for part, in structure, position, and embryologic origin. In the embryo, the genital protuberance appears identical in both sexes. The embryo is characteristically female initially and does not differentiate until fetal androgens begin to masculinize tissues (7th to 12th weeks of pregnancy). Thus it is not surprising that the mature analogous organs function similarly.

In the male, sympathetic (adrenergic) impulses produce ejaculation by causing contraction of the prostate and seminal vesicles along with effects on the bulbocavernosus and ischiocavernosus muscles. **Impotence,** or impotency, is the inability of the adult male to achieve or maintain a penile erection and decreased sexual function.

Drugs that block adrenergic impulses may affect ejaculatory function through sympathetic blockade. Parasympathetic (cholinergic) stimulation controls penile erection. This response results from congestion of the vascular sinuses in the penile corpora caused by parasympathetic nerve action in the venous channels. Drugs that interfere with parasympathetic nerve transmitters (cholinergic nerves) can cause defects in erection. In addition, ganglionic blocking agents, which may block both sympathetic and parasympathetic nerve transmission, can cause complete impotence and impaired sexual functioning.

In the female, parasympathetic (cholinergic) impulses cause arterial dilation and venoconstriction, which produce clitoral erection and vasocongestion of the vulva, transudation (oozing of a fluid through pores) of lubricating secretions from the vaginal walls, and swelling of the introitus (vaginal opening). Continued stimulation of the clitoris or the Graefenberg spot, which is located on the anterior wall of the vagina, may then produce orgasm and, for some, a miniature facsimile of ejaculation from glands that surround the female urethra.

DRUGS THAT IMPAIR LIBIDO AND SEXUAL GRATIFICATION

Antihypertensives

Central acting $alpha_2$ agonists such as methyldopa (Aldomet), clonidine (Catapres), guanabenz (Wytensin), and guanfacine (Tenex) have been associated with more frequent reports of impotency and sexual dysfunction. Difficulty in ejaculation has been reported with guanethidine (Ismelin), and reserpine (Serpasil) may induce impotency or a decreased interest in sex.

Anticholinergic drugs, especially those with ganglionic blocking activity, may also produce impotence and other untoward effects on sexual function. Guanethidine falls into this category. Other agents include mecamylamine (Inversine) and trimethaphan (Arfonad), which are used as antihypertensive agents. Since these drugs may block both sympathetic and parasympathetic innervation of the sex organs, both erectile capability and ejaculatory function may be affected during their use.

Diuretics

The thiazide diuretics may induce sexual dysfunction, and spironolactone (Aldactone) has been associated with a decrease in libido, impotency, and gynecomastia. Spironolactone has considerably more sexual dysfunction reports than the thiazides; this effect appears to be dose related.

Antihistamines

Antihistaminic drugs act as competitive inhibitors of histamine at physiologic receptor sites to prevent histamine effects. Well-known examples of such drugs include diphenhydramine (Benadryl), promethazine (Phenergan), and chlorpheniramine (Chlor-Trimeton). These drugs are consumed by millions as antiemetics, as mild sedatives, and for the control of allergy symptoms. Most antihistamines display anticholinergic effects such as dry mouth, urinary retention, and constipation. Continuous use of these drugs may interfere with sexual activity. This effect is presumably mediated by the blockade of parasympathetic nerve impulses to the sex glands and organs.

Antianxiety and Psychotropic Drugs

A wide variety of central acting agents affect sexual interest and capability both directly and indirectly. The benzodiazepines, phenothiazines, and short-acting barbiturates are often associated with sexual dysfunction.

Phenothiazines such as chlorpromazine (Thorazine), prochlorperazine (Compazine), thioridazine (Mellaril), and mesoridazine (Serentil) are commonly prescribed agents that often induce a sedative effect, which may partly account for decreased sexual interest of persons undergoing phenothiazine therapy.

In addition to their central nervous system effects, the peripheral effects of phenothiazines may contribute to inhibition of sexual function. These drugs decrease skeletal muscle tone and block cholinergic synapses at both muscarinic and nicotinic receptors. Various adrenergic impulses may be inhibited as well. Impotence, decreased libido, ejaculation disorders, and prolonged amenorrhea have been reported in individuals taking phenothiazines. Failure to ejaculate has been reported in men treated with thioridazine, although erection and orgasm do not appear to be affected. Therapy with thioridazine, which has a significantly greater peripheral alpha-adrenergic blocking effect than the other phenothiazines, results in a higher incidence of this side effect. Ejaculation problems have also been reported with the use of chlorprothixene (Taractan) and mesoridazine (Serentil).

Benzodiazepine compounds are commonly prescribed antianxiety medications. Diazepam (Valium) is used for treating anxiety and alcoholism and as a skeletal muscle relaxant. The sedative and relaxing effects of this drug may account for the decreased interest in sexual activity. There have been several reports of anorgasmia in males and females and ejaculation failure (Thompson, 1995). Alternatively, the judicious use of these tranquilizers has been considered of value in the treatment of sexual impotence and other problems involving sexual performance when excessive anxiety was a factor in decreased sexual performance.

Several other types of drugs used in the treatment of psychologic problems depress sexual activity in human beings. Haloperidol (Haldol), an antipsychotic, can adversely affect libido in men. Failure to ejaculate without concomitant alteration of erection or orgasm has been reported in individuals treated with phenoxybenzamine (Dibenzyline), an alpha-adrenergic blocking agent once used to supplement psychiatric therapy. This drug has been referred to as the male contraceptive. Interestingly enough, this product has been used successfully in males with premature ejaculation problems (Ruggiero, 1995).

Antidepressants

Depression is often associated with diminished sexual interest, drive, and activity (see Chapter 13). The drugs used to treat depression often compound these negative effects on sexual function. While antidepressants generally elevate mood and thus increase sexuality, they can cause impotence and influence sexual behavior adversely. The effect of the tricyclic antidepressants on sexuality may be related to peripheral anticholinergic effects, such as those produced by some antihypertensives. Examples of these drugs include imipramine (Tofranil) and amitriptyline (Elavil). Although monoamine oxidase (MAO) inhibitors may be used as antihypertensives and antidepressants, the impotence that can result may be caused by their tendency to block peripheral ganglionic nerve transmission.

Ethyl Alcohol

Ethyl alcohol is considered for its effects on human sexual function and behavior as a drug of individual and unique notoriety. Revered for centuries as a sexual stimulant and cure of all ills, alcohol is in fact a depressant and is recognized today to have far greater social than therapeutic value. Although a sedative, alcohol in moderate amounts may enhance sexual activity by relieving anxieties and loosening the inhibitions that often shroud sexual behavior.

Beyond a certain limit, however, neither desire nor potency will overcome the depressed physical capability that occurs under its influence. Studies on the pharmacologic action of alcohol show that the central nervous system is more affected by alcohol than is any other system of the body. Electrophysiologic studies suggest that alcohol first depresses the part of the brain responsible for integrating the various activities of the nervous system. The result is that various processes related to thought and motor activities become disrupted.

The first mental processes affected are related to sobriety and self-restraint, producing a less inhibited and less restrained approach to sexual behavior and other activities normally inhibited by previous training or experience. With continued consumption of alcohol, however, the brain becomes narcotized, reflexes become slowed, blood vessels are dilated, and the capacity for sexual function is diminished. In addition, alcohol produces a severe diuretic effect, which may also interfere with sexual function.

Typically, the male alcoholic experiences delayed ejaculation during intoxication and impotence after years of chronic alcoholism. Vascular changes, peripheral neuropathy, and lower testosterone levels because of liver damage are thought to cause the impotence. Body image changes such as testicular atrophy and gynecomastia compound the problem.

Barbiturates

Barbiturates, such as amobarbital (Amytal), pentobarbital (Nembutal), secobarbital (Seconal), and thiopental (Pentothal), are sedative-hypnotic drugs that have general depressant effects on all nervous tissues. As with alcohol, these drugs in prescribed dosage produce relaxation, hypnosis, and sleep with depression of various body functions, including sexual performance and ability. With prolonged use or overdose barbiturates can cause respiratory failure and death. Withdrawal after long-term heavy consumption of barbiturates may result in convulsions. There is no rationale for their use in altering sexual behavior in human beings.

H_2 Receptor Antagonists

H_2 receptor antagonists such as cimetidine (Tagamet) and ranitidine (Zantac) have been reported to cause antiandrogenic effects (impotency and gynecomastia) when administered in high doses for a prolonged time period.

Hormones and Derivatives

Sex hormones act on the central nervous system and other body organs to influence sexual and aggressive behavior, as well as mood and emotional outlook. Thus variations in female hormones may produce the anxiety, irritability, and depression associated with **premenstrual syndrome (PMS)**, whereas male hormones are associated with aggression and increased sexual interest. Evidence indicates that sexual drive may be influenced by sex hormone treatment.

The anabolic steroids are derived from or related to the male sex hormone testosterone. They have been misused by athletes and other postpubertal persons to promote muscle growth and endurance. But when used by normally developed, well-nourished individuals, the effects of these drugs on strength and development are questionable. Considerable evidence indicates these drugs cause virilization, hirsutism, libido changes, and clitoral enlargement in females and testicular atrophy, impotence, chronic priapism, and oligospermia in males (see Chapter 6).

Additional Medications

A number of other medications have been reported to cause sexual dysfunctions. Ketoconazole (Nizoral), an antifungal agent, may cause oligospermia and decreased libido in males (Cleary et al, 1995). Propranolol (Inderal), a beta-adrenergic blocking agent, has been associated with decreased libido and erectile dysfunction. Nifedipine (Adalat, Procardia), diltiazem (Cardizem), and verapamil (Calan, Isoptin) are calcium channel blocking agents that may cause erectile dysfunction. Opioids have also been associated with sexual dysfunction (Thompson, 1995).

DRUGS THAT ENHANCE LIBIDO AND SEXUAL GRATIFICATION

Substances to increase sexual potency or drive have been sought throughout history. Inscriptions in the ruins of ancient cultures have described the preparation of "erotic potions," and an endless number of "aphrodisiacs" have been described since then. In contemporary society many drugs and chemicals that modify mood and behavior are claimed to have aphrodisiac properties.

In reality, no known drugs specifically increase libido or sexual performance, and chemicals taken for this purpose without medical advice and especially in combination with other drugs pose the danger of adverse reactions, drug interaction, or overdose. However, many pharmacologically active agents temporarily modify both physiologic responsiveness and subjective perception to enhance the enjoyment, if not the fulfillment, of the sex act. Some of these agents are considered in this section.

cantharis [kan thar is′]

Cantharis (cantharidin, Spanish fly), a legendary sexual stimulant, is a powerful irritant and potent systemic poison. It is not an effective sexual stimulant. A powder made from dried beetles *(Cantharis vesicatoria)* found in southern Europe, cantharis can produce severe illness characterized by vomiting, diarrhea, abdominal pain, and shock. When taken internally, it causes irritation and inflammation of the genitourinary tract and dilation of the blood vessels of the penis and clitoris, sometimes producing prolonged erections (priapism) or engorgement, usually without increased sexual desire. Deaths have been reported from the promiscuous use of cantharis as an aphrodisiac. It is currently recognized that cantharis is not an effective sexual stimulant, and it is seldom used in modern medical practice.

yohimbine [yo him been′]

Another natural substance with purported aphrodisiac properties is yohimbine, an alkaloid derived from the west African tree *Corynanthe yohimbe.* Yohimbine produces a competitive alpha-adrenergic block of limited duration and antidiuresis, probably from the release of antidiuretic hormone. Although yohimbine stimulates the lower spinal nerve centers controlling erection, there is no convincing evidence that it acts as a sexual stimulant. It currently has no therapeutic uses.

opioids and psychoactive agents

The use of drugs such as morphine, heroin, cocaine, marijuana, lysergic acid diethylamide (LSD), and amphetamines as aphrodisiacs has become widespread in contemporary society. These agents can, under certain circumstances, enhance the enjoyment of the sexual experience for some. More commonly, however, sexual behavior decreases. Responsiveness varies because these agents have no particular properties that specifically increase sexual potency, but rather they tend to affect the user according to expectations. Thus the user's state of mind and the amount consumed contribute considerably to the effect achieved. Like alcohol, these drugs act on the central nervous system to weaken inhibitions, which are often the cause of problems involving sexual behavior. Taken in excess or too often, however, these drugs have the opposite effect and inhibit sexual drive and function. Because of these variations, researchers are skeptical of their value.

Marijuana (cannabis), an extract of the *Cannabis sativa* plant, is considered by many to be a sexual stimulant. However, like alcohol, its effect results indirectly from relaxation and release of inhibitions surrounding sexual activity. The active ingredient in marijuana is tetrahydrocannabinol. The pharmacologic effects resulting from smoking marijuana depend on the expectations and personality of the user, the dose, and the prevailing circumstances. Usually the effects of marijuana are time distortion and enhanced suggestibility, producing the illusion that sexual climax is somewhat prolonged. Thus the expectation that marijuana is an aphrodisiac may enhance enjoyment of the sex act. Studies on the properties of marijuana for a specific effect on sexual behavior, however, have shown that it has no such properties. On the contrary, there is evidence that marijuana smokers have a higher incidence of decreased libido and impaired potency than nonusers. In addition, chronic intensive use of marijuana depresses plasma testosterone levels in healthy males and produces gynecomastia in some users. Chromosomal breaks have also occurred.

LSD is another drug that, although considered an aphrodisiac by some, has potentially untoward effects on sexual function and behavior. Like marijuana, any alteration of sexual performance produced by LSD is principally subjective. This drug acts almost entirely on the central nervous system. Little response, if any, has been noted in other organ systems that can be attributed to a direct effect of LSD, and no biochemical or pharmacologic evidence supports the contention that LSD or similar drugs contain any sex-stimulating properties. On the other hand, the repeated use of LSD may produce serious psychologic problems, which could overall adversely affect sexual interest or activity. Uses of LSD during pregnancy may have a higher rate of malformed babies or stillbirths than nonusers.

Amphetamines such as Dexedrine have also been used to stimulate sexual function. These drugs have a powerful central stimulant action in addition to peripheral alpha and beta sympathomimetic effects. The main effects are wakefulness and alertness, mood elevation, increased motor and speech activity, and often elation and euphoria. Physical performance is usually improved, and fatigue can be prevented or reversed. The effects of amphetamines on sexual performance, however, are inconsistent.

Amphetamines, along with other psychoactive agents, do little to promote the enjoyment of sexual activity and over time may produce adverse psychologic and physical effects that reduce sexual interest and capability.

Drugs That Stimulate Sexual Behavior

Various clinically used or experimental drugs enhance sexual interest or potency as a side effect in both humans and laboratory animals.

levodopa [lee voe doe′ pah] (L-dopa)

Levodopa (L-dopa) is a natural intermediate in the biosynthesis of catecholamines in the brain and peripheral adrenergic nerve terminals. In the biologic sequence of events it is converted to dopamine, which in turn serves as a substrate of the neurotransmitter norepinephrine. Levodopa is used successfully in the treatment of Parkinson's syndrome, a disease characterized by dopamine deficiency. When levodopa is administered to an individual with this syndrome, the symptoms are ameliorated, presumably because the drug is converted to dopamine, thereby counteracting the deficiency.

Individuals treated with levodopa, especially elderly men, have been observed to have a sexual rejuvenation. This effect has led to the belief that levodopa stimulates sexual powers. Consequently, studies with younger men complaining of decreased erectile ability have shown that levodopa increases libido and incidence of penile erections. Overall, however, these effects have been short-lived and do not reflect continued satisfactory sexual function and potency. Thus levodopa is not a true aphrodisiac, but the increased sexual activity experienced by parkinsonian patients treated with levodopa may reflect improved well-being and partial recovery of normal sexual functions impaired by Parkinson's disease.

amyl nitrite [am′ il]

Amyl nitrite, a drug used in the past to treat angina pectoris, is alleged to enhance sexual activity in humans. As a vasodilator and smooth muscle stimulant, amyl nitrite has been reported to intensify the orgasmic experience for men if inhaled at the moment of orgasm. This effect is probably the result of relaxation of smooth muscles and consequent vasodilation of the genitourinary tract. No effects of amyl nitrite on libido have been reported, but loss of erection or delayed ejaculation may result. Women generally experience negative effects on orgasm when taking this drug.

vitamin E

Much has been said about the positive effects of vitamin E (alpha-tocopherol) on sexual performance and ability in human beings. Unfortunately, little scientific rationale substantiates such claims. The primary reasons for attributing a positive role in sexual performance to vitamin E come from experiments on vitamin E deficiency in laboratory animals. In such experiments the principal manifestation of this deficiency is infertility, although the reasons for this condition differ in males and females. In female rats there is no loss in ability to produce apparently healthy ova or any defect in the placenta or uterus. However, fetal death occurs shortly after the first week of embryonic life, and fetuses are reabsorbed. This situation can be prevented if vitamin E is administered any time up to the fifth or sixth day of embryonic life. In the male rat the earliest observable effect of vitamin E deficiency is immobility of spermatozoa, with subsequent degeneration of the germinal epithelium. However, secondary sex organs are not altered and sexual vigor is not diminished, although vigor may decrease if the deficiency continues.

Because of experimental results such as these, vitamin E has been conjectured to restore potency, or preserve fertility, sexual interest, and endurance in humans. No evidence supports these contentions, but since sexual performance is often influenced by mental attitude, a person who believes vitamin E may improve sexual prowess may actually find improvement. The only established therapeutic use for vitamin E is for the prevention or treatment of vitamin E deficiency, a condition that is rare in humans.

sildenafil [sil den′ afil] (Viagra)

A new product released in 1998, sildenafil (Viagra) is the first oral medication approved by the Food and Drug Administration to treat impotency. The mechanism of action is secondary to sexual stimulation, which increases the release of nitric oxide and increases the levels of cyclic guanosine monophosphate (cGMP), a smooth muscle relaxant. Sildenafil also enhances the nitric oxide effects by inhibiting phosphodiesterase 5, a substance found primarily in the penis that degrades cGMP. Therefore the increased levels of cGMP in the corpus cavernosum enhance the smooth muscle relaxation, inflow of blood, and erection. Sildenafil will have no effect in the absence of sexual stimulation (Viagra, 1998).

Since sildenafil's release and public acceptance, postmarketing information indicates a number of adverse reaction reports, and approximately 16 reports of fatality have been associated with its usage (Viagra Postmarketing Information, 1998). According to this report, the FDA still supports the safety of this drug, as concomitant medications and/or disease states may have been involved in the outcome. The manufacturer (Pfizer, 1998) sent a letter to physicians to warn them that ". . . the only contraindication for taking Viagra is the concomitant administration of an organic nitrate." The company also issued a list of organic nitrate products to remind the prescriber about the products that should not be combined with sildenafil. This contraindication is based on the combination causing severe hypotension and possibly a decrease in coronary perfusion, which may result in myocardial ischemia and infarction.

The healthcare professional should be aware that a male without a history of angina who takes sildenafil for sexual impotency and develops his first angina attack should not receive any nitrate products in the emergency room. This includes nitroglycerin and nitroprusside.

Drug interactions

Do not use with nitrite preparations as discussed previously. As the usage of this product expands, more drug interactions may be reported so the student is urged to monitor current literature closely.

Side effects and adverse reactions

These include headache, nausea, facial flushing, nasal congestion, gastric distress, back pain, flu syndrome, arthralgia, allergic reaction, and cardiovascular events (e.g., angina pectoris, tachycardia, and hypotension). At higher dosages, the drug may cause some visual changes including a blue color tinge in the field of vision for some men.

Warnings

Use with caution in patients with cardiac disease, bleeding disorders, Peyronie's disease, and conditions that predispose to priapism, such as multiple myeloma, leukemia, and sickle cell anemia.

Contraindications

Avoid use in persons with sildenafil hypersensitivity or concurrent use of organic nitrates.

Dosage and administration

The usual adult dose is 50 mg, taken about 1 hour before sexual activity.

SUMMARY

Many medications, both legal and illegal, may affect sexuality and sexual behavior. Healthcare professionals need to aware of their patients' needs and, when necessary, provide the appropriate medical intervention necessary to help their patients.

REVIEW QUESTIONS

1. Describe the effect of ethyl alcohol on sexual function and behavior.
2. What effects do H_2 receptor antagonists have when they are administered in large doses for an extended time period?
3. Discuss the effects of ketoconazole, propranolol, nifedipine, diltiazem, and verapamil on sexual function.
4. Name three drugs discussed in this chapter and describe their effects in enhancing libido and sexual gratification.

REFERENCES

Cleary JD, Chapman SW, Clark A, Lucia H: Fungal infections. In Young LY, Koda-Kimble MA, editors: *Applied therapeutics: the clinical use of drugs,* ed 6, Vancouver, Wash, 1995, Applied Therapeutics, Inc.

Pfizer, Inc: U.S. Food and Drug Administration, retyped text of letter from Pfizer, Inc, http://www.fda.gov/medwatch/safety/1998/viagra.htm (July 4, 1998).

Ruggiero RJ: Contraception. In Young LY, Koda-Kimble MA, editors: *Applied therapeutics: the clinical use of drugs,* ed 6, Vancouver, Wash, 1995, Applied Therapeutics, Inc.

Thompson JF: Geriatric urological disorders. In Young LY, Koda-Kimble MA, editors: *Applied therapeutics: the clinical use of drugs,* ed 6, Vancouver, Wash, 1995, Applied Therapeutics, Inc.

Viagra Postmarketing Information: Sildenafil citrate (Viagra): synopsis of fatal outcome reports submitted to the FDA regarding Viagra use, http://www.fda.gov/cder/news/viagrapostmarket.htm (July 4, 1998).

Viagra (sildenafil citrate), package information, http://www.viagra.com (July 4, 1998).

ADDITIONAL REFERENCES

Abramowicz M, editor: Drugs that cause sexual dysfunction: an update, *Med Lett* 34(876):73, 1992.

Anderson KN et al, editors: *Mosby's medical, nursing, and allied health dictionary,* ed 5, St Louis, 1998, Mosby.

Mosby: *Mosby's GenRx,* St Louis, 1998, Mosby.

UNIT XIII

Drugs Used in Neoplastic Diseases

CHAPTER 48

Antineoplastic Chemotherapy

CHAPTER FOCUS

Although progress in antineoplastic chemotherapy has helped many persons with a cancer diagnosis, the primary cancers of lung, colon and rectum, female breast, prostate, and pancreas are the leading causes of cancer death in the United States (Facts and Figures, 1998). The antineoplastic agents are usually extremely potent; therefore they possess both desirable effects and undesirable side effects and adverse reactions. A thorough knowledge of antineoplastic chemotherapy is very important for the healthcare professional.

OBJECTIVES

After reading and studying this chapter, the student should be able to do the following:

1. *Define and discuss the key terms.*
2. *Identify the reproductive cycles for normal and cancer cells and name a drug or drug classification that is effective in each cycle or phase.*
3. *Name the three principles of antineoplastic chemotherapy.*
4. *Describe the difference between a common side effect, adverse reaction, and specific dose-limiting drug effect.*
5. *Name and describe the most common side effects of antineoplastic chemotherapy.*
6. *Discuss age-related considerations for cancer in elderly and pediatric patients.*

KEY TERMS

cancer, (p. 616)
combination chemotherapy, (p. 618)
dose-limiting effects, (p. 619)
Gompertzian growth, (p. 617)
metastasis, (p. 617)
micrometastases, (p. 618)

Cancer refers to a group of over 300 diseases that is characterized by uncontrolled growth and spread of abnormal cells. It has been estimated that approximately 40% to 45% of Americans will develop cancer during their lifetime (Finley et al, 1995a). Many people fear cancer because it is difficult to accept that a small lump or mole that has the potential for rapid growth may lead to serious illness or death. Therefore education and early treatment are imperative to win the battle against cancer, which is second only to cardiovascular disease as a cause of death.

Statistically, the chances of developing cancer and dying from cancer are greater now than ever before. When a 20-year trend of cancer death rates from all sites was compared (from 1972 to 1974 and 1992 to 1994), the death rate for males increased by 5%, while that for females increased by 7% (Facts and Figures, 1998). While some gains in survival were noted for particular cancers, such as a 60% decrease in the death rate from Hodgkin's disease, Facts and Figures (1998) reported that the lung cancer death rate increased 147% in females and 48% in males. Therefore the reported incidence of cancer deaths compared with past years is increased for cancer overall and for particular cancers.

This chapter discusses the principles of antineoplastic chemotherapy and the use of chemotherapeutic drugs in the treatment of cancer. However, to better understand the mechanisms and sites of action of the cancer chemotherapeutic agents, it is important to understand the kinetics of both normal cells and cancer cells.

CELL KINETICS

The reproductive cycles of normal and cancer cells are essentially the same (Fig. 48-1). In the presynthesis phase (G_1), ribonucleic acid (RNA) and protein synthesis may occur. Also during this phase, the decision for cell replication or cell differentiation is determined. The cell progresses to the synthesis phase (S), which is the replication phase; deoxyribonucleic acid (DNA) doubles in preparation for cell division. During the postsynthesis or premitotic phase (G_2), DNA synthesis ceases, but RNA and protein synthesis continue to prepare the cell for mitosis (M), or spindle formation. During the M-phase, cells divide into two completely new cells that may leave the cell cycle to do the following: (1) develop into differentiated cells that perform a specialized function (such as neuron or epithelium), which means that these cells can no longer undergo cell division; or (2) become either temporarily or permanently nonproliferative (G_0-phase). Cells in the G_0-phase (or resting phase)

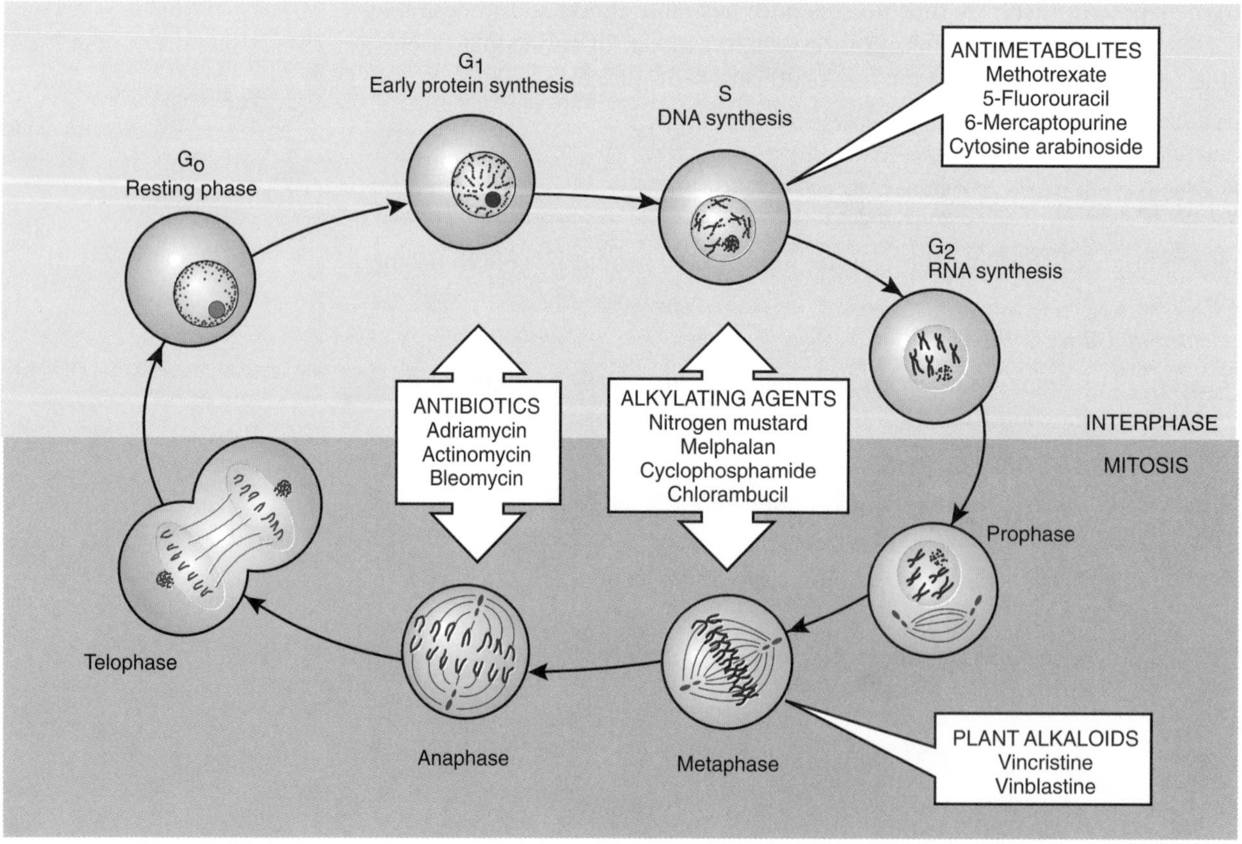

FIGURE 48-1
Phases of a cell cycle. Drugs are identified by where they exert their effects. *(From Beare, Myers, 1998.)*

may remain in this phase, may reenter the cell cycle in time, or may mature and die.

The anticancer agents have different sites of action on the dividing cell cycle. Agents that are most effective in one specific phase are referred to as cell cycle-specific agents. For example, methotrexate is more active in the S-phase of the cell cycle, so it is considered an S-phase cell cycle-specific agent. Antineoplastic agents that are active against both proliferating and resting cells are called cell cycle-nonspecific agents. An example of this group is the alkylating agents (see Table 49-1). Antineoplastic classifications are an important consideration in selecting the appropriate drug or drugs for the specific cancerous state. Methotrexate, an agent active predominantly in the S-phase of the cell cycle, would be much less effective in treating large tumor masses, which generally have slowly dividing cancer cells.

Normal cells grow and divide in an orderly fashion. The body process of cell adhesion inhibits the movement of the newly formed cells, and the body's homeostatic mechanisms control the entire cell growth process. Cancer cells may evolve from a hereditary or genetic predisposition plus contact with certain environmental conditions. Generally such neoplastic cells lack the cellular differentiation of the tissues in which they originate and therefore are unable to function like the normal cells around them. Cancer growth is enhanced by an increased rate of cell proliferation that lacks the normal body control system on cellular growth patterns. Cancer cells, because of the genetic differences, lack the cell adhesive property of normal cells, which may lead to **metastasis,** or spread of the cancer.

The growth of a cancer is usually rapid in the early stages, but as the tumor enlarges, it nearly outgrows its blood and nutrient supply, and the growth rate pattern decreases or reaches the plateau phase for the tumor. This is referred to as **Gompertzian growth** kinetics (Box 48-1). A cell burden of 10^9 is usually the smallest tumor burden (quantitative size) that is physically detectable (palpated). At this point, the individual has approximately 1 billion cancer cells, which is equal to a tumor about the size of a small grape and weighing 1 g. This is the point at which clinical symptoms usually first appear.

The Papanicolaou (Pap) smear is a cytologic test capable of detecting carcinoma of the cervix and endometrium in the subclinical stages. Early detection and treatment of small cancer lesions that are not detectable by visual examination have dramatically reduced the mortality associated with cancer of the cervix in the United States and Canada.

Animal studies have shown that chemotherapeutic drugs given in adequate doses to the host will kill a constant fraction of the cancer cells. For example, a drug or drug combination capable of killing 99.9% of the cells would only reduce a 10^{10} cell burden to 10^7 cancer cells. Each course of chemotherapy may reduce cancer cells to levels that may eventually be controlled by the patient's immune system (Fig. 48-2). This reduction may produce a remission, but if further therapies are not instituted or the immune system is inadequate, the remaining cells may grow into another detectable tumor.

PRINCIPLES OF CHEMOTHERAPY

To obtain optimal therapeutic effects with an antineoplastic agent or with combination cancer chemotherapies, the following principles should be considered:

1. Cancer chemotherapy is most effective against small tumors because they usually have an efficient blood supply

BOX 48-1 Cancer Cell Growth (Gompertzian)

	Number of cells present	
10^0	1	
10^1	10	
10^2	100	
10^3	1000	Subclinical disease (undetectable by physical examination)
10^4	10,000	
10^5	100,000	
10^6	1,000,000	
10^7	10,000,000	
10^8	100,000,000	
10^9	1,000,000,000	(1 g) Clinical symptoms appear
10^{10}	10,000,000,000	Regional spread
10^{11}	100,000,000,000	
10^{12}	1,000,000,000,000	Metastases
10^{13}	10,000,000,000,000	Lethal

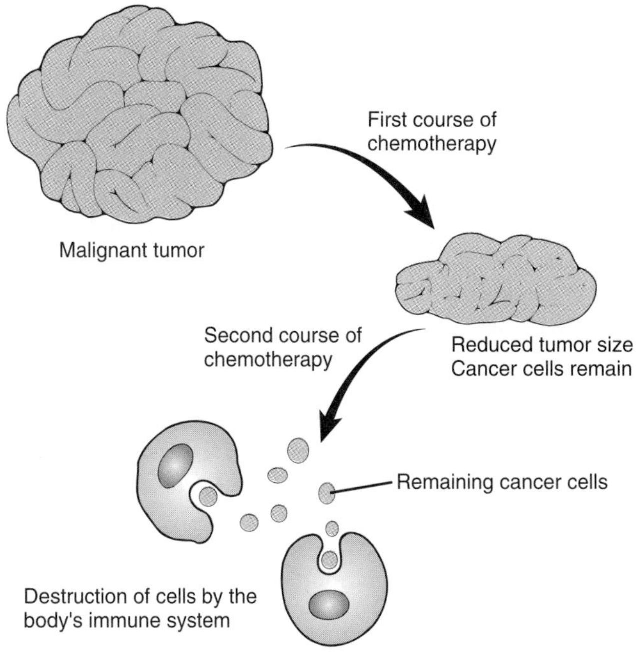

FIGURE 48-2
Cancer cell response to chemotherapy. *(From Beare, Myers, 1998.)*

and therefore drug delivery to the cancer site is increased. Also, small tumors generally have a higher percentage of proliferating cells so that a higher cell-kill factor is possible.

2. The removal of large localized tumors by surgery reduces the tumor cell burden and thus contributes to the success of the adjuvant chemotherapy. The major use of adjuvant chemotherapy is to help eradicate the **micrometastases** (the migration of cancer cells via the bloodstream or lymphatic system to grow in organs, bone, or tissues, far from the primary site) of cancer after surgery or radiation.
3. In general, combination cancer chemotherapeutic agents have a higher cancer cell-kill than treatment with a single drug agent.

COMBINATION CHEMOTHERAPY

In the late 1960s, **combination chemotherapy,** the use of two or more anticancer drugs at the same time, was initiated for the treatment of acute lymphoblastic leukemia and Hodgkin's disease. When the complete response rates for single agents were compared with the response rates for combination drugs, the results were enlightening. The response rates for the MOPP treatment of advanced Hodgkin's disease is a classic illustration, as follows:

DRUG	COMPLETE RESPONSE RATES
M mustine (Mustargen)	20%
O vincristine (Oncovin)	<10%
P procarbazine	<10%
P prednisone	<5%
MOPP combination	80%

The following considerations are used to select the drugs for combination chemotherapy:

1. Each drug when used alone should be active against the specific cancer.
2. Each drug should have a different site of action and act at a different point of the cell cycle (specificity).
3. Each drug should have a different organ toxicity, or if the toxic effect is similar, it should occur at different times after drug administration.

When the preceding principles are applied to the MOPP drug therapy, the concept of combination chemotherapy can be understood. First, the previous list illustrates the effectiveness of each drug against Hodgkin's disease. Second, the sites of major activity for each antineoplastic agent are believed to be different.

1. Mustine (Mustargen) is an alkylating agent that can interfere with the replication, transcription, and translation of DNA.
2. Vincristine (Oncovin) inhibits mitosis by interfering with the mitotic spindle.
3. Procarbazine is a weak monoamine oxidase (MAO) inhibitor, and its antineoplastic action is believed to occur during the S-phase. It inhibits the synthesis of DNA, RNA, and protein.
4. Prednisone has lympholytic properties and may produce an antifibrotic effect that would be useful in treating cancer metastases surrounded by fibrous materials. It also improves appetite and general feelings of well-being.

The third principle, that of different organ toxicity or toxicities that occur at different times, has also been substantiated for the MOPP combinations. The dose-limiting toxicity of bone marrow suppression is a property of both mustine and procarbazine, but the nadir, or the lowest depression point for this effect, occurs approximately 10 days after drug administration for mustine and 21 days after for procarbazine. Thus additive myelosuppressive effects from this combination are essentially avoided. Also, vincristine does not have bone marrow suppression effects but does exhibit a dose-limiting neurotoxicity. Prednisone does not demonstrate bone marrow suppression or neurotoxicity. Therefore the third principle of combination drug therapy is fulfilled.

Oncologists frequently use combination therapy in antineoplastic treatment. Table 48-1 lists other commonly prescribed drug combinations.

TOXIC EFFECTS

Most of the currently available antineoplastic agents appear to act on similar metabolic pathways in both normal and malignant cells. A major limitation of cancer drugs is their lack of tumor specificity. Drug toxicities or side effects may be divided into (1) common side effects, (2) adverse reactions, and (3) specific dose-limiting drug effects. A dose-limiting effect is a response to a drug that indicates that the maximum permissible dose has been reached, and the drug should be decreased or discontinued.

TABLE 48-1 Combination Chemotherapeutic Regimens

Cancer	*Acronym*	*Drug*
Breast	CMF	cyclophosphamide methotrexate fluorouracil
	CFPT	cyclophosphamide flourouracil prednisone tamoxifen
Colon	FLe	flourouracil levamisole
	F-Cl	flourouracil calcium leucovorin
Lung	CAV	cyclophosphamide doxorubicin (Adriamycin) vincristine
	COPE	cyclophosphamide vincristine (Oncovin) cisplatin (Platinol) etoposide

The most common side effects are alopecia (hair loss), nausea, vomiting, anorexia, diarrhea, and stomatitis (inflammation of the mouth). Cancer chemotherapy is most active or effective against dividing cells, but they are not capable of differentiating between cancer cells and normal dividing body cells. Therefore the most rapidly dividing cells in the body, which are in the bone marrow, hair follicles, and gastrointestinal tract, are generally the most affected by the anticancer drugs. See Box 48-2 for selected chemotherapeutic agents and their emetic potential.

The most common adverse reactions that can lead to serious and even life-threatening infections are leukopenia, thrombocytopenia, and anemia. Bone marrow suppression is the major dose-limiting property most frequently encountered in cancer chemotherapy.

Specific **dose-limiting effects** are adverse reactions that should indicate to the prescriber that the maximum permissible dose has been delivered, and the drug needs to be discontinued. Fortunately, this occurs with only certain drugs. For example, drugs that can produce hepatotoxicity include methotrexate (Mexate, Folex), mercaptopurine (Purinethol), lomustine (CCNU, CeeNu), dacarbazine (DTIC-Dome), doxorubicin (Adriamycin), and carmustine (BCNU, BiCU).

BOX 48-2 Selected Chemotherapeutic Agents: Emetic Potential

High Emetic Potential
cisplatin
dicarbazine (DTIC)
nitrogen mustard
streptozocin
actinomycin D
doxorubicin
daunorubicin
nitrosoureas (BCNU, CCNU)
procarbazine
cyclophosphamide (IV)
etoposide
mitomycin
methotrexate (high dose)

Low Emetic Potential
5-FU
vincristine
vinblastine
methotrexate
bleomycin
chlorambucil
melphalan
busulfan
cyclophosphamine (oral)
6-mercaptopurine

From Lane et al, 1991.

Cyclophosphamide (Cytoxan) is associated with hemorrhagic cystitis. (Since dehydration increases the risk factor, adequate fluid intake is important when this agent is administered.) Methotrexate is associated with tubular necrosis, which can be prevented by prehydrating with normal saline and alkalinizing the urine to increase the elimination of the drug. Cisplatin (Platinol) is associated with tubular necrosis. Prehydration with 1 to 2 L of intravenous fluid and adequate fluids after drug administration helps to reduce this adverse reaction. Nephrotoxicity, ototoxicity, and peripheral neuropathy have been reported with cisplatin. Cardiac toxicity is reported with both doxorubicin (Adriamycin) and daunorubicin (Cerubidine). Cardiotoxicity increases in patients who receive more than 550 mg/m^2 of body surface (total accumulated dosage given throughout therapy). Toxicity is also greater in geriatric patients and children younger than 2 years of age. Since this effect is cumulative if either drug is given, the amount of one drug already received by the person must be considered when planning therapy with the other drug.

Neurologic toxicity may range from tingling of the hands and feet and loss of deep tendon reflexes to ataxia, footdrop, confusion, and personality changes. Drugs reported to produce neurologic effects include vincristine (Oncovin), vinblastine (Velbane, Velsar), and methotrexate (Folex).

AGE-RELATED CONSIDERATIONS

Cancer in the Elderly

Cancer in the elderly is a serious disease, and its incidence increases sharply with age. About 50% of all cases of cancer in the United States occur in persons older than 65 years of age (Patel, Koeller, 1993). When compared with younger cancer victims, the elderly have more concurrent illnesses, which may decrease their ability to withstand the effects of cancer or the antineoplastic therapies. In addition, decreased pulmonary and renal function and decreased bone marrow cellularity may interfere with treatment. Other factors to be considered when managing regimens for elderly persons are the possibility of reduced income and loss of loved ones and family support.

Often, compromises in treatment are made because of a person's advanced age; however, data suggest that a dosage reduction of chemotherapy based on age alone is not always appropriate. A treatment approach should be based on the individual cancer and the biologic and physiologic differences noted in the elderly person. More clinical trials are also needed to further examine the relationship between cancer chemotherapy responsiveness and the person's age.

Cancer in Children

Although cancer in children is relatively uncommon, the most common cause of death of children in the United States between the ages of 1 and 14 years is cancer. Acute leukemias are the most common pediatric cancers. Carcinomas, which are common in adults, are rare in children, while sarcomas are much more common in children (Finley et al,

1995b). Because tumors in children grow rapidly, childhood cancer is generally more responsive to chemotherapy than is cancer in an adult. Children also tend to tolerate the acute side effects of chemotherapy better than adults. Fifty percent of children with cancer are long-term survivors or are actually cured.

SUMMARY

Cancer has been and still is a major health issue today. More people then ever are being cured of cancer, but the cancer death rates for all sites is still increasing. Early detection and treatment are crucial to combating cancer. An understanding of the phases of a cell cycle, cell kinetics, and combination antineoplastic therapies and information on the drug's side effects and adverse reactions are essential for the healthcare professional.

REVIEW QUESTIONS

1. Explain the Gompertzian growth kinetics in cancer. Approximately how many cancer cells are present before clinical symptoms first appear?
2. Describe three considerations used to select drugs for combination antineoplastic chemotherapy. Discuss the MOPP treatment for advanced Hodgkin's disease and how it meets the principles for combination chemotherapy.
3. Name the specific dose-limiting effect for methotrexate, cyclophosphamide, vincristine, and doxorubicin. Discuss methods of management for these toxicities.

REFERENCES

Beare PG, Myers JL: *Adult health nursing,* ed 3, St Louis, 1998, Mosby.

Facts and Figures: Cancer death rates, graphical data, American Cancer Society (http://www.cancer.org/statistics/cff98/graphicaldata.html (July 2, 1998).

Finley RS, LaCivita CL, Lindley CM: Neoplastic disorders and their treatment: General principles. In Young LY, Koda-Kimble MA, editors: *Applied therapeutics: the clinical use of drugs,* ed 6, Vancouver, Wash, 1995a, Applied Therapeutics, Inc.

Finley RS, Lindley CL, Henry DW: Solid tumors. In In Young LY, Koda-Kimble MA, editors: *Applied therapeutics: the clinical use of drugs,* ed 6, Vancouver, Wash, 1995b, Applied Therapeutics, Inc.

Lane M et al: Dronabinol and prochlorperazine in combination for treatment of cancer chemotherapy-induced nausea and vomiting, *J Pain Sympt Manage* 6(6):352, 1991.

Patel NH, Koeller J: Cancer chemotherapy in the elderly, *Highlights Antineoplas Drugs* 11(4):58-64, 1993.

ADDITIONAL REFERENCES

McCance KL, Huether SE: *Pathophysiology: the biologic basis for disease in adults and children,* ed 3, St Louis, 1998, Mosby.

Melmon KL et al: *Melmon and Morelli's clinical pharmacology,* ed 3, New York, 1992, McGraw-Hill.

Parker SL, Tong T, Bolden S, Wingo PA: Cancer statistics, 1996, *Cancer J Clin* 46(1):5-28, 1996.

Sagraves R, Letassy NA, Barton TL: Obstetrics. In Young LY, Koda-Kimble MA, editors: *Applied therapeutics: the clinical use of drugs,* ed 6, Vancouver, Wash, 1995, Applied Therapeutics, Inc.

CHAPTER 49

Antineoplastic Agents

KEY DRUGS

cyclophosphamide, (p. 627)
doxorubicin, (p. 629)
methotrexate, (p. 624)
vincristine, (p. 630)

KEY TERMS

alkylating agents, (p. 622)
antibiotic antitumor agents, (p. 622)
antimetabolites, (p. 622)
leucovorin, (p. 626)
leucovorin rescue, (p. 626)
mitotic inhibitors, (p. 622)

CHAPTER FOCUS

Cancer is a leading cause of death in the United States, second only to death from cardiac disease. The three primary methods of treating cancer include surgery, radiation, and antineoplastic chemotherapy. Solid tumors are generally treated with surgery and/or radiation, while disseminated cancers plus a few localized cancers are treated with the antineoplastic agents. Many new antineoplastic agents are released annually; therefore the healthcare professional should be well informed on the pharmacology, toxicity, and therapeutic management of these drugs.

OBJECTIVES

After reading and studying this chapter, the student should be able to do the following:

1. *Define and describe the key terms and key drugs.*
2. *Describe the mechanisms of action of the antimetabolites, alkylating agents, antibiotic antitumor agents, and mitotic inhibitors.*
3. *Discuss the use of hormones, antihormones, and corticosteroids in the treatment of cancer.*
4. *Review the common side effects and major adverse reactions of antineoplastic agents.*
5. *Name and describe the significant drug interactions of methotrexate.*

The antineoplastic agents do not directly kill tumor cells; they act by interfering with cell reproduction or replication at some point in the cell cycle. (See Chapter 48 for a discussion of the cell cycle.) For cells to proliferate, the genetic material deoxyribonucleic acid (DNA) must be replicated once every cell cycle. DNA is the genetic substance in body cells that transfers information, resulting in the production of the ribonucleic acid (RNA) necessary to produce enzymes and protein synthesis (Fig. 49-1). The enzymes determine the structure, biochemical activity, growth rate, and functions of the cell. The antineoplastic agents are divided into various classes based on their probable major mechanisms of action. See headings under Generic (brand name) in Table 49-1 for classifications.

OVERVIEW OF DRUG EFFECTS

The formation of the nucleic acids, DNA and ultimately RNA, requires pyrimidines and purines (nitrogen compounds) as the basic building block materials. **Antimetabolites** have a structure similar to a necessary building block for the formation of DNA. This substance is accepted by the cell as the necessary ingredient for cell growth, but because it is an impostor, it interferes with the normal production of DNA. **Alkylating agents** are drugs that substitute an alkyl chemical structure for a hydrogen atom in DNA. This results in a cross-linking of each strand of DNA, thus preventing cell division. Alkylator-like drugs are chemically different agents that are believed to have an action similar to the alkylating agents.

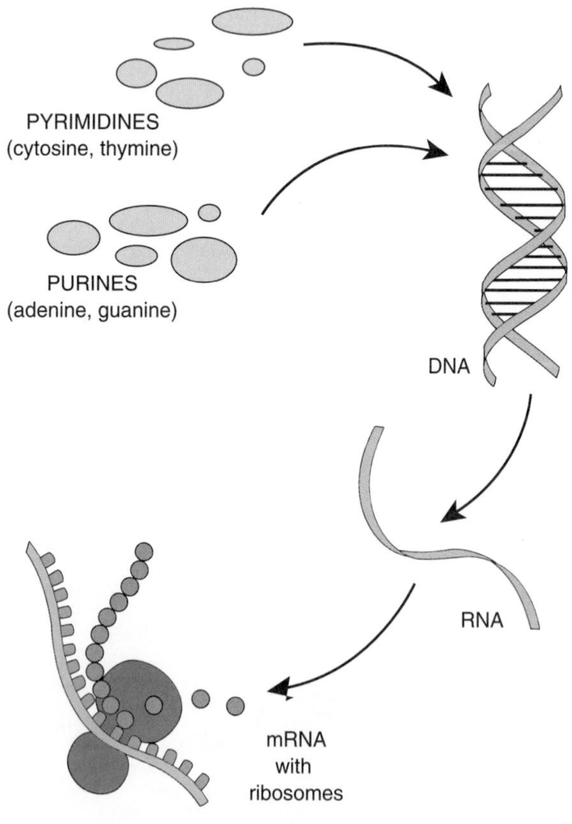

FIGURE 49-1
Protein synthesis.

Antibiotic antitumor agents interfere with DNA functioning by blocking the transcription of new DNA or RNA. In addition, they delay or inhibit mitosis.

The **mitotic inhibitors,** vinblastine and vincristine, are plant alkaloids that block cell division in metaphase. Vinorelbine (Navelbine) is a semisynthetic vinca alkaloid that also has antitumor activity in metaphase. These agents probably have other major sites of action because they differ from each other pharmacologically and in therapeutic application. Vinblastine has been used in the treatment of various lymphomas and carcinoma of the breast and testes; vincristine is frequently used to treat acute leukemias and Hodgkin's disease while vinorelbine is indicated for non–small-cell lung cancer.

Hormones, antihormones, corticosteroids, and various other agents are classified in the miscellaneous section of this chapter.

ANTIMETABOLITE DRUGS

The antimetabolite classification contains fluorouracil, floxuridine, fludarabine, methotrexate, cytarabine, mercaptopurine, and thioguanine. Two of the most common agents prescribed, fluorouracil and methotrexate, are reviewed in this section although the primary indications and major adverse effects of each drug will be found in Table 49-1. In this table, the common side effects as noted in Chapter 48 will only be repeated if the effect is considered a major problem. The antidote leucovorin will also be discussed.

fluorouracil [flure oh yoor′ a sill] (Adrucil, 5-FU)

Fluorouracil is a pyrimidine antagonist that interferes with the synthesis of DNA and RNA. It is a cell cycle-specific agent that produces its effect in the S-phase of cell division. It is indicated for palliative treatment of carcinomas of the colon, rectum, breast, stomach, and pancreas.

Pharmacokinetics

Fluorouracil is metabolized rapidly (within 1 hour) in the tissues to its active metabolite floxuridine. The final metabolic degradation occurs in the liver. The drug is distributed throughout the body and also crosses the blood-brain barrier. The half-life for the alpha phase is 10 to 20 minutes; for the beta phase half-life is prolonged up to 20 hours because of tissue storage of metabolites. Excretion is primarily respiratory as carbon dioxide (60% to 80%).

Drug interactions

A significant drug interaction occurs if fluorouracil is administered with other bone marrow depressants; a dosage reduction of one or both drugs may be necessary. The administration of any live virus vaccine concurrently with flu-

TABLE 49-1 Antineoplastic Medications

Generic (Brand Name)	*Primary Indications*	*Major Toxicities*
Alkylating Agents		
Nitrogen Mustards		
chlorambucil (Leukeran)	CLL, Hodgkin's and non-Hodgkin's lymphomas	Bone marrow suppression
cyclophosphamide* (Cytoxan)	See drug monograph in text	Bone marrow suppression, hemorrhagic cystitis
ifosfamide (IFEX)	Testicular tumors	Bone marrow suppression, nausea, vomiting, encephalopathy
mechlorethamine* (Mustargen)	See drug monograph in text	Bone marrow suppression, severe nausea, and vomiting
melphalan (Alkeran)	Multiple myeloma, ovarian cancer	Bone marrow suppression, allergic reactions
uracil mustard (Uracil Mustard)	CLL, CML, non-Hodgkin's lymphomas, mycosis fungoides	Leukopenia, thrombocytopenia
Nitrosureas		
carmustine (BiCNU)	Primary brain tumors, multiple myeloma	Bone marrow suppression, lung fibrosis, nephrotoxicity
lomustine* (CeeNU)	See drug monograph in text	Bone marrow suppression, anorexia, nausea, vomiting
streptozocin (Zanosar)	Pancreatic cancer	Nephrotoxicity, nausea, vomiting
Other		
busulfan (Myleran)	CML	Bone marrow suppression, hyperpigmentation, gynecomastia
Carboplatin (Paraplatin)	Ovarian carcinoma	Bone marrow suppression, nausea, vomiting, neurotoxicity, neuropathies, ototoxicity
cisplatin* (Platinol)	See drug monograph in text	Nephrotoxicity, severe nausea and vomiting, bone marrow suppression
pipobroman (Vercyte)	CGL, polycythemia vera	Bone marrow suppression, nausea, vomiting, diarrhea
thiotepa (Thioplex)	Breast, ovarian, bladder cancers, lymphomas, malignant effusions	Bone marrow suppression
Antimetabolites		
cytarabine (Cytosar-U)	AML, ALL	Bone marrow suppression, anorexia, oral and GI ulceration
fluorouracil* (Adrucil)	See drug monograph in text	Diarrhea, stomatitis, bone marrow suppression
floxuridine (FUDR)	GI adenocarcinoma with liver metastasis	Bone marrow suppression, stomatitis, anaphylaxis
fludarabine (Fludara)	CLL	Bone marrow suppression, fever, chills, nausea, vomiting, infection
mercaptopurine (Purinethol)	ALL, AML	Bone marrow suppression, anorexia, cholestasis
methotrexate* (Folex)	See drug monograph in text	Bone marrow suppression, diarrhea, stomatitis
thioguanine (Thioguanine)	ANLL	Bone marrow suppression
Antibiotics		
bleomycin (Blenoxane)	Squamous cell carcinoma, lymphomas, testicular cancer	Chills, fever, pneumonitis, mucositis, lung fibrosis, hyperpigmentation
dactinomycin (Cosmegen)	Wilms' tumor, Ewing's sarcoma, choriocarcinoma, rhabdomyosarcoma	Bone marrow suppression
daunorubicin liposomal (DaunoXome)	HIV-Kaposi's sarcoma	Bone marrow suppression, cardiomyopathy, severe mucositis
doxorubicin* (Adriamycin)	See drug monograph in text	Same as daunorubicin

Continued

Table 49-1 Antineoplastic Medications—cont'd

Generic (Brand Name)	Primary Indications	Major Toxicities
Antibiotics—cont'd		
idarubicin (Idamycin)	AML	Severe bone marrow suppression, infection, alopecia, nausea, vomiting, hemorrhage
mitomycin (Mutamycin)	Disseminated adenocarcinoma of pancreas or stomach	Bone marrow suppression
mitoxantrone (Novantrone)	ANLL	Cardiotoxicity, severe myelosuppression
pentostatin (Nipent)	Hairy cell leukemia	Bone marrow suppression, renal toxicity, rash
plicamycin (Mithracin)	Testicular tumors, hypercalcemia	Epistaxis, hemorrhage, nausea, bone marrow suppression, stomatitis, vomiting, diarrhea
Mitotic Inhibitors		
etoposide (VePesid)	Refractory testicular tumors, small cell lung cancer	Bone marrow suppression, alopecia
teniposide (Vumon)	ALL	Bone marrow suppression, mucositis, alopecia
vinblastine* (Velban)	see drug monograph in text	leukopenia, alopecia, muscle pain, hyperuricemia
vincristine * (Oncovin)	See drug monograph in text	Mild to severe paresthesias, jaw pain, ataxia, muscle wasting, constipation
vinorelbine (Navelbine)	Non–small-cell lung cancer	Bone marrow suppression, nausea, vomiting, asthenia

*Drug monograph in text.
ALL, acute lymphoblastic leukemia; AML, acute myelogenous leukemia; ANLL, acute nonlymphocytic leukemia; CLL, chronic lymphocytic leukemia; CML, chronic myelocytic leukemia; CGL, chronic granulocytic leukemia.

orouracil should only be done with very close supervision of the oncologist. Fluorouracil will suppress the patient's normal defense mechanisms and thus may increase the virus's replication and adverse effects. It is usually recommended that live virus vaccines not be administered until months after chemotherapy has been discontinued. Persons in close contact with the patient should not receive immunization with the oral poliovirus vaccine because the live virus is excreted by the person receiving it and can be transmitted to the immunocompromised individual.

Side effects and adverse reactions

These include diarrhea, esophagopharyngitis, leukopenia, thrombocytopenia, gastrointestinal (GI) tract ulceration (severe nausea and vomiting, black stools, and abdominal cramps), dermatitis on the extremities (less often on the trunk), anorexia, weakness, loss of hair, and dry skin. See Table 49-1 for primary indications and major toxicities.

Warnings

Use with caution in patients with chickenpox (recent or current), herpes zoster, liver or kidney function impairment, bone marrow suppression, infection, and tumor cell infiltration in the bone marrow. See the box for Food and Drug Administration (FDA) pregnancy safety classifications.

Contraindications

Avoid use in persons with fluorouracil hypersensitivity.

Dosage and administration

The usual adult dose is 7 to 12 mg/kg of body weight daily intravenously for 4 days; if no toxicity occurs during the following 3 days, a dosage of 7 to 10 mg/kg of body weight is then administered every 3 to 4 days for a total course of 2 weeks. For alternate schedules, see a current package insert or drug reference. The maximum dosage for adults is 800 mg/day or 400 mg/day for the high-risk patient. Investigational protocols may use higher dosages than stated in the product's package insert. Review Chapter 2 for legal implications.

Topical fluorouracil preparations (Efudex, Fluoroplex) are used for treatment of skin cancer (basal cell carcinomas) and precancerous skin lesions.

methotrexate [meth oh trex' ate] (Mexate, Folex)

Methotrexate is an antimetabolite that is cell cycle-specific for the S-phase. To synthesize DNA, folic acid must be reduced to tetrahydrofolate by the enzyme dihydrofolate reductase. Methotrexate binds with dihydrofolate reductase, thus inhibiting the synthesis of DNA and RNA. Because malignant cellular growth is usually greater than cell growth of

PREGNANCY SAFETY

Category	Drug
B	amifostine, mesna
C	aldesleukin, anastrozole, asparaginase, dacarbazine, dactinomycin, dexrazoxane, interferon alfa-2a, interferon alfa-2b, levamisole, pegaspargase, testolactone, streptozocin
D	altretamine, busulfan, carboplatin, carmustine, chlorambucil, cladribine, cyclophosphamide, cytarabine, daunorubicin, docetaxel, doxorubicin, etoposide, fludarabine, fluorouracil, flutamide, goserelin, idarubicin, ifosfamide, lomustine, mechlorethamine, mercaptopurine, methotrexate, mitoxantrone, paclitaxel, pentostatin, pipobroman, procarbazine, tamoxifen, teniposide, thioguanine, tretinoin, vinblastine, vincristine, vinorelbine
X	leuprolide, plicamycin

normal tissues, cancer growth may be impaired by methotrexate.

Indications

Methotrexate is indicated for the following:

- Treatment of breast, head and neck, and lung cancers; trophoblastic tumors; renal, ovarian, bladder, and testicular carcinomas; and acute lymphocytic leukemia and non-Hodgkin's lymphomas.
- Prevention and treatment of meningeal leukemia.
- Treatment of advanced cases of mycosis fungoides and osteosarcoma.
- Treatment for some noncancerous conditions such as selected cases of severe psoriasis and rheumatoid arthritis that are unresponsive to standard therapies.

Pharmacokinetics

Methotrexate is administered orally or parenterally (IM, IV, and intrathecal). The oral preparation reaches peak serum levels within 1 to 2 hours. Limited amounts of methotrexate can cross the blood-brain barrier, but significant quantities pass into the systemic circulation after intrathecal drug administration. It is metabolized intracellularly and in the liver with unchanged drug excreted by the kidneys.

Drug interactions

The following effects may occur when methotrexate is given with the drugs listed below:

Drug	Possible effect and management
Alcohol or hepatotoxic drugs	Increased risk of hepatotoxicity. Avoid or a potentially serious drug interaction may occur.
acyclovir injection	Neurologic complications may occur with the use of intrathecal methotrexate. Avoid or a potentially serious drug interaction may occur.
asparaginase	Cell replication is inhibited by asparaginase, thus impairing the therapeutic effects of methotrexate. If asparaginase is administered 9 to 10 days before or within 24 hours after methotrexate, this effect is not reported. The major side effects of methotrexate—GI and hematologic (blood components suppression)—may also be reduced in this drug administration schedule. Avoid or a potentially serious drug interaction may occur.
Bone marrow depressants or radiation	Bone marrow-depressant effects may be increased. Avoid or a potentially serious drug interaction may occur. If necessary to give concurrently, a decrease in drug dosage is usually indicated.
Nonsteroidal antiinflammatory drugs (NSAIDs)	Concurrent administration may result in severe methotrexate toxicity. Avoid or a potentially serious drug interaction may occur. Refer to manufacturer's recommendations on individual NSAIDs to reduce this possibility.
probenecid or salicylates	May interfere with excretion of methotrexate, which results in elevated serum levels. Salicylates may also displace methotrexate from its protein-binding sites, also resulting in increased, and possibly toxic, serum levels. Avoid or a potentially serious drug interaction may occur. If necessary to use in combination, monitor serum methotrexate levels closely. The methotrexate dosage level should be decreased and the patient closely monitored for signs of toxicity.
Vaccines, live oral	May result in a decrease in antibody response along with an increase in side effects and adverse reactions. Avoid or a potentially serious drug interaction may occur.

Color type indicates an unsafe drug combination.

Side effects and adverse reactions

These include nausea, vomiting, anorexia, acne, boils, skin rash or itching, loss of hair, GI ulcers and bleeding, leukopenia, infections, thrombocytopenia, stomatitis, pharyngitis, and, with prolonged daily therapy, liver toxicity, pneumonitis, or pulmonary fibrosis. With high-dose drug therapy, renal failure, hyperuricemia, and cutaneous vasculitis may occur.

See Table 49-1 for primary indications and major toxicities.

Warnings

Use with caution in patients with aciduria (a urine pH below 7), gout, GI obstruction, a history of kidney stone formation, nausea, and vomiting (which may increase the potential for dehydration) and in dehydrated patients.

Contraindications

Avoid use in persons with methotrexate hypersensitivity, ascites, pleural effusions, liver or kidney function impairment, bone marrow suppression, chickenpox (recent or current), herpes zoster, infection, peptic ulcer or ulcerative colitis, and oral mucositis.

Dosage and administration

The adult and pediatric methotrexate dosage varies according to the indication and course of treatment. Generally, the antineoplastic adult dosage orally is 15 to 30 mg daily for 5 days, repeated from three to five times with a 7- to 14-day interval between each course. The pediatric oral dosage is 20 to 40 mg/m^2 once a week. For other indications and recommended parenteral doses, see a current package insert or USP DI.

leucovorin [loo koe vor′ in] (folinic acid, Wellcovorin)

Leucovorin, or folinic acid, is a form of folic acid that does not require dihydrofolate reductase to produce folic acid. Therefore it is used to prevent or treat toxicity induced by folic acid antagonists.

Indications

Leucovorin is indicated for the following:

- Use as an antidote (prophylaxis and treatment) for folic acid antagonists, such as methotrexate, pyrimethamine, and trimethoprim. **Leucovorin rescue** is a term used to describe the use of leucovorin to reduce the time that sensitive (normal) cells are exposed to the toxic effects of high-dose methotrexate treatments.
- Treatment of megaloblastic anemia caused by nutritional deficiencies, sprue, or pregnancy, and whenever oral folic acid therapy is not appropriate.

Pharmacokinetics

Leucovorin is rapidly absorbed orally and converted by the intestinal mucous membrane and liver to 5-methyltetrahydrofolate, an active metabolite. The onset of action orally is between 20 and 30 minutes, intramuscularly between 10 and 20 minutes, and intravenously less than 5 minutes. The duration of action by all routes is between 3 and 6 hours. It is primarily excreted by the kidneys.

Drug interactions

No significant drug interactions are reported with leucovorin.

Side effects and adverse reactions

These include allergic reactions, (rash, hives, itching, and wheezing) and convulsions. See Table 49-1 for primary indications and major toxicities.

Warnings

Use with caution in patients with aciduria (urine pH below 7), ascites, GI obstruction, pleural effusion, and nausea and vomiting (decrease hydration may result in an increase in methotrexate toxicity) and in dehydrated patients.

Contraindications

Avoid use in persons with leucovorin hypersensitivity and kidney function impairment.

Dosage and administration

As an antidote to the toxic effect of folic acid antagonists, the adult oral dose is 10 mg/m^2 every 6 hours, until methotrexate blood levels fall to less than 5×10^{-8} M. For additional dosing recommendations, see a current reference or package insert.

ALKYLATING DRUGS

Alkylating drugs are frequently used as anticancer agents and are believed to be the first class of medications applied clinically in the modern era of antineoplastic drug therapy. Various groups of alkylating agents are available, which include the nitrogen mustards and nitrosoureas. See Table 49-1 for specific drugs, primary indications, and major toxicities for this classification.

This chapter reviews mechlorethamine (Mustargen) and cyclophosphamide (Cytoxan) from the nitrogen mustard category, lomustine (CeeNU) from the nitrosoureas, and cisplatin (Platinol), an alkylator-like drug.

mechlorethamine [me klor eth′ a meen] (Mustargen)

The cell cycle-nonspecific agent mechlorethamine is an alkylating agent capable of cross-linking DNA and RNA and also inhibiting protein synthesis.

Indications

Mechlorethamine is indicated for the treatment of lung carcinoma, Hodgkin's and non-Hodgkin's lymphomas, chronic leukemia, malignant effusions, mycosis fungoides, and polycythemia vera.

Pharmacokinetics

It may be administered intravenously or by the intracavitary route (such as intrapleurally or intraperitoneally). A topical preparation is also available to treat cutaneous manifestations of mycosis fungoides.

Mechlorethamine's onset of action is nearly immediate (within seconds or minutes), and it is also rapidly deactivated in body tissues.

Drug interactions

The following effects may occur when mechlorethamine is given with the drugs listed below:

Drug	Possible effect and management
Bone marrow depressants or radiation	Increased bone marrow depression may occur. Avoid or a potentially serious interaction may occur. If necessary to use concurrently, a decrease in drug dosage is usually indicated.
probenecid or sulfinpyrazone	Hyperuricemia and gout may occur. The prescriber may adjust the antigout medications or prescribe allopurinol. The latter is often preferred to prevent drug-induced hyperuricemia.
Vaccines, live viral	See methotrexate drug interactions.

Color type indicates an unsafe drug combination.

Side effects and adverse reactions

These include nausea, vomiting, diarrhea, anorexia, a metallic taste in the mouth, neurotoxicity, weakness, hair loss, leukopenia, thrombocytopenia, precipitation of herpes zoster, ototoxicity, hyperuricemia, and gonadal suppression or missing menstrual periods. Rarely, peripheral neuropathy, allergic reaction, peptic ulcer, and liver toxicity are reported. See Table 49-1 for primary indications and major toxicities.

Warnings

Use with caution in patients with a history of gout or urate kidney stones.

Contraindications

Avoid use in persons with mechlorethamine hypersensitivity, bone marrow suppression, chickenpox (recent or current), herpes zoster, infection, and tumor infiltration of bone marrow.

Dosage and administration

The usual adult total dose is 0.4 mg/kg IV in single or divided doses. If patients have previously received chemotherapy or radiation, this dosage should not exceed 0.2 to 0.3 mg/kg of body weight. For additional dosing recommendations, see a current reference or package insert.

cyclophosphamide [sye kloe foss' fa mide] (Cytoxan, Procytox)

Cyclophosphamide is a cell cycle-nonspecific agent that cross-links DNA and RNA strands and also inhibits the protein synthesis.

Indications

Cyclophosphamide is indicated for acute and chronic leukemias, carcinomas of the ovary and breast, neuroblastomas, retinoblastomas, Hodgkin's and non-Hodgkin's lymphomas, multiple myeloma, and mycosis fungoides and as an immunosuppressant in corticosteroid-resistant nephrotic syndrome.

Pharmacokinetics

The drug is well absorbed orally and has limited crossing of the blood-brain barrier. Cyclophosphamide undergoes hepatic metabolism to active and inactive metabolites, Its half-life is between 3 to 12 hours and excretion is primarily via the kidneys.

Drug interactions

The following effects may occur when cyclophosphamide is given with the drugs listed below:

Drug	Possible effect and management
Bone marrow depressants or radiation	Increased bone marrow depression may occur. Avoid or a potentially serious drug interaction may occur. If necessary to use concurrently, a decrease in drug dosage is usually indicated.
cocaine	Inhibition of cholinesterase activity by cyclophosphamide reduces cocaine metabolism and excretion and may lead to cocaine toxicity. Avoid or a potentially serious drug interaction may occur.
cytarabine (Cytosar)	Concurrent use in preparation for bone marrow transplant may result in increased cardiomyopathy with subsequent death. Avoid or a potentially serious drug interaction may occur.
probenecid (Benemid) or sulfinpyrazone (Anturane)	Hyperuricemia and gout may occur. The prescriber may adjust antigout medications. Allopurinol is not indicated since it may increase the bone marrow toxicity of cyclophosphamide. If drugs are given concurrently, monitor closely for toxicity.

Immunosuppressant agents including azathioprine (Imuran), chlorambucil (Leukeran), corticosteroids, cyclosporine (Sandimmune), mercaptopurine (Purinethol), and muromonab-CD3 (Orthoclone OKT3)	Increased risk of infections and further development of neoplasms. Avoid or a potentially serious drug interaction may occur.
Vaccines, live viral	See methotrexate drug interactions.

Color type indicates an unsafe drug combination.

Side effects and adverse reactions

These include nausea, vomiting, anorexia, darkening of the skin and nails, diarrhea, abdominal pain, flushing of the face, headache, increased sweating, swollen lips, rash, hair loss, gonadal suppression or missing menstrual periods, leukopenia, anemia, and thrombocytopenia. With high-dose therapies or long-term treatments, cardiotoxicity, hemorrhagic cystitis, hyperuricemia, nephrotoxicity, pneumonitis or interstitial pulmonary fibrosis, and a syndrome that resembles the syndrome of inappropriate antidiuretic hormone (SIADH) secretion (confusion, agitation, increased weakness, and dizziness) may occur. Rare adverse effects include anaphylaxis, hepatitis, hyperglycemia, hemorrhagic colitis, and stomatitis. See Table 49-1 for primary indications and major toxicities.

Warnings

Use with caution in patients with adrenalectomy (toxicity or cyclophosphamide increases) and a history of gout or urate kidney stones.

Contraindications

Avoid use in persons with cyclophosphamide hypersensitivity, bone marrow suppression, chickenpox (current or recent), herpes zoster, liver or kidney function impairment, infection, and tumor cell infiltration in bone marrow.

Dosage and administration

The usual adult antineoplastic dosage is 1 to 5 mg/kg orally daily; the intravenous dose is 40 to 50 mg/kg in divided doses over 2 to 5 days. The pediatric intravenous dosage is 2 to 8 mg/kg in divided doses for 6 or more days.

NITROSOUREAS

Nitrosoureas are highly lipophilic, alkylating agents that easily cross the blood-brain barrier. These agents are generally very useful for the treatment of primary brain tumors. See Table 49-1 for other nitrosoureas, primary indications, and major toxicities.

lomustine [loe mus′ teen] (CeeNU)

Lomustine is used to treat primary brain tumors and Hodgkin's lymphomas.

Pharmacokinetics

It is well absorbed orally, has a half life of approximately 90 minutes (active metabolites half-life is 16 to 48 hours), and is metabolized in the liver and excreted primarily by the kidneys.

Drug interactions

Significant drug interactions occur with bone marrow suppressants, radiation therapy, or live virus vaccines. See methotrexate.

Side effects and adverse reactions

The most common side effects include anorexia, nausea, and vomiting, while bone marrow depression (leukopenia, thrombocytopenia, and anemia), neurotoxicity, nephrotoxicity and, rarely, hepatotoxicity, pulmonary infiltrates, and/or fibrosis are the adverse reactions reported with lomustine. Drug toxicity is cumulative; thus drug dosage is adjusted regularly, based on the nadir blood count from the previous dose administered. Because of the seriousness of this effect, blood counts are closely monitored. Current reference sources should be reviewed when monitoring a patient who is receiving nitrosourea agents.

Warnings

Use with caution in patients with bone marrow suppression, chickenpox (current or recent), herpes zoster, infection, and lung or kidney impairment.

Contraindications

Avoid use in persons with lomustine hypersensitivity.

ALKYLATOR-LIKE DRUGS

The alkylator-like drugs are chemically different from the alkylating agents, but they are believed to have a similar action.

cisplatin [sis′ pla tin] (Platinol)

Although the exact mechanism of action of cisplatin is unknown, it is believed to be a cell cycle-nonspecific agent that has an action similar to that of the alkylating agents. It cross-links DNA, thus interfering with its function.

Indications

It is indicated for the treatment of bladder, ovarian, and testicular carcinomas.

Pharmacokinetics

Cisplatin administered intravenously does not significantly cross the blood-brain barrier. Its half-life is biphasic: alpha phase is 25 to 49 minutes and beta phase is 58 to 73 hours. It is metabolized to inactive metabolites that are renally excreted after 5 days, although platinum has been detected in body tissues for 4 months or longer.

Drug interactions

The following effects may occur when cisplatin is given with the drugs listed below:

Drug	Possible effect and management
Bone marrow depressants or radiation	Increased bone marrow depression may occur. Avoid or a potentially serious interaction may occur. If necessary to use concurrently, a decrease in drug dosage is usually indicated.
probenecid (Benemid) or sulfinpyrazone (Anturane)	Hyperuricemia and gout may occur. The prescriber may adjust the antigout medications or prescribe allopurinol. The latter is often preferred to prevent drug-induced hyperuricemia.
Nephrotoxic or ototoxic drugs	Concurrent or sequential administration is not recommended. The risk for nephrotoxicity and ototoxicity is increased, especially in patients with renal impairment. Avoid or a potentially serious drug interaction may occur.
Vaccines, live viral	See methotrexate drug interactions.

Color type indicates an unsafe drug combination.

Side effects and adverse reactions

These include severe nausea and vomiting, anorexia, bone marrow suppression (anemia, leukopenia, and thrombocytopenia), nephrotoxicity, ototoxicity, neurotoxicity (peripheral neuropathies), anaphylaxis, extravasation (pain or redness at the injection site, which can result in tissue cellulitis, fibrosis, and necrosis). Rare adverse reactions include optic neuritis, blurred vision, SIADH secretion (agitation, confusion, dizziness, hallucinations, anorexia, depression, convulsions, insomnia, and unconsciousness). See Table 49-1 for primary indications and major toxicities.

Warnings

Use with caution in patients with a history of gout or urate kidney stones, bone marrow suppression, chickenpox (current or recent), herpes zoster, hearing impairment, infection, and kidney function impairment.

Contraindications

Avoid use in persons with cisplatin hypersensitivity.

Dosage and administration

The adult dosage varies according to the site of cancerous growth; for example, for advanced bladder cancer the dose is 50 to 70 mg/m^2 IV every 3 to 4 weeks. Recommended dosages vary according to cancer and protocol and also whether therapy is initial or maintenance. Check a current reference for information.

ANTIBIOTIC ANTITUMOR DRUGS

The antitumor antibiotics are cytotoxic agents that directly bind DNA, thus inhibiting DNA and RNA synthesis. The early agents in this class caused the clinically limiting adverse effect of irreversible cardiomyopathy. Newer agents are being sought that lack this cardiac toxicity. See Table 49-1 for the drugs in this classification, primary indications, and major toxicities.

doxorubicin [dox oh roo′ bi sin] (Adriamycin)

Doxorubicin is an antineoplastic cell cycle-specific agent for the S-phase of cell division.

Indications

It is indicated for the treatment of acute leukemia, Wilms' tumor, soft tissue and bone sarcomas, Hodgkin's disease, lymphomas, and breast and various other carcinomas.

Pharmacokinetics

Doxorubicin does not cross the blood-brain barrier and is highly tissue bound. It is metabolized in the liver to produce the active metabolite, adriamycinol. The half-life of doxorubicin is biphasic: 0.6 hour and 16.7 hours. The active metabolite has a biphasic half-life of 3.3 hours and 31.7 hours. It is metabolized in the liver and excreted primarily in bile.

Drug interactions

Significant drug interactions are reported with other bone marrow depressant drugs or radiation, with probenecid (Benemid) or sulfinpyrazone (Anturane), and with live virus vaccines. See mechlorethamine above.

In addition, the use of doxorubicin in patients who have received daunorubicin (Cerubidine) increases the risk of inducing cardiotoxicity. Both drugs have cumulative maximum dosing limits that must be followed: a total dose of 550 mg/m^2 from either drug alone or both drugs together. If the patient has received previous chest radiation or other cardiotoxic drugs, the maximum dose is reduced to 400 mg/m^2.

Side effects and adverse reactions

These include severe nausea and vomiting, darkening of soles, palms, or nails (especially in children and black patients), diarrhea, red urine, loss of hair, leukopenia, thrombocytopenia, stomatitis, esophagitis, cardiotoxicity (usually congestive heart failure), extravasation leading to cellulitis or tissue necrosis, hyperuricemia, nephropathy, and dark or red skin.

Warnings

Use with caution in patients with a history of gout or urate kidney stones, bone marrow suppression, chickenpox (current or recent), herpes zoster, cardiac disease, liver function impairment, and tumor cell infiltration in the bone marrow.

Contraindications

Avoid use in persons with doxorubicin hypersensitivity and who have had excessive total dosage, as previous discussed.

Dosage and administration

The usual adult dose is 60 to 75 mg/m^2 intravenously, repeated every 3 weeks. The pediatric dosage is 30 mg/m^2 of body surface daily on 3 consecutive days every month.

MITOTIC INHIBITORS

The primary mitotic inhibitors vinblastine and vincristine (vinca alkaloids derived from a periwinkle plant) are cell cycle-specific agents that inhibit mitosis during the M-phase. Vinorelbine is a semisynthetic vinca alkaloid. Although these agents are similar chemically, they have different therapeutic indications and different side effects and adverse reactions. See Table 49-1 for primary indications and major toxicities.

vinblastine [vin blas′ teen] (Velban)
vincristine [vin kris′ teen] (Oncovin)

Vinblastine is used to treat breast and testicular carcinoma, Hodgkin's and non-Hodgkin's lymphomas, Kaposi's sarcoma, and mycosis fungoides. Vincristine is used to treat acute lymphoblastic leukemia, Hodgkin's and non-Hodgkin's lymphomas, rhabdomyosarcoma, neuroblastoma, Wilms' tumor, and various other carcinomas.

Pharmacokinetics

Both drugs are administered intravenously and do not cross the blood-brain barrier. They are highly tissue bound with a triphasic half-life of 3.7 minutes, 1.6 hours, and 25 hours for vinblastine and 0.07 hour, 2.27 hours, and 85 hours for vincristine. They are metabolized in the liver and excreted primarily in bile.

Drug interactions

Both drugs may have significant drug interactions with probenecid (Benemid), sulfinpyrazone (Anturane), and live virus vaccines. See mechlorethamine above. In addition, vinblastine and to a lesser extent vincristine, have a drug interaction with bone marrow suppressants and radiation therapy (see mechlorethamine above).

In addition, the following interactions may occur when vincristine is given with the drugs listed below:

Drug	Possible effect and management
asparaginase (Elspar)	When given concurrently with vincristine, an increase in neurotoxicity may result. To reduce the possibility of this interaction, asparaginase should be given only after vincristine is administered, not concurrently or before vincristine.
doxorubicin (Adriamycin)	If administered with vincristine and prednisone, an increase in bone marrow-depressant effects may occur. Avoid or a potentially serious drug interaction may occur.

Color type indicates an unsafe drug combination.

Side effects and adverse reactions

These include neurotoxicity as the major dose-limiting side effect for vincristine, whereas bone marrow suppression is the major undesirable effect for vinblastine.

In addition with vinblastine, muscle pain, nausea, vomiting, hair loss, extravasation at the injection site and cellulitis, hyperuricemia, stomatitis, rectal bleeding, and hemorrhagic colitis have been noted.

Vincristine may also induce anorexia, nausea, vomiting, rash, autonomic toxicity (abdominal cramping, constipation, bed-wetting, increased, decreased or painful urination, orthostatic hypotension, and lack of sweating), hyperuricemia, a progressive neurotoxicity (blurred or double vision, difficulty in walking, drooping eyelids, headache, jaw pain, numbness and pain in fingers and toes, and weakness), and SIADH secretion (see cisplatin). See Table 49-1 for primary indications and major toxicities.

Warnings

Use both drugs with caution in patients with chickenpox (current or recent), herpes zoster, a history of gout or urate kidney stones, infection, and liver function impairment. In addition, use vinblastine with caution in patients that have tumor cell infiltration in bone marrow and use vincristine with caution in patients with leukopenia and neuromuscular disease.

Contraindications

Avoid use in persons with vinblastine or vincristine hypersensitivity.

Dosage and administration

The adult antineoplastic dosage for vinblastine is 0.1 mg/kg IV weekly, adjusting dosages according to tumor size response and leukocyte counts. The vincristine adult dosage is 0.01 to 0.03 mg/kg as a single dose weekly. For various dosage schedules, see a current package insert or drug reference.

MISCELLANEOUS ANTINEOPLASTIC AGENTS

Miscellaneous agents are those that cannot be classified by their mechanism of action into any of the previous groups. In this section, hormones and miscellaneous, cytoprotective, and immunomodulator agents are discussed.

HORMONES

Hormonal agents are used in the treatment of neoplasms sensitive to hormonal growth controls in the body. Their exact mechanism of action against neoplasms is unknown, but apparently they interfere with growth-stimulating receptors on target tissues. Such agents are more selective and less toxic than other antineoplastic medications and include corticosteroids, androgens and antiandrogens, estrogens and antiestrogens, progestins, and gonadotropin-releasing hormone.

Corticosteroids retard lymphocytic proliferations; therefore their greatest value lies in the treatment of lymphocytic leukemias and lymphomas. They are also used in conjunction with radiation therapy to decrease the occurrence of radiation edema in critical areas such as the superior mediastinum, brain, and spinal cord.

Prednisone and dexamethasone are corticosteroids that are often prescribed for patients with cancer. Prednisone has a lympholytic and antiinflammatory effect that is useful in the treatment of leukemias, lymphomas, and breast carcinomas. Steroids, especially dexamethasone, are useful in reducing cerebral edema induced by the increasing growth of a brain tumor or from radiation therapy. Individual drugs belonging to this category are discussed in Chapter 41.

Androgens such as testosterone and fluoxymesterone (Halotestin) are used to treat advanced breast carcinoma if surgery, radiation, and other therapies are inappropriate or ineffective.

Antiandrogens

bicalutamide [bik ah loot′ ah mide] (Casodex)

Bicalutamide competitively inhibits androgens from receptor binding in target tissues. It is indicated in combination with a luteinizing hormone-releasing hormone for treatment of advanced prostate cancer. Clinical trials indicate that it is comparable to flutamide combination therapy in survival time (Olin, 1998).

flutamide [floo′ ta myde] (Eulexin)

An oral antiandrogen product, flutamide inhibits the uptake and/or the binding of androgens at the target site. The result is suppression of ovarian and testicular steroidogenesis, thus inducing a medical castration. It is used in combination with leuprolide (Lupron), a luteinizing hormone-releasing hormone agonist, to treat metastatic prostate carcinomas. This combination has been reported to prolong survival by at least 25% compared with leuprolide therapy alone. Side effects and adverse reactions include diarrhea, impotency, and hepatotoxicity.

nilutamide [nye lut′ amide] (Nilandron)

Nilutamide is an antiandrogen used in conjunction with surgery or chemical castration for the treatment of metastatic prostate cancer. It blocks testosterone effects at the androgen receptor in vitro, while in vivo it interacts with the androgen receptor to prevent normal androgen responses. For maximum effect it must be started on the same day as surgical castration (Olin, 1998).

goserelin [goe′ se rel in] (Zoladex)

A palliative agent used in the treatment of advanced prostate carcinoma, goserelin is also a luteinizing hormone-releasing hormone. It is a potent inhibitor of pituitary gonadotropins; with long-term administration, the serum levels of testosterone usually drop to the range seen in surgically castrated men within 2 to 4 weeks after initiation of drug therapy. A 3.6 mg dose is implanted subcutaneously in the upper abdominal wall every 28 days. Adverse reactions reported generally are related to the lowered testosterone levels and may include hot flashes, sexual dysfunction, and decreased erections.

Estrogens

Estrogens may be used to treat androgen-sensitive prostatic carcinomas or advanced breast carcinoma in postmenopausal women. For example, estrogens such as diethylstilbestrol (DES, Stilphostrol), polyestradiol (Estradurin), ethinyl estradiol (Estinyl), and estramustine (Emcyt) are used to treat advanced prostatic carcinoma. The latter drug is a combination of estradiol and nitrogen mustard that provides both a weak hormone effect and alkylating action. In this combination, estrogen helps to carry the drug into estrogen receptor cells, thus enhancing the nitrogen mustard cytotoxic effects in these cells.

The main precaution in monitoring estramustine therapy is an increased risk of inducing thrombosis, especially in persons with a history of thrombophlebitis or thromboembolic disease. Avoid immunizations unless specifically ordered by the prescriber. The patient and others in the household should avoid immunization with oral poliovirus vaccine.

Estramustine is taken orally (14 mg/kg/day in divided doses), preferably 1 hour before meals with water. Avoid concurrent consumption of milk, dairy products, or any calcium-containing products.

Antiestrogens

tamoxifen [ta mox′ i fen] (Nolvadex, Nolvadex-D ♣)

Tamoxifen is a synthetic antiestrogen preparation with both agonist and antagonist effects that has replaced both androgens and estrogens as the initial approach in breast cancer therapy (Chabner et al, 1996). It is believed to bind to estrogen receptors in breast cancer cells; thus it acts as a competitive inhibitor of estrogen. It is effective for tumors that contain high concentrations of estrogen receptors. In addition, it is an estrogen agonist in the liver, which has desirable effects on serum lipids in postmenopausal women. It also helps to preserve bone mineral density, which may decrease the osteoporosis risk in these women (Robinson et al, 1996).

Side effects and adverse reactions

These include nausea, vomiting, and headache, hot flashes and weight gain in females, and impotency in males. Other rare adverse reactions include an increased risk for endometrial carcinoma, thromboembolism, and ocular toxicity (Robinson et al, 1996).

raloxifene (Evista)

While currently used to prevent postmenopausal osteoporosis, raloxifene (Evista) is also being studied for the treatment of breast cancer. An initial study indicates it may have decreased the number of new breast cancer incidents by 50%, but further studies are necessary to validate these results and to compare raloxifene to tamoxifen (Tarlach, 1998).

toremifene [tor remy′ fen] (Fareston)

Toremifene is an antiestrogen product released in 1998 for the treatment of metastatic breast cancer in postmenopausal women. Toremifene is similar to tamoxifen chemically and has a similar pharmacologic effect. The major difference between the products is that chronic use of large doses of tamoxifen is hepatotoxic in rats whereas toremifene does not produce this effect. Both products have a hypocholesterolemic effect after chronic administration, but the effect of toremifene on bone mineral density, thromboembolic events, and the risk for endometrial cancer is unknown due to the lack of long-term clinical studies (Buzdar, Hortobagyi, 1998).

anastrozole [a nahs′ troe zole] (Arimidex)
testolactone [tes tah lack′ tone] (Teslac)

These agents inhibit steroid aromatase, thus reducing estrone synthesis in the adrenal glands, the major source of estrogen in postmenopausal women. They are indicated for palliative therapy of advanced breast cancer in postmenopausal women. Testolactone is also used in premenopausal women with nonterminated or terminated ovarian function.

Progestins

Progestins such as medroxyprogesterone (Depo-Provera) and megestrol (Megace) are used to treat advanced endometrial cancer. This is primarily a palliative approach that seeks tumor regression and an increase in the patient's survival time. Megesterol is also indicated for advanced carcinoma of the breast, and medroxyprogesterone is also used in patients with advanced renal carcinoma.

Other Agents

altretamine [al tret′ a meen] (Hexalen)

Altretamine is a cytotoxic agent for the palliative treatment of persistent or recurrent ovarian cancer. Its mechanism of action is unknown although chemically it resembles the alkylating agents. Clinically, however, it is effective for ovarian tumors that are resistant to the previously marketed alkylating agents. Side effects and adverse reactions include nausea and vomiting, neurotoxicity, myelosuppression, and central nervous system (CNS) changes (ataxia, dizziness, and mood alterations). The most significant drug interactions to avoid include cimetidine (increases half-life of altretamine) and monoamine oxidase (MAO) inhibitors (severe hypotension).

topotecan [to poe′ ti kan] (Hycamtin)

Topotecan, a topoisomerase inhibitor, is indicated for the treatment of relapsed or refractory metastatic carcinoma of the ovary after failure of other therapies. Its action may be due to inhibition of topoisomerase activity in DNA during DNA synthesis. This product should only be administered to women with adequate bone marrow reserves, that is, neutrophil counts of at least 1500 cells/mm^3 and platelet counts of 100,000/mm^3 or greater. Side effects and adverse reactions include neutropenia (a dose-limiting toxicity), leukopenia, thrombocytopenia, anemia, headache, diarrhea, stomach pain, nausea, vomiting, alopecia, tiredness, dyspnea, and neuromuscular pain. The usual dose is 1.5 mg/m^2 by IV infusion over 30 minutes daily for 5 days. See a current package insert for detailed information on this product.

MISCELLANEOUS AGENTS

asparaginase [a spare′ a gi nase] (Elspar, Kidrolase ♣)

Asparaginase reduces asparagine to aspartic acid in the body. Asparagine is necessary for cell survival, and because normal body cells are capable of synthesizing adequate supplies of asparaginase, they are not affected by an asparaginase deficiency. Certain cancer cells, however, depend on a circulating supply of asparaginase within the blood and when it is decreased, cancer cells will die. Asparaginase is used to treat acute lymphocytic leukemia. Side effects and adverse reactions include hyperammonemia (headache, anorexia, nausea, vomiting, and abdominal cramps), a decrease in the blood clotting factors, allergic reactions, liver toxicity, pancreatitis, and anaphylaxis.

cladribine [kla dri been′] (Leustatin)

Cladribine is used to treat hairy cell leukemia. Cladribine enters the cell and is phosphorylated to a deoxyadenosine concentration that accumulates in these cells, interfering with DNA repair and eventually resulting in cell death. Side effects and adverse reactions include severe anemia, infection, skin rash, bleeding or bruising, anorexia, headache, nausea, vomiting, and fatigue.

dacarbazine [da kar′ ba zeen] (DTIC-Dome)

Dacarbazine is a cell cycle-nonspecific agent that inhibits DNA and RNA synthesis and appears to be more active in the late G_2-phase of the cell cycle. It is indicated for the treatment of malignant melanoma and Hodgkin's disease. Side effects and adverse reactions include a flu-like syndrome, anorexia, nausea, vomiting, and diarrhea.

docetaxel [dok i tax′ el] (Taxotere)

Docetaxel is a taxoid, that is, a semisynthetic product originating from the yew plant. It may produce its effect by binding and stabilizing microtubule bundles, thus inhibiting cell mitosis. It is indicated for the treatment of advanced breast cancer. Side effects and adverse reactions include bone marrow suppression, nausea, diarrhea, stomatitis, fever, skin reactions, and myalgia.

gemcitabine [gem sit′ a been] (Gemzar)

Gemcitabine interferes with cell synthesis (S-phase) and also blocks cell progression through the G_1/S-phase of the cycle. It is indicated for treatment of adenocarcinoma of the pancreas in persons with nonresectable or metastatic pancreatic cancer who have been previously treated with 5-FU. Side effects and adverse reactions include dyspnea, peripheral edema, a flu-like syndrome, nausea, vomiting, diarrhea, rash, paresthesia, and stomatitis. Gemcitabine is administered intravenously; the adult dose is 1000 mg/m^2 given over 30 minutes. See current literature for additional information (Olin, 1998).

hydroxyurea [hye drox ee yoo ree′ ah] (Hydrea)

Hydroxyurea inhibits DNA synthesis without affecting the synthesis of RNA or protein. It is indicated for the treatment of head, neck, and ovarian carcinoma, chronic myelocytic leukemia, and malignant melanoma. Side effects and adverse reactions include bone marrow suppression, diarrhea, anorexia, nausea, vomiting, and drowsiness.

irinotecan [i rin′ oe tek an] (Camptosar)

Irinotecan is the first of a new class of oncolytic agents indicated for the treatment of metastatic colorectal cancer or rectal cancer that has occurred or progressed after 5-FU chemotherapy. This product is a topoisomerase 1 inhibitor that binds to the topoisomerase 1-DNA complex, resulting in double-stranded DNA breaks that cause tumor cell death. Irinotecan may cause severe diarrhea, which requires immediate treatment with loperamide (Imodium). Severe myelosuppression, nausea, and vomiting may also occur (Camptosar, 1996).

levamisole [lee vam′ i sol] (Ergamisol)

A biologic response modifier (immunostimulant), levamisole is used in combination with 5-FU to treat colorectal carcinoma (Dukes C adenocarcinoma). This combination has resulted in an increased survival time (decreased mortality) and decreased risk of cancer recurrence. Significant side effects and adverse reactions include bone marrow suppression, nausea, diarrhea, a metallic taste, arthralgia, and a flu-like syndrome.

mitotane [mye′ toe tane] (Lysodren)

Mitotane is an adrenal gland-suppressing agent indicated for the treatment of an inoperable carcinoma of the adrenal cortex. Administered orally, it is distributed throughout the body but is mainly stored in fat. The onset of effect is reported within 48 to 72 hours of starting therapy; tumor response is usually within 6 weeks. Significant side effects and adverse reactions include adrenal gland insufficiency, dark skin, diarrhea, anorexia, depression, nausea, vomiting, weakness, drowsiness, and lightheadedness.

paclitaxel [pa kli tax′ el] (Taxol)

A natural substance extracted from the yew tree, paclitaxel is marketed for the treatment of metastatic ovarian cancer refractory to other drug treatments. It is an antimicrotubule agent that stabilizes microtubule bundles, therefore interfering with the late G_2-phase of the mitotic cell cycle and resulting in inhibition of cell replication. It is also used for the treatment of metastatic breast cancer, and some studies indicate it should be used earlier, such as immediately after surgery, as it then produces better effects than chemotherapy alone (Tarlach, 1998). Side effects and adverse reactions include severe allergic reactions (prevented by pretreatment with a steroid and an H_1 and H_2 antagonist), bone marrow suppression, peripheral neuropathy, muscle pain, alopecia, and gastric distress.

pegaspargase [peg as′ per gase] (Oncaspar)

Pegaspargase is a modification of the L-asparaginase enzyme that is used in combination chemotherapies for acute lymphoblastic leukemia in persons unable to take L-asparaginase. Side effects and adverse reactions include hypersensitivity reactions, hepatotoxicity, and coagulopathies.

procarbazine [pro kar′ ba zeen] (Matulane)

Procarbazine is an alkylating agent and a weak MAO inhibitor that is cell cycle-specific for the S-phase of cell division. It is believed to inhibit DNA, RNA, and protein synthesis. It is commonly prescribed for the treatment of Hodgkin's disease. Side effects and adverse reactions include bone marrow suppression, pneumonitis, nausea, vomiting, weakness, drowsiness, myalgia, muscle twitching, insomnia, nightmares, and increased nervousness.

tretinoin [tret′ i noyn] (Vesanoid)

Vesanoid is a retinoid that appears to enhance maturation of primitive promyelocytes from the leukemic clone, which is followed by reseeding the bone marrow and blood with normal blood cells. It is used to treat acute promyelocytic leukemia. Side effects and adverse reactions include headaches, fever, increased weakness, malaise, shivering, infections, hemorrhage, and peripheral edema.

CYTOPROTECTIVE COMBINATIONS

An antineoplastic drug combination is ifosfamide [eye foss′ fa mide] (IFEX) with mesna [mess′ na] (Mesnex). This product is used for the treatment of germ cell testicular tumors. Ifosfamide, an alkylating agent, has been studied since the early 1970s, but its adverse effect of hemorrhagic cystitis (urotoxicity) has limited its usefulness. Mesna has been discovered to be a specific antidote for this type of toxicity. Thus using both drugs in combination allows for more aggressive therapy, while reducing the potential of ifosfamide-induced hematuria and cystitis.

Amifostine [am i foss′ teen] (Ethyol) is a cytoprotective agent administered before cisplatin to reduce the potential for renal toxicity. Dexrazoxane [dex ra zock′ zain] (Zinecard) is a cardioprotective substance used with doxorubicin administration to reduce drug-induced cardiomyopathy. It is an intracellular chelating agent although its mechanism of action is not clearly defined. There are some reports that the use of this product with the 5-FU, doxorubicin (Adriamycin), and cyclophosphamide (FAC) regimen used to treat breast cancer resulted in a lower response rate to therapy. For this reason, it was recommended that dextrazoxane be used only in individuals who have received the cumulative 300 mg/m^2 dose of doxorubicin and are continuing on this product (Olin, 1998). Side effects and adverse reactions include myelosuppression effects of alopecia, nausea, vomiting, tiredness, anorexia, stomatitis, fever, diarrhea, neurotoxicity, phlebitis, and dysphagia. See a current package insert for detailed dosing and other information.

IMMUNOMODULATOR AGENTS

Interferons

Interferon alfa-2a, recombinant (Roferon-A), and interferon alfa-2b, recombinant (Intron A), are manufactured by the process of recombinant DNA technology, resulting in highly purified proteins that have an effect similar to the interferon alfa subtypes produced by human leukocytes.

Interferons are released by the body in response to viral infections or substances that induce their release. Interferons have antiviral (inhibit virus replication), antiproliferative (decrease cell proliferation), and immunomodulatory (enhance phagocyte activity and assist the cytotoxicity properties of lymphocytes for target cells) properties. Their mechanism of action as antineoplastic agents is unknown but may be the result of one or more of the three properties identified. For example, in some types of cancer, interferon appears to have a dual effect of both cytotoxic and immune stimulation. Some patients demonstrate an increase in hematologic factors, granulocytes, platelets, and hemoglobin serum levels.

Interferon alfa-2a and alfa-2b are indicated for the treatment of hairy cell leukemia, genital warts, acquired immunodeficiency syndrome (AIDS)-related Kaposi's sarcoma, bladder cancer, and chronic active hepatitis. Toxicities reported include a flu-like syndrome that includes fever, chills, muscle pain, loss of appetite, and lethargy. At higher doses, myelosuppression, nausea, vomiting, neurotoxicity, and cardiotoxicity may occur. For additional information, see the section on drugs affecting the immunologic system in Chapter 56.

aldesleukin [al dess loo′ kin] (Proleukin, interleukin 2)

Aldesleukin is another cytokine biologic product that stimulates immune function and is nearly identical in chemical structure and action to human interleukin 2. It is indicated for the treatment of renal cell carcinoma. This substance appears to stimulate T cell proliferation and is a cofactor in developing cytotoxic T lymphocyte activity against tumors. Its cytotoxic action may be caused by its enhancing growth of the body's natural killer cells and the lymphokine-activated killer cells. Side effects and adverse effects of aldesleukin include edema, anemia, thrombocytopenia, and hypotension.

granulocyte-macrophage colony-stimulating factor (GM-CSF; sargramostim) *granulocyte colony-stimulating factor* (G-CSF; filgrastim [Neupogen])

Granulocyte-macrophage colony-stimulating factor (GM-CSF; sargramostim) and granulocyte colony-stimulating factor (G-CSF; filgrastim, [Neupogen]) are immunomodulator agents with a variety of approved and investigational uses. GM-CSF is used to accelerate myeloid recovery in persons with acute lymphoblastic anemic, Hodgkin's disease, and non-Hodgkin's lymphoma undergoing bone marrow transplantation. Complete blood counts are performed to monitor the hematologic response to this drug. Investigationally this drug has been used to increase white blood cell counts in AIDS patients receiving zidovudine (AZT) and to correct neutropenia in aplastic anemia. Closely monitor patients who are receiving lithium or corticosteroids concurrently because the myeloproliferative action of this drug may be increased.

G-CSF (Neupogen)

G-CSF (Neupogen) is used to decrease the potential for infection in persons receiving myelosuppressive agents that are associated with severe neutropenia and fever. Neutrophil counts are closely monitored; the drug should be discontinued when the absolute neutrophil count is 10,000/mm^3 or more after the nadir induced by the chemotherapy. The major side effects and adverse reactions include nausea, vomiting, hair loss, diarrhea, fevers, mucositis, anorexia, and fatigue. Bone pain has been reported about 2 to 3 days before the increase in neutrophil count. This pain is usually controlled with nonopioid-type analgesics. The usual starting dose is 5 μg/kg/day by SC or IV injection.

rituximab [re tux′ e mab] (Rituxan)

Rituximab is a genetically made monoclonal antibody that is directed against an antigen (CD20) located on the surface of both normal and malignant B lymphocytes. The CD20 antigen governs the early steps in cell cycle initiation and differentiation, and it is found on >90% of B cell non-Hodgkin's lymphomas. It is indicated for the treatment of patients who have relapsed or have a refractory low-grade or follicular, CD20-positive, B-cell, non-Hodgkin's lymphoma. Side effects and adverse reactions include fever, chills, weakness, headache, angioedema, hypotension, myalgia, nausea, vomiting, leukopenia, pruritus, and rash.

CANCER CHEMOTHERAPY RESEARCH

Cancer chemotherapy research is a priority area of study in the United States and Canada. Many new drugs are being studied with the hope of improving the treatment and survival of cancer patients and patients with AIDS-induced cancer (AIDS is reviewed in Chapter 56). The reader is encouraged to monitor professional literature for information on the release of new drugs for the treatment of cancer and for other related research.

Another promising area of study is liposomes as a delivery system to hold lipid-soluble drugs. Drugs encapsulated in a liposome capsule can be distributed differently in the body than free drugs. Liposomes accumulate at sites of inflammation and infection, as well as in some solid tumors. Thus they are under study for the treatment of systemic fungal infections (amphotericin B) and for the treatment of specific cancers. Doxorubicin (Adriamycin), cisplatin (Platinol), and methotrexate (Folex) are just a few of the antineoplastic agents currently undergoing clinical testing. Doxorubicin in liposome administration has been reported to deliver the drug more directly to the site of action, resulting in fewer cardiac and other side effects and adverse reactions. Cisplatin in liposomes has been reported to cause much less kidney damage than cisplatin alone. If studies of liposome drug therapy continue to report that in addition to a decrease in side effects and adverse reactions, the therapeutic outcome is also efficacious, then the potential exists for liposomes to be an exciting new avenue of drug delivery in the next few years.

Another drug in phase III trials is trastuzumab (Herceptin), a drug that treats a protein produced by an altered gene (known as HER-2/neu) found in approximately 30% of women with breast cancer. This gene-produced protein triggers tumor growth by inducing overproduction of the growth-stimulating hormones; therefore it produces a very aggressive cancer. Herceptin is an anti-HER-2 monoclonal antibody that slows breast cancer progression and increases tumor reduction in women with this altered gene (Tarlach, 1998).

See Box 49-1 for investigational drug classifications.

BOX 49-1 Investigational Drug Classifications

Investigational drugs are agents that have not been released for marketing by the Food and Drug Administration. While responsibility for regulating drugs rests with the FDA, the National Cancer Institute (NCI) is the largest developer of antineoplastic agents in the United States. The NCI has established stringent regulations to monitor the receipt, use, and disposal of investigational drugs. It also requires that investigators report adverse reactions on an established time schedule. For example, anaphylactic reactions to an investigational drug must be reported by phoning a specific branch office that is available on a 24-hour basis. This call must be followed up with a written report within 10 working days.

Investigational drugs are divided into three groups:

	Drug Group	Purpose
Phase I	A	To determine maximum tolerated dosage To detect toxicities associated with various dosage schedules To determine pharmacokinetics and optimum dosing schedule
Phase II	B	To identify antineoplastic activity in specific cancers affecting humans To determine patient's response to various drug dosages and schedules
Phase III	C	New agent now compared with previously marketed drugs to ascertain effectiveness, effect on quality of life, and mortality, and morbidity

SUMMARY

The use of antineoplastic agents in the treatment of cancer is based on the individual drug's effects in interfering with cell reproduction or replication at some point in the cell cycle. These drugs are classified according to their potential mechanisms of action: antimetabolites, alkylating agents, mitotic inhibitors, antibiotic antitumor agents, hormones, cytoprotective and immunomodulator agents, and miscellaneous agents. Antineoplastic medications are usually nonselective; therefore they can affect normal body cells, especially those with a high rate of growth, such as those in the GI tract, bone marrow, and hair follicles. As a result, these very potent drugs may cause many side effects and, at times, serious adverse reactions. A thorough knowledge of these drugs is necessary for safe administration and monitoring of patients.

REVIEW QUESTIONS

1. Describe the reason(s) why live virus vaccines should not be administered to patients receiving antineoplastic drug therapy.
2. What is leucovorin, its primary indications, and leucovorin rescue?
3. Name the primary indications for cyclophosphamide and a method of reducing the adverse effects of hemorrhagic cystitis.
4. What is the major toxicity with the use of doxorubicin? What effect does daunorubicin have on this toxicity and how can it be managed?
5. What is the dose-limiting toxicity with the use of vincristine? Describe the progressive toxicity.

REFFERENCES

Buzdar AU, Hortobagyi, GN: Tamoxifen and toremifene in breast cancer: comparison of safety and efficacy. *J Clin Oncol* 16(1):348-353, 1998, http://www.medscape.com/server-java/MedPage?med98-99+97360+(tamoxifen+drug+review+) (April 18, 1998).

Camptosar, package insert, #816 907 000, 1996, Pharmacia and Upjohn.

Chabner BA, Allegra CJ, Curt GA, Calabresi P: Antineoplastic agents. In Hardman JG, Limbird LE, editors: *Goodman & Gilman's the pharmacological basis of therapeutics,* ed 9, New York, 1996, McGraw-Hill.

Olin BR: *Facts and comparisons.* Philadelphia, 1998, JB Lippincott.

Robinson E, Kimmick GG, Muss HB: Tamoxifen in postmenopausal women: a safety perspective, *Drugs Aging* 8(5):329-337, 1996, http://www.medscape.com/server-java/MedPage?med95-97+593452+(tamoxif en+drug+review) (April 18, 1998).

Tarlach GM: New advances hold promise in battle against cancer, *Hosp Pharmacist Rep* 12(6):17, 20, 1998.

ADDITIONAL REFERENCES

American Hospital Formulary Service: *AHFS drug information '98,* Bethesda, Md, 1998, American Society of Hospital Pharmacists.

Anderson KN et al, editors: *Mosby's medical, nursing, and allied health dictionary,* ed 5, St Louis, 1998, Mosby.

Mosby: *Mosby's GenRx,* St Louis, 1998, Mosby.

Patterson W, Perry MC: Chemotherapeutic toxicities: a comprehensive overview, *Contemp Oncol* 3(7):56-64, 1993.

United States Pharmacopeial Convention: *USP DI: drug information for the health care professional,* ed 18, Rockville, Md, 1998, The Convention.

UNIT XIV

Drugs Used in Infectious Diseases and Inflammation

CHAPTER 50

Overview of Infections, Inflammation, and Fever

CHAPTER FOCUS

Fever, inflammation, and infection have been a concern to those caring for the ill and injured since ancient times. The majority of patients have experienced these symptoms, not only as a direct result of their injuries or illnesses, but also as the indirect consequence of multiple invasive devices, surgical procedures, and immunosuppression. Healthcare professionals have the responsibility of assessment, palliation of symptoms, and evaluation of therapies with these patients. The following key terms and objectives are important for a good understanding of this chapter.

OBJECTIVES

After reading and studying this chapter, the student should be able to do the following:

1. *Define and describe the key terms*
2. *Describe the inflammatory response to injured tissue.*
3. *Define and describe complement and its effects.*
4. *Explain the body temperature regulation mechanism.*
5. *Identify and describe the five different types of fever.*
6. *Relate the goal and various mechanisms of action for antimicrobial therapy.*
7. *Describe antimicrobial agent-induced allergic or hypersensitivity reactions.*

KEY TERMS

bacteremia, (p. 640)
bactericidal agents, (p. 644)
bacteriostatic agents, (p. 644)
colonization, (p. 640)
infection, (p. 640)
inflammation, (p. 640)
microorganisms, (p. 640)
phagocytosis, (p. 640)
resistance, (p. 646)
sepsis, (p. 640)
septicemia, (p. 640)
superinfection, (p. 645)

INFECTIONS

Infectious diseases comprise a wide spectrum of illnesses caused by pathogenic microorganisms. Some common pathogens and their most likely sites of infection in the body are listed in Table 50-1. These pathogens cause pneumonia, urinary tract infections, upper respiratory tract infections, gastroenteritis, venereal disease, vaginitis, tuberculosis, and candidiasis.

Infection, the invasion and multiplication of pathogenic microorganisms in body tissues causing disease by local cellular injury, secretion of a toxin, or antigen-antibody reaction in the host, is classified primarily as either local or systemic. A localized infection involving the skin or internal organs may progress to a systemic infection. A systemic infection involves the whole body rather than a localized area of the body. Several terms describe the degree of local or systemic infection.

Colonization is the localized presence of microorganisms in body tissues or organs, which can be pathogenic or part of the normal flora. Colonization alone is not necessarily an infection but rather it signifies the potential for infection depending on the multiplication of the microorganisms or an alteration in the individual's host defense mechanisms. When flora at its normal colonization site is altered (e.g., by the administration of an antibiotic that affects pathogens and some but not all normal microorganisms), unaffected microorganisms within that environment may grow uninhibited and cause a secondary infection.

Inflammation is a protective mechanism of body tissues in response to invasion or toxins produced by colonizing microorganisms. This reaction consists of cytologic and histologic tissue responses for the localization of phagocytic activity and destruction or removal of injurious material leading to repair and healing.

Bacteremia is the presence of viable bacteria in the circulatory system. **Septicemia** refers to a systemic infection caused by microorganism multiplication in the circulation. Although bacteremia may lead to septicemia in the immunocompromised host, it is (depending on the pathogen) usually a short-lived, self-limited process. In the immunocompromised host, bacteremia may rapidly produce an overwhelming systemic disease. **Sepsis** is a syndrome involving multiple system organ involvement that is a result of microorganisms or their toxins circulating in the blood.

For nonpathogenic organisms colonizing humans or causing transient bacteremias without tissue invasion, antibiotic therapy is rarely required in the immunocompetent host, whereas prophylactic antibiotic therapy may be required in immunocompromised hosts. In most cases of localized inflammation, such as wound infections, pneumonia, or urinary tract infections, antimicrobials reduce the number of viable pathogens. This permits the immune system to eliminate microorganisms. Antimicrobials are also an essential part of the treatment of septicemia and sepsis.

Microorganisms are divided into several groups: bacteria, mycoplasmas, spirochetes, fungi, and viruses. Bacteria are classified according to their shape, such as bacilli, spirilla, and cocci, and their capacity to be stained. Specific identification of bacteria requires a Gram stain and culture with chemical testing. A Gram stain is a sequential procedure involving crystal violet and iodine solutions followed by alcohol, which allows the rapid identification of organisms into groups, such as gram-positive or gram-negative rods or cocci. The culture procedures identify specific organisms, but they require 24 to 48 hours for completion.

Often the initial or empiric antibiotic selection is based on the prescriber's clinical impression plus the Gram stain procedure; the antibiotic may be changed once culture and sensitivity results are available.

INFLAMMATION

Inflammation is the reaction of body tissues to injury, such as physical trauma, foreign bodies, chemical substances, surgery, radiation, and electricity. The area affected will undergo a series of changes as the body processes attempt to wall off, heal, and/or replace the injured tissue. For example, after an injury occurs, the body will release chemical substances into the tissue that form a wall called a chemotactic gradient. Fluids and cells will begin to move toward this area.

Blood vessels dilate within 30 minutes of the insult, which provides for an increase in blood flow and exudation of fluid from blood vessels into the injured tissues. The exudate includes protein-rich fluids high in fibrinogen that will attract other substances to the area, such as complement, antibodies, and leukocytes. Fluids collecting in this area will result in edema or swelling. Generally, this occurs within 4 hours of the injury.

During the cellular phase, granulocytes will migrate to the area from the dilated blood vessels at the site. The granulocytes will migrate toward the chemotactic site and accumulate in the area of injury. If the injury is a foreign substance or bacteria, they will engulf and destroy the foreign material (**phagocytosis**). Neutrophils, monocytes (macrophages), and lymphocytes (which arrive later) are the granulocytes that affect the injured area. The phagocytosis process tends to localize or wall off the foreign material to prevent its spread through the tissues. Large numbers of phagocytes lead to pus accumulation and the eventual destruction and removal of the foreign material.

Some pathogens are resistant to destruction and are only walled off, such as tuberculosis bacilli, which can live for many years within the confined cells in the body. Others may transform from a local infection into a systemic infection, thus requiring antimicrobial or antibiotic treatment.

MEDIATORS OF THE INFLAMMATORY SYSTEM

The complement system is composed of complement components (18 distinct proteins and their cleavage products) present in the blood in the form of inactive proteins called zymogens. Complement is essential in responding to an

TABLE 50-1 Primary Organisms and Common Sites of Infection

Organism	*Infection Site*
Gram-Positive Cocci	
Staphylococcus aureus Non-penicillinase producing Penicillinase producing *Staphylococcus epidermidis* Non-penicillinase producing Penicillinase producing Methicillin resistant	Burns, skin infections, decubital and surgical wounds, paranasal sinus and middle ear (chronic sinusitis and otitis), lungs, lung abscess, pleura, endocardium, bone (osteomyelitis), joints
Streptococcus pneumoniae	Paranasal sinus and middle ear, lungs, pleura
Streptococcus pyogenes (group A β-hemolytic)	Burns, skin infections, decubitus and surgical wounds, paranasal sinus and middle ear, throat, bone (osteomyelitis), joints
Streptococcus, viridans group	Endocardium
Gram-Positive Bacilli	
Clostridium tetani (anaerobe)	Puncture wounds, lacerations, and crush injuries; toxins affecting nervous system
Corynebacterium diphtheriae	Throat, upper part of the respiratory tract
Gram-Negative Cocci	
Neisseria gonorrhoeae	Urethra, prostate, epididymis and testes, joints
Neisseria meningitidis	Meninges
Enteric Gram-Negative Bacilli	
As a group (*Bacteroides, Enterobacter, Escherichia coli, Klebsiella pneumoniae, Proteus mirabilis,* other *Proteus, Salmonella, Serratia, Shigella)*	Peritoneum, biliary tract, kidney and bladder, prostate, decubital and surgical wounds, bone
Bacteroides	Brain abscess, lung abscess, throat, peritoneum
Enterobacter	Peritoneum, biliary tract, kidney and bladder, endocardium
Escherichia coli	Peritoneum, biliary tract, kidney and bladder
Klebsiella pneumoniae	Lungs, lung abscess
Other Gram-Negative Bacilli	
Haemophilus influenzae	Meninges, paranasal sinus and middle ear, lungs, pleura
Pseudomonas aeruginosa	Burns, paranasal sinus and middle ear (chronic otitis media), decubital and surgical wounds, lungs, joints
Acid-Fast Bacilli	
Mycobacterium tuberculosis *Mycobacterium avium*	Lungs, pleura, peritoneum, meninges, kidney and bladder, testes, bone, joints
Mycoplasmas	
Mycoplasma pneumoniae	Lungs
Spirochetes	
Treponema pallidum (syphilis)	Any tissue or vascular organ of the body
Fungi	
Aspergillus	Paranasal sinus and middle ear, lungs
Candida species	Skin infections, throat, lungs, endocardium, kidney and bladder, vagina
Cryptococcus	
Viruses	
Herpes virus or varicella-zoster virus	Skin infections (herpes simplex or zoster)
Enterovirus, mumps virus, and others	Meninges, epididymis, and testes
Respiratory viruses (including Epstein-Barr virus)	Throat, lungs
Anaerobes	
Gram-positive *Clostridium difficile* *Clostridium perfringens* *Peptococcus* species *Peptostreptococcus* species Gram-negative *Bacteroides fragilis* *Fusobacterium* species	Deep wounds, gut

acute inflammatory reaction caused by bacteria, some viruses, and immune complex diseases. Complement enhances chemotaxis, increases blood vessel permeability, and eventually causes cell lysis.

Histamine, prostaglandins, arachidonic acid, and leukotrienes are other mediators capable of producing local reactions, smooth muscle contraction, increased chemotaxis, blood vessel vasodilation, and other inflammatory effects. When the foreign agent is destroyed, the resulting debris will be removed by the macrophages and neutrophils, thus resolving the inflammatory reaction.

FEVER

The hypothalamus sets the point at which body temperature is maintained, but body temperature regulation depends on a balance between the heat production and loss. Fever may be the result of infection or an inflammatory process. It may be caused by the release of endogenous pyrogens from the macrophages. These pyrogens, or fever-producing substances, will interfere with the temperature-regulating centers located in the hypothalamus, raising the thermostat set point. The body may respond to the pyrogens by increasing cytokine formation, which in turn increases the synthesis of prostaglandin E_2, which then increases the hypothalamic set point (Insel, 1996). The body will react by conserving heat through vasoconstriction, piloerection (goose flesh), and shivering—all factors that increase the body temperature.

The normal body temperature is 98.6 °F (37 °C), and the normal range is 97 °F to approximately 99 °F when measured orally. Rectally, a person's body temperature is 1 °F higher than orally. Hyperthermia occurs when the body's temperature rises above normal. When the body temperature reaches 106 °F, convulsions may result. If the body's thermoregulatory mechanisms have trouble returning the body temperature to a normal setting, body metabolism may increase so rapidly that the body cannot regulate its own heat production. At 108 °F tissue damage occurs, and cells begin to die, resulting in irreversible brain damage.

Several types of fever are known. For example, a constant fever rises or falls only a few degrees above or below a specified point; an example is typhoid fever. An intermittent fever may return to normal once or several times in 24 hours. This type of fever is associated with pyogenic infections, abscesses, lymphomas, tuberculosis, and drug reactions. A remittent fever fluctuates but does not usually return to normal; this occurs in many viral and bacterial infections. Relapsing fever consists of afebrile episodes of one or more days between fevers, such as in malaria and Hodgkin's disease.

Fever of unknown origin (FUO) has been described as a temperature greater than 103 °F recorded daily for more than 2 weeks in a person with an uncertain diagnosis after a week's evaluation in a hospital setting. Most patients with FUO are later found to have an infection, neoplasm, or connective tissue disease.

Body temperature is regulated by nervous system feedback mechanisms through a temperature-regulating center in the hypothalamus. When the hypothalamus is no longer in contact with the pyrogens, it will reset the temperature to the normal set point. Prostaglandins of the E series produced in response to endogenous pyrogens act on the anterior hypothalamus to increase the set point, resulting in fever. Drugs that inhibit the synthesis of E prostaglandins have antipyretic activity (acetaminophen and salicylates). For example, salicylates reduce raised body temperatures by causing the hypothalamic center to reestablish a normal set point. Heat production will not be inhibited, although heat loss will be increased by an increase in cutaneous blood flow and sweating, caused by the lowered thermostat (Fig. 50-1). Antibiotics indirectly reduce temperature by destroying the bacteria causing the fever.

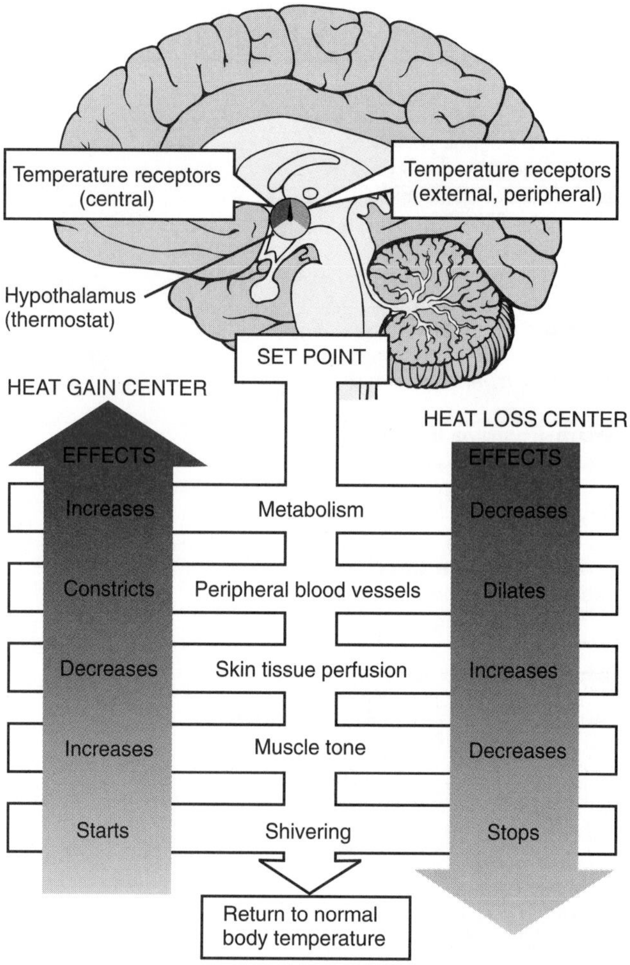

FIGURE 50-1
Set point temperature mechanism.

ANTIMICROBIAL THERAPY

The treatment of an infectious disease depends on the microorganism group; different groups of antimicrobial agents are used to treat different groups of microorganisms. Table 50-2 lists some antimicrobial agents used in the treatment

TABLE 50-2 Antimicrobial Drugs of Choice

Organism	***Drug(s)***
Gram-Positive Cocci	
Staphylococcus aureus	
Non-penicillinase producing	penicillin G or V, first-generation cephalosporins, vancomycin
Penicillinase producing	first-generation cephalosporins, cloxacillin, dicloxacillin, methicillin
Methicillin resistant	vancomycin ± gentamicin ± rifampin
Streptococcus pneumoniae	penicillin G or V
Streptococcus pyogenes (group A)	penicillin G or V
Streptococcus (group B)	penicillin G, ampicillin
Streptococcus viridans	penicillin G ± gentamicin
Gram-Positive Bacilli	
Bacillus anthracis	penicillin G, erythromycin
Corynebacterium diphtheriae	erythromycin
Corynebacterium, JK strain	vancomycin, erythromycin
Listeria monocytogenes	amikacin, gentamicin
Gram-Negative Cocci	
Neisseria gonorrhoeae	ceftriaxone, cifixime
Neisseria meningitidis	penicillin G, cefotaxime
Gram-Negative Enteric Bacilli	
Escherichia coli	cefotaxime, ceftizoxime
Klebsiella pneumoniae	same as *E coli*
Proteus mirabilis	ampicillin, cephalosporin
Salmonella species	ceftriaxone, fluoroquinolone
Other Bacilli	
Pseudomonas aeruginosa	fluoroquinolone, carbenicillin
Anaerobes	
Gram-positive	
Clostridium difficile	metronidazole
Clostridium perfringens	penicillin G, metronidazole
Clostridium tetani	penicillin G, tetracycline
Gram-negative	
Bacteroides (gastrointestinal strains)	metronidazole, clindamycin
Mycoplasmas	
Mycoplasma pneumoniae	erythromycin, tetracycline, clarithyromycin
Spirochetes	
Treponema pallidum (syphilis)	penicillin G
Fungi	
Aspergillus, Candida species	amphotericin B, fluconazole, itraconazole
Viruses	
Herpes simplex	vidarabine, acyclovir

of infectious diseases. Antimicrobial drugs can help cure or control most infections caused by microorganisms but they alone do not necessarily produce the cure. They are adjuncts to methods such as surgical incision and drainage and wound debridement for removal of nonviable infected tissue.

The first major antimicrobial agents were the sulfonamides while the second group of antimicrobials were true antibiotics such as penicillin. Antibiotics are natural substances derived from certain organisms (bacteria, fungus, and others) that are used against infections caused by other organisms. As a result of research, there are now many synthetic and semisynthetic antibiotics. Other antimicrobial agents include the urinary tract antiseptics and the antimycobacterial, antifungal, and antiviral agents.

Mechanism of action

The goal of antimicrobial therapy is to destroy or to suppress the growth of infecting microorganisms so that normal host defense and other supporting mechanisms can control the infection, resulting in its cure. To exert their effects, antimicrobial agents must first gain access to target sites. Usually this can be accomplished by absorption and distribution of the drug into and by way of the circulatory system. More specific antibiotics or antimicrobial agents are capable of penetrating to the site and having an affinity for the bacterial target proteins. Sometimes, as in the case of infections of the skin and eyes, local application to the infected area may be necessary. Once the drug has reached its site of action, it can have bactericidal or bacteriostatic effects, depending on its mechanisms of action.

Bacteriostatic agents inhibit bacterial growth, allowing host defense mechanisms additional time to remove the invading microorganisms. **Bactericidal agents,** on the other hand, cause bacterial cell death and lysis. Antimicrobial agents may be divided into bacteriostatic and bactericidal categories, with the sulfonamides as an example of the former and the penicillins the latter. Such categorization is not always valid or reliable, however, because the same antimicrobial agent may have either effect depending on the dose administered and the concentration achieved at its site of action. Tetracycline, for example, is generally bacteriostatic but may be bactericidal in high concentrations. Chloramphenicol, which is often listed as a bacteriostatic drug, has bactericidal effects against *Streptococcus pneumoniae* and *Haemophilus influenzae* in the cerebrospinal fluid.

Antimicrobial agents may exert their bacteriostatic or bactericidal effects in one of four major ways:

1. Inhibit bacteria cell wall synthesis. Unlike host cells, bacteria are not isotonic with body fluids; thus their contents are under high osmotic pressure and their viability depends on the integrity of the cell walls. Any compound that inhibits any step in the synthesis of this cell wall causes it to be weakened and the cell to lyse. Antimicrobial agents having this mechanism of action are bactericidal.
2. Disrupt or alter membrane permeability, resulting in leakage of essential bacterial metabolic substrates. Agents causing the effects can be either bacteriostatic or bactericidal.
3. Inhibit protein synthesis. Antimicrobial agents may induce the formation of defective protein molecules; such agents are bactericidal in their action. Antimicrobial agents that inhibit specific steps in protein synthesis are bacteriostatic.
4. Inhibit synthesis of essential metabolites. Antimicrobial agents that work in this manner structurally resemble physiologic compounds and act as competitive inhibitors in a metabolic pathway. Generally, they are bacteriostatic agents. (Box 50-1)

BOX 50-1 Antimicrobials: Classification by Mechanism of Action

Inhibit Cell Wall Synthesis
penicillins
cephalosporins
vancomycin
bacitracin
cycloserine

Alter Membrane Permeability
amphotericin B
nystatin
polymyxin
colistin

Inhibit Protein Synthesis
Impede Replications of Genetic Information
nalidixic acid
griseofulvin
novobiocin
rifampin
pyrimethamine

Impair Translation of Genetic Information
chloramphenicol
tetracycline
erythromycin
aminoglycosides
lincomycins

Antimetabolites
sulfonamides
paraaminosalicylic acid (PAS)
isoniazid (INH)
ethambutol

Side effects and adverse reactions

Although the development of antimicrobial agents represents one of the most important advances in drug therapy, these drugs can have adverse and toxic effects. The list of side effects and toxic effects of each specific drug group is long and varied. Table 50-3 identifies some of the major allergic and toxic effects of a few antimicrobial agents. All antimicrobial agents, however, are capable of producing two general types of adverse reactions of which the healthcare professional must be aware.

Allergic or hypersensitivity reactions. Allergic or hypersensitivity reactions may occur with all available antimicrobial agents. Hypersensitivity is a state of altered reactivity in which the body reacts with an exaggerated immune response. Such responses include rash, fever, urticaria with pruritus, chills, a generalized erythema, anaphylaxis, and the Stevens-Johnson syndrome. Stevens-Johnson syndrome is a form of toxic epidermal necrolysis in which the epidermis separates from the dermis, leaving the patient with a skin loss similar to a second-degree burn.

A minor rash may be easily tolerated, but an individual with a generalized rash or erythema accompanied by chills and fever needs medical intervention. For example, an allergic response to a rapid infusion of vancomycin can result in a generalized red skin reaction, fever, and chills; to mitigate

TABLE 50-3 Antimicrobial Drugs: Selected Allergic and Toxic Effects

Effect	*Drug*
Anaphylaxis	penicillin
Hematologic effects	chloramphenicol (low incidence but high mortality) sulfonamides (low incidence)
Nephrotoxicity	polymyxins aminoglycosides sulfonamides (low incidence with newer drugs)
potential for neuromuscular blockade	polymyxins aminoglycosides
Injury to eighth cranial nerve	aminoglycosides

this reaction, antihistamines would need to be given. Some rashes fade with continued treatment, as with some individuals receiving ampicillin; however, other symptoms may become more severe, necessitating discontinuing the medication. Respiratory distress (wheezing) or anaphylaxis is a medical emergency requiring immediate attention to prevent a fatal outcome. Sensitization has occurred through indirect exposure to a drug, such as drinking milk from cows treated with antibiotics or eating poultry or beef from livestock treated with antimicrobials. Previous topical application of antimicrobials may also cause sensitization.

Treatment of allergic reactions includes the use of antihistamines and epinephrine, which block or counteract the effects of the vasoactive mediators of allergy, and the use of corticosteroids, which may reduce tissue injury and edema in the inflammatory response. The use of steroids is controversial in the face of systemic infection because of their prolonged inhibition of normal host defense responses.

Superinfection. Superinfection is an infection that occurs during the course of antimicrobial therapy delivered for either therapeutic or prophylactic reasons. Most antibiotics reduce or eradicate the normal microbial flora of the body, which are then replaced by resistant exogenous or endogenous bacteria. If the number of these replacement organisms is large and the host conditions favorable, clinical superinfection can occur.

Approximately 2% of persons treated with antibiotics get superinfections. The risk is greater when large doses of antibiotics are given, when more than one antibiotic is administered concurrently, and when broad-spectrum drugs are used. Some specific antimicrobials are more commonly associated with superinfection than others. For example, *Pseudomonas* organisms frequently colonize in and infect individuals taking cephalosporins. In a similar manner, persons taking tetracyclines may become infected with *Candida albicans.* Generally, superinfections are caused by microorganisms that are resistant to the drug the patient is receiving. In the past penicillinase-producing staphylococci were the most common cause of superinfection. *Staphylococcus aureus* and *Staphylococcus epidermidis* superinfections, especially with methicillin-resistant strains, are again on the rise. Gram-negative enteric bacilli and fungi are the most common offenders. The proper management of superinfections includes (1) discontinuing the drug being given or replacing it with another drug to which the organism is sensitive, (2) culturing the suspected infected area, and (3) possibly administering an antimicrobial agent effective against the new offending organism.

General guidelines for use

Several important principles guide the judicious and optimal use of the antimicrobial agents. Causes of adverse reactions to antimicrobial agents and therapeutic failures are often related to lack of adherence to the following principles of antimicrobial therapy.

Identification of infecting organism. Because most antimicrobial agents have a specific effect on a limited range of microorganisms, the prescriber must formulate a specific diagnosis about the potential pathogens or organisms most likely causing the infectious process. The drug most likely to be specifically effective against the suspected microorganism can then be selected.

This objective is most reliably accomplished by obtaining specimens from the infected area if possible (e.g., urine, sputum, and wound drainage) or by obtaining venous blood specimens and sending them to the laboratory for culture and identification of the causative organism. The recovery of a specific microorganism from appropriate specimens is a significant factor in the determination of antimicrobial therapy. When a significant microorganism has been isolated, laboratory tests for antimicrobial susceptibility to various antimicrobial agents are performed.

It is desirable to receive culture and sensitivity reports before initiating antimicrobial therapy. In some situations, however, it is not practical to wait for these laboratory results. For example, antimicrobial therapy must be initiated without delay in acute, life-threatening situations, such as peritonitis, septicemia, or pneumonia. In such situations the choice of antimicrobial agent for initial use must be based on a tentative identification of the pathogen and Gram stain. It is known, for example, that microorganisms commonly isolated in acute adult infections of the lung include pneumococci, *Haemophilus* strain streptococci, and staphylococci. Antimicrobial agents specifically toxic to those organisms may be administered temporarily. The drugs can then be changed, if necessary, after laboratory reports have been received.

When even tentative identification is difficult, either broad-spectrum antibiotics, which are effective against a wide range of microorganisms, can be prescribed or several antimicrobial agents may be prescribed for simultaneous administration.

Some infections are most effectively treated with the use of only one antibiotic. In other situations combined antimicrobial drug therapy may be indicated. Indications for the simultaneous use of two or more antimicrobial agents include (1) treatment of mixed infections, in which each drug may act on a separate portion of a complex microbial flora, (2) the need to delay the rapid emergence of bacteria resistant to one drug, and (3) the need to reduce the incidence or intensity of adverse reactions by decreasing the dose of a potentially toxic drug. Indiscriminate use of combined antimicrobial drug therapy should be avoided because of expense, toxicity, and higher incidence of superinfections and resistance.

Sensitivity and resistance of microorganisms. Frequently, a discrepancy exists between the in vitro testing and the activity of the drug within the body. This depends on a number of variables such as affinity for antibiotic active sites and penetration into the bacteria, pH, temperature, and ability of the drug to reach the site of an infection. For example, in the case of meningitis it would be inappropriate to use a drug that does not cross the blood-brain barrier even though the organism tested may be sensitive to the drug.

Resistance refers to the ability of a particular microorganism to resist the effects of a specific antibiotic. Resistance occurs in one of three ways:

1. The antibiotic is unable to reach the potential target site of its action. Some organisms, such as *Pseudomonas,* form a protective membrane (a glycocalyx or slime) that prevents the antibiotic from reaching the cell wall.
2. The microorganism may produce an enzyme that acts to reduce or eliminate the toxic effect of the antibiotic to the cell wall. Examples of these enzymes are the beta-lactamases that cleave the beta-lactam ring on penicillins and cephalosporins, forming inactive compounds, acylases that acetylate chloramphenicol to yield inactive derivatives, and enzymes that inactivate aminoglycosides by phosphorylation, adenylation, and acetylation.
3. The microorganism may also be altered in the individual through several biochemical changes. The changes occur in such a way that the target site for the antibiotic no longer accommodates the drug. In this case a specific organism is said to have "become resistant" to a previously susceptible antibiotic. As a rule, microorganisms resistant to a certain drug will tend to be resistant to other chemically related antimicrobial agents, a phenomenon known as cross-resistance. For example, bacteria unresponsive to tetracycline will also be resistant to oxytetracycline and chlortetracycline.

Role of host defense mechanisms. No antimicrobial agent will effect the cure of an infectious process if host defense mechanisms are inadequate. Such drugs act only on the causative organisms of infectious disease and have no effect on the defense mechanisms of the body, which need to be assessed and supported. Many infections do not require drug therapy and are adequately combatted by individual defense mechanisms, including antibody production, phagocytosis, interferon production, fibrosis, or gastrointestinal rejection (vomiting and diarrhea). However, host defense mechanisms may be diminished, for example, in persons with diabetes mellitus, neoplastic disease, and immunologic suppression. In addition, the very ill patient may require supportive care to ensure adequate oxygenation, fluid and electrolyte balance, and optimal nutrition for antimicrobial therapy to be effective. In some situations surgical intervention is also necessary. In general, in the presence of a substantial amount of pus, necrotic tissue, or a foreign body, the most effective treatment is a combination of an antimicrobial agent and an appropriate surgical procedure.

The status of the host's defense mechanisms will also influence choice of therapy, route of administration, and dosage. If an infection is fulminating, for example, parenteral (preferably intravenous) administration of a bactericidal drug will be selected rather than oral administration of a bacteriostatic drug. Large "loading" doses of antimicrobial agents are often administered at the beginning of treatment of severe infections to achieve maximum blood concentrations rapidly. However, factors influencing drug dosage are also related to the status of a patient's renal function. Because many antimicrobial agents are metabolized and/or excreted by the kidneys, a major management problem exists with individuals who have compromised renal function. Drug dosages are then generally reduced in parallel with the person's creatinine clearance levels. Hemodialysis may further alter the therapeutic regimen. In some disease states (such as burns) antibiotic dosage may need to be increased to achieve therapeutic levels. In short, the administration of an antimicrobial agent specifically toxic to the isolated microorganism is not the only important measure in antimicrobial therapy. An additional and very important determinant of the effectiveness of an antimicrobial agent is the functional state of the host's defense mechanisms.

Dosage and duration of therapy. Administering antimicrobial drugs for therapeutic purposes in adequate dosage and for long enough periods of time is an important principle of infectious disease therapy. Fortunately, serum levels of some of the more potent antibiotics can be monitored to prevent or minimize the risk of toxicity, for example, aminoglycosides.

Failures of antimicrobial therapy are frequently the result of drug doses being too small or being given for too short a period of time. Generally, antimicrobial therapy should not be discontinued until the individual has been afebrile and clinically well for 48 to 72 hours. Follow-up cultures should be obtained to assess the effectiveness of therapy.

Inadequate drug therapy may lead to remissions and exacerbations of the infectious process and may contribute to the development of resistance. When antibiotics are used prophylactically, they usually are given for short periods of time to enhance host defense mechanisms. For example, with perioperative antibiotics a loading dose is given immediately before surgery and continued for 48 hours after surgery.

Antimicrobial agents currently being used are discussed as chemically related groups of drugs. The healthcare professional should be familiar with the general characteristics of each drug group or category and with one or two prototype drugs in each group. Because the dosage for any given antibiotic varies with the type of infection, the site of infection, and the age of the patient, only general dosages or dose ranges are given in this text. It is recommended that the manufacturer's package insert or a formulary be consulted for specific dosages.

SUMMARY

This chapter reviews fever, inflammation, and infection, symptoms that are involved with many illnesses caused by bacteria or pathogenic microorganisms. Pathogenic microorganisms include bacteria, mycoplasmas, spirochetes, fungi, and viruses. Inflammation is a protective mechanism in the body, a response to invading toxins and physical, chemical, and thermal injuries. The body temperature regulating system involving the hypothalamus, set point, and heat gain and heat loss centers was also discussed. Fever is a sign of infection or inflammation, which must be evaluated and addressed by the healthcare professional.

Antimicrobial therapy may include bacteriostatic (inhibiting bacterial growth) or bactericidal (causing bacterial cell death and lysis) drugs or drugs that have both effects, depending on the concentration at the site of action. They produce their effects by inhibiting the bacterial cell wall synthesis, altering the membrane permeability, inhibiting protein synthesis, or inhibiting the synthesis of essential metabolites. Such medications are generally well tolerated, although the complications of an allergic or hypersensitive response, a superinfection, or a serious adverse effect may also occur during or as a result of the drug therapy.

REVIEW QUESTIONS

1. Describe the four ways that bacteriostatic or bactericidal medications produce their effect against infecting microorganisms. Name a drug from each category.
2. Describe superinfection, typical organisms that occur and/or persist, and suggested management.
3. Discuss the three mechanisms postulated for the development of drug resistance.
4. Define loading dose, broad-spectrum antibiotics, and mixed infections.

REFERENCES

Insel PA: Analgesic-antipyretic and antiinflammatory agents and drugs employed in the treatment of gout. In Hardman JG, Limbird LE, editors: *Goodman & Gilman's the pharmacological basis of therapeutics,* ed 9, New York, 1996, McGraw-Hill.

ADDITIONAL REFERENCES

Abramowicz M: The choice of antibacterial drugs, *Med Lett* 36(925):53-60, 1994.

Anderson KN et al, editors: *Mosby's medical, nursing, and allied health dictionary,* ed 5, St Louis, 1998, Mosby.

Balk RA, Parrillo JE: Prognostic factors in sepsis: the cold facts, *Crit Care Med* 20(10):1373-1374, 1992.

Bone RC: The search for a magic bullet to fight sepsis, *JAMA* 269 (17):2266, 1993.

Foster MT: Septicemia, *Hosp Pract* 26(suppl 5):43-46, 1991.

Grimes D: *Infectious diseases,* St Louis, 1991, Mosby.

McCance KL, Huether SE: *Pathophysiology: the biologic basis for disease in adults and children,* ed 3, St Louis, 1998, Mosby.

Melmon KL et al: *Melmon and Morelli's clinical pharmacology,* ed 3, New York, 1992, McGraw-Hill.

Chapter 51

Antibiotics

KEY DRUGS

ciprofloxacin (p. 660)
erythromycin (p. 655)
gentamicin, (p. 657)
penicillin G (p. 649)
trimethoprim-
  sulfamethoxazole (p. 663)
vancomycin, (p. 657)

KEY TERMS

aminoglycosides, (p. 657)
antibiotics, (p. 649)
bactericidal, (p. 649)
bacteriostatic, (p. 655)
cephalosporins, (p. 651)
fluoroquinolones, (p. 660)
macrolide antibiotics,
  (p. 655)
penicillins, (p. 649)
superinfection, (p. 651)
tetracyclines, (p. 658)

CHAPTER FOCUS

The discovery of sulfonamides and penicillin in the 1940s revolutionized the treatment of infectious diseases. Since then many antibiotics or anti-microbial agents have been discovered and released for patient usage. Although many infections have been controlled with these medications, their usage has resulted in the occurrence of drug-resistant strains of microorganisms and the opportunistic bacterial infections that accompany the human immunodeficiency virus (HIV). Healthcare professionals need to be informed on the benefits and potential problems with the use of antibiotics.

OBJECTIVES

After reading and studying this chapter, the student should be able to do the following:

1. *Define and discuss the key terms and key drugs.*
2. *List the mechanisms of action for penicillins, cephalosporins, macrolides, lincomycins, aminoglycosides, tetracyclines, and quinolones.*
3. *Present the four classifications of penicillins, listing one drug example from each.*
4. *Compare the effectiveness of penicillins with cephalosporins.*
5. *Name the six aminoglycosides and present their mechanisms of action and primary indications.*
6. *Discuss the mechanisms of action and indications for the tetracyclines.*
7. *Compare and contrast the role of antibiotics, sulfonamides, urinary antiseptics, and urinary tract analgesics in the treatment of urinary tract infections.*

Antibiotics are chemical substances produced from various microorganisms (bacteria and fungus) that kill or suppress the growth of other microorganisms. This term is also used for synthetic antimicrobial agents such as sulfonamides and quinolones. Although hundreds of antibiotics are available that vary in antibacterial spectrum, mechanism of action, potency, toxicity, and pharmacokinetic properties, this chapter is divided into penicillins and related antibiotics, cephalosporins, macrolides, lincomycins, vancomycin, aminoglycosides, tetracyclines, chloramphenicol, quinolones, miscellaneous antimicrobials, and urinary tract antimicrobials. An understanding of the general principles of antibiotic therapy, as discussed in Chapter 50, is essential for the healthcare professional.

PENICILLINS AND RELATED ANTIBIOTICS

Penicillins are antibiotics derived from a number of strains of common molds often seen on bread or fruit (Fig. 51-1). Introduced into clinical practice in the 1940s, penicillin and related antibiotics constitute a large group of antimicrobial agents that remain the most effective and least toxic of all available antimicrobial drugs.

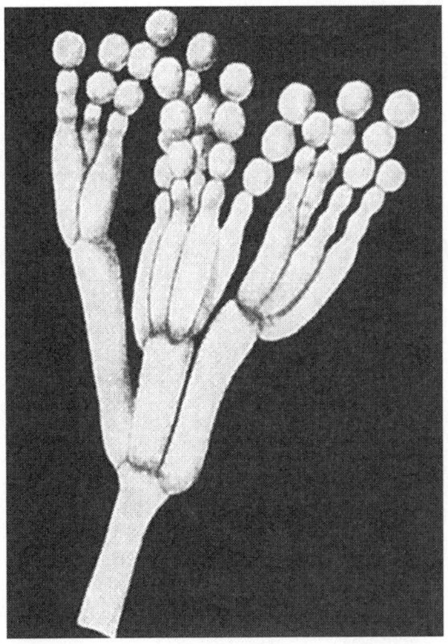

FIGURE 51-1
Typical penicillus of *Penicillium notatum*, Flemming's strain. *(From Raper, Alexander, 1945.)*

Bacteria cell walls are permeable and rigid to protect cellular cytoplasm. Penicillins weaken the cell wall by inhibition of transpeptidase enzymes responsible for cross-linking the cell wall strands, which results in cell lysis and death. Therefore penicillins are **bactericidal** because they inhibit bacterial cell wall synthesis.

Penicillin is not useful in the presence of bacterial enzymes capable of destroying penicillins, such as penicillinase strains of the beta-lactamase enzymes. There are now four different classifications of antibiotics that contain the beta-lactam ring: penicillins, cephalosporins, monobactams, and carbapenems. Alteration of the beta-lactam rings (depending on the antibiotic and specific bacteria) has resulted in the formulation of drugs more active against gram-negative cell wall organisms and a decrease in susceptibility to beta-lactamases that inactivate the antibiotic. For example, the beta-lactam altered penicillins, aztreonam and imipenem, are stable in the presence of beta-lactamases while ampicillin and amoxicillin must be combined with beta-lactamase inhibitors, such as clavulanate, sulbactam or tazobactam to improve their effectiveness.

Although most penicillins are much more active against gram-positive than gram-negative bacteria, ticarcillin, carbenicillin, aztreonam, imipenem, and the combination of penicillins with beta-lactamase inhibitors are more effective against gram-negative bacteria (*Escherichia coli, Klebsiella pneumoniae,* and others). Prophylactically, penicillin is indicated for the prevention of diphtheria, bacterial endocarditis, and rheumatic fever. Penicillins are divided into the following:

1. Natural penicillins include penicillin G and penicillin V. Penicillin G and penicillin V are comparable therapeutically, but oral penicillin V is more stable in stomach acid; therefore it reaches higher serum levels than oral penicillin G. Penicillin G is available orally, IM, and IV in various salt formulations, sodium penicillin G, potassium penicillin G, procaine penicillin G, benzathine penicillin G, and a parenteral combination of the latter two formulations. The active substance in all formulations is penicillin G.
2. Penicillinase-resistant penicillins include cloxacillin, dicloxacillin, methicillin, nafcillin, and oxacillin. A chemical alteration of the penicillin structure resulted in penicillins resistant to beta-lactamase inactivation thus they are used to treat penicillinase-producing staphylococcus. These antibiotics though are not effective against methicillin-resistant bacteria.
3. Aminopenicillins or broader-spectrum penicillins include amoxicillin, amoxicillin and potassium clavulanate, ampicillin, ampicillin and sulbactam, and bacampicillin. Although these antibiotics have the spectrum of activity of penicillin in addition to efficacy against selected gram-negative bacteria, the single agents are usually not very effective against *Staphylococcus aureus* (beta-lactamase-producing) bacteria. When combined with beta-lactamase inhibitors, such as potassium clavulanate and sulbactam, the penicillin is protected from inactivation by beta-lactamase enzymes.
4. Extended-spectrum penicillins include carbenicillin, mezlocillin, piperacillin, piperacillin and tazobactam, ticarcillin, and ticarcillin and potassium clavulanate. These antibiotics have a broader spectrum of antimicrobial activity that includes *Pseudomonas aeruginosa, Enterobacter, Proteus,* and others. Only the combination antibiotics in this category, though, are effective against *S aureus* (beta-lactamase-producing) bacteria.

The healthcare professional should be aware that reducing or eliminating the normal bacteria flora with antibiotic

TABLE 51-1 Penicillins: Pharmacokinetics and Usual Adult Dosing

Classification	*Pharmacokinetics*			
Drug(s)	***Oral Absorption (%)***	***Peak Serum (hr)****	***Renal Excretion (%)†***	***Usual Adult Dose***
Natural Penicillins				
penicillin G 🔑				
oral	15-30	1-2	20	200,000-500,000 U q4-6h
IV	—	—	60-90	1-5 mU q4-6h
IM	—	B-24	60-90	1.2-2.4 mU single dose
		P-4	60-90	600,000 U—1.2 mU daily
penicillin V				
oral	60-73	0.5-1	20-40	125-500 mg q6-8h
Penicillinase-Resistant Penicillins				
cloxacillin (Tegopen)				
oral	50	1-2	30-60	250-500 mg q6h
IV 🍁	—	E of I	30-60	250-500 mg q6h
dicloxacillin (Dynapen)				
oral	37-50	0.5-1	50-70	125-250 mg q6h
methicillin (Staphcillin)				
IM	—	0.5-1	60-80	1 g q4-6h
IV	—	E of I	60-80	1 g q6h
nafcillin (Unipen)				
oral	Erratic	1-2	10-30	250 mg-1 g q4-6h
IM	—	0.5-1	10-30	500 mg q4-6h
IV	—	E of I	10-30	0.5-1.5 g q4h
oxacillin (Prostaphlin)				
oral	30-35	0.5-1	55-60	0.5-1 g q4-6h
IM	—	0.5-1	55-60	250 mg-1 g q4-6h
IV	—	E of I	55-60	250 mg-1 g q4-6h
Aminopenicillins (Broader-Spectrum)				
amoxicillin (Amoxil)				
oral	75-90	1-2	60-75	250-500 mg q8h
amoxicillin + clavulanate (Augmentin, Clavulin 🍁)				
oral	90	1-2	50-78	500 mg q8h
ampicillin (Polycillin)				
oral	35-50	1-1.5	75-90	250-500 mg q6h
IM	—	1	75-90	250-500 mg q6h
IV	—	E of I	75-90	250-500 mg q6h
ampicillin + sulbactam (Unasyn)				
IM	—	—	75-85	1.5-3 g q6h
IV	—	E of I	—	1.5-3 g q6h
bacampicillin (Spectrobid)				
oral	35-50‡	0.5-1‡	70-75‡	400-800 mg q12h
Extended-Spectrum Penicillins				
carbenicillin (Geocillin)				
oral	30	0.5-1	36	0.5-1 g q6h
IM	—	0.5-1	—	50-83.3 mg/kg q4h
IV	—	E of I	75-95	50-83.3 mg/kg q4h
mezlocillin (Mezlin)				
IM	—	0.5-1	55-60	33.3-58.3 mg/kg q4h
IV	—	E of I	55-60	33.3-58.3 mg/kg q4h
piperacillin (Pipracil)				
IM	—	0.5	60-80	3-4 g q4-6h
IV	—	E of I	60-80	3-4 g q4-6h
piperacillin + tazobactam (Zosyn, Tazocin 🍁)				
IV	—	E of I	68	3.375-4.5 g q6-8h
ticarcillin (Ticar)				
IM	—	0.5-1	60-80	1 g q6h
IV	—	E of I	60-80	1-4 g q6h
ticarcillin + clavulanate (Timentin)				
IV	—	E of I	60-70	33.3-50 mg q4h

From *USP DI*, 1998.
*Time to peak serum level (hours); †renal excretion of active drug (%, percent excreted unchanged); ‡as ampicillin.
B, benzathine, and *P*, procaine dosage forms; *mU*, million units; *E of I*, end of infusion.

therapy may provide an environment that is conducive to growth of undesirable microorganisms, such as bacteria or fungus. This is a condition known as **superinfection** and may present as diarrhea from altered gastrointestinal flora or a candida fungal infection vaginally.

Table 51-1 lists penicillin pharmacokinetics and usual adult dosages.

Drug interactions

The following effects may occur when penicillins are given with the drugs listed below:

Drug	Possible effect and management
Angiotensin-converting enzyme (ACE) inhibitors, potassium-sparing diuretics, potassium-containing drugs, or potassium supplements	If given concurrently with parenteral penicillin G potassium, serum potassium levels may increase, causing hyperkalemia. Monitor closely; dosage adjustments may be necessary.
Anticoagulants, oral coumarin or indanedione, heparin, or thrombolytic agents	Increased risk of bleeding when given with high doses of parenteral carbenicillin or ticarcillin, as these drugs inhibit platelet aggregation. Monitor closely for signs of bleeding. Concurrent use of these penicillins with thrombolytic agents also increases the risk for severe bleeding. Avoid or a potentially serious drug interaction may occur.
Nonsteroidal antiinflammatory drugs (NSAIDs), platelet aggregation inhibitors (such as salicylates, dextran, dipyridamole [Persantine], valproic acid [Depakote], and sulfinpyrazone [Anturane])	With high doses of carbenicillin or ticarcillin (parenteral dosage forms), an increased risk for bleeding or hemorrhage exists. These drugs inhibit platelet function, and large doses of salicylates may induce hypoprothrombinemia and also gastrointestinal ulcers (from NSAIDs, salicylates, or sulfinpyrazone), all adding to the potential risk of hemorrhage. Avoid or a potentially serious drug interaction may occur.
cholestyramine (Questran) or colestipol (Colestid)	May decrease absorption of oral penicillin G if given concurrently. Advise patients to take the antibiotic first and other medications 3 hours later.
Estrogen-containing contraceptives	When used concurrently with ampicillin, amoxicillin, or penicillin V, the effectiveness of the oral contraceptives may be decreased because of an increase in estrogen metabolism or a reduction in enterohepatic circulation of estrogens. Advise patients to use an alternate method of contraception while taking these antibiotics.
methotrexate (Folex)	Concurrent use with penicillins decreases methotrexate clearance and may result in methotrexate toxicity. Monitor closely. Leucovorin rescue doses may need to be increased and given for a longer period of time.
probenecid (Benemid)	Decreased renal tubular secretion of penicillins, resulting in elevated serum levels and an increase in half-life. It may also increase toxicity. Several combinations of penicillin and probenecid are marketed to take advantage of this effect.

Color type indicates an unsafe drug combination.

Side effects and adverse reactions

For penicillins these include diarrhea, nausea, vomiting, headache, sore mouth or tongue, oral and vaginal candidiasis, allergic reactions, anaphylaxis, serum sickness-type reaction (rash, joint pain, and fever), hives, and pruritus. Rare adverse effects include hepatotoxicity with some penicillins, especially cloxacillin, dicloxacillin, flucloxacillin, and oxacillin; leukopenia or neutropenia; mental disturbances (with large dosages of procaine penicillin); convulsions (with high dosages of penicillin and/or in persons with advanced renal function impairment); and interstitial nephritis. The latter is seen primarily with methicillin and to a lesser degree with nafcillin and oxacillin, but the this effect may occur with any penicillin. Platelet dysfunction has been reported with carbenicillin, piperacillin, and ticarcillin, especially in patients with renal impairment.

Warnings

Use with caution in patients with general allergies, carnitine deficiency, and hypertension.

Contraindications

Avoid use in persons with penicillin hypersensitivity (see Fig. 51-2), bleeding disorders, congestive heart failure, cystic fibrosis, gastrointestinal (GI) disease (especially antibiotic-associated colitis as penicillins may cause pseudomembranous colitis), mononucleosis, and kidney function impairment.

See the box for Food and Drug Administration (FDA) pregnancy safety classifications for all of drugs in this chapter. Also see the Pediatric Implications box for appropriate antibiotic therapy in children and Box 51-1 for the effect of food on oral penicillin absorption.

CEPHALOSPORINS AND RELATED PRODUCTS

Cephalosporins and related products are chemical modifications of the penicillin structure. These modifications create compounds with different microbiologic and pharmacologic activities. To classify the differences in antimicrobial activity, cephalosporins are divided into four generations.

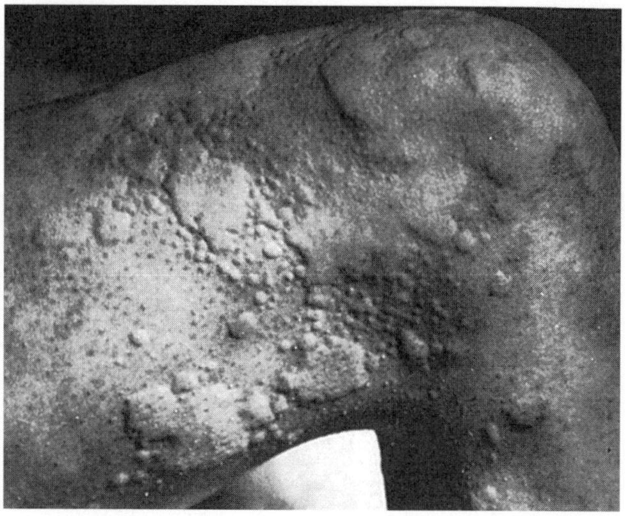

FIGURE 51-2
Urticaria such as that seen in individuals sensitive to penicillin.

PREGNANCY SAFETY

Category	Drug
B	aztreonam, azithromycin, cephalosporins, metronidazole, nitrofurantoin, penicillins, phenazopyridine
C	cinoxacin, clarithromycin, dirithromycin, fluoroquinolones, gentamicin, imipenam/cilastatin, methenamine, sulfonamides, vancomycin
D	amikacin, kanamycin, netilmicin, streptomycin, tetracyclines, tobramycin
Unclassified	chloramphenicol (not recommended at term or during labor), clindamycin, lincomycin, nalidixic acid (not recommended in pregnancy), spectinomycin, troleandomycin

Loracarbef (Lorabid, a carbacephem), a drug that is chemically similar drug to second-generation cephalosporins, is included in this section. Initially the prototype drug for this category was cephalothin (Keflin); this product was taken off the market in 1998.

Cephalosporins inhibit cell wall synthesis similar to penicillin and are also bactericidal. They are effective in numerous situations, but until the third-generation cephalosporins were marketed, the majority were not considered to be drugs of choice for any serious infection. The first-generation cephalosporins are primarily active against gram-positive bacteria whereas the second-generation drugs (cefamandole and others) had increased activity against gram-negative microorganisms. The third-generation drugs are more active against gram-negative bacteria (ceftazidime and cefoperazone are also effective against *P aeruginosa*) and beta-lactamase-producing microbial strains. However, the third-generation cephalosporins are less effective against gram-positive cocci. Cefepime is a fourth-generation cephalosporin that has antimicrobial effects comparable to those of third-generation cephalosporins and is also more resistant to some beta-lactamases (Mandell, Petri, 1996).

Initially the advantage of cephalosporins over penicillins was their resistance to enzymatic degradation by penicillinase (beta-lactamase). However, drug resistance has been reported to drugs from all three generations, possibly through four mechanisms: (1) a microorganism lacking an outer cell membrane permeability, causing poor drug penetration in the bacteria; (2) bacteria lacking a receptor for

PEDIATRIC IMPLICATIONS

Antibiotic Therapy

To assess the appropriateness of antibiotic therapy in children, the following criteria are generally accepted:

1. In choosing empiric therapy, the selected antimicrobial should have documentation of both adequate penetration at the site and proven effectiveness against the common organisms usually isolated from that specific site.
2. If a broad range of possible microorganisms is suspected or if multiple organisms have been isolated from an infection site, then multiple drug therapy may be indicated. Whenever possible, though, the minimal number of drugs necessary to treat the infection should be used.
3. If no contraindication is present, the drug of first choice should be selected. The drug dosage regimen should be within the accepted range of current usage for the individual, taking into account the child's body surface area (height and weight), organ function, and concurrent disease processes.
4. Unless the benefit far outweighs the risk, no antibiotic should be used in patients with prior documentation of an allergic or adverse reaction to the specific medication.
5. Children receiving potent and potentially dangerous drugs, such as gentamicin, amikacin, tobramycin, or vancomycin, for more than 2 days, should have blood drawn for steady-state drug serum concentrations at the appropriate times for evaluation.
6. Whenever possible, samples for culture should be taken before initiation of antibiotic therapy. Usual sites cultured include sputum, urine, blood, wound, or nonhealing topical sites.
7. Antibiotic therapy should be continued until infection is no longer present. Time periods, though, should not exceed the usual treatment time established for the suspected infection. Prophylactic antibiotic therapy given after uncomplicated surgery is usually discontinued within 48 hours with few exceptions, such as cardiac surgery.

BOX 51-1 Effect of Food on Oral Penicillin Absorption*

Drug	Food Effect
amoxicillin	None
amoxicillin and clavulanate	None
ampicillin	Decreased
bacampicillin tablet	None
carbenicillin indanyl sodium	Increased
cloxacillin	Decreased
dicloxacillin	Decreased
nafcillin	Decreased
oxacillin	Decreased
penicillin G benzathine	Decreased
penicillin V potassium	Decreased slightly

*Penicillins whose absorption decreases after food intake are generally acid labile; therefore administer with a full glass of water with an empty stomach 1 hour before or 2 hours after meals.

the specific drug; (3) bacteria producing a beta-lactamase enzyme that can split the beta-lactam ring in the cephalosporins (many such enzymes have been isolated); or (4) development of a type of bacteria tolerance, that is, bacterial strains that are inhibited but not killed by the cephalosporins. The reason for this latter effect is the lack of, or deficiency in, autolytic enzymes in the bacterial cell wall (Katzung, 1992). Also this class of drugs has been overused and thus reports of bacterial resistance have increased.

Cephalosporin antibiotics are often prescribed for patients allergic to penicillins. The possibility of a cross-reaction is 5% to 15%; however, if the individual reports a serious reaction or anaphylaxis to penicillin, cephalosporins should not be used (Beringer, Middleton, 1995).

Because cephalosporins inhibit cell wall synthesis, cell division and growth, rapidly dividing bacteria are most affected by them. These agents are indicated for the treatment of a variety of infections and also as presurgery prophylactic agents. Combinations of third-generation cephalosporins and aminoglycosides are used synergistically to treat *P aeruginosa, Serratia marcescens,* and other susceptible organisms.

Table 51-2 lists cephalosporin pharmacokinetics and usual adult dose.

Drug interactions

The following effects may occur when cephalosporins are given with the drugs listed below:

Drug	Possible effect and management
Alcohol	Not recommended with cefamandole, cefmetazole, cefoperazone, or cefotetan. An increase in acetaldehyde in the blood may result, producing a disulfiram (Antabuse)-type reaction such as stomach pain, nausea, vomiting, headaches, low blood pressure, tachycardia, respiratory difficulties, increased sweating, or flushing of the face. Patients should avoid drinking alcohol-containing beverages, taking medications containing alcohol, or using intravenous alcohol solutions during the administration of these drugs and for 3 days afterward.
Anticoagulants, coumarin or indanedione, heparin, or thrombolytic agents	Increased risk of bleeding and hemorrhage when given concurrently with cefamandole, cefmetazole, cefoperazone, or cefotetan. These cephalosporins interfere with vitamin K metabolism in the liver, resulting in hypoprothrombinemia. Dosage adjustments of the anticoagulants may be necessary during and after administration of these drugs. Avoid concurrent use of these drugs with thrombolytic agents because of the increased risk of serious bleeding and hemorrhage.
NSAIDs, especially aspirin, inhibitors, and sulfinpyrazone (Anturane)	When given with cefamandole, cefoperazone, or cefotetan, an increased risk of hemorrhage exists because of the additive effect on platelet inhibition. Also, high dosages of salicylates and the specified antibiotics may induce hypoprothrombinemia, and the potential for GI ulcers or hemorrhage with NSAIDs or salicylates may increase when used with the previously mentioned cephalosporins. Avoid or a potentially serious drug interaction may occur.
probenecid (Benemid)	Probenecid decreases renal tubular secretion of the cephalosporins that are excreted by this mechanism, which can result in increased serum levels, extended half-life, and increased potential for toxicity. Probenecid does not affect the secretion of cefoperazone, ceftazidime, or ceftriaxone. Cephalosporins and probenecid are also used concurrently to treat specific infections such as sexually transmitted diseases, in which a high serum level and prolonged effect are desirable.

Color type indicates an unsafe drug combination.

Side effects and adverse reactions

These include diarrhea, abdominal cramps or distress, oral and/or vaginal candidiasis, rash, pruritus, redness,

TABLE 51-2 Cephalosporins: Pharmacokinetics and Usual Adult Dose

	Pharmacokinetics			
Drug	**Oral Absorption (%)**	**Peak Serum (hr)***	**Renal Excretion (%/hr)†**	**Usual Adult Dose**
First Generation				
cefadroxil (Duricef)	95	PO: 1.5-2	93/24	500 mg q12h
cefazolin (Ancef)	—	IM: 1-2 IV: E of I	56-89/6 80-100/24	IM 1 g presurgery IV infusion: 0.25-1.5 g q6-8h
cephalexin (Keflex)	95	PO: 1	80/6 90/8	250-500 mg q6h
cephapirin (Cefadyl)	—	IM: 0.5-1 IV: E of I	70/6	IM/IV: 0.5-1 g q4-6h
cephradine (Velosef, Anspor)	95	PO: 1 IM: 0.8-2 IV: E of I	60-80/6	250-500 mg PO q6h IM/IV: 0.5-1 g q6h
Second Generation				
cefaclor (Ceclor)	95	PO: 0.5-1	60-85/8	250-500 mg q8h
cefamandole (Mandol)	—	IM: 0.5-2 IV: E of I	65-85/8	IM/IV: 500 mg q6h
cefmetazole (Zefazone)	—	IV: E of I	71/24	IV: 2 g q6-12h
cefonicid (Monocid)	—	IM: 1 IV: E of I	99/24	IM/IV: 0.5-1 g q24h
cefotetan (Cefotan)	—	IM: 1-3 IV: E of I	50-80/24	IM/IV: 1-2 g q12h
cefoxitin (Mefoxin)	—	IM: 0.3-0.5 IV: E of I	85/6	IV: 1-2 g q6-8h
cefprozil (Cefzil)	95	PO: 1.5	60/8	500 mg q12h
cefuroxine (Zinacef)	pc-52 fasting-37	PO: 2-3.6 IM: 0.75 IV: E of I	32-48/12	250-500 mg q12h IM/IV: 0.75-1.5 g q8h
loracarbef (Lorabid)	90	PO: 0.5-1.2	87-97	200-400 mg q12h
Third Generation				
cefixime (Suprax)	40-50	PO: 2-6	50/24	200 mg q12h
cefoperazone (Cefobid)	—	IM: 1-2 IV: E of I	20-30/12‡	IV infusion: 1-2 g q12h
cefotaxime (Claforan)	—	IM: 0.5 IV: E of I	60/6	IV infusion: 1-2 g q4-12h
cefpodoxime (Vantin)	50	PO: 2-3	29-33/12	200 mg q12h
ceftazidime (Fortaz)	—	IM: 1 IV: E of I	80-90/24	IM/IV: 0.5-2 g q8-12h
ceftibuten (Cedax)	—	PO: N/A	56	400 mg daily
ceftizoxime (Cefizox)	—	IM: 1 IV: E of I	85-95/24	IV: 1-2 g q8-12h
ceftriaxone (Rocephin)	—	IM: 2-3 IV: E of I	33-67/24	IV: 1-2 g q24h
Fourth Generation				
cefepime (Maxipime)	—	IM: N/A IV: E of I	N/A	IM/IV: 0.5-1 g q12h

*Time to peak serum level (hours); †renal excretion, percent excreted unchanged/hr; ‡majority excreted unchanged in bile.
E of I, end of infusion; *pc,* after meals, *N/A,* not available.
From Olin, 1998; *USP DI,* 1998.

edema, allergic reaction, anaphylaxis, Stevens-Johnson syndrome, hemolytic anemia, renal toxicity, convulsions, thrombophlebitis, hypoprothrombinemia (mostly with cefamandole, cefmetazole, cefoperazone and cefotetan), and pseudomembranous colitis. In addition, an increase in bleeding episodes and bruising due to hypoprothrombinemia is reported with cefamandole, cefmetazole, cefoperazone, and cefotetan.

Warnings

Use with caution in patients with phenylketonuria (cefprozil suspension contains phenylalanine).

Contraindications

Avoid use in persons with reports of anaphylaxis to penicillin, penicillin derivatives, penicillamine or cephalosporins, bleeding disorders, GI disease, and liver or kidney function impairment.

MACROLIDE ANTIBIOTICS

The **macrolide antibiotics** are **bacteriostatic,** since they inhibit ribonucleic acid (RNA)-dependent protein synthesis, but in high concentrations with selected organisms, they may be bactericidal. Currently the macrolide antibiotics include azithromycin (Zithromax), clarithromycin (Biaxin), erythromycin, dirithromycin (Dyna-bac), and troleandomycin (TAO). Dirithromycin is a prodrug that is activated during intestinal absorption to an active metabolite, erythromycylamine. Erythromycin is the first macrolide and key drug from this classification.

With the exception of troleandomycin, these agents have similar antimicrobial action (against gram-positive and selected gram-negative microorganisms) and are used for respiratory, GI tract, skin and soft tissue infections when betalactam antibiotics are contraindicated (Olin, 1998). Troleandomycin is only indicated for the treatment of *Streptococcus pneumoniae* and *Streptococcus pyogenes.*

Drug interactions

The following effects may occur when the macrolide antibiotics are given with the drugs listed below:

Drug	Possible effect and management
alfentanil (Alfenta)	May increase plasma levels and action of alfentanil. Monitor closely if given in combination.
carbamazepine (Tegretol)	Carbamazepine metabolism may be inhibited, leading to elevated serum levels and, possibly, toxicity. Monitor closely.
chloramphenicol (Chloromycetin) or lincomycins	May antagonize the therapeutic effects of chloramphenicol and lincomycin. Avoid concurrent administration.
cyclosporine (Sandimmune)	Concurrent administration with erythromycin may increase cyclosporine serum levels and increase risk for nephrotoxicity. Monitor closely if given concurrently.
Hepatotoxic medications	Increased possibility for liver toxicity. Monitor liver function studies closely if given concurrently.
terfenadine (Seldane) and astemizole (Hismanol)	Concurrent drug administrations may increase risk of cardiotoxicity. Avoid or a potentially serious drug interaction may occur.
warfarin (Coumadin)	May result in decreased warfarin metabolism and excretion, leading to an increased risk of bleeding or hemorrhage. Dosage adjustments of coumarin may be necessary during and after treatment with erythromycin. Monitor prothrombin times closely.
Xanthines, such as aminophylline, caffeine, oxtriphylline, and theophylline (exception, dyphylline)	An increase in theophylline levels and toxicity is reported with this combination of drugs. This effect is usually seen at approximately the sixth day of erythromycin therapy, because it appears to be related to the peak erythromycin serum level. Monitor the serum levels of xanthines closely, as dosage adjustments of xanthines may be necessary during and after erythromycin therapy.
zidovudine (AZT)	Concurrent administration with clarithromycin may result in delayed time to peak zidovudine concentrations. Administer doses of these two drugs at least 4 hours apart.

Color type indicates an unsafe drug combination.

Side effects and adverse reactions

These are as follows:

- azithromycin: stomach pain, nausea, vomiting, diarrhea, dizziness, headache and, rarely, allergic reactions and acute interstitial nephritis
- clarithromycin: anorexia, headache, nausea, vomiting, lethargy, severe anemia, fever, infection, rash, headache, abnormal taste sensations, and, rarely, *Clostridium difficile* colitis, hepatotoxicity, hypersensitivity, and thrombocytopenia
- dirithromycin: stomach pain, headache, nausea, diarrhea, dizziness, and *C difficile* colitis
- erythromycin: abdominal cramps, diarrhea, nausea, vomiting, oral and/or vaginal candidiasis, and, rarely, hypersensitivity, cardiac toxicity, hearing loss, pancreatitis, and hepatotoxicity

TABLE 51-3 Macrolide: Pharmacokinetics and Usual Adult Dose

Drug	Pharmacokinetics			Usual Adult Dose
	Oral Absorption (%)	Peak Serum (hr)*	Renal Excretion (%)†	
azithromycin (Zithromax)	Good	2-4	4.5/72‡	500 mg first day then 250 mg daily thereafter
clarithromycin (Biaxin)	Good	2-3	20-30/–	250-500 mg q12h
erythromycin	30-65	2-4	2-5/–‡	250 mg q6h IV infusion: 250-500 mg q6h
dirithromycin (Dynabac)	10	—	2/–‡	500 mg daily
troleandomycin (TAO)	—	2	20/–	250-500 mg qid

*Time to peak serum level (hr); †renal excretion, percent excreted unchanged/hr; ‡primarily excreted unchanged in bile; —unavailable.
From Olin, 1998, *USP DI*, 1998.

▼ troleandomycin: stomach cramps and discomfort, nausea, vomiting, diarrhea, skin rash, jaundice and, rarely, allergy or anaphylaxis

For macrolide pharmacokinetics and usual adult dose, see Table 51-3.

Warnings

Use with caution in patients with severe liver function impairment. In addition, use erythromycin cautiously in patients with hearing loss and clarithromycin cautiously in persons with severe kidney function impairment.

Contraindications

Avoid use in persons with individual drug hypersensitivity; also avoid use of erythromycin in persons with cardiac dysrhythmias.

LINCOMYCINS

clindamycin [klin da mye' sin] (Cleocin, Dalacin C ♣)

lincomycin [lin koe mye' sin] (Lincocin)

Lincomycin inhibits protein synthesis by binding to bacterial ribosomes and preventing peptide bond formation. It is primarily bacteriostatic, although it may be bactericidal in high doses with selected organisms. It was used to treat serious streptococci, pneumococci, and staphylococci infections but has been replaced by safer and more effective antibiotics.

Clindamycin, which is a semisynthetic derivative of lincomycin, has a similar mechanism of action as lincomycin but it is more effective. It is indicated for the treatment of bone and joint, pelvic (female) and intraabdominal, and skin and soft tissue infections, bacterial septicemia, and pneumonia caused by susceptible bacteria.

Pharmacokinetics

Oral clindamycin is well absorbed and should be administered with food or with a full glass (8 oz) of water. It is rapidly distributed to most body fluids and tissues with the exception of cerebrospinal fluid with the highest concentrations noted in bone, bile, and urine. The half-life of clindamycin in adults is 2 to 3 hours. It reaches peak blood levels within ¾ to 1 hour after oral administration in adults, within 1 hour in children, and within 3 hours after intramuscular injection and by the end of the infusion by intravenous injection. It is metabolized in the liver and excreted primarily by the kidneys.

Drug interactions

The following effects may occur when clindamycin is given with the drugs listed below:

Drug	Possible effect and management
Anesthetics, such as chloroform, enflurane (Ethrane), halothane (Fluothane), isoflurane (Forane), methoxyflurane (Penthrane), trichloroethylene, or the neuromuscular blocking agents	May result in enhanced neuromuscular blockade, skeletal muscle weakness, respiratory depression, or paralysis if this cyclopropane combination is used during or immediately after surgery. Avoid or a potentially serious drug interaction may occur.
Antidiarrheals, adsorbent type (kaolins, attapulgite)	Decreases absorption of oral lincomycins. Avoid concurrent usage or advise patient to take the antidiarrheal 2 hours before or 3 to 4 hours after the oral lincomycins.
chloramphenicol (Chloromycetin) or erythromycin	May antagonize the therapeutic effect of lincomycins. Avoid concurrent administration.

Color type indicates an unsafe drug combination.

Side effects and adverse reactions

These include GI distress (stomach pain, diarrhea, nausea, vomiting, oral and/or vaginal candidiasis, hypersensitivity, neutropenia, and thrombocytopenia. In addition, a significant adverse and limiting effect for both drugs is antibiotic-associated pseudomembranous colitis (AAPMC).

Warnings

Use with caution in patients with GI disorders, especially ulcerative colitis, antibiotic-induced colitis, and regional enteritis.

Contraindications

Avoid use in persons with clindamycin or lincomycin hypersensitivity.

Dosage and administration

The usual adult clindamycin dose is 150 to 300 mg (PO, IM, or IV), every 6 hours. In infants 1 month of age and older; the oral dosage is 2 to 5 mg/kg of body weight every 6 hours.

VANCOMYCIN

vancomycin [van koe mye′ sin] (Vancocin)

Vancomycin inhibits bacterial cell walls by binding to a cell wall precursor, a mechanism that differs from penicillin or cephalosporins. This action leads to cell lysis, so it is bactericidal for many organisms. Vancomycin may also inhibit RNA synthesis. Oral vancomycin is indicated for the treatment of AAPMC *(C difficile)* and the treatment of staphylococcal enterocolitis. Parenteral vancomycin is not recommended for use in AAPMC. Instead it is indicated for bone and joint infections, for bacterial septicemia caused by *Staphylococcus* species, and for the prevention and treatment of bacterial endocarditis caused by *Staphylococcus,* including methicillin-resistant strains.

Pharmacokinetics

Vancomycin's absorption from the intestinal tract is poor. It is excreted mainly in the feces. Parenteral vancomycin has a half-life of 6 hours in adults and about 2 to 3 hours in children. It is excreted primarily by the kidneys.

Drug interactions

The following effects may occur when vancomycin is given with the drugs listed below:

Drug	Possible effect and management
Aminoglycosides, amphotericin B parenteral (Fungizone), aspirin, bacitracin parenteral, bumetanide (Bumex), capreomycin (Capastat), cisplatin (Platinol), cyclosporine (Sandimmune), ethacrynate sodium parenteral (Edecrin), furosemide parenteral (Lasix), paromomycin (Humatin), polymyxins, or streptozocin (Zanosar)	Increased potential for ototoxicity and nephrotoxicity. In patients with pseudomembranous colitis or severe kidney impairment, the serum levels of vancomycin may be increased, thus leading to an increased potential for toxicity. Avoid or a potentially serious drug interaction may occur.
cholestyramine (Questran) or colestipol colestipol	When given concurrently with the oral dosage form, a reduction in vancomycin antibacterial activity is reported. Avoid this combination if possible. If not, give oral vancomycin several hours apart from the other medications.

Color type indicates an unsafe drug combination.

Side effects and adverse reactions

Side effects for oral dosing include nausea, vomiting, anorexia, hearing loss, tinnitus, and taste alterations; and less frequent or rare parenteral adverse effects include ototoxicity and nephrotoxicity. The "red-neck syndrome" is reported after bolus or too rapid drug injection, which results in histamine release and chills, fever, tachycardia, pruritus, rash, or red face, neck, upper body, back, and arms (USP DI, 1998).

Contraindications

Avoid use in persons with vancomycin hypersensitivity, deafness or history of hearing loss, and kidney disease.

Dosage and administration

The oral adult dosage of vancomycin for the treatment of *C difficile* colitis or diarrhea is 125 to 500 mg every 6 hours for 5 to 10 days, repeated if necessary. In children, the dosage is 10 mg/kg (up to 125 mg) every 6 hours for 5 to 10 days, repeated if necessary. By IV infusion the dose is 7.5 mg/kg every 6 hours.

AMINOGLYCOSIDES

Aminoglycosides are potent bactericidal antibiotics that are usually reserved for serious or life-threatening infections. They are very effective against many bacteria (gram-positive and gram-negative), but are generally reserved for gram-negative infections. Safer and less toxic agents are available to treat the majority of gram-positive infections. Currently available aminoglycosides include the following.

amikacin [am ih kay′ sin] (Amikin)
gentamicin [jen ta mye′ sin] (Garamycin)
kanamycin [kan ah mye′ sin] (Kantrex)
netilmicin [ne til mye′ sin] (Netromycin)
streptomycin [strep toe mye′ sin]
tobramycin [toe bra mye′ sin] (Nebcin)

The mechanism of action for aminoglycosides is to irreversibly bind ribosomes of susceptible bacteria, thus inhibiting protein synthesis (interferes with the complex between messenger RNA and the bacteria ribosomes), leading to eventual cell death (bactericidal). They are indicated for the treatment of serious or life-threatening infections when other agents are ineffective or contraindicated. They are used with penicillins, cephalosporins, or vancomycin for their synergistic effects and are especially useful for the treatment of gram-negative infections such as those caused by *Pseudomonas* sp., *E coli, Proteus* sp., *Klebsiella* sp., *Serratia* sp., and others.

Pharmacokinetics

Aminoglycosides are poorly absorbed from an intact intestinal tract, but are rapidly absorbed intramuscularly. Local topical application or irrigation may lead to absorption from most areas of the body with the exception of the urinary bladder.

Ranges of therapeutic aminoglycoside serum levels (μg/ml) are as follows:

amikacin	15-25
gentamicin	4-10
kanamycin	15-30
tobramycin	4-10

Drug interactions

The following effects may occur when aminoglycosides are given with the drugs listed below:

Drug	Possible effect and management
Other aminoglycosides (two or more concurrently) or capreomycin (Capastat)	Potential for ototoxicity, nephrotoxicity, and neuromuscular blockade is enhanced. Hearing loss may progress to deafness even after the drug is stopped. In some cases, hearing loss may be reversed. Avoid or a potentially serious drug interaction may occur.
amphotericin B parenteral (Fungizone), aspirin, bacitracin, parenteral, bumetanide parenteral (Bumex), cisplatin (Platinol), cyclosporine (Sandimmune), ethacrynate sodium parenteral (Edecrin), furosemide parenteral (Lasix), paromomycin (Humatin), streptozocin (Zanosar), or vancomycin (Vancocin)	Increased potential for ototoxicity and/or nephrotoxicity. Hearing loss may be permanent if drugs are given concurrently. Vancomycin and aminoglycosides may be ordered to prevent bacterial endocarditis or to treat specific infections such as carditis caused by organisms such as streptococci and corynebacteria. In these instances, frequent determinations of drug serum levels and renal function are recommended, because dosage adjustments or other interventions may be necessary.
Anesthetics (halogenated hydrocarbon) or citrate-anticoagulated blood by massive transfusions or neuromuscular blocking agents	May increase neuromuscular blockade. Avoid or a potentially serious drug interaction may occur.
methoxyflurane (Penthrane) or polymyxins, parenteral	Increased possibility for nephrotoxicity and/or neuromuscular blockade. Avoid or a potentially serious drug interaction may occur.

Color type indicates an unsafe drug combination.

Side effects and adverse reactions

These include nausea, vomiting, tinnitus, increase or decrease in urinary frequency, ataxia, dizziness, nephrotoxicity, neurotoxicity, ototoxicity (auditory and vestibular), hypersensitivity, peripheral neuritis, and, rarely, neuromuscular blockade (difficulty breathing, increased sedation, and weakness).

Warnings

Use with caution in dehydrated patients.

Contraindications

Avoid use in persons with a known aminoglycoside allergic reaction or hypersensitivity, myasthenia gravis, parkinsonism, kidney disease, eighth cranial nerve impairment, and infant botulism.

Dosage and administration

The usual adult dosages of aminoglycosides are the following: amikacin, 5 mg/kg IM/IV every 8 hours; gentamicin, 1 to 1.7 mg/kg IM or by IV infusion every 8 hours; kanamycin, 3.75 mg/kg IM every 6 hours; netilmicin 1.3 to 2.2 mg/kg IM/IV every 8 hours; streptomycin (tuberculosis adult dose), 1g IM daily given in combination with other antimycobacterials; and tobramycin 0.75 mg to 1.25 mg/kg IM or IV infusion every 6 hours. For additional dosing recommendations, see a current package insert or reference.

TETRACYCLINES

Tetracyclines were the first broad-spectrum antibiotics released in the United States. They include a large group of drugs that have a common basic structure and similar chemical activity.

demeclocycline [de me kloe sye′ kleen] (Declomycin)
doxycycline [dox i sye′ kleen] (Doxychel, Vibramycin)
minocycline [mi noe sye′ kleen] (Minocin)
oxytetracycline [ox i tet ra sye′ kleen] (Terramycin)
tetracycline [tet ra sye′ kleen] (Achromycin V, Novotetra 🍁)

Tetracyclines are bacteriostatic for many gram-negative and gram-positive organisms; they exhibit cross-sensitivity and cross-resistance. Tetracyclines inhibit protein synthesis by blocking the binding of transfer RNA to the messenger RNA ribosome and therefore inhibiting protein synthesis.

TABLE 51-4 Tetracycline: Half-life and Usual Adult Dose

	Half-life (hr)		
Drug	**Normal**	**Anuric**	**Usual Adult Dose**
democlocycline (Declomycin)	10-17	40-60	150 mg q6h
doxycycline (Vibramycin)	12-22	12-22	100 mg bid on first day, then 100 to 200 mg daily (PO or IV infusion)
minocycline (Minocin)	11-23	11-23	200 mg initially, then 100 mg q12h (PO or IV infusion)
oxytetracycline (Terramycin)	6-10	47-66	250-500 mg PO q6h or 250-500 mg every 12 hours by IV infusion
tetracycline	6-11	57-108	250-500 mg PO q6h or 150 mg IM q12h

From USP DI, 1998.

Demeclocycline also is used to treat the syndrome of inappropriate diuretic hormone secretion because it inhibits the ADH-induced water reabsorption in the kidneys resulting in diuresis.

The tetracyclines have been commonly used to treat many infections such as acne vulgaris, actinomycosis, anthrax, bacterial urinary tract infections, bronchitis, and numerous systemic bacterial infections sensitive to the tetracyclines.

Pharmacokinetics

Oral tetracyclines are fairly well absorbed and distributed to most body fluids. Cerebrospinal fluid levels vary and can range from 10% to 25% of the plasma drug concentration after parenteral administration. Tetracyclines localize in teeth, liver, spleen, tumors, and bone. Doxycycline can reach clinical concentrations in the eye and prostate whereas minocycline reaches in high levels in saliva, sputum, and tears. Doxycycline and minocycline are inactivated in the liver, but most tetracyclines are excreted via the kidneys.

Table 51-4 lists tetracycline half-life and usual adult dose.

Drug interactions

The following effects may occur when tetracycline is given with the drugs listed below:

Drug	Possible effect and management
Antacids, calcium supplements, choline and magnesium salicylates, iron supplements, magnesium salicylate or magnesium laxatives, foods containing milk and milk products	May result in nonabsorbable complex, thus reducing the absorption and serum levels of choline and the antibiotic. Also, antacids may increase gastric pH, which decreases the absorption of tetracyclines. If given concurrently, advise patients to separate medications by 1 to 3 hours from the oral tetracyclines.
colestipol (Colestid) and cholestyramine (Questran)	May bind oral tetracyclines, thus decreasing their absorption. Separate drugs by at least 2 hours.
Estrogen-containing oral contraceptives	Concurrent long-term therapy may reduce contraceptive effectiveness and also may result in breakthrough bleeding. Avoid concurrent drug usage.

Color type indicates an unsafe drug combination.

Side effects and adverse reactions

These include dizziness, ataxia, GI distress, photosensitivity, discoloration of infants' or children's teeth (do not give to children up to 8 years of age), nephrogenic diabetes insipidus with demeclocycline, skin and mucous membrane pigmentation with minocycline, oral, rectal, or genital fungus, dark or discolored tongue, and, rarely, hepatotoxicity, pancreatitis, and benign intracranial hypertension.

Warnings

Use with caution in patients with liver impairment.

Contraindications

Avoid use in persons with tetracycline or "caine" local anesthetic (e.g., lidocaine and procaine) hypersensitivity, nephrogenic diabetes insipidus, and kidney function impairment.

CHLORAMPHENICOL (CHLOROMYCETIN)

Chloramphenicol, a broad-spectrum antibiotic, is a potent inhibitor of protein synthesis. It is a bacteriostatic agent for a wide variety of gram-negative and gram-positive organisms; however, because it is has the potential to be seriously toxic to bone marrow (aplasia leading to aplastic anemia and possibly death), its approved indications are limited.

Although chloramphenicol is usually bacteriostatic, in high doses with highly susceptible organisms, it may be bactericidal. It penetrates bacteria cell membranes and reversibly prevents peptide bond formation, thus inhibiting protein synthesis.

It is indicated for the treatment of meningitis *(Haemophilus influenzae, Streptococcus pneumoniae,* and *Neisseria meningitidis),* paratyphoid fever, Q fever, Rocky Mountain spotted fever, typhoid fever *(Salmonella typhi)*, typhus infections, brain abscesses, and bacterial septicemia.

Pharmacokinetics

Chloramphenicol has good oral and parenteral bioavailability with the highest concentrations reported in the liver and kidneys. Concentrations of up to 50% of serum levels have been noted in cerebrospinal fluid. Chloramphenicol is metabolized in the liver to the inactive glucuronide, but in utero and in neonates an immature liver cannot conjugate chloramphenicol, which may result in toxic levels or accumulation of the active drug ("gray syndrome": blue-gray skin, hypothermia, irregular breathing, coma, and cardiovascular collapse).

The half-life of chloramphenicol in an adult is 1.5 to 3.5 hours; in infants (1 to 2 days of age) it is 1 to 2 days or more. In infants 10 to 16 days of age it is 10 hours. Peak serum levels are reached in 1 to 1.5 hours via the intravenous route. Chloramphenicol is excreted mainly by the kidneys.

Drug interactions

The following effects may occur when chloramphenicol is given with the drugs listed below:

Drug	Possible effect and management
alfentanil (Alfenta)	May result in increased alfentanil blood levels, prolonging its effect. Monitor closely.
Anticonvulsants (hydantoin), blood dyscrasia-causing drugs, bone marrow depressants, and radiation therapy	May result in enhanced bone marrow-depressant effects. Dosage reduction may be necessary. Monitor complete blood counts closely for leukopenia.
Antidiabetic oral agents	May inhibit antidiabetic drug metabolism resulting in increased serum levels and hypoglycemic effects of tolbutamide and chlorpropamide. Monitor blood glucose levels closely because dosage adjustment may be necessary.
clindamycin, erythromycin, or lincomycin	Therapeutic action of chloramphenicol and these drugs may be antagonized. Avoid this drug combination.
phenobarbital (Luminal), phenytoin (Dilantin), or warfarin (Coumadin)	Concurrent drug administration may result in elevated drug serum levels and toxicity of these agents. Monitor all drugs metabolized by the liver enzyme system (chloramphenicol inhibits the cytochrome P-450 system), because toxicity may result.

Side effects and adverse reactions

These include diarrhea, nausea, vomiting, blood dyscrasias, Gray syndrome in neonates, hypersensitivity, neurotoxic reactions (delirium, confusion, and headaches), peripheral neuritis, optic neuritis, and, possibly, irreversible bone marrow depression that may result in aplastic anemia.

Warnings

Use with extreme caution in patients who have had antineoplastic chemotherapy or radiation therapy.

Contraindications

Avoid use in persons with chloramphenicol hypersensitivity, bone marrow suppression, and liver function impairment.

Dosage and administration

Chloramphenicol oral dosage forms were withdrawn from the market in 1998. The intravenous adult dosage is 12.5 mg/kg every 6 hours. The pediatric intravenous dosage for premature and full-term infants up to 2 weeks of age is 6.25 mg/kg every 6 hours. For infants 2 weeks of age and older, it is 12.5 mg/kg every 6 hours (USP DI, 1998). Chloramphenicol is not recommended for use during pregnancy or during breastfeeding.

FLUOROQUINOLONES

The **fluoroquinolones** are synthetic, broad-spectrum agents that have bactericidal activity. They alter deoxyribonucleic acid (DNA) by interfering with DNA gyrase, an enzyme that is necessary for the duplication, transcription, and repair of bacterial DNA. Some examples of quinolones include ciprofloxacin [sip ro flocks′ a sin] (Cipro), enoxacin [a nocks′ a sin] (Penetrex); lomefloxacin [lome flocks′ a sin] (Maxaquin); norfloxacin [nor flocks′ a sin] (Noroxin); and ofloxacin [o flocks′ a sin] (Floxin).

The fluoroquinolones are indicated for the treatment of bone and joint infection, bronchitis, gastroenteritis, gonorrhea, pneumonia, urinary tract infections, and many other infections caused by susceptible microorganisms. Individual fluoroquinolones may vary in their spectrum of activity; for example, all five drugs are indicated for the treatment of urinary tract infections but only ciprofloxacin is approved to treat bone and joint infections.

Pharmacokinetics

The oral bioavailability of fluoroquinolones is good, and they are widely distributed in the body with the following half-lives: ciprofloxacin, 4 hours; enoxacin, 3 to 6 hours; lomefloxacin, 7 to 8 hours; norfloxacin, 3 to 4 hours; and ofloxacin, 4 to 7 hours. They are metabolized in the liver (minimally for ofloxacin and lomefloxacin) and excreted primarily by the kidneys.

Drug interactions

The following effects may occur when fluoroquinolones are given with the drugs listed below:

Drug	Possible effect and management
Antacids, ferrous sulfate or sucralfate	May decrease absorption of ciprofloxacin, reducing drug effectiveness. Administer fluoroquinolone at least 2 hours before these medications.
theophylline and other xanthines	Fluoroquinolones (with the possible exception of lomefloxacin and ofloxacin) may result in increased theophylline plasma levels and toxicity. Monitor theophylline plasma levels closely because dosage adjustments may be necessary.
warfarin (Coumadin)	May result in increased anticoagulant effect and potential for bleeding. While not currently reported with all quinolones, it is recommended that prothrombin time (PT) be monitored closely whenever these drugs are administered concurrently.

Side effects and adverse reactions

These include dizziness, drowsiness, restlessness, stomach distress, diarrhea, nausea, vomiting, photosensitivity, and, rarely, central nervous system (CNS) stimulation (psychosis, confusion, hallucinations, and tremors), hypersensitivity (skin rash, redness, Stevens-Johnson syndrome, face or neck swelling, and shortness of breath), and interstitial nephritis. In addition, Achilles tendinitis and tendon rupture injuries have been reported.

Warnings

Use with caution in patients with liver disease and CNS disorders, including epilepsy and arteriosclerosis.

Contraindications

Avoid use in persons with fluoroquinolone hypersensitivity.

Dosage and administration

Usual adult doses for the fluoroquinolones are the following: ciprofloxacin, 500 to 750 mg PO every 12 hours for 1 to 2 weeks and 400 mg IV every 12 hours; enoxacin, 200 to 400 mg every 12 hours for 1 to 2 weeks; lomefloxacin, 400 mg daily for 10 to 14 days; norfloxacin, 400 mg every 12 hours for 72 hours; ofloxacin, 300 to 400 mg PO or IV every 12 hours for 10 days. Fluoroquinolones are not recommended for use in infants and children.

MISCELLANEOUS ANTIBIOTICS

This section includes a monobactam (aztreonam), a carbapenem (imipenem-cilastatin), metronidazole, and spectinomycin. Other antibiotics in current use are primarily topical agents, which are discussed in Chapter 58.

aztreonam [az tree′ oh nam] (Azactam)

Aztreonam, the first drug in a monobactam class of antibiotics is a synthetic bactericidal antibiotic with activity similar to that of penicillin. It binds to the penicillin-binding protein, resulting in inhibition of bacterial cell wall synthesis, cell lysis, and death. It is active against many gram-negative microorganisms and is used in the treatment of urinary tract, bronchitis, intraabdominal, gynecologic, and skin infections.

Pharmacokinetics

Aztreonam is well absorbed after IM injection and reaches peak serum level in 0.6 to 1.3 hours. Its half-life in adults with normal renal function is 1.4 to 2.2 hours, and it is eliminated primarily by the kidneys.

Drug interactions

No significant drug interactions are reported.

Side effects and adverse reactions

These include gastric distress, diarrhea, nausea, vomiting, hypersensitivity, and thrombophlebitis at the site of injection.

Contraindications

Avoid use in persons with aztreonam hypersensitivity, cirrhosis, and kidney function impairment.

Dosage and administration

Administered by IV infusion, the adult dose is 0.5 to 2 g every 8 to 12 hours, or 1 to 2 g may be administered IV or IM every 8 to 12 hours.

imipenem-cilastatin [i mi pen′ em-sye la stat′ in] (Primaxin IM, Primaxin IV)

Imipenem-cilastatin, a member of a new class of antibiotics (carbapenem) related to the beta-lactam antibiotics, has a wide spectrum of activity against gram-positive and gram-negative aerobic and anaerobic organisms. Imipenem binds to penicillin-binding proteins, thus inhibiting bacterial cell wall synthesis. It is very resistant to degradation by beta-lactamases. Cilastatin inhibits renal dihydropeptidase and blocks the tubular secretion of imipenem, thus preventing renal metabolism of this drug. Therefore cilastatin is combined with imipenem to prevent its inactivation by renal dihydropeptidase.

This antibiotic is indicated for the treatment of bone, joint, skin, and soft tissue infections, bacterial endocarditis, intraabdominal bacteria infections, pneumonia, urinary tract and pelvic infections, and bacterial septicemia when caused by susceptible organisms.

Pharmacokinetics

Administered intramuscularly, imipenem's time to peak serum level is within 2 hours with a half-life of 2 to 3 hours. Intravenously, the half-life is about 60 minutes. Excretion is primarily by the kidneys.

Drug interactions

No significant drug interactions have been reported to date with this product.

Side effects and adverse reactions

These include gastric distress, diarrhea, nausea, vomiting, allergic-type reactions, confusion, lightheadedness, convulsions, and tremors. Pseudomembranous colitis has also been reported with this product.

Contraindications

Avoid use in persons with imipenem, cilastatin or other beta-lactam (e.g., penicillin and cephalosporin) hypersensitivity, kidney impairment, and CNS disorders (e.g., a history of convulsions and brain lesions).

Dosage and administration

The usual adult IV infusion dosage is 250 to 500 mg every 6 hours for mild infections up to 500 mg every 6 to 8 hours for moderate to severe infections. The maximum dose is 50 mg/kg daily. The IM adult dosage is 500 to 750 mg every 12 hours up to a maximum of 1500 mg of imipenem per day. The dosage for children up to the age of 12 is not determined; older children may receive the adult dose.

The second carbapenem released is meropenem (Box 51-2).

metronidazole [me troe ni′ da zole]

(Flagyl, Flagyl I.V.)

Metronidazole is reduced intracellularly to a short-acting, cytotoxic agent that interacts with DNA, thus inhibiting bacteria synthesis and resulting in cell death (microbicidal). It is active against many anaerobic bacteria and protozoa.

BOX 51-2 Meropenem (Merrem IV)

Meropenem (Merrem IV) is a bactericidal, broad-spectrum carbapenem antibiotic. It inhibits cell wall synthesis and is indicated for the treatment of susceptible intraabdominal infections (complicated appendicitis and peritonitis) and bacterial meningitis.

Pseudomembranous colitis, hypersensitivity, and side effects and adverse reactions of diarrhea, nausea, vomiting, headache, and rash have been reported. Adult dose is 1 g IV every 8 hours (Olin, 1998).

Indications

Metronidazole is indicated for the treatment of amebiasis (intestinal and extraintestinal), AAPMC, bone infections, brain abscesses, CNS infections, bacterial endocarditis, genitourinary tract infections, septicemia, trichomoniasis, and other infections caused by organisms susceptible to metronidazole's action.

Pharmacokinetics

Oral metronidazole is well absorbed and distributed throughout the body. It reaches peak serum levels within 1 to 2 hours and has a half life of 8 hours. It is metabolized in the liver and primarily excreted in the kidneys.

Drug interactions

The following effects may occur when metronidazole is given with the drugs listed below:

Drug	Possible effect and management
Alcohol	Metronidazole interferes with the metabolism of alcohol, leading to an accumulation of acetaldehyde. This may result in disulfiram (Antabuse)-type effects: flushing, headaches, nausea, vomiting, and abdominal distress. Avoid or a potentially serious drug interaction may occur.
Anticoagulants (coumarin or indanedione)	May enhance anticoagulant effects by inhibiting their metabolism. Monitor closely with prothrombin testing as dosage adjustments may be necessary.
disulfiram (Antabuse)	Avoid concurrent use or use within 14 days of disulfiram administration in alcoholic patients. Adverse reactions such as confusion and psychosis have been reported.

Color type indicates an unsafe drug combination.

Side effects and adverse reactions

These include dizziness, headache, gastric distress, diarrhea, anorexia, nausea, vomiting, dry mouth, taste alterations, dark urine, peripheral neuropathy, CNS toxicity, hypersensitivity, leukopenia, thrombophlebitis, vaginal candidiasis, and convulsions (with high drug doses).

Warnings

Use with caution in patients with cardiac disease.

Contraindications

Avoid use in persons with metronidazole hypersensitivity, blood dyscrasias, severe liver disease, and active organic CNS disease.

Dosage and administration

The usual adult oral dose is 7.5 mg/kg up to maximum of 1 g every 6 hours for a week or longer. The adult IV infusion dose is 15 mg/kg initially, then 7.5 mg/kg up to a maximum of 1 g every 6 hours for a week or longer. Maximum daily dose is 4 g.

spectinomycin [spek ti noe mye′ sin] (Trobicin)

Spectinomycin's therapeutic indication is the treatment of infections caused by *Neisseria gonorrhoeae.* It is bacteriostatic because it inhibits protein synthesis in the bacteria cell. It is for intramuscular use only and generally is recommended as an alternate regimen for individuals with gonorrhea who have antibiotic resistance or cannot take ceftriaxone.

It is not effective for treating syphilis and should not be used for mixed infections (gonorrhea and syphilis), since it can mask the symptoms of syphilis.

Pharmacokinetics

Spectinomycin is rapidly absorbed after IM injection and reaches peak serum levels in 1-2 hours (after a 2 to 4 g IM dose). Its half-life is 1 to 3 hours with elimination via the kidneys.

Drug interactions

No significant drug interactions are noted.

Side effects and adverse reactions

These include hypersensitivity (chills and fever), nausea, dizziness, urticaria, and pain at site of injection.

Dosage and administration

The usual adult dose for gonorrhea is 2 g IM as a single dose.

URINARY TRACT ANTIMICROBIALS

Urinary tract infections (UTIs) are the most common bacterial infections reported in the United States. Between 10% and 20% of women will experience at least one urinary tract infection in their lifetime. The incidence of UTIs increases in institutional settings, up to as much as 35% to 40% of the population in extended stay hospitals (Sahai, 1995). See Box 51-3 for predisposing risk factors for UTIs.

BOX 51-3 Predisposing Risk Factors for UTIs

Risk Factors	*Frequency Reported*
Urinary tract instrumentation (urethral and ureteral catheterization)*	Up to 67%
Pregnant women	4%-10%
Nonpregnant women	2%-5%

*After a week of indwelling catheterization, up to 100% colonization and bacteriuria (Ahronheim, 1992).

Differentiation between an upper UTI (pyelonephritis) and lower UTI (cystitis) infection is usually based on the presenting signs and symptoms. The upper UTI usually causes pain in the lower back, flank, or stomach plus fever, sweating, nausea, vomiting, weakness, and headache. A lower UTI presents with complaints of a pattern of frequent but small amounts on urination, urgency, dysuria, and, perhaps, incontinence. However, in approximately one third of patients with UTIs, the infection may be present in both the upper and lower urinary tract. UTIs are primarily caused by bacteria.

In community-acquired infections, most UTIs are caused by gram-negative aerobic bacilli from the intestinal tract, such as *E coli.* It has been reported that *E coli* may cause up to 90% of all community-acquired, uncomplicated UTIs (Sahai, 1995). Hospital-acquired infections are often complicated and difficult to treat. Organisms involved include *P aeruginosa, Serratia, Enterobacter,* and other gram-negative microorganisms.

Drug therapies for lower UTIs are often started before culture and sensitivity reports are known. The most probable infecting organism and the antibiotic sensitivity can be predicted from previous information.

Today with the increasing development of antibiotic resistance, the medications that are most effective for UTIs are the sulfonamides, such as trimethoprim-sulfamethoxazole (TMP-SMX) and cephalosporins. Alternate medications include the urinary tract antiseptics, aztreonam, and fluoroquinolones, whereas phenazopyridine (Pyridium) is used primarily as a urinary tract analgesic.

SULFONAMIDES

Sulfonamides (TMP-SMX is most commonly used) are among the most widely used antibacterial agents in the world, particularly for UTIs. These agents are primarily bacteriostatic, in concentrations that are normally useful in controlling infections in humans rather than bactericidal. All of the sulfonamides used therapeutically are synthetically produced, and because they are structurally similar to paraaminobenzoic acid (PABA), they inhibit a bacterial enzyme (dihydropteroate synthetase) necessary to incorporate PABA into dihydrofolic acid.

The blocking of dihydrofolic acid synthesis results in a decrease in tetrahydrofolic acid, which interferes with the synthesis of purines, thymidine, and DNA in the microorganism. Therefore bacteria most sensitive to sulfonamides are those that synthesize their own folic acid. The presence of pus, necrotic tissue, and serum interferes with the activities of the sulfonamides because PABA is present in such materials. Among the microorganisms highly susceptible to sulfonamides are group A beta-hemolytic streptococci, pneumococci, *N meningitides, N gonorrhoeae, E coli, Pasteurella pestis, Bacillus anthracis, Shigella* species, *H influenzae,* and *Pneumocystis carinii.*

Pharmacokinetics

The absorption of sulfonamides is good, with peak serum levels reached between 2 and 6 hours for the majority of them and 6 and 12 hours for sulfamethoxazole, the intermediate-acting sulfonamide. These agents are acetylated in the liver and excreted primarily by the kidneys.

Although the newer sulfonamides, such as sulfisoxazole and sulfacetamide, are quite soluble (even in acid urine), it is recommended that individuals increase their fluid intake to maintain a urine output of at least 1200 ml/day.

Drug interactions

The following effects may occur when sulfonamides are given with the drugs listed below:

Drug	Possible effect and management
Anticoagulants, such as coumarin or indanedione derivatives, anticonvulsants (hydantoin), oral antidiabetic agents, or methotrexate	These agents are highly protein bound; concurrent drug administration may displace them from their protein-binding sites, resulting in increased serum levels and possible toxicity. Metabolism of these agents may also be inhibited by sulfonamides. Monitor closely for signs of toxicity, which indicate the need for dosage adjustment.
Hemolytics, other hepatotoxic medications	Increased potential for toxicity. With these agents an increased risk of inducing liver toxicity exists. Monitor closely for symptoms, such as yellow eyes or skin.
methenamine (Mandelamine)	Methenamine requires an acid urine to be active and effective. It may precipitate if given with a sulfonamide and result in crystalluria. Do not administer concurrently.

Contraindications

Avoid use in persons with spectinomycin hypersensitivity.

Table 51-5 lists side effects and adverse reactions and usual adult dose ranges for urinary tract agents.

URINARY TRACT ANTISEPTICS

Cinoxacin, methenamine mandelate, nalidixic acid, and nitrofurantoin are the primary urinary tract antiseptics. Urinary tract antiseptics are drugs that exert antibacterial activity in the urine but have little or no systemic antibacterial effects. Their usefulness is limited to the treatment of UTIs.

cinoxacin [sin ox′ a sin] (Cinobac)

Cinoxacin inhibits replication of bacterial DNA, thus producing urinary bactericidal effects.

Pharmacokinetics

It is absorbed well orally; its serum levels are usually low, whereas its urinary levels are high. This product does cross the placenta. The time for peak serum levels is between 2 and 3 hours. Cinoxacin is metabolized in the liver and excreted by the kidneys.

For side effects and adverse reactions and usual adult dose ranges of urinary tract agents, see Table 51-5.

Contraindications

Avoid use in persons with cinoxacin or other quinolone hypersensitivity and kidney impairment.

methenamine mandelate [meth en′ a meen] (Mandelamine)
methenamine hippurate
[Hiprex, Urex, Hip-Rex ✱]

Methenamine, which is used to treat UTIs, combines the action of methenamine and mandelic acid or hippurate acid salts. Its effectiveness depends on the release of formaldehyde, which requires an acid medium. The acids released from the mandelate or hippurate salts contribute to this acidity. Formaldehyde may be bactericidal or bacteriostatic, and its effects are believed to be the result of denaturation of bacteria protein. It is ineffective in alkaline urine. Because of its fairly wide bacterial spectrum, low toxicity, and low incidence of resistance, methenamine has often been the drug of choice in long-term suppression of infections.

Pharmacokinetics

Methenamine is absorbed orally and takes ½ to 2 hours to reach peak urinary formaldehyde levels at a urinary pH of 5.6, while the enteric-coated methenamine mandelate reaches its urinary peak in 3 to 8 hours. Excretion is via the kidneys.

Drug interactions

The following effects may occur when methenamine is given with the drugs listed below:

Drug	Possible effect and management
Urinary alkalizers, such as antacids (calcium and/or magnesium) carbonic anhydrase inhibitors, citrates, sodium bicarbonate, or thiazide diuretics	May result in an alkaline urine, thus inhibiting methenamine's conversion to formaldehyde and rendering it ineffective. Avoid concurrent drug administration.
sulfamethizole (Thiosulfil Forte)	In acid urine, the formaldehyde produced may precipitate with certain sulfonamides, which increases the potential for crystalluria. Avoid or a potentially serious drug interaction may occur.

Color type indicates an unsafe drug combination.

TABLE 51-5 Urinary Tract Agents: Side/Adverse Effects and Usual Adult Dose

Drug	Usual Adult Dose	Side Effects and Adverse Reactions
Sulfonamides		*Common:* anorexia, diarrhea, nausea, vomiting, dizziness, headaches, pruritus, rash
sulfadiazine (generic)	2-4 g PO initially, then 1 g q4-6h	
sulfamethizole (Thiosulfil Forte)	0.5-1 g PO q6-8h	*Less common:* muscle and joint pain, fever, sore throat, Stevens-Johnson syndrome, pain on urination, increased bleeding tendencies
sulfamethoxazole (Gantanol)	2 g PO initially, then 1 g q8-12h	
sulfisoxazole (Gantrisin)	2-4 g PO initially, then 0.75 to 1.5 g q4h	
Antiseptics		
cinoxacin (Cinobac)	250 mg PO q hs	*Less common:* nausea, rash, pruritus, diarrhea, anorexia, vomiting, photosensitivity, tinnitus, insomnia
methenamine mandelate (Mandelamine)	1 g PO qid	*Less common:* nausea, rash, stomach distress, painful urination, low back pain
methenamine hippurate (Hiprex)	1 g PO bid	
nalidixic acid (NegGram)	1 g PO q6h	*Common:* diarrhea, nausea, vomiting, rash, pruritus, headache, drowsiness *Less common:* visual disturbances, such as double or blurred vision, halos, or very bright appearance around lights
nitrofurantoin (Furadantin)	50-100 mg PO q6h	*Common:* stomach distress, diarrhea, anorexia, nausea, vomiting, pneumonitis
Analgesic		
phenazopyridine (Pyridium, Phenazo 🍁)	200 mg PO tid	*Less common:* stomach cramps or distress, headache *Rare:* hemolytic anemia, renal failure, hepatotoxicity, aseptic meningitis

Warnings

Use with caution in severely dehydrated patients.

Contraindications

Avoid use in persons with severe liver or kidney impairment.

For side effects and adverse reactions and usual adult dose ranges of urinary tract agents, see Table 51-5.

nalidixic acid [nal i dix′ ik] (NegGram)

Nalidixic acid appears to inhibit bacterial DNA synthesis by interfering with the polymerization of DNA. Resistance usually develops rapidly during treatment with this drug. This drug is indicated for the treatment of UTIs caused by the *Proteus, Klebsiella, Enterobacter,* and *E coli* species.

Pharmacokinetics

Nalidixic acid is well absorbed orally and reaches peak serum levels in 1 to 2 hours and peak urine levels in 3 to 4 hours. It is metabolized in the liver with approximately 30% converted to the active metabolite, hydroxynalidixic acid. Excretion is via the kidneys.

Drug interactions

Nalidixic acid, when given with oral anticoagulants (e.g., coumarin and dicumarol), may displace the anticoagulants from their protein-binding sites, resulting in enhanced anticoagulant action. Dosage adjustments may be necessary, so monitor the patient's risk for injury related to an increase in bleeding tendency if concurrent therapy is necessary.

Warnings

Use with caution in patients with glucose-6-phosphate dehydrogenase (G6PD) deficiency, severe kidney impairment, and advanced cerebral arteriosclerosis.

Contraindications

Avoid use in persons with nalidixic acid or guinolone hypersensitivity, history of convulsions, and liver disease.

For side effects and adverse reactions and usual adult dose ranges of urinary tract agents, see Table 51-5.

nitrofurantoin [nye tro fyoor′ an toyn] (Furadantin, Macrodantin)

Nitrofurantoin is a broad-spectrum bactericidal agent at therapeutic serum levels. It is reduced by bacteria to reactive substances that inactivate or alter bacterial ribosomal proteins. It is indicated for the treatment of urinary tract infections caused by organisms such as *E coli, S aureus, Klebsiella, Enterobacter,* and *Proteus* species.

Pharmacokinetics

After oral administration nitrofurantoin is absorbed and has a half-life of 20 to 60 minutes. Approximately 65% of the drug is rapidly metabolized and inactivated in the liver and body tissues and excreted by the kidneys.

Drug interactions

The following effects may occur when nitrofurantoin is given with he drugs listed below:

Drug	Possible effect and management
Hemolytic agents	Increased possibility of toxic side effects. Monitor blood counts for anemia closely if concurrent therapy is necessary.
Neurotoxic medications	Increased risk of inducing neurotoxicity. Monitor closely for dizziness, drowsiness, or headache if concurrent therapy is necessary.
probenecid (Benemid) or sulfinpyrazone (Anturane)	Tubular secretion of nitrofurantoin will be inhibited, leading to increased serum levels and possible toxicity. A decrease in urinary concentrations and effectiveness may also result. Dosage adjustment of probenecid may be required.

Contraindications

Avoid use in persons with nitrofurantoin hypersensitivity, G6PD deficiency, peripheral neuropathy, lung disease, and kidney function impairment.

For side effects and adverse reactions and usual adult dose ranges of urinary tract agents, see Table 51-5.

AZTREONAM AND THE FLUOROQUINOLONES

Aztreonam and fluoroquinolones (ciprofloxacin, norfloxacin, and ofloxacin) are potent drugs used in the treatment of UTIs. Aztreonam is effective against many gram-negative bacteria and appears to be a safer agent than aminoglycoside therapy in the seriously ill person. Generally, the fluoroquinolones are preferred agents when antibiotic-resistant bacteria are suspected. Refer to the previous sections for information on these medications.

URINARY TRACT ANALGESIC

phenazopyridine [fen az oh peer′ i deen] (Pyridium)

Phenazopyridine's exact mechanism of action is unknown, but it appears to have a topical analgesic or local anesthetic effect on the mucosa of the urinary tract. Phenazopyridine is used for urinary tract irritation, such as pain and burning on urination and urinary frequency. It is only indicated for short-term use because the underlying reason for the irritation should be determined and treated appropriately.

Pharmacokinetics

Phenazopyridine is metabolized by the liver and other body tissues and is excreted by the kidneys.

Drug interactions

No significant drug interactions are reported.

Warnings

Use with caution in patients with hepatitis and kidney function impairment.

Contraindications

Avoid use in persons with phenazopyridine hypersensitivity and G6PD deficiency.

For side effects and adverse reeactions and usual adult dose ranges of urinary tract agents, see Table 51-5.

SUMMARY

Antibiotics are chemical substances produced from microorganisms or synthetically that kill or suppress the growth of microorganisms. Penicillin was originally discovered in molds and then found to be bactericidal (inhibiting the synthesis of the bacterial cell wall). There are now four generations of cephalosporins, which are a modification of the penicillin chemical structure and are also bactericidal. The macrolide antibiotics, or primary erythromycin, is a bacteriostatic agent that inhibits protein synthesis and in high serum levels, is bactericidal for selected microorganisms. The lincomycins are primarily bacteriostatic, whereas vancomycin is bactericidal for many organisms and bacteriostatic for enterococci.

The aminoglycosides are very potent bactericidal antibiotics that are primarily indicated for serious or life-threatening infections. Tetracyclines are bacteriostatic, and the fluoroquinolones inhibit bacterial RNA synthesis and are bactericidal. Metronidazole is a short-acting cytotoxic agent that affects DNA; therefore it is effective against anaerobic bacteria and protozoa.

Drug therapy for urinary tract infections may include sulfonamides, antiseptics, fluoroquinolones, and urinary tract analgesics.

Although many antibiotic products are available, the healthcare professional should be alert to the development of new pathogens and drug resistance (superinfection).

REVIEW QUESTIONS

1. Describe the four generations of cephalosporins as to mechanism of action and indications.
2. Discuss the alcohol and cefamandole (or cefmetazole, cefoperazone, or cefotetan) drug interaction. How can this reaction be avoided?
3. Name and describe the major drug interactions reported with vancomycin and the aminoglycosides.
4. Describe the drug interaction between tetracycline and estrogen-containing oral contraceptives.
5. Discuss the red-neck syndrome reported with vancomycin. How can it be avoided?

REFERENCES

Ahronheim JC: *Handbook of prescribing medications for geriatric patients,* Boston, 1992, Little, Brown.

Beringer PM, Middleton RK: Anaphylaxis and drug allergies. In Young LY, Koda-Kimble MA, editors: *Applied therapeutics: the clinical use of drugs,* ed 6, Vancouver, Wash, 1995, Applied Therapeutics, Inc.

Katzung BG: *Basic and clinical pharmacology,* ed 5, Norwalk, Conn, 1992, Appleton & Lange.

Mandell GL, Petri WA Jr: Antimicrobial agents. In Hardman JG, Limbird LE, editors: *Goodman & Gilman's the pharmacological basis of therapeutics,* ed 9, New York, 1996, McGraw-Hill.

Olin BR: *Facts and comparisons.* Philadelphia, 1998, JB Lippincott.

Raper KB, Alexander DF: *J Elsiha Mitchell Sci Soc* 61:74, 1945.

Sahai JV: Urinary tract infections. In Young LY, Koda-Kimble MA, editors: *Applied therapeutics: the clinical use of drugs,* ed 6, Vancouver, Wash, 1995, Applied Therapeutics, Inc.

United States Pharmacopeial Convention: *USP DI: drug information for the health care professional,* ed 18, Rockville, Md, 1998, The Convention.

ADDITIONAL REFERENCES

American Hospital Formulary Service: *AHFS drug information '98,* Bethesda, Md, 1998, American Society of Hospital Pharmacists.

Anderson KN et al, editors: *Mosby's medical, nursing, and allied health dictionary,* ed 5, St Louis, 1998, Mosby.

Cunha BA: The urologic uses of aminoglycosides, *Emerg Med* 24(7):299, 1992.

Danziger LH, Itokazu GS: Gastrointestinal infections. In Young LY, Koda-Kimble MA, editors: *Applied therapeutics: the clinical use of drugs,* ed 6, Vancouver, Wash, 1995, Applied Therapeutics, Inc.

Doughty DB, Jackson DB: *Gastrointestinal disorders,* St Louis, 1993, Mosby.

Grimes D: *Infectious disease,* St Louis, 1991, Mosby.

Just PM: Overview of the fluoroquinolone antibiotics, *Pharmacotherapy* 13(2, part 2):4S, 1994.

Melmon KL et al: *Clinical pharmacology,* ed 3, New York, 1992, McGraw-Hill.

Mosby: *Mosby's GenRx,* St Louis, 1998, Mosby.

Mullenix T et al: Urinary tract infections and prostatitis. In DiPiro JT, Talber R et al, editors: *Pharmacotherapy, a pathophysiologic approach,* ed 2, Norwalk, Conn, 1993, Appleton & Lange.

Mylotte JM et al: Staying on top of hospital infections, *Patient Care* 27(2):116, 1993.

Semla TP et al: *Geriatric dosage handbook,* Cleveland, 1993, American Pharmaceutical Association.

Williams SR: *Basic nutrition and diet therapy,* ed 11, St Louis, 1999, Mosby.

CHAPTER 52

Antifungal and Antiviral Drugs

KEY DRUGS

acyclovir, (p. 673)
amphotericin B, (p. 669)
indinavir, (p. 681)
ketoconazole, (p. 670)
zidovudine, (p. 680)

KEY TERMS

candidiasis, (p. 669)
chemoprophylactic, (p. 672)
fungi, (p. 669)
fungistatic agent, (p. 671)
mycoses, (p. 669)
onychomycosis, (p. 672)

CHAPTER FOCUS

The extensive use of antibiotics (especially broad-spectrum) for the treatment of infections has often resulted in the development of a superinfection. In addition, immunosuppressed patients, as the result of a transplant or antineoplastic therapy, corticosteroids, and persons with acquired immunodeficiency syndrome (AIDS) are also at increased risk for a superinfection with fungal or viral microorganisms. The need for more potent and effective antifungal and antiviral agents to treat these devastating infections has resulted in early or fast-track Food and Drug Administration (FDA) approval of these agents. The healthcare professional needs to have current knowledge about the use and monitoring of the antifungal and antiviral drugs.

OBJECTIVES

After reading and studying this chapter, the student should be able to do the following:

1. *Define and describe the key terms and key drugs.*
2. *List and discuss the four commonly used antifungal agents, including their mechanisms of action and indications.*
3. *Name and describe four major adverse reactions with the use of amphotericin B and the azole antifungals.*
4. *Define the terms tinea capitis, tinea corporis, tinea cruris, and tinea pedis.*
5. *Explain why effective antiviral drug therapy is limited compared with other antibacterial therapies.*
6. *Compare the effects of a reverse transcriptase inhibitor with a protease inhibitor, including mechanisms of action, indications, and significant drug interactions.*

ANTIFUNGAL DRUGS

Human infections by **fungi** can be caused by any of about 50 species of plantlike, parasitic microorganisms. These simple, parasitic plants, lacking chlorophyll, are unable to make their own food and so are dependent on other life forms. Infections by fungi, termed **mycoses,** can range from mild and superficial to severe and life threatening. Infecting organisms can be ingested orally or become implanted under the skin after injury or inhaled if the fungal spores are airborne. One species of fungi, *Candida albicans,* is usually part of the normal flora of the skin, mouth, intestines, and vagina; overgrowth and systemic infection from it may result from antibiotic, antineoplastic, and corticosteroid drug therapy. This is referred to as an opportunistic infection. Oral **candidiasis** (thrush) is common in newborn infants and immunocompromised patients, whereas vaginal candidiasis is more common in pregnant women, women with diabetes mellitus, or in women who take oral contraceptives. The prevalence of mycoses as an opportunistic infection in persons with AIDS is increasing, as the incidence of AIDS increases. Nonopportunistic fungal infections such as blastomycosis, histoplasmosis, and others are usually rare.

The lag in the development of antifungal chemotherapy is related to the high chemical concentrations of antifungal agents necessary, which cannot be tolerated by the human host. Therefore only a few antifungal compounds are available for systemic use. Topical antifungal preparations are discussed in Chapter 58. The following discussions include only systemic agents. See the box for FDA pregnancy safety classifications of antifungal drugs.

amphotericin B [am foe ter′ i sin] (Fungizone Intravenous)

Amphotericin B can be fungistatic or fungicidal, depending on the concentrations achieved clinically. This drug does not have a therapeutic effect on bacteria or viruses. Amphotericin B binds to sterols in the fungus cell membrane to increase cell permeability, which results in a loss of potassium and other elements from the cell.

Amphotericin B is effective for treating aspergillosis, blastomycosis, candidiasis (moniliasis), coccidioidomycosis, cryptococcosis, fungal endocarditis, histoplasmosis, cryptococcal meningitis, fungal septicemia, and many other systemic fungal infections.

PREGNANCY SAFETY

Category	Drug
B	amphotericin B, didanosine, famciclovir, nelfinavir, ritonavir, saquinavir, valacyclovir
C	acyclovir, amantadine, cidofovir, delavirdine, fluconazole, flucytosine, foscarnet, ganciclovir, indinavir, itraconazole, ketoconazole, lamivudine, miconazole, nevirapine, rimantadine, stavudine, zalcitabine, zidovudine
X	ribavirin

Pregnancy safety for griseofulvin is not established, although it is recommended that this drug not be taken during pregnancy because of reported teratogenic effects.

Pharmacokinetics

Administered parenterally, amphotericin B is widely distributed in the body. It has a initial half-life in adults of 24 hours, and the terminal half-life is approximately 15 days. The site of metabolism is unknown, but excretion is via the kidneys. About 40% of the drug is excreted over 7 days, but it has still been detected in the urine for at least 7 weeks after the drug was discontinued.

Drug interactions

The following effects may occur when amphotericin B is given with the drugs listed below:

Drug	Possible effect and management
Adrenocorticoids, glucocorticoids, and mineralocorticoids (ACTH)	May result in severe hypokalemia; if given concurrently, frequent serum potassium determinations should be performed. May decrease adrenal cortex response to corticotropin (ACTH)
bone marrow depressants and radiation therapy	May produce increased bone marrow-depressant effects; monitor blood cell counts closely because dosage adjustments may be necessary if the anemia, leukopenia, or thrombocytopenia increases.
Digitalis glycosides	Amphotericin B-induced hypokalemia may increase the potential for digitalis toxicity. Monitor closely for dysrhythmias, anorexia, nausea, vomiting, or other indications of possible toxicity.
Nephrotoxic medications and potassium-depleting diuretics	Increased risk of nephrotoxicity; monitor closely for edema or decrease in urination, as drug dosage adjustments may be necessary.

Side effects and adverse reactions

With the IV infusion of amphotericin B these include headache, gastrointestinal (GI) distress, anemia, hypokalemia, infusion reaction (fever, chills, nausea, vomiting, and hypotension), renal impairment, anemia, hypokalemia, thrombophlebitis at the infusion site, blurred vision, cardiac dysrhythmias, rash, leukopenia, peripheral neuropathy, convulsions, and thrombocytopenia.

Contraindications

Avoid use in persons with amphotericin B hypersensitivity and kidney function impairment.

Dosage and administration

The adult dose for systemic fungus infection is usually a 1 mg test dose in 5% dextrose solution administered over 10 to 30 minutes. This is followed by increments of 5 to 10 mg of amphotericin B infusion (up to 50 mg/day), administered over 2 to 6 hours, depending on the infection and the individual's tolerance of the medication. The pediatric dose is initially, a 0.25 mg/kg daily in 5% dextrose administered over 6 hours, increased gradually (up to 1 mg/kg/day), depending on the infection and the child's tolerance of this medication.

Amphotericin B lipid complex injection (Abelcet) is a liposomal encapsulation of amphotericin used to treat aspergillosis in persons that are refractory to or unable to tolerate standard amphotericin B therapy. The liposome formulation provides a therapeutic effect with significantly less nephrotoxicity than amphotericin B. The most common side effects and adverse reactions include fever, chills, nausea, hypotension, vomiting, dyspnea, and respiratory failure.

The usual daily dose for adults and children is 5 mg/kg by single infusion, at a rate of 2.5 mg/kg/hr. See current references for additional information on this product (Abelcet, 1996).

AZOLE ANTIFUNGALS

fluconazole [floo koe′ na zole] (Diflucan)
itraconazole [eye trah koe′ na zole] (Sporanox)
ketoconazole [kee toe koe′ na zole] (Nizoral)
miconazole [my kon′ a zole] injection (Monistat IV)

The azole antifungals may be fungistatic or fungicidal agents, depending on dosage and systemic levels achieved. Ergosterol is the primary sterol in fungus cell membranes. These agents affect the biosynthesis of the fungal sterols by interfering with the cytochrome P-450 enzyme system. The result is impaired or depleted ergosterol biosynthesis, inhibiting fungus growth.

Fluconazole and itraconazole have a greater affinity for fungal P-450 activity than for the human liver cytochrome P-450 system. Fluconazole has good penetration in cerebrospinal fluid (CSF); thus it is used for the treatment of cryptococcal meningitis, whereas itraconazole has poor CSF penetration but is widely distributed in the body and is indicated for treatment of aspergillosis, blastomycosis, and histoplasmosis.

Ketoconazole is well distributed in body fluids (saliva, bile, urine, breast milk, and inflamed joint fluid), tendons and other body tissues. It is indicated for the treatment of disseminated and mucocutaneous candidiasis, paracoccidioidomycosis, and recalcitrant tinea infections. Miconazole is also widely distributed in body tissues, but neither ketoconazole nor miconazole adequately crosses the blood-brain barrier. Miconazole is primarily indicated for the treatment of disseminated and chronic mucocutaneous candidiasis.

Pharmacokinetically, fluconazole, itraconazole, and ketoconazole are administered orally, while fluconazole and miconazole may be administered intravenously. Oral administration rates are good if fluconazole is administered in the fasting state, while itraconazole and ketoconazole should be administered with food. Ketoconazole requires an acid medium for dissolution and absorption; therefore achlorhydria, hypochlorhydria, or an increase in stomach pH caused by medications will impair absorption of ketoconazole.

For pharmacokinetics and usual adult dose of azole antifungals, see Table 52-1.

Drug interactions

The following effects may occur when an azole antifungal agent is given with the drugs listed below:

Drug	Possible effect and management
Alcohol or hepatotoxic drugs	Concurrent use increases the risk for hepatotoxicity. Also, use of alcohol and ketoconazole is reported to cause a disulfiram-like reaction.

TABLE 52-1 Azole Antifungals: Pharmacokinetics and Usual Adult Dose

	Pharmacokinetics		
Drug	***Peak Serum (hr)****	***Half-life (hr)†***	***Usual Adult Dose***
fluconazole (Diflucan)	1-2	Adults: 30 Children: 14-20	100-200 mg PO/IV daily
itraconazole (Sporanox)	3-4	Single dose: 21 Steady state: 64	200 mg PO once or twice a day
ketoconazole (Nizoral)	1-4	8	200 to 400 mg PO daily
miconazole (Monistat IV)	E of I	20-25	0.2 to 1.2 g/IV infusion

From Olin, 1998, USP DI, 1998.
*Time to peak serum concentration. †Half-life for normal renal function. E of I, end of infusion.

Antacids, anticholinergics, histamine H receptor antagonists, omeprazole (Prilosec), sucralfate (Carafate), or didanosine (ddI) (Videx)	These drugs increase GI pH, thereby reducing the absorption of itraconazole and ketoconazole. Administer the drugs at least 2 hours apart.
Antidiabetic agents, oral (chlorpropamide [Diabinese], glyburide [DiaBeta], glipizide [Glucotrol], tolbutamide [Orinase])	May cause increased serum concentrations of these antidiabetic agents, resulting in hypoglycemia. Monitor blood glucose closely levels if drugs are given concurrently because a dosage adjustment of the antidiabetic agents may be necessary.
astemizole (Hismanal) or terfenadine* (Seldane)	Concurrent use results in elevated plasma levels of astemizole or terfenadine by inhibiting their metabolic pathway, which may result in cardiac dysrhythmias and death. Avoid or a potentially serious drug interaction may occur.
carbamazepine (Tegretol)	Concurrent use decreases itraconazole levels; may lead to treatment failures.
cyclosporine (Sandimmune)	Monitor plasma cyclosporine levels closely; they have been reported to increase in some individuals receiving both drugs concurrently.
digoxin (Lanoxin)	Itraconazole increases serum digoxin levels, leading to digoxin toxicity. Monitor digoxin levels carefully.
phenytoin (Dilantin)	Closely monitor phenytoin levels because increased serum levels are reported in patients receiving both drugs concurrently.
rifampin (Rifadin) or rifabutin (Mycobutin)	Concurrent drug administration may result in increased fluconazole metabolism. Monitor closely; the fluconazole dose may need to be increased.
warfarin (Coumadin)	May result in a decrease in warfarin metabolism, resulting in an increase in prothrombin time (PT). Closely monitor PTs in patients receiving both drugs concurrently.

Color type indicates an unsafe drug combination.
*No longer available in the United States but may be available in other countries.

Side effects and adverse reactions

For azole antifungals these include nausea, vomiting, stomach distress, diarrhea, flushing, drowsiness, dizziness, headache, and hypersensitivity (fever, chills, and rash). Miconazole has caused redness, swelling, or pain at injection site. Rarely, ketoconazole may cause gynecomastia and impotency due to inhibition of adrenal steroid and testosterone synthesis, menstrual irregularities, and photophobia. Other rare effects include liver toxicity, anemia, agranulocytosis and exfoliative skin disorders such as Stevens-Johnson syndrome (for fluconazole), and thrombocytopenia for fluconazole and miconazole.

Contraindications

Avoid use in persons with azole antifungal hypersensitivity, achlorhydria, or hypochlorhydria (reduces drug absorption, especially itraconazole and ketoconazole), alcoholism, and liver or kidney function impairment.

flucytosine capsules [floo sye′ toe seen] (Ancobon, Ancotil 🍁)

Flucytosine enters fungus cells, where it is converted to fluorouracil, an antimetabolite. It interferes with pyrimidine metabolism, thus preventing nucleic acid and protein synthesis. It has selective toxicity against susceptible strains of fungi because the body cells do not convert significant quantities of this drug into fluorouracil.

Flucytosine is indicated for the treatment of fungal endocarditis (caused by *Candida* species), fungal meningitis (caused by *Cryptococcus* species), and fungal pneumonia, septicemia, or urinary infections caused by *Candida* or *Cryptococcus* species.

Pharmacokinetics

It is well absorbed orally and widely distributed in the body including CSF, the latter being approximately 60% to 90% of serum concentrations. Flucytosine, with a half-life of 2.5 to 6 hours, is not significantly metabolized but is excreted via the kidneys, mostly as unchanged drug.

Drug interactions

Concurrent use in patients who are receiving bone marrow suppressants or radiation therapy may result in an increased bone marrow-depressant effect. Monitor closely as drug dosage reduction may be necessary.

Side effects and adverse reactions

These include confusion, hallucinations, photosensitivity, headache, dizziness, sedation, gastric distress, anemia, hepatitis, hypersensitivity, and bone marrow suppression (leukopenia and thrombocytopenia)

Dosage and administration

The adult and pediatric oral dosage is 12.5 to 37.5 mg/kg every 6 hours.

GRISEOFULVIN PRODUCTS

griseofulvin microsize [gri see oh ful′ vin] (Grisactin, Grifulvin V, Fulvicin-U/F, Grisovin-FP 🍁)

griseofulvin tablets, ultramicrosize (Fulvicin P/G)

Griseofulvin is a **fungistatic agent;** it inhibits fungus cell mitosis during metaphase. It is also deposited in the keratin precursor cells in skin, hair, and nails, thus inhibiting fungal invasion of the keratin. When infested keratin is shed, healthy keratin will replace it. Griseofulvin is indicated for the treatment of susceptible organisms for **onychomycosis** (nail fungus), tinea barbae (fungal infection of bearded section of face and neck), tinea capitis (fungal infection of scalp, ringworm), tinea corporis (fungal infection of nonhairy skin), tinea cruris (fungal infection in groin), and tinea pedis (fungal infection of foot, athlete's foot).

Pharmacokinetics

The oral absorption of microsize griseofulvin varies from 25% to 70% of the oral dose, while the ultramicrosize form is nearly completely absorbed. If griseofulvin is administered with or after a fatty meal, absorption is significantly enhanced. Griseofulvin is distributed in keratin layers in the skin, hair, and nails with very little being distributed in body tissues and fluids. It has a half-life of 24 hours and reaches peak serum levels in about 4 hours. Metabolism is in the liver, and it is primarily excreted unchanged in feces.

Drug interactions

The following effects may occur when griseofulvin is given with the drugs listed below:

Drug	Possible effect and management
Anticoagulants, oral (coumarin or indanedione)	Decreased anticoagulant effect may be noted; monitor prothrombin times closely until a stable serum level is achieved. Dosage adjustments may be required during and after griseofulvin administration.
Contraceptives, estrogen-containing, oral	Chronic, long-term use of griseofulvin may decrease the effectiveness of oral contraceptives. Intercycle menstrual bleeding, amenorrhea, or pregnancy may be seen. Advise the patient to use an alternate method of contraception when taking griseofulvin.
Other hepatic enzyme-inducing agents	May increase the potential for toxicity; monitor closely for dark urine, jaundice, yellow sclera, and changes in hepatic function studies.

Side effects and adverse reactions

These include headache, dizziness, gastric distress, insomnia, weakness, confusion, hypersensitivity (rash or hives), photosensitivity, and, rarely, leukopenia, hepatitis, and peripheral neuritis.

Warnings

Use with caution in patients with lupus erythematosus or lupus-like syndromes.

Contraindications

Avoid use in persons with griseofulvin hypersensitivity, liver disease, and porphyria.

Dosage and administration

The oral adult microsize dose is 500 mg orally daily or divided in two doses. To treat tinea pedis or onychomycosis, the dose is 500 mg twice daily. The pediatric dosage is 5 mg/kg every 12 hours (USP DI, 1998). The ultramicrosize adult dose is 250 to 375 mg daily.

nystatin lozenges [nye stat′ in] (Mycostatin)
nystatin (Mycostatin, Nilstat, Nadostine ♣)

Nystatin is an antibiotic primarily used to treat cutaneous or mucocutaneous infections caused by the monilial organism *C albicans.* Nystatin adheres to sterols in the fungal cell membrane, altering cell membrane permeability, which results in loss of essential intercellular contents.

Pharmacokinetics

Nystatin is not absorbed from the GI tract, producing a local antifungal effect. It is excreted in the feces.

Side effects and adverse reactions

These are uncommon, mainly gastric distress.

Contraindications

Avoid use in persons with nystatin hypersensitivity.

Dosage and administration

The usual oral adult dose for candidiasis is 200,000 to 400,000 unit lozenges dissolved slowly in the mouth four or five times daily. The oral suspension dose is 400,000 to 600,000 units orally four times daily, and the tablet dose is 500,000 to 1,000,000 units orally three times daily.

ANTIVIRAL DRUGS

Chemotherapy for viral diseases has been more limited than chemotherapy for bacterial diseases because development and clinical application of antiviral drugs are difficult. In many viral infections, the replication of the virus in the body reaches its peak before any clinical symptoms appear. By the time signs and symptoms of illness appear, the multiplication of the virus is ending, and the subsequent course of the illness has been determined. Therefore to be clinically effective, antiviral drugs must be administered in a **chemoprophylactic** manner as preventive agents before disease appears.

A second factor limiting the development of antiviral drugs is that viruses are true parasites; they replicate within the mammalian cell and use the host cells' enzyme systems. Thus drugs that would inhibit virus replication would also disturb the host cells and may therefore be too toxic for use.

The protease inhibitors are currently the most potent antiviral agents available. These agents have suppressed viral replication for up to a year in clinical trials and administering them in combination therapies has decreased viral loads and increased CD4 counts (MacDonald, Kazanjian, 1996). Studies of various combinations of these agents and their effect on human immunodeficiency virus (HIV) infection and AIDS complications and disease progression are currently being investigated (Fig. 52-1).

The antivirals reviewed here include acyclovir (Zovirax) ⚷, amantadine (Symmetrel), famciclovir (Famvir), foscarnet (Foscavir), ganciclovir (Cytovene), ribavirin (Virazole), rimantadine (Flumadine), and valacyclovir (Valtrex). In addition, antivirals in current use (alone or in combination) for the treatment of HIV infection are divided into (1) reverse transcriptase inhibitors (nucleoside analogs), (2) protease inhibitors, and (3) non-nucleoside reverse transcriptase inhibitors. The reverse transcriptase inhibitors include didanosine (Videx), lamivudine (3TC, Epivir), stavudine (D4T, Zerit), zalcitabine (ddC, Hivid), and zidovudine (AZT, Retrovir) ⚷. Protease inhibitors include indinavir (Crixivan) ⚷, ritonavir (Norvir), and saquinavir (Invirase). The non-nucleoside reverse transcriptase inhibitor is nevirapine (Viramune).

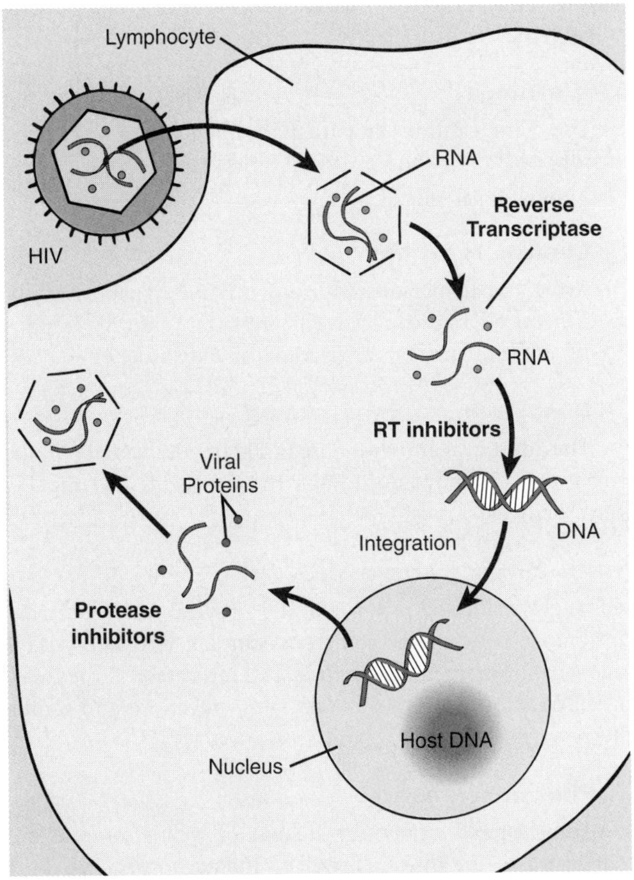

FIGURE 52-1
Inhibition sites for HIV replication. The HIV redundant genes are composed of RNA, which are translated to DNA by reverse transcriptase (RT) enzyme to reproduce. The RT inhibitors interfere with virus production at this site. When integrated DNA becomes part of the cell, the cell produces viral proteins requiring protease enzyme for the production of new HIVs. The protease inhibitors block this enzyme to prevent the release of new viruses into the bloodstream. As a result, combination therapies can reduce the viral load of new HIV produced in the body.

acyclovir [ay sye' kloe ver] (Zovirax) ⚷

Acyclovir is selectively taken up by herpes simplex virus (HSV)-infected cells and is eventually converted via a number of cellular enzymes to an active triphosphate form that is incorporated into growing DNA chains produced by the virus, resulting in inhibition of viral DNA replication.

Indications

Oral acyclovir is used in the prophylaxis and treatment of genital herpes infections in immunocompromised and non-immunocompromised patients. It is also used to treat varicella (chickenpox) infections in non-immunocompromised children if used within 24 hours of the rash appearance. Injectable acyclovir is used to treat initial severe herpes genitalis in immunocompromised and non-immunocompromised patients unable to take or absorb the oral dose form. The parenteral dose form is also used to treat herpes simplex encephalitis and herpes zoster infections, the latter caused by the varicella-zoster virus.

Pharmacokinetics

The oral dose form is poorly (15% to 30%) absorbed, but serum levels achieved are therapeutic. It is widely disseminated to various body fluids and tissues including CSF, and herpetic vesicular fluid. CSF levels are approximately 50% of the serum drug concentration.

The half-life is approximately 2.5 hours. The drug is metabolized by the liver and excreted primarily in the urine.

Drug interactions

Concurrent use of acyclovir intravenously with nephrotoxic medications may increase the risk for nephrotoxicity. Monitor closely, especially if the patient has kidney disease or impairment.

Side effects and adverse reactions

These include gastric distress, headache, dizziness, nausea, diarrhea, and vomiting with the oral dosage form. With the parenteral form phlebitis at the injection site, acute renal failure with rapid injection or, rarely, encephalopathic alterations such as confusion, hallucinations, convulsions, tremors, and coma may occur.

Warnings

Use with caution in patients with neurologic abnormalities or history of prior neurologic reactions to cytotoxic medications.

Contraindications

Avoids use in persons with acyclovir or ganciclovir hypersensitivity and kidney function impairment or in dehydrated persons.

Dosage and administration

The usual oral adult dose for herpes genital infection is 200 mg orally every 4 hours during waking hours (five times daily) for 10 days. For chronic suppression of recurrent infection, the dose is 400 mg orally twice a day. The dose for varicella in children 2 to 12 years of age is 20 mg/kg up to 800 mg/dose four times daily for 5 days.

The parenteral adult dosage for severe genital herpes is 5 mg/kg every 8 hours for 5 days. For other dosage recommendations, see A current package insert.

amantadine [a man′ ta deen] (Symmetrel, Symadine)

Amantadine appears to block the uncoating of the influenza A virus and the release of viral nucleic acid into host respiratory epithelial cells. It also increases dopamine release and inhibits the reuptake of dopamine and norepinephrine centrally. Therefore amantadine is indicated for the prevention and treatment of influenza A, for treatment of Parkinson's disease, and for the treatment of drug-induced extrapyramidal reactions.

Pharmacokinetics

Amantadine is rapidly absorbed orally and distributed to saliva and nasal secretions and crosses the blood-brain barrier. It has a half-life of 11 to 15 hours, reaching a peak serum level within 2 to 4 hours. Its onset of action as an antidyskinetic is usually within 2 days. It is excreted mostly unchanged by the kidneys.

Drug interactions

The following effects may occur when amantadine is given with the drugs listed below:

Drug	Possible effect and management
Alcohol	Increased risk for central nervous system (CNS) side effects such as dizziness, fainting episodes, confusion, or circulatory problems reported. Avoid or a potentially serious drug interaction may occur.
Anticholinergics	May result in an increase in anticholinergic side effects, such as hallucinations, dry mouth, blurred vision, confusion, and nightmares. Monitor closely, as dosage adjustment of amantadine may be required.
CNS-stimulating agents	May cause increased CNS stimulation, resulting in insomnia, increased irritability, and nervousness. Cardiac dysrhythmias and convulsions may also occur. Avoid or a potentially serious drug interaction may occur. If given concurrently, be sure to monitor pulse rate and neurologic status closely.

Color type indicates an unsafe drug combination.

Side effects and adverse reactions

These include CNS toxicity, gastric distress, and with chronic therapy, livedo reticularis (a vasospastic disorder worsened by exposure to cold that is evidenced by a reddish blue mottling of the legs and sometimes arms), anticholinergic side effects (dry mouth, constipation, blurred vision, confusion, and difficult urination), vomiting, and orthostatic hypotension.

Warnings

Use with caution in patients with eczema rash (or a history of), psychosis, or in individuals with severe psychoneurosis.

Contraindications

Avoid use in persons with amantadine hypersensitivity, peripheral edema, congestive heart failure, kidney impairment, and epilepsy or other convulsive disorders.

Dosage and administration

The adult oral antiviral dose is 200 mg orally daily or 100 mg every 12 hours. Antidyskinetic dosage is 100 mg PO once or twice a day.

famciclovir [fam sye′ kloe veer] (Famvir)

Famciclovir, an oral prodrug of the antiviral penciclovir, has inhibitory action against herpes simplex viruses (types 1 and 2) and varicella-zoster virus. It is indicated for the treatment of acute herpes zoster (shingles) infections and genital herpes (Mosby, 1998).

Pharmacokinetics

Administered orally, famciclovir is well absorbed and converted in the intestinal wall to the active penciclovir. It reaches its peak serum level in about 1 hour, its half life is 2 to 3 hours, and it is excreted unchanged primarily in urine and feces.

Side effects and adverse reactions

These include headaches, weakness, gastric distress (nausea, vomiting, and diarrhea), and fatigue.

Contraindications

Avoid use in persons with kidney function impairment.

Dosage and administration

The usual adult dose is 500 mg PO every 8 hours for 1 week.

foscarnet [fos car' net] (Foscavir)

Foscarnet is a virustatic agent; that is, it inhibits viral replication of all known herpes viruses in vitro, which includes cytomegalovirus (CMV), herpes simplex virus types 1 and 2, Epstein-Barr virus, and varicella-zoster virus. It acts by selective inhibition at the pyrophosphate binding site of viral DNA polymerase. If the drug is discontinued, viral replication will resume. It is currently used to treat cytomegalovirus retinitis in patients with AIDS.

Pharmacokinetics

This drug is administered by intravenous infusion, has an elimination half-life of 3.3 to 6.8 hours, reaches peak serum level at the end of the infusion, is not metabolized, and is excreted primarily unchanged in the urine.

Drug interactions

The following effects may occur when foscarnet is given with the drugs listed below:

Drug	Possible effect and management
Nephrotoxic medications	May result in increased risk of renal toxicity. Monitor renal status closely if drugs such as acyclovir (Zovirax), aminoglycosides, amphotericin B (Fungizone), or other nephrotoxic medications are administered concurrently.
pentamidine (Pentam 300)	Concurrent administration of IV pentamidine with foscarnet may result in severe hypocalcemia, hypomagnesemia, and nephrotoxicity. Avoid or a potentially serious drug interaction may occur.

Color type indicates an unsafe drug combination.

Side effects and adverse reactions

These include nephrotoxicity, gastric distress, neurotoxicity, anemia, leukopenia, and phlebitis or pain at injection site.

Warnings

Use with caution in patients with anemia.

Contraindications

Avoid use in persons with foscarnet hypersensitivity and kidney impairment and in dehydrated persons.

Dosage and administration

For induction, the usual adult dose by IV infusion is 60 mg/kg administered over a minimum of 1 hour by infusion pump, every 8 hours for 2 to 3 weeks. The maintenance dosage is 90 to 120 mg/kg daily.

ganciclovir [gan sye' kloe vir] (Cytovene, Cytovene-IV)

Ganciclovir is converted intracellularly to the triphosphate form, which is the active, antiviral agent. In the presence of the cytomegalovirus, ganciclovir is rapidly phosphorylated to ganciclovir-triphosphate, which then inhibits viral DNA polymerase, suppressing viral DNA synthesis. If ganciclovir is discontinued, viral replication will resume.

Pharmacokinetics

Ganciclovir is administered by IV infusion or by intravitreal injection. The serum half-life is 2.5 to 3.6 hours, and the vitreous fluid half-life is about 13 hours. This drug is excreted unchanged primarily by the kidneys.

Oral ganciclovir is indicated only for maintenance of CMV retinitis in persons who had resolution of active retinitis after induction therapy with parenteral ganciclovir. The oral dosage form has a half-life of 3 to 5.5 hours and reaches peak serum concentration in 3 hours if administered with food. An intravitreal ganciclovir implant (Vitasert Implant) is in phase III studies, and thus far, it has been found to be more effective in delaying the progression of retinitis than IV ganciclovir (Hitchens, 1996).

Drug interactions

The following effects may occur when ganciclovir is given with the drugs listed below:

Drug	Possible effect and management
Bone marrow-depressant drugs	Concurrent use may result in increased bone marrow-suppressant effects. Monitor blood closely for neutropenia and thrombocytopenia.
zidovudine (AZT)	May result in severe hematologic toxicity. Avoid or a potentially serious drug interaction may occur.

Color type indicates an unsafe drug combination.

Side effects and adverse reactions

After IV or oral administration these include granulocytopenia, thrombocytopenia, anemia, gastric distress, CNS effects (e.g., anxiety and tremors), hypersensitivity, and phlebitis or pain at the injection site. After intravitreal administration, a variety of ophthalmic disorders may result, such as retinal detachment, scleral induration, subconjunc-

BOX 52-1 Additional Antifungal Agents

Drug	Indication	Comments
cidofovir (Vistide)	Treatment of cytomegalovirus retinitis	Selectively inhibits viral DNA polymerase. Adult dose: 5 mg/kg, administered by IV infusion over 1 hour once weekly for 2 weeks, then every 2 weeks thereafter. Probenecid (2 g) is given 3 hours before each cidofovir dose, and 1 g is administered 2 and 8 hours after the infusion. SE/AR include weakness, GI distress, headache, nephrotoxicity, neutropenia, fever, and, rarely, ocular hypotony. Contraindicated in patients with cidofovir or probenecid hypersensitivity or severe kidney function impairment.
delavirdine (Rescriptor)	Antiviral for HIV infection	A non-nucleoside reverse transcriptase inhibitor, it is used alone or in combination with other antiviral agents. Adult dose is 400 mg PO three times a day. SE/AR include diarrhea, weakness, headache, nausea, vomiting, severe skin rash, conjunctivitis, fever, joint and muscle aches, oral lesions in mouth, and, rarely, dyspnea. Numerous significant drug interactions are reported; check a current reference. A decrease in gastric pH from H_2 receptor antagonists (cimetidine and others) or concurrent antacids will decrease absorption of delavirdine. Avoid chronic use of these medications and separate antacid dosing by at least 1 hour. Contraindicated in patients with liver function impairment.
nelfinavir (Viracept)	Antiviral for HIV infection	Inhibits HIV protease. Cross-resistance with the reverse transcriptase inhibitors is unlikely as different enzymes are involved. More study is needed in this area. Oral powder is only used in children 2 to 13 years of age, 20 to 30 mg/kg three times daily with food. SE/AR include diarrhea, gas, nausea, skin rash, diabetes, or hyperglycemia and ketoacidosis. Many significant drug interactions are noted; check a current reference. (The cytochrome P450 enzyme CYP3A system is involved.) It also interferes with oral contraceptives and rifampin; alternate medical approaches are recommended. Contraindicated in patients with nelfinavir hypersensitivity and liver impairment.

SE/AR, side effects and adverse reactions.

tival hemorrhage, conjunctival scarring, and bacterial endophthalmitis.

Contraindications

Avoid use in persons with acyclovir or ganciclovir hypersensitivity, an absolute neutophil count <500 cells/mm^3, a platelet count <25,000 cells/mm^3, and kidney function impairment.

Dosage and administration

The usual adult dose by IV infusion for induction is 5 mg/kg every 12 hours for 2 to 3 weeks. The maintenance dosage is 5 mg/kg daily. The maintenance dose with oral ganciclovir is 1000 mg three times daily with food.

See Box 52-1 for information on additional antifungal agents.

ribavirin for inhalation [rye ba vye′ rin] (Virazole)

Ribavirin is virustatic with a mechanism of action that is diverse and not completely understood. It rapidly penetrates virus-infected cells and is believed to reduce intracellular guanosine triphosphate (GTP) storage. It inhibits viral ribonucleic acid (RNA) and protein synthesis, thus inhibiting viral duplication, spread to other cells, or both. It is indicated for serious viral pneumonia caused by respiratory syncytial virus.

Pharmacokinetics

After oral inhalation, it is well absorbed and rapidly distributed to plasma, respiratory tract secretions, and erythrocytes. Its half-life is 9.5 hours after oral inhalation and approximately 40 days in erythrocytes. Ribavirin is metabolized in the liver and excreted primarily by the kidneys.

Drug interactions

In vitro studies indicate that ribavirin and zidovudine are antagonistic and should not be administered concurrently.

Side effects and adverse reactions

These are uncommon and may include skin rash or irritation (inhalation product), CNS effects (insomnia, headache, and lethargy) with IV and oral dosages, and gastric distress (anorexia and nausea), and anemia (usually with higher dosages). The healthcare professional or provider should use caution in administering this medication as side effects of headache, itching, swelling, or red eyes have been reported.

Warnings

Use with caution in patients with severe anemia.

Contraindications

Avoid use in persons with ribavirin hypersensitivity.

Dosage and administration

The adult dosage for ribavirin as an inhalation aerosol has not been established. For viral pneumonia in children, administer by oral inhalation via a Viratek small-particle aerosol generator, using a 20 mg/ml ribavirin concentration in the reservoir. Administer over 12 to 18 hours/day for 3 to 7 days. Although an unapproved indication in the United States, the oral and parenteral dosage forms, respectively, may be indicated to prevent and treat Lassa fever.

rimantadine [ri man′ ti deen] (Flumadine)

Rimantadine, an analog of amantadine, inhibits viral replication by blocking or reducing the uncoating of viral RNA in host cells. It is indicated for the treatment and prevention of influenza type A respiratory tract infections.

Pharmacokinetics

This product is well absorbed orally. It reaches a peak concentration in 1 to 4 hours and has a half life of 13 to 38 hours in children (4 to 8 years of age), 25 to 30 hours in younger adults (22 to 44 years of age), and 32 hours in the elderly (71 to 79 years of age). It is metabolized in the liver and excreted primarily by the kidneys.

Side effects and adverse reactions

These are uncommon with the elderly having a higher incidence of side effects than younger adults. They include CNS effects (difficulty in concentration and sleeping, headache, anxiety, weakness, and dizziness), and gastric distress (dry mouth, anorexia, nausea, vomiting, and abdominal pain).

Warnings

Use with caution in patients with liver dysfunction.

Contraindications

Avoid use in persons with amantadine or rimantadine hypersensitivity, epilepsy or other convulsive disorders, and severe kidney disease or renal failure.

Dosage and administration

For rimantadine prophylaxis and treatment in children older than 10 years of age and adults, the dose is 100 mg twice a day. For elderly nursing home patients or persons with liver or renal impairment, the recommended dose is 100 mg daily.

valacyclovir [va la sye′ kloe veer] (Valtrex)

Valacyclovir is a prodrug that is converted to acyclovir by first-pass intestinal and liver metabolism. It is indicated for the treatment of herpes zoster (shingles) caused by varicella-zoster virus in immunocompetent persons. When compared with acyclovir, valacyclovir was reported to be more effective in reducing the pain and postherpetic neuralgia associated with herpes zoster in persons older that 50 years of age. Valacyclovir has not been studied in children, immunocompromised individuals, or in persons with disseminated zoster (USP DI, 1998).

Pharmacokinetics

Administered orally, valacyclovir is well absorbed and converted to acyclovir, the active substance. It reaches peak serum levels in 1.6 to 2 hours; its half-life is 2.5 to 3.3 hours. Valacyclovir is converted to inactive metabolites by alcohol and aldehyde dehydrogenase and excreted primarily in urine.

Side effects and adverse reactions

No serious adverse reactions for valacyclovir have been reported to date. Side effects may include nausea, headache, weakness, gastric distress (constipation, diarrhea, anorexia, abdominal pain, and vomiting), and dizziness.

Warnings

Use with caution in patients with liver dysfunction.

Contraindications

Avoid use in persons with valacyclovir or acyclovir hypersensitivity, bone marrow or kidney transplantation, advanced HIV infections, and kidney function impairment.

Dosage and administration

The usual adult dose is 1 g three times daily for 1 week.

REVERSE TRANSCRIPTASE INHIBITORS

didanosine [dye dah′ noe seen] (ddI, Videx)

Didanosine is converted intracellularly to its active form ddA-triphosphate, which in turn inhibits HIV deoxyribonucleic acid (DNA) reverse transcriptase. This action results in suppression of HIV replication. Didanosine is indicated for the treatment of AIDS and advanced HIV infection in patients exhibiting a decreased response to or persons who are unable to take zidovudine.

Pharmacokinetics

This product, which is available in oral dosage forms, is considered to be acid labile. Therefore oral formulations are buffered to increase gastric pH to protect didanosine from gastric acid destruction. Didanosine crosses the blood-brain barrier; has a half-life of 1.5 hours in adults, and reaches peak serum concentration in 30 to 60 minutes. Excretion is primarily via the kidneys.

Drug interactions

The following effects may occur when didanosine is given with the drugs listed below:

Drug	Possible effect and management
Alcohol, asparaginase (Elspar), azathioprine (Imuran), estrogens, furosemide (Lasix), nitrofurantoin (Furadantin), pentamidine IV (Pentam 300), sulfonamides, sulindac (Clinoril), tetracyclines, thiazide diuretics, or valproic acid (Depakene), or other drugs associated with pancreatitis	Concurrent drug use may result in pancreatitis. Avoid or a potentially serious drug interaction may occur. If combination therapy is necessary, use extreme caution.
chloramphenicol, (Chloromycetin), cisplatin (Platinol), dapsone (Avlosulfon), ethambutol (Myambutol), ethionamide (Trecator-SC), hydralazine (Apresoline), isoniazid (INH), lithium, metronidazole (Flagyl), nitrofurantoin (Furadantin), nitrous oxide, phenytoin (Dilantin), stavudine (Zerit), vincristine (Oncovin), or zalcitabine (Hivid), or other drugs associated with peripheral neuropathy	May increase the potential for peripheral neuropathy. Avoid or a potentially serious drug interaction may occur. If one of these drugs must be used, monitor closely for numbness and tingling in the fingers and toes.
dapsone (Avlosulfon), itraconazole (Sporanox), or ketoconazole (Nizoral)	May result in decreased absorption of dapsone or ketoconazole because they require an acidic media for absorption. Administer these drugs at least 2 hours before didanosine.
fluoroquinolone antibiotics such as ciprofloxacin (Cipro), norfloxacin (Noroxin), and ofloxacin (Floxin), or tetracyclines	Concurrent drug administration may reduce absorption of these antibiotics because didanosine chewable tablets and pediatric powder contain magnesium and aluminum antacids that may chelate the antibiotics, thus reducing absorption. If both drugs are prescribed, give antibiotics at least 2 hours before or after didanosine. The buffered didanosine powder for solution has a citrate buffer that does not interfere with the antibiotics; therefore its use would reduce the risk of this interaction.

Color type indicates an unsafe drug combination.

Side effects and adverse reactions

These include peripheral neuropathy, CNS toxicity (e.g., headache, anxiety, increase irritability and insomnia), gastric distress (stomach pain, nausea, and diarrhea), and dry mouth. Less frequent and rare adverse effects include pancreatitis, cardiomyopathy, blood disorders (anemia, leukopenia, or thrombocytopenia), hepatitis, convulsions, hypersensitivity, and retinal depigmentation.

Warnings

Use with caution in patients with gouty arthritis, liver dysfunction, phenylketonuria, and kidney function impairment.

Contraindications

Avoid use in persons with hypertriglyceridemia, pancreatitis, alcoholism, peripheral neuropathy, and any conditions that require sodium restriction (such as heart failure, cirrhosis or severe liver disease, and hypertension). Two didanosine chewable or dispersible tablets contain 529 mg of sodium whereas each single dose packet of the buffered powder contains 1380 mg of sodium (USP DI, 1998).

Dosage and administration

The usual adult dosage for patients weighing <60 kg is 167 mg orally every 12 hours; for patients weighing >60 kg the dose is 250 mg every 12 hours. For the pediatric dosing schedule, check a current package insert or drug reference for didanosine for buffered oral suspension.

lamivudine [la mi′ vue deen] (3TC, Epivir)

Lamivudine is used in combination with zidovudine for the treatment of HIV infection, based on evidence of disease progression. It is converted in the body to an active metabolite, lamivudine triphosphate (L-TP), which then inhibits HIV reverse transcription by terminating the viral DNA chain. It also inhibits RNA- and DNA-dependent DNA polymerase functions of reverse transcriptase. A combination dosage form has since been released that contains 150 mg of lamivudine and 300 mg of zidovudine (Combivir) (Olin, 1998).

Pharmacokinetics

Rapidly absorbed after oral administration, lamivudine reaches a peak serum level in 1 hour (fasting state) and 3.2

hours (with food). L-TP has an intracellular half-life of 10 to 15 hours and is excreted unchanged by the kidneys.

Drug interactions

Check the patient's drug regimen to determine the potential for concurrent drug interactions such as increased blood levels of lamivudine with trimethoprim/sulfamethoxazole (Bactrim, TMP/SMX) or elevated zidovudine (AZT) serum levels. Monitor drug combinations closely.

Side effects and adverse reactions

For lamivudine these include headaches, dizziness, fatigue, fever, nausea, vomiting, diarrhea, gastric pain or distress, anorexia, neuropathy, insomnia, depression, cough, skeletal muscle pain, pancreatitis, paresthesias, and peripheral neuropathy, and, rarely, anemia, rash, and neutropenia.

Warnings

Use with caution in patients with pancreatitis and peripheral neuropathy, including those with a history of these conditions.

Contraindications

Avoid use in persons with lamivudine hypersensitivity and kidney function impairment.

Dosage and administration

The usual dose of lamivudine for adolescents (12 to 16 years of age) and adults is 150 mg PO twice a day.

stavudine [stav′ yoo deen] (d4T, Zerit)

Stavudine is an antiviral agent indicated for the treatment of advanced HIV infection or AIDS in persons who have not responded to or are unable to take zidovudine and other proven therapeutic agents. Stavudine is converted to stavudine triphosphate, which then competes with deoxythymidine triphosphate, resulting in inhibition of HIV replication and DNA synthesis.

Pharmacokinetics

Oral stavudine is rapidly absorbed and reaches a peak serum level in 0.5 to 1.5 hours. It has a half-life of 1 to 1.6 hours and is excreted primarily unchanged by the kidneys.

Drug interactions

The following effects may occur when stavudine is given with the drugs listed below:

Drug	Possible effect and management
Drugs that cause peripheral neuropathy, such as chloramphenicol (Chloromycetin), cisplatin (Platinol), dapsone (Avlosulfon), didanosine (Videx), ethambutol (Myambutol), ethionamide (Trecator-SC), hydralazine (Apresoline), isoniazid (INH), lithium, metronidazole (Flagyl), nitrofurantoin (Furadantin), phenytoin (Dilantin), vincristine (Oncovin), or zalcitabine (Hivid)	Stavudine can cause peripheralneuropathy; therefore whenever possible avoid other drugs that can also cause peripheral neuropathy.

Color type indicates an unsafe drug combination.

Side effects and adverse reactions

These include dose-related peripheral neuropathy and anemia. Other adverse effects include arthralgia, hypersensitivity, myalgia, pancreatitis, weakness, GI distress, headache, and insomnia.

Warnings

Use with caution in patients with liver function impairment or alcoholism.

Contraindications

Avoid use in persons with peripheral neuropathy and kidney function impairment.

Dosage and administration

The usual adult oral dose of stavudine is 30 mg every 12 hours for persons weighing <60 kg and 40 mg every 12 hours for persons weighing >60 kg.

zalcitabine [zal sye′ ta bean] (ddC, Hivid)

The antiviral agent zalcitabine is converted by cellular enzymes to its active form, ddC-triphosphate, which inhibits viral reverse transcriptase, inhibiting viral replication. In vitro studies, zalcitabine has been reported to be approximately 10 times more potent than zidovudine against HIV (USP DI, 1998).

Indications

Zalcitabine is indicated for the treatment of advanced HIV infection and AIDS in persons who either cannot take zidovudine or have disease progression while taking zidovudine.

Pharmacokinetics

Administered orally, zalcitabine is metabolized intracellularly to ddC-triphosphate. It reaches peak serum levels in 1 to 2 hours and has a half-life of 1 to 3 hours. It is excreted primarily via the kidneys.

Drug interactions

The following effects may occur when zalcitabine is given with the drugs listed below:

Drug	Possible effect and management
Alcohol, asparaginase (Elspar), azathioprine (Imuran), furosemide (Lasix), methyldopa (Aldomet), nitrofurantoin (Furadantin), pentamidine IV (Pentam 300), sulfonamides, sulindac (Clinoril), tetracyclines, thiazide diuretics, or valproic acid (Depakene)	Concurrent use increases the potential risk of pancreatitis. Avoid or a potentially serious drug interaction may occur. If given, monitor for estrogens, abdominal pain, anorexia, and nausea and vomiting and perform serum amylase determinations.
Aminoglycosides, parenteral, amphotericin B (Fungizone), and foscarnet (Foscavir)	May decrease renal excretion of zalcitabine, which may result in toxicity. Monitor serum levels of the drug closely.
chloramphenicol (Chloromycetin), cisplatin (Platinol), dapsone (Avlosulfon), ethionamide (Trecator-SC), hydralazine (Apresoline), isoniazid (INH), lithium, metronidazole (Flagyl), nitrofurantoin (Furadantin), nitrous oxide, phenytoin (Dilantin), or vincristine (Oncovin)	Concurrent drug administration may result in increased potential for peripheral neuropathy. Avoid or a potentially serious drug interaction may occur. If given, monitor patient closely for numbness and tingling in the fingers and toes.

Color type indicates an unsafe drug combination.

Side effects and adverse reactions

These include peripheral neuropathy, arthralgia, hypersensitivity, myalgia, mouth and throat ulcers, gastric distress (stomach pain, diarrhea, and nausea), headache, and, rarely, hepatotoxicity, leukopenia, and pancreatitis.

Warnings

Use with caution in patients with kidney function impairment.

Contraindications

Avoid use in persons with hypertriglyceridemia and pancreatitis (or a history of), alcoholism, liver function impairment, and peripheral neuropathy.

Dosage and administration

The usual adult oral dosage for zalcitabine is 0.75 mg alone or in combination with 200 mg of zidovudine every 8 hours.

zidovudine [zye doe′ vue deen] (AZT, Retrovir)

Zidovudine is an antiviral agent (virustatic) that intracellularly is converted to monophosphate, diphosphate, and then zidovudine triphosphate by cellular enzymes. The triphosphate form competes with natural thymidine triphosphate for incorporation in growing chains of viral RNA-dependent DNA polymerase (reverse transcriptase), thus inhibiting viral DNA replication. It has a greater affinity for retroviral reverse transcriptase than for the human alpha-DNA polymerase; thus it selectively inhibits viral replication.

Indications

Zidovudine is indicated for the treatment of HIV infection and AIDS in adults with a CD4 lymphocyte count of $500/mm^3$ or less. Zalcitabine may be used in combination with zidovudine, especially when the CD4 count is $300/mm^3$ or less.

Pharmacokinetics

Administered orally, zidovudine is rapidly absorbed and distributed in plasma and CSF, reaches a peak serum level in 0.5 to 1.5 hours, and has a half-life of approximately 1 hour (in serum, 3.3 hours intracellularly). It is metabolized in the liver and excreted by the kidneys.

Drug interactions

The following effects may occur when zidovudine is given with the drugs listed below:

Drug	Possible effect and management
Bone marrow depressants, radiation therapy	May exacerbate bone marrow depression and toxicity. Dosage reductions may be necessary. Monitor complete blood counts closely for leukopenia and anemia.
clarithromycin (Biaxin)	Concurrent drug administration has been reported to result in a lower peak plasma level of zidovudine. Monitor serum concentrations of the drug closely.
ganciclovir (Cytovene)	Concurrent use has been reported to result in synergistic myelosuppressive toxicity. As this is a serious hematologic toxicity, avoid or a potentially serious drug interaction may occur.
probenecid (Benemid)	May cause decreased liver metabolism of zidovudine, resulting in increased serum levels and an increased risk of toxicity. There is also a high incidence of rash (USP DI, 1998). Monitor serum drug levels closely if drugs are administered concurrently.

Color type indicates an unsafe drug combination.

Side effects and adverse reactions

These include nausea, myalgia, insomnia, severe headaches, bone marrow depression (anemia and leukopenia), hepatotoxicity, myopathy, neurotoxicity, and hyperpigmentation of nails.

Warnings

Use with caution in patients with folic acid or vitamin B_{12} deficiency; such deficiencies increase the risk of anemia.

Contraindications

Avoid use in persons with zidovudine hypersensitivity, bone marrow depression, and liver function impairment.

Dosage and administration

The adult oral dose for treatment of symptomatic HIV infection is 100 mg every 4 hours around the clock (600 mg daily). For asymptomatic HIV infection, the adult dose is 100 mg every 4 hours while awake (500 mg daily). For children 3 months to 12 years of age, the oral dose is 90 to 180 mg/m^2 every 6 hours.

The parenteral adult dose for symptomatic HIV infection is 1 mg/kg by IV infusion administered over 60 minutes every 4 hours around the clock, until oral therapy can be used. The pediatric dosage is 120 mg/m^2 every 6 hours.

PROTEASE INHIBITORS

indinavir [in din′ a veer] (Crixivan)

Indinavir was released under the Food and Drug Administration's accelerated review for the treatment of HIV infection in adults. Although its complete mechanism of action is unknown, indinavir appears to inhibit the replication of retroviruses (HIV type 1 and 2) by interfering with HIV protease. Indinavir affects the replication cycle of HIV and is active in both acute and chronically infected cells, which are generally not affected by the dideoxynucleoside reverse transcriptase inhibitors, such as didanosine, lamivudine, stavudine, zalcitabine, and zidovudine. Thus this product has a virustatic effect due to its HIV protease inhibitor effects (AHFS Suppl A, 1996).

Pharmacokinetics

Administered orally, indinavir reaches a peak serum level in approximately 1 hour. It is metabolized in the liver and excreted primarily in feces.

Drug interactions

The following effects may occur when indinavir is given with the drugs listed below:

Drug	Possible effect and management
astemizole (Hismanal), cisapride (Propulsid), midazolam (Versed), terfenadine* (Seldane), or triazolam (Halcion)	Indinavir and these drugs are metabolized in the liver by the cytochrome P-450 (CYP3A4) enzyme. Concurrent use may result in a decreased metabolism of these drugs and toxicity. Avoid or a potentially serious drug interaction may occur.
didanosine (Videx)	When given concurrently, space drugs at least 1 hour apart and take on an empty stomach. Indinavir needs an acidic pH for absorption, and didanosine needs a buffer to increase pH to prevent acid from destroying it.
ketoconazole (Nizoral)	Concurrent use results in an increased serum level of indinavir. Reduce the dose of indinavir to 600 mg every 8 hours if administered with ketoconazole.
rifabutin (Mycobutin)	Concurrent use results in an increased serum level of indinavir. Reduce the dose of rifabutin to 400 mg every 8 hours if administered concurrently with indinavir.
rifampin (Rifadin)	Rifampin increases CYP3A4 (a potent inducer), which may decrease the serum levels of indinavir. Avoid concurrent use.

Color type indicates an unsafe drug combination.
*No longer available in the United States but may be available in other countries.

Side effects and adverse reactions

These include gastric distress, nausea, vomiting, diarrhea, headache, dizziness, fatigue, insomnia, changes in taste sensation, kidney stones, fever, flu-like syndrome, and, rarely, diabetes or hyperglycemia and ketoacidosis.

Warnings

Use with caution in patients with hemophilia.

Contraindications

Avoid use in persons with indinavir hypersensitivity or liver function impairment.

Dosage and administration

The usual adult dose is 800 mg every 8 hours.

ritonavir [ri ton′ a veer] (Norvir)

Ritonavir is an inhibitor of HIV-1 and HIV-2 protease that interferes with the production of the HIV virus. Use of this product results in the production of noninfectious, immature HIV substances (Olin, 1998).

Pharmacokinetics

Administered orally, ritonavir reaches peak serum levels within 2 or 4 hours (fasting or nonfasting). Five metabolites have been identified with ritonavir, but only the M-2 metabolite has antiviral activity. It has a half-life of 3 to 5 hours and is excreted primarily in feces.

Drug interactions

The following effects may occur when ritonavir is given with the drugs listed below:

Drug	Possible effect and management
alprazolam (Xanax), clorazepate (Tranxene), diazepam (Valium), estazolam (ProSom), flurazepam (Dalmane), midazolam (Versed), triazolam (Halcion), or zolpidem (Ambien)	These drugs increase the liver enzyme cytochrome P-450 (CYP3A) activity, which will increase the metabolism of ritonavir, decreasing the plasma levels. In addition, ritonavir's affinity for various cytochrome P-450 isoform systems may produce a large increase in serum levels of these medications, which may result in excessive sedation and respiratory depression. Do not administer these drugs concurrently with ritonavir, as a potentially serious drug interaction may occur.
amiodarone (Cordarone), astemizole (Hismanal), bepridil (Vascor), bupropion (Wellbutrin), cisapride (Propulsid), clozapine (Clozaril), dihydroergotamine (D.H.E. 45), ergotamine (Ergostat), flecainide (Tambocor), meperidine (Demerol), pimozide (Orap), piroxicam (Feldene), propafenone (Rythmol), propoxyphene (Darvon products), quinidine, rifabutin (Mycobutin), or terfenadine* (Seldane)	Do not administer these medications concurrently with ritonavir, as large increases in the serum levels of these medications may occur. This increases the potential for dysrhythmias, hematologic disorders, convulsions, and other serious adverse effects. Avoid or a potentially serious drug interaction may occur.
clarithromycin (Biaxin)	Concurrent use may increase serum levels of clarithromycin. Drug dosage adjustments are only necessary in patients with impaired renal function.
Contraceptives, oral, containing estrogen	When contraceptives containing ethinyl estradiol are given concurrently with ritonavir, a decrease in estrogen serum level occurs. It is suggested that a oral contraceptive with a higher estrogen amount or an alternative contraception method should be used.
theophylline	Concurrent use reduced theophylline serum levels by up to 40%. Monitor theophylline levels closely, as drug dosage adjustment may be necessary.

Color type indicates an unsafe drug combination.
*No longer available in the United States, but may be available in other countries.

Side effects and adverse reactions

For ritonavir these include weakness, nausea, vomiting, diarrhea, stomach distress, taste alterations, peripheral paresthesias, allergic reactions, back or chest pain, chills, facial edema, dizziness, headache, drowsiness, alterations in taste perception, numbness or tingling around mouth (circumoral paresthesia), peripheral paresthesia, flu symptoms, and, rarely, diabetes, hyperglycemia, and ketoacidosis.

Warnings

Use with caution in patients with hemophilia and liver function impairment.

Contraindications

Avoid use in persons with ritonavir hypersensitivity.

Dosage and administration

The usual dose is 600 mg twice a day, with meals.

saquinavir [sa kwin' a veer] (Invirase)

Saquinavir inhibits HIV protease, preventing the cleavage of viral polyproteins. It is used in combination with the nucleoside analogs to treat advanced HIV infection in selected individuals. For example, it may be prescribed concurrently with zidovudine (AZT) in untreated persons or with zalcitabine (ddC) in persons who were previously treated with extended zidovudine (AZT) therapy. Clinical studies based on disease progression and survival are underway to determine the clinical benefits of combination therapy.

Pharmacokinetics

Administered orally, saquinavir has extensive first-pass metabolism, is highly protein bound, is metabolized in the liver, and is excreted primarily in the feces.

Drug interactions

The following effects may occur when saquinavir is given with the drugs listed below:

Drug	Possible effect and management
rifampin (Rifadin), rifabutin (Mycobutin), carba	These drugs are potent metabolic inducers of cytochrome P-450 enzymes; therefore concurrent use

mazepine (Tegretol), dexamethasone, phenobarbital, or phenytoin (Dilantin)	may reduce serum levels of the drugs and possibly saquinavir. Avoid concurrent drug administration.
terfenadine* (Seldane), or astemizole (Hismanal)	Saquinavir may increase blood levels of these drugs and increase the risk of cardiovascular toxicities. Avoid or a potentially serious drug interaction may occur.
Calcium channel blockers, clindamycin (Cleocin), dapsone (Avlosulfon), quinidine, or triazolam (Halcion)	Saquinavir may increase blood levels of these drugs because the drugs are substrates of the cytochrome P-450 CYP3A4 enzyme systems. Monitor patients closely if concurrent drug therapy is used.

Color type indicates an unsafe drug combination.
*No longer available in the United States, but it may be available in other countries.

Side effects and adverse reactions

These are usually mild and include diarrhea, abdominal distress, headache, weakness, and, rarely, paresthesia, skin rash, confusion, ataxia, Stevens-Johnson syndrome, seizures, thrombocytopenia, anemia, and hepatotoxicity (Olin, 1998).

Contraindications

Avoid use in persons with saquinavir hypersensitivity.

Dosage and administration

The usual dose in combination with a nucleoside analog (such as zalcitabine or zidovudine) is 600 mg three times a day, administered within 2 hours of a full meal.

NON-NUCLEOSIDE, REVERSE TRANSCRIPTASE INHIBITOR

nevirapine [ne veer′ a peen] (Viramune)

Nevirapine is a nonnucleoside antiviral agent that binds directly to reverse transcriptase to block the RNA- and DNA-dependent DNA polymerase activity. This drug can cause resistant HIV if given alone; therefore it should be administered in combination with at least another antiretroviral agent.

Pharmacokinetics

Administered orally, nevirapine is well absorbed. It reaches peak serum levels in 4 hours and is distributed in CSF (45% or serum concentration). Nevirapine is metabolized in the liver and is also an inducer of hepatic cytochrome P-450 metabolic enzymes; thus auto-induction or an increased clearance and a decrease in drug half-life occurs within 2 to 4 weeks of therapy

Drug interactions

The following effects may occur when nevirapine is given with the drugs listed below:

Drug	Possible effect and management
Contraceptives, oral, containing estrogen; protease inhibitors such as indinavir (Crixivan), ritonavir (Norvir), and saquinavir (Invirase)	Nevirapine increases cytochrome P-450 CYP3A action, which will decrease the serum levels of the oral contraceptives and the protease inhibitors. Concurrent use is not recommended.
rifabutin (Mycobutin) or rifampin (Rifadin)	Nevirapine-induced induction of cytochrome P-450 CYP3A may decrease serum levels of these drugs. If used concurrently, monitor closely.

Side effects and adverse reactions

These include nausea, headache, diarrhea, fever, hepatitis, ulcerative stomatitis, and life-threatening skin reactions such as Stevens-Johnson syndrome. Nevirapine should be discontinued in individuals who develop a severe rash or a rash accompanied with other symptoms such as fever, myalgia, fatigue, oral lesions, and conjunctivitis.

Warnings

Use with caution in patients with kidney function impairment.

Contraindications

Avoid use in persons with nevirapine hypersensitivity and liver function impairment.

Dosage and administration

Initial therapy is 200 mg PO daily for 2 weeks; the maintenance dose is 200 mg twice daily in combination with another antiretroviral agent.

SUMMARY

Systemic fungus and viral infections can be very serious and life-threatening to the individual. Fungal infections are often superinfections; that is, they occur after prolonged or high-dose usage of broad-spectrum antibiotics or after immunosuppression from transplantation or antineoplastic chemotherapy or from corticosteroid therapy. The systemic antifungal agents are very potent and potentially toxic medications. They include amphotericin B, fluconazole, flucytosine, griseofulvin, itraconazole, ketoconazole, miconazole, and nystatin. Drugs that are either systemic fungistatic and fungicidal agents are used to treat a wide variety of mycotic infections.

With viral infections, by the time symptoms appear the multiplication of the virus has reached its peak; even though the signs and symptoms of illness are present, viral replication is now on the decline. Therefore antiviral therapy is much more limited than other therapies, and antiviral medications would need to prophylactically administered to be effective. Many antiviral agents are discussed in this chapter, including acyclovir, amantadine, famciclovir, foscarnet, ganciclovir, nevirapine, ribavirin, and others, as well as the reverse transcriptase inhibitors, protease inhibitors, and the non-nucleoside reverse transcriptase inhibitor.

REVIEW QUESTIONS

1. Describe the difference in absorption rates between the oral azole antifungal agents. Which agents require an acid medium, a fasting state, or food for absorption?
2. Discuss the mechanism of action of griseofulvin in the treatment of onychomycosis or nail fungus.
3. What is the action of acyclovir in the treatment of herpes simplex virus? Name the primary drug interactions, side effects and adverse reactions, and contraindications with the use of this product.
4. Name two antiviral drugs that should not be used in patients with peripheral neuropathy. Name five other drugs that may also cause peripheral neuropathy.
5. Explain the drug interaction between the protease inhibitors and astemizole, cisapride, terfenadine, or triazolam. What interaction occurs between the benzodiazepines (alprazolam and others) and ritonavir? Explain.

REFERENCES

Abelcet package insert, #1-1001-41-US-D, 1996, The Liposome Co, Inc.

American Hospital Formulary Service: *AHFS drug information: current developments, Supplement A,* Bethesda, Md, 1996, American Society of Hospital Pharmacists.

Hitchens K: New eye implant for treating cytomegalovirus, *Hosp Pharm Rep* 10(4):20, 1996.

MacDonald L, Kazanjian P: Antiretroviral therapy in HIV infection: an update. *Hosp Formulary* 31(9):780-804, 1996.

Mosby: *Mosby's GenRx,* St Louis, 1998, Mosby.

Olin BR: *Facts and comparisons.* Philadelphia, 1998, JB Lippincott.

United States Pharmacopeial Convention: *USP DI: drug information for the health care professional,* ed 18, Rockville, Md, 1998, The Convention.

ADDITIONAL REFERENCES

American Hospital Formulary Service: *AHFS drug information '98,* Bethesda, Md, 1998, American Society of Hospital Pharmacists.

Anderson KN et al, editors: *Mosby's medical, nursing, and allied health dictionary,* ed 5, St Louis, 1998, Mosby.

Hayden FG: Antimicrobial agents: antiviral agents. In Hardman JG, Limbird LE, editors: *Goodman & Gilman's the pharmacological basis of therapeutics,* ed 9, New York, 1996, McGraw-Hill.

Melmon KL et al: *Clinical pharmacology,* ed 3, New York, 1992, McGraw-Hill.

Project Inform: PI perspective: cidofovir approved, San Francisco, 1996, The Project.

CHAPTER 53

Other Antimicrobial Drugs and Antiparasitic Drugs

KEY DRUGS

chloroquine, (p. 688)
isoniazid, (p. 671)
pyrazinamide, (p. 696)
rifampin, (p. 697)

CHAPTER FOCUS

This chapter reviews the various antimicrobial or antiparasitic medications used to treat malaria, tuberculosis, amebiasis (protozoan parasite infestation), toxoplasmosis, trichomoniasis, and helminthiasis (flatworms, roundworms, and pinworms), and leprosy. These diseases are prevalent throughout the world and their control has peaked and waned, depending on the potency and availability of medications, patient compliance with specific drug therapies, and, with tuberculosis, the development of drug-resistant strains. The control of such infestations is important and challenging to the healthcare professional.

KEY TERMS

amebiasis, (p. 698)
cestodes, (p. 700)
Hansen's disease, (p. 704)
helminths, (p. 700)
leprosy, (p. 704)
malaria, (p. 686)
toxoplasmosis, (p. 700)
trichomoniasis, (p. 700)
tuberculosis, (p. 691)

OBJECTIVES

After reading and studying this chapter, the student should be able to do the following:

1. *Define and describe the key terms and key drugs.*
2. *Describe the life cycle of the malarial parasite and ameba in the human body.*
3. *Name one drug from each classification reviewed and discuss the mechanism of action for each drug.*
4. *Relate the epidemiology, pathogenesis, and treatment of tuberculosis.*
5. *Discuss the indications and mechanisms of action for the antiamebiasis agents.*
6. *Describe the anthelmintic agents and the drugs used to treat leprosy.*

Antimicrobial and antiparasitic agents include antimalarial, antituberculous, amebicidal, anthelmintic, and leprostatic medications. Sulfonamides are reviewed in Chapter 51.

MALARIA

Malaria has been and still is a prevalent disease despite efforts to control the causative parasite and insect vector. Although it is endemic to the tropics, in 1988 approximately 1000 cases of malaria were diagnosed in the United States and Canada (Anandan, 1995). Four species of the genus *Plasmodium* are responsible for human malaria: *Plasmodium vivax, Plasmodium malariae, Plasmodium ovale,* and *Plasmodium falciparum. P ovale,* which is found in West Africa, is considered rare. *P falciparum* malaria is the most lethal form of malaria and is usually resistant to chloroquine.

Malaria is transmitted to humans by the bite of an infected female Anopheles mosquito, as well as by blood transfusion (usually *P malariae*), congenitally, or by contaminated needles commonly used by drug abusers.

Life Cycle of the Malarial Parasite

To understand the chemotherapy of malaria, it is essential to review the life cycle of the malarial parasite, the plasmodium. Fig. 53-1 presents the cycle in seven basic steps.

Plasmodia have two interdependent life cycles: the sexual cycle, which takes place in the mosquito, and the asexual cycle, which occurs in the human body.

Sexual Cycle

The sexual cycle is noted in step 7 of Fig. 53-1. The female Anopheles mosquito becomes the carrier of the parasite by drawing blood containing male and female forms from an infected person. These sexual forms of the parasite are known as gametocytes. In the stomach of the mosquito the female gametocytes are fertilized by the males; zygotes form, which result in numerous cell divisions that develop into sporozoites. The formation of sporozoites in the mosquito completes the sexual cycle. Sporozoites then migrate to the salivary glands of the infected mosquito and are injected into the bloodstream of the human by the bite of the female insect (step 1, Fig. 53-1).

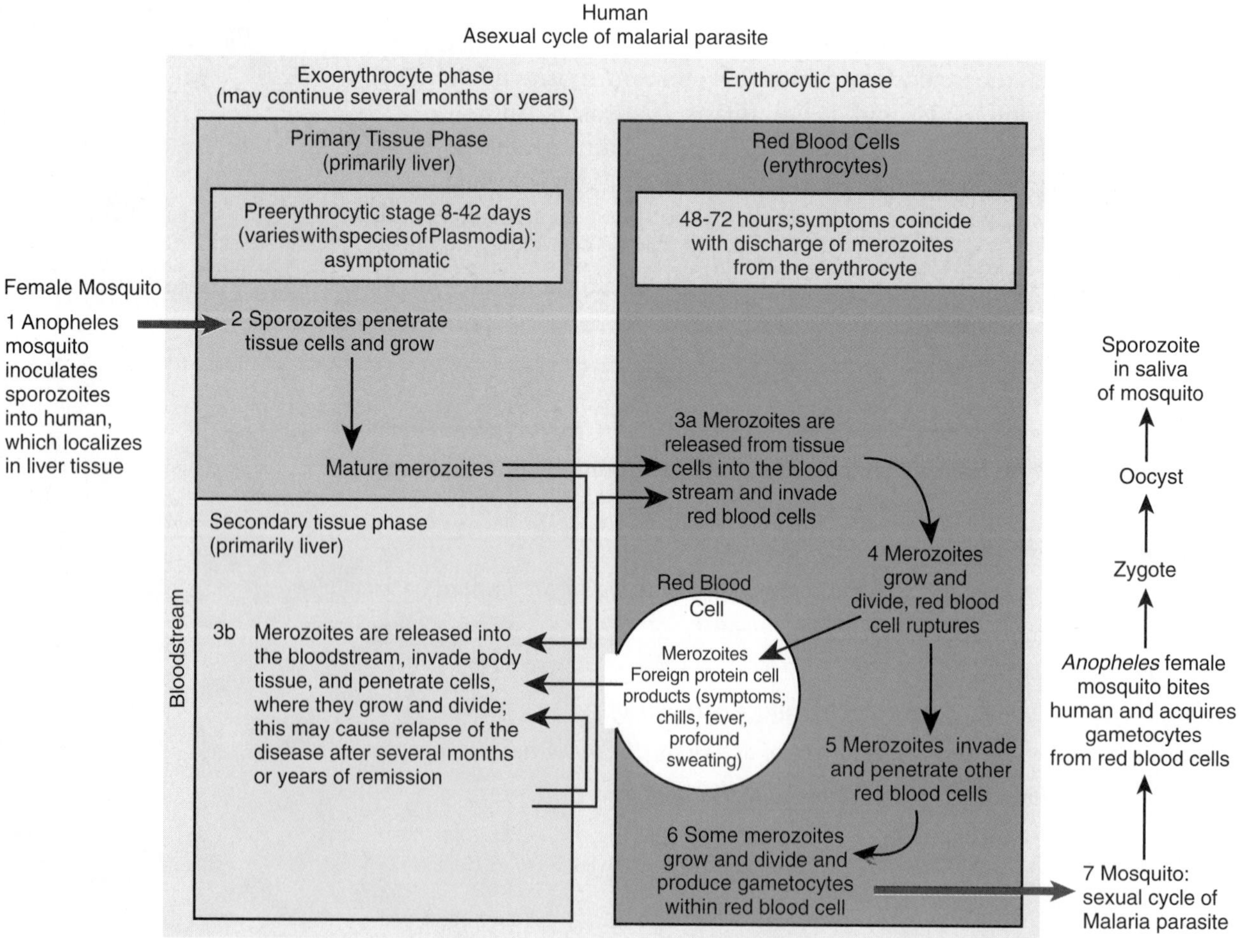

FIGURE 53-1
Life cycle of the malarial parasite.

Asexual Cycle

In the human the asexual cycle of the plasmodium consists of the exoerythrocytic phase and the erythrocytic phase.

Exoerythrocytic phase

Shortly after the introduction of the sporozoites into the circulation of the human, they leave the blood and enter fixed tissue cells (reticuloendothelial cells) of the liver, where multiplication and maturation take place (step 2). For a period of time (8 to 42 days), which varies with different plasmodia, the individual exhibits no symptoms, no parasites are found in erythrocytes, and the blood is noninfective. This phase is known as the preerythrocytic stage. The parasites are called primary tissue schizonts, or preerythrocytic forms. After this stage, the young parasites burst from the liver cells as merozoites.

Erythrocytic phase

When merozoites enter the bloodstream, they penetrate the erythrocytes and begin the erythrocytic phase of their existence (step 3a). In the case of *P vivax* (but not *P falciparum*) some of the merozoites invade other tissue cells to form secondary exoerythrocytic forms (step 3b). The relapses in *P vivax* and other forms of malaria are believed to be caused by the successive formations of merozoites produced by various secondary exoerythrocytic forms of the parasite. Drugs affecting malarial parasites in the bloodstream do not always destroy those in the exoerythrocytic, or tissue, stage.

After the merozoites bore into red blood cells, they again multiply, but this time asexually, and erythrocytic schizonts are formed. The erythrocytic phase is completed when the parasitized red blood cells rupture, setting free many more merozoites that are formed from the schizonts. Pyrogenic substances are also liberated, causing a rapid rise in body temperature (step 4). Some of the merozoites may be destroyed in the plasma of the blood by leukocytes and other agents, but some enter other erythrocytes to repeat the cycle (step 5). The recurring chills, fever, and prostration that are prominent clinical symptoms of malaria occur when the red blood cells rupture and release the young parasites with foreign protein and cell products. The erythrocytic phase lasts 48 to 72 hours, depending on the plasmodium involved. After a few cycles, some of the asexual forms of the malarial parasites develop into sexual forms called gametocytes (step 6). When the mosquito bites a person infected with malarial parasites and ingests the sexual forms, the cycle begins again.

P vivax is the most common form of malaria; this infestation is usually mild, drug resistance is uncommon, and it can easily be suppressed with antimalarial medications. The *P falciparum* strain of malaria is less common but much more severe than the *P vivax* form. Drug-resistant strains of *P falciparum* are reported, and the symptoms with this infestation occur at irregular intervals and can cause very serious complications. If untreated or treatment is delayed, the disease may progress to irreversible cardiovascular shock and death. Although relapses are reported with *P vivax* malaria, once the *P falciparum* form is eliminated, no dormant forms are in the liver; therefore no relapses are reported with *P falciparum*.

Persons who harbor the sexual forms of plasmodia are called carriers, since it is from carriers that mosquitoes receive the parasite forms that perpetuate the disease. The asexual forms cause the clinical symptoms of malaria. Carriers should avoid giving blood, since it is possible that the recipient of this blood will contract malaria or become a carrier. An increasing number of malaria cases (some fatal) have occurred from transfusions of infected blood. Some of the infected individuals who donated blood may have once lived in a malarious area. Any person who has had malaria or has been exposed to the disease by visiting a region where it is prevalent must be disqualified as a blood donor.

ANTIMALARIAL MEDICATIONS

The choice of a drug for treatment of malaria is based on the particular malarial strain involved and the stage of the plasmodium life cycle. Therefore drugs (schizonticides) are classified according to the type of therapy they provide, which is as follows:

1. Travelers to endemic areas should receive malaria chemoprophylaxis. Calling the Centers for Disease Control and Prevention ([404] 332-4555 for computer-assisted information) can verify malaria prophylaxis and also if chloroquine-resistant *P falciparum* has been reported in a specific country (Anandan, 1995). Chloroquine, which suppresses the asexual erythrocytic forms, is effective against all species of malaria except drug-resistant *P falciparum*.
2. In chloroquine-resistant *P falciparum* areas, mefloquine is used for prophylaxis or, if the person cannot take mefloquine, doxycycline is recommended.
3. Clinical cure of an acute malaria attack occurs when multiplication of the parasites within the erythrocyte is interrupted, thereby terminating the malarial symptoms of the attack. If chloroquine-resistant *P falciparum* is present, then combination therapies such as pyrimethamine and a sulfonamide (sulfadoxine) may be necessary.
4. For eradication of latent forms of *P vivax* that persist and may cause infection relapse, primaquine therapy may be recommended. This drug is usually started after an acute attack or during the last few weeks of chloroquine prophylaxis. To induce a radical cure requires medications that destroy both the exoerythrocytic and erythrocytic parasites to prevent relapsing malaria; therefore primaquine is given with chloroquine, which suppresses the erythrocytic cycle.

The emergence of drug-resistant strains of malaria, particularly that caused by *P falciparum*, poses a major public health problem throughout the world. Despite the combined efforts of many countries to eradicate malaria, it remains the most devastating infectious disease in the world because of the many lives lost and the economic burdens it imposes. Fortunately, in the United States and Canada, endemic malaria has been completely eradicated.

It is essential that travelers contemplating a trip to malarious areas of the world be aware of the need to obtain information from their healthcare provider about measures for reducing exposure to the disease. Malaria exists in Haiti, Mexico, Central and South America, the Middle East, and many other countries.

chloroquine [klor′ o kwin] (Aralen)
hydroxychloroquine [hye drox ee klor′ oh kwin] (Plaquenil)

The mechanisms of action of antiprotozoal agents to treat malaria are unknown but may be a result of their ability to bind or alter DNA properties. They increase the pH of acid vesicles, thus interfering with its functions. During suppressive therapy, they inhibit the erythrocytic stage of development of plasmodia whereas in acute malarial attacks, they interfere with erythrocytic schizogony of parasites.

As the drugs selectively accumulate in parasitized erythrocytes, they have a selective toxicity in the erythrocytic stages of plasmodial infestation.

Indications

These agents are indicated for the prevention and treatment of malaria for the four strains of plasmodium. Curing *P vivax* and *P ovale* malaria requires primaquine administration also. Hydroxychloroquine is also approved for the treatment of rheumatoid arthritis and for discoid and systemic lupus erythematosus, and chloroquine is also used to treat amebic liver abscess, usually in combination with a primary intestinal amebicide.

Pharmacokinetics

The drugs are fairly well absorbed orally, widely distributed in body tissues, and reach peak serum levels in approximately 3 to 3.5 hours. The terminal half-life of chloroquine is 1 to 2 months while the terminal half-life for hydroxychloroquine in blood is approximately 50 days and in plasma 32 days. Both drugs are partially metabolized in the liver and excreted by the kidneys.

Side effects and adverse reactions

These are usually dose-related and reversible. Gastric distress, headaches, pruritus, blurred vision, difficulty in reading, headache, itching (reported mostly in black patients), hair loss or bleaching of hair, a blue-black discoloration of skin, nails, or inside mouth, rash, corneal opacities, keratopathy, retinopathy, and, rarely, blood disorders (agranulocytosis, neutropenia, or thrombocytopenia), hypotension, cardiac dysrhythmia, mood alterations, psychosis, ototoxicity, muscle weakness, and convulsions have been reported for both drugs.

Warnings

Use with caution in patients with severe gastrointestinal (GI) disorders, porphyria, psoriasis, and glucose-6-phosphate dehydrogenase (G6PD) deficiency. Be aware that approximately 10% of African Americans and 5% to 10% of Sephardic Jews, Greeks, Iranians, Chinese, Filipinos, and Indonesians have a G6PD deficiency. This deficiency is transmitted as an X-linked trait, and without G6PD, red blood cell metabolism is impaired by chloroquine and other antimalarials.

It these drugs are administered, an acute intravascular hemolysis may occur (Kudzma, 1992).

Contraindications

Avoid use in persons with chloroquine or hydroxychloroquine hypersensitivity, severe blood dyscrasias, liver function impairment, severe neurologic disorders (both drugs may cause ototoxicity, polyneuritis, convulsions, or neuromyopathy), or retinal or visual field changes.

Dosage and administration

The usual oral chloroquine adult dose to suppress malaria is 500 mg daily every 7 days. The pediatric dosage is 8.3 mg/kg PO daily (not exceeding adult dose) every 7 days. The parenteral adult dose is 200 to 250 mg IM repeated in 6 hours if needed. Do not exceed 1000 mg in the first day.

The hydroxychloroquine adult oral dose is 400 mg daily every 7 days. The pediatric dosage is 6.4 mg/kg PO daily, repeated weekly.

Additional comments

Both medications should be taken with meals or milk to reduce the potential for GI distress. When prescribed to treat rheumatoid arthritis, if improvement is not documented within 6 months of therapy, the medication should be discontinued.

mefloquine [me′ floe kwin] (Lariam)

Mefloquine is a blood schizonticide; it prevents the replication of asexual erythrocytic parasites but has no effect on the gametocytes of *P falciparum.* Its exact mechanism of action is unknown, although it is believed to inhibit protein synthesis (bind deoxyribonucleic acid [DNA]) and increase the intravascular pH of acid vesicles in the parasite, and it may have a variety of other actions. However, it is not effective in eliminating the exoerythrocytic or intrahepatic stages of *P vivax* or *P ovale* infections.

Indications

It is indicated for the prevention and treatment of chloroquine-resistant malaria and multiple drug-resistant strains of *P falciparum.* It is also used to prevent malaria caused by *P vivax, P ovale,* and *P malariae.*

Pharmacokinetics

Mefloquine is well absorbed orally and widely distributed in the body, reaching peak serum levels in 7 to 24 hours. It has an elimination half-life of 13 to 33 days, is partially metabolized in the liver, and is excreted primarily in bile and feces.

Drug interactions

The following effects may occur when mefloquine is given with the drugs listed below:

Drug	Possible effect and management
Beta blockers, calcium channel blocking agents, quinidine or quinine	Concurrent use may result in an increase risk of dysrhythmias, cardiac arrest, and seizures (the latter especially with quinine). Avoid or a potentially serious drug interaction may occur. If concurrent use cannot be avoided, monitor closely, and also advise patients to take mefloquine at least 12 hours after a dose of quinidine or quinine.
chloroquine (Aralen)	May increase seizure activity. Monitor closely.
divalproex (Depakote) or valproic acid (Depakene)	Decreased serum levels of valproic acid are reported with loss of seizure control. Monitor serum levels if concurrent drug therapy is necessary.

Color type indicates an unsafe drug combination.

Side effects and adverse reactions

These generally are dose related and occur more commonly in therapeutic rather than prophylactic drug regimens. Side effects include nausea, vomiting, headache, dizziness, insomnia, gastric distress, diarrhea, visual disturbances, and, rarely, bradycardia, and central nervous system (CNS) toxicity (depression, hallucinations, convulsions, psychosis, anxiety, and confusion).

Warnings

Use with caution in patients with epilepsy or history of convulsive disorders.

Contraindications

Avoid use in persons with heart block (first or second degree), a history of psychiatric problems (psychosis, hallucinations, anxiety, and depression), and a profession that requires coordination and spatial discrimination such as neurosurgeons and airline pilots.

Dosage and administration

The usual adult dose for prophylaxis is 250 mg once a week, beginning 1 week before travel, then weekly during traveling and for 1 month after leaving the endemic areas. The therapeutic dose for chloroquine-resistant *P falciparum* malaria is 1250 mg orally as a single dose.

primaquine [prim′ a kween]

Primaquine's mechanism of action is unknown, but it can bind and alter DNA. It is very effective in the exoerythrocytic stages of *P vivax* and *P ovale* malaria and against the primary phase (exoerythrocytic stage) of *P falciparum* malaria. It is also effective against the sexual forms (gametocytes) of plasmodia (especially *P falciparum*). It is indicated to prevent malaria relapses (radical cure) caused by *P vivax* and *P ovale* and is also effective against gametocytes of *P falciparum.*

Pharmacokinetics

Primaquine is absorbed orally and reaches peak level within 2 to 3 hours. With a half-life of approximately 6 hours, it is rapidly metabolized in an unspecified site and a small amount is excreted via the kidneys.

Drug interactions

The following effects may occur when primaquine is given with the drugs listed below:

Drug	Possible effect and management
Other hemolytic agents	May increase the risk for myelotoxic effects; monitor for muscle weakness and diminished deep tendon reflexes closely. Avoid or a potentially serious drug interaction may occur.
quinacrine (Antabrine)	This combination drug use is not recommended as an increase in primaquine toxicity is reported. Avoid or a potentially serious drug interaction may occur.

Color type indicates an unsafe drug combination.

Side effects and adverse reactions

These include gastric distress (stomach cramps or pain, nausea, and vomiting), hemolytic anemia (anorexia, back, leg or abdominal pain, dark urine, pale skin, weakness, and fever), methemoglobinemia (cyanosis, dizziness, respiratory difficulty, and weakness), and, rarely, leukopenia.

Warnings

Use with caution in patients with history (personal or family) of acute hemolytic anemia or a nicotinamide adenine dinucleotide (NADH) methemoglobin reductase deficiency.

Contraindications

Avoid use in persons with primaquine hypersensitivity or G6PD deficiency (primaquine may cause hemolytic anemia especially in G6PD-deficient persons).

Dosage and administration

The adult oral dose is 26.3 mg daily for 2 weeks. The pediatric dosage is 680 μg/kg daily for 2 weeks. Use of primaquine during pregnancy is not recommended.

quinine [kwye′ nine]

Quinine was the first drug used to treat malaria. As a schizonticidal agent it concentrates in parasitized erythrocytes, which may be why it has selective toxicity during the erythrocytic stages of plasmodial infections. It can also bind to DNA, thus inhibiting RNA synthesis and DNA replication.

Quinine sulfate is indicated in combination with other drugs (tetracycline, doxycycline, clindamycin, pyrimethamine plus sulfadiazine or, pyrimethamine plus sulfadoxine) for the treatment of chloroquine-resistant malaria caused by chloroquine-resistant, *P falciparum,* but today it is rarely used because more effective and less toxic drugs are available. Quinine has been reported to cause congenital malformations and stillbirths; therefore this drug should not be taken by pregnant women (see the Pregnancy Safety box).

Drug interactions

The following effects may occur when quinine is given with the drug listed below:

Drug	Possible effect and management
mefloquine (Lariam)	When used concurrently an increased incidence of convulsions and electrocardiogram (ECG) abnormalities have been reported. This predisposes the persons to cardiac dysrhythmias. If possible, avoid this combination. If not, then administer mefloquine at least 12 hours after the last dose of quinine. If both drugs must be given concurrently, the patient should be hospitalized and closely monitored for cardiac dysrhythmias and seizure activity.

PREGNANCY SAFETY

Category	Drug
B	rifabutin, niclosamide, praziquantel
C	capreomycin, clofazimine, cycloserine, dapsone, isoniazid, mebendazole, mefloquine, oxamniquine, pyrazinamide, pyrimethamine, rifampin, thiabendazole
D	streptomycin
X	primaquine, quinine
Unclassified*	aminosalicylates, chloroquine, diethylcarbamazine, hydroxychloroquine, ethambutol, ethionamide, iodoquinol, paromomycin, piperazine, pyrantel

*Risk-to-benefit ratio should be carefully evaluated before use.

Side effects and adverse reactions

These include cinchonism (changes in color vision or blurred vision, headache, very severe nausea and vomiting, tinnitus, and transient hearing loss), GI distress (stomach pain or cramps, diarrhea, nausea, and vomiting), and, rarely, hemolytic uremic syndrome (hemolytic anemia, thrombocytopenia, disseminated intravascular coagulation, and acute renal failure), hypoglycemia, hypersensitivity, and hepatotoxicity.

Warnings

Use with caution in patients with or history of cardiac dysrhythmias and G6PD deficiency.

Contraindications

Avoid use in persons with quinine or quinidine hypersensitivity or a history of Blackwater fever or thrombocytopenic purpura, hypoglycemia, and myasthenia gravis.

Dosage and administration

The adult dose for chloroquine-resistant *P falciparum* malaria is 600 to 650 mg PO every 8 hours for 3 days along with other medications as previously mentioned.

pyrimethamine tablets [peer i meth′ a meen] (Daraprim)
pyrimethamine with sulfadoxine (Fansidar)

Pyrimethamine is an antiprotozoal agent used to treat malaria and toxoplasmosis. It binds to and inhibits the protozoal enzyme dihydrofolate reductase, thus inhibiting the conversion of dihydrofolic acid to tetrahydrofolic acid. This results in a depletion of folate, which is essential for nucleic acid synthesis and protein production. Pyrimethamine in combination with mefloquine and sulfadoxine is indicated for the treatment of chloroquine-resistant *P falciparum* malaria. The drug is also combined with a sulfapyrimidine sulfonamide to treat toxoplasmosis caused by *Toxoplasma gondii.*

Pharmacokinetics

Pyrimethamine is orally absorbed and widely distributed in the body, although it concentrates mainly in blood cells, kidneys, liver, and spleen. It reaches peak plasma levels in 3 hours and has a half-life of 80 to 123 hours. It is metabolized in the liver and excreted via the kidneys.

Drug interactions

When pyrimethamine is administered concurrently with other bone marrow depressants, an increase in leukopenia and/or thrombocytopenia may result. Monitor complete blood counts closely.

Side effects and adverse reactions

These are usually rare, but in high dosages gastric distress (anorexia, nausea, vomiting, and diarrhea), atrophic glossitis (pain, burning or inflamed tongue, and changes or a loss in taste sensation), and blood dyscrasias (such as agranulocytosis, megaloblastic anemia, and thrombocytopenia) may be seen.

Warnings

Use with caution in patients with liver function impairment.

Contraindications

Avoid use in persons with pyrimethamine hypersensitivity, anemia, bone marrow suppression, and a history of convulsive disorders.

Dosage and administration

The adult oral dose in specific world areas, such as Southeast Asia, East Africa, or the Amazon, is 75 mg of pyrimethamine in combination with 750 mg of mefloquine and 1.5 g of sulfadoxine as a single dose. For additional dosing recommendations, see a current package insert or the USP DI.

TUBERCULOSIS

The incidence of **tuberculosis** (TB), a chronic granulomatous infection caused by the acid-fast bacillus, *Mycobacterium tuberculosis,* declined in the United States until 1985 when an increased incidence was noted in native-born Americans. Worldwide, approximately 8 million new cases of TB are diagnosed annually and 2.9 million persons die from this disease each year (Cali, 1995). Nursing home residents account for nearly 25% of TB cases in the United States (Yoshikawa, 1995). The increased incidence of tuberculosis is largely attributed to the increasing numbers of individuals with AIDS, persons living on the street or homeless persons, drug abusers, undernourished or malnourished persons, and persons taking immunosuppressant drugs or suffering from cancer. Thus persons at high risk are groups living in crowded facilities with less than optimum healthcare, some of which include prisons, homeless shelters, and human immunodeficiency virus (HIV) clinics and wards (Posey, 1996).

It has been reported that "tuberculosis is now the single biggest infectious killer of women in the world, according to an international research meeting on TB and gender in Sweden" (World Health Organization [WHO] Global, 1998, p. 1). Women who die from TB worldwide now constitute 9% of all deaths of women between the ages of 15 to 44. When compared with other causes of death in this age group, HIV is reported at 3% and heart disease at 3%. This is unfortunate, because the DOTS plan for tuberculosis (discussed below), if implemented, would definitely improve this situation (WHO Global, 1998).

M tuberculosis, the bacteria that causes tuberculosis, most commonly affects the lungs, but other body areas can also be infected, such as bones, joints, skin, meninges, or genitourinary tract. This bacteria is an aerobic bacillus that needs a highly oxygenated organ site for growth; thus the lungs, growing ends of bones, and cerebral cortex are ideal sites. Tubercle bacilli may be transmitted by airborne droplets but cannot be transmitted on objects such as dishes, clothing, or sheets and bedding (Fig. 53-2). Sharing an enclosed environment with an infected person creates a high risk of developing this infection (Ebert, 1993).

The development of drug-resistant tuberculosis is a major concern today. It has been estimated that there is approximately a 9% incidence of drug-resistant organisms in the United States (Ward, 1995). Resistance to two or more drugs (multidrug-resistant [MDR] TB) has resulted in outbreaks in institutional facilities. The WHO reported that individuals in the United States with MDR TB has decreased, but the number of states that report drug-resistant TB increased from 13 to 42 over a 6-year period (WHO MDR, 1998). The WHO recommends the DOTS (directly observed treatment short-course) program as the approach to TB control and cure in 85% of all new cases. The DOTS program is basically a strategy that includes five steps and involves the health system in the steps to a cure. The five steps include the following:

1. D, directly. Community resources should be focused on identification of persons with sputum-positive TB so treatment can be started. In other words, identify and treat the persons with the worse cases of tuberculosis first so reduce the disease spread.
2. O, observed. Observe that patients actually swallow each dose of medication prescribed, which is especially critical during the first 2 months of treatment. At this time, the patient is usually more seriously ill and infectious to others and is also at a greater risk of acquiring a drug resistance. While it may not be possible to actually monitor each dose, the healthcare professional can institute an individual plan concerning observation of treatment and should follow-up on patients who do not keep their appointments. The specified observer must be accountable to the healthcare service and also be accessible to the patient.
3. T, treatment. This is a two-step process that includes treatment and monitoring. Patients with contagious disease should have their sputum examined by microscope for TB bacilli after 2 months and at the end of treatment. The goal is to achieve a TB bacilli-free result. Monitor and report on each TB patient so that a healthcare service can identify and intervene in communities that are not obtaining a 85% cure rate. Additional resources such as support and training may be necessary.
4. S, short-course. The right drug combination and dosage should be used for the proper length of time to kill the tuberculosis bacilli. The drugs may include isoniazid, rifampin, pyrazinamide, streptomycin, and ethambutol; they are typically prescribed for 6 or 8 months of therapy.
5. DOTS! This program needs government support and funding to achieve long-term TB control. According to

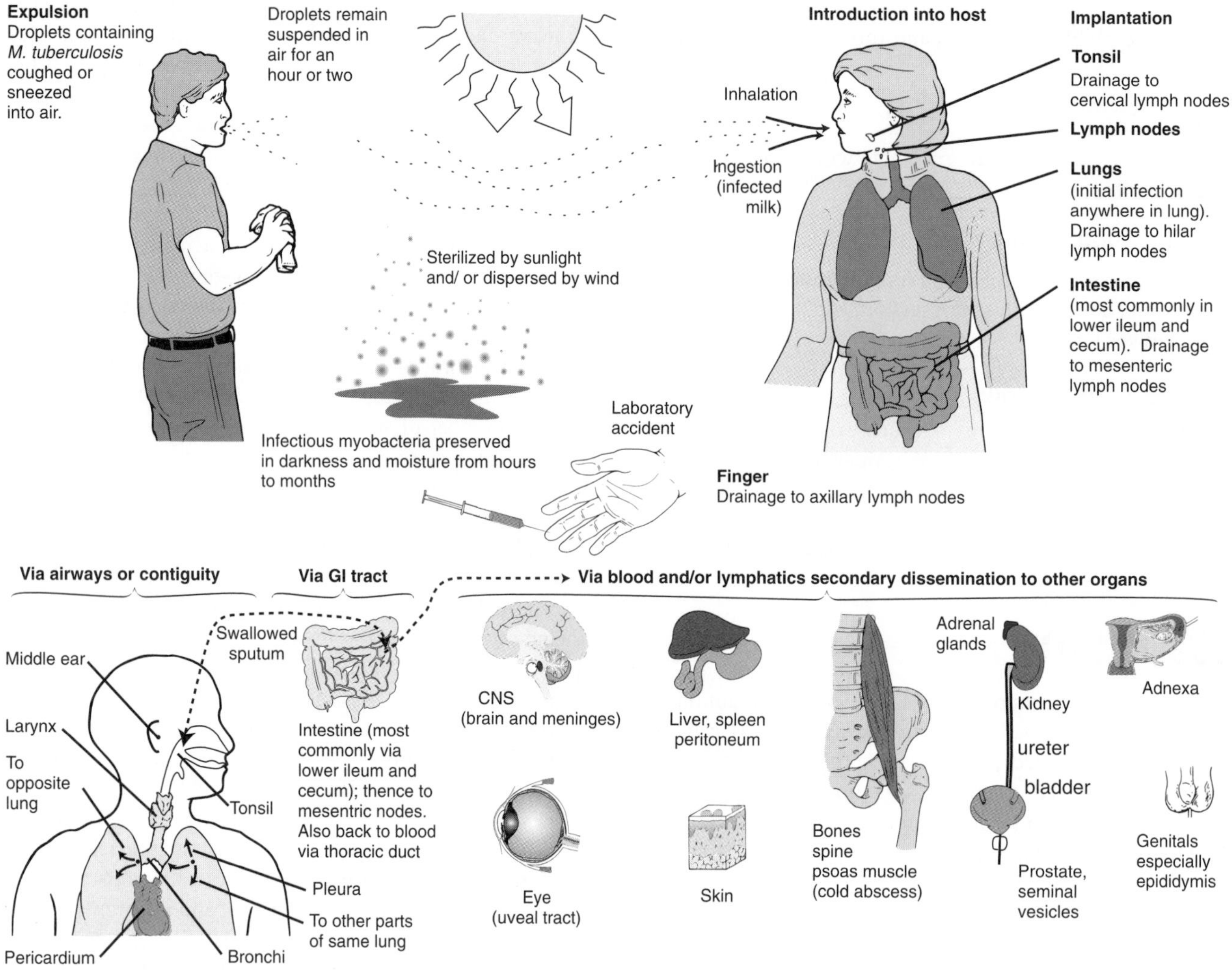

FIGURE 53-2
Dissemination of tuberculosis.

the WHO, only 10% of all TB patients were treated in 1997 under the DOTS strategic plan (WHO DOTS, 1998). The lack of instituting such a plan is obvious: increased number of cases of TB, MDR TB, and deaths.

Pathogenesis

Tubercle bacilli droplets are transmitted when an infected person coughs or sneezes. Persons producing sputum generally have many bacilli and are more infectious than the infected person who does not cough. Three types of tubercle bacilli are pathogenic to humans: human to human, bovine to human, and avian to human. Avian TB is rare in the United States and Canada, and with the pasteurization of milk and testing of cows, bovine TB is much less prevalent. Thus the primary source of transmission is human to human. Fig. 53-2 illustrates dissemination of tuberculosis.

When the tubercle bacilli enter the lungs, infection can spread to other body organs through the blood and lymph system. Usually, however, the infection may become dormant and be walled off by calcified and fibrous tissues. The bacilli become inactive, perhaps for the lifetime of the host. If host defenses break down, however, or if the host receives an immunosuppressive drug, the bacilli may be reactivated.

Drug Treatment Regimens

Effective drug regimens are available to treat tuberculosis. Drug selection is based on the development of drug-resistant organisms and drug toxicity. General guidelines include:

1. To avoid the development of drug-resistant organisms, all individuals in whom TB is diagnosed (isolated *M tuberculosis*) should have drug susceptibility tests on their first isolation.
2. In most instances, the result of the in vitro susceptibility test is unknown when drug therapy is started. It is recommended that a four-drug regimen be instituted (especially in areas where primary isoniazid resistance occurs) because this regimen provides an adequate drug regimen that will be at least 95% effective, even in the presence of

drug-resistant organisms. The recommended drugs are isoniazid, rifampin, pyrazinamide, and ethambutol or streptomycin (CDC, 1993; Mandell, Petri, 1996).

3. When drug susceptibility results are available, the drug regimen can be adjusted.
4. Monitor the prescribed therapy regimen closely to support patient compliance, to detect side effects or adverse reactions, and to register progress of the treatment program.

ANTITUBERCULOUS AGENTS

aminosalicylate [a mee noe sal i′ si late] (PAS, Tubasal, Nemasol ✤)

Aminosalicylate is a bacteriostatic agent closely related to aminobenzoic acid (PABA); thus it competitively inhibits folic acid formation resulting in suppression of the growth and reproduction of *M tuberculosis.* In combination with other antitubercular agents, it is indicated for the treatment of *M tuberculosis,* pulmonary and extrapulmonary.

Pharmacokinetics

Aminosalicylate is well absorbed orally and distributed to various body fluids with high levels accumulating in pleural fluids, kidney, lungs, and liver tissues. Its half-life is between 45 and 60 minutes, although patients with impaired renal function may have a half-life of up to 23 hours. Peak serum level is reached within 1 to 2 hours. This drug is metabolized in the liver and excreted by the kidneys.

Drug interactions

The concurrent use of aminosalicylate with aminobenzoates (Potaba) is not recommended because the aminobenzoate may be absorbed by the bacteria in preference to aminosalicylate, which results in antagonism of the bacteriostatic effects of aminosalicylate.

Side effects and adverse reactions

For aminosalicylate therapy these include gastric distress (stomach pain, nausea, vomiting, anorexia, and diarrhea), hypersensitivity reactions (fever, joint pain, rash, increased weakness, and leukopenia), goiter or myxedema, crystalluria, hemolytic anemia, hepatitis, and infectious mononucleosis-type syndrome.

Warnings

Use with caution in patients with G6PD deficiency and in severe liver or kidney disease.

Contraindications

Avoid use in persons with aminosalicylates, other salicylates or sulfonamide hypersensitivity, congestive heart failure, and gastric ulcer.

Dosage and administration

The adult oral dose given in combination with other antimycobacterial agents is 3.3 to 4 g every 8 hours up to a maximum daily dose of 20 g. The pediatric dose in combination with other antimycobacterial agents is 50 to 75 mg/kg PO every 6 hours. If gastric distress occurs, take medication with or after meals or with an antacid.

capreomycin [kap ree oh mye′ sin] (Capastat)

Capreomycin is an antimycobacterial agent with an unknown mechanism of action. It is indicated in combination therapy for the treatment of pulmonary tuberculosis caused by *M tuberculosis* after primary medications (streptomycin, isoniazid, rifampin, pyrazinamide, and ethambutol) fail or when these medications cannot be used because of resistant bacilli or drug toxicity.

Pharmacokinetics

Administered parenterally, capreomycin has a half-life between 3 to 6 hours and reaches a peak serum level in 1 to 2 hours after IM administration. It is excreted by the kidneys primarily unchanged.

Drug interactions

When capreomycin is given with any of the following drugs, very serious reactions may result. Avoid if possible.

Drug	Possible effect and management
Aminoglycosides	Increased risk for developing ototoxicity, nephrotoxicity, and neuromuscular blockade. Hearing loss may progress to deafness, even after the drug is stopped. This can be a very dangerous combination. Avoid concurrent drug administration.
amphotericin B parenteral (Fungizone), bacitracin parenteral, bumetanide parenteral (Bumex), cisplatin (Platinol), cyclosporine (Sandimmune), ethacrynic acid (Edecrin) or furosemide parenteral (Lasix), paromomycin (Humatin), streptomycin, or vancomycin (Vancocin)	Concurrent or even sequential use of capreomycin with any of these drugs can increase the risk of ototoxicity and nephrotoxicity. Hearing loss may occur and progress to deafness, even if drugs are stopped. Avoid if at all possible
methoxyflurane (Penthrane) or polymyxins, parenteral	The potential for nephrotoxicity and neuromuscular blockade is increased, which may lead to respiratory depression or paralysis. Avoid concurrent or sequential drug administration.

Neuromuscular blocking agents	May result in increased neuromuscular blocking effects, causing respiratory depression or paralysis. Monitor closely, especially during surgery or in the post-operative period. If possible, avoid this combination. If not, closely monitor and keep anticholinesterase agents or calcium salts on hand to reverse the blockade.

Color type indicates an unsafe drug combination.

Side effects and adverse reactions

These include nephrotoxicity, hypokalemia, neuromuscular blockade, ototoxicity (auditory: hearing loss, and ringing or buzzing noise; vestibular: ataxia, dizziness, nausea, and vomiting), hypersensitivity, and pain, soreness, or hardness at the injection site.

Warnings

Use with caution in dehydrated patients.

Contraindications

Avoid use in persons with capreomycin hypersensitivity, eighth cranial nerve damage, myasthenia gravis, Parkinson's disease, or kidney function impairment.

Dosage and administration

The adult dose in combination with other antitubercular agents is 1 g IM daily for 2 to 4 months followed by 1 g two or three times weekly.

cycloserine [sye kloe ser′ een] (Seromycin)

This is a broad-spectrum antibiotic that can be bacteriostatic or bactericidal, depending on drug concentration at infection site and organism susceptibility. It is an antimycobacterial agent that interferes with bacterial cell wall synthesis. In combination with other drugs, it is indicated for the treatment of active pulmonary and extrapulmonary tuberculosis after failure of the primary antitubercular medications.

Pharmacokinetics

Cycloserine is well absorbed orally and is widely distributed in body tissues and fluids. It reaches a peak serum level between 3 and 4 hours and has a half-life of 10 hours. About 35% of cycloserine is metabolized with excretion primarily via the kidneys.

Drug interactions

The following effects may occur when cycloserine is given with the drugs listed below:

Drug	Possible effect and management
Alcohol	In chronic alcohol abusers, it may increase the risk of seizures. Avoid or a potentially serious drug interaction may occur.
ethionamide (Trecator-SC)	May increase CNS side effects such as seizures. Monitor closely, as dosage adjustments may be necessary.

Color type indicates an unsafe drug combination.

Side effects and adverse reactions

These include headache, dose-related CNS toxicity (confusion, dizziness, sedation, irritability, restlessness, depression, tremors, nightmares, mood alterations, speech problems, anxiety, and thoughts of suicide), hypersensitivity, peripheral neuropathy, and convulsions.

Warnings

Use with caution in patients with severe anxiety, depression, or psychosis.

Contraindications

Avoid use in persons with cycloserine hypersensitivity, kidney impairment, and history of convulsive disorders.

Dosage and administration

The adult oral dose used in combination with other drugs is 250 mg every 12 hours for 2 weeks, then the dose is increased as necessary up to 250 mg every 6 to 8 hours. The maximum daily dose is 1 g. The pediatric dosage is 10 to 20 mg/kg daily in divided doses.

Additional comments

If gastric distress occurs, administer medications after meals. Be aware that CNS toxicity increases with drug dosages more than 500 mg/day. Monitor serum levels closely and keep the range between 25 and 30 μg/ml to treat tuberculosis.

ethambutol [e tham′ byoo tole] (Myambutol, Etibi 🍁)

This antitubercular agent is bacteriostatic; it is believed to diffuse into the mycobacteria bacilli and suppress RNA synthesis. It is effective only against actively dividing mycobacteria. It is indicated in combination with other drugs for the treatment of tuberculosis.

Pharmacokinetics

Ethambutol is absorbed orally and distributed to most body tissues and fluids with the exception of cerebrospinal fluid. High concentrations are found in the kidneys, lungs, saliva, urine, and erythrocytes. The time to peak serum level is 2 to 4 hours, and the half-life is between 3 and 4 hours. Ethambutol is metabolized in the liver and excreted by the kidneys.

Drug interactions

There is an increased risk for neurotoxicity such as optic and peripheral neuritis when ethambutol is administered concurrently with other neurotoxic medications. Monitor closely if concurrent therapy is instituted.

Side effects and adverse reactions

These include gastric distress, confusion, disorientation, headache, optic neuritis, peripheral neuritis, hypersensitivity, and acute gouty arthritis.

Warnings

Use with caution in patients with acute gouty arthritis as ethambutol may increase uric acid levels.

Contraindications

Avoid use in persons with ethambutol hypersensitivity, optic neuritis, and kidney function impairment.

Dosage and administration

The adult oral dose in combination with other agents is 15 to 25 mg/kg daily. Take medication with food if gastric distress occurs. Instruct the patient to report any visual changes to the physician as soon as possible.

ethionamide [e thye on am′ ide] (Trecator-SC)

Ethionamide is an antimycobacterial agent indicated for the treatment of tuberculosis after failure of the primary antitubercular agents (streptomycin, isoniazid, rifampin, and ethambutol). Its mechanism of action is unknown, but it is believed to inhibit peptide synthesis.

Pharmacokinetics

Ethionamide is well absorbed orally and distributed to most body tissues and fluids, including cerebrospinal fluid. It has a half-life of 2 to 3 hours and may be metabolized in the liver and excreted primarily by the kidneys.

Drug interactions

Concurrent use of cycloserine will increase the risk for CNS toxicity, especially seizures. The patient should be monitored closely for CNS toxicity as drug dosage adjustments may be necessary.

Side effects and adverse reactions

These include gastric distress, orthostatic hypotension, peripheral neuritis, hepatitis, psychiatric disorders (depression, confusion, and mental alterations), and, rarely, goiter or hypothyroidism, hypoglycemia, optic neuritis, and rash.

Contraindications

Avoid use in persons with ethionamide hypersensitivity, diabetes mellitus, and liver function impairment.

Dosage and administration

The adult oral dose in combination with other agents is 250 mg every 8 to 12 hours. The pediatric dosage is 4 to 5 mg/kg orally every 8 hours. If gastric distress occurs, take medication with or after meals.

isoniazid [eye soe nye′ a zid] (Nydrazid, INH)

Isoniazid is an antimycobacterial (bactericidal) agent that affects mycobacteria in the division phase. Its exact mechanism of action is unknown, but it is believed to inhibit mycolic acid synthesis and cause cell wall disruption in susceptible organisms. Isoniazid is indicated for the treatment and prevention of tuberculosis.

Pharmacokinetics

Isoniazid is well absorbed orally and is widely distributed throughout the body. The time to peak serum level is 1 to 2 hours for fast drug acetylators (metabolism) or 4 to 6 hours for slow drug acetylators. Its half-life in fast acetylators is 0.5 to 1.6 hours and in slow acetylators is 2 to 5 hours. Isoniazid is metabolized in the liver, primarily by acetylation to inactive metabolites, some of which may be hepatotoxic. The rate of acetylation by the liver is genetically determined; slow acetylators have a decrease in hepatic N-acetyltransferase. Excretion is primarily via the kidneys.

Be aware that slow acetylators may need lower drug dosages and are more apt to develop adverse reactions, particularly peripheral neuritis. The incidence of slow acetylators is highest in Egyptian, Israeli, Scandinavian, other Caucasian, and black populations, while the lowest is in Eskimo, Oriental, and Native American populations.

Drug interactions

The following effects may occur when isoniazid is given with the drugs listed below:

Drug	Possible effect and management
Alcohol	Daily use of alcohol may result in increased isoniazid metabolism and increased risk of hepatotoxicity. Monitor patients because a drug dose adjustment may be necessary.
alfentanil (Alfenta)	Isoniazid inhibits liver metabolism, which may decrease alfentanil metabolism, leading to increased alfentanil serum levels and prolonging its duration of action. Monitor serum levels closely.

carbamazepine (Tegretol)	May result in increased carbamazepine serum levels and toxicity. Monitor serum levels closely.
disulfiram (Antabuse)	May increase the incidence of CNS side effects such as ataxia, irritability, dizziness, or insomnia. Monitor closely for these symptoms because dosage reduction or even discontinuation of disulfiram may be required.
Hepatotoxic drugs	May increase potential for hepatotoxicity. Avoid or a potentially serious drug interaction may occur.
ketoconazole (Nizoral), miconazole (Monistat IV) (parenteral), or rifampin (Rifadin)	Isoniazid with ketoconazole may decrease serum levels of ketoconazole; if both isoniazid and rifampin are given with ketoconazole, the serum levels of ketoconazole or rifampin have been reported to be undetectable. Therefore the combination of isoniazid or rifampin together or individually with ketoconazole or parenteral miconazole is not recommended. Rifampin with isoniazid may increase the potential for hepatotoxicity, especially in patients with liver impairment and in fast acetylators of isoniazid. Monitor closely for hepatotoxicity, especially during the first 90 days of therapy.
phenytoin (Dilantin)	May result in impaired phenytoin metabolism, leading to increased serum levels and toxicity. The phenytoin dose may need to be adjusted. Monitor serum phenytoin closely.

Color type indicates an unsafe drug combination.

Side effects and adverse reactions

These include gastric distress, anorexia, nausea, vomiting, weakness, hepatitis, peripheral neuritis, and, rarely, blood dyscrasias, hypersensitivity, and optic neuritis.

Warnings

Use with caution in patients with severe kidney disease and convulsive disorders.

Contraindications

Avoid use in persons with isoniazid, ethionamide, pyrazinamide, niacin, and nicotinic acid hypersensitivity and liver function impairment, and in alcoholics.

Dosage and administration

The adult oral and parenteral (IM) prophylactic dose of isoniazid is 300 mg daily. The parenteral (IM) treatment dosage when administered in combination with other agents is 5 mg/kg up to 300 mg once daily. The oral treatment dosage when given in combination with other agents to treat tuberculosis is 300 mg daily. The pediatric dosage for prophylaxis orally and parenterally (IM) is 10 mg/kg up to 300 mg daily.

Additional comments

If gastric distress occurs, this medication may be taken with meals or an antacid, although aluminum antacids should be separated by at least 1 hour from isoniazid. Be aware though that oral absorption is decreased when food or antacids are given concurrently. Also, pyridoxine may be prescribed concurrently to prevent peripheral neuritis, although it is usually not necessary for children if their dietary intake of vitamins is adequate.

isoniazid combinations

For ease of drug administration, isoniazid has been combined with rifampin (Rifamate) and in dual packs (Rimactane/INH). See individual headings (isoniazid and rifampin) for additional information.

pyrazinamide [peer a zin′ a mide] (pms Pyrazinamide ♣, Tebrazid ♣)

Pyrazinamide is an antimycobacterial agent with an unknown mechanism of action. Depending on concentration at the site of action and susceptibility of the mycobacteria, this drug can be bacteriostatic or bactericidal. It is indicated in combination with other agents for the treatment of tuberculosis.

Pharmacokinetics

Pyrazinamide is well absorbed orally and is widely distributed in the body. The time to peak serum level is 1 to 2 hours, and elimination half-life is 9 to 10 hours. Pyrazinamide is primarily metabolized in the liver and excreted by the kidneys.

Side effects and adverse reactions

These include arthralgia related to hyperuricemia, pruritus, rash, and, rarely, gouty arthritis and hepatotoxicity.

Warnings

Use with caution in patients with gout.

Contraindications

Avoid use in persons with pyrazinamide, ethionamide, isoniazid, niacin, or nicotinic hypersensitivity and severe liver disease.

Dosage and administration

The adult oral dose when given in combination with other agents is 15 to 30 mg/kg daily, up to a maximum dose of 2 g daily.

rifabutin [riff′ a byoo tin] (Mycobutin)

Rifabutin is an antimycobacterial agent indicated for the prophylaxis of disseminated *Mycobacterium avium* complex

(MAC) in persons with advanced HIV infection. It inhibits DNA-dependent RNA polymerase in susceptible *Escherichia coli* and *Bacillus subtilis,* and in vitro it has activity against many strains of *M tuberculosis.* It is used in combination with isoniazid for the prophylaxis of tuberculosis and MAC.

Pharmacokinetics

It is absorbed from the GI tract, reaches peak serum levels in 2 to 4 hours, and has a terminal half-life of 45 hours. Rifabutin is highly lipophilic so it crosses the blood-brain barrier and cerebrospinal fluid levels are approximately 50% of the corresponding serum level. It is metabolized in the liver (five metabolites have been identified) and excreted primarily by the kidneys.

Drug interactions

When rifabutin is administered concurrently with zidovudine (AZT), some studies indicate that the mean zidovudine serum level may decrease. Monitor closely if combination therapy is used.

Side effects and adverse reactions

These include nausea, vomiting, skin rash, and, rarely, joint pain, a change in taste sensations, myalgia, neutropenia, pseudojaundice (yellow tinge skin), and uveitis.

Contraindications

Avoid use in persons with rifabutin or rifampin hypersensitivity and active tuberculosis.

Dosage and administration

The usual adult dose is 300 mg daily, preferably on an empty stomach. It gastric distress occurs, then split the dose (150 mg twice a day) and take it with food. If patient cannot swallow the capsule, its contents can be mixed with applesauce before administration (USP DI, 1998).

rifampin [rif' am pin] (Rifadin, Rofact)

Rifampin is a broad-spectrum bactericidal antibiotic (antimycobacterial) that blocks RNA transcription. It is indicated for the treatment of tuberculosis and for asymptomatic meningococcal carriers of *Neisseria meningitidis.* It is well absorbed orally and widely distributed in the body.

Pharmacokinetics

Rifampin is lipid soluble; thus it may reach and kill intracellular and extracellular susceptible bacteria. The time to reach peak serum level is 1.5 to 4 hours; elimination half-life is up to 5 hours. It is metabolized in the liver to a number of metabolites, including an active metabolite (25-*O*-desacetylrifampin), and excreted primarily in the feces.

Drug interactions

The following effects may occur when rifampin is given with the drugs listed below:

Drug	Possible effect and management
Alcohol	Daily use of alcohol may increase the risk of rifampin-induced hepatotoxicity and increase the rate of rifampin metabolism. Monitor hepatic function studies closely, as dosage adjustments may be necessary.
Antidiabetic agents (oral)	Concurrent use enhances the metabolism of the antidiabetic drugs; dosage adjustment may be indicated.
Corticosteroids, glucocorticoids, and mineralocorticoids, anticoagulants, oral, warfarin (Coumadin) or indanedione, digitalis glycosides, disopyramide (Norpace), mexiletine (Mexitil), tocainide (Tonocard), quinidine, azole antifungals, phenytoin (Dilantin), or chloramphenicol (Chloromycetin)	Rifampin increases levels of liver-metabolizing enzymes and therefore may decrease the effectiveness of these medications, which are metabolized by the liver. Monitor serum levels of these drugs closely to ensure therapeutic levels because dosage adjustments may be needed.
Estrogen-containing oral contraceptives, estramustine, or estrogens	Decreased effectiveness due to increased liver metabolism of estrogen. May result in menstrual irregularities, spotting, and unplanned pregnancies. Advise patient of the possible effects when these drugs are combined and suggest alternative contraception.
Hepatotoxic drugs, other	Increases the risk of hepatotoxicity. Avoid or a potentially serious drug interaction may occur.
isoniazid (INH) or ketoconazole (Nizoral) oral or miconazole parenteral (Monistat IV)	Increases risk for hepatotoxicity. Avoid concurrent drug administration.
methadone	May decrease the effectiveness of methadone and may induce methadone withdrawal in dependent patients. Monitor closely; dosage adjustments may be necessary during and after rifampin therapy.
verapamil, oral	Accelerates the metabolism of oral verapamil, decreasing blood levels and decreasing its cardiovascular effects.

Xanthenes, aminophylline, oxtriphylline, and theophylline	Increases the metabolism of these drugs thus increasing drug clearance. Monitor with serum levels of the patient's xanthene drug.

Color type indicates an unsafe drug combination.

Side effects and adverse reactions

These include gastric distress, hypersensitivity, a flu-like syndrome, red-orange discoloration of urine, feces, saliva, sputum, sweat, and tears (soft contact lenses can be discolored by rifampin), fungal overgrowth, and, rarely, blood dyscrasias, hepatitis, and interstitial nephritis.

Contraindications

Avoid use in persons liver function impairment and in alcoholics.

Dosage and administration

The rifampin adult oral dose in combination with other agents (for tuberculosis) is 600 mg daily. To treat asymptomatic meningococcal carriers, the dose is 600 mg orally twice daily for 2 days. For children 1 month of age and older, the dose to treat tuberculosis (with other antitubercular agents) is 10 to 20 mg/kg daily. For asymptomatic meningococcal carriers, the dose is 5 mg/kg orally every 12 hours for 2 days.

Additional comments

Rifampin should be taken with a full glass of water (8 oz) on an empty stomach, that is, 1 hour before or 2 hours after a meal to obtain the maximum absorption. If gastric distress is a problem though, it may be taken with food. For patients who have difficulty swallowing the capsule, the contents of the capsules may be mixed with applesauce before administration. Concurrent alcohol consumption should be avoided. Blood counts should be monitored and dental procedures deferred until blood counts are normal.

streptomycin injection [strep toe mye' sin]

Streptomycin is a aminoglycoside antibiotic that is poorly absorbed from the GI tract; therefore it is given intramuscularly. It was one of the first effective agents used in the late 1940s to treat tuberculosis, and it still is an important agent in managing severe tuberculosis. Like the other aminoglycosides, its major toxicities include ototoxicity and nephrotoxicity, especially when given to patients with impaired renal function or with other medications with the same toxicities. See Chapter 51 for detailed information on the aminoglycosides.

The adult dose for streptomycin is 1 g IM daily. As soon as possible, reduce the dose to 1 g two or three times weekly. For geriatric patients, the dose is 500 to 750 mg daily, in combination with other antitubercular agents. For children, the dose is 20 mg/kg daily, in combination with other antitubercular agents. The maximum daily dose is 1 g.

AMEBIASIS

Amebiasis is an infection of the large intestine produced by a protozoan parasite, *Entamoeba histolytica.* This infestation is found worldwide but is prevalent and severe in tropical areas. It also has been detected in poorly sanitized areas including some rural communities, Native American reservations, and migrant labor farm camps and is also common in homosexual males (Anandan, 1995). Transmission is usually through ingestion of cysts (fecal to oral route) from contaminated food or water or from person-to-person contact. Poor personal hygiene can increase the spread of this parasite.

Life Cycle of Ameba

The protozoan has two stages in its life cycle: (1) the trophozoite (vegetative ameba), which is the active, motile form, and (2) the cyst, or inactive, drug-resistant form that appears in intestinal excretion. The trophozoite stage is capable of ameboid motion and sexual activity. Because of its susceptibility to injury, it generally succumbs to an unfavorable environment. However, under certain circumstances, the trophozoite protects itself by entering the cystic stage. During this phase the protozoan becomes inactive by surrounding itself with a resistant cell wall within which it can survive for a long time, even in an unsuitable environment.

The complete life cycle of the ameba occurs in humans, the main host. It begins by ingestion of cysts that are present on hands, food, or water contaminated by feces. On reaching the stomach the hydrochloric acid does not destroy the swallowed cysts, but instead they pass unharmed into the small intestine. The digestive juices penetrate the cystic walls, and the trophozoites are released. The motile amoebae later pass into the colon, where they live and multiply for a time, feeding on the bacterial flora of the gut.

The presence of bacteria is essential for their survival. Finally, before excretion, the trophozoites move toward the terminal end of the bowel and again become encysted. After the cysts are eliminated in the feces, they remain viable and infective. Unfortunately, the cycle may begin again when the cysts appearing in fecal excretion are ingested through contamination of food or water.

The parasite causing amebiasis replicates in three major locations: (1) the lumen of the bowel, (2) the intestinal mucosa, and (3) extraintestinal sites. Thus amebiasis is classified according to its primary site of action: intestinal amebiasis, where amebic activity is restricted to the bowel lumen or intestinal mucosa, or extraintestinal amebiasis, where parasitic invasion occurs outside the intestine.

Intestinal Amebiasis

Intestinal amebiasis may be manifested as an asymptomatic intestinal infection or a symptomatic intestinal infection that may be mild, moderate, or severe.

Asymptomatic intestinal amebiasis

In asymptomatic intestinal amebiasis the action of the parasite is restricted to the lumen of the bowel. The individual is asymptomatic but becomes a carrier of the disease by passing mature cysts of the parasite in formed stools. Outside the body the cysts can live for several weeks, surviving dry, freezing, or high temperature conditions. By this means the infection is transmitted from person to person by flies or contaminated food or water. Ordinary concentrations of chlorine in water purification do not destroy the cysts. If the carrier fails to follow any drug treatment, serious gastrointestinal pathologic problems eventually develop. Occasionally mild symptoms exist including vague abdominal pain, nausea, flatulence, fatigue, and nervousness.

Symptomatic intestinal amebiasis

Symptomatic amebiasis occurs when the trophozoites in the lumen of the bowel penetrate the mucosal lining of the colon. After they multiply and thrive on bacterial flora, a large infestation occurs, producing diarrhea and abdominal pain. The increased loss of fluid may cause prostration. In addition, ulcerative colitis may result. This state of the disease is called intestinal amebiasis and is usually diagnosed as mild, moderate, or severe according to the intensity of the symptoms and the extent of the disease.

Extraintestinal amebiasis

The term "extraintestinal amebiasis" means the parasites have migrated to other parts of the body, such as the liver or occasionally the spleen, lungs, or brain. When the parasites are in the liver, necrotic foci develop because of the parasites' destructive effect on tissues. When there is liver involvement, the terms "liver abscess" and "hepatic amebiasis" are usually used.

ANTIAMEBIASIS AGENTS

Drugs for the treatment of amebiasis are classified according to the site of the previously described amebic action. Luminal amebicides act primarily in the bowel lumen and are generally ineffective against parasites in the bowel wall or tissues. Tissue amebicides are drugs that act primarily in the bowel wall, liver, and other extraintestinal tissues. No single drug is effective for both types of amebiasis; therefore a luminal and extraluminal (tissue) amebicide or combination therapy is often prescribed. The intestinal amebicides are considered to be iodoquinol, metronidazole, and paromomycin; the extraintestinal amebicides are chloroquine and metronidazole.

iodoquinol [eye oh do kwin′ ole] (diiodohydroxyquin, Yodoxin)

Iodoquinol is an antiprotozoal agent with an unknown mechanism of action. It is poorly absorbed from the intestinal tract; thus it produces its effect against the trophozoites of *E histolytica* at the site of intestinal infestation. It is indicated for the treatment of intestinal amebiasis in asymptomatic carriers of *E histolytica.*

Pharmacokinetics

After administration and local effect, iodoquinol is excreted in the feces.

Side effects and adverse reactions

These include gastric distress, hypersensitivity, fever, chills, headache, pruritus in the rectal area, thyroid gland enlargement, and with chronic high-dose drug administration (especially in children), optic atrophy or neuritis, peripheral neuropathy, and subacute myelo-optic neuropathy.

Warnings

Use with caution in patients with preexisting optic neuropathy or thyroid disease.

Contraindications

Avoid use in persons with liver or kidney disease.

Dosage and administration

The adult oral dose is 650 mg three times a day, after meals for 20 days. The pediatric dosage is 40 mg/kg orally in three divided doses after meals for 20 days. Take the drug after meals to reduce gastric distress.

paromomycin [par oh moe mye′ sin] (Humatin)

Paromomycin is both an amebicidal and an antibacterial agent. The drug is an aminoglycoside antibiotic with antibacterial properties similar to those of neomycin. Paromomycin acts directly on intestinal amebae and on bacteria such as *Salmonella* and *Shigella.* Because the drug is poorly absorbed from the gastrointestinal tract, it exerts no effect on systemic infections such as extraintestinal amebiasis. It is indicated for the treatment of acute and chronic intestinal amebiasis and for adjunct therapy in management of hepatic coma.

Pharmacokinetics

Paromomycin is poorly absorbed from the intestinal tract; thus most of the drug is excreted in the feces.

Drug interactions

See aminoglycosides in Chapter 51.

Side effects and adverse reactions

These include nausea, diarrhea, and gastric distress. Paromomycin is an aminoglycoside; therefore the drug interactions possible with this family of medications may also occur with paromomycin. See the discussion of aminoglycoside antibiotics in Chapter 51.

Warnings and contraindications

See aminoglycosides in Chapter 51.

Dosage and administration

The adult and pediatric dosage to treat intestinal amebiasis is 25 to 35 mg/kg daily in three divided doses given with meals for 5 to 10 days. To manage hepatic coma, the adult dosage is 4 g daily in divided doses at regular intervals for 5 or 6 days.

Other Drugs

Metronidazole (Flagyl) is an antibacterial, antiprotozoal, and anthelmintic agent. It is used for treatment of extraintestinal and intestinal amebiasis. When used in the treatment of invasive amebiasis, the recommendation is that it be administered with a luminal amebicide, such as iodoquinol or paromomycin.

Its mechanism of action appears to be due to an interaction between the intracellular reduced metronidazole (which is cytotoxic) and DNA, which results in inhibition of nucleic acid synthesis and cell death. For additional drug information, see Chapter 51.

Chloroquine (Aralen) is used to treat amebic liver abscess, usually in combination with other drugs. See the drug discussion earlier in this chapter for further information on this drug.

Dehydroemetine (Mebadin) and diloxanide furoate (Furamide) are also antiinfective agents used to treat amebiasis but are available only from the Centers for Disease Control and Prevention (Parasitic Disease Drug Service, Division of Host Factors, Center for Infectious Disease, Atlanta, GA, 30333), because they are considered investigational agents.

OTHER PROTOZOAN DISEASES

Several other protozoan diseases are widespread throughout the world and may be encountered in clinical practice in the United States and Canada. In this section, each disease and the primary antiprotozoan agent used in its treatment will be described.

TOXOPLASMOSIS

Toxoplasmosis is caused by an intracellular parasite, *Toxoplasma gondii.* This parasite is found worldwide and infests a variety of animals, including humans. It is often harbored in the host with no evidence of the disease. Toxoplasmosis is contracted by ingesting cysts found in inadequately cooked raw meat or by accidentally ingesting cysts from cat feces.

The most common form of the disease in the United States and Canada is usually subclinical. Symptomatically the individual may experience lymphadenopathy, fever, and occasionally a rash on the palms and soles. The most serious complication of toxoplasmosis is meningoencephalitis. Toxoplasmosis is treated with a combination of sulfadiazine and pyrimethamine, both of which alter the folic acid cycle of the *Toxoplasma* organism, resulting in its death. The oral dosage of pyrimethamine is 25 mg/day for 3 to 4 weeks; the dosage of sulfadiazine is 1 to 4 g/day for 1 to 3 weeks.

TRICHOMONIASIS

Trichomoniasis is a disease of the vagina caused by *Trichomonas vaginalis.* Its characteristic presentation consists of a wet, inflamed vagina, a "strawberry" cervix, and a thin, yellow, frothy malodorous discharge. Usually both sexual partners are infected by this organism, which can be identified microscopically from semen, prostatic fluid, or exudate from the vagina. Infections often recur, which indicates that the protozoans persist in extravaginal foci, male urethra, or the periurethral glands and ducts of both sexes.

Metronidazole (Flagyl) is the drug of choice, and treatment must be given simultaneously to both partners involved for cure.

HELMINTHIASIS

The disease-producing **helminths** are classified as metazoa, or multicellular animal parasites. Unlike the protozoa, they are large organisms that have a complex cellular structure and that feed on host tissue. They may be present in the gastrointestinal tract, but several types also penetrate the tissues, and some undergo developmental changes during which they wander extensively in the host. Because most anthelmintics used today are highly effective against specific parasites, the organism must be accurately identified before treatment is started, usually by finding the parasite ova or larvae in the feces, urine, blood sputum, or tissues of the host.

Parasitic infestations do not necessarily cause clinical manifestations, although they may be injurious for a number of reasons:

1. Worms may cause mechanical injury to the tissues and organs. Roundworms in large numbers may cause obstruction in the intestine, filariae may block lymphatic channels and cause massive edema, and hookworms often cause extensive damage to the wall of the intestine and considerable loss of blood.
2. Toxic substances produced by the parasite may be absorbed by the host.
3. The tissues of the host may be traumatized by the presence of the parasite and made more susceptible to bacterial infections.
4. Heavy infestation with worms will rob the host of food. This is particularly significant in children.

Helminths that are parasitic to humans are classified as (1) Platyhelminths (flatworms), which include two subclasses, cestodes (tapeworms) and trematodes (flukes), and (2) Nematoda (roundworms).

Platyhelminths (Flatworms)

Cestodes

Cestodes are tapeworms, of which there are four varieties: (1) *Taenia saginata* (beef tapeworm), (2) *Taenia solium* (pork tapeworm), (3) *Diphyllobrothrium latum* (fish tapeworm), and (4) *Hymenolepis nana* (dwarf tapeworm). As indicated by the name of the worm, the parasite enters the intestine by way of improperly cooked beef, pork, or fish or from contaminated food, as in the case of the dwarf tapeworm.

The cestodes are segmented flatworms with a head or scolex, which has hooks or suckers that are used to attach to tissues, and a number of segments, or proglottids, which in some cases may extend for 20 to 30 feet in the bowel. Drugs affecting the scolex allow expulsion of the organisms from the intestine. Each of the proglottids contains both male and female reproductive units. When filled with fertilized eggs, they are expelled from the worm into the environment. Upon ingestion, the infected larvae develop into adults in the small intestine of the human. The larvae may travel to extraintestinal sites and enter other tissues such as the liver, muscle, and eye. The tapeworms, with the exception of the dwarf tapeworm, spend part of their life cycle in a host other than humans: pigs, fish, or cattle. The dwarf tapeworm does not require an intermediate host.

The tapeworm has no digestive tract; it depends on the nutrients that are intended for the host. Subsequently, the victim suffers by eventually developing nutritional deficiency.

Trematodes

Trematodes, or flukes, are flat, nonsegmented parasites with suckers that attach to and feed on host tissue. The life cycle begins with the egg, which is passed into fresh water after fecal excretion from the body of the human host. The egg containing the embryo forms into a ciliated organism, the miracidium. In the presence of water the miracidium escapes from the egg and enters the intermediate host, the freshwater snail, which exists extensively in rice paddies and irrigation ditches. After entry, the fluke forms a cyst in the lungs of the snail. In the cyst, many organisms develop. They can penetrate other parts of the snail and grow into worms called cercariae. Eventually, the cercariae are released from the snail into the water, attaching themselves to blades of grass to encyst. A human, the final host, then becomes infected by the parasite.

When encysted organisms in snails or even fish and crabs are swallowed by humans, they develop into adult flukes in different structures of the body. The flukes therefore are classified according to the type of tissues they invade. After ingestion, the eggs of *Schistosoma haematobium* appear in the urinary bladder and cause inflammation of the urogenital system. This can result in chronic cystitis and hematuria. Infestations with *Schistosoma japonicum* and *Schistosoma mansoni* produce intestinal disturbance with resultant ulceration and necrosis of the rectum. *S japonicum* is more concentrated in the veins of the small intestine. If the liver and spleen become infected, the disease is usually fatal. *S mansoni* prefers the portal veins that drain the large intestine, particularly the sigmoid colon and rectum. Unlike the other parasites, the cercariae of *S mansoni* are not ingested but burrow through the skin, especially between the toes of the human host who is standing in contaminated water. They then make their way to the portal system, where they mature into adult flukes.

Schistosomiasis (bilharziasis) is endemic to Africa, Asia, South American, and the Caribbean islands. The disease can be controlled largely by eliminating the intermediate host, the snail.

Travelers to these areas must avoid contact with contaminated water for drinking, bathing, or swimming. Unfortunately, the disease has been introduced in the United States and Canada by immigrants or individuals who have traveled to the endemic areas.

Nematoda (Roundworms)

Nematoda are nonsegmented, cylindrical worms that consist of a mouth and complete digestive tract. The adults reside in the human intestinal tract; there is no intermediate host. Two types of nematode infection exist in the human: the egg form and the larval form.

Egg Infective Form

Ascaris lumbricoides is a large nematode (about 30 cm in length) and is known as the "roundworm of humans."

The adult *Ascaris* usually resides in the upper end of the small intestine of the human, where it feeds on semidigested foods. The fertilized egg, when excreted with feces, can survive in the soil for a long time. When inadvertently ingested by another host, the embryos escape from the eggs and mature into adults in the host. To prevent the disease, proper sanitary conditions and meticulous personal habits must be observed.

Infection with *Enterobius vermicularis,* or pinworm, is highly prevalent among children and adults in the United States. Adult pinworms reside in the large intestine. However, the female migrates to the anus, depositing her eggs around the skin of the anal region. This causes intense itching and can be noted especially in children.

Diagnosis is made with the Graham sticky tape method. Ingestion of excreted eggs can infect an individual. In addition, eggs that contaminate clothing, bedding, furniture, and other items may be responsible for continuing the reinfection of an individual and initiating the infection of others.

Larval Infective Form

Necator americanus (New World) or *Ancylostoma duodenale* (Old World) hookworms are somewhat similar in action. They reside in the small intestine of humans. When the eggs are excreted in the feces, the larvae hatch in the soil. The larvae can penetrate the skin of humans, particularly through the soles of the feet, producing dermatitis (ground itch). On entry into the small intestine, they develop into adult worms. During the process they extravasate blood from the intestinal vessels and cause a profound anemia in the victim. The presence of eggs in the feces indicates a positive test for hookworm disease. This infection can be avoided by wearing shoes.

Trichinella spiralis is a small pork roundworm that causes trichinosis. In humans the disease begins by ingestion of insufficiently cooked pork or bear meat. On entry of encysted meat into the small intestine, the larvae are released from the cysts.

After maturation, the females develop eggs that later form into larvae. They then migrate by the bloodstream and the lymphatic system to the skeletal muscles and encyst. Encapsulation and eventually calcification of the cysts occur. Diagnosis of trichinosis is made by muscle biopsy, whereby microscopic examination reveals the presence of larvae. The disease is prevented by thoroughly cooking pork and bear meat before eating.

ANTHELMINTIC AGENTS

Anthelmintic drugs are used to rid the body of worms (helminths). Anthelmintics are among the most primitive types of chemotherapy. It has been estimated that one third of the world's population is infested with these parasites.

diethylcarbamazine [dye eth il kar′ ba ma zeen] (Hetrazan)

Diethylcarbamazine has a microfilaricidal and a macrofiaricidal effect. The microfilaricidal action is to increase the loss of microfilariae and inhibit the rate of embryogenesis from nematodes. It has no sterilizing effect on adult worms. It is indicated for the treatment of Bancroft's filariasis, loiasis, onchocerciasis, and tropical eosinophilia.

Pharmacokinetics

It is absorbed after oral administration and is distributed to nonfatty tissues. Its peak serum level is reached in 1 to 2 hours with a half-life of 8 hours. Excretion is via the kidneys.

Side effects and adverse reactions

These include joint pains, increased weakness, headache, dizziness, nausea, vomiting, facial swelling, especially around the eyes, pruritus, fever, rash, and painful, tender glands especially in the neck, armpits, or groin area. Also, visual disturbances such as vision loss, night blindness and tunnel vision has also been reported.

Contraindications

Avoid use in persons with diethylcarbamazine hypersensitivity.

Dosage and administration

The adult dosage is 2 to 3 mg/kg PO three times daily. For tropical eosinophilia the dose is 6 mg/kg PO daily for 4 to 7 days. This product should be taken after meals.

mebendazole [me ben′ da zole] (Vermox)

Mebendazole is a vermicidal and may also be ovicidal for most helminths. It causes degeneration of a parasite's cytoplasmic microtubules, which results in blocking glucose uptake in the helminth, leading to death of the parasite. It is indicated for the treatment of *Trichuriasis* (whipworm), *Enterobiasis* (pinworm), *Ascariasis* (roundworm), *Ancylostoma* (common hookworm), and *Necator* (American hookworm), singly or in mixed infestations.

Pharmacokinetics

Mebendazole oral absorption is increased if given with fatty foods. It is distributed to serum, cyst fluid, liver, hepatic cysts, and muscle tissues, with a half-life of 2.5 to 5.5 hours. It is metabolized in the liver and excreted primarily in feces.

Side effects and adverse reactions

These are uncommon and include gastric distress, diarrhea, nausea, vomiting, alopecia, dizziness, headache, and, rarely, hypersensitivity and neutropenia.

Warnings

Use with caution in patients with Crohn's ileitis and ulcerative colitis.

Contraindications

Avoid use in persons with mebendazole hypersensitivity and liver function impairment.

Dosage and administration

The adult and pediatric dosage (children 2 years of age and older) is 100 mg PO twice daily for 3 days. If necessary, this dosage may be repeated in 2 to 3 weeks. These tablets can be chewed, crushed, mixed with food, or swallowed whole and if high-dose therapy is used, taken with meals, especially fatty ones to increase absorption and serum levels.

niclosamide [ni kloe′ sa mide] (Niclocide)

Niclosamide is an anthelmintic agent that affects the mitochondria of the cestode, inhibiting aerobic and possibly anaerobic metabolism, on which many cestodes depend for survival. Contact with the drug results in destruction of the scolex and proximal segments of the organism, the proglottids. The scolex, when loosened from the intestinal wall, is usually digested in the intestine. Consequently, identification of the worm in the feces cannot be made.

Indications

Niclosamide is indicated for the treatment of *T saginata* (beef tapeworm), *D latum* (fish tapeworm), *Hymenolepis nana* (dwarf tapeworm), *Dipylidium caninum* (dog and cat tapeworm), and *T solium* (pork tapeworm) infestations.

Pharmacokinetics

Because niclosamide is poorly absorbed from the intestinal tract, this drug can exert its effect on intestinal helminths, the site of its action. Excretion is in the feces.

Side effects and adverse reactions

These include stomach pain or distress, anorexia, nausea, vomiting, rectal itching, dizziness, sedation, rash, and a bad taste in the mouth.

Contraindications

Avoid use in persons with niclosamide hypersensitivity.

Dosage and administration

Niclosamide tablets should be thoroughly chewed and taken with water. The adult dosage for fish and beef tapeworms is four tablets (2 g) as single dose; for dwarf tapeworm the dose is four tablets (2 g) daily for 1 week. Preferably this drug should be taken after a light meal such as breakfast or on an empty stomach. For additional dosing recommendations, see a current package insert or drug reference.

oxamniquine [ox am′ ni kwin] (Vansil)

Oxamniquine is schistosomicidal against both immature and mature worms, and it produces its effect by causing worms to shift from the mesenteric veins to the liver, where they are then destroyed. Male schistosomes appear to be more susceptible to this drug than females, but after a successful treatment with this agent, the female schistosomes stop laying eggs. Oxamniquine is indicated for the treatment of schistosomiasis.

Pharmacokinetics

Oxamniquine is well absorbed orally with a time to peak serum level of 1 to 1.5 hours. It is metabolized in the liver and excreted by the kidneys.

Side effects and adverse reactions

These include gastric distress, dizziness, sedation, headaches, red-orange urine discoloration, and, rarely, fever, hallucinations, convulsions, and rash or hives.

Contraindications

Avoid use in persons with oxamniquine hypersensitivity, epilepsy, or a history of other convulsive disorders.

Dosage and administration

The pediatric and adult oral dose is 15 mg/kg twice a day for 1 or 2 days, depending on the strain of organism. Take this product after meals to decrease the potential for side effects.

piperazine [pi′ per a zeen] (Entacyl)

Piperazine is an anthelmintic agent that affects the worm muscle (paralysis), possibly by blocking the stimulating effects of acetylcholine at the myoneural junction. The muscle paralysis of roundworms makes them unable to maintain their position in the host; they are dislodged and expelled as a result of normal peristalsis.

Indications

Piperazine is indicated for treatment of enterobiasis (pinworms) and ascariasis (roundworm).

Pharmacokinetics

It is absorbed orally, reaching a peak serum level in 2 to 4 hours. It is partially metabolized in the liver and primarily excreted by the kidneys.

Drug interactions

The following effects may occur when piperazine is given with drugs listed below:

Drug	Possible effect and management
Phenothiazines (especially chlorpromazine)	The administration of high doses of piperazine may increase phenothiazine (especially chlorpromazine) effects and increase the risk of convulsions. Avoid or a potentially serious drug interaction may occur.
pyrantel (Antiminth)	Concurrent use may antagonize piperazine's anthelmintic effects. Avoid concurrent drug administration.

Color type indicates an unsafe drug combination.

Side effects and adverse reactions

These include gastric distress, and rarely, CNS toxic effects, headaches, dizziness, ataxia, trembling, and blurred vision, choreiform movements, paresthesia, and hypersensitivity.

Contraindications

Avoid use in persons with piperazine hypersensitivity, liver or kidney function impairment, and a history of epilepsy or seizures.

Dosage and administration

The adult dose is 3.5 g PO daily for 2 days for ascariasis. For children the dosage is 75 mg/kg (up to 3.5 g) daily for 2 days. For adults and children the dose for enterobiasis is a single daily dose of 65 mg/kg (maximum daily dose is 2.5 g) for 7 consecutive days.

praziquantel [pray zi kwon′ tel] (Biltricide)

Praziquantel is an anthelmintic agent that penetrates cell membranes and increases cell permeability in susceptible worms. This results in an increased loss of intracellular calcium, contractions, and muscle paralysis of the worm. The drug also disintegrates the schistosome tegument (covering). Subsequently, phagocytes are attracted to the worm and ultimately kill it.

Indications

Praziquantel is indicated for the treatment of schistosomiasis, opisthorchiasis (liver flukes), and clonorchiasis (Chinese or Oriental liver fluke) infestations.

Pharmacokinetics

Praziquantel is absorbed orally and reaches a peak serum level in 1 to 3 hours. Half-life is 0.8 to 1.5 hours for praziquantel and 4 to 6 hours for its metabolites. It is excreted by the kidneys and is generally well tolerated.

Side effects and adverse reactions

These include headache, lightheadedness, gastric distress, sweating, rash, pruritus, dizziness, drowsiness, fever, increased sweating, and GI distress including bloody diarrhea.

Warnings

Use with caution in patients with severe liver disease.

Contraindications

Avoid use in persons with praziquantel hypersensitivity and ocular cysticercosis.

Dosage and administration

For clonorchiasis the adult or pediatric dosage for children 4 years of age and older is 25 mg/kg three times a day for 1 day. Swallow tablets whole with water during meals.

pyrantel [pi ran′ tel] (Antiminth, Combantrin ♣)

Pyrantel is an anthelmintic agent that is a depolarizing neuromuscular blocking agent; it causes contraction and then paralysis of the helminth muscles. The helminths are dislodged and then expelled from the body by peristalsis. Pyrantel is indicated for the treatment of ascariasis, enterobiasis, and helminth infestations.

Pharmacokinetics

This product is poorly absorbed from the GI tract. Pyrantel reaches peak serum level in 1 to 3 hours and is primarily excreted in the feces.

Drug interactions

Concurrent use with piperazine may antagonize pyrantel's anthelmintic effects. Avoid concurrent drug administration.

Side effects and adverse reactions

These include gastric distress, CNS side effects, and hypersensitivity.

Contraindications

Avoid use in persons with pyrantel hypersensitivity.

Dosage and administration

The adult and pediatric (2 years of age and older) dose of pyrantel for ascariasis and enterobiasis is 11 mg/kg PO as a single dose. If necessary, it may be repeated in 2 to 3 weeks.

thiabendazole [thye a ben′ da zole] (Mintezol)

Thiabendazole's mechanism of action is unknown, but it has been reported to inhibit specific enzymes (fumarate reductase) in the helminth. It is vermicidal. Thiabendazole is indicated for the treatment of cutaneous and visceral larva migrans (creeping eruption), strongyloidiasis, and trichinosis.

Pharmacokinetics

Thiabendazole is rapidly absorbed orally reaching a peak serum level in 1 to 2 hours. Its half-life ranges from 0.9 to 2 hours with metabolism in the liver and excretion via the kidneys.

Drug interactions

Concurrent use with theophylline may reduce the elimination of theophylline by up to 50%, possibly resulting in toxic serum levels. Monitor theophylline serum levels closely.

Side effects and adverse reactions

These include gastric distress, neuropsychiatric and CNS side effects, dry mouth and eyes, hypersensitivity, and, rarely, crystalluria, intrahepatic cholestasis, ocular disorders, convulsions, and Stevens-Johnson syndrome.

Warnings

Use with caution in patients with kidney function impairment.

Contraindications

Avoid use in persons with thiabendazole hypersensitivity and liver function impairment.

Dosage and administration

The adult and pediatric (weighing 13.6 kg and more) dose of thiabendazole for cutaneous larva migrans is 25 mg/kg PO twice a day after meals (breakfast and supper) for 2 days. If lesions are still present, the dosage may be repeated 2 days after the completion of the initial treatment. For other dosing recommendations, see a current package insert or USP DI.

LEPROSY

Leprosy, or **Hansen's disease,** is caused by *Mycobacterium leprae* in humans. Although estimates indicate that nearly 15 million people have leprosy worldwide, in the United States it is more frequently found in Hawaii and areas of Texas, Louisiana, and Florida. Leprosy has also been seen in foreign-born patients, especially those from the Philippines, Mexico, and Vietnam. It is more prevalent in males than females (3 to 1) in some areas.

Although the precise mode of transmission is unknown, the incubation period for leprosy is a few months to decades. Large numbers of leprosy bacilli are generally shed from skin ulcers, nasal secretions, the gastrointestinal tract, and, perhaps, biting insects.

M leprae is a bacillus that in humans first presents as a skin lesion: a large plaque or macule that is erythematous or hypopigmented in the center. More numerous lesions, peripheral nerve trunk involvement, and the common complications of plantar ulceration of the feet, footdrop, loss of hand function, and corneal abrasions may follow.

Most cases can be arrested, if not cured, by appropriate therapy and management. The drugs of choice are dapsone and clofazimine.

dapsone [dap′ sone] (DDS, Avlosulfon)

Dapsone is an antibacterial (antileprosy) agent that is bacteriostatic with an action similar to that of the sulfonamides. It may also be a dihydrofolate reductase inhibitor. Dapsone is effective against *M leprae,* the cause of leprosy; therefore it is indicated for the treatment of all types of leprosy and for dermatitis herpetiformis.

Pharmacokinetics

Dapsone is absorbed orally, distributed throughout the body, and found in fluids and in all body tissues. The time to peak serum level is 2 to 6 hours; its half-life is approximately 30 hours. It is acetylated by *N*-acetyltransferase in the liver; thus slow acetylators are more apt to develop higher serum levels and adverse reactions than fast acetylators. Excretion is via the kidneys.

Drug interactions

The following effects may occur when dapsone is given with the drugs listed below:

Drug	Possible effect and management
dideoxyinosine (ddI)	Concurrent drug administration may reduce absorption of dapsone. Dapsone requires an acid media for absorption while ddI is given with a buffer to neutralize stomach acid to increase absorption. Administer dapsone a minimum of 2 hours before ddI.
Hemolytic agents	Concurrent drug use increases the potential for a serious adverse effect. Avoid or a potentially serious drug interaction may occur.

Color type indicates an unsafe drug combination.

Side effects and adverse reactions

These include hypersensitivity, hemolytic anemia, methemoglobinemia, and, rarely, CNS side effects, gastric distress, blood disorders, exfoliative dermatitis, hepatic damage, mood alterations, peripheral neuritis, and the sulfone syndrome (fever, tiredness, exfoliative dermatitis, jaundice, lympadenopathy, anemia, and methemoglobinemia).

Warnings

Use with caution in patients with liver function impairment.

Contraindications

Avoid use in persons with dapsone or sulfonamide hypersensitivity, severe anemia, G6PD deficiency, or methemoglobin reductase deficiency.

Dosage and administration

The adult dapsone antileprosy dose (given in combination with other antileprosy drugs) is 50 to 100 mg orally daily. As a suppressant for dermatitis herpetiformis, the adult dose is 50 mg PO daily initially, increased as necessary until symptoms are controlled. The dosage for children as an antileprosy agent is 1.4 mg/kg PO daily.

clofazimine [kloe fa′ zi meen] (Lamprene)

Clofazimine's antileprosy mechanism of action is unknown; it has a slow bactericidal effect on *M leprae,* inhibits mycobacterial growth and tends to bind preferentially to mycobacterial DNA. It is indicated as a secondary drug for the treatment of leprosy, especially in the dapsone-resistant type of leprosy.

Pharmacokinetics

Clofazimine has a variable oral absorption and is distributed primarily in fatty tissues and cells. Macrophages take up this drug and further distribute it throughout the body. Its half-life is about 2 to 3 months with chronic therapy, and its time to peak serum level is between 1 and 6 hours. It is excreted primarily in feces.

Side effects and adverse reactions

These include gastric distress, ichthyosis, and discoloration (red and brown-black) of skin, feces, sweat, tears, and urine, a change in taste sensations, dry, burning, itching, or irritated eyes, photosensitivity, and, rarely, GI bleeding, hepatitis, and depression.

Warnings

Use with caution in patients with liver function impairment.

Contraindications

Avoid use in persons with clofazimine hypersensitivity or a history of gastrointestinal disorders.

Dosage and administration

The adult dose in dapsone-resistant leprosy, in combination with one or more other agents, is 50 to 100 mg PO daily, taken with meals or milk.

SUMMARY

Malaria and tuberculosis are still prevalent diseases throughout the world. Malaria is endemic in more than 100 countries, and it has been reported that worldwide between 200,000 to 300,000 million individuals have these diseases. Approximately 8 million new cases of tuberculosis are diagnosed and nearly 3 million individuals die from this disease annually. In 1998, the World Health Organization has reported that TB is the single, largest infectious killer of women between the ages of 15 to 44 years in the world; this number is three times the number of deaths in women from cardiac disease or from HIV infection.

The incidence of tuberculosis is increasing because of the increasing numbers of persons with AIDS, persons living in the street or homeless, drug abusers, malnourished individuals, and those taking immunosuppressant drugs. The World Health Organization has recommended the DOTS approach for the control of tuberculosis and has projected that the use of this system would result in a 85% cure of all new cases. This system and the various drugs used in treatment are reviewed in this chapter.

Knowledge about the various drugs available alone and in combination (when applicable) to treat malaria, tuberculosis, leprosy, amebiasis, and helminthiasis is vital information for the healthcare professional. An informed professional can then institute a proper patient treatment plan that includes patient teaching, close monitoring of the prescribed medications, patients' compliance, and their individual therapeutic response.

REVIEW QUESTIONS

1. How is a drug selected for the treatment of malaria? Name the four types of therapy according to drug classification.
2. Present the World Health Organization DOTS five-step plan for the treatment of tuberculosis. If properly implemented, what is the expected outcome?
3. Discuss drug selection for tuberculosis. What are the general guidelines for the drug regimens?
4. Define luminal and tissue amebicides and name one drug from each category.
5. List four reasons why parasitic infestations are dangerous to the individual. Name the human parasitic helminths and the drugs that are usually used to treat these infestations.

REFERENCES

Anandan JV: Parasitic infections. In Young LY, Koda-Kimble MA, editors: *Applied therapeutics: the clinical use of drugs,* ed 6, Vancouver, Wash, 1995, Applied Therapeutics, Inc.

Cali TJ: Tuberculosis: implications for the 1990s and beyond, *Clin Consult* 14(12):1-12, 1995.

Centers for Disease Control and Prevention: Initial therapy for tuberculosis of the era of multidrug resistance: Recommendations of the Advisory Council for the Elimination of Tuberculosis, *MMWR* 42(RR-7):1-8, 1993.

Ebert SC: Tuberculosis. In DiPiro JT, Talber R et al, editors: *Pharmacotherapy, a pathophysiologic approach,* ed 2, Norwalk, Conn, 1993, Appleton & Lange.

Kudzma EC: Drug response: all bodies are not created equal, *Am J Nurs* 92(12):48, 1992.

Mandell GL, Petri AW Jr: Drugs used in the chemotherapy of tuberculosis, *Mycobacterium avium* complex disease, and leprosy. In Hardman JG, Limbird LE, editors: *Goodman & Gilman's the pharmacological basis of therapeutics,* ed 9, New York, 1996, McGraw-Hill.

World Health Organization DOTS: Global tuberculosis programme, DOTS: directly observed treatment short-course, World Health Organization, http://www.who.ch/gtb/dots/index.htm (July 15, 1998).

World Health Organization Global: Global tuberculosis programme, TB is single biggest killer of young women, http://www.who.ch/gtb/press/gender__release.htm (July 15, 1998).

World Health Organization MDR: Global tuberculosis programme, press release WHO/74 (Oct 22, 1997), http://www.who.ch/gtb/press/who74.htm (July 15, 1998).

Yoshikawa TT: Tuberculosis in the nursing home, *Nurs Home Med* 3(9):207-213, 1995.

ADDITIONAL REFERENCES

American Hospital Formulary Service: *AHFS drug information '98,* Bethesda, Md, 1998, American Society of Hospital Pharmacists.

Anderson KN et al, editors: *Mosby's medical, nursing, and allied health dictionary,* ed 5, St Louis, 1998, Mosby.

Centers for Disease Control and Prevention: *Prescription drugs for malaria,* Document No 221010, Atlanta, 1996, The Centers.

Centers for Disease Control and Prevention: Guidelines for preventing the transmission of *Mycobacterium tuberculosis* in health-care facilities, *MMWR* 43(RR-13):1-132, 1994.

Grimes D: *Infectious diseases,* St Louis, 1991, Mosby.

Levy RA: *Ethnic and racial differences in response to medicines: preserving individualized therapy in managed pharmaceutical programs,* Reston, Va, 1993, National Pharmaceutical Council.

Lordi GM, Reichman LB: Drug-resistant tuberculosis: the new face of an old enemy, *Drug Ther* Mar 17-28, 1993.

Malseed RT, Wilson BA: Isoniazid and rifampin therapy for tuberculosis: what patients need to know, *MedSurg Nurs* 2(3):236-238, 1993.

Meyer UA: Drugs in special patient groups: Clinical importance of genetics in drug effects. In Melmon KL et al: *Clinical pharmacology,* ed 3, New York, 1992, McGraw-Hill.

Mosby: *Mosby's GenRx,* St Louis, 1998, Mosby.

Olin BR: *Facts and comparisons.* Philadelphia, 1998, JB Lippincott.

Posey LM: Tuberculosis: new problems from an old disease, *Consult Pharm* 11(1):27-28, 31, 1996.

United States Department of Health and Human Services: *Health information for international travelers,* Washington, DC, 1988, DHHS.

United States Pharmacopeial Convention: *USP DI: drug information for the health care professional,* ed 18, Rockville, Md, 1998, The Convention.

United States Public Health Service Task Force on Prophylaxis and Therapy for *Mycobacterium avium* complex: Recommendations on prophylaxis and therapy for disseminated *Mycobacterium avium* complex for adults and adolescents infected with human immunodeficiency virus, *MMWR* 42(42):14-20, 1993.

Ward ES Jr: Tuberculosis. In Young LY, Koda-Kimble MA, editors: *Applied therapeutics: the clinical use of drugs,* ed 6, Vancouver, Wash, 1995, Applied Therapeutics, Inc.

UNIT XV

Drugs Affecting the Immunologic System

CHAPTER 54

Overview of the Immunologic System

CHAPTER FOCUS

The first lines of defense in the body are the anatomical barriers, the skin and mucous membranes. However, when a chemical, foreign body, or microorganism penetrates this defense, the body tries to contain and eliminate it by the inflammatory response and the immune system. The human has a complex immune system that consists of specialized lymphoid structures—lymph nodes, spleen, tonsils, and thymus gland—and billions of circulating cells, mainly lymphocytes and plasma cells, that may influence all other systems in the body. A thorough knowledge of the immune system is essential for the healthcare professional.

OBJECTIVES

After reading and studying this chapter, the student should be able to do the following:

1. *Define and discuss the key terms.*
2. *Identify and describe the functions of the lymphoid organs of the immune system.*
3. *Name the immunocompetent cells that are involved in the immune response.*
4. *Describe and contrast the functions of the T cells, B cells, and antibodies in the body.*
5. *Name the five classes of antibodies and describe their functions.*
6. *Define humoral and cell-mediated immunity.*
7. *Describe natural and acquired immunity and active and passive immunity.*

KEY TERMS

acquired immunity, (p. 711)
antibodies, (p. 712)
B lymphocytes (B cells), (p. 711)
complement system, (p. 713)
immunity, (p. 712)
passive immunity, (p. 713)
T lymphocytes (T cells), (p. 710)

The immunologic system is composed of cells and organs that defend the body against invasion by foreign biologic and/or chemical substances. The immunocompetent cells in the body have an inherent ability to distinguish foreign protein substances from the body's own cells. This chapter reviews the organs and tissues of the immune system, the immunocompetent cells, and the types of immunity.

THE IMMUNE SYSTEM

The spleen, tonsils, lymph nodes, and thymus are the lymphoid organs located in the body. The lymphoid tissues are mainly lymphocytes and plasma cells, which travel freely throughout the human system. The two major classes of lymphocytes are T-cell and B-cell lymphocytes, which are discussed below under Immunocompetent Cells. Fig. 54-1 identifies the organs and tissues of the immune system.

Spleen

The spleen, the largest lymphatic organ in the body, is located on the left side in the extreme superior, posterior corner of the abdominal cavity and performs two main functions. It is: (1) a storage site or reservoir for blood and (2) a processing station for red blood cells (i.e., the red blood cells near the end of their life cycle will break down in the spleen). Macrophages lining the pulp and sinuses of the spleen remove cellular debris and process hemoglobin in the red pulp area of the spleen. The white pulp area of the spleen contains lymphocytes and plasma cells that are involved in the immune process. The spleen intercepts foreign matter or antigens that have reached the bloodstream.

Tonsils

The tonsils are an accumulation of lymphoid tissue, named according to their location: lingual, palatine, and pharyngeal tonsils. They intercept foreign bodies or antigens that enter the body by way of the respiratory tract. Similar lymphoid tissue is located in the submucosal areas of the gastrointestinal tract (Peyer's patches) to intercept antigens (bacteria and viruses) entering from the gut. Other lymphoid tissues are located in the bone marrow and help to intercept antigens in the blood and in the lymph nodes.

Lymph Nodes

The lymph nodes are capsulated organs located throughout the body that are involved with lymph circulation. The outer portion of the lymph node is the cortex, and the inner portion is the medulla. The thymus-dependent zone exists in the deep area or middle cortex. This area contains mainly **T lymphocytes (T cells),** lymphocytes formed or seeded from the thymus gland, which when exposed to an antigen divide rapidly and produce large numbers of new T cells sensitized to that antigen.

Lymph nodes are essentially a row of in-line filters, which screen the lymph flowing through it. Many lymphocytes and macrophages are located throughout the lymph nodes,

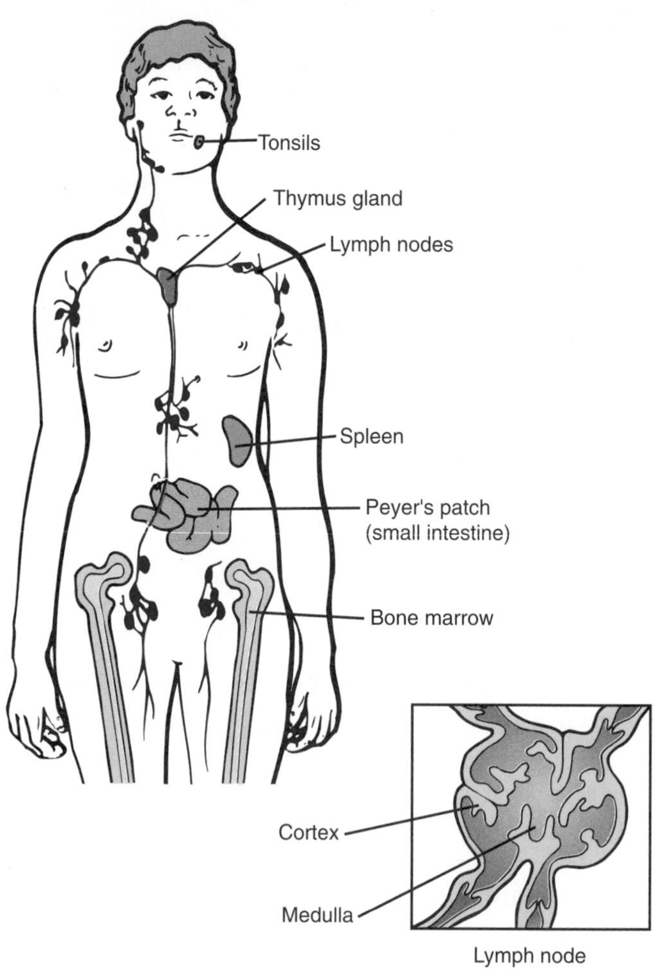

FIGURE 54-1
Location of organs and tissues of the immune system; inset shows cross-section of lymph node.

especially in the cortical, paracortical, and medullary areas. T lymphocytes are located mainly in the paracortical region, whereas plasma cells are found in the medullary sinuses.

Thymus Gland

The thymus gland is located in the mediastinal area. It processes lymphocytes, and in the early years up to puberty, it rapidly produces lymphocytes. The immune system is developed when immature lymphocytes from the bone marrow are processed in the thymus gland and then sent to the spleen, the lymphatic system, and other tissues and organs in the body to mature. The lymphocytes are active against some bacteria and viruses, allergens, fungus infections, and foreign tissue.

At birth, the thymus gland is larger than it is in an adult. By the time a person reaches puberty, the thymus has grown to nearly six times its original size. After puberty this gland undergoes involution, and in the elderly, it is usually a small mass of reticular fibers with some lymphocytes and connective tissue. Although its importance was largely discounted over the years, today it is one of the most important areas for medical research.

Scientists are searching for answers to the many questions about the thymus gland and its relationship to the other tissues and organs in the immune system.

IMMUNOCOMPETENT CELLS

Mononuclear T and B cells and the polymorphonuclear leukocytes (PMLs) are involved in the immune response, although only mononuclear T and B cells are immunocompetent cells, cells with the ability to mobilize and deploy antibodies and other responses to stimulation by an antibody. The PMLs are nonspecific cells that interact with lymphocytes to produce an inflammatory response, whereas B and T cells are capable of recognizing specific antigens and initiating the immune response.

In humans, stem cells from the bone marrow are transformed to T cells or T lymphocytes in the thymus gland and B cells or B lymphocytes elsewhere in the body. The T lymphocytes then migrate to lymphoid tissue and organs as reviewed in the previous section. When in contact with an antigen, T lymphocytes will form specialized cells to provide cellular immunity. The **B lymphocytes (B cells)**, a type of small agranulocytic leukocyte, form antibodies that search out, identify, and bind with specific antigens to provide humoral immunity.

T Lymphocytes (T Cells)

T cells are generally long-lived. When they are not in their special areas, they circulate continuously through the body by way of the bloodstream and lymphatic system. They are involved with the B lymphocytes (B cells) in that they can cooperate with them (helper T cells) or inhibit them (suppressor T cells). The B cells do not interact with the thymus. Clones are groups of lymphocytes capable of forming one specific antibody (B cell or T cell) to respond to a specific type of antigen; only the specific antigen can activate the specialized clones.

When the T cells first contact an antigen, the lymphocytes that recognize the foreign substance will proliferate, thus giving rise to larger numbers of cells that have the capacity to recognize and respond to this antigen. Some of the cells will go on to produce antibody or cell-mediated immune-type responses, whereas others will increase the population of antigen-sensitive memory cells. This is called **acquired immunity**, an immunity that is not innate but obtained during life. The second exposure to this antigen will provoke a more powerful response by the specific T cells.

Three major groups of T cells identified in the past few years include (1) cytotoxic T cells, (2) helper T cells, and (3) suppressor T cells.

Cytotoxic T Cells

This type of cell can bind tightly to organisms or cells that contain their binding-specific antigen. Then the T cells release cytotoxic (probably lysosomal) enzymes directly into the cell. Cytotoxic T cells are capable of killing microorganisms, cancer cells, viruses, heart transplant cells, and other cells that are foreign to the person's body. Body tissue that contains viruses or foreign cells may also be attacked by the killer cells.

Helper T Cells

These compose the majority of the T cells and help the immune system in many ways. They increase the activation of B cells, cytotoxic T cells, and suppressor T cells by antigens. Helper T cells clones are activated by very small amounts of antigens, quantities that may not activate the previously mentioned B cells, cytotoxic T cells, or suppressor T cells. Once the helper T cells are activated, they secrete lymphokines, which are chemical factors that attract macrophages to the site of infection or inflammation and increase the response of these three lymphoid cells to the antigen.

Helper T cells may also secrete interleukin 2, a lymphokine that is capable of stimulating the action of other T cells, such as cytotoxic T cells and some suppressor T cells.

Helper T cells also secrete macrophage migration inhibition factor, another lymphokine. This substance slows or stops the migration of macrophages into the affected area and will also activate the macrophages present to be more effective phagocytotic agents. The activated macrophages can attack and destroy a vastly increased number of the invading organism.

Acquired immunodeficiency syndrome (AIDS) is the final outcome of an infection with the human immunodeficiency virus (HIV). This virus binds to protein on the cell membranes of the helper T lymphocytes (T4 cells), monocytes, macrophages, and colorectal cells. The helper T cells are destroyed by the virus, which leads to the immunodeficiency known as AIDS. See additional information on this disease and treatment in Chapter 56.

Suppressor T Cells

Less is known about these cells than the others, but it is known that they can suppress the function of both cytotoxic and helper T cells. This suppression may be useful in preventing excessive immune reactions that can cause severe body damage. These cells are often called regulatory T cells.

B Lymphocytes (B Cells)

B-lymphocyte clones are dormant in lymphoid tissue until a foreign antigen appears. The macrophages in the lymphoid tissue phagocytize the foreign substance, and the adjacent B lymphocytes and perhaps the T cells are activated. B cells specific for the antigen will enlarge, and some will differentiate to form plasmablasts, a plasma cell precursor, and memory cells. The plasmablasts proliferate and divide, so that in 4 days, approximately 500 plasma cells will be present for each original plasmablast. The plasma cells rapidly produce gamma globulin antibodies that are secreted into the lymph and transported by the blood.

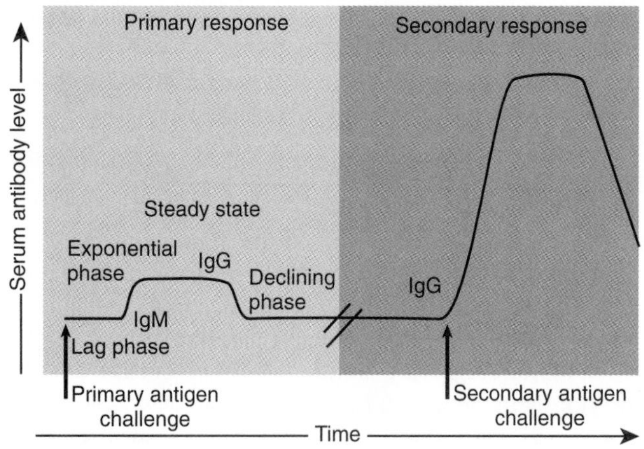

FIGURE 54-2
Primary and secondary immune responses. *(From Mudge-Grout, 1992.)*

Cells similar to those in the original clone are called memory cells. A second exposure to the same antigen will cause a more rapid and potent antibody response. The first response to an antigen may be slow, weak, and of short duration. The second response will be much more rapid, far more potent and prolonged, and antibodies will be formed for months rather than only for a few weeks. This is the reason why vaccination using several doses given at periods of weeks or months apart is so effective (Fig. 54-2).

ANTIBODIES

Antibodies are gamma globulins (a type of protein), called immunoglobulins, that are specific for particular antigens. They are produced by lymphoid tissue in response to antigens. At the present time, five classes of antibodies have been identified: IgG, IgM, IgA, IgD, and IgE. (The "Ig" stands for immunoglobulin, and the other letters designate the classes.)

IgG is the major immunoglobulin in the blood (about 75% to 80% of the total antibodies in the normal person) and is capable of entering tissue spaces, coating microorganisms, and activating the complement system, thus accelerating phagocytosis. It is the only immunoglobulin capable of crossing the placenta to provide the fetus with passive immunity until the infant can produce its own immune defense system.

IgM is the first immunoglobulin produced during an immune response. It is located primarily in the bloodstream and develops in response to an invasion of bacteria or viruses. IgM activates complement and can destroy foreign invaders during the initial antigen exposure. Its level decreases in approximately 1 week, while IgG levels are progressively increasing.

IgA is located primarily in external body secretions—saliva, sweat, tears, mucus, bile, and colostrum—and it is found in respiratory tract mucosa and in plasma. It helps to provide a defense against antigens on exposed surfaces and antigens that enter the respiratory and gastrointestinal tracts. The plasma cells in the intestinal area secrete IgA and secretory component to defend the body against bacteria and viruses.

The function of IgD is unknown. It is in the plasma and has been located on lymphocyte surfaces together with IgM, so it may be associated with binding antigens to the cell surface. Although levels of IgD are increased in chronic infections, IgD does not appear to have a particular affinity for specialized antigens.

IgE binds to histamine-containing mast cells and basophils. It can mediate the release of histamine in immune response to parasites (helminths) and in some allergic conditions. It is often called the reaginic antibody because of its involvement in immediate hypersensitivity reactions. Concentrations of it are low in the serum because the antibody is firmly fixed on tissue surfaces. Once activated by an antigen, it will trigger the release of the mast cell granules, resulting in the signs and symptoms of allergy and anaphylaxis.

IMMUNITY

Links in the chain of the infectious disease may be broken at many points. One link can be broken by attacking the pathogen (human disease-causing organism) with antimicrobial or antiinfective therapy. Another can be broken by augmenting human resistance by using biologic agents such as vaccines and serums, which artificially supply antibodies or catalyze the ability of the immune system to produce its own. An immunologic reaction that destroys or resists foreign cells or their products (antigens) is termed **immunity.** The most successful antigens, or immunogens, are protein or polysaccharide macromolecules that are usually bacterial, viral, fungal, or rickettsial in origin.

The primary types of immunity are humoral immunity and cell-mediated immunity.

Humoral Immunity

Antigens may be recognized by T-helper cells that activate specific B cells, by a strong B-cell response to the invasion of certain antigens (such as large polymers, *Escherichia coli,* and dextrans) or by a macrophage intermediary. Macrophage interactions often enhance the antigen recognition by both T and B cells in the body. Humoral response is described as primary or secondary immune response.

Primary Response

The foreign antigen in the body will bind to specific B cells to produce specialized antibody-producing plasma cells. Usually within 6 days, antibodies that are specific to the antigen can be found in the blood. Initially the immunoglobulin is IgM, which increases in quantity for up to 2 weeks; then production declines so that very little IgM is present in a few weeks. After the initial IgM evaluation, IgG antibodies start to appear at approximately day 10, peak in several weeks, and maintain high levels for a much longer time period (Fig. 54-2).

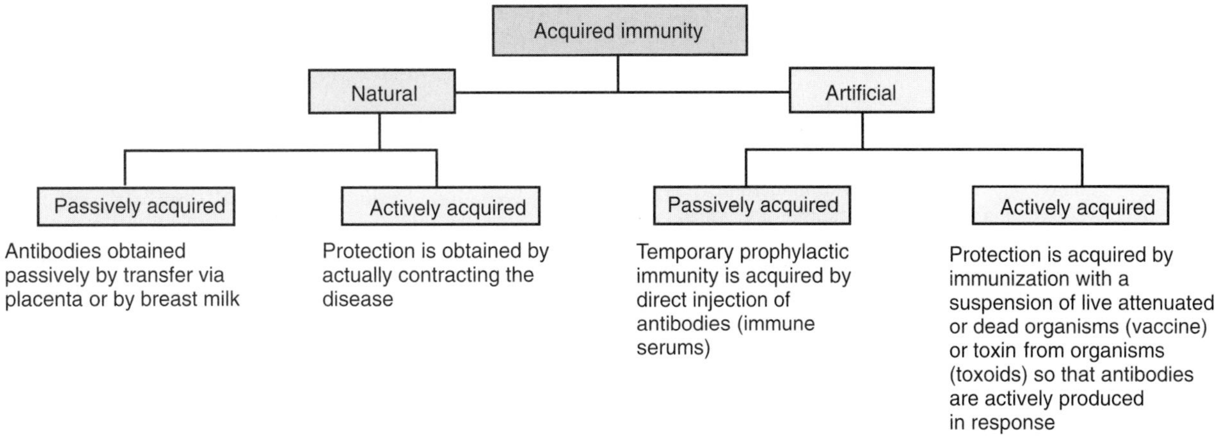

FIGURE 54-3
The process of acquired immunity.

Secondary Response

This response is often called the memory response, because the immune system responds so much faster to the second exposure to the same antigen. Both T and B memory cells are involved in beginning immediate production of antibodies in large amounts.

The second part of humoral immunity is activation of the **complement system,** a series of approximately 20 proteins that circulate in the blood in an inactive form. When an antigen-antibody complex triggers complement, each component in the cascade is activated in precise order. This reaction causes the mast cell release of substances that produce redness, increased heat, and edema of inflammation. It may also cause bacterial cell death and damage to normal tissue that surrounds the affected area.

Cell-Mediated Immunity

Cell-mediated immunity is the result of contact between T cells and antigens. Receptors on the T-cell surface are capable of recognizing foreign antigens, and antigen destruction may occur through one of two processes: (1) directly, by injecting chemical compounds into the target cell membrane (killer activity by cytotoxic T cells) or (2) by secreting lymphokines. The lymphokines can enhance or suppress the action of other lymphocytes, or they can create a chemotactic gradient in the area that will attract macrophages (and eosinophils, basophils, and neutrophils) to the site. Cell-mediated immunity (delayed hypersensitivity) involves only the direct action of T cells without humoral assistance.

Natural and Acquired Immunity

The body has certain inherited and innate abilities to resist encounters with antigens. This ability is known as natural resistance or natural immunity, which is not to be confused with naturally acquired immunity. Some general defenses inherent to natural resistance come from factors familiar to the focus of healthcare; for example, adequate rest, nutrition, exercise, and freedom from undue stress. Physiologic factors, which discourage proliferation of microbes, include the acidity of gastric secretions, respiratory tract cilia, and bactericidal lysozymes in tears. During a lifetime an individual may also acquire further immune capabilities through both natural and artificial means. This type of acquired immunity is conferred by either active or passive action (Fig. 54-3).

Unbroken skin is extremely effective in barring entry to microorganisms, but a barrage of defenses is mounted by the inflammatory response if invasion does succeed. The immune system identifies the threatening antigens or allergens and creates specific gamma globulins destructive to the particular species of antigen. These gamma globulins, or antibodies or immunoglobulins (Ig), are proteins that are chemically complementary and specifically configured to lock into the foreign antigen, inactivating it.

Antibodies also activate cellular defenses to phagocytize the invading microorganisms. Custom-made gamma globulins, or antibodies, provide acquired immunity to the specific type of antigen for varying lengths of time. Those antibodies will then gradually disappear from the serum, but the potential for their rapid replication in response to a repeat challenge by that specific antigen continues to exist after the initial exposure. Consequently, the result, known as naturally acquired immunity, is a process of active immunity because of the body's active involvement in creating the antibodies. Naturally acquired immunity can also result from a process of **passive immunity** when antibodies made by the mother's body are passively transferred by means of the placenta or by breast milk (especially colostrum, the breast milk produced shortly after delivery) to the fetus or infant.

On the other hand, artificial induction of the immune state, artificially acquired immunity, is initiated purposefully for protection of the susceptible individual. It may also be induced either actively or passively. Artificially acquired active immunity is evoked by the deliberate administration of antigens, either live partially modified organisms, killed or-

TABLE 54-1 Comparison of Active and Passive Immunity

	Active Immunity	*Passive Immunity*
Source	Individual	Other human or animal
Efficacy	High	Low to moderate
Method	Contracting disease Immunization with vaccines or toxoids	Administer preformed antibody by injection, maternal transplacental transfer or in breast milk
Time to develop	5-21 days	Immediate effect
Duration	Long, up to years	Usually shorter in time
Ease of reactivation	Easy with booster dose	Can be dangerous; anaphylaxis may occur, especially if animal sources are used
Purpose	Prophylaxis	Prophylaxis and therapeutic

ganisms, or their toxins. The parenteral route is the predominant mode of administration. Periodic reactivation of actively acquired artificial immunity against certain organisms by booster doses (e.g., tetanus) is sometimes necessary. Artificially acquired passive immunity is conferred by the parenteral administration of antibody-containing immune serum from immune humans or animals (Fig. 54-3).

Artificially acquired active immunity generally secures protection for a longer duration than any kind of passive immunity and is usually the prophylactic treatment of choice for populations at potential risk. Side effects may include local pain at the injection site and headache with mild to moderate fever. Because of the agents used, active immunity results in fewer adverse effects than passive immunity. Artificially acquired passive immunity is often chosen for susceptible individuals after a known exposure. A combination of active and passive approaches is also occasionally used. A number of products used in artificial passive immunization have caused adverse reactions because of individual hypersensitivities to animal products, especially horse serum or eggs, to the preservative used in a medication, or to an antibiotic. The products of bacterial metabolism are the agents responsible for other adverse reactions.

The presence of a mild to moderate upper respiratory tract infection or pregnancy does not always prohibit immunization; however, an immunosuppressed state (as a result of cancer chemotherapy or disease) may. Current manufacturers' instructions should always be consulted. Table 54-1 makes a direct comparison of the capabilities and effects of active and passive immunities.

SUMMARY

When the first line of defense is penetrated by a chemical, foreign body, or microorganism, the human's inflammatory response and immune system respond to contain and/or eliminate the foreign invader. The immune system is complex and contains the lymphoid organs, the spleen, tonsils, lymph nodes, and thymus, as well as the immunocompetent cells, i.e., T lymphocytes (T cells), B lymphocytes (B cells), and antibodies, the body's defense mechanisms against invasion of foreign biologic and chemical substances.

Immunity may be natural or artificial, active or passive. An understanding of this system is necessary for the health-care professional in clinical practice.

REVIEW QUESTIONS

1. Name and describe the three major groups of T cells. Which cell is compromised in acquired immunodeficiency syndrome (AIDS)?
2. Describe the functions of the B lymphocytes or B cells.
3. What effect does the complement system have in the human body?
4. Present the contrasting features of active immunity and passive immunity.

REFERENCES

Mudge-Grout CL: *Immunologic disorders,* St Louis, 1992, Mosby.

ADDITIONAL REFERENCES

Anderson KN et al, editors: *Mosby's medical, nursing, and allied health dictionary,* ed 5, St Louis, 1998, Mosby.

Guyton AC: *Textbook of medical physiology,* ed 8, Philadelphia, 1990, WB Saunders.

Klein DM, Witek-Janusek L: Advances in immunotherapy of sepsis, *Dimens Crit Care Nurs* 11(2):75, 1992.

McCance KL, Huether SE: *Pathophysiology: the biologic basis for disease in adults and children,* ed 3, St Louis, 1998, Mosby.

McIntyre WJ, Tami JA: Immunology for the consultant pharmacist, *Consult Pharm* 8(4):376, 1993.

Seeley RR, Stephens TD, Tate P: *Anatomy and physiology,* ed 3, New York, 1995, McGraw Hill.

Thibodeau GA, Patton KT: *Anatomy and physiology,* ed 4, St Louis, 1999, Mosby.

Van Wynsberghe D, Noback CR, Carola R: *Human anatomy and physiology,* ed 3, New York, 1995, McGraw-Hill.

CHAPTER 55

Serums, Vaccines, and Other Immunizing Agents

CHAPTER FOCUS

The serums, vaccines, and other immunizing agents discussed in this chapter have dramatically reduced the number of persons who get infectious diseases and the serious complications that such diseases produce. Before the polio vaccine, between 13,000 to 20,000 new cases of paralytic poliomyelitis were reported annually in the United States. In 1996, only 3,500 cases were reported throughout the entire world. Therefore the global efforts for immunization have tremendously reduced the incidence of polio and polio epidemics today. Other devastating diseases have also been improved with the immunizing agents; these include measles, *Haemophilus influenzae* type b (Hib) meningitis, whooping cough, and rubella to name a few (CDC, 1998). Knowledge of these agents is important information for healthcare professionals in practice today.

OBJECTIVES

After reading and studying this chapter, the student should be able to do the following:

1. *Define and discuss the key terms.*
2. *Discuss the previous and present status of measles,* Haemophilus influenzae *type b meningitis, and pertussis.*
3. *State the recommended guidelines for spacing live and killed antigens.*
4. *Discuss the risks of vaccination in premature infants and in pregnant and breastfeeding women.*
5. *Relate the recommended immunization schedule for children up to 2 years of age.*
6. *Describe the recommended use of tetanus toxoid and tetanus immune globulin in wound management.*
7. *List side effects and adverse reactions of immunizations and correlate them with patient education.*
8. *Compare the advantages and disadvantages of live attenuated and inactivated biologic products.*

KEY TERMS

active immunity, (p. 716)
anaphylactic reactions, (p. 719)
antibody titer, (p. 716)
passive immunity, (p. 716)

The body's first defense against invasion by potentially lethal microorganisms is intact skin and mucous membranes. The antiinflammatory process and a competent immune system are the body's defenses against microbes that break this barrier.

Active immunity exists when the body is capable of producing specific antibodies to combat infections caused by specific antigens or microbes. This immunity may be referred to as "naturally acquired active immunity," in that a person who recovers from an infectious disease produces antibodies and memory cells against that specific antigen. The next time the body is in contact with the same antigen, the immune system will be primed to destroy the antigen.

Passive immunity occurs when antibodies are transferred from a human or animal to a susceptible person. Newborn infants usually have passive acquired immunization that is naturally acquired from their mothers. However, this type of immunity protects only for short periods of time (weeks to several months).

Vaccines and toxoids are available to provide artificially acquired active immunity; vaccines contain whole microbes (dead or attenuated) that are not pathogenic but can induce antibody formation. Toxoids contain detoxified microbe by-products, which are antigenic and also induce antibody production. Sera and antitoxins contain exogenous antibodies and are used to provide artificially acquired passive immunity.

OVERVIEW

The critical age period for immunization is from birth through grade school entry and during the school years (many states now require maintenance of immunizations as a criterion for remaining in the school system). Certain groups are found to be at high risk: adolescents, new parents (unimmunized or with waning immunity, who are exposed to childhood illness or vaccines), debilitated persons, and healthcare providers. Other groups such as migrant workers and recent immigrants to the United States and Canada are predictably at high risk for infectious diseases.

International political and economic upheavals and the refugee influx to the United States and Canada have illustrated the major problems with diseases encountered in other countries: diphtheria, measles, hepatitis B, tuberculosis, and malaria carrier status. Immunization programs that are taken for granted in the United States, Canada, and other countries are not as well funded in developing countries.

As a group, adolescents also seem to be at high risk for preventable infections. Of these, certain subgroups may be particularly in need of immunization, such as athletes, heavy drug users, runaways, foreign travelers, and those isolated from or rejecting traditional healthcare. Several million children are not immunized against measles, polio, rubella (German measles), mumps, diphtheria, pertussis (whooping cough), and tetanus.

Newspapers and television news coverage have reported the adverse reactions associated with the pertussis and other vaccines, which has served to bias some individuals against vaccination. In patient teaching, it is important to stress that the vaccines are not without some risks but that the serious risks associated with not being vaccinated and actually contracting the disease are greater still. Box 55-1 discusses the impact of diseases before immunizations. Diphtheria, tetanus, polio, and the other diseases can cause crippling and death, and most of these diseases are very contagious. Schedules for immunizations for these diseases have been developed as guidelines for the practitioner and for parents to ensure adequate protection for their children (Table 55-1).

A valid history of clinical disease or obtaining an **antibody titer,** the concentration of antibodies in the serum, for some of these diseases is useful in determining disease exposure and immunity. However, proven exposure to the disease does not always guarantee immunity. Therefore timely immunizations are even more important if the potential for development of the disease is imminent or increased, as it is for persons traveling to foreign countries where some diseases are endemic, indigenous to a geographic area or population. Required and recommended immunizations for foreign travel are constantly changing and are best obtained before travel from the local department of health.

Any time a traumatic wound (especially a puncture wound) is encountered, the individual's tetanus immunization status must be assessed. If the person has not been fully immunized within the past 10 years, or if the wound is contaminated and an immunization is more than 5 years old, a booster dose of tetanus toxoid may be in order. In adults, tetanus and diphtheria toxoid is recommended because the individual's diphtheria protection will be enhanced by this combination (McCormack, Brown, 1996).

Most new parents today are too young to remember the fear engendered by the very mention of childhood illnesses a few decades ago. For example, measles, the most common childhood disease, can cause pneumonia, encephalopathy, deafness, blindness, and seizures in 1 of every 1000 children with the disease (McCormack, Brown, 1996). If parents are not convinced, outbreaks of diseases (e.g., poliomyelitis) may make the argument for us. Complacency about childhood illnesses and their current and potential threats must be shaken. The initial effects of childhood illnesses can be very serious, and more potential future hazards are currently being discovered (e.g., the possible association of mumps with eventual diabetes and of chickenpox with shingles).

A request for exemption from required immunizations for school entry on medical grounds can be obtained from the child's physician. A model form for exemption on religious grounds can be obtained from the Christian Science Committee on Publications. However, it is theoretically possible that the right to exempt certain children could interfere with "herd immunity" by sustaining a continued pool of susceptible children, thereby maintaining a hazard that would be unacceptable to other parents who might apply legal and other pressures.

BOX 55-1 Impact of Selected Diseases before Immunizations

Disease	Comments
Measles	Before vaccinations nearly everyone in the United States got measles (an estimated 3 to 4 million cases yearly). The average annual number of measles-related deaths was 450 (1953 to 1963). A low rate of vaccination in preschool children in 1995 resulted in >55,000 cases, 11,000 hospitalizations, and 120 deaths. Risk for measles in African-American and Hispanic children was 8 to 10 times greater than in white children, because of lower vaccination rates in these children.
Haemophilus influenzae type b (Hib) meningitis	Before release of this vaccine in December 1987, Hib was the most common cause of meningitis in U.S. infants and children. Approximately 8,000 new cases were seen annually with 600 deaths, and many survivors were left with deafness, convulsions, or mental retardation. Since the vaccine was released, the incidence of Hib meningitis decreased 97% to 99% from previous reports.
Pertussis (whooping cough)	Before the vaccine, 150,000 to 260,000 children had pertussis annually with approximately 9,000 deaths. This is a serious illness that can cause prolonged coughing and vomiting that can last weeks. Infants may contract pneumonia and pertussis may also cause convulsions, brain damage and mental retardation. The new acellular pertussis (DTaP) vaccine is safer than the older, whole-cell diphtheria, tetanus toxoid, and pertussis (DTP) vaccine. It has been available since 1991 in the United States. Countries report epidemics of pertussis when immunization levels declined; for example, Japan's immunization dropped from 80% to 20% from 1974 to 1979 and in 1979, a pertussis epidemic resulted in 13,000 new cases and 41 deaths.
Rubella	This is usually a mild disease in children and adults but a serious problem in pregnant women during the first trimester. Adverse effects may occur in up to 90% of babies born; that is, they may contract congenital rubella syndrome (CRS), which causes heart defects, cataracts, deafness, and mental retardation. During 1964 to 1965 before rubella vaccination was regularly used in the United States, a rubella epidemic of nearly 20,000 infants were born with CRS, 2,100 died, 11,250 miscarriages were reported. Of the 20,000 infants with CRS, 11,600 were born deaf, 3,580 blind, and 1,800 mentally retarded.

From CDC, 1998.

All healthcare professionals as well as teachers, the local public health departments, the Department of Health and Human Services, and the World Health Organization need to work together to share their expertise in public education, current case reports, screening techniques, and mass immunization programs.

CURRENT ISSUES

Refinements and developments in clinical immunology field are advancing with the Centers for Disease Control and Prevention (1994) issuing the following general recommendations.

Spacing of Immunizations

When multiple doses of a particular immunization are recommended to achieve an adequate antibody response, the time interval between dosages should be followed. While a time that is longer than the recommended interval is acceptable and does not require starting over, shorter intervals are not acceptable. This is because the overall antibody response will be decreased and some persons will have an increased frequency in local or systemic adverse reactions (CDC, 1994). Although live vaccines such as the oral polio and yellow fever vaccines can be given at any time with an immune globulin, there is some evidence that high doses of immune globulin can inhibit the immune response to measles vaccine for over a 3-month period. There are instances when an inactivated vaccine interferes with other killed or live antigens. See Tables 55-2 and 55-3 for the recommended guidelines for spacing the administration of live and killed antigens and immune globulin.

The following guidelines cover vaccination in special situations (CDC, 1994).

- Premature infants should be vaccinated on the same chronological age schedule as full-term infants with the same recommended vaccine dose.
- There is no contraindication to vaccinations during breastfeeding.
- The decision of whether to vaccinate during pregnancy depends on weighing the potential risk of the vaccine to

TABLE 55-1 Recommended Schedule for Routine Active Vaccination of Infants and Children

Vaccine	*Birth*	*1 mo*	*2 mo*	*4 mo*	*6 mo*	*12 mo*	*15 mo*	*18 mo*	*4-6 yr*	*11-12 yr*	*13 yr*
Diphtheria, tetanus toxoid, and pertussis vaccine*			X	X	X		├— X	—┤	X		
Poliovirus vaccine, oral†			X	X	├——	—— X	——	——┤	X		
Measles, mumps, and rubella vaccine‡						├— X	—┤		X	or X	
Haemophilus influenzae type b vaccine§			X	X	X	├— X	—┤				
Hepatitis B¶											
HBsAg positive	X	├— X	—┤		X						
HBsAg negative	├——	X	——┤	See below							
Varicella vaccine‖						├——	——	——	X	——	——┤

From CDC Recommendations, 1998; DiGuiseppi, 1998; MedicineNet, 1998; Poon, Lavelle, 1998.
*Diphtheria, tetanus toxoid, and acellular pertussis (DTaP) vaccine is the preferred vaccine for all doses. An acceptable alternative is the whole cell diphtheria, tetanus toxoid, and pertussis (DTP) vaccine.
†Two poliovirus vaccines are available in the United States: inactivated poliovirus vaccine (IPV) and oral poliovirus vaccine (OPV). Both are acceptable, but OPV is preferred for most children. Alternate options for this immunization includes (1) two doses of IPV followed by two doses of OPV and (2) four doses of IPV, both on the same schedule as outlined above. IPV is the recommended vaccine for immunocompromised children and their household contacts.
‡The second dose of measles, mumps, and rubella (MMR) vaccine is usually recommended at either 4 to 6 or 11 to 12 years of age but can be administered during any visit provided that (1) it is at least 1 month or more since the first dose and (2) both doses are started after 12 months of age and completed by the time the child reaches 11 or 12 years of age.
§Three *H influenzae* type b (Hib) conjugate vaccines are available in the United States. If the PRP-OMP (PedvaxHIB, Merck) is used, the 6-month dose is not required.
¶Hepatitis B vaccine schedule is determined by the mother's status, that is, hepatitis B surface antigen (HBsAg) positive or negative. For HBsAg negative, the first dose is administered by 2 months of age, the second dose 1 month later, and the third dose at 6 months of age.
‖Varicella vaccine (chickenpox) may be administered to susceptible children at any visit after their first birthday, between 1 and 13 years of age. If given to children older than 13 years of age, two doses should be administered, from 4 to 8 weeks apart. This is a live attenuated virus that is contraindicated in human immunodeficiency virus (HIV)-infected, pregnant or lactating women, children of pregnant mothers, and women who are planning to become pregnant within 1 month of receiving the vaccine.

TABLE 55-2 Guidelines for Spacing the Administration of Live and Killed Antigens

Antigen Combination	*Recommended Minimum Interval between Doses*
≥2 Killed antigens	None. May be administered simultaneously or at any interval between doses.*
Killed and live antigens	None. May be administered simultaneously or at any interval between doses.†
≥2 Live antigens	4-week minimum interval if not administered simultaneously.§ However, oral polio vaccine can be administered at any time before, with, or after measles-mumps-rubella, if indicated.

From Centers for Disease Control and Prevention, 1994.
*If possible, vaccines associated with local or systemic side effects (e.g., cholera, parenteral typhoid, and plague vaccines) should be administered on separate occasions to avoid accentuated reactions.
†Cholera vaccine with yellow fever vaccine is the exception. If time permits, these antigens should not be administered simultaneously, and at least 3 weeks should elapse between administration of yellow fever vaccine and cholera vaccine. If the vaccines must be administered simultaneously or within 3 weeks of each other, the antibody response may not be optimal.
§If oral live typhoid vaccine is indicated (e.g., for international travel undertaken on short notice), it can be administered before, simultaneously with, or after oral poliovirus vaccine.

the disease exposure. For example, tetanus and diphtheria toxoids are routinely used for susceptible pregnant women; hepatitis B vaccine, influenza, and pneumococcal vaccines are also recommended for pregnant women at risk for the infection or from complications of the disease.

- Contraindications to all vaccines include a history of anaphylaxis to the individual vaccine or a component of it or the presence of moderate to severe illness with or without a fever. Generally, immunocompromised individuals should not receive any live vaccines. Special exceptions for the immunocompromised person and specific recommendations for their household contacts are available.

AIDS Vaccine

Acquired immunodeficiency syndrome (AIDS), which often results in fatal, unusual malignancies and opportunistic infections, has been recognized as an immunodeficiency state that results from an infection with a human retrovirus, the human immunodeficiency virus (HIV). While new drugs have been released to treat AIDS, the search for an HIV vaccine has not been productive (Santiago, 1996).

Two HIV envelope protein gp120 vaccines were tested in HIV-positive persons, but in 1994 the development of infections after administration of the vaccines resulted in cancellation of the major clinical trials (McCann, 1994). While trials with this vaccine are continuing in Thailand, other re-

TABLE 55-3 Guidelines for Spacing the Administration of Immune Globulin Preparations* and Vaccines

Simultaneous Administration		*Nonsimultaneous Administration*		
		Immunobiologic Administered		*Recommended Minimum Interval between Doses*
Immunobiologic Combination	*Recommended Minimum Interval between Doses*	*First*	*Second*	
Immune globulin and killed antigen	None. May be given simultaneously at different sites or at any time between doses.	Immune globulin Killed antigen	Killed antigen Immune globulin	None None
Immune globulin and live antigen	Should generally not be administered simultaneously.† If simultaneous administration of measles-mumps-rubella (MMR), measles-rubella, and monovalent measles vaccine is unavoidable, administer at different sites and revaccinate or test for seroconversion after the recommended interval.	Immune globulin Live antigen	Live antigen Immune globulin	Dose related†,§ 2 weeks

From Centers for Disease Control and Prevention, 1994.
*Blood products containing large amounts of immune globulin (such as serum immune globulin, specific immune globulins [e.g., TIG and HBIG], intravenous immune globulin [IGIV], whole blood, packed red cells, plasma, and platelet products).
†Oral polio virus, yellow fever, and oral typhoid (Ty21a) vaccines are exceptions to these recommendations. These vaccines may be administered at any time before, after, or simultaneously with an immune globulin-containing product without substantially decreasing the antibody response.
§The duration of interference of immune globulin preparations with the immune response to the measles component of the MMR, measles-rubella, and monovalent measles vaccine is dose-related (Table 8 of original document).

searchers believe an HIV vaccine such as ALVAC, which stimulates both a cellular and a humoral response, may hold some promise. It is still in phase I trials but may be approved for investigational trials in the United States in the future. Some investigators are looking at a completely new vaccine, one that prevents the disease but not the infection itself.

Many viral vaccines work by preventing the acute illness from developing and not by preventing the infection itself. This method though may be risky with HIV, but investigators are looking into this possibility currently by testing in primates (Santiago, 1996). See Chapter 56.

SIDE EFFECTS AND ADVERSE REACTIONS

As important as protection from debilitating infectious disease is, immunization is not without some risk. Side effects (i.e., slight fever, sore injection site, or minor rash) are usually mild and transient; occasionally, more serious effects (i.e., encephalitis and convulsions) are reported.

Although serious, the incidence of these effects—when weighed against the effects of diseases preventable through immunization—usually tips the balance in favor of immunization, particularly for those at high risk.

Joint pains and malaise may also be seen, especially after certain live and inactivated vaccines. Rarely, allergy to the egg protein providing the culture medium for the organism involved, to antiserums or antitoxins, to the mercury preservative, or to contained antibiotics causes a reaction, which is usually controllable by antihistamines. When any unusual or severe reaction occurs, the family, nurse, or healthcare professional should contact the prescriber and an informational form should be sent to the Centers for Disease Control and Prevention. Vaccinees should be given a contact's name in case they become sick and should visit a physician, hospital, or clinic within 4 weeks after immunization.

Monitoring any adverse reactions is part of a surveillance system to detect uncommon, severe, previously unrecognized, and rare reactions to vaccination. Past examples are the Guillain-Barré syndrome accompanying a small percentage of influenza vaccinations, encephalitis after measles vaccine, and peripheral neuropathy after rubella vaccinations; these are all very rare occurrences.

Even though uncommon, a large number of benign, expected reactions could indicate a "hot" lot of vaccine. Data are collected by the CDC for comparison with national data and are published in the Quarterly Adverse Reaction Report.

Minor expected reactions can be treated with acetaminophen (if the prescriber approves) and rest. Severe fevers (more than 103° F) can be treated with acetaminophen and sponge baths to reduce the temperature; occasionally a convulsion may accompany a high temperature, and parents need to be advised. Serum sickness sometimes occurs after repeated serum injections; it consists of rash, urticaria, arthritis, adenopathy, and fever starting hours or even days after the injection. Treatment consists of analgesics, antihistamines, or corticosteroids.

Rare but serious **anaphylactic reactions** can cause urticaria, dyspnea, cyanosis, shock, or unconsciousness that occurs within minutes of injection. This is not normal; it is an emergency situation. Therefore the healthcare professional or a responsible individual should observe any recipient of immunotherapy for up to ½ hour after therapy. Treatment for anaphylaxis may require administration of epinephrine.

TABLE 55-4 Biologic Agents for Active Immunization

Active immunization uses either inactivated (K or killed) material or live (L) attenuated agents.
Advantages: Usually higher levels of antibody are induced, and it is not necessary to repeat the procedure frequently.
Disadvantages: Adverse effects may occur, such as allergic reactions, that are not usually seen with passive immunization.
See Box 55-3 for advantages and disadvantages of live attenuated and inactivated biologic products.

Product	Route of Administration	Primary Immunization Schedule	Comments	Contraindications, Precautions, Side Effects, and Administration
Cholera vaccine	(K) bacteria SC, IM	Two doses, 1-4 wk apart (adult dose)	Provides 50% protection for about 6 mo.	Contraindications: acute illness; severe reaction or allergic response to previous dose; pregnancy evaluated individually Precautions: review of hypersensitivity history Side effects: redness, induration, pain at site; occasionally malaise, headache, mild to moderate temperature elevations Administration: IM in the deltoid muscle to adults and children older than 3 yr of age. Have epinephrine 1:1000 on hand.
Haemophilus influenzae	IM	See Table 55-1.	Efficacy improved if given to child younger than 2 yr of age.	Contraindications, immunosuppression, acute illnesses, and febrile states Administration: Shake vial well. Store in refrigerator. May be given at the same time as DPT but at different sites. Reconstitute with diluent provided. Record date on vial. Refrigerate; stable 30 days. Have epinephrine 1:1000 available.
Hepatitis B	(K) IM	See Table 55-1.	Provides >90% protection.	Contraindications/precautions: hypersensitivity. Safety and efficacy not yet established for children younger than 3 mo of age and in pregnant or breastfeeding women. Clinical judgement would probably weigh the risk of the disease higher than the potential risks caused by the vaccine's secondary effects. Delay giving vaccine in persons with serious active infection or in presence of severely compromised cardiopulmonary status. Side effects: injection site soreness; occasionally 101° F fevers are reported; infrequently malaise, headache, nausea, myalgias, arthralgias Administration: Shake before drawing up suspension; inspect for particles; do not dilute. Store opened and unopened vials in the refrigerator.
Influenza	(K) IM	One dose; split doses used in persons younger than 13 years of age (lower incidence of side effects)	Give annually by November.	Contraindications: hypersensitivity to egg products; individuals who are immunosuppressed; acute febrile illness; do not inject intravenously. Precautions: pregnancy; keep epinephrine on hand; not effective against all possible strains of influenza virus; resterilize jet injection apparatus if contaminated with blood; complete immunizations by November. Toxic drug reactions may occur (especially with phenytoin, warfarin, or theophylline) after viral infection or vaccination. Side effects: local tenderness, redness, induration; fever, malaise, myalgia; rarely allergic skin and respiratory reactions and Guillain-Barré syndrome; very rarely encephalopathy. Administration: Inject IM into deltoid or lateral midthigh or gluteus. Refrigerate. Have epinephrine 1:1000 available.

TABLE 55-4 Biologic Agents for Active Immunization—cont'd

Product	Route of Administration	Primary Immunization Schedule	Comments	Contraindications, Precautions, Side Effects, and Administration
Measles virus vaccine	(L) SC	One dose at 12 to 15 mo; earlier if epidemic occurs. See Table 55-1.	If given before 15 mo, may need to reimmunize. Also may prevent disease if given within 72 hr of exposure to measles.	Contraindications: neomycin or chicken product hypersensitivity; active febrile infection; active untreated tuberculosis; immunosuppression or immunodeficiency; bone marrow or lymphatic deficiencies; pregnancy (pregnancy should also be avoided for 3 mo after vaccination). Precautions: give no sooner than 3 mo after transfusion of blood/plasma/human immune serum globulin of more than 0.02 ml/lb body weight. Give with or after TB skin test. Do not give within 1 mo of immunization by other live virus vaccines except one of the MMR type or combination Side effects: moderate fever to 102° F, rash (in 5-12 days); rarely fever more than 103° F with convulsions; 1 per million occurrences encephalitis or subacute sclerosing panencephalitis; previous recipients of killed virus vaccine—local swelling, redness, vesiculation Administration: Refrigerate before reconstitution and afterward. Use within 8 hr; avoid light at all times. Inject 0.5 ml of reconstituted vaccine subcutaneously. Solution may be pink or yellow but must be clear. Discard cloudy solutions. Have epinephrine 1 : 1000 available.
Meningococcal meningitis vaccine	SC	One dose. If a household disease, antibiotic prophylaxis (rifampin) should be given for several days, since antibody response requires at least 5 days.	Used in epidemics.	Contraindications: immunosuppression; acute illness Precautions: pregnancy Side effects: mild, local erythema Administration: Administer in a single parenteral dose. Do not give IV. Have epinephrine 1 : 1000 available.
Mumps vaccine	(L) SC	One dose	If administered before 1 year old, reimmunization may be necessary.	Contraindications and precautions: same as for measles vaccine with following exceptions in side effects. Side effects: mild fever; low incidence of parotitis, orchitis, purpura, allergic reactions (urticaria); very rarely encephalitis and other nervous system reactions. Administration: Same as measles vaccine.
Pertussis (in DTP)	(K) IM	As per DTP. See Table 55-1.	Use only whole-cell DTP for first three doses. See Table 55-1.	Contraindications: acute infection; previous reactions to an initial dose (all three antigens or only pertussis may be omitted then) such as fever greater than 103° F (39° C), convulsions, altered consciousness, focal neurologic signs, "screaming fits," shock/collapse, purpura; preexisting neurologic disorder; immunosuppression; older than 6 yr (give tetanus toxoid and diphtheria [Td] instead). Precautions: reactions to DTP call for reevaluation and possibly administration of Td only. Side effects: usually local redness, induration, and possible tenderness; possible abscess; mild to moderate fever Administration: IM. Shake before using. Refrigerate. Have epinephrine 1 : 1000 available.
Pneumococci polyvalent vaccine	SC, IM	See current literature.	Not used in children younger than 2 yr of age.	Contraindications: hypersensitivity, revaccination, pregnancy, intradermal administration, and IV administration. Will not protect against specific antigens not included. Within 10 days of start of chemotherapy of Hodgkin's disease, vaccine is contraindicated.

Continued

TABLE 55-4 Biologic Agents for Active Immunization—cont'd

Product	Route of Administration	Primary Immunization Schedule	Comments	Contraindications, Precautions, Side Effects, and Administration
Pneumococci polyvalent vaccine—cont'd				Precautions: active infection; younger than 2 yr of age; immunosuppression; severely compromised cardiac or pulmonary function; history of pneumococcal infection. Keep epinephrine on hand. Side effects: local redness and soreness, induration, fever greater than 100.9° F; rarely anaphylactoid reactions.
Poliomyelitis vaccine	(L) oral	See Table 55-1.		Contraindications: never administered parenterally; acute illness; advanced, debilitated condition; persistent vomiting or diarrhea; immunodeficient or immunosuppressed states. Precautions: will not modify/prevent existing or incubating disease Side effect: rarely paralytic disease after vaccination or after contact with vaccinee (advise unimmunized close contacts of vaccinee to seek immunization as needed). Administration: Store frozen, thaw before use, and agitate before giving 2 drops orally, in chlorine-free water, simple syrup, or milk, or on bread, cake, or cube sugar (usually dropper supplied). See package insert for specific storage advice. Change of color from pink to yellow is not remarkable.
Rabies vaccine Rabies	(K) IM	Preexposure: two doses a week apart followed by a third dose in between 21-28 days. Postexposure: see current literature for guidelines.		Precautions: History of hypersensitivity dictates cautious use of rabies vaccine. Administration: Flush and cleanse wound; possible initial prophylaxis with tetanus and antibiotic therapy. Have epinephrine 1:1000 available. Discontinue corticosteroids during immunization.
Rubella vaccine	(L) SC	One dose. See Table 55-1.	Give between 12-15 mo of age. Do not give during pregnancy. Woman must not become pregnant for 3 mo after injection. Contraceptive counseling may be needed.	Contraindications and precautions as for Attenuvax with the following exceptions: postpubertal females with rubella titers of more than 1:8; pregnancy (pregnancy also to be avoided for 3 mo after vaccine) Precautions: theoretical possibility of live virus transmission from nose/throat of vaccinees. Side effects: occasionally mild symptoms of naturally acquired rubella (lymphadenopathy, urticaria, rash, malaise, sore throat, fever, headache, polyneuritis, arthralgias, local pain, swelling, redness; fever rarely more than 103° F); very rarely encephalitis. Administration: Same as for measles vaccine
Tetanus toxoid	IM	Included in DTP. See Table 55-1.	DTP is preferred for children while Td is preferred for adults. Tetanus toxoid is usually used to test cell-mediated immunity.	Contraindications: not for treatment of an actual tetanus infection; any acute infection; immunosuppression. Precautions: hypersensitivity; keep epinephrine on hand; history of cerebral damage, neurologic disorders, or febrile convulsions should be evaluated individually. Side effects: occasionally Arthus-type response to high levels of tetanus antibody (antitoxin) in those receiving regular or frequent tetanus toxoid boosters (thus the recommended 10-yr interval between Td booster). Response may include significant local symptoms of redness, edema resembling a giant "hive," axillary lymphadenopathy; systemic symptoms can include low fever, malaise, aches and pains, general urticaria, tachycardia, and hypotension. Prolonged intervals between primary immunizing doses has no effect on eventual immunity status. Administration: Shake well and give deep IM. Refrigerate, but do not freeze. Have epinephrine 1:1000 available.

BOX 55-2 RespiGam

Respiratory syncytial virus intravenous immune globulin (RespiGam) was approved to prevent the serious lower respiratory tract infection caused by respiratory syncytial virus (RSV) in children younger than 2 years of age who were either born prematurely or have bronchopulmonary dysplasia. This product reduces the incidence and duration of RSV hospitalizations and also the severity of the disease in high-risk infants. It is infused once a month during the RSV period from November through April (Pharmacy News, 1996).

BOX 55-3 Live versus Inactivated Products

The advantages of live attenuated-type immunization are the long-lasting immunity and the similarity of the resistance that occurs to that which is produced by the natural disease. The disadvantages with live immunization are an increased risk of inducing disease, plus the fact that a mild disease state is usually needed to induce immunity. One also has a higher risk of the vaccine being contaminated, and finally, the product is more labile, requiring special storage.

The inactivated (killed) biologic product is easier to ship and store. It is usually highly purified, and there is little risk of inducing a disease from infection. The disadvantage is that it provides a short-acting immunity so that the person often needs reimmunization. It may or may not simulate protective type factors, and it may not prevent a reinfection without the actual disease having been present.

Vasopressors and intermittent positive pressure breathing (IPPB) oxygen, antihistamines, and corticosteroids may help. Immunization therapy may cautiously be resumed after all signs of anaphylaxis are gone.

A description of biologic agents (active and passive) used for immunization and their secondary effects may be found in Table 55-4. Box 55-2 contains information on RespiGam, used to prevent lower respiratory tract infections. Also see Box 55-3 for a comparison of live versus inactivated products.

Sources of Information

Sources of information on immunization include primarily the Public Health Service Advisory Committee on Immunization Practices (ACIP), which advises the public health agencies, and the Committee on Control of Infectious Diseases (the Red Book Committee), which is drawn from the members of the American Academy of Pediatrics and advises the private health sector. The ACIP can be contacted through the Centers for Disease Control and Prevention in Atlanta. Because the two groups maintain a slightly different perspective, minor inconsequential variations in recommendations may occasionally be noted. Other sources include local public health departments and printed package inserts included with the vaccine or serum. Biologic preparations and accompanying inserts are regulated by the Bureau of Biologics of the Food and Drug Administration (FDA). The state of the art of immunotherapy is in rapid flux. Keeping up to date with current immunization practice requires effort on the part of the healthcare professional through reading current journals, attending seminars, and consulting with experts in the field.

SUMMARY

Immunization is needed to protect children and adults from dangerous diseases that have serious complications. Vaccines may have side effects (fever, rash, and soreness at injection site), and in some individuals, they have caused serious reactions. However, the risks from not vaccinating though are much greater than the risks of a serious reaction. The previously reported epidemics of polio, measles, *H influenzae* meningitis, pertussis, and rubella have nearly been eliminated in populations that are immunized. Vaccines are also available for other infectious diseases such as yellow fever, hepatitis B, rabies, cholera, typhoid, and plague. Healthcare professionals must be informed on this topic so that they can educate their patients on the advantages provided by immunization.

REVIEW QUESTIONS

1. Name four side effects/adverse reactions of immunization and the recommendations for management.
2. What is the difference (advantages and disadvantages) between live and inactivated vaccines? Name two vaccines from each category.
3. Why is a 10-year interval recommended between tetanus and diphtheria (Td) booster injections? Describe the reaction.
4. Why is it important to teach women not to become pregnant for 3 months after receiving a rubella vaccine immunization?

REFERENCES

Centers for Disease Control and Prevention: General recommendations on immunization: Recommendations of the Advisory Committee on Immunization Practices (ACIP), *MMWR* 43(RR-1):1-38, 1994.

Centers for Disease Control and Prevention: What would happen if we stopped vaccinations? http://www.cdc.gov/nip/vacsafe/valuefs.htm (July 17, 1998).

Centers for Disease Control and Prevention Recommendations: Recommended childhood immunization schedule, United States, January-December, 1998, http://www.cdc.gov/nip/child.htm (July 17, 1998).

DiGuiseppi C: Childhood immunizations, guide to clinical preventive services, ed 2, immunizations and chemoprophylaxis, http:¢pmcnet.columbia.edu/tests/gcps0075.html (July 18, 1998).

McCann J: Researchers tout triple therapy for HIV/AIDS, *Hosp Pharm Rep* 8(9):18, 1994.

McCormack JP, Brown G: Traumatic skin and soft tissue infections. In Young LY, Koda-Kimble MA, editors: *Applied therapeutics: the clinical use of drugs,* ed 6, Vancouver, Wash, 1995, Applied Therapeutics, Inc.

MedicineNet: Immunizations (vaccinations), http://www.medicinenet.com/Art.asp?li=MNI&ag=Y&ArticleKey=394 (July 18, 1998).

Pharmacy News: Drug updates, *J Am Pharm* NS36(4):225, 1996.

Poon CY, Lavelle M: Childhood immunization: recent changes and new recommendations, *US Pharmacist* 24(6), 1998.

Santiago L: Slow progress on HIV vaccines, *GMHC Treat Iss: Newslett Exp AIDS Ther* 10(4):1-4, 1996.

ADDITIONAL REFERENCES

Abramowicz M, editor: Routine immunization for adults, *Med Lett* 32(819):54, 1990.

Anderson KN et al, editors: *Mosby's medical, nursing, and allied health dictionary,* ed 5, St Louis, 1998, Mosby.

DiPiro JT, Talber R et al, editors: *Pharmacotherapy, a pathophysiologic approach,* ed 2, Norwalk, Conn, 1993, Appleton & Lange.

Keane V et al: Perceptions of vaccine efficacy, illness, and health among inner-city parents, *Clin Pediatr* 32(1):2-7, 1993.

Merenstein GB, Kaplan DW, Rosenberg AA: *Handbook of pediatrics,* ed 17, Norwalk, Conn, 1994, Appleton & Lange.

Mosby: *Mosby's GenRx,* St Louis, 1998, Mosby.

National Institutes of Allergy and Infectious Diseases (NIAID): Evolution of vaccine development, *Neonatal Netw* 11(4):43-44, 1992.

National Institutes of Allergy and Infectious Diseases (NIAID): Vaccines in clinical trials, *Neonatal Netw* 11(4):45-47, 1992.

Olin BR: *Facts and comparisons.* Philadelphia, 1998, JB Lippincott.

CHAPTER 56

Immunosuppressants and Immunomodulators

KEY DRUG

azathioprine, (p. 727)

CHAPTER FOCUS

This chapter reviews the drugs used to prevent rejection of kidney, liver, and heart transplants, i.e., the immunosuppressant agents. Also discussed are the immunomodulating agents, or drugs that may activate the body's immune defense or modify a biological response to an unwanted stimulus. The latter drugs have been used primarily to treat human immunodeficiency virus (HIV) infection and acquired immunodeficiency syndrome (AIDS), but as new agents are discovered, the treatment of other viral diseases and various cancers may also be discovered. This area of study has enormous potential for growth and may contribute the knowledge needed to solve the mysteries of specific disease states.

KEY TERMS

acquired immunodeficiency syndrome (AIDS), (p. 731)
human immunodeficiency virus (HIV), (p. 731)
immunocompromised state, (p. 726)
immunomodulating agent, (p. 730)
immunosuppressant agents, (p. 726)

OBJECTIVES

After reading and studying this chapter, the student should be able to do the following:

1. *Define and describe the key terms and key drug.*
2. *Name the four factors that can lead to an immunocompromised state.*
3. *Name the six immunosuppressant drugs. Discuss the primary indications, drug interactions, and major side effects and adverse reactions of the primary immunosuppressant agents azathioprine, cyclosporine, daclizumab, and tacrolimus.*
4. *Describe the etiology, patient survival, and current treatment approaches for acquired immunodeficiency syndrome.*

The rejection of kidney, liver, and heart allogenic transplants has led to the development of **immunosuppressant agents,** or agents that decrease or prevent an immune response. A foreign substance or organ transplant in the body activates an immune response by the release of macrophages to phagocytize and process the foreign substance. In addition, interleukin 1 production increases, which activates helper T cells containing a surface receptor or CD3. The activated T cell stimulates production of killer or cytotoxic T lymphocytes and B lymphocytes in part by producing interleukin 2. T cells are necessary for cellular immunity (attack the foreign substance directly and with released toxic substances), and the B lymphocytes are responsible for humoral immunity or the production of antibodies. The primary sites of action of the immunosuppressant agents are illustrated in Fig. 56-1.

Immunodeficiency or immunosuppression may also occur from a genetic or an acquired disorder of the immune system. Although genetic disorders such as agammaglobulinemia or severe combined immune deficiency syndrome (SCIDS) are usually diagnosed shortly after birth, acquired disorders may occur at any time throughout life. Acquired immunodeficiency may be induced by a variety of drugs such as chemotherapeutic and immunosuppressant agents, by radiation therapy, or through viral infections such as acquired immunodeficiency syndrome (AIDS). Because AIDS often has devastating complications and a fatal outcome, much research interest has been directed toward the development of immunomodulating or immunostimulating medications.

An **immunocompromised state** may result from one or more of the following: (1) inhibition of granulocyte formation leading to severe neutropenia; (2) impairment of synthesis and antibody production; (3) loss of mucocutaneous barriers that permit bacteria or microorganisms access to internal organs, which may occur in a variety of therapeutic situations, such as after the use of medical devices (central venous catheters, Foley catheters, and endotracheal tubes) or after chemotherapy; (4) impairment of cellular immunity such as macrophages and T-cell lymphocytes (usually seen in patients who receive immunosuppressive agents, e.g., corticosteroids or cyclosporine, in patients with certain types of cancer [e.g., Hodgkin's lymphoma], or organ transplant recipients).

In the majority of patients, combinations of these defects are common because several immune functions may be affected at the same time. For example, chronic therapy with antineoplastic medications will affect granulocytes and cellular immunity. Chemotherapy may result in the loss of mucocutaneous barriers or the development of mucositis and ulcers in the mouth and gastrointestinal tract. These individuals are at a greater risk for the development of bacterial, fungal, or viral infections. This chapter reviews some of

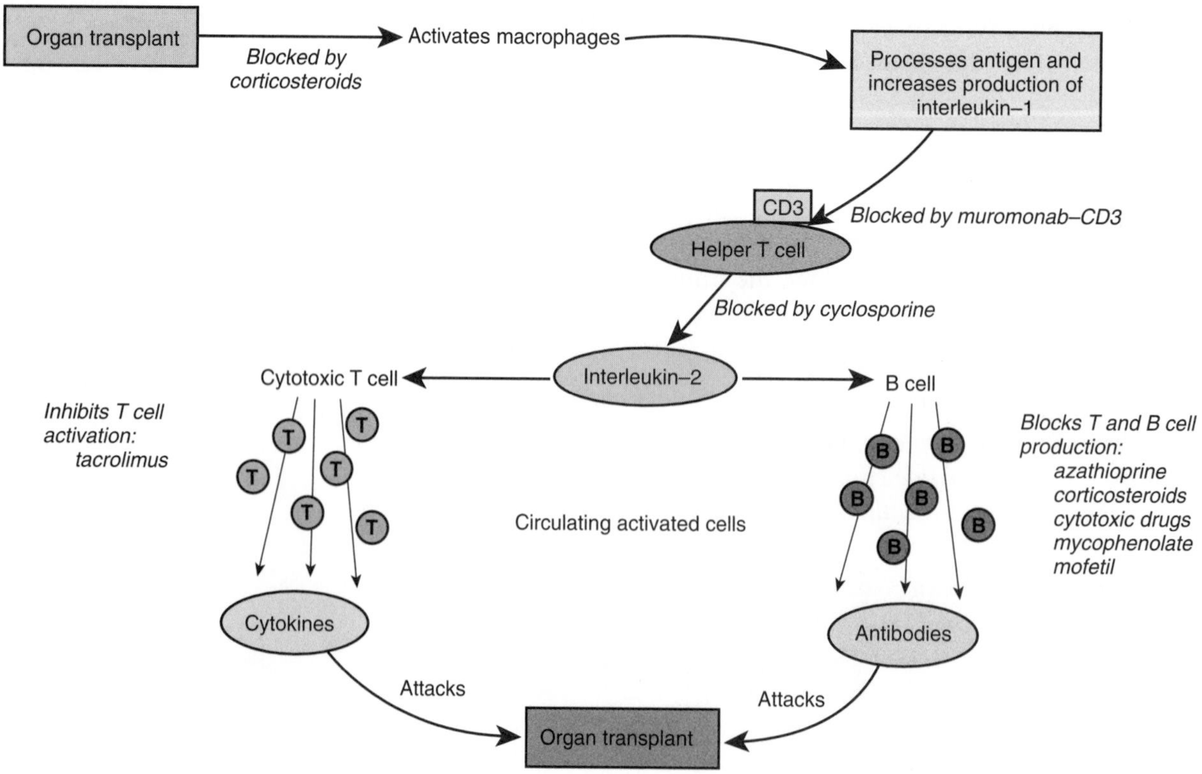

FIGURE 56-1
Sites of action for immunosuppressive agents.

the primary agents that suppress, modify, or stimulate the human immune system.

IMMUNOSUPPRESSANTS

The primary immunosuppressant drugs are azathioprine (Imuran), cyclosporine (Sandimmune), daclizumab (Zenapax), muromonab-CD3 (Orthoclone OKT3), mycophenolate mofetil (CellCept), and tacrolimus (FK506, Prograf).

azathioprine [ay za thye' oh preen] (Imuran)

Azathioprine is indicated as an adjunct medication to prevent rejection in renal organ transplant recipients and for severe, active rheumatoid arthritis in persons who have not responded to other therapies. The mechanism of action for azathioprine is unknown but it appears to suppress T-and B-ell production primarily; that is, it suppresses cell-mediated hypersensitivity and antibody production. In combination with steroids, it appears to have a steroid-conserving effect; a lower dose of steroid may be used to treat chronic inflammatory processes when given with azathioprine.

Pharmacokinetics

Azathioprine is available in oral and parenteral dosage forms. Orally it is well absorbed from the intestinal tract. It has a half-life of 5 hours, with an onset of action of 6 to 8 weeks in rheumatoid arthritis and perhaps 4 to 8 weeks in other inflammatory disease states. It is metabolized in the liver to active metabolites (6-mercaptopurine and 6-thioinosinic acid) with further metabolism by xanthine oxidase. It is primarily excreted via the biliary system.

Drug interactions

The following effects may occur when azathioprine is given with the drugs listed below:

Drug	Possible effect and management
allopurinol	Allopurinol inhibits xanthine oxidase, which may result in increased azathioprine activity and toxicity. Avoid or a potentially serious drug interaction may occur. If it is absolutely necessary to give both drugs concurrently, reduce the dosage of azathioprine to 1/4 to 1/3 of the usually prescribed dosage; monitor closely and adjust dosage as needed.
Immunosuppressant agents, other (glucocorticoids, cyclophosphamide, and cyclosporine)	May increase the risk for developing infections and/or neoplasms. Avoid or a potentially serious drug interaction may occur.
Vaccines, live virus	Immunization with live vaccines should be postponed in persons receiving this drug and also in close family members. The use of a live virus vaccine in immunosuppressed patients may result in increased replication of the vaccine virus, may increase side effects and adverse reactions to the vaccine virus, and may possibly cause a decrease in the patient's antibody response to the vaccine. Avoid or a potentially serious drug interaction may occur.

Color type indicates an unsafe drug combination.

Side effects and adverse reactions

These include anorexia, nausea, vomiting, leukopenia or infection, megaloblastic anemia (the patient is usually asymptomatic but may also have fever, chills, cough, low back or side pain, pain on urination, or increased weakness), hepatitis, thrombocytopenia, hypersensitivity, pancreatitis, pneumonitis, sores in the mouth and on the lips, and skin rash. The risk of hepatotoxicity is greater when the dosage of azathioprine exceeds 2.5 mg/kg daily.

Warnings

Use with caution in patients with pancreatitis and in individuals who have received antineoplastic chemotherapy or radiation. See the box for Food and Drug Administration (FDA) pregnancy safety classifications.

Contraindications

Avoid use in persons with azathioprine hypersensitivity, chickenpox, herpes zoster, gout, liver or kidney function impairment, infection, and severe xanthine oxidase deficiency.

Dosage and administration

The pediatric and adult immunosuppressant dose is 3 to 5 mg/kg orally 1 to 3 days before or at the time of surgery, or if given intravenously, before, during, or immediately after surgery. The maintenance dosage is 1 to 2 mg/kg. For rheumatoid arthritis, the adult oral dose is 1 mg/kg daily, adjusted every 1 to 2 months as necessary.

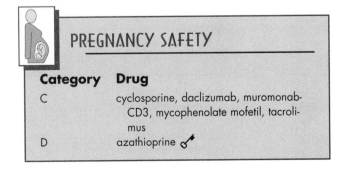

PREGNANCY SAFETY

Category	Drug
C	cyclosporine, daclizumab, muromonab-CD3, mycophenolate mofetil, tacrolimus
D	azathioprine

cyclosporine [sye′ klow spor een] (Sandimmune)

Cyclosporine is a potent immunosuppressant used for the prevention of organ (renal, hepatic, or cardiac allografts) transplant rejection. It is usually administered in combination with corticosteroids. Its mechanism of action is unknown, but studies indicate that it inhibits the formation and release of interleukin 2, the substance necessary to induce a cytotoxic T lymphocyte response to an antigenic challenge. It does not cause significant myelosuppression or bone marrow depression.

Pharmacokinetics

Cyclosporine is available in oral and parenteral dosage forms. Orally, its bioavailability is variable (about 30%), which may improve with increasing doses and chronic administration. Absorption may decrease after a liver transplant or in patients with liver impairment or gastrointestinal dysfunction, such as diarrhea or vomiting. It has a half-life of approximately 7 hours in children and 19 hours in adults; orally it reaches peak serum levels in 3.5 hours. It is extensively metabolized in the liver and excreted primary in bile and feces.

Drug interactions

The following effects may occur when cyclosporine is given with the drugs listed below:

Drug	Possible effect and management
Androgens, cimetidine (Tagamet), danazol, (Danocrine), diltiazem (Cardizem), estrogens, erythromycin, ketoconazole (Nizoral), or miconazole (Monistat IV)	May result in increased serum levels of cyclosporine, increasing the potential risk for hepatotoxicity and nephrotoxicity. If drugs must be administered concurrently, use extreme caution and monitor closely.
Diuretics, potassium-sparing (amiloride, spironolactone, or triamterene) or potassium supplements or salt substitutes	May increase the risk of hyperkalemia. Monitor serum levels and signs and symptoms of hyperkalemia (confusion; irregular heart rate; paresthesias of hands, feet, or lips; respiratory difficulties; increased weakness; and feeling of weak or heavy legs).
Immunosuppressants	Increases the risk of developing infection or other lymphoproliferative-type disorders (e.g., lymphomas). Use extreme caution if given concurrently.
lovastatin (Mevacor)	When used in heart transplant patients, it may increase the risk of developing rhabdomyolysis and acute renal failure. Monitor closely if concurrent therapy is necessary.
Vaccines, live virus	See azathioprine.

Side effects and adverse reactions

These are dose related and include hirsutism, tremors, acne or oily skin, headache, leg cramps, nausea, vomiting, gingival hyperplasia (swollen, bleeding gums), nephrotoxicity, seizures, hepatotoxicity, severe hypertension (usually associated with 25 to 50 mg/kg doses of cyclosporine), and, rarely, anaphylaxis, hemolytic-uremic syndrome, hyperkalemia, pancreatitis, and renal toxicity. Lymphomas, skin malignancies, and other lymphoproliferative-type disorders have been reported; some have regressed when the drug is stopped (USP DI, 1998). Gingival hyperplasia, a common problem with the use of this drug, is generally reversible about 6 months after cyclosporine is discontinued.

Warnings

Use with caution in patients with hyperkalemia and malabsorption.

Contraindications

Avoid use in persons with cyclosporine hypersensitivity, chickenpox, herpes zoster, infection, and liver or kidney function impairment.

Dosage and administration

The pediatric and adult oral dose is 12 to 15 mg/kg daily, starting 4 to 12 hours before surgery and continuing for 7 to 14 days afterward. The dose is then decreased weekly until the maintenance dose of 5 to 10 mg/kg daily is reached. Children may need higher or more frequent dosing because they seem to metabolize this drug rapidly. The IV dose is 2 to 6 mg/kg daily until the patient can take oral medication.

daclizumab [da kle′ zoo mab] (Zenapax)

Daclizumab is a monoclonal antibody immunosuppressant that is used in combination with cyclosporine and corticosteroids to prevent acute rejection of transplanted kidneys. This drug is an interleukin 2 (IL-2) receptor antagonist, that is, it binds to the alpha subunit of the IL-2 receptor complex thus inhibiting IL-2 binding. This inhibition results in a decreased activation of lymphocytes and an impaired immune system response to antigens.

Pharmacokinetics

Administered parenterally, daclizumab has a half-life (elimination) of 11 to 38 days and a therapeutic serum level between 5 to 10 μg/ml.

Side effects and adverse reactions

These include joint pain, constipation, diarrhea, dizziness, heartburn, headache, insomnia, myalgia, chest pain, dyspnea, fever, hypertension, peripheral edema, pulmonary edema, tachycardia, tremors, weakness, wound infection, and, rarely, hypoglycemia.

Warnings

Use with caution in patients with diabetes mellitus, infection, and a history of or current malignancy.

Contraindications

Avoid use in persons with daclizumab hypersensitivity.

Dosage and administration

The usual adolescent and adult dose is 1 mg/kg administered by IV infusion over 15 minutes every 2 weeks. Do not begin infusion before 24 hours after transplantation.

muromonab-CD3 [myoo roe moe′ nab-CD3] (Orthoclone OKT3)

Muromonab-CD3 is a monoclonal antibody that reacts with CD3 receptor on the surface of T lymphocytes. It blocks the activation and functions of the T cells in response to an antigenic challenge. Thus it functions as an immunosuppressant and does not cause myelosuppression.

Indications

Muromonab-CD3 is indicated for the treatment of acute renal organ transplant rejection and is usually given in combination with azathioprine, cyclosporine, or corticosteroids. It is also administered to treat acute rejection (steroid-resistant) in cardiac and hepatic transplant patients.

Pharmacokinetics

Available parenterally, it acts to reduce activated T cells within minutes after administration. It reaches steady-state plasma levels in about 3 days and has a duration of action of about 7 days. In other words, the number of circulating CD3-positive T cells will return to baseline levels within a week after discontinuation of muromonab-CD3.

Drug interactions

Concurrent use with other immunosuppressant agents may increase the risk of infection and perhaps the development of lymphoproliferative diseases. A reduced dose of corticosteroids and azathioprine is recommended when muromonab is started. Monitor closely. For interactions with live viral vaccines, see azathioprine above.

Side effects and adverse reactions

The most frequent adverse reactions of muromonab-CD3 occur with the first course. The first-dose effect consists of lightheadedness, elevated temperature, chills, nausea, vomiting, diarrhea, headache, dyspnea, chest pain, and tremors, and trembling. These effects may be repeated to a lesser degree after the second dose but are rarely encountered with later doses. Fever and chills that occur later may be caused by infection. Anaphylaxis, hypersensitivity, encephalopathy, convulsions, cerebral edema, and aseptic meningitis syndrome are reported less frequently.

Warnings

Use with caution in patients with history of thrombosis.

Contraindications

Avoid use in persons with muromonab-CD3 hypersensitivity, unstable angina, fever greater than 100° F, fluid overload, uncompensated heart failure, cerebrovascular disease, chronic obstructive pulmonary disease, symptomatic ischemic heart disease, recent myocardial infarction, neuropathy, pulmonary edema, septic shock, chickenpox, herpes zoster, and a history of convulsions.

Dosage and administration

The adult dose is 5 mg daily for 10 to 14 days. Children younger than 12 years of age receive 0.1 mg/kg/day for 10 to 14 days.

mycophenolate mofetil

[mye koe fee′ noe late moe′ fe tyl] (CellCept)

Mycophenolate used in conjunction with cyclosporine and corticosteroids is indicated for the prophylaxis of renal transplant rejection. Mycophenolate is metabolized to MPA, an active metabolite that inhibits the response of T and B lymphocytes to mitogenic and allospecific stimulation. Therefore this drug has a cytostatic effect on lymphocytes. It also suppresses antibody formation by B-lymphocytes and may inhibit the influx of leukocytes into inflammatory and graft rejection sites.

Pharmacokinetics

Available orally, it is rapidly metabolized to the active metabolite, MPA and other inactive metabolites. MPA's half-life is 18 hours with excretion primarily in the kidneys.

Drug interactions

The following effects may occur when mycophenolate is given with the drugs listed below:

Drug	Possible effect and management
Immunosuppressant agents, other (azathioprine, glucocorticoids, cyclophosphamide, and cyclosporine)	May increase the risk for developing infections and neoplasms.
acyclovir (Zovirax) or ganciclovir (Cytovene)	These drugs compete with mycophenolate for renal excretion and may increase each others' toxicity. Avoid or a potentially serious drug interaction may occur. If used concurrently, monitor patient closely.
Antacids (magnesium and aluminum hydroxide); cholestyramine (Questran), colestipol (Colestid)	These drugs decrease the absorption of mycophenolate. Administer mycophenolate 1 hour before or 2 hours after antacids and bile acid sequestrants.

Color type indicates an unsafe drug combination.

Side effects and adverse reactions

These include abdominal pain, constipation or diarrhea, nausea, vomiting, dizziness, acne, insomnia, rash, anemia, chest pain, cough, dyspnea, hematuria, hypertension, leukopenia, peripheral edema, dysrhythmia, arthralgia, colitis, gastrointestinal (GI) bleeding, gingival hyperplasia, gingivitis, myalgia, oral moniliasis, pancreatitis, thrombocytopenia, and tremors.

Warnings

Use with caution in patients with posttransplant, delayed renal graft function.

Contraindications

Avoid use in persons with mycophenolate hypersensitivity, active GI system disease, and severe kidney function impairment.

Dosage and administration

The oral dose administered within 3 days of transplantation is 1 g twice a day with cyclosporine and corticosteroids.

tacrolimus [tak roe lye' mus] (FK506, Prograf)

Tacrolimus in conjunction with corticosteroids is indicated for the prophylaxis of organ (liver) rejection. It inhibits activation of T lymphocytes and although its exact mechanism of action is unknown, it is believed to bind to FKBP-12 protein and form complexes that prevent T-lymphocyte activation.

Pharmacokinetics

It is available orally and parenterally. Oral absorption is variable, reaching a peak blood level in 0.5 to 4 hours with an elimination half-life of 11 to 40 hours. Tacrolimus is metabolized in the liver (primarily by the cytochrome P-450 3A system) to a number of metabolites, including several active ones; less than 1% is excreted in the urine.

Drug interactions

The following effects may occur when tacrolimus is given with the drugs listed below:

Drug	Possible effect and management
Aminoglycoside antiinfectives, amphotericin B (Fungizone), cisplatin (Platinol), or cyclosporine (Sandimmune)	Concurrent use increases the risk of nephrotoxicity. Allow 24 hours to pass after discontinuing cyclosporine before starting tacrolimus. Monitor renal function studies carefully.
Angiotensin-converting enzyme inhibitors, potassium-sparing diuretics	Concurrent use increases the risk of hyperkalemia. Monitor serum potassium levels.
Antifungals, bromocriptine (Parlodel), calcium channel blockers, cimetidine (Tagamet), clarithromycin (Biaxin), cyclosporine (Sandimmune), danazol (Danocrine), erythromycin, methylprednisolone, or metoclopramide (Reglan)	Concurrent use increases tacrolimus blood levels. Observe patient for symptoms of toxicity.
phenobarbital, phenytoin (Dilantin), carbamazepine (Tegretol), or rifamycins	Concurrent use decreases tacrolimus blood levels. Monitor tacrolimus blood levels frequently. Dosage adjustments may be necessary.
Vaccines, live	Avoid concurrent use. Other than live vaccines may be less effective if given concurrently.

Color type indicates an unsafe drug combination.

Side effects and adverse reactions

These include weakness, blood disorders, GI distress, anorexia, hyperglycemia, hyperkalemia, hypomagnesemia, nephrotoxicity, neurotoxicity, headaches, insomnia, tremors, convulsions, paresthesia, pleural effusion, peripheral edema, pruritus, rash, cardiac disorders (e.g., cardiomyopathy and hypertension), neuropathy, muscle cramps, osteoporosis, sweating, tinnitus, blurred vision, and rarely, anaphylaxis, and hepatotoxicity.

Warnings

Use with caution in patients with diabetes mellitus, liver or neurologic function impairment, hepatitis B or C infection, and hyperkalemia.

Contraindications

Avoid use in persons with tacrolimus or polyoxyl 60 hydrogenated castor oil hypersensitivity, current cancer, chickenpox, herpes zoster, infection, and kidney function impairment.

Dosage and administration

By IV infusion, the adult dose is 0.05 to 1 mg/kg/day, converted to oral as soon as possible, usually in 2 to 3 days of therapy. The initial oral adult dose is 0.15 to 0.3/mg/kg/day. For adults, the lower dose range is used initially, whereas children need and tolerate a higher dose of this product.

IMMUNOMODULATING AGENTS

Biotechnology refers to the development of new agents that can either activate the body's immune defenses or modify a biologic response to an unwanted stimulus, such as an antitumor response. These agents are called **immunomodulat-**

ing agents. With the advent of recombinant deoxyribonucleic acid (DNA) technology in the early 1980s, new agents were made available in larger quantities for clinical trials and investigations. Although still in its infancy, this area of study has the potential for solving some of the mysteries about disease that have eluded researchers for centuries and may also provide pharmaceuticals that control the devastation, pain, and suffering induced by many viral diseases, AIDS, and cancer.

ACQUIRED IMMUNODEFICIENCY SYNDROME

A pathogenic retrovirus known as **human immunodeficiency virus (HIV)** is the etiologic agent in **acquired immunodeficiency syndrome (AIDS)** (Box 56-1). AIDS is one of the leading causes of death in Americans between the ages of 25 and 44. From 1987 to 1994, deaths associated with the AIDS virus increased an average of 16% per year but then in 1995 and 1996, this number dropped 26% (Wall Street Journal, 1997). The progress reported, though, is largely due to new drugs (protease inhibitors and others) and, perhaps, more effective prevention programs.

According to the Reuters NewMedia (1998), the Centers for Disease Control and Prevention (CDC) reported a decline of 15% in deaths in males, but there was an increased death rate in females (3%). In addition, deaths from AIDS have decreased by 18% in homosexual males while an increase has been reported (3%) in persons infected through heterosexual contacts.

BOX 56-1 AIDS Overview

Human immunodeficiency virus (HIV)

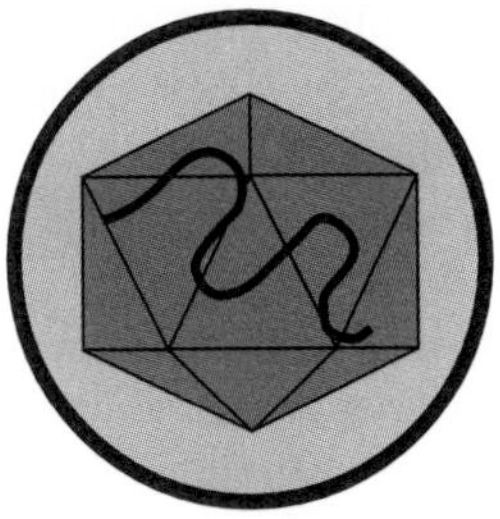

T cell and macrophage infiltration and destruction

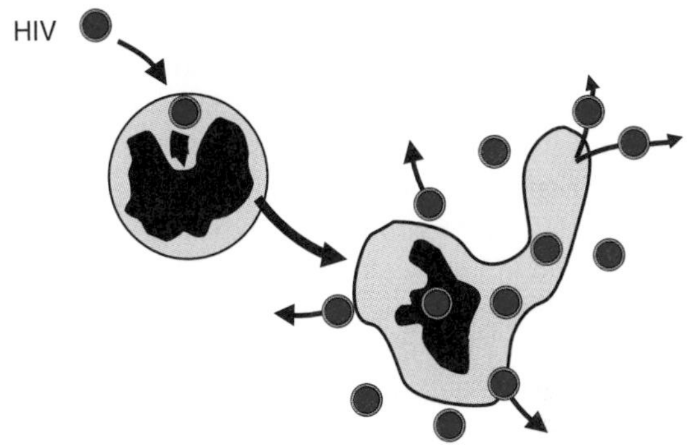

HIV virus enters T cells and macrophages, which, ironically, are the cells the body sent to destroy the virus. By reproduction the virus eventually kills them.

AIDS has no cure. Note that:
- The HIV reproduces faster than any other virus.
- It is present in the bloodstream in very small amounts; thus it is currently hard to target with medications.

AIDS has been diagnosed in:
- All races
- Men, women, and children
- Homosexuals and heterosexuals

AIDS in the Elderly:
- 10% of cases are persons older than 50 years of age; in 1992, 10,000 were older than 60 years of age.
- Majority of patients between the ages of 50 to 59 are homosexual/bisexual; older persons were infected by blood transfusions.
- Older persons with AIDS have much shorter lifespans after diagnosis than younger persons.
- Nearly 50% of all elderly patients with AIDS develop symptoms of dementia (e.g., personality changes, impaired concentration, and apathy [Cowan, 1993]).

AIDS may be acquired by:
- Intravenous drug use with an infected or contaminated needle.
- Sexual contact with an infected person. The virus is transmitted in blood products, semen, breast milk, and vaginal secretions. A small tear in the rectum lining or in the vagina can provide an entrance for the virus.
- AIDS can be transmitted during birth or during breastfeeding, if the mother is AIDS infected.
- HIV-infected persons are not always sick, but they can still transmit the AIDS virus.

Patient Counseling:

To reduce the possibility of infection:
- Allow no exchange of body fluids
- Do not share needles
- Use latex condoms or nonoxynol-9 cream with a condom

Symptoms of HIV infection:
- Fever
- Chills
- Skin rash
- Sore or aching muscles
- Enlarged glands
- Headache
- Weight loss
- Women: chronic vaginal infections; may not have fever, chills, or loss of weight

While the early spread of HIV disease was primarily among homosexual men, IV drug abusers, and persons receiving contaminated blood products, in the last few years disease progression in these populations has declined, and an increased incidence has been reported in heterosexuals, especially females and infants. Most of the pediatric AIDS cases were caused by perinatal transmission. Although AIDS can affect all racial groups, current statistics indicate that the epidemiology of pediatric cases is much more common in black and Hispanic children than in white children (Morse et al, 1996).

The HIV virus is transmitted sexually, via blood and blood products, or from a mother with AIDS to her child during birth. Commercial blood transfusion transmission is considered rare today, but transmission via IV drug abuse is still very common. Current evidence indicates that the AIDS virus is not transmitted by shaking hands, hugging, social kissing, coughing, sneezing, or sharing meals. It is also not contracted from swimming pools, toilet seats, hot tubs, dishes, or via food prepared by persons infected with the AIDS virus. HIV is transmitted by intimate contact with the body fluids of an infected person, which can occur through sex, through sharing of contaminated needles and syringes (drug addicts), from blood or blood product transfusions, and from mother to child before, during, or shortly after birth.

Because healthcare workers with documented invasive exposure to HIV may test positive for the HIV antibody, the CDC has issued guidelines for healthcare workers to follow to minimize the possibility of virus exposure and transfer (Gilden, 1996; Reuters Health Information, 1998). The following is a summary of the recommendations:

- Chemoprophylaxis is recommended when healthcare personnel are exposed to HIV in the workplace, and it is a high-risk exposure (punctured skin). Zidovudine should be included in any antiretroviral regimen with treatment starting promptly, preferably within 1 or 2 hours of exposure.
- A three-drug combination is recommended after exposure to HIV-contaminated blood, that is, zidovudine, lamivudine and indinavir. If the exposure presents a lower degree of risk, such as contact with mucous membrane or skin or exposure to contaminate body fluids other than blood, then two drugs (zidovudine and lamivudine) may be used.
- Information is limited on the effectiveness and toxicity with the use of drugs in postexposure prophylaxis; therefore a consultation with a healthcare professional knowledgeable about these drugs and HIV transmission is suggested, as then risk to benefit can be ascertained.

Of special concern is the finding of a rare AIDS strain (HIV-1 group 0) in a African woman in California (Cooper, 1996). This is the first time this strain was discovered in the United States, and there are fewer than 100 patients known worldwide who are or have been infected with this strain. This strain has mostly been identified in infected people from western or central Africa. The virus that caused the global AIDS epidemic is HIV-1, group M. When compared with the group M population, the group 0 strain does not appear to be different in modes of transmission, progression of disease, or the types of opportunistic infections reported. Additional information about this strain, though, is limited.

As AIDS is a deadly disease and there is no known cure for it at this time, patient teaching should focus on disease prevention.

HIV LIFE CYCLE

Although the pathogenesis of AIDS is not fully understood, HIV infection is an intracellular infection that primarily infests CD4 T lymphocytes. The virus is a retrovirus that has ribonucleic acid (RNA) in its core; therefore after it binds to $CD4^+$ T-lymphocyte receptor cells in the body, it releases its RNA into the cytoplasm. It also has the potential of infecting monocytes and macrophages. Reverse transcriptase, an enzyme carried by HIV, assists in transcribing the HIV RNA into viral DNA strands in the host body. Thereafter activation of this DNA will result in production of viral substances that infect other $CD4^+$ T-lymphocyte cells, leading to the eventual loss of functioning CD4 lymphocytes.

The destroying of the $CD4^+$ helper cells by the virus eventually leads to the immunodeficiency disease known as AIDS. The $CD4^+$ cells are needed directly and indirectly for proper functioning of the human immune system. Both the humoral immune response, which involves antibodies produced by B lymphocytes, and the cellular immune response, which involves stimulation of the cytotoxic T cells (or T8 cells), are mediated by the helper-inducer T cells (Wong, 1993). Therefore a severe decline or destruction of CD4 cells by the HIV is responsible for the multiple symptoms of AIDS: severe suppression of the immune system leading to opportunistic infections and cancers. See Box 56-2 for functions of a T4 helper cell and Fig. 56-2 for T-cell effects in the body.

The revised CDC classification for HIV infection emphasizes the importance of the $CD4^+$ T-lymphocyte count. The system includes all symptomatic and asymptomatic persons with a CD4 count <200 $CD4^+$ T-lymphocytes/µl or a $CD4^+$ T-lymphocyte percentage of total lymphocytes of $<14\%$. This expanded definition has been estimated to result in an increased number of AIDS cases reported initially, thus allowing for better surveillance and earlier interventions for this devastating disease state. Three clinical conditions, pulmonary tuberculosis, recurrent pneumonia, and invasive cervical cancer, have also been added to the previously identified AIDS conditions (CDC, 1992) (Table 56-1).

As the number of $CD4^+$ T lymphocytes declines, the risk and severity of opportunistic infections increase; therefore the use of this system helps to identify persons in need of close medical attention. Instituting antiviral therapy and antimicrobial prophylaxis in correlation with HIV immunosuppression levels as measured by the $CD4^+$ T-lymphocytes has slowed the rate of progression from HIV positive status to AIDS-defined clinical conditions (CDC, 1992). Zidovudine (AZT) was the first antiretroviral agent for treatment of AIDS, but mutations of HIV have developed that resulted in resistance to this drug. The second class of antiretroviral agents, the protease inhibitors, includes ritonavir (Norvir), indinavir (Crixivan), and saquinavir (Invirase).

Ongoing trials with drug combinations (such as AZT and saquinavir or AZT/zalcitabine (ddC) and a protease inhibitor) have shown that these combinations appear to be more effective than the individual drugs alone and may help to delay resistance to the individual agents. Unusual symptoms have been reported since protease inhibitors were added to the drug regimen; they include hyperglycemia or exacerbated cases of diabetes, elevated levels of triglycerides and cholesterol (in some cases, excessive elevations), and changes in body composition, that is, lipodystrophy or abnormal fat accumulations in the back (buffalo hump), breast, and stomach. Patients typically seem to have muscle wasting in the arms, chest, and legs along with their fatty growths in areas such as the upper back and neck (lipomas). Most persons start to develop this condition soon after starting the triple combination drug regimen with protease inhibitors, especially indinavir. Approximately 20 cases of hemolytic anemia have also been reported with indinavir (Huff, 1997/1998). Additional studies will be necessary to determine the short-term and long-term effects of these agents.

The prognosis of HIV disease is variable, with some persons remaining in a fairly stable state for many years. But in the later stages, the breakdown in cellular immunity results in the development of opportunistic infections in the body. (See Table 56-2 for drugs of choice for AIDS-related infections.) In advanced stages of AIDS, most patients usually

BOX 56-2 Functions of a T4 Helper Cell

T4 cells are responsible for a variety of immune functions, some of which include:

1. Release of colony-stimulating factors and lymphokines to stimulate production of leukocytes, such as macrophages and eosinophils.
2. Activation of the natural killer cells (cytotoxic NK cells), which are large lymphocytes in the blood that have non-antigen–specific antitumor and antibacterial properties.
3. T4 helper-inducer cells can activate the T8 suppressor cells, which will stop antibody production, or the T4 suppressor-inducers can activate T8 cytotoxic T cells and stimulate B cells to increase production of antibodies.

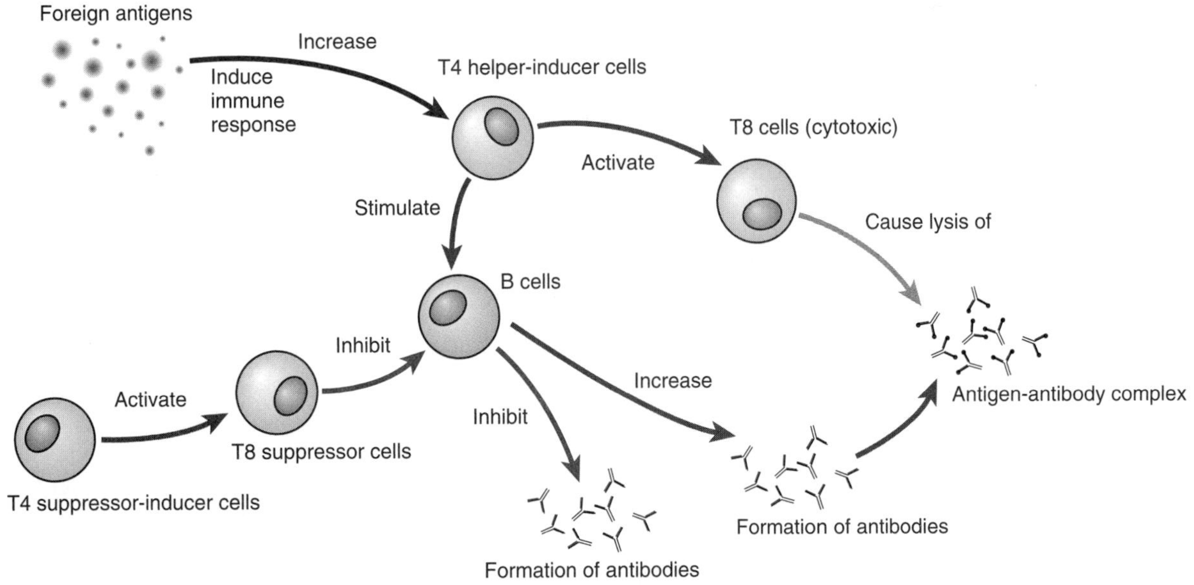

FIGURE 56-2
T4 cell effects in the body. T4 cells are mainly the helper-induces type of cells. They increase when antigens are present. T4 suppressor-inducer cells do not respond to antigens. They act indirectly to suppress antibody function.

TABLE 56-1 1992 Revised Criteria for HIV Classification and AIDS Surveillance*

	CD4+ T-cell Categories		
Clinical categories	**≥500/μl**	**200-499/μl**	**<200/μl**
A. Asymptomatic HIV infection or persistent generalized lymphadenopathy or acute HIV infection with	A1	A2	A3
B. Symptomatic conditions due to HIV infection not in C, i.e.	B1	B2	B3
Bacillary angiomatosis			
Candidiasis, oropharyngeal			
Candidiasis, vulvovaginal (persistent, responds poorly to treatment)			
Cervical dysplasia			
Fever (38.5° C) or diarrhea lasting >1 month			
Hairy oral leukoplakia			
Herpes zoster, two distinct episodes			
Idiopathic thrombocytopenic purpura			
Listeriosis			
Pelvic inflammatory disease (PID)			
Peripheral neuropathy			
C. AIDS indicators	C1	C2	C3
Candidiasis of bronchi, trachea, or lungs			
Candidiasis, esophageal			
Cervical cancer, invasive			
Coccidioidomycosis, disseminated or extrapulmonary			
Cryptococcosis, extrapulmonary			
Cryptosporidiosis, chronic, intestinal (>1 month)			
Cytomegalovirus disease (other than liver, spleen, or nodes)			
Cytomegalovirus retinitis (with vision loss)			
Encephalopathy, HIV related			
Herpes simplex: chronic ulcer(s) (>1 month); or bronchitis, pneumonitis or esophagitis			
Histoplasmosis, disseminated or extrapulmonary			
Isosporiasis, chronic intestinal (>1 month)			
Kaposi's sarcoma			
Lymphoma, Burkitt's, immunoblastic, or primary of brain			
Mycobacterium avium complex or *Mycobacterium kansasii,* disseminated or extrapulmonary			
Mycobacterium tuberculosis, any site			
Mycobacterium other species, disseminated or extrapulmonary			
Pneumocystis carinii pneumonia			
Pneumonia, recurrent			
Progressive multifocal leukoencephalopathy			
Salmonella septicemia, recurrent			
Toxoplasmosis of brain			
Wasting syndrome due to HIV			

*CDC (1992) criteria for persons 13 years of age or older with two or more positive tests for HIV antibodies in addition to a specific antibody supplemental test (e.g., Western blot, immunofluorescence assay), virus isolation test, HIV antigen detection, or positive results from any other highly specific licensed HIV test. The 1993 revised classification system for HIV infection and AIDS surveillance includes the classifications A, B, and C plus numbers 1, 2, or 3. Categories A, B, and C are described under the clinical categories, whereas A3, B3, C1, C2, and C3 are AIDS-indicator conditions. The numbered letters refer to the CD4+ T-cell counts (CDC, 1992).

have a very low helper T-cell count, and the majority die within a few years. Box 56-3 discusses the most common opportunistic infection, *Pneumocystis carinii* pneumonia (PCP).

IMMUNOTHERAPY

Lymphokines (interleukins 1 and 2), interferons (primarily alpha), and granulocyte or granulocyte-macrophage colony-stimulating factors (G-CSF or filgrastim [Neupogen] or GM-CSF-Leukine, [Leucomax]) are under investigation to help the compromised immune system. Lymphokines are protein substances released by sensitized lymphocytes when in contact with specific antigens to activate macrophages to stimulate humoral and cellular immunity for the host. Interleukins have been called the chemical messengers of immune cell communication. Interleukin 2 is believed to be a T-cell growth factor that promotes the long-term survival and growth of the T lymphocytes, which is necessary for the continuation of the immune response and is also involved in the rejection of transplanted organs. Although some persons have been helped with these therapies, to date the data on their effectiveness are conflicting and, at least in some instances, adjuvant therapies were required (Morse et al, 1996).

TABLE 56-2 Drugs of Choice for AIDS-related Infections

AIDS-related Infections	*Syndrome*	*Drugs*
Fungal Infections		
Candidiasis (oral thrush)	Presents as white plaque-type lesions on sides of tongue; may present as sore throat, difficulty swallowing, and pain near sternum	nystatin suspension, troches or clotrimazole (Mycelex) or ketoconazole (Nizoral)
Cryptococcus meningitis	Headache, fever, nausea, vomiting, photophobia, stiff neck, seizures, mental status changes	amphotericin B (Fungizone IV) plus flucytosine (Ancobon)
Viral Infections		
Cytomegalovirus (CMV)	Serious infection; can be life-threatening; affects eyes (can cause blindness), CNS, lungs and GI tract	ganciclovir (Cytovene) and foscarnet (Foscavir)
Herpes simplex virus (HSV)	Persistent or recurrent disseminated skin ulceration; encephalitis, perioral, and perianal lesions may occur	acyclovir (Zovirax) or vidarabine (Vira-A)
Mycobacterial Infections		
Mycobacterium avium complex (MAC)	Common infection in AIDS; may be asymptomatic or symptomatic with GI symptoms, fever, weight loss, anemia	multidrug therapy such as clarithromycin (Biaxin) and ethambutol (Myambutol)
Mycobacterium tuberculosis	Pulmonary and extrapulmonary tuberculosis seen in this population	multidrug therapy with isoniazid, pyrazinamide, rifampin (Rifadin), and ethambutol (Myambutol)
Protozoal Infections		
Pneumocystis carinii pneumonia (PCP)	See Box 56-3	
Toxoplasmosis gondii	Encephalitis, brain abscess, focal neurologic problems, seizures, headaches, lethargy	sulfadiazine, pyrimethamine

BOX 56-3 *Pneumocystis carinii* pneumonia (PCP)

Pneumocystis carinii pneumonia is a common infection in persons with bone marrow transplants and AIDS. Untreated PCP has a high mortality rate.

Symptoms

Fever; dry, persistent, nonproductive cough; shallow breathing; progressive shortness of breath; weight loss; night sweats.

Treatment

Active Infection

TMP-SMX*, IV or PO: 15 to 20 mg TMP/kg/day and 75 to 100 mg/kg/day SMX in four divided doses for 2 to 3 weeks. Pentamidine IV (Pentam 300): 4 mg/kg/day administered over 60 to 90 minutes for 2 to 3 weeks. Atovaquone (Mepron): 750 mg every 8 hours for 3 weeks. Trimetrexate (Neutrexin), a dihydrofolate reductase inhibitor: 45 mg/m^2 every 6 hours for 3 weeks. This product may be given with sulfadiazine: 1 g every 6 hours for 3 weeks.

Prophylaxis

TMP-SMX PO: 160 mg of TMP with 800 mg of SMX daily twice a day or three times a week (Morse et al, 1996).
Pentamidine inhalation (NebuPent): 300 mg once a month (Olin, 1998).

*TMP-SMX, trimethoprim-sulfamethoxazole (Co-Trimoxazole).

SUMMARY

Immunosuppressants and immunomodulators are agents that decrease or modify an immune system response. Research in this area is ongoing and extensive with the potential for release of many more new pharmacologic agents in the next few years. Healthcare professionals must strive to remain current in this area, as the disease states discussed in this chapter may be devastating and even fatal for the individual.

REVIEW QUESTIONS

1. Describe the body's response to the introduction of a foreign substance or an organ transplant. What cells are necessary for cellular immunity and for antibody production?
2. Explain why live virus vaccines should be avoided in patients receiving an immunosuppressant drug.
3. Describe gingival hyperplasia. Which drug in this chapter is reported to cause it? What advice might you give a patient concerning this adverse effect?
4. Present the three recommendations issued by the CDC for the treatment of healthcare workers exposed to HIV.
5. Name and describe the unusual symptoms reported since protease inhibitors have been added to drug combinations used to treat HIV/AIDS.

REFERENCES

Centers for Disease Control and Prevention (CDC): 1993 revised classification for HIV infection and expanded surveillance case definition for AIDS among adolescents and adults, *MMWR* 41(RR-17):1, 1992.

Cooper, M: Rare AIDS strain found for first time in U.S., AEGIS (AIDS Education Global Information System), http://www.aegis.com/aegis/news/re/re1996/re960729.html (July 21, 1998).

Gilden D: Post-exposure prophylaxis for health care workers, *GMHC Treat Iss Newslett Exp AIDS Ther* 10(6/7):20, 1996.

Huff A: Protease inhibitor side effects take people by surprise, *GMHC Treat Iss Newslett Exp AIDS Ther* 12(1):25-27, 1997/1998.

Morse GD, Shelton MJ, O'Donnell AM: Human immunodeficiency virus (HIV) infection. In Young LY, Koda-Kimble MA, editors: *Applied therapeutics: the clinical use of drugs,* ed 6, Vancouver, Wash, 1995, Applied Therapeutics, Inc.

Olin BR: *Facts and comparisons.* Philadelphia, 1998, JB Lippincott.

Reuters Health Information Sustems: New CDC guidelines for occupational HIV exposure, AEGIS (AIDS Education Global Information System), http://www.aegis.com/aegis/news/re/re1996/re960630.html July 21, 1998).

Reuters NewMedia: U.S. reports first-ever decline in AIDS deaths, AEGIS (AIDS Education Global Information System), http://www.aegis.com/aegis/news/re/re1997/re970294.html and re970292.html (July 21, 1998).

United States Pharmacopeial Convention: *USP DI: drug information for the health care professional,* ed 18, Rockville, Md, 1998, The Convention.

Wall Street Journal: AIDS study shows drop of 26% in mortality rate, *Wall Street Journal,* September 23, 1997, AEGIS (AIDS Education Global Information System), http://www.aegis.com/aegis/news/wsj/wj1997/wj970902.html (July 21, 1998).

Wong RJ: Treating HIV infection: What pharmacists need to know, *Am Pharm* NS33(5):57, 1993.

ADDITIONAL REFERENCES

American Hospital Formulary Service: *AHFS drug information '98,* Bethesda, Md, 1998, American Society of Hospital Pharmacists.

Anderson KN et al, editors: *Mosby's medical, nursing, and allied health dictionary,* ed 5, St Louis, 1998, Mosby.

Cowan K: AIDS in the elderly, *Geriatr Med Curr* 14(1):4, 1993.

Gilden D: Protease inhibitor new math, *GMHC Treat Iss Newslett Exp AIDS Ther* 10(5):3-6, 1996.

Henahan S: Resistance fighters, *Drug Top* 139(16):32-33, 1995.

Jahansouz F, Kriett JM: Transplantation: a review of immunosuppressive agents, *Crit Care Nurs Q* 15(4):13-22, 1993.

Mosby: *Mosby's GenRx,* St Louis, 1998, Mosby.

Mudge-Grout CL: *Immunologic disorders,* St Louis, 1992, Mosby.

Project Inform: The new era in AIDS treatment, *PI Perspect* 18:1-8, 1996.

Tartaglione TA et al: Principles and management of the acquired immunodeficiency syndrome. In DiPiro JT, Talber R et al, editors: *Pharmacotherapy, a pathophysiologic approach,* ed 2, Norwalk, Conn, 1993, Appleton & Lange.

UNIT XVI

Drugs Affecting the Integumentary System

CHAPTER 57

Overview of the Integumentary System

CHAPTER FOCUS

The skin is the largest organ of the body. It is combined with hair, nails, and glands to form the integumentary system. The primary function of the skin is to serve as a barrier with the environment; that is, it protects the body from microorganisms, ultraviolet light, and loss of body fluids. It also helps in the regulation of body temperature and the production of vitamin D, and topical medications are administered via skin application. The healthcare professional must know the structure and function of the skin to understand the topical agents used in treatment.

KEY TERMS

apocrine glands, (p. 740)
dermis, (p. 740)
eccrine glands, (p. 740)
epidermis, (p. 740)
exocrine glands, (p. 740)
melanin, (p. 740)
sebaceous glands, (p. 740)

OBJECTIVES

After reading and studying this chapter, the student should be able to do the following:

1. *Define and describe the key terms.*
2. *Describe the structure of the skin.*
3. *Name and describe the three types of exocrine glands.*
4. *Relate the five major functions of the skin.*
5. *Name three skin appendages.*

The skin (or integument) has been described as the largest organ in the body. In most disease states, medications are administered at a site that is distant from the target organ, but in dermatology, medications can be directly applied to the target site. Because skin functions are vital to an individual's survival and also quite diverse, this chapter reviews the structure of the skin, functions of the skin, and skin appendages (Fig. 57-1).

STRUCTURE OF THE SKIN

The skin is made up of two layers, the epidermis and the dermis. The **epidermis,** or outer skin layer, consists of four strata or layers.

1. Stratum corneum (horny layer). This layer consists of outer dead cells that have been converted to keratin, a water-repellent protein and forms a protective cover for the body. It will desquamate or shed and be replaced by new cells from the bottom layers.
2. Stratum lucidum or clear layer. This area contains translucent flat cells; keratin is formed here.
3. Stratum granulosum or granular layer. Granules are located in the cytoplasm of these cells. Cells die in this layer of skin.
4. Stratum germinativum. This has been divided into two layers in some references; the top layer is the stratum spinosum, and the innermost layer is the stratum basale. The latter two names were devised to describe the cellular structure of the two layers: stratum spinosum contains spinelike cells, whereas stratum basale has column-shaped cells. The cells in the latter area germinate; they undergo cellular mitosis to generate new cells for the skin.

Melanocytes, which are responsible for synthesizing **melanin,** a skin color pigment that occurs naturally in the hair and skin, are also located deep in the stratum germinativum. The more melanin that is present, the deeper the brown skin color. Melanin also is a protective agent; it blocks ultraviolet rays, thus preventing injury to underlying dermis and tissues.

The epidermis has no direct blood supply of its own; it is nourished only by diffusion. The **dermis** lies between the epidermis and subcutaneous fat. It is approximately 40 times thicker than the epidermis, and it contains and provides skin support from its blood vessels, nerves, lymphatic tissue, and elastic and connective tissues. The two main divisions of the dermis are the papillary dermis and the reticular dermis. Sweat glands, sebaceous glands, and hair follicles originate in the reticular dermis, and their structures branch out in the papillary dermis.

Below the dermis layer is the hypodermis or subcutaneous layer, which contributes flexibility to the skin. Subcutaneous fat tissue is an area for thermal insulation, nutrition, and cushioning or padding.

The skin contains three types of **exocrine glands:** sebaceous, eccrine, and apocrine. These exocrine glands are multicellular glands that open on the surface of the skin through ducts in the epithelium.

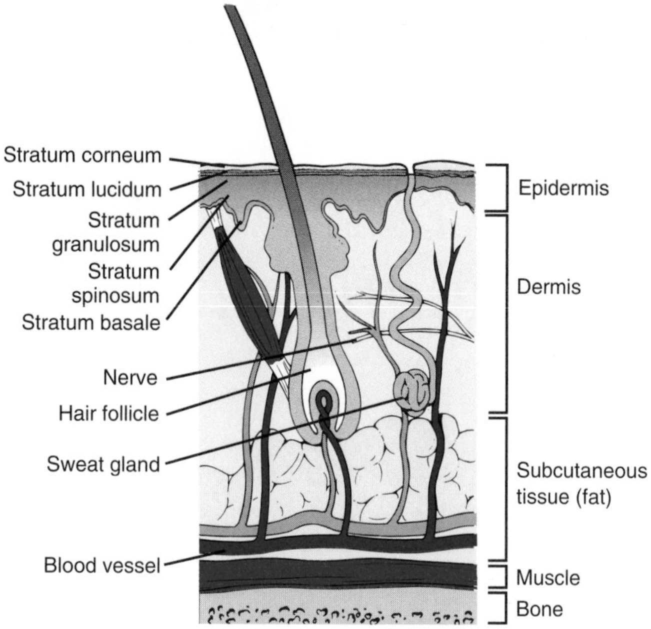

FIGURE 57-1
Structures of the skin.

Sebaceous glands are large, lipid-containing cells that produce sebum, the oil or film layer that covers the epidermis, especially abundant in the scalp, face, anus, and external ear. This protects and lubricates the skin, so it is not only water repellent but also has some antiseptic effects. The sebaceous fluid travels by way of a short duct (sebaceous duct) to the hair follicles in the upper dermis. Thus hair, which is located everywhere on the skin except the palms, soles, and mucous membrane tissues, is lubricated.

The **eccrine glands,** or sweat glands, are also widely distributed on the skin surface, including the soles and palms. These glands help to regulate body temperature by promoting cooling by evaporation of their secretion and also help to prevent excessive skin dryness.

The **apocrine glands** are located mainly in the axillae, genital organs, and breast areas. They are odoriferous and are believed to represent scent or sex glands.

Normal skin pH is 4.5 to 5.5, which is weakly acidic. This acid mantle is a protective mechanism because microorganisms grow best at pH 6 to 7.5. Infected areas of the skin usually have a higher pH.

FUNCTIONS OF THE SKIN

The skin serves many functions in the body. Some of the major functions are listed here.

- *Protective function.* The skin forms a protective covering for the entire body. It protects the internal organs and their environment from external forces. Thus it is a barrier against microorganism and chemical body invasion.
- *Organ of sensation.* Nerve endings permit the transfer of stimuli sensations, such as heat, cold, pressure, and pain.

- *Body temperature regulator.* It maintains a body temperature homeostasis by regulating heat loss or heat conservation. Blood vessels in the dermis area can dilate, and perspiration increases when the body temperature is elevated. If the body temperature is below normal, the skin blood vessels constrict, and perspiration is decreased to conserve body heat.

Skin excretes fluid and electrolytes (sweat glands), stores fat, synthesizes vitamin D (when skin is exposed to sunlight or ultraviolet rays, the steroid 7-dehydrocholesterol, which is normally present in the skin, is converted to vitamin D_3), and provides a site for drug absorption. Fat-soluble vitamins (A, D, E, and K), estrogens, corticoid hormones, and some chemicals can be absorbed through skin.

Skin contributes to the concept of body image and a feeling of well-being. A disfiguring skin condition can lead to emotional problems, and a chronic skin condition may also lead to depression.

APPENDAGES OF THE SKIN

The appendages of the skin are the hair, nails, and skin glands. These areas are discussed when drug therapy is specific for these sites.

SUMMARY

The skin combined with hair, nails, and glands forms the integumentary system. The largest organ of the body, it consists of two layers and serves as a barrier to the external environment. It also helps in body temperature regulation and production of vitamin D and serves as the site for topical drug application for the treatment of a variety of dermatologic problems. These drugs will be discussed in the next chapter.

REVIEW QUESTIONS

1. Describe how the skin protects the individual from a high temperature on a hot summer day.
2. What other protective functions are provided by the skin?
3. What is the skin's pH? Microorganisms grow best at what pH?

REFERENCES

Anderson KN et al, editors: *Mosby's medical, nursing, and allied health dictionary,* ed 5, St Louis, 1998, Mosby.

McCance KL, Huether SE: *Pathophysiology: the biologic basis for disease in adults and children,* ed 3, St Louis, 1998, Mosby.

Thibodeau GA, Patton KT: *Anatomy and physiology,* ed 4, St Louis, 1999, Mosby.

Van Wynsberghe D, Noback CR, Carola R: *Human anatomy and physiology,* ed 3, New York, 1995, McGraw-Hill.

CHAPTER 58

Dermatologic Drugs

CHAPTER FOCUS

As the skin is the largest organ in the body, skin disorders are common and can involved both physical and biochemical alterations. Numerous preparations are available to treat and, in some instances, prevent the skin reaction or disorder. This chapter reviews the various topical products available such as sunscreen preparations and therapeutic agents used to treat specific skin problems.

KEY TERMS

antipruritic, (p. 756)
ectoparasites, (p. 756)
keratolytics, (p. 753)
sun protection factor (SPF), (p. 749)

OBJECTIVES

After reading and studying this chapter, the student should be able to do the following:

1. *Define and describe the key terms.*
2. *Relate the principles of skin absorption.*
3. *Describe six different types of lesions and the conditions or diseases associated with them.*
4. *Discuss the general goals of therapy.*
5. *Name and describe the three life-threatening drug-induced eruptions.*
6. *Describe the general properties of dermatologic preparations and their indications, including baths, soaps, solutions, lotions, and cleansers.*
7. *Define and name a topical keratolytic, acne, and ectoparasiticidal agent.*
8. *Name three drugs that reportedly cause photosensitivity. Define photosensitivity.*

Many dermatologic preparations are available to treat the numerous common skin disorders. Often particular ointments, creams, powders, or specific vehicles provide a desired effect without the addition of an active ingredient. For example, for the person with dry, scaly skin found in psoriasis or dry eczema, an ointment with an occlusive emollient effect is desired, such as lanolin or a synthetic base. The person with a moist or dry skin condition may receive a cooling emollient preparation that is also moisturizing, such as a cream formulation.

The individual with an acute inflammation that is weeping or oozing often needs a drying and soothing lotion, such as a saline solution, aluminum acetate solution, or calamine lotion. A lichenified, oozing skin problem (eczema) may need a protective and drying agent such as coal tar paste, Lassar's paste, or zinc compound paste. If the skin problem is sore, wet, and located on an elbow or knee, then a dusting powder such as talcum or starch may be appropriate to reduce friction and help dry the area.

SKIN DISORDERS

Reactions or disorders of the skin are manifested by symptoms such as itching, pain, or tingling and by signs such as swelling, redness, papules, pustules, blisters, and hives. Some common dermatologic disorders in the United States and Canada include acne vulgaris (cystic acne and acne scars), atopic dermatitis, eczema, folliculitis, fungus infections, herpes simplex, lichen simplex chronicus, psoriasis, seborrheic dermatitis, verruca (warts), and vitiligo.

A reaction of the skin that makes the individual uncomfortable or unsightly may be due to sensitivity to drugs, allergy, infection, emotional conflict, genetic disease (e.g., atopic eczema or psoriasis), hormonal imbalance, or degenerative disease. Sometimes the cause of the skin disorder is unknown and the treatment may be empiric in the hope that the right remedy will be found.

Dermatologic diagnosis includes physical assessment, personal and family medical history, drug history including over-the-counter (OTC) medications, and laboratory tests, cytodiagnosis, and biopsy.

When the nature of the lesion has been established, its characteristics should be defined according to size, shape, surface, and color (Box 58-1).

The next step is to discover the distribution of the condition because a diagnosis can at times be made from the distribution alone. However, it should not be inferred that because a disease is not found in its usual pattern of distribution, it can be ruled out as a possible diagnosis. For example, psoriasis is commonly found on the extensors, but occasionally it will be seen as a solitary lesion in the external ear. A basal cell carcinoma is most common on the face, but occasionally it occurs on the trunk. On the other hand, rosacea only attacks those areas of the face that flush.

Box 58-2 is a summary of the vast number of dermatologic reactions caused by drugs and their characteristic lesions and sequelae. Some may even be life-threatening. See Table 58-1 for the most common drugs involved in life-threatening drug-induced skin eruptions.

The healthcare professional always needs to be cognizant of the patient's drug history and current therapy to relate such lesions and sequelae to the appropriate cause because simply discontinuing a particular drug often resolves a complicated dermatologic problem or sequelae of unknown origin.

1. Eczema and dermatitis are noninfectious inflammatory dermatoses. Contact dermatitis has clinical features that include skin rash with eczema (red, thick, crusty, fissured, suppurating area) in various stages. The causes may be contact with a primary irritant (acids, oils, and soaps) in the environment, home, or work place or a delayed allergic reaction (as seen with poison ivy contact).
2. Atopic dermatitis appears as a general eczema dermatitis usually on the flexor body surfaces; it has genetic associations with hay fever or asthma.
3. Seborrheic dermatitis often appears on the scalp, eyebrows, ears, or sternum as a brown to red scaly rash.
4. Stasis dermatitis, often preceding a venous stasis ulcer, is found on the lower legs secondary to venous stasis and poor vascularity and is brown and eczematous in appearance.
5. Papulosquamous eruptions are noninfectious inflammatory dermatoses that include urticaria (hives), psoriasis, pityriasis rosea, lichen planus, and exfoliative dermatitis. The healthcare professional will see acute urticaria as an insidious-appearing, itchy erythematous wheal resulting from an allergen. Chronic urticaria appears as a large hive without the sensation of itch or pruritus and is often accompanied by angioneurotic edema.
6. Psoriasis often appears as erythematous plaques and orange-red-brown lesions covered with silvery scales. Psoriasis is often found on the scalp and extensor surfaces of the limbs and neck. Often the nails become thick and irregular.
7. Pityriasis rosea is a self-limited oval salmon-colored patch that follows the axis of skin cleavage lines. The major patches appear on the trunk, and smaller scales appear on the peripheral areas.
8. Infectious inflammatory dermatoses include viral diseases (verruca [wart], herpes simplex, and varicella zoster/chickenpox), bacterial diseases (impetigo, folliculitis, and furuncle [boil]), and fungal diseases. Herpes simplex and infectious inflammatory dermatoses appear as vesicles with an inflamed base and have an incubation period of up to 2 weeks in the primary infection. Late antibody development occurs. The herpes virus type 1 affects skin and the oral cavity while herpes virus type 2 affects the skin of neonates and genital mucosa. The recurrent infection is a reactivation of the older infection or new infection; antibodies appear early.
9. Fungal diseases, which include tinea or dermatophytosis, appear in the following various clinical classifications: tinea capitis (caused by either a *Trichophyton* or *Micros-*

BOX 58-1 Different Types of Lesions and Some Conditions Associated with Them

Macule: flat; nonpalpable; circumscribed; less than 1 cm in diameter; brown, red, purple, white, or tan in color
Examples: freckles; flat moles; rubella; rubeola; drug eruptions

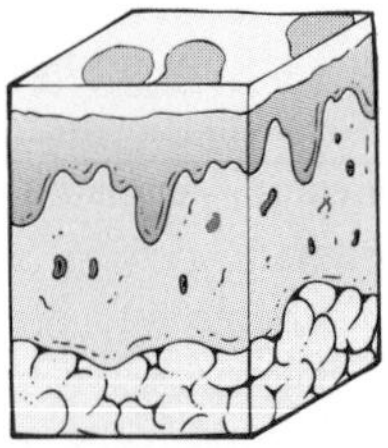

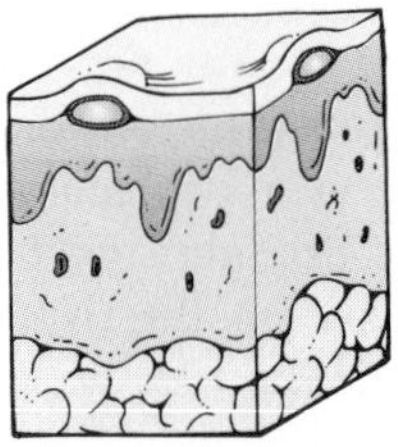

Vesicle: elevated; circumscribed; superficial; filled with serous fluid; less than 1 cm in diameter
Examples: blister; varicella

Papule: elevated; palpable; firm; circumscribed; less than 1 cm in diameter; brown, red, pink, tan, or bluish red in color
Examples: warts; drug-related eruptions; pigmented nevi; eczema

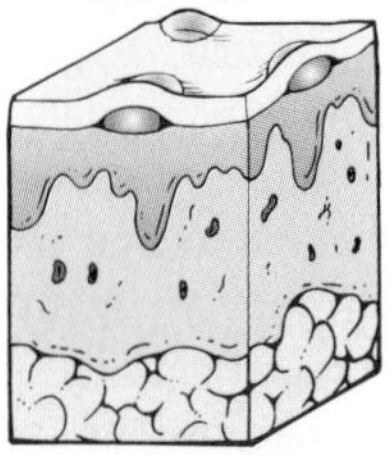

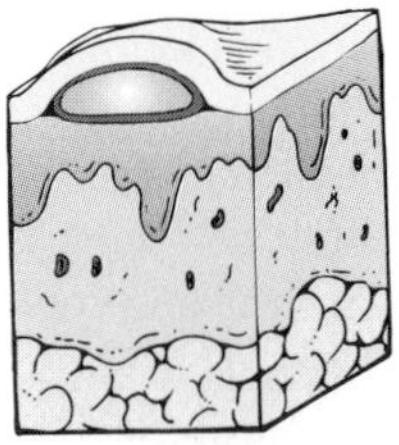

Bulla: vesicle greater than 1 cm in diameter
Examples: blister; pemphigus vulgaris

Plaque: elevated; flat topped; firm; rough; superficial papule greater than 1 cm in diameter, may be coalesced papules
Example: psoriasis; seborrheic and actinic keratoses; eczema

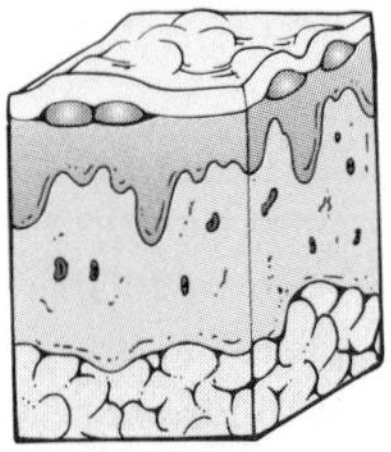

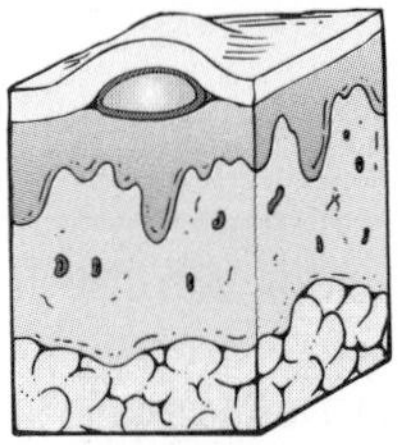

Pustule: elevated; superficial; similar to vesicle but filled with purulent fluid
Examples: impetigo; acne; variola; herpes zoster

Wheal: elevated, irregular-shaped area of cutaneous edema; solid, transient, changing variable diameter; pale pink in color
Examples: urticaria; insect bites

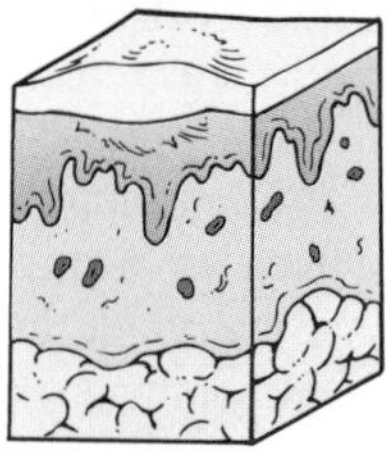

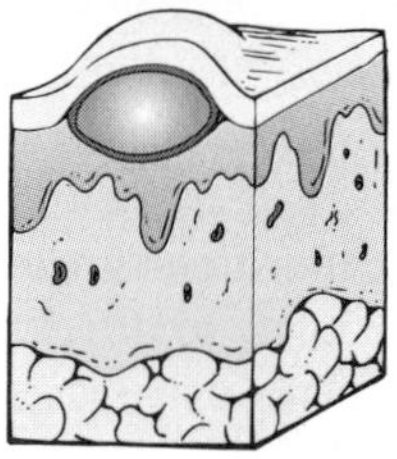

Cyst: elevated; circumscribed; palpable; encapsulated; filled with liquid or semisolid material
Example: sebaceous cyst

Nodule: elevated; firm; circumscribed; palpable; deeper in dermis than papule; 1 to 2 cm in diameter
Examples: erythema nodosum; lipomas

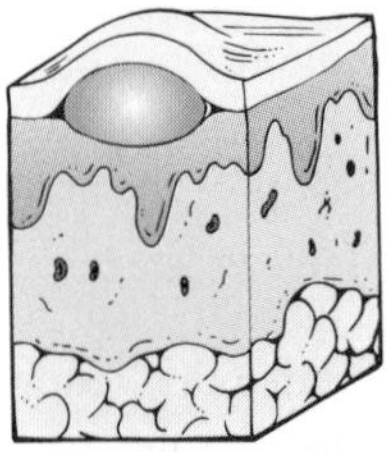

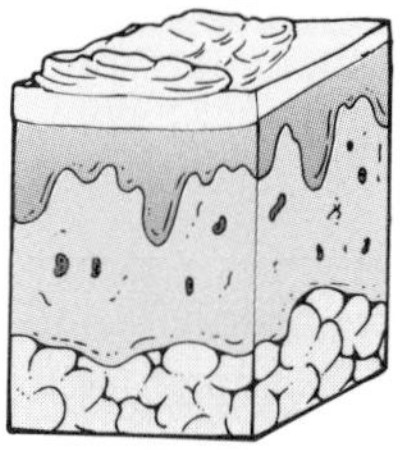

Scale: heaped-up keratinized cells; flaky exfoliation; irregular; thick or thin; dry or oily; varied size; silver, white, or tan in color
Examples: psoriasis; exfoliative dermatitis

Tumor: elevated; solid; may or may not be clearly demarcated; greater than 2 cm in diameter; may or may not vary from skin color
Example: neoplasms

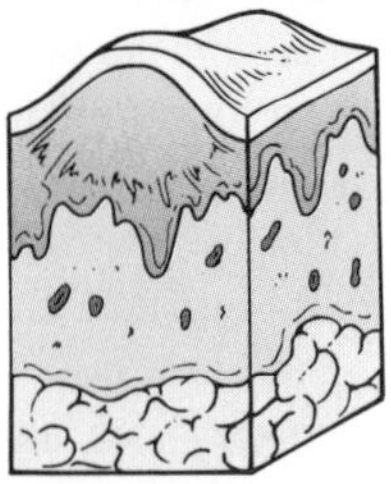

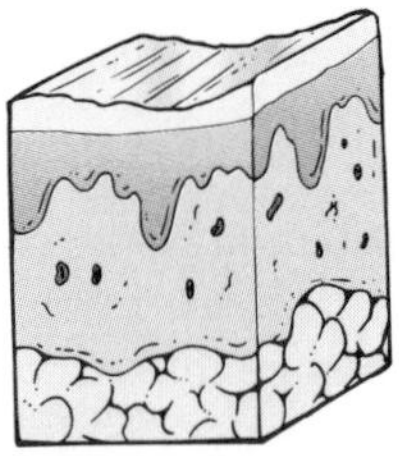

Lichenification: rough, thickened epidermis; accentuated skin markings due to rubbing or irritation; often involves flexor aspect of extremity
Example: chronic dermatitis

From Beare, Myers, 1998.

porum fungal infection in children or adults); tinea corporis (or *Microsporum* in children; *Trichophyton* in adults); tinea cruris *(Epidermophyton* or *Trichophyton);* and tinea pedis; onychomycosis *(Trichophyton);* and tinea versicolor *(Malassezia furfur).* Tinea or dermatophytosis often appears as a scaly erythematous circular lesion. Tinea versicolor appears as a brown discoloration. Breaking of the hair is seen in tinea capitis or tinea barbae, and with onychomycosis the patient has thick, discolored nails.

As previously stated, so many dermatologic products are available that it would be difficult to discuss them all in this

BOX 58-2 Common Drug-Induced Dermatologic Conditions

Drugs Causing an Acneform Reaction

ACTH
androgenic hormones
corticosteroids
cyanocobalamin
hydantoins
iodides
methyltestosterone
oral contraceptives

Drugs Causing Purpura

ACTH
allopurinol
amitriptyline
anticoagulants
barbiturates
carbamides
chloral hydrate
chlorothiazide
chlorpropamide
chlorpromazine
corticosteroids
digitalis
fluoxymesterone
gold salts
griseofulvin
iodides
meprobamate
penicillin
quinidine
rifampin
sulfonamides
thiazides
trifluoperazine

Drugs Causing Urticaria

ACTH
amitriptyline
barbiturates
chloramphenicol
dextran
enzymes
erythromycin
griseofulvin
hydantoins
insulin
iodides
meperidine
meprobamate
mercurials
nitrofurantoin
opioids
penicillin
penicillinase
pentazocine
phenolphthalein
phenothiazines
propoxyphene
rifampin
salicylates
serums
streptomycin
sulfonamides
tetracyclines
thiouracil

Drugs Causing Alopecia

alkylating agents
anticoagulants
antimetabolites
bleomycin
mephenytoin
methimazole
methotrexate
norethindrone acetate
quinacrine
oral contraceptives
warfarin
trimethadione

Drugs Causing Morbilliform Reactions

anticonvulsants
anticholinergics
antihistamines
barbiturates
chloral hydrate
chlordiazepoxide
chlorothiazide
gold salts
griseofulvin
hydantoins
insulin
meprobamate
mercurials
p-aminosalicylic acid
penicillin
phenothiazines
quinacrine
salicylates
serums
streptomycin
sulfonamides
sulfones
tetracyclines
thiouracil

Drugs Causing Lichenoid Reactions

chloroquine
gold salts compounds
p-aminosalicylic acid
quinacrine
quinidine
thiazides

Drugs Causing Fixed Eruptions

acetylsalicylic acid
amphetamine sulfate
anthralin
antipyrine
barbiturates
belladonna
bismuth salts
chloral hydrate
chloroquine
chlorothiazide and sun
chlorpromazine
chlortetracycline
dextroamphetamine
diethylstilbestrol
digitalis
dimenhydrinate
diphenhydramine
disulfiram and alcohol
ephedrine
epinephrine
ergot alkaloids

Continued

BOX 58-2 Common Drug-Induced Dermatologic Conditions—cont'd

Drugs Causing Fixed Eruptions—cont'd

erythrocin
eucalyptus oil
gold compounds
griseofulvin
iodine
ipecac
karaya gum
magnesium hydroxide
meprobamate
mercury salts
methenamine
opioids
oxytetracycline
p-aminosalicylic acid
penicillin
phenobarbital
phenolphthalein
phenytoin
potassium chlorate
quinacrine
quinidine
quinine
reserpine
salicylates
saccharin
scopolamine
sodium salicylate
streptomycin
sulfadiazine
sulfapyridine
sulfathiazole
sulfisoxazole
sulfonamides
tetracyclines
tripelennamine
vaccines and immunizing agents

Drugs Causing Contact Dermatitis

antihistamines
atabrine
bacitracin
benzocaine
bleomycin
chloramphenicol
chlorhexidine
chlorphenesin
chlorpromazine
diphenhydramine
ephedrine
formaldehyde
iodine
isoniazid
lanolin
meprobamate
mercurials
neomycin
nitrofurazone
novobiocin
p-aminosalicylic acid
parabens
penicillin
peru balsam
phenindamine
phenol
procaine and other anesthetics
promethazine
quinacrine
quinine
resorcin
streptomycin
sulfonamides
tetracyclines
thiamine
thimerosal

Photosensitizers

acetohexamide
aminobenzoic acid
anesthetics (procaine group)
antimalarials
barbiturates
benzene
bergamot (perfume)
carbamazepine
carbinoxamine d-form
carrots, wild
cedar oil
celery
chlorophyll
citrus fruits
clover
coal tar
contraceptives, oral
corticosteroids, topical
cyproheptadine
desipramine
diethylstilbestrol
digalloyl trioleate (sunscreen)
dill
diphenhydramine
disopyramide
dyes (methylene blue, toluidine blue)
estrone
fennel
fluorescein dyes
5-fluorouracil
gold salts
grass (meadow)
griseofulvin
haloperidol
lavender oil
lime oil
9-mercaptopurine
methotrimeprazine
methoxsalen
methoxypsoralen
mustards
nalidixic acid
naphthalene
oral contraceptives
parsley
parsnips
phenolic compounds
phenothiazines
phenytoin
porphyrins
promethazine
pyrazinamide
quinethazone
quinidine
quinine
salicylanilides
salicylates
sandalwood oil (perfume)
silver salts
sulfonamides
sulfonylureas (antidiabetics)
tetracyclines
thiazide diuretics
tolbutamide
toluene
tricyclic antidepressants
tridione
trimethadione
vanillin oils
xylene

TABLE 58-1 Life-threatening Drug-induced Skin Eruptions

Skin Eruption	***Description***	***Drugs Involved***
Exfoliative dermatitis	Entire surface of skin is red and scaly and will eventually slough off. Hair and nails may also be affected. Eruption may take weeks or months to resolve after causative agent is stopped. If not resolved, it may be fatal.	barbiturates, carbamazepine, demeclocycline, furosemide, gold, griseofulvin, penicillin, phenothiazines, phenytoin, sulfonamides, tetracyclines
Stevens-Johnson syndrome (erythema multiforme)	Severe form that involves widespread eruptions or lesions usually on face, neck, arms, legs, hands, and feet. May also involve mucosa, may produce fever and malaise. Syndrome may last months and is life-threatening.	May result from use of many drugs, especially carbamazepine, penicillin, phenytoin, sulfonamides, tetracyclines
Lupus erythematosus	Erythematous rash that may be flat or elevated (butterfly) on cheek (malar), and across nose. Joint swelling and pain, rash, oral ulcers, serositis, renal, hematologic, pulmonary, and other systems may be affected. Reversible when drug is stopped.	hydantoins, hydralazine, isoniazid, procainamide, quinidine, trimethadione

BOX 58-3 Principles of Skin Absorption

Keratin in the outer skin layer provides a waterproof barrier. To enhance drug absorption, the epidermis, or keratin skin layer, needs to be hydrated. Therefore some medications are placed under an occlusive dressing (such as plastic wrap) or administered in an occlusive type of ointment (petroleum jelly) because both will trap and prevent water loss (sweat) from the skin, thus increasing epidermis hydration.

Fat- or lipid-soluble drugs are better absorbed through skin than water-soluble drugs.

In specific body areas, the skin is very thin (eyelids, scrotum area, or the skin of a child) or very thick. The palms of the hands or soles of feet are nearly impenetrable by topical agents.

Products with alcohol content may be administered for drying effects.

Steroid products thin the skin and many are contraindicated for the face, groin, and axillae. Fluorinated steroids should not be used for these areas. If a steroid is necessary, hydrocortisone is generally recommended.

BOX 58-4 General Goals of Therapy

Identify and remove the cause of the skin disorder, if possible.

Institute measures to restore and maintain the structure and normal function of the skin.

Relieve symptoms that are produced by the disorder, such as itching, dryness, pain, and infection.

chapter. For the sake of simplicity, this chapter discusses three selected groups of dermatologic products: general, prophylactic agents, and therapeutic agents. Some general dermatologic products include those previously discussed, as well as solutions, baths, soaps, wet dressings, and soaks. See Box 58-3 for the principles of skin absorption and Box 58-4 for general goals of therapy.

Prophylactic agents include sunscreens, protectives, and antiseptics and disinfectants. Therapeutic agents include antiinfectives, antiinflammatory corticosteroids, keratolytic agents, acne products, stimulants and irritants, topical anesthetics, burn products for second- and third-degree burns, antiaging products, and ectoparasiticidal topical drugs.

GENERAL DERMATOLOGIC PREPARATIONS

This section refers to single and combination formulations used as bath preparations, cleansers, soaps, solutions and lotions, emollients, skin protectants, wet dressings and soaks, and rubs and liniments.

BATHS

Baths may be used to cleanse the skin, medicate, or reduce temperature. The usual method of cleansing the skin is by the use of soap and water, but this may not be tolerated in skin diseases. In some cases even water is not tolerated, and inert oils must be substituted. Persons with dry skin should bathe less frequently than those with oily skin. Frequent bathing tends to stimulate oil production, causing oily skin to remain oily. It is possible to keep the skin clean without a daily bath. For dry skin, an oily lotion is preferable to alcohol (isopropyl or ethyl).

To render baths soothing in irritative conditions, oatmeal, starch, or gelatin may be added; usually 1 to 2 oz per gallon of water. Oils such as Alpha-Keri and oilated oatmeal in a proportion of 1 oz to a tub of water decrease the drying effect of water and helps relieve the itching of a sensitive, xerotic skin. A lubricating topical medication or bland emollient should be applied immediately after the bath while the skin is still moist because this increases absorption and hydration.

SOAPS

Ordinary soap, the sodium salt of palmitic, oleic, or stearic acids alone or in a mixture, is made by saponifying fats or oils with alkalies. The oil used for castile soap is supposed to be olive oil; some soaps are made with coconut oil. The consistency of the soap depends on the major acid and alkali used.

Although all soaps are relatively alkaline, an excess of free alkali or acid is a potential source of skin irritation. Medicated soaps contain antiseptics, but soaps per se are antiseptic only to the degree that they mechanically clean the skin. Many people believe that soap and water are bad for the complexion, which is erroneous because a clean skin helps to promote a healthy skin. The soap used in maintaining a clean skin should be mild and contain a minimum of irritating materials. Perfumed or medicated soaps may be harmful if the skin is extrasensitive to soap products, if the soap is not adequately rinsed off the skin, if it stimulates excess production of natural skin oils, or if it dries the skin excessively. Soaps are irritating to mucous membranes, and they are used in enemas mainly because of this action.

SOLUTIONS AND LOTIONS

Soothing preparations may be liquids that carry an insoluble powder or suspension, or they may be mild acid or alkaline solutions, such as boric acid solution, limewater, or aluminum acetate used as wet dressings and soaks. The bismuth salts and starch are also commonly used for their soothing effect.

Aluminum Acetate Solution (Burow's Solution, Modified Burow's Solution)

Aluminum acetate solution is a mild astringent that coagulates bacterial and serum protein. It is diluted with 10 to 40 parts of water before application.

Calamine Lotion

Calamine lotion contains calamine, zinc oxide, bentonite magma, and glycerin in a calcium hydroxide solution. It is a soothing lotion used for the dermatitis caused by poison ivy, insect bites, and prickly heat.

CLEANSERS

Cleansers are usually free of soap or are modified soap products that are recommended for persons with sensitive, dry, or irritated skin, or those who may have had a previous reaction to a soap product. These cleansers are less irritating, may contain an emollient substance, and may also have been adjusted to a slightly acidic or neutral pH. Included in this category are Aveeno Cleansing Bar, Lowila Cake, and others.

EMOLLIENTS

Emollients are fatty or oily substances that may be used to soften or soothe irritated skin and mucous membrane. An emollient is often used as a vehicle for other medicinal substances. Examples of emollients include lanolin, petroleum jelly (Vaseline), vitamin A and D ointment, vitamin E, and cold cream. Examples of emollient products on the market include Panthoderm, vitamin E topical products, vitamin A and D topical products, Lubriderm, Dermassage, Nivea Skin, and many more.

SKIN PROTECTANTS

Skin protectants are used to coat minor skin irritations or to protect the person's skin from chemical irritants. Some commercially available products include AeroZoin, Benzoin, and Benzoin Compound.

WET DRESSINGS AND SOAKS

Wet dressings and soaks include some of the preparations discussed under solutions and lotions. These liquids are either a wet or an astringent type of dressing used to treat inflammatory skin conditions, such as insect bites and poison ivy. Aluminum acetate solution, Domeboro Powder, and others are available for this use.

RUBS AND LINIMENTS

Rubs and liniments are indicated for pain relief for intact skin. Pain caused by muscle aches, neuralgia, rheumatism, arthritis, and sprains is the type of pain that usually responds to these products. The ingredients in the preparations may include a counterirritant (e.g., camphor, oil of cloves, or methyl salicylate), an antiseptic (chloroxylenol, eugenol, or thymol), a local anesthetic (benzocaine), or analgesics (salicylate-containing substances). Examples from this category include Aspercreme, Ben-Gay, and Icy Hot.

For information on capsaicin topical, see Chapter 8.

PROPHYLACTIC AGENTS

PROTECTIVES

Protectives are soothing, cooling preparations that form a film on the skin. To be useful they must not macerate the skin or prevent drying of the tissues and must keep out light, air, and dust. Nonabsorbable powders are usually listed as protectives, but they are not particularly useful because they stick to wet surfaces and have to be scraped off and do not stick to dry surfaces at all. Nonabsorbable powders include zinc stearate, zinc oxide, certain bismuth preparations, talcum powder, and aluminum silicate.

Collodion is a 5% solution of pyroxylin in a mixture of ether and alcohol. When collodion is applied to the skin, the ether and alcohol evaporate, leaving a transparent film that adheres to the skin to protect it. Flexible collodion is a mixture of collodion with 2% camphor and 3% castor oil. The addition of the latter makes the resulting film elastic and more tenacious. Styptic collodion contains 20% tannic acid and therefore is astringent, as well as protective.

Although it is safe to say that no substances known at present can stimulate healing at a more rapid rate than is normal under optimal conditions, preparations that act as bland protectives may help by preventing crusting and trauma. In some instances they may reduce offensive odors.

SUNSCREEN PREPARATIONS

Extended exposure to the sun, whether from sunbathing or as a normal consequence of an outdoor occupation, may lead to sunburn and/or premature aging of the skin (photoaging). Certain chemicals (e.g., tetracyclines, sulfonamides, thiazides, and phenothiazines), plants, cosmetics, and soaps may cause a phototoxic reaction. Photosensitivity or phototoxicity occurs when an ultraviolet wavelength substance (UVA absorbing compound) is present on the skin in sufficient amounts and is also exposed to a particular sunlight wavelength. The substance absorbs the offending wavelength, energy is transferred, and the result is destructive to surrounding tissues. The exposed skin rapidly becomes red, painful, prickling, or burning with peak skin reaction reached within 24 to 48 hours of exposure. This reaction does not involve the immune system.

A photoallergy reaction is different from a phototoxic reaction; it is less common and requires prior exposure to the photosensitizing agent. The immune system is involved and when the photosensitizers react with UVA, a delayed hypersensitivity reaction occurs. The reaction occurs several days after exposure and presents as severe pruritus and a rash that can spread to skin areas that were not exposed to sunlight (Mailloux, 1995).

Excessive exposure to ultraviolet rays (UVR) may result in skin damage that progresses from minor irritations to a precancerous skin condition and, perhaps, to skin cancer later in life. Cutaneous malignant melanoma has been associated with excessive sun exposure, especially during childhood; whereas large cumulative UVR doses over a lifetime appear to increase the incidence of nonmelanoma skin cancers. See Box 58-5 on skin cancer.

Sunscreen preparations are applied either to absorb or reflect the sun's harmful rays. Absorbing agents are chemicals such as aminobenzoic acid (*p*-aminobenzoic acid, or PABA), benzophenones, cinnamates, and anthranilates; reflectors are physical agents such as titanium dioxide and zinc oxide. The latter agents are opaque (i.e., they look like thick paste) and must be applied heavily; thus they are not cosmetically acceptable to most persons.

BOX 58-5 Skin Cancer

Incidence

Nonmelanoma skin cancer is the most prevalent cancer in the United States. Skin cancers are composed essentially of nonmelanoma (basal and squamous cell carcinomas) and malignant melanoma. The American Cancer Society has predicted 1 million cases of skin cancer for 1998 (Hill, Ferrini, 1998; McDonald, 1998). Melanoma is the most common cause of death from skin cancer.

Preventive Measures

Sun protection is necessary because of the 10- to 20-year period between the ultraviolet (UV) light exposure (especially UVB) and the appearance of the skin cancer.

- The primary source of protection is to avoid sunburns, especially in childhood and adolescence. If possible, avoid outdoor activities when the sun is strongest (10 or 11 AM to 3 PM), wear protective clothing (hat and long sleeves), and if exposed to sun, use a sunscreen that blocks exposure to UV light (SPF 15 or 30). Reapply every 1 to 2 hours and after swimming.
- UV radiation can also affect the eyes, increasing the risk for cataracts and other eye disorders, and it can also suppress the immune system. It is recommended that sunglasses that block 99% to 100% of UV radiation be worn (Strange, 1995).

The spectrum for ultraviolet radiation includes UVA, UVB, and UVC. UVA, or long-wave radiation, has a wavelength of 320 to 400 nm (nanometers) and is the closest to visible light. UVB has also been determined to be responsible for skin cancer induction, although the carcinogenic properties of UVB appear to be augmented by UVA. Approximately 90% of UVB radiation is blocked by the earth's ozone layer, with the balance absorbed by the epidermal skin layer. UVB has a wavelength between 290 and 320 nm, which causes erythema and is also associated with vitamin D_3 synthesis. The UVC radiation from the sun does not appear to reach the earth's surface; therefore this type of radiation is usually emitted by artificial ultraviolet sources. UVC can cause some erythema but will not stimulate tanning.

The **sun protection factor (SPF)** is a ratio between the exposures to ultraviolet wavelengths required to cause erythema with and without a sunscreen. This is expressed as MED, or the minimal erythemal dose. Therefore if a person experiences 1 MED with 25 units of UV radiation (in an unprotected state), and if after application of a sunscreen the person requires 250 units of radiation to produce 1 MED, then this product would be given an SPF rating of 10. The higher the SPF, the longer it takes to develop a tan. If a person normally burned with 1 MED within 30 minutes, then applying a sunscreen with an SPF of 6 would allow that person to stay in the sun six times longer, or for nearly 3 hours, before reaching 1 MED. The following is the recommended SPF for various skin types (DeSimone, 1996):

TYPE	DESCRIPTION	SPF RECOMMENDED
1	Always burns very easily, never tans	20-30
2	Always burns easily, tans minimally	12-<20
3	Moderate burn, tans gradually	8-<12
4	Minimal burn, always tans well	4-<8
5	Burns rarely, tans profusely	2-<4
6	Pigmented person, never burns	—

The best way to choose a sunscreen agent is according to your skin type, the length of time spent in the sun, the usual intensity of the sun's rays in your geographic area, and the type of preparation or formulation you prefer. For example, if your skin gets red after being in the sun for 10 minutes, the use of a SPF of 15 would permit you to stay in the sun 15 × 10 or 150 minutes. An SPF of 30 is recommended for use in the tropics (Weil, 1998).

Two categories of sunscreens have been proposed, which are based on the products' active ingredients. A product with ingredients that absorb at least 85% of the radiation in the UV wavelength from 290 to 320 nm is known as a sunscreen with active ingredients. An opaque agent that reflects or scatters (prevents or minimizes suntan and sunburn) all radiation in the UV range from 290 to 777 nm is a sunscreen-opaque sunblock agent.

A topical sunscreen can be either chemical (absorb and block UV radiation) or physical (opaque, reflect and scatter UV radiation but do not absorb it). Most products are a combination of these categories and the primary difference between a preventive agent and a suntanning agent might be the concentration of the active ingredient.

The efficacy of a sunscreen agent depends on its ability to remain effective during vigorous exercise, sweating, and swimming. Two categories established are water resistant and very water resistant (waterproof), which are defined as follows:

A water-resistant product maintains its sun protection for at least 40 minutes in water; very water-resistant products maintain sun protection for at least 80 minutes in water. In addition, some products may have dual sun protective factors on the label, which refers to the SPF measured under dry conditions and the SPF under a water-testing condition. For example, the product be SPF 30 (before sweating or going into the water) and SPF 20 (after 40 minutes of sweating or water activity).

Application

Generally sunscreens should be liberally applied to all exposed body areas (except eyelids) and reapplied as frequently as recommended to achieve the maximum effectiveness. It has been recommended that sunblock be applied a half-hour before exposure as it takes approximately that long before it fully protects (Weil, 1998). Reapplication will depend on the product used (the SPF and water-resistant category) and the planned activity of the individual. It is recommended that individuals stay out of the sun when the UV rays are at the highest intensity, usually between 10 or 11 AM to 3 PM.

TABLE 58-2 Selected Sunscreen Preparations

Sunscreen Preparation	*SPF*
Hawaiian Tropic Baby Faces Sunblock	25
Coppertone Moisturizing Sunblock	30 or 45
PreSun Active	15 or 30
Blistex Ultra Protection	30
Coppertone Sport	4, 8, 15, or 30

Be aware that very little UV radiation is blocked by the cloud cover, although infrared radiation that contributes to the sensation of heat is usually reduced, which may give the person a false sense of security against a sunburn. Also, be aware of reflective surfaces: the sun's rays can be reflected on skin from water, concrete, snow, and sand. Keep infants out of the sun; sunscreens should always be used on children older than 6 months of age, preferably a product with a SPF 15 to SPF 30. It has been projected that the use of an SPF 15 from 6 months of age through 18 years of age will result in a 78% reduction in the incidence of skin cancer over a person's lifetime (DeSimone, 1996).

See Table 58-2 for examples of sunscreen agents, including their SPFs.

THERAPEUTIC AGENTS

TOPICAL ANTIINFECTIVES

Antiinfectives include topical antibiotic, antiviral, and antifungal agents.

Antibiotics

The most frequent causative organisms of skin infections (exodermas) are *Streptococcus pyogenes* and *Staphylococcus aureus.* Folliculitis, impetigo, furuncles, carbuncles, and cellulitis often result from these organisms. These common skin disorders are infections for which topical prophylaxic antibiotics may be applied. Some of these agents are discussed next; other topical antibiotics are discussed in sections on acne products, antifungals, and antivirals.

bacitracin [bass i tray′ sin]

Bacitracin is very useful in the local treatment of infectious lesions. The ointment form (Baciguent) is most commonly used, although bacitracin has also been used in solution to moisten wet dressings or as a dusting powder. It is odorless

TABLE 58-3 Spectrums of Antimicrobial Activity of Topical Antibiotics

	Spectrum of Activity		
Antibiotic	***Gram +***	***Gram −***	***Broad Spectrum***
bacitracin ointment		X	
chlortetracycline ointment			X
chloramphenicol cream			X
erythromycin liquid or ointment	X		
gentamicin cream and ointment			X
neomycin cream and ointment			X

and nonstaining, and its use seldom results in sensitizing; however, allergic contact dermatitis has occurred.

neomycin [nee oh mye′ sin]

Neomycin has been used successfully in the treatment of infections of the skin and mucous membrane. Applied topically, it occasionally irritates the skin, and allergic contact dermatitis is reported, especially when neomycin is used on stasis ulcers. An ointment (Mycitracin), which combines neomycin, bacitracin, and polymixin B, may be more efficacious in mixed infections than when these agents are used singly.

For conditions where absorption of neomycin may occur (including burns and trophic ulceration), there is the potential for nephrotoxicity, ototoxicity, and neomycin hypersensitivity reactions. This risk is seen more frequently in persons with compromised renal function, in persons with extensive burns, and in patients using other aminoglycoside antibiotics. Sensitization may occur to any of the antibiotic ingredients, and prolonged use may produce superinfection as an overgrowth of nonsusceptible organisms such as fungi. Photosensitivity is reported with topical gentamicin.

The possibility of hypersensitivity occurs when chloramphenicol is used topically, as does the additional risk of bone marrow hypoplasia, blood dyscrasias, itching, burning, angioneurotic edema, urticaria, and vesicular and maculopapular dermatitis. Tetracyclines may stain clothing and cause erythema, irritation, and swelling locally. See Table 58-3 for a list of topical antibiotics and their spectrums of activity. Eythromycin generally has activity against gram-positive organisms, and it is also approved for the treatment of acne vulgaris.

mupirocin [myoo peer′ oh sin] (Bactroban)

Mupirocin is a topical antibacterial preparation indicated for the treatment of impetigo caused by *S aureus* and other beta-hemolytic streptococci. It is usually applied to affected areas three times daily.

Many topical preparations and antibiotic combinations available over the counter are labeled as first-aid products to help prevent infection in minor cuts, burns, or injuries. They cannot be recommended to treat known infections. Prescription antibiotic ointments are generally indicated for the treatment of minor or surface bacterial infections.

Antivirals

acyclovir [ay sye′ kloe ver] (Zovirax Ointment 5%)

Acyclovir inhibits the viral enzymes necessary for deoxyribonucleic acid (DNA) synthesis. Topical acyclovir is used for the treatment of herpes simplex (non-life-threatening) in immunocompromised patients. However, in many instances systemic acyclovir is much more effective and may be the preferred formulation.

Side effects and adverse reactions include local pain, rash, pruritus, or stinging. The dosage is adequate covering of the lesions with ointment every 3 hours six times daily for 7 days.

Antifungals

There are few fungi that produce keratinolytic enzymes to provide for their existence on skin. Three infectious fungi can cause local fungal infections without systemic effects: *Microsporum, Trichophyton,* and *Epidermophyton.* The possibility of a mixed infection with these fungi must never be overlooked.

Fungi exist in a moist, warm environment, preferably in dark areas such as skin areas covered by shoes and socks (tinea pedis or athlete's foot). Immunologic mechanisms may have an important role in fungal control. The triad for suspicion for fungal infections is an immunologic deficit, a specific fungal involvement, and the skin condition.

The stratum corneum is a layer of dead desquamated cells that are shed normally or are dissolved in sebum. The fungi invade this layer and cause inflammation and induce sensitivity when they penetrate the epidermis and dermis. Because the stratum corneum is shed daily, the ability to spread or transmit the fungi is by contact.

Side effects and adverse reactions with the use of the topical antifungals include local irritation, pruritus, burning sensation, scaling, erythema, blistering, stinging, peeling, and urticaria. General irritation may occur with products like clotrimazole.

The primary topical antifungal agents include undecylenic acid products (Desenex and others), clioquinol (Vioform), miconazole (Micatin), econazole (Spectazole), ciclopirox (Loprox), clotrimazole (Lotrimin), oxiconazole (Oxistat), triacetin (Fungoid), haloprogin (Halotex), tolnaftate (Tinactin), nystatin, gentian violet, and a variety of antifungal combination ointments, powders, and liquids. See Table 58-4 for the generic name, trade name, status of (OTC or prescription), and comments on the products.

CORTICOSTEROIDS

Topical corticosteroids are generally indicated for relief of inflammatory and pruritic dermatoses. They also offer the

TABLE 58-4 Topical Antifungal Agents

Name	Prescription Drug	Over-the-counter	Special Comments
amphotericin B (Fungizone)	X		Equivalent to nystatin against *Candida albicans* (Monilia) infections
ciclopirox olamine (Loprox)	X		Broad-spectrum antifungal; used for tinea pedis, tinea cruris, tinea corporis, candidiasis caused by *C albicans,* and tinea versicolor caused by *M. furfur*
clioquinol (Vioform)		X	Antibacterial and antifungal; may cause staining of clothes, skin, or hair
clotrimazole (Lotrimin, Mycelex)	X	X	Broad-spectrum antifungal agent
econazole nitrate (Spectrazole)	X		Broad-spectrum antifungal agent
haloprogin (Halotex)	X		Broad-spectrum synthetic antifungal agent
ketoconazole (Nizoral)	X		Broad-spectrum synthetic antifungal agent
miconazole (Micatin)		X	Used for tinea pedis (athlete's foot), tinea cruris, tinea corporis, and tinea versicolor
(Monistat-Derm)	X		Lotion preferred for intertriginous areas
nystatin (Mycostatin, Nilstat)	X		Antifungal antibiotic with both fungicidal and fungistatic effects
tolnaftate (Tinactin, Aftate)		X	Used for topical fungus skin infections
triacetin (Fungoid)	X		Treats athlete's foot and other topical fungus infections
undecylenic acid (Desenex)		X	Antifungal and antibacterial agent for athlete's foot and ringworm, with exception of nails and hairy sites; also used for diaper rash, prickly heat, minor skin irritations, jock itch, excessive perspiration, and skin irritation in the groin area

benefit of less systemic side effects and allow direct contact with the localized lesion.

The effectiveness of the topical corticosteroids is a result of their antiinflammatory, antipruritic, and vasoconstrictor actions. Topical corticosteroids may also stabilize epidermal lysosomes in the skin, and fluorinated steroids are antiproliferative.

Fluorinated topical corticosteroids (fluocinonide, betamethasone, and others) are used for the treatment of dermatologic disorders such as psoriasis because of their antiinflammatory, antipruritic, and vasoconstrictive actions, as well as their ability to decrease cell proliferation. They are very potent agents and are less likely to cause sodium retention.

A correlation exists between the potency and the therapeutic efficacy of corticosteroids (Box 58-6). The vehicle (aerosol, cream, gel, lotion, ointment, solution, or tape) in which the corticosteroid is placed may alter the vasoconstrictor property and therapeutic efficacy. Corticosteroid skin penetration is enhanced by the following vehicles (in decreasing order of effectiveness): ointments, gels, creams, and lotions.

Ointment bases and propylene glycol both enhance the penetration of the corticosteroid and its vasoconstrictor effects. As a result of their occlusive nature ointments hydrate the stratum corneum, permitting granular steroid penetration. Lotions are well suited for hairy areas or for lesions that are oozing and wet. Creams and ointments are well suited for dry, scaling, thickened, and pruritic areas. Sprays, lotions, and gels are suited for the scalp or hairy areas. Sprays are esthetically suitable for acute weeping lesions, are cooling, and have antipruritic effects. All these vehicles influence absorption and therapeutic effect.

The rate of percutaneous penetration after application also influences therapeutic efficacy. Steroid percutaneous penetration increases with its vehicle base solubility. It is limited by three factors: rate of dissolution, rate of passive diffusion, and drug penetration rate (the skin itself is a barrier, and the stratum corneum is a rate-limiting membrane). The skin is selectively permeable by regional variations in absorptive capacity. Because most topical corticosteroids are in suspension vehicles (ointments, creams, and lotions), the addition of a solvent (propylene glycol) to the product can enhance drug dissolution, which may improve absorption. The sebum, enzymes, and perspiration of the skin convert topical suspensions partially to solutions needing the inclusion of a solvent, surfactant, or emulsifier in the vehicle to increase the rate of dissolution and distribution. Inflamed skin absorbs topical steroids to a greater degree than thick or lichenified skin.

Side effects and adverse reactions for topical corticosteroids include acneiform eruptions, allergic contact dermatitis, burning sensations, dryness, itching, hypopigmentation, purpura, hirsutism (usually facial), folliculitis, round and

BOX 58-6 **Potencies of Topical Steroid Products**

The following list compares relative potencies of the topical corticosteroid products.

Most Potent
clobetasol (Temovate 0.05%)
halobetasol (Ultravate 0.05%)

High Potency
amcinocide (Cyclocort)
betamethasone dipropionate (Diprosone 0.05%)
desoximetasone (Topicort 0.25%)
fluocinolone (Lidex 0.05%)

Moderate Potency
betamethasone (Benisone 0.025%)
betamethasone valerate (Valisone 0.1%)
desoximetasone (Topicort 0.05%)
flurandrenolide (Cordran 0.025%)
triamcinolone (Aristocort)

Less Potency
desomide (Tridesilon)
fluocinolone acetonide (Synalar 0.01%)
hydrocortisone 0.25% to 2.5%

swollen face, alopecia (usually of scalp), overgrowth of bacteria, fungus, and virus, and immunosuppression.

The adult dosage is one or two applications daily as directed. Application frequency depends on site, response of the cutaneous eruption to medication, and application technique.

KERATOLYTICS

Keratolytics (keratin dissolvers) are drugs that soften scales and loosen the outer horny layer of the skin. Salicylic acid and resorcinol are drugs of choice. Their action makes the penetration of other medical substances possible by cleaning the involved lesions. Salicylic acid is particularly important for its keratolytic effect in local treatment of scalp conditions, warts, corns, fungous infections, acne, and chronic types of dermatitis. It is used up to 20% in ointments, plasters, or collodion for this purpose.

ACNE PRODUCTS

Acne vulgaris is a skin disease that involves increased sebum production and abnormal keratinization that leads to the formation of a keratin plug at the base of the pilosebaceous follicle; it affects up to 90% of adolescents (Seaton, 1995). The reduction and removal of sebum and bacteria, specifically *Propionibacterium acnes,* are the targets of acne vulgaris therapy.

Treatment of acne may include (1) removal of keratin plugs, (2) decreasing the number of *P acnes,* (3) lowering the amounts of free fatty acid and decreasing its formation, (4) decreasing the sebum production, and (5) effectively improving the appearance of the individual for psychosocial benefits.

Of the many treatment modalities in acne therapy, only the topical forms of benzoyl peroxide, tetracycline, erythromycin, clindamycin, tretinoin, and isotretinoin will be discussed here.

benzoyl peroxide

Benzoyl peroxide slowly and continuously liberates active oxygen, producing an antibacterial, keratolytic and drying effect. The release of oxygen into the pilosebaceous and comedone area creates unfavorable growth conditions for *P acnes* and reduces the release of the fatty acids from sebum. Additionally, the drying vehicle aids in shrinking the papules or pustules but does not have an effect on comedones or cysts. Benzoyl peroxide is used in the treatment of acne vulgaris.

Benzoyl peroxide is absorbed and metabolized in the skin to benzoic acid. Approximately 5% of the benzoic acid is absorbed and excreted in the kidneys. Acne improvement is usually noted in 4 to 6 weeks of therapy.

Side effects and adverse reactions are infrequent and include dry or peeling skin, red skin, or sensation of warmth of the skin, severe redness, pruritus, blisters, and burning or swelling of skin caused by an allergic reaction. No significant drug interactions are reported.

In adults and children 12 years of age and older, benzoyl peroxide lotion (5% or 10%) is applied one to four times daily.

Topical Antibiotics

Topical and systemic antibiotics used in the treatment of acne have an unknown mechanism of action. Acne is not an infection nor is it contagious, but *P acnes* appears to convert comedones to inflamed pustules or papules. The antibiotics may decrease the colonization of *P acnes,* thus decreasing the formation of sebaceous fatty acid byproducts and preventing the formation of new acne lesions. The antibiotics used include clindamycin, erythromycin, and tetracycline. Topical erythromycin and clindamycin are most commonly prescribed for mild to moderate acne while oral antibiotics (tetracyclines) are generally reserved for individuals with severe acne and for those who are intolerant or whose acne did not respond to topical agents. Treatment failures have been associated with antibiotic resistance (Seaton, 1995).

clindamycin [klin da mye′ sin]
(Cleocin T topical solution)

Topical clindamycin may be as effective as low-dose, oral tetracycline therapy for inflammatory acne. This is one of the most widely used topical antibiotics indicated for in the treatment of acne vulgaris.

Pharmacokinetically, about 1.7% is absorbed after twice daily topical dosing. Tissue phosphatases hydrolyze the inactive clindamycin phosphate to active clindamycin base, which is excreted by the kidneys.

Side effects/adverse reactions include dry, scaly, and peeling skin; stinging or burning sensation, contact dermatitis or hypersensitive skin reaction, gastrointestinal (GI) distress, and, rarely, pseudomembranous colitis.

erythromycin topical solution

[er ith roe mye′ sin] (A/T/S, EryDerm)

Erythromycin topical solution is also indicated for the treatment of acne vulgaris.

Side effects and adverse reactions include skin reactions such as erythema, desquamation, tenderness, dryness, pruritus, burning, oiliness, and acne.

Erythromycin is also available in combination with benzoyl peroxide (Benzamycin), which is also indicated for topical treatment of acne vulgaris. Improvement is usually seen within 3 to 4 weeks but it may take up to 2 or 3 months before the full therapeutic effect is seen. This product is dispensed in two separate medications with specific instructions for mixing them together and applying to the affected area. After application, the patient needs to wait at least 1 hour before applying another topical medication for acne.

tetracycline topical solution [tet ra sye′ kleen] (Topicycline)

Topical tetracycline, which is believed to suppress *P acnes* growth, is directly applied to the pilosebaceous units (hair follicle and sebaceous gland), which are most numerous on the face, back, chest, and upper arms.

Side effects and adverse reactions include dry, scaly skin, stinging, pain, redness, or swelling at the site of application.

Low-dose oral tetracycline (usually 250 mg/day) is usually reserved for severe acne as reviewed previously. This dose may be increased for acute acne flare-ups but should be decreased to maintenance dosing within 1 month or so. Although low-dose therapy has been continued for years, it has been recommended that the antibiotic be discontinued periodically (Seaton, 1995). This may help reduce the potential for side effects and adverse reactions and possibly drug resistance.

tretinoin [tret′ i noyn]

(retinoic acid, vitamin A acid, Retin-A)

Tretinoin is an irritant that stimulates epidermal cell turnover, which causes skin peeling; this reduces the free fatty acids and horny cell adherence within the comedone. Tretinoin is used in the treatment of acne vulgaris in which comedones, pustules, and papules predominate.

Side effects and adverse reactions of tretinoin include red and edematous blisters, crusted, stinging or peeling skin, and temporary alterations in skin pigmentation. Concomitant topical use with drying or peeling agents such as benzoyl peroxide, resorcinol, salicylic acid, and sulfur may result in excessive keratolytic and peeling effects.

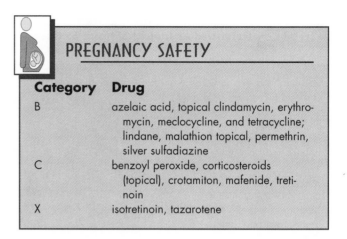

PREGNANCY SAFETY

Category	Drug
B	azelaic acid, topical clindamycin, erythromycin, meclocycline, and tetracycline; lindane, malathion topical, permethrin, silver sulfadiazine
C	benzoyl peroxide, corticosteroids (topical), crotamiton, mafenide, tretinoin
X	isotretinoin, tazarotene

Tretinoin emollient cream (Renova) was released to treat facial wrinkles caused by age or the sun. This product contains 0.05% tretinoin and is the first prescription with this indication (Olin, 1998).

isotretinoin [eye soe tret′ i noyn] (Accutane)

Isotretinoin is a systemic product indicated for the treatment of severe recalcitrant cystic acne. This product inhibits sebaceous gland activity and thus decreases sebum formation and secretion. It also has antikeratinizing and antiinflammatory effects. It is reserved to treat severe acne and has induced prolonged remissions in severe cystic acne.

Women who are pregnant or are planning to become pregnant should not use this preparation. Many spontaneous abortions have been reported in pregnant women, as well as major abnormalities (hydrocephalus, microcephalus, and external ear and cardiovascular problems) in the fetus at birth (see the Pregnancy Safety box).

Because some drug interactions have been reported with isotretinoin, carefully check the patient's medication regimen for the following drugs. The use of isotretinoin is not recommended with etretinate, tretinoin, or vitamin A because additive toxicity may result. The use of tetracyclines with isotretinoin increases the risk for the development of pseudotumor cerebri (a condition characterized by increased intracranial pressure, headache, blurring of the optic disc margins, vomiting, and papilledema without neurologic findings, except palsy of the sixth cranial nerve).

Side effects and adverse reactions include dry eye, mouth, nose, or skin, pruritus, red, itching or inflamed eye, nosebleeds, inflammation of lips, depression, skin infection, rash, headache, photosensitivity, myalgia, peeling of skin from palms of hands or soles of feet, GI distress, weakness, and, rarely, bleeding gums, cataracts or other eye disorders, hepatitis, inflammatory bowel disease, optic neuritis, and mood alterations.

The usual adolescent and adult dose for severe recalcitrant cystic acne is 0.5 to 1 mg/kg of body weigh daily, given in two divided doses for 4 to 5 months.

Several other acne products are available, including azelaic acid (Azelex Cream) and tazarotene (Tazorac). For azelaic acid, which has a low pH, skin irritation (burning, stinging, or pruritus) may occur if it is applied on broken skin. Tazarotene is a retinoid prodrug that is converted to its active form (cognate carboxylic acid of tazarotene) after application to the skin. This product is used to treat mild to moderate facial acne vulgaris and psoriasis.

BURN PRODUCTS

Burn injuries range from mild and superficial to very severe with extensive skin loss associated with systemic and metabolic complications. Approximately 12,000 Americans die annually of thermal injury (Mailloux, 1995). The chief cause of death is shock, a fact of considerable significance in any effective plan of treatment.

Burns cause lesions of the skin accompanied by pain. The burn may be caused by heat (thermal burn), chemical cauterizing agents (chemical burns), or electricity (electrical burns). Sources may be friction, lightning, or electromagnetic energy sources (ultraviolet light, x-rays, lasers, or atomic explosion). The types of burns that result from various sources are relatively specific and diagnostic.

Consideration of what takes place in the damaged tissues clarifies many points of treatment. At first capillary permeability is altered in the local injured area: permeability is increased, resulting in a loss of plasma and weeping of the surface tissues. If the burn is at all extensive, considerable amounts of plasma fluid may be lost in a relatively short time.

This depletes the blood volume and causes decreased cardiac output and diminished blood flow. Unless the situation is rapidly brought under control, irreparable damage may result from rapidly developing tissue anoxia. The lack of sufficient oxygen and accumulation of waste products from inadequate oxidation results in loss of tone in the minute blood vessels. The increased capillary permeability then extends to tissues remote from those suffering the initial injury. Thus a generalized edema often develops, and the vicious cycle once established tends to be self-perpetuating. One of the aims of the treatment of burns is therefore to stop the loss of plasma and to replenish that which is lost as quickly as possible.

Partial- or full-thickness burns must be thought of as open wounds with the accompanying danger of infection. The infection must be prevented or treated. The treatment, however, must be such that it will not cause any further destruction of tissue or of the small islands of remaining epithelium from which growth and regeneration can take place.

Burns are classified by degree, which is determined by the depth of skin involved within a geographic designation. First-degree burns involve only the epidermis, causing erythema with characteristic dry, painful reddening and edema without blistering or vesiculation (e.g., overexposure to sun or flash burn). Second-degree burns involve the epidermis extending into the dermis and may be superficial or involve deep dermal necrosis. Epithelial regeneration may extend from the deep skin appendages such as hair follicles and sebaceous glands that penetrate the dermis. This burn is characterized by a moist, blistered, very painful surface (e.g., flash or scald burns from nonviscous liquids). Third-degree burns involve destruction of the entire dermis and epidermis characterized by white, lustrous, or opaque skin; dry, leathery skin; or coagulated, charred skin without sensation as a result of the destruction of nerve endings (e.g., flame burns or hot viscous liquids). Fourth-degree burns extend into subcutaneous fat, muscle, or bone, appear black and dry in appearance, and cause scarring.

The severity of electrical burns depends on the amount of voltage received, the condition of the skin (e.g., cuts, abrasions, and moisture, which lower resistance), and contraction of flexor muscles, which inhibits release from the power source. Electrical burns result in necrosis of more tissue than thermal burns and are of three types. In type I burns, the electrical current causes effects on blood vessels such as occlusion, thrombosis, or tissue destruction. Type II electrical burns from high-tension currents (e.g., an electrical arc) produce a crater in the skin. Type III electrical burns are similar to flame burns because the arc flame ignites the person's clothes.

Chemical burns occur after contact with acid or alkali; the initial treatment is water irrigation of the affected area followed by neutralization. Chemical burns may occur in the mouth and appear as a white slough owing to necrosis of the epithelium and underlying connective tissues.

First-Aid Treatment of Burns

An important first-aid treatment for minor and major burns regardless of cause (chemical, electric, or thermal) is to immediately cool the wound to remove irritants, decrease inflammation, and constrict blood vessels; this reduces the permeability of the blood vessels and checks edema formation. Cold tap water can be used to flush the wound thoroughly and to cool hot clothing. The more quickly the wound is cooled, the less tissue damage there is likely to be, and the more rapid will be the recovery. No greasy ointments, lard, butter, or dressings should be applied, since these agents will inhibit loss of heat from the burn, which will increase both discomfort and tissue damage. The burn may be left exposed to the air, or cold wet compresses may be applied until the person can be transported for medical attention.

Burn victims treated in an emergency room or burn unit will be stabilized with intravenous fluids, given analgesics for pain, and sedated if necessary. Such individuals are immunized with tetanus toxoid and/or tetanus immunoglobulin, depending on their immunization status. Catheterization may be necessary to measure urinary output, depending on the patient's status. After stabilization, the burn wound is cleaned with a mild soap and water and a sterile, nonadherent gauze dressing with hydrophilic petrolatum is applied to the wound. In some settings, synthetic dressings (Duoderm, Opsite) may be used. Topical antiinfective therapy may also be indicated. Silver sulfadiazine is usually preferred because of its broad-spectrum activity and also because this product is easy and painless to apply and remove from the burn. Povidone iodine was commonly used in some centers, and it also penetrates eschar. However, povidone iodine causes pain on application and when dry, will harden the eschar area (Mailloux, 1995).

silver sulfadiazine [sul fa dye′ a zeen] (Silvadene)

Silver sulfadiazine is an antiinfective agent with broad antimicrobial activity against many gram-negative and gram-positive bacteria, similar to mafenide. It acts only on the cell membrane and cell wall to produce its bactericidal effect.

Silver sulfadiazine is used in second- and third-degree burns for the prevention and treatment of sepsis. It softens eschar, facilitating its removal and preparation of the wound for grafting.

Silver sulfadiazine is available as a 1% cream to be applied topically to cleansed, debrided burn wounds once or twice daily. It should be applied with a sterile gloved hand to a thickness of about 1.5 mm. Burn wounds should be continuously covered with the cream. Daily bathing and debriding are important, and a dressing may or may not be used.

Therapy is usually continued until satisfactory healing has occurred or the wound is ready for grafting. Because silver sulfadiazine inhibits bacterial growth, delayed eschar separation may occur, necessitating escharotomy to prevent contractures. Pain, burning, and itching occur infrequently after application of the silver sulfadiazine cream.

Silver sulfadiazine may cause a hypersensitivity reaction; if this occurs, the drug should be discontinued. Hemolysis may occur in persons with glucose-6-phosphate dehydrogenase deficiency. When silver sulfadiazine is applied to extensive areas of the body, significant amounts of the drug may be absorbed, reaching therapeutic serum levels and producing adverse reactions characteristic of the sulfonamides. Renal function in these patients should be monitored and the urine examined for sulfa crystals.

mafenide [ma′ fe nide] (Sulfamylon)

Mafenide (sulfonamide), a broad-spectrum, antibacterial (bacteriostatic) topical agent, penetrates eschar even in the presence of pus and serum. It is a carbonic anhydrase inhibitor, though, that can alter acid-base balance, resulting in metabolic acidosis. In contrast to silver sulfadiazine, it is usually painful on application.

On application, mafenide rapidly diffuses through partial (second-degree) and full-thickness (third-degree) burns and has proved to be an effective means for preventing and retarding bacterial invasion in burn wounds. While relatively nontoxic, burning or pain on application and allergic reactions have been reported. It is rapidly metabolized to a metabolite and eliminated by way of the kidneys.

TOPICAL ANTIPRURITICS

Antipruritic agents are given to allay itching of skin and mucous membranes. There is less need for these preparations as the constitutional treatment of persons with skin disorders is better understood. Dilute solutions containing phenol have been widely used. Dressings wet with potassium permanganate 1:4000, aluminum subacetate 1:16, boric acid, or physiologic saline solution may cool and soothe and thus prevent itching. Lotions such as calamine or calamine with phenol (phenolated calamine), and cornstarch or oatmeal baths may also be used to relieve itching.

Local anesthetics such as dibucaine and benzocaine may decrease pruritus, but their use is not recommended because of their high sensitizing and irritating effects. The application of hydrocortisone in a lotion or ointment in a strength of 0.5% to 1% has proven to be one of the best methods of relieving pruritus and decreasing inflammation. An additional advantage is its low sensitizing index.

TOPICAL ECTOPARASITICIDAL DRUGS

Ectoparasites are insects that live on the outer surface of the body. Ectoparasiticides are drugs used against those animal parasites. For human use, these drugs are more frequently referred to as pediculicides and scabicides (miticides), reflecting the parasite treated with each group.

Pediculosis is a parasite infestation of lice on the skin of a human. Lice are transmitted from one person to the next by close contact with infested persons, clothing, combs, and towels. There are three different varieties of infestations: (1) pediculosis pubis, caused by *Phthirus pubis* (pubic or crab louse), (2) pediculosis corporis, caused by *Pediculus huma-*

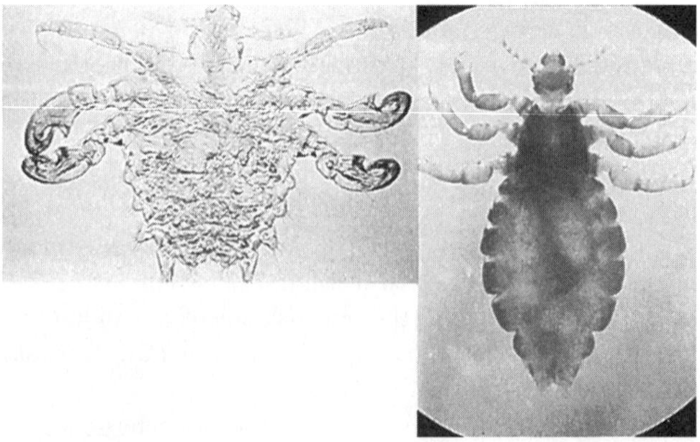

FIGURE 58-1
Left, Pubic louse *(Phthirus pubis); right,* body louse *(Pediculus humanus).* Notice that the first pair of legs on the pubic louse are thinner than the second and third pairs. Also, the abdomen is shorter. On the body louse, all legs are approximately the same length and the abdomen is longer.

nus corporis (body louse), and (3) pediculosis capitis, caused by *Pediculus humanus capitis* (head louse) (Fig. 58-1). A characteristic finding of pediculosis corporis, except in heavily infested individuals, is that the parasite is absent from the body but inhabits seams of clothing that come in contact with the axillae or that are in the beltline or collar.

Common findings in a person who is infested include pruritus, nits (eggs of louse) on hair shafts, lice on skin or clothes, and, with pubic lice, occasionally sky-blue macules on the inner thighs or lower abdomen. The drug of choice is the pediculicide lindane (gamma-benzene hexachloride).

Scabies is a parasitic infestation caused by the itch mite, *Sarcoptes scabiei.* It is transmitted from one person to the next by close contact, such as sleeping next to an infested individual. It bores into the horny layers of the skin in cracks and folds, causing irritation and pruritus. Itching occurs almost exclusively at night. The adult infestation is usually generalized over the body, especially in web spaces between fingers, wrists, elbows, and buttocks. The drug of choice is permethrin cream because it is considered more effective than crotamiton and lindane (Anandan, 1995).

lindane [lin′ dane]
(gamma-benzene hexachloride, Kwell)

Lindane is both a scabicide and a pediculicide because it is effective in the treatment of both lice and mite infestations. It is available in a 1% cream, lotion, and shampoo. For the treatment of pediculosis pubis and infestations of *P humanus capitis,* the cream or lotion is applied in a sufficient quantity to cover the skin and hair of the infected and surrounding areas, left on for 12 hours, and then thoroughly washed. It seldom needs to be applied more than once. The shampoo is worked into the hair and left on for 4 minutes. Then the hair is rinsed and dried, and nits (eggs) are combed from the hair shafts. Retreatment is usually not necessary.

For the treatment of scabies, the cream or lotion is used. If crusted lesions are present, a warm bath preceding the application of lindane is recommended. Lindane is applied over the entire body from the neck down. It is left on for 8 hours and then washed off. Usually one application is sufficient. It is common to have pruritus after application, but this does not indicate a need for reapplication unless live mites can be demonstrated.

Lindane occasionally will cause an eczematous skin rash. It penetrates human skin and has a potential for central nervous system toxicity (e.g., seizures, increased irritability, and dizziness), especially in children.

crotamiton [kroe tam′ i tonn] (Eurax)

Crotamiton is indicated for the treatment of scabies, it is rubbed into the skin from the chin down, particularly in the folds and creases of the body and moist areas, such as underarms and groin. It is reapplied in 24 hours, and 48 hours after the second application it is washed from the body surface. Two applications of crotamiton usually eradicate most infestations. In resistant cases it may be applied again 1 week later.

Crotamiton, available as a 10% cream or lotion, may cause an occasional skin rash on application.

permethrin [per meth′ rin] (Nix)

Permethrin acts on the nerve cell membranes of lice, ticks, mites, and fleas. It disrupts the sodium channel repolarization, thus paralyzing the parasites. It has a high cure rate (up to 99%) in treating head lice after only a single application. The most common side effects and adverse reactions include pruritus, mild burning on application, transient erythema, edema, and rash.

malathion [mal′ i thye one] (Ovide)

Malathion is an organophosphate cholinesterase inhibitor available for the treatment of head lice and ova. This product is usually effective in lice-infested individuals within 24 hours and is well tolerated. Malathion lotion is rubbed into the scalp and left to air dry. Because the drug is flammable, the individual must be warned to avoid open flames and smoking, and not to use a hairdryer. The hair should be shampooed 8 to 12 hours after application; dead lice are combed out.

SUMMARY

Although there are numerous dermatologic agents available to treat skin disorders, three major groups of preparations are discussed in this chapter, i.e., general, prophylactic, and therapeutic agents. The general preparations include bath substances, cleansers, soaps, solutions and emollients, skin protectants, wet dressings and soaks, and rubs and liniments while the prophylactic topicals block the skin from sun, light, or foreign substance damage. Therapeutic agents may include antiinfectives (antibiotics, antivirals, and antifungals), corticosteroids, keratolytics, acne products, burn products, antipruritics, and ectoparasiticidal drugs. Understanding the effects of topical agents is important in the care of patients with skin disorders.

REVIEW QUESTIONS

1. Define the sun protection factor (SPF) and how it is derived. What sunscreen SPF would you recommend or a person who burns easily and never tans?
2. What is the definition of a water-resistant and very water-resistant sunscreen product? What should the consumer know about a sunscreen product that states it has SPF 30 and SPF 20 on the label?
3. Discuss first-aid treatment of minor and major burns. Name one drug used to treat burns and describe its mechanism of action, directions, and side effects and adverse reactions.
4. Name and describe the three varieties of pediculosis. Name one drug and describe its indications and use as a pediculicide.

REFERENCES

Beare PG, Myers JL: *Adult health nursing,* ed 3, St Louis, 1998, Mosby.

DeSimone EM II: Sunscreen and suntan products. In Covington TR, editor: *Handbook of nonprescription drugs,* ed 11, Washington, DC, 1996, American Pharmaceutical Association.

Hill L, Ferrini RL: Skin cancer prevention and screening: summary of the American College of Preventive Medicine's Practice Policy Statements. *CA Cancer J Clin* 48:232-235, 1998.

Mailloux AT: Photosensitivity and burns. In Young LY, Koda-Kimble MA, editors: *Applied therapeutics: the clinical use of drugs,* ed 6, Vancouver, Wash, 1995, Applied Therapeutics, Inc.

McDonald CJ: American Cancer Society perspective on the American College of Preventive Medicine's Policy Statements on Skin Cancer Prevention and Screening, *CA Cancer J Clin* 48:229-231, 1998.

Olin BR: *Facts and comparisons.* Philadelphia, 1998, JB Lippincott.

Seaton TL: Acne. In Young LY, Koda-Kimble MA, editors: *Applied therapeutics: the clinical use of drugs,* ed 6, Vancouver, Wash, 1995, Applied Therapeutics, Inc.

Strange CJ: Twarting skin cancer with sun sense, *FDA Consumer* 29(6), July-Aug 1998, http://www.fda.gov/fdac/features/695_skincanc.html (July 23, 1998).

Weil A: Best method to block out sunburn, http://cgi.pathfinder.com/drweil/archiveqa/1,2283,1313,00.html (July 23, 1998).

ADDITIONAL REFERENCES

Anandan JV: Parasitic infections. In Young LY, Koda-Kimble MA, editors: *Applied therapeutics: the clinical use of drugs,* ed 6, Vancouver, Wash, 1995, Applied Therapeutics, Inc.

Anderson KN et al, editors: *Mosby's medical, nursing, and allied health dictionary,* ed 5, St Louis, 1998, Mosby.

Bhawan J et al: Effects of tretinoin on photodamaged skin: a histologic study, *Arch Dermatol* 127:666, 1991.

Dicken CH et al: Retinoids: what role in your practice? *Patient Care* 26(10):18-19, 25-28, 31-32, 34, 37, 41-45, 1992.

Fitzpatrick TB et al: *Dermatology in general medicine,* ed 4, vols I and II, New York, 1993, McGraw-Hill.

Gupta MA et al: Treatment of mildly to moderately photoaged skin with topical tretinoin has a favorable psychosocial effect: a prospective study, *J Am Acad Dermatol* 24:780, 1991.

McCance KL, Huether SE: *Pathophysiology: the biologic basis for disease in adults and children,* ed 3, St Louis, 1998, Mosby.

Mosby: *Mosby's GenRx,* St Louis, 1998, Mosby.

Seeley RR, Stephens TD, Tate P: *Anatomy and physiology,* ed 3, New York, 1995, McGraw-Hill.

United States Pharmacopeial Convention: *USP DI: drug information for the health care professional,* ed 18, Rockville, Md, 1998, The Convention.

CHAPTER 59

Debriding Agents

CHAPTER FOCUS

Pressure sores (bedsores) often occur in bedridden and handicapped persons who are not rotated or shifted to a new position on a regular basis. These skin ulcers are the result of skin pressure against a bony area of the body such as the heels or hips. The damage from untreated pressure sores can be extensive, as they can penetrate muscle and bone resulting in a serious infection. This chapter reviews identification, cleansing, and debridement of these wounds. The best treatment for them, of course, is prevention.

OBJECTIVES

After reading and studying this chapter, the student should be able to do the following:

1. *Define and describe the key terms.*
2. *Discuss the impact of and causes contributing to pressure sores in patient care.*
3. *List the four basic principles for developing a treatment plan for pressure sores.*
4. *Name and describe the significant drug interactions with the use of collagenase.*
5. *Describe the procedure for use of dextranomer.*
6. *Name one enzymatic and nonenzymatic agent used to treat pressure sores.*

KEY TERMS

debridement, (p. 760)
eschar, (p. 760)
granulation tissue, (p. 761)
proteolytic enzymes, (p. 761)
pressure sore, (p. 760)

This chapter covers debriding agents, which are agents used to remove dirt, foreign objects, damaged tissue, and cellular debris from a wound or burn to prevent infection and promote healing. In treatment of a wound, **debridement** is the first step in cleansing it; debridement also allows examination of the extent of the injury.

PRESSURE SORES

The **pressure sore** (bedsore or decubitus ulcer) is a break in the skin and underlying subcutaneous and muscle tissue caused by abnormal, sustained pressure or friction exerted over the bony prominences of the body by the object on which the body part rests. It results in vascular insufficiency and ischemic necrosis, and it most frequently affects debilitated, comatose, immobilized, or paralyzed patients. According to the Agency for Health Care Policy and Research (AHCPR), the prevalence of pressure ulcers ranges from 9.2% in acute care facilities to 33% in critical care patients and up to 23% in skilled care facilities and nursing homes (Bergstrom et al, 1994). In addition to the human suffering of patients and their families, the total cost of treating such wounds was estimated as exceeding $1.335 billion (Bergstrom et al, 1994).

There are many causes contributing to this condition that must be addressed. Local and systemic causes include the following: obesity or malnutrition; debilitation; a pressure and shearing force on the lower body if the head of the bed is raised more than 30°; a loss of sensation of pressure or pain; muscle atrophy and motor paralysis; a reduction in the amount of adipose tissue between skin and underlying bone; emaciation and dehydration; poor nutrition because of inadequate intake of vitamins, minerals, and trace elements (such as copper and zinc); friction; local anatomic defects; trauma; incontinence; edema; infections; heat and moisture (maceration); hypertension; septicemia; and local circulatory interference.

The bacterial flora of pressure sores (present in stages II, III, and IV) are both gram-negative and gram-positive organisms, which include *Staphylococcus aureus, Streptococcus* groups A and D, *Escherichia coli, Clostridium tetani,* and *Bacteroides, Proteus, Pseudomonas, Klebsiella,* and *Citrobacter* organisms. Parenteral antibiotics (adequate levels in granulating wounds are not reached) may be needed in difficult-to-treat infected pressure sores as an adjunct to surgical management just before and at the time of surgery.

An individual with a full-thickness loss of skin may be a candidate for surgical intervention either to cover the ulcer area or to stabilize the wound. Decisions to perform surgery include the following considerations: the underlying disease, the ability of the patient to withstand surgery, and the condition or prognosis of the pressure sore (especially those in which all soft tissue is destroyed, exposing bone).

PHARMACOLOGIC MANAGEMENT

A treatment plan for pressure sores should take into consideration four basic principles: (1) assessment and interventions to improve the patient's general health, which may help to reduce factors contributing to the problem, such as incontinence, anemia, or edema; (2) reduction of pressure sites by positioning or the use of padding, special beds, and other items, thus increasing blood flow to the site; (3) maintenance of a clean wound site; and (4) use of an appropriate agent for treatment or stimulation of granulation tissue.

The treatment of pressure sores depends on the stage of the ulcer and the condition of the wound bed. In many instances, cleansing and debridement prevent bacterial colonization from progressing to an infection. If a clean ulcer has exudate or does not heal after 2 to 4 weeks of treatment, a 2 week trial with topical antibiotics should be considered. The topical agent should be effective against gram-positive, gram-negative, and anaerobic bacteria, such as a triple antibiotic or silver sulfadiazine (Bergstrom et al, 1994).

If the ulcerated area does not respond, a tissue biopsy and bacterial culture are recommended in addition to an evaluation for osteomyelitis. Systemic antibiotics are necessary for sepsis, osteomyelitis, bacteremia, and advancing cellulitis (Bergstrom et al, 1994).

Saline solutions are considered safe and effective for cleaning most pressure sores. Avoid the use of povidone iodine, iodophor, Dakin's solution, acetic acid, and hydrogen peroxide because they are reported to be cytotoxic, that is, toxic to fibroblasts and interfering with the granulation process (Eastman, 1995).

Pressure sores have been classified into four grades or stages (Fig. 59-1):

- Stage I: a red area that overlies a bony or tendinous (tendons) site that remains even when the pressure is relieved
- Stage II: a partial-thickness skin loss involving epidermis and/or dermis
- Stage III: skin ulcer extending into exposed subcutaneous tissue that may include necrotic tissue, sinus tract formation, exudate, and/or infection
- Stage IV: deep skin ulcer that exposes muscle and bone; usually the body enzymes separate the eschar, sloughing of tissue results in an ulcer; may include necrotic tissue, sinus tract formation, exudate, and/or infection

Table 59-1 is a recommended treatment protocol based on the previous staging system.

Before the application of topical enzymes, the wound should be thoroughly but gently cleansed to flush away necrotic debris and exudates, with a solution that does not inactivate the enzyme (preferably normal saline or sterile distilled water). All previously applied ointment should be removed before the new ointment is applied.

An area that is dense, dry and thick, an **eschar,** or crust, should be cross-hatched by the physician with a blade so that adequate contact with the enzyme can be assured. The ointment is applied directly to the wound with a gauze pad,

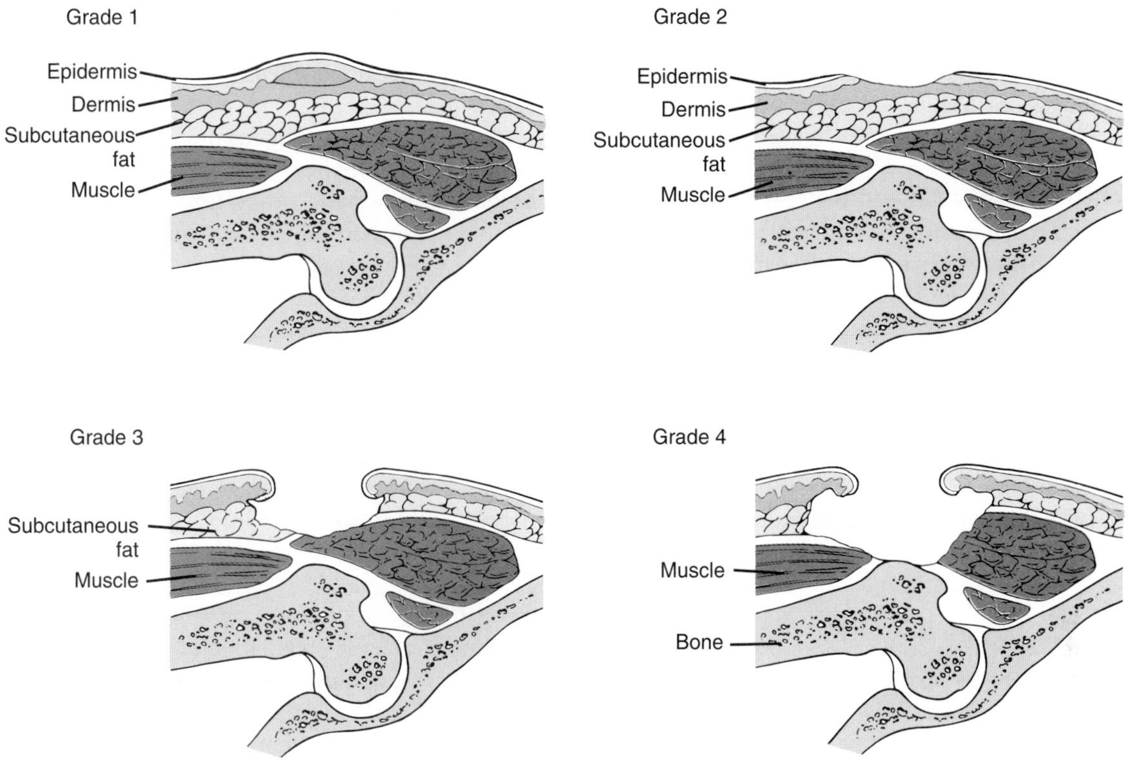

FIGURE 59-1
The four grades of pressure sores.

TABLE 59-1 Decubitus Ulcers: Recommended Treatment Protocol

Staging	*Typical Treatment Modalities*
Stage I or II	Silicone spray, transparent or hydrocolloidal dressing
Stage III	Wet to dry dressings, enzymatic debridement, hydrocolloidal dressing
Stage IV	Wet to dry dressings, enzymatic debridement, surgical debridement

sterile tongue depressor, or spatula and covered with sterile gauze. Bandage or tape is applied to hold the dressing in place. Confine application of the preparations to the wound only, protecting the surrounding healthy tissue from the enzyme (zinc oxide paste may be used for this purpose). Keep the treated lesion moist and protect it from drying.

To avoid delaying the healing, discontinue the enzyme when the wound is clean and debrided and **granulation tissue** (pink, healthy, soft new tissue) is present. A secondary skin closure or grafting may be necessary after the debridement. Be aware that debriding may increase the risk for bacteremia in debilitated persons, so monitor for infection. Also, monitor for allergic or hypersensitivity type reactions such as dermatitis and fever.

PROTEOLYTIC (DEBRIDING) ENZYMES

Debridement is used to remove necrotic and sloughing tissue in a pressure ulcer. This tissue delays healing and provides a media for bacterial infestation. Although commonly used for debridement, wet-to-dry saline dressings can be irritating, painful, and disruptive to healthy tissue. **Proteolytic enzymes** are used for chemical debridement; they digest or liquefy necrotic tissue. The drawback with these preparations is that 2 or 3 days are usually needed to get rid of an eschar. However, their use is appropriate for noninfected necrotic sites and for persons unable to tolerate surgical intervention. If used for infected necrosis tissue, a systemic antibiotic may also be necessary.

The enzyme preparation should be discontinued when granulation tissue is evident, or if bleeding occurs during gentle cleansing (Chamberlain et al, 1992). In very serious ulceration, or if complications are present (osteomyelitis), surgical debridement may be required.

Most enzymes contain the suffix "ase" in their name plus the name of the substrate on which they act. For example, collagenase acts on and degrades collagen; hyaluronidase acts on hyaluronic acid, a ground substance of connective tissue. Enzymes are also grouped according to the reactions they catalyze. For example, proteolytic enzymes hasten the hydrolysis of proteins. Because enzymes are proteins, they may be antigenic and cause toxic reactions of an immunologic type.

The enzymes discussed in this chapter are used topically for medical or chemical debridement: the removal, by enzymatic digestion, of necrotic and injured tissue, clotted blood, purulent exudates, or fibrinous accumulations in wounds. This action cleans the wounds and facilitates healing.

collagenase [kole′ a jen aze] (Santyl)

Collagenase, an enzymatic debriding agent, is capable of degrading both native and denatured collagen. Other proteolytic enzymes act only on denatured collagen. Thus it is claimed that collagenase produces more effective debridement by acting on collagen at the wound edges where necrotic slough is anchored. This product is used to debride necrotic lesions and severe burns.

This ointment should be applied only within the area of the lesion, since a transient erythema has been reported as a cutaneous reaction on the wound surface or the area adjacent to the lesion. This reaction may be prevented by applying a protectant (e.g., zinc oxide paste) around the lesion.

Drug interactions

The following effects may occur if collagenase is used with the following products:

Drug	Possible effect and management
Burow's solution and other acidic solutions	Collagenase can be inactivated by irrigating the lesion with acidic solutions such as Burow's (pH 3.6 to 4.4). The optimal pH range for collagenase is 6 to 8; a pH outside this range will decrease the enzyme's activity.
Detergents, soaps, cleansing agents, heavy metal ions (mercury and silver) antiseptics (e.g., iodine, hexachlorophene, and benzalkonium chloride), and boric acid	Activity of collagenase is inhibited.

Directions

Collagenase is usually applied once daily. If the wound is shallow, a gauze pad may be used for application whereas a deep wound requires application with a wooden tongue depressor or spatula.

fibrinolysin and desoxyribonuclease [fye bri nol′ ih sin/des ock see rye bo nu′ klee aze] (Elase)

The proteolytic enzymes fibrinolysin and desoxyribonuclease have individual effects: fibrinolysin digests fibrin or blood clots and desoxyribonuclease digests deoxyribonucleic acid (nucleic acids). Because purulent exudates are composed mainly of fibrin and nucleic acids, this product produces its effects on denatured proteins (devitalized tissue), while the protein elements of living cells are unaffected.

An ointment that contains the two enzymes in combination with chloramphenicol is also available. The added antibiotic bacteriostatic properties inhibit bacterial protein synthesis in infected lesions. Systemic antibiotics are also indicated when clinical infection has been verified by positive culture results.

This product is used to debride inflamed and/or infected lesions, including surgical wounds, ulcerative lesions, second- and third-degree burns, and wounds resulting from circumcision or episiotomy. The combination product with antibiotic is preferred for infected lesions. This product is also used for treatment of vaginitis and cervicitis (intravaginal use), and irrigation of infected wounds and superficial hematomas not adjacent to or near fatty tissue.

sutilains [soo′ ti lains] (Travase)

Sutilains is a sterile preparation of proteolytic enzymes that digests necrotic soft tissues and purulent exudates. It aids in the selective removal of only nonviable protein in necrotic soft tissue and of purulent exudate from open wounds and ulcers resulting from second- and third-degree burns, decubitus ulcers, peripheral vascular disease, and wounds (incisions, trauma, and pyogens).

Side effects are mild; they include mild, transient pain (managed with a mild analgesic), local paresthesia, bleeding, and transient dermatitis.

TOPICAL ENZYME COMBINATION PRODUCTS

Trypsin and papain (proteolytic enzymes), balsam Peru (mild antibacterial agent that aids in improving circulation in the wound area by stimulating the capillary bed), castor oil (protective covering that improves epithelialization), urea (emollient and keratolytic), and chlorophyll derivatives (aid in controlling wound odor and healing) have been formulated into various combinations and marketed. For example, Granulex contains trypsin, balsam Peru, and castor oil, whereas Panafil contains papain, urea, and chlorophyll derivatives.

Such products may be ordered for administration once or twice daily. The wound area should be cleansed by flushing with physiologic saline before application each time. Be aware that hydrogen peroxide solution can inactivate papain activity.

NONENZYMATIC AGENTS

dextranomer [dex tran′ oh mer] (Debrisan)

Dextranomers are hydrophilic beads placed in the wound to absorb exudate, bacteria, and other matter. It is used for cleansing only a wet or secreting wound (not dry wounds), and the action continues until all the beads are saturated. The assumption of a grayish-yellow color by the beads indicates that they are saturated and ready for removal.

Therapy with dextranomer is continued until healthy granulation is evident. Monitor patients who have diabetes mellitus or immunosuppression closely as they are more susceptible to the development of severe infections.

flexible hydroactive dressings and granules (Duo-Derm)

The control of wound fluid exudate absorption is a function of the rate at which the dressing interacts with the exudate. These dressings are indicated for necrotic wounds only after the thick eschar at the wound margin is removed. They provide local management of venous stasis ulcers and ulcers secondary to arterial insufficiency, diabetes mellitus, trauma, pressure sores, and superficial wounds. The granule form is for local management of exudating dermal ulcers in association with the dressings.

metronidazole [me troe ni′ da zole] (Flagyl)

Metronidazole is an antiinfective systemic agent used investigationally (orphan drug) to treat grade III and IV anaerobic-bacteria infested decubitus ulcers (Olin, 1998). An approved topical metronidazole (MetroGel) is used to treat acne rosacea in adults.

SUMMARY

The best treatment for pressure sores is prevention, as when they do occur they may be painful and require extensive care, perhaps even hospitalization. They are usually treated with proteolytic enzyme or nonenzymatic preparations, depending on the wound.

REVIEW QUESTIONS

1. Describe the four stages of classification for pressure sores. What stage(s) would require a proteolytic enzyme?
2. Explain the procedure for application of a proteolytic enzyme to a pressure sore and name two proteolytic enzyme products.
3. What products are used to improve circulation in the wound area? Name and discuss the reason for the five ingredients they may contain.

REFERENCES

Bergstrom N, Bennett MA, Carlson CE et al: *Treatment of pressure ulcers: clinical practice guidelines No 15,* AHCPR Pub No 95-0652, Rockville, Md, 1994, Agency for Health Care Policy and Research, US Department of Health and Human Services. Public Health Service.

Chamberlain TM et al: Assessment and management of pressure sores in long-term care facilities, *Consul Pharm* 7(12):1328-1340, 1992.

Eastman SR: Prevention and treatment of pressure ulcers: interpretation and practical application of AHCPR guidelines: Part 1. *Clin Consul* 14(10):1-8, 1995.

Olin BR: *Facts and comparisons.* Philadelphia, 1998, JB Lippincott.

ADDITIONAL REFERENCES

Anderson KN et al, editors: *Mosby's medical, nursing, and allied health dictionary,* ed 5, St Louis, 1998, Mosby.

Mosby: *Mosby's GenRx,* St Louis, 1998, Mosby.

United States Pharmacopeial Convention: *USP DI: drug information for the health care professional,* ed 18, Rockville, Md, 1998, The Convention.

Zanowiak P: Safe and effective management of pressure ulcers, *US Pharm: Skin Care Suppl* 6:6, 1996.

UNIT XVII

Intravenous and Nutritional Therapy

CHAPTER 60

Vitamins and Minerals

CHAPTER FOCUS

Vitamins and mineral preparations are essential compounds for specific body functions, particularly growth, maintenance, and reproduction. The healthcare professional should be informed on the proper use of these agents, their recommended dosages, and the side effects and adverse reactions and toxicity that occur when they are used inappropriately.

KEY TERMS

avitaminosis, (p. 768)
fat-soluble vitamins, (p. 768)
hypervitaminosis, (p. 768)
vitamins, (p. 768)
water-soluble vitamins, (p. 768)

OBJECTIVES

After reading and studying this chapter, the student should be able to do the following:

1. *Define and describe the key terms.*
2. *Name and discuss the factors that might contribute to inadequate intake of vitamins and/or iron.*
3. *Describe the difference between a fat-soluble and water-soluble vitamin and name the vitamins in each category.*
4. *Name the effects reported with a deficiency of each vitamin.*
5. *Name and describe the significant drug interactions reported with vitamins and iron.*

The nutritional needs of the individual are best met by adequate oral ingestion of fluids and regular balanced meals. Breast milk or formula meets the normal nutrition needs of the infant; strained and chopped table foods are added to the diet as tolerated by the growing child. Throughout life, challenges to nutrition status can occur that necessitate nutrient, vitamin, mineral, electrolyte, and fluid replacement or supplementation. Debilitation from nutritional deprivation may impair wound healing; reduce collagen, hormone, and enzyme synthesis; and decrease essential protein production, reducing circulating albumin, fibrinogen, and hemoglobin. Malnutrition or mild-to-moderate starvation produces serious cellular biochemical changes, including diminished liver glycogen stores, that start the first day of deprivation. Diminished protein stores are supplemented via gluconeogenesis because amino acids are converted into glucose as an energy source. Tissue proteins are depleted and short-lived in the intestinal mucous membranes, liver, pancreas, and kidney tubular epithelia. Muscle proteins are converted to provide energy, and adipose tissues are metabolized to produce free fatty acids for energy substrates. The byproducts of fatty acid oxidation (ketones) are used as energy for the brain if starvation is prolonged.

Unusual or abnormal circumstances necessitating administration of the various nutritional modalities, such as vitamin replacement and enteral or parenteral feedings, are discussed in the following sections.

VITAMINS

Vitamins are organic compounds that help maintain normal metabolic functions, growth, and tissue repair. Mechanisms of action, specific indications for use, and pharmacokinetics are not well understood for all vitamins, nor have dosages been established for all vitamins. However, vitamin supplement therapy may be essential during periods of nutritional challenge, typically during rapid growth, pregnancy, lactation, or convalescence. Other challenges to nutrition occur with inadequate nutrient ingestion, malabsorption syndromes, and increased nutrient requirements caused by specific disease states, such as celiac sprue and ulcerative colitis. An increase in cellular proliferation in the latter conditions may result in key nutrient depletion, such as of folic acid.

Insufficient dietary intake of vitamins and other essential nutrients occasionally may be traced to impoverished diets resulting from cultural, religious, or personal beliefs; fad diets; alcoholism; poverty; ignorance; or lack of available food. Mild forms of **avitaminosis** (vitamin deficiency), however, are more common in the United States and Canada (often as a result of alcoholism) than the pronounced deficiency states of beriberi, pellagra, rickets, or scurvy. The potential for iatrogenic starvation, however, exists because of ignorance or oversight on the part of the healthcare personnel who routinely fail to assess their patients' nutrition status or do not know how to correct it when necessary. Many medical procedures, such as nothing by mouth (NPO) orders to prepare the person for various gastrointestinal (GI) x-ray studies and procedures, may also potentially contribute to a person's malnutrition.

A commonly prescribed intravenous solution of dextrose 5% in water only delivers 170 calories/L and purely in the form of a carbohydrate. Multiple cleansing enemas or prolonged gastrointestinal suction rob the body of essential electrolytes. Only perfunctory medical assessment may be made of the effects of intraoperative blood losses or of wound drainage on nutrition needs, and surgery always is accompanied by increased nitrogen excretion.

Vitamin preparations and other, more aggressive, supportive nutrition therapies are needed for the hospitalized patient more often than is recognized because only a few vitamins are synthesized in the body. Vitamin K is formed by bacteria in the gut, vitamin D is produced when skin is exposed to sunlight, and small, insufficient amounts of vitamin B also are made in the gut. Thus most vitamins must either be ingested in food or taken as dietary supplements. There are two schools of thought concerning the consumption of vitamin supplements. Nutrition experts generally believe that the average American diet contains adequate vitamins and that additional supplements are unnecessary. Others, though, refer to surveys that indicate specific segments of our society—the elderly, smokers, nursing home residents, and teenagers—who reportedly do not consume the recommended daily allowance (RDA) levels of all vitamins and minerals. The most effective approach to correct such deficiencies is through diet, perhaps with the help of a dietitian. However, there are some circumstances in which a vitamin or nutritional supplement is indicated. Table 60-1 reviews vitamins and RDAs.

Hypervitaminosis is also of concern today, especially with the large consumption of vitamins in the United States. Hypervitaminosis is defined as an abnormal condition that results from consumption of high or excessive amounts of one or more vitamins, usually over an extended time period. The effects produced are discussed under the individual vitamin monographs. See the box on p. 771 for Food and Drug Administration (FDA) pregnancy safety categories.

Vitamins are classified as being fat soluble or water soluble. The **fat-soluble vitamins** are A, D, E, and K. They are stored in the liver and fatty tissue in large amounts, and a deficiency in these vitamins occurs only after long deprivation from an adequate supply or disorders preventing their absorption. **Water-soluble vitamins** include the B complex group and C. These vitamins are not stored in the body in large amounts, and short periods of inadequate intake can lead to a deficiency. Vitamins are important components of enzyme systems that catalyze the reactions for protein, fat, and carbohydrate metabolism.

Many multivitamin capsules and tablets vary in their contents. "Optional vitamins" (E, B_6, folic acid, pantothenic acid, and B_{12}) may or may not be included as ingredients in

TABLE 60-1 Vitamin Review

Vitamin	*Sources*	*Adverse Effects**	*Deficiency Effects*	*RDA†*
Fat Soluble				
A	Fish-liver oil, liver, butter, yellow fruit, green leafy vegetables, milk	Acute: confusion, irritation, diarrhea, dizziness, visual alterations, skin peeling, severe vomiting Chronic: bone pain, dry, cracked skin or lips, fever, increased urination, anorexia, loss of hair, seizures, vomiting	Night blindness, xerophthalmia, keratomalacia, skin lesions	Infant: 375 μg Child‡: 400-700 μg Male: 1000 μg Female: 800 μg Pregnant: 800 μg
D	Fish-liver oil, fortified milk, fish, exposure to sunlight	Early with hypercalcemia: constipation (mostly in children), diarrhea, headache, increased thirst and urination, metallic taste, nausea, vomiting Late: bone and muscle pain, increased blood pressure, pruritus, lethargy, mood alterations, pancreatitis	Bone and muscle pain, weakness, softening of bones that may result in fractures	Infant: 7.5-10 μg Child‡: 10 μg Male: 5-10 μg Female: 5-10 μg Pregnant: 10 μg
E	Nuts, green leafy vegetables, wheat and rice germ	Acute: visual disturbances, headache, nausea, stomach pain, weakness, blurred vision Chronic: increased bleeding tendencies in vitamin K-deficient clients, altered thyroid metabolism, impaired sexual function	Hyporeflexia, ataxia, myopathy, anemia, may increase cancer risk	Infant: 3-4 μg Child‡: 6-7 μg Male: 10 μg Female: 8 μg Pregnant: 10 μg
K	Liver, green leafy vegetables	Hypersensitivity (flushing, dyspnea, chest pain), taste alterations	Increased bleeding (e.g., ecchymoses, hematuria, GI bleeding)	Infant: 5-10 μg Child‡: 15-30 μg Male: 45-80 μg Female: 45-65 μg Pregnant: 65 μg
Water Soluble				
B_1 (thiamine)	Whole grain and enriched cereals, beef, pork, peas, beans, nuts	Low oral toxicity	Peripheral neuritis, loss of muscle strength, depression, memory loss, anorexia, poor memory, dyspnea	Infant: 0.3-0.4 mg Child‡: 0.7-1 mg Male: 1.2-1.5 mg Female: 1 mg Pregnant: 1.5 mg
B_2 (riboflavin)	Milk, cheese, eggs, green leafy vegetables, whole grain and enriched cereals and breads, organ meats	Low toxicity	Sore throat, stomatitis, red, painful or swollen tongue, facial dermatitis, anemia	Infant: 0.4-0.5 mg Child‡: 0.8-1.2 mg Male: 1.4-1.8 mg Female: 1.2-1.3 mg Pregnant: 1.6 mg
B_3 (niacin)	Meats, eggs, milk, dairy products	Flushing, pruritus, feelings of warmth High doses: dizziness, dysrythmias, dry skin, hyperglycemia, myalgia, nausea, vomiting, diarrhea	Skin eruptions, stomatitis, diarrhea, enteritis, headache, dizziness, insomnia, memory impairment, dementia	Infant: 5-6 mg Child‡: 9-13 mg Male: 15-20 mg Female: 13-15 mg Pregnant: 17 mg

*Adverse effects will include acute and chronic or early and late overdose symptoms, when available.
†RDA is the recommended daily allowance recommended from dietary sources.
‡Child; 1 to 10 yr of age.
From Allen, 1996; Marcus, Coulston, 1996a, 1996b; USP DI, 1998.

Continued

TABLE 60-1 Vitamin Review—cont'd

Vitamin	*Sources*	*Adverse Effects**	*Deficiency Effects*	*RDA†*
Water Soluble—cont'd				
B_6 (pyridoxine)	Liver, meats, whole-grain bread/ cereals, soybeans, eggs, vegetables	Acute: low toxicity Chronic high doses: neurotoxicity—ataxia, numb feet, clumsiness	Seborrhea-like skin lesions, stomatitis, seizures, peripheral neuritis	Infant: 0.3-0.6 mg Child‡: 1-1.4 mg Male: 1.7-2 mg Female: 1.4-1.6 mg Pregnant: 2.2 mg
B_9 (folic acid)	Liver, fresh green vegetables, yeast, some fruits	Allergic reaction, red skin, fever, skin rash, pruritus	Megaloblastic anemia	Infant: 25-35 μg Child‡: 50-100 μg Male: 150-200 μg Female: 150-180 μg Pregnant: 400 μg
B_{12} (cyanocobalamin)	Fish, egg yolk, milk, fermented cheeses	No toxicity	Irreversible nervous system damage (paresthesia, ataxia), memory loss, confusion, dementia, abnormal hematopoiesis	Infant: 0.3-0.5 μg Child†: 0.7-1.4 μg Male: 2 μg Female: 2 μg Pregnant: 2.2 μg
C (ascorbic acid)	Citrus fruits, tomatoes, potatoes, strawberries, cabbage	Kidney stones, dizziness High doses: diarrhea, red skin, headache, nausea, vomiting	Scurvy (loosening of teeth, gingivitis), anemia Infants: irritability, pain if touched	Infant: 30-35 mg Child‡: 40-45 mg Male: 50-60 mg Female: 50-60 mg Pregnant: 70 mg

*Adverse effects will include acute and chronic or early and late overdose symptoms, when available.
†RDA is the recommended daily allowance recommended from dietary sources.
‡Child; 1 to 10 yr of age.
From Allen, 1996; Marcus, Coulston, 1996a, 1996b; USP DI, 1998.

PREGNANCY SAFETY

Category	Drug
A	thiamine, pyridoxine, folic acid
C	vitamin D, cyanocobalamin (vitamin B_{12}), ascorbic acid (vitamin C), iron
X	vitamin A
Unclassified	niacin, riboflavin, vitamin K, vitamin E

over-the-counter (OTC) multivitamin preparations. However, the most popular OTC multivitamin preparations contain all the vitamins needed by humans. Most OTC vitamin preparations are designed to meet daily body needs completely without regard for the amounts of various vitamins contained in the daily diet.

FAT-SOLUBLE VITAMINS

vitamin A [Aquasol A]

Vitamin A, the fat-soluble, growth-promoting vitamin, is essential for growth in the younger age groups, for normal function of the retina, and for maintenance of health at all ages. Vitamin A (retinol) is derived from animals, whereas the provitamin A carotenoids are found in plants. Beta-carotene, the most active carotenoid from plants, is hydrolyzed in the body to form two molecules of vitamin A. Animal fats, such as those found in butter, milk, eggs, and fish liver, are sources of the carotenoids that were originally derived from plants and stored in animal tissues.

Vitamin A is essential in promoting normal growth and development of bones and teeth and maintaining the health of epithelial tissues of the body. Its function in relation to normal vision and the prevention of night blindness has been studied carefully. Vitamin A actually is part of one of the major retinal pigments, rhodopsin, and thus is required for normal "rod vision" in the retina of human beings and many animals.

Vitamin A has the following indications:

1. It is used to treat or relieve symptoms associated with a deficiency of vitamin A, such as night blindness (nyctalopia), hyperkeratosis, retarded growth, xerophthalmia, keratomalacia, weakness, and increased susceptibility of mucous membranes to infection.
2. An analog (tretinoin) is used to treat acne (see Chapter 58).
3. Vitamin requirements increase during pregnancy and during breastfeeding; when possible, these needs are best met with food rather than with drugs. However, prescribers may recommend vitamin supplementation especially in women who may not consume a proper diet or those in a high-risk category, such as heavy cigarette smokers, alcohol or substance abusers, or women pregnant with more than one fetus. Consuming excessive amounts of vitamins, especially of the fat-soluble vitamins, may be dangerous to both the mother and fetus. Large doses of vitamin A may cause neurologic and skin damage in adults, and excessive doses are known to produce highly toxic effects in rats and in young children.

Vitamin A and carotene are readily absorbed from the normal gastrointestinal tract. Efficient absorption depends on fat absorption and therefore on the presence of adequate bile salts in the intestine. Certain conditions such as obstructive jaundice, some infectious diseases, and the presence of mineral oil in the intestine may result in vitamin A deficiency despite the amount ingested being normal.

Vitamin A is stored to a greater extent in the liver than elsewhere. The liver also functions in changing carotene to vitamin A; this function is inhibited in persons with liver diseases and diabetes. The amount of vitamin A stored depends on the dietary intake. When intake is high or excessive, the stores formed in the liver may be sufficient to last several years. Vitamin A is metabolized by the liver and excreted by the feces and kidneys. For adverse and deficiency effects plus the RDA, see Table 60-1.

The vitamin A dosage depends on the age, sex, and condition of the individual and on the purpose (prophylaxis or treatment). See a current reference for dosing information.

vitamin D

The term "vitamin D" is applied to two substances that affect the proper usage of calcium and phosphorus in the body. Both substances have the ability to prevent or cure rickets. The plant vitamin D is referred to as vitamin D_2 or ergocalciferol; the natural form of vitamin D is produced in the skin by ultraviolet irradiation of 7-dehydrocholesterol and is referred to as vitamin D_3 or cholecalciferol. Although ergocalciferol contains a chemical double bond and an extra methyl group, the difference is not significant physiologically.

Both cholecalciferol and ergocalciferol are metabolized in the liver to calcifediol, which is then transported to the kidney where it is converted to calcitriol, which is believed to be the most active analog (Marcus, 1996).

Calcitriol appears to bind to a receptor in the intestinal mucosa and is incorporated into the cell nucleus, resulting in the formation of a calcium-binding protein that increases calcium absorption from the intestine. Parathyroid hormone and calcitriol both act to control the transfer of calcium ions from bones into the extracellular fluid; therefore they maintain a calcium homeostasis effect in the extracellular fluid. Although an essential vitamin, vitamin D is found in only a few foods of the average American/Canadian diet (see Table 60-1).

Other vitamin D analogs available include alfacalcidol (One-Alpha 🍁), calcitriol (Rocaltrol), and dihydrotachysterol (Hytakerol). They are preferred in certain situations, such as for the person in renal failure, as they do not require required conversion for their action. They also have shorter half-lives so any toxic adverse effects would be easier to manage. Calcifediol (Calderol) appears to have some vitamin D activity in addition to its conversion to the active metabolite calcitriol.

Vitamin D is necessary for the absorption and use of calcium and phosphorus in the body and for the normal calcification of bone. In the absence of vitamin D (even if the calcium and phosphate intake is adequate) rickets in children and osteomalacia in adults may result. Vitamin D is used to treat and prevent nutritional rickets, osteomalacia, hypoparathyroidism, and osteoporosis (Marcus, 1996).

The incidence of rickets is low in the United States and Canada, but it can occur in young children who are restricted to vegetarian diets without milk supplementation or in infants who are breastfed by mothers who did not take prenatal vitamins nor drink milk. A vitamin D deficiency results in an inadequate intake and perhaps an excessive loss of calcium from the body.

Vitamin D is absorbed from the small intestine (ergocalciferol requires the presence of bile salts for absorption). It is protein bound and stored mainly in fat and in the liver.

Pharmacokinetics

The serum half-life of calcifediol is about 16 days, of calcitriol is from 3 to 6 hours, and of ergocalciferol is within 19 to 48 hours, but the latter can be stored in fat sites for longer periods. The onset of the hypercalcemic effect for calcitriol is within 3 to 6 hours; for dihydrotachysterol within hours, although the maximum effect is seen in 7 to 14 days; and for ergocalciferol within 12 to 24 hours, although a therapeutic response may not be seen until 10 to 14 days later.

The duration of effect after oral administration for calcifediol is 15 to 20 days, for calcitriol 3 to 5 days, for dihydrotachysterol up to 9 weeks, and for ergocalciferol up to 6 months. Excretion is via the bile and kidneys. For adverse and deficiency effects plus the RDA, see Table 60-1.

Drug interactions

The following effects may occur when vitamin D products are given with the drugs listed below:

Drug	Possible effect and management
Antacids containing magnesium	May result in hypermagnesemia, especially in patients with chronic renal failure. Avoid concurrent administration if possible; if not, monitor closely for diminished reflexes, muscle weakness, drowsiness, confusion, lethargy, bradycardia, and hypotension.
Calcium preparations in high doses or thiazide diuretics	Increases risk for hypercalcemia. Monitor closely for drowsiness, lethargy, weakness, muscle flaccidity, hypertension, anorexia, nausea, constipation, polyuria, and flank pain.
Vitamin D, other products	Increased risk of toxicity. Avoid or a potentially serious drug interaction may occur.

Color type indicates an unsafe drug combination

Dosage and administration

The usual adolescent and adult dose for alfacalcidol is 1 μg/day for calcifediol 50 to 100 μg/day, for calcitriol 0.25 mg/day, and for dihydrotachysterol 125 μg to 2 mg/day. Dosages are adjusted periodically as necessary. Pediatric dosages vary. See a current reference for recommendations.

vitamin E (α-tocopherol)
vitamin E capsules (Aquasol E)

Vitamin E is a fat-soluble vitamin that is present in margarine made from plant oils such as cottonseed oil, as well as in green, leafy vegetables and whole grains. Although a number of compounds have been found to exhibit vitamin E activity, the most active of these is α-tocopherol as it is the substance used to calculate the food content of vitamin E.

Studies have reported a significant decrease in coronary artery disease in persons consuming large doses of vitamin E. The hypothesis is that oxidation of lipoproteins reduces atherogenesis (Steinberg, 1993).

Rimm et al (1993) studied 39,910 male healthcare professionals in the United States for 4 years and assessed their intake of various nutrients, including vitamin E. They found that men who consumed a high intake of vitamin E had a lower risk of developing coronary artery heart disease. Stampfer et al (1993) followed 87,245 female nurses between the ages of 34 to 59 years for up to 8 years. They reported similar findings in women: middle-aged women using vitamin E supplements for more than 2 years had a reduced risk of developing coronary heart disease. In both studies, the participants excluded anyone with a history of cardiovascular disease. Further studies are necessary to evaluate the vitamin E dosages necessary to produce this effect and also the potential risk of toxicity from long-term consumption of large doses of vitamin E.

Vitamin E is an essential nutrient, but its exact function is unknown. It has been reported to have antioxidant properties when used in conjunction with dietary selenium, to prevent the effects of peroxidase on unsaturated bonds in the cell membranes, and to protect red blood cells from hemolysis. It is also known to be a cofactor for several enzyme systems in the body.

Pharmacokinetics

The absorption of vitamin E from the GI tract requires the presence of bile salts, dietary fats, and normal pancreatic functioning. Vitamin E binds to beta-lipoproteins in the blood and is stored in all body tissues, especially in fat depots (which contain up to a 4-year requirement of this vitamin). It is metabolized in the liver and excreted in bile and kidneys. For adverse and deficiency effects and the RDA, see Table 60-1.

Drug interactions

When vitamin E is given concurrently with large doses of iron supplements, vitamin E oxidation increases, which increases the daily requirement for vitamin E. If given concurrently, monitor closely to determine an appropriate intervention.

Dosage and administration

The usual adult dose for vitamin E deficiency is 100 to 400 units daily. Pediatric dosages vary. See a current reference for recommendations.

WATER-SOLUBLE VITAMINS

The water-soluble vitamins are ascorbic acid (vitamin C) and B vitamins. The B vitamins are often found together in food and are referred to as vitamin B complex. However, they are chemically dissimilar and have different metabolic functions. This B grouping is largely based on their having been discovered in sequential order. A sensible and increasingly popular trend promotes discarding such names as vitamin B_1 and B_2 and referring to these vitamins as thiamine and riboflavin. The vitamin B complex includes thiamine, riboflavin, nicotinic acid, pyridoxine, folic acid, pantothenic acid, biotin, choline, inositol, and vitamin B_{12} (cyanocobalamin).

This discussion will be limited to the B vitamins that are associated with deficiency states and for which information on therapeutic application is available: thiamine (vitamin B_1), riboflavin (vitamin B_2), niacin (nicotinic acid), pyridoxine (vitamin B_6), cyanocobalamin (vitamin B_{12}), and folic acid.

thiamine [thye′ a min]
(vitamin B_1, Biamine, Bewon ♣)

Thiamine in combination with adenosine triphosphate (ATP) results in thiamine pyrophosphate coenzyme, a substance necessary for carbohydrate metabolism. Thiamine is used to prevent and treat thiamine deficiency, which can result in beriberi or Wernicke's encephalopathy.

Pharmacokinetics

Thiamine is well absorbed from the GI tract, except in malabsorption syndrome or in the presence of alcohol, which inhibits absorption. It is metabolized in the liver and excreted by the kidneys. Side effects are usually rare. Skin rash, pruritus, or respiratory difficulties (wheezing) may occur rarely after a large intravenous dose is administered (anaphylactic reaction).

Dosage and administration

The usual adult dose is determined by age, sex, and degree of vitamin deficiency and ranges from 5 to 30 mg/day. For the recommended pediatric dose, see a current reference.

riboflavin [rye′ boo flay vin] (vitamin B_2)

Riboflavin is converted in the body into two coenzymes: flavin mononucleotide (FMN) and flavin adenine dinucleotide (FAD), substances necessary for normal tissue respiration. Riboflavin is also necessary to activate pyridoxine and convert tryptophan to niacin and may also be connected to maintenance of erythrocyte integrity.

Riboflavin is indicated for the prevention and treatment of riboflavin deficiency; usually this deficiency does not occur in healthy persons but may be detected as a result of malnutrition or intestinal malabsorption.

Pharmacokinetics

Riboflavin is well absorbed in the GI tract and has a half-life of approximately 1 to 1.5 hours. It is metabolized in the liver and excreted by the kidneys. Side effects are rare. No significant drug interactions have been reported with riboflavin.

Dosage and administration

The usual adult dose to treat riboflavin deficiency ranges from 5 to 10 mg. See a current reference for additional dosing information.

niacin [nye′ a sin] (nicotinic acid)
niacin extended release (Nicobid, Slo-Niacin)
niacinamide tablets/injection

Niacin is converted to niacinamide in the body and is part of two coenzymes, nicotinamide adenine dinucleotide (NAD) and nicotinamide adenine dinucleotide phosphate (NADP), necessary for glycogenolysis, tissue respiration, and lipid, protein, and purine metabolism. As an antihyperlipidemic agent, niacin lowers serum cholesterol and triglyceride levels by reducing very-low-density lipoprotein (VLDL) synthesis. VLDL is the precursor to low-density lipoprotein, the main carrier of cholesterol in the blood.

Niacin and niacinamide are indicated for the prevention and treatment of vitamin B_3 deficiency conditions. A niacin deficiency may result in pellagra. Only niacin is indicated as a treatment adjunct for hyperlipidemia, but its usefulness may be limited by its side effects, especially its vasodilating effects. Niacinamide does not cause direct peripheral vasodilation.

Pharmacokinetics

With the exception of the malabsorption syndromes, both niacin and niacinamide are readily absorbed orally and have a half-life of 45 minutes. Whereas onset of action to reduce triglyceride serum levels is several hours, to reduce cholesterol levels takes several days. Niacin is metabolized by the liver and excreted in the kidneys. For adverse and deficiency effects and the RDA, see Table 60-1. No significant drug interactions are reported with its use.

Dosage and administration

For antihyperlipidemia, the usual adult dose for niacin is 1 g PO daily, increased every 2 to 4 weeks as necessary. As dose of niacin and niacinamide vary according to age and sex of the individual, check current reference for additional information.

pyridoxine [peer i dox′ een] (vitamin B_6)
pyridoxine extended release (Rodex)

Pyridoxine is taken up by erythrocytes and converted into pyridoxal phosphate, a coenzyme necessary for many metabolic functions that affect proteins, carbohydrates, and lipid usage in the body. Pyridoxine is also involved with the conversion of tryptophan to niacin or serotonin.

Pyridoxine is indicated to treat or prevent pyridoxine deficiency. A deficiency state can lead to sideroblastic anemia, neurologic disturbances, seborrheic dermatitis, cheilosis, and xanthurenic aciduria.

Pharmacokinetics

Oral pyridoxine is well absorbed from the jejunum and converted in erythrocytes to pyridoxal phosphate, which is totally protein bound in the plasma. It has a half-life of 15 to 20 days and is metabolized by the liver and excreted in the kidneys. Side effects and adverse reactions are very rare. Side effects are seen only when dosages of 200 mg/day are given for more than a month, resulting in a dependency-type syndrome. Megadoses can cause problems (see Table 60-1).

Dosage and administration

The usual pyridoxine dose varies according to age, sex, and degree of vitamin deficiency. See a current reference for dosing recommendations.

cyanocobalamin [sye an oh koe bal′ a min] (vitamin B_{12})
hydroxocobalamin [hye drox oh koe bal′ a min] (Alphamin)

Cyanocobalamin is a coenzyme for a variety of metabolic functions including protein synthesis, and fat and carbohydrate metabolism. It is also needed for growth, cell replication, hematopoiesis, and nucleoprotein and myelin synthesis.

Cyanocobalamin is used to treat pernicious anemia (caused by lack of intrinsic factor) and to prevent and treat vitamin B_{12} deficiency caused by malabsorption or strict vegetarianism. Vitamin B_{12} deficiency can lead to macrocytic megaloblastic anemia and irreversible neurologic damage.

Pharmacokinetics

For vitamin B_{12} to be absorbed orally, the intrinsic factor must be present in the intestinal tract. It is highly protein bound with a half-life of 6 days and reaches its peak serum level in 8 to 12 hours. It is metabolized (and stored) by the liver and excreted in bile and urine. After parenteral injection, anaphylactic reactions are possible but rare (see Table 60-1). No significant drug interactions are reported.

Dosage and administration

The usual dose varies according to age, sex, and degree of vitamin deficiency. See Box 60-1 for information on the nasal spray form of vitamin B_{12}. See a current reference for dosing recommendations.

BOX 60-1 Vitamin B_{12} Nasal Spray

Nascobal, a vitamin B_{12} nasal spray, was approved as a maintenance drug for persons in remission after IM therapy for conditions such as pernicious anemia. The dose is usually 500 μg intranasally once a week. A warning on the product states that if the person's condition is not properly maintained on this spray, resumption of intramuscular vitamin B_{12} is necessary.

Side/adverse effects include infection, headache, glossitis, nausea, and rhinitis (FDA News and Product Notes, 1997).

folic acid (vitamin B_9)
folic acid (Folvite, Apo-Folic ♣)

Folic acid is converted to tetrahydrofolic acid in the body, which is necessary for normal erythropoiesis, metabolism of amino acids, and nucleoprotein synthesis.

Folic acid is used to treat and prevent folic acid deficiency. Folic acid should not be administered until pernicious anemia has been ruled out as a potential diagnosis. If administered to patients with undiagnosed pernicious anemia, it will correct the hematologic changes and mask pernicious anemia while the underlying neurologic damage progresses.

A folic acid deficiency may result in megaloblastic and macrocytic anemias and glossitis. A deficiency of maternal folic acid is associated with neural tube defects.

Pharmacokinetics

Folic acid is absorbed mostly from the upper duodenum; it is highly protein bound, metabolized (and stored) in the liver, and excreted by the kidneys. Folic acid in the presence of vitamin C (ascorbic acid) is converted in the liver and serum to its active form, tetrahydrofolic acid, by dihydrofolate reductase.

Side effects and adverse reactions

These are rare. An allergic reaction (elevated temperature and rash) or yellow discoloration of urine may occur. The usual folic acid dose varies according to age, sex, and degree of vitamin deficiency. See a current reference for dosing recommendations.

ascorbic acid (vitamin C)

Ascorbic acid is necessary for collagen formation in fibrous tissue including bone and in the development of teeth, blood vessels, and blood cells. It also plays a role in carbohydrate metabolism. It is believed to stimulate the fibroblasts of connective tissue and thus promote tissue repair and the healing of wounds. It also may help maintain the integrity of the intercellular substance in the walls of blood vessels; the capillary fragility associated with scurvy is explained on this basis. It may be necessary for the metabolism of phenylalanine, tyrosine, folic acid, norepinephrine, histamine, and iron.

The effectiveness of ascorbic acid in preventing or relieving cold symptoms or in the treatment of cancer, infertility, aging, or peptic ulcer is primarily unproven. Studies performed over the years have not substantiated these claims (USP DI, 1998).

Pharmacokinetics

Ascorbic acid is well absorbed from the GI tract and stored in plasma and cells, with the highest concentration found in glandular sites. It is metabolized in the liver and excreted by the kidneys. See Table 60-1 for additional information.

Drug interactions

Concurrent administration of ascorbic acid with deferoxamine may increase tissue iron, especially in the heart, causing cardiac decompensation. If absolutely necessary to give ascorbic acid, then the oral dose of ascorbic acid should be given 1 to 2 hours after the deferoxamine infusion.

Dosage and administration

The adult dosage as a nutritional supplement is 50 to 100 mg daily. To treat a vitamin C deficiency the dosage varies according to age and severity of vitamin deficiency.

MULTIPLE-VITAMIN PREPARATIONS

Numerous multivitamin preparations are available in the United States and Canada. Supplemental preparations should provide 100% of the United States RDA to meet the needs of the vast majority of patients. Extra-potency or high-potency vitamins are rarely necessary for routine supplementation. In addition, the healthcare professional should be aware that many preparations contain chemicals that are not yet known to be associated with any known deficiency states.

MINERALS

Although many minerals are available, this discussion is limited to iron, the most commonly prescribed mineral for iron-deficiency anemia. Other minerals are reviewed in other sections of this book.

iron supplements

Iron is an essential mineral for the proper functioning of many biologic systems in the body. It functions as an oxygen carrier in hemoglobin and myoglobin, for tissue respiration, and for many enzyme reactions in the body. It is also stored in various body sites, such as the liver, spleen, and bone marrow. Iron deficiency is the most common nutritional deficiency in the United States resulting in anemia. Young children and women, especially pregnant women, are most frequently affected.

Iron is supplied through diet (lean red meats) and iron supplements. Ingested iron is converted to the ferrous state by gastric juices, which is then more readily absorbed in the body. The absorption of iron will be increased if it is taken with ascorbic acid (vitamin C), orange juice, veal, and other animal tissues. Coffee, tea, milk, eggs, whole grain breads, and cereals decrease iron absorption.

Iron is indicated for the treatment of iron-deficiency anemia.

Pharmacokinetics

In iron deficiency, between 10% to 30% of iron is absorbed while in normal individuals, about 5% to 15% is usually absorbed. Ferrous iron is absorbed better than the ferric dosage form. Iron binds to transferrin and is transported to bone marrow to aid in red blood cell production. Iron is not eliminated physiologically by the body. Excess iron intake can result in accumulation and iron toxicity. Small amounts are lost daily in shedding of skin, nails, hair, breast milk, urine, and menstrual blood. In healthy adults the daily iron loss is approximately 1 mg/day for men and postmenopausal women and 1.5 to 2 mg/day in healthy premenopausal women.

Drug interactions

The following effects may occur when iron salts are given with the drugs listed below:

Drug	Possible effect and management
acetohydroxamic acid (Lithostat)	Iron may be chelated by the acetohydroxamic acid, resulting in reduced absorption of both drugs. If iron therapy is necessary for a patient receiving acetohydroxamic acid, it is suggested that iron be administered parenterally.
calcium supplements, milk or dairy products, coffee, fiber, or selected food products (see previous section)	Decreased iron absorption may result. Schedule iron supplements at least 1 hour before and 2 hours after administration of these substances.
dimercaprol (BAL in oil)	A toxic complex may result if iron and dimercaprol are given concurrently. Postpone daily administration of iron for at least 24 hours after dimercaprol is discontinued. If a severe iron deficiency occurs while the patient is receiving dimercaprol, a blood transfusion may be indicated.
etidronate (Didronel)	May result in decreased absorption of oral etidronate. Teach patients to avoid consumption of iron products within 2 hours of etidronate.

Tetracyclines, oral	Decreases absorption of tetracycline, which may result in reduced antibiotic effectiveness. May impair hematologic effectiveness of the iron supplement. Administer iron supplements 2 hours after tetracyclines.
vitamin E	Concurrent administration with iron may reduce the patient's hematologic response to iron therapy. If larger iron doses are administered, vitamin E requirements may also need to be increased. Close monitoring is suggested when concurrent therapy is administered.

Color type indicates an unsafe drug combination

Side effects and adverse reactions

For iron therapy these include nausea, vomiting, constipation (diarrhea, less frequently reported), and abdominal cramps. For treatment of iron toxicity, see the box on Management of Drug Overdose.

SUMMARY

Maintaining an adequate vitamin and iron intake is best accomplished by the regular consumption of a balanced diet. Vitamins are necessary for maintaining normal metabolic functions, growth, and repair of body tissues. Vitamin deficiencies, when they occur, are usually multiple (more than a single vitamin) and result from impoverished diets perhaps due to alcoholism, poverty, fads, ignorance, a number of chronic diseases, and cancer. They occur most frequently in the elderly, smokers, and teenagers. Replacement vitamin therapy is necessary in such persons. This chapter reviewed the recommended daily dosages of the individual vitamins (fat and water soluble) and iron in addition to the signs and symptoms of deficiency or excessive use of these agents. Supplement therapy is practical, but, as in all nutritional deficiencies, the best remedy is dietary intake.

MANAGEMENT OF DRUG OVERDOSE

Iron Supplements

- **Early signs of acute toxicity:** diarrhea that may contain blood, fever, severe abdominal cramps/pain, vomiting
- **Late signs:** pale, cold skin; convulsions; increased weakness; sedation; blue-tinted lips, fingernails, and palms of hands; irregular heart beat; hypotension, metabolic acidosis; cardiovascular collapse
- **Treatment:** Seek medical attention immediately. Induce emesis with ipecac syrup or lavage containing sodium bicarbonate, depending on condition of the individual.
- Maintain fluid and electrolyte balance.
- Antidote (deferoxamine) is used for severe iron toxicity. Avoid antidote if person has renal failure.
- Monitor laboratory tests (e.g., serum iron, hemoglobin, hematocrit, electrolytes, blood gases, blood glucose, total iron-binding capacity, and complete blood counts) closely.
- If necessary, an exchange transfusion may be given.

REVIEW QUESTIONS

1. Why is vitamin supplementation recommended for persons who are hospitalized for extended time-periods? Assume the individual is receiving dextrose in water, 2 L/24 hr. Discuss your answer.
2. Name the different forms of vitamin D. How does the body process this vitamin? Name two indications for vitamin D.
3. Discuss the function and indications for niacin, cyanocobalamin, pyridoxine, ascorbic acid, folic acid, and vitamin E in the body.

REFERENCES

Allen LV Jr: Nutritional products. In Covington TR, editor: *Handbook of nonprescription drugs,* ed 11, Washington, DC, 1996, American Pharmaceutical Association.

FDA News and Product Notes: New formulations/combinations, *Formulary* 32(1):23-24, 1997.

Marcus R: Agents affecting calcification and bone turnover. In Hardman JG, Limbird LE, editors: *Goodman & Gilman's the pharmacological basis of therapeutics,* ed 9, New York, 1996, McGraw-Hill.

Marcus R , Coulston AM: Fat-soluble vitamins. In Hardman JG, Limbird LE, editors: *Goodman & Gilman's the pharmacological basis of therapeutics,* ed 9, New York, 1996a, McGraw-Hill.

Marcus R , Coulston AM: Water-soluble vitamins, In Hardman JG, Limbird LE, editors: *Goodman & Gilman's the pharmacological basis of therapeutics,* ed 9, New York, 1996b, McGraw-Hill.

Rimm EB et al: Vitamin E consumption and the risk of coronary heart disease in men, *N Engl J Med* 328(20):1450, 1993.

Stampfer MJ et al: Vitamin E consumption and the risk of coronary disease in women, *N Engl J Med* 328(20):1444, 1993.

Steinberg D: Antioxidant vitamins and coronary heart disease, *N Engl J Med* 328(20):1487, 1993.

United States Pharmacopeial Convention: *USP DI: drug information for the health care professional,* ed 18, Rockville, Md, 1998, The Convention.

ADDITIONAL REFERENCES

American Hospital Formulary Service: *AHFS drug information '98,* Bethesda, Md, 1998, American Society of Hospital Pharmacists.

Anderson KN et al, editors: *Mosby's medical, nursing, and allied health dictionary,* ed 5, St Louis, 1998, Mosby.

Covington TR, editor: *Handbook of nonprescription drugs,* ed 11, Washington, DC, 1996, American Pharmaceutical Association.

Fawzi WW et al: Vitamin A supplementation and child mortality, *JAMA* 269(7):898, 1993.

Katzung BG: *Basic and clinical pharmacology,* ed 5, Norwalk, Conn, 1992, Appleton & Lange.

Mosby: *Mosby's GenRx,* St Louis, 1998, Mosby.

CHAPTER 61

Fluids and Electrolytes

CHAPTER FOCUS

The administration of intravenous fluids and electrolytes is commonly done today in hospitals, in outpatient departments, and in the home setting. An understanding of the different solutions and electrolytes available, composition, dosage, and proper administration is vital information for the healthcare professional.

OBJECTIVES

After reading and studying this chapter, the student should be able to do the following:

1. *Define and describe the key terms.*
2. *List at least five reasons for the use of intravenous solutions.*
3. *Describe the importance and uses of water in human beings.*
4. *Explain water transport in the body, including intake, loss, and transport.*
5. *Name the four categories of parenteral solutions, and give two examples of solutions in each category.*
6. *Identify one condition or disease state for the use of each category of parenteral solutions.*
7. *Name and describe the differences between the three types of dehydration.*
8. *Relate the normal serum level, dietary sources, functions, and problems associated with a deficiency or excess of sodium, potassium, and calcium.*

KEY TERMS

dehydration, (p. 778)
extracellular fluid, (p. 778)
intracellular fluid, (p. 778)
milliequivalent (mEq), (p. 787)
osmolality, (p. 779)
osmosis, (p. 779)
overhydration, (p. 778)

The intravenous administration of parenteral fluids has become more prevalent during the past 50 years. Initially, the problems associated with the use of unsafe solutions were caused by pyrogens. Once this issue was resolved, the advances in the technology of intravenous therapy have resulted in products that have significantly improved patient safety (Box 61-1).

INTRODUCTION

There has also been a vast increase in outpatient and home administration of IV medications, hyperalimentation, and fluids. New sophisticated delivery systems have been developed, and different methods of application are constantly being conceived. Intravenous solutions are infused for various therapeutic reasons, including the following:

- Replace fluids and electrolytes
- Correct acid-base imbalance
- Administer medications
- Maintain ready access to the venous system if any of the first three measures is anticipated
- Measure changes in venous pressure
- Measure the kidneys' excretory capabilities by diagnostic test
- Administer essential nutrients

Blood and its components are transfused intravenously to (1) replace blood volume or plasma fractions; (2) restore the blood's capabilities for oxygen carrying, clotting, or oncotic pressure; or (3) cleanse the plasma of harmful constituents by exchanges. Intravenous hyperalimentation or parenteral nutrition solutions are infused to complement or supplement dietary intake of individuals in deprived nutrition states.

Box 61-1 Intravenous Therapy: 1930s to Today

Early 1930s

Intravenous injections were reserved for only seriously ill patients.

Only a physician could perform the venipuncture.

1940s

Massachusetts General Hospital became one of the first hospitals to assign a nurse to intravenous therapy.

The job description included administering intravenous solutions and blood transfusions, cleaning the infusion sets for reuse, and cleaning and sharpening needles for reuse.

The primary responsibility was of a technical nature: administering and maintaining the infusions and keeping the equipment clean and functional.

1950s to 1990s

Improvements and innovations in equipment (such as pumps and monitors), needles (Intracaths, and so forth), tubing, development of plastic and disposable equipment, and an increased variety of commercially prepared intravenous fluids increased the safety of intravenous therapy.

The development of intravenous filters prevents particulate matter, bacteria, or fungus from entering the bloodstream.

The intravenous route is used to administer many medications and hyperalimentation fluids, in addition to intravenous fluids.

FLUIDS

Depending on the amount of adipose tissue present, water comprises from 45% to 75% of the total human body weight. Infants and young children have more water per unit of body weight than adults, and female adults have less water content than male adults. The greatest amount of body water (up to 45% of body weight) is found in the intracellular fluid; the remainder of body water is located in the extracellular fluid. **Intracellular fluid** is the fluid inside the cells, where the chemical reactions of all metabolism essential to life occur. **Extracellular fluid** is the fluid surrounding the cells: plasma, interstitial fluid, and lymph, as well as extracellular portions of dense connective tissue, cartilage, and bone. The volume of fluid in the two body fluid compartments varies with age and differs in the sexes. In this fluid, metabolic exchanges between cells and tissues and the external environment occur.

The importance of body water is highlighted by two facts: (1) it is the medium in which all metabolic reactions occur, and (2) precise regulation of volume and composition of body fluid is essential to health. In the healthy individual, body water remains remarkably constant, maintained by a balance between intake and excretion—the water gained each day is equal to the water lost. If the water gained exceeds the water lost, fluid volume excess, or **overhydration,** and edema will occur. If the water lost exceeds the water gained, fluid volume deficit, or **dehydration,** will occur. If 20% to 25% of body water is lost, death usually occurs.

Water, an excellent solvent that permits many substances to be dispersed through it, also has a high dielectric constant that permits ionization of electrolytes. These electrolytes are important in maintaining any physiologic processes and body fluid volume and distribution. They include the cations sodium (Na^+) for extracellular fluid, potassium (K^+) and magnesium (Mg^{++}) for intracellular fluid, the anions chloride (Cl^-) and bicarbonate (HCO_3^-) for extracellular fluid, and phosphate ($PO_4^{\equiv}$) and protein for intracellular fluid.

Intracellular ions also occur in the extracellular fluid but in smaller amounts. Water is also an excellent lubricant between membranes, and it functions well as a heat insulator and heat exchanger.

Daily intake of water in some form is essential to maintain water balance. During starvation, human beings can go several weeks without food but can survive only a few days without water. The average volume of water consumed daily is 120 to 150 ml/kg of body weight in neonates and infants, 120 to 130 ml/kg in children, and 30 ml/kg in adults.

Thirst, the subjective desire to ingest water, helps maintain water balance. Although thirst is complex and not well understood, a decrease in saliva and dryness of the mouth and throat induce it. Dehydration of thirst receptors may lead to their stimulation.

Water intake occurs primarily by (1) drinking fluids, (2) ingesting food containing moisture (most foods contain a high percentage of water), and (3) absorbing water formed by the oxidation of hydrogen in the food during metabolic processes, which produces about 0.5 L of water per day.

Water is lost from the body in five principal ways: (1) by way of the kidneys as urine, (2) through the skin as insensible perspiration and sweat, (3) through expired air as water vapor, (4) through feces, and (5) through the excretion of tears and saliva. Urine excretion accounts for 50% to 60% of the total daily water loss. Urine output, of course, varies with the amount of water ingested.

Water loss by the kidney varies with the solute (molecular ions or particles) load and the antidiuretic hormone (vasopressin) level. If an increase in solute load occurs (as in diabetes mellitus or following ingestion of excessive amounts of food, especially those that generate solutes, such as sodium from salty foods), the kidney excretes sufficient urine to transport the solutes into the bladder. The reabsorption of water in the distal convoluted tubules is controlled by vasopressin, the antidiuretic hormone (ADH). An increase in ADH levels will lead to an increase in water reabsorption, which produces a more concentrated urine. ADH (vasopressin) is secreted by the posterior pituitary gland. This secretion is regulated by osmoreceptors located in the supraoptic nucleus. ADH has an action on specific vasopressin receptors on the medullary tubular cell to stimulate cyclic 3,′5′-adenosine monophosphate (cAMP) production in this cell. The cAMP activates an enzyme that alters protein structure in the cell membrane to increase tubular cell permeability to water. This will increase water resorption and increase urine osmolality.

WATER TRANSPORT IN THE BODY

Water travels from less concentrated areas to areas with higher concentrations of solutes or dissolved substances by **osmosis.** The solutes may be electrolytes, such as potassium chloride or sodium chloride, which, when dissolved in water, yield potassium cations and chloride anions (a chemical balance is maintained) or nonelectrolytes, such as dextrose, urea, or creatinine. Each fluid compartment in the body, intracellular and extracellular, has its own electrolyte composition (Table 61-1). Disturbances in electrolyte composition can be reflected in clinical symptoms in the patient.

Osmolality refers to the total solute concentration usually expressed per liter of serum. The osmotic pressure is decided by the number of solutes in solution. For example, if the extracellular fluid contained a large amount of dissolved particles and the intracellular fluid had a small amount of dissolved particles, then the osmotic pressure from the intracellular fluid would force water to pass from the less concentrated area to the more concentrated extracellular area. This would occur until both concentrations were equal. Therefore deciding on the appropriate intravenous therapy for a person would necessitate knowing the electrolyte values. The level of sodium, the principal electrolyte in the extracellular fluid, is essential to know, although potassium levels are also important, along with serum osmolality, current disease state or illnesses, specific laboratory values if appropriate, and the initial signs and symptoms.

TABLE 61-1 Normal Body Electrolyte Distribution*

Electrolytes	Extracellular (mEq/L) Plasma	Extracellular (mEq/L) Interstitial	Intracellular (mEq/L)
sodium (Na^+)	142	146	15
potassium (K^+)	5	5	150
calcium (Ca^{++})	5	3	2
magnesium (Mg^{++})	2	1	27
chloride (Cl^-)	103	114	1
bicarbonate (HCO_3^-)	27	30	10

*In addition, phosphates, sulfates, and other substances are located in the extracellular and intracellular fluids.

PARENTERAL SOLUTIONS

Parenteral solutions generally may be divided into four categories: (1) hydrating solutions, (2) isotonic solutions, (3) maintenance solutions, and (4) hypertonic solutions (Table 61-2).

Hydrating solutions include dextrose 2.5%, 5%, or higher in water or in 0.2% to 0.5% normal saline (hypotonic saline; note that full strength normal saline is not included in this category). Hydrating solutions are used to hydrate or to prevent dehydration. They are often used to assess kidney status before specific electrolytes are ordered as replacement and maintenance therapy and also to help increase diuresis in dehydrated individuals.

Dextrose is a source of calories (1 L of 5% dextrose = approximately 170 calories) that is rapidly metabolized in the body. Dextrose solutions are considered isotonic or more than isotonic in the bottle; but internally, dextrose is metabolized leaving water that decreases the osmotic pressure of the plasma, easily transfers to body cells, and provides water immediately to dehydrated tissues.

Isotonic solutions are usually prescribed to replace extracellular fluid losses that occur from blood loss, severe vomiting episodes, or any situation in which the chloride loss is equal to or greater than the sodium loss. Isotonic or normal saline is also used before and after a blood transfusion. The reason is that hemolysis of red blood cells, which occurs with dextrose in water, is avoided by using this product.

Isotonic sodium chloride is also used to treat metabolic alkalosis, especially when it occurs in the presence of fluid loss. The increased administration of chloride ions will help to decrease the number of bicarbonate ions in the indi-

TABLE 61-2 Four Categories of Selected Parenteral Solutions*

	Na^+	K^+	Mg^{++}	Ca^{++}	Cl^-	Osmolarity
Hydrating Solutions						
dextrose 2.5%, 5%, 10%						126,252,505
dextrose 2.5% in 0.45% NaCl injection†	56				56	280
dextrose 5% in 0.45% NaCl injection‡	7				77	405
Isotonic Solutions						
normal saline or sodium chloride injection (0.9% NaCl)	154				154	310
Ringer's injection	147	4		4	155	310
lactated Ringer's injection	130	4		3	109	275
Maintenance Solutions						
PlasmaLyte 56	40	13	3		40	111
PlasmaLyte 148 (or Normosol-R, Isolyte S)	140	5		3	98	295
Hypertonic Solutions						
sodium chloride, 3% injection	513				513	1025
sodium chloride, 5% injection	855				855	1710

*Normal plasma contains (in mEq/L) Na^+ (136-145), K^+ (3.5-5), Mg^{++} (1.5-2.5), Ca^{++} (4.3-5.3), Cl^- (100-106), and HCO_3^- (27); osmolarity (280-300 mOsm/L).
†Dextrose 2.5% = 25 g dextrose/L or 85 calories.
‡Dextrose 5% = 50 g dextrose/L or 170 calories.

vidual. Other solutions considered isotonic preparations include Ringer's injection and lactated Ringer's injection. A major difference between Ringer's injection and lactated Ringer's injection is the 28 mEq of lactate, a precursor of bicarbonate, in the lactated injection. Thus lactated Ringer's is preferred for individuals with metabolic acidosis perhaps caused by burns or infections. Ringer's injection, however, has more chloride ions; thus it is more useful in treating dehydration from reduced water intake, vomiting, or diarrhea or for patients with hypochloremia.

Maintenance solutions or multiple electrolyte solutions have been formulated to replace daily electrolyte and extracellular needs and water. Such solutions may also be indicated to replace electrolytes and water loss from severe vomiting or diarrhea. With these preparations, the extracellular replacement is usually achieved within 2 days (usually 1 to 3 L/day is administered), and this should be closely monitored by laboratory tests. If maintenance solutions are continued after the patient's deficits have been corrected, the excess sodium may lead to circulatory overload, pulmonary edema, and heart failure. Examples of maintenance solutions include PlasmaLyte and Normosol.

Hypertonic solutions are used to treat hypotonic expansion (water intoxication) when the increased body fluid volume is caused by water only. This can happen under several different circumstances: (1) hospitalized patients who receive large amounts of dextrose 5% in water or electrolyte-free solutions to replace fluid and electrolytes lost from vomiting, diarrhea, diuresis, or gastric suction, or (2) most likely in elderly patients during the postoperative period when water is retained in response to stress (endocrine response to stress).

When behavioral changes, such as lethargy, confusion, and, perhaps, disorientation occur postoperatively in the elderly person, overhydration or hypotonic expansion should be considered. Central nervous system signs and symptoms have been noted, such as increased tiredness, muscle twitching, headaches, nausea, vomiting, and even seizures. Weight gain is always present and the blood pressure may be normal or elevated.

In milder cases, the treatment usually includes withholding all fluids until excess fluids are excreted. In severe cases of hyponatremia, small quantities of hypertonic sodium chloride are administered to (1) increase the osmotic pressure, (2) increase the water flow from body cells to the extracellular compartment, and (3) to enhance excretion of the fluids by the kidneys.

The typical hypertonic saline is a 3% or 5% solution that, when ordered, must be administered slowly with close supervision (to prevent pulmonary edema). Close monitoring of laboratory tests for electrolytes is also required.

FLUID-ELECTROLYTE BALANCE

A dynamic relationship exists in the body between water and sodium. Abnormal states of hydration can be classified as (1) dehydration (volume depletion), (2) overhydration (hypervolemia or volume excess), (3) loss of water in excess of sodium (hypernatremia), and (4) loss of sodium in excess of water (hyponatremia). The second abnormal state is over hydration or volume excess, which was reviewed under the description of hypertonic solutions in the preceding section. The other three abnormal states may be viewed as various types of dehydration.

TABLE 61-3 Differences Among Three Types of Dehydration

	Hypotonic	*Isotonic*	*Hypertonic*
Cause	Loss of salt (NaCl)	Blood loss	Water loss or lack of sufficient fluid intake
Effect on ICF and ECF compartments	Volume ICF↑ Volume ECF↓	Decrease in ECF volume	Decrease in ICF and ECF volume
Significant signs			
Rate of water elimination	Increased	Decreased	Decreased
Thirst			Early warning, because of cell dehydration
Pulse rate	Increased, weak, thready	Regular	Regular in early stages
Behavioral signs	May see vomiting, abdominal cramps		Confusion, irritability, agitation
Late stages	Skin turgor Weak pulse, lethargy, confusion, death owing to circulatory failure	Shock, weak Weak, thready	Skin turgor Dry, furrowed tongue; death
Clinical laboratory results			
Hematocrit	Increased	Increased	Increased
Hemoglobin	Increased	Increased	Increased
Sodium levels	Decreased		Increased

ICF, intracellular fluid; ECF, extracellular fluid.

TABLE 61-4 Hypertonic Dehydration Symptoms

Clinical Grading	*Symptoms*
Mild or early	Increased thirst. Usually a 2% body weight loss.
Moderate to severe	Very dry mouth, difficulty in swallowing, scant urine output (highly concentrated urine), increased pulse rate and body temperature, poor skin turgor; an approximate 6% body weight loss.
Extreme or very severe	All previous symptoms plus impaired mental and physical capabilities, rectal temperature very high, respiratory difficulties (hyperventilation that may lead to tetany), cyanosis, severe oliguria or anuria, circulatory failure, loss of more than 7% in body weight. Usually coma and death occur when approximately 15% of body weight is lost.

Dehydration

Table 61-3 illustrates the differences between the three types of dehydration. Note that the causes of the three dehydration states are different, as are the effects on fluid compartments in the body and some of the initial signs and laboratory values, especially sodium concentration. This is very important information because it will aid the physician not only in diagnosing the initial condition but also in choosing an appropriate intravenous therapy for the individual patient.

Hypertonic dehydration caused by heat exhaustion that results from water depletion can occur on land or sea. Many cases of boaters lost at sea or refugees fleeing their countries for another country run out of water for days before being rescued or reaching land. Such persons require intensive care for their dehydration, and some may die from this deprivation (Table 61-4).

The healthcare professional should be aware that geriatric patients with decreased renal function will be more vulnerable to dehydration and electrolyte imbalance. As a result of the aging process, the additional physiologic changes experienced by the elderly may also make them more susceptible to the adverse effects of fluid and electrolyte administration, such as overhydration or decreased renal excretion of exogenous potassium or magnesium with resultant toxic accumulation in the body.

ELECTROLYTES

The major electrolytes in the body are sodium, potassium, calcium, and magnesium. This section will review the normal requirements, sources, specific functions, and problems associated with an excess or deficiency of the electrolyte.

SODIUM

Sodium is the major electrolyte in the extracellular fluid; the normal range is from 136 to 145 mEq/L of plasma. The sodium content in the body is regulated by sodium consumption (dietary) and sodium excretion by the kidneys. In the average person with normal renal function, sodium excretion will closely match sodium intake. This aids in keeping sodium content in the body at a constant level even if sodium intake is somewhat varied. Major dietary sources of sodium are table salt (sodium chloride), catsup, mustard, cured meats and fish, cheese, peanut butter, pickles, olives, potato chips, and popcorn. The typical American diet provides between 3 to 6 g of sodium per day (Johnson, Lalonde, 1993), while the recommended dietary sodium allowance is much less. Sodium is necessary for control of body water; for the electrophysiology of nerve, muscle, and gland cells; and for the regulation of pH and isotonicity.

Hyponatremia

Hyponatremia may be detected when the serum level falls below 135 mEq/L. It may be induced by excessive sweating with replacement of only the water, infusion of large quantities of nonelectrolyte parenteral fluids, and adrenal insufficiency or gastrointestinal (GI) suctioning with replacement fluids limited to water by mouth.

Symptoms include lethargy, hypotension, stomach cramps, vomiting, diarrhea, and, possibly, seizures. Deficiency states are usually treated with Ringer's solution or normal saline injection.

Hypernatremia

Hypernatremia is seen when the serum sodium levels are higher than normal, usually >150 mEq/L. This excess may be induced by excessive use of saline infusions, inadequate water consumption (as described previously), or excess fluid loss without a corresponding loss of sodium.

Signs and symptoms include edema; hypertonicity; red, flushed skin; dry, sticky mucous membranes; increased thirst; temperature elevation; and a decrease in or absence of urination. Treatment includes reducing salt intake and using dextrose in water intravenously to promote diuresis and increase the excretion of both salt and water from the blood.

POTASSIUM

Potassium is the major electrolyte in the intracellular fluids. The amount of potassium in the intracellular fluid is approximately 150 mEq/L, whereas the amount in the plasma is between 3.5 and 5 mEq/L. Even though this plasma amount appears to be low, it is of great importance, since serum potassium must be maintained between 3.5 and 5 mEq/L for survival. The diet of most individuals contains from 35 to 100 mEq of potassium daily, and normally any excess potassium is excreted by the kidney in the urine. Potassium plays an important part of (1) muscle contraction, (2) conduction of nerve impulses, (3) enzyme action, and (4) cell membrane function.

Hypokalemia

Hypokalemia, or potassium deficit, may be caused by chronic administration of intravenous solutions containing little or no potassium; diuretic therapy with potassium-depleting medications; reduced dietary intake (e.g., in persons on "starvation diets"); poor absorption because of steatorrhea, regional enteritis, or short-bowel syndrome; loss of GI secretions, which are very rich in potassium, due to vomiting, diarrhea, GI suction, or fistula drainage; extensive burn conditions; or the presence of excessive amounts of adrenocortical hormone.

Unlike sodium, which is reabsorbed when the serum sodium level is low, potassium ions continue to be excreted in the urine when the serum potassium level is low. As potassium loss continues, the individual's condition deteriorates unless potassium intake is increased, and normal levels are reestablished.

With hypokalemia, impaired skeletal muscle function may cause profound weakness or paralysis, including paralysis of the respiratory muscles, while impaired smooth muscle function may result in ileus. Cardiac effects of hypokalemia include increased sensitivity to digitalis with potential toxicity and electrocardiogram (ECG) changes. Early potassium deficiency may be detected by the use of the ECG as the T wave tends to flatten when serum potassium levels are less than 3.5 mEq/L while it tends to elongate vertically when the serum potassium level is 5.8 mEq/L or higher. Atrioventricular block and cardiac arrest may occur.

Hypokalemia also causes movement of Na^+ and H^+ from extracellular fluid and the excretion of H^+, which may elevate plasma pH, resulting in metabolic alkalosis. Other effects are decreased water reabsorption in the renal tubule, resulting in polyuria, and hypochloremia.

Treat hypokalemia by replacing potassium orally or parenterally. However, be aware that a hazard of parenteral correction is potassium poisoning, or hyperkalemia.

Parenteral or Intravenous Administration

The dose of potassium supplements depends on individual requirements and needs close supervision. Intravenous potassium must always be diluted and administered slowly. Potassium generally is given only to individuals with a documented adequate urine flow. In dehydrated patients, it is best to give a potassium-free fluid first to hydrate the individual and determine urinary output.

It is recommended that parenteral fluids should not contain more than 40 mEq/L of potassium and the rate of administration should not be more than 20 mEq/hr (AHFS, 1998). Whenever possible, the oral preparations or consumption of foods high in potassium should replace the intravenous potassium solutions (see Chapter 28).

The parenteral potassium salts are available as acetate, chloride, and phosphate salts. Generally, the potassium chloride is the preferred preparation, since the chloride will help to correct the hypochloremia that often is seen with hypokalemia. In general, the alkalinizing potassium salts (acetate, bicarbonate, citrate, or gluconate) may be necessary to treat hypokalemia associated with metabolic acidosis (a rare situation).

Oral Administration

Potassium salts available include acetate, bicarbonate, chloride, citrate, and gluconate alone or in combinations for oral administration. Liquid preparations are generally preferred for oral therapy and most contain 10, 20, or 40 mEq of potassium per 15 ml. These preparations must be diluted with fruit juice or water before ingestion and taken after meals with a full glass of water to minimize gastrointestinal irritation. For powder preparations, closely follow the manufacturer's instructions. The uncoated and enteric-coated (no longer available in the United States) dosage forms of potassium have caused intestinal and gastric ulcers with bleeding episodes (AHFS, 1998). Although still available, they are rarely used medically; instead liquid, effervescent, powders, and extended-release dosage forms (wax matrix or microencapsulated) are currently the preferred products. Be aware that ulceration has also been reported with the extended-release products (although much less frequently than with the other products), and these preparations should be reserved for patients who cannot or will not take the liquid or effervescent potassium.

If the individual complains of stomach pain, swelling, or severe vomiting or if gastrointestinal bleeding is noted, the extended-release potassium should be stopped immediately, and the prescriber should be contacted. Potassium supplements are contraindicated in patients with severe renal impairment, untreated chronic adrenocortical insufficiency (Addison's disease), hyperkalemia, and severe burn conditions or acute dehydration. They should also be avoided or used with extreme caution in persons taking potassium-sparing diuretics or angiotensin-converting enzyme (ACE) inhibitors. Solid dosage forms of potassium should not be administered to patients with esophageal compression caused by an enlarged left atrium or other anatomic variation, resulting in increased compression in this area. In such cases, ingestion of potassium-rich foods may also be helpful. (See Box 28-1 for foods rich in potassium.)

The dosage of potassium supplements depends on individual requirements. The approximate daily allowance for adults is 40 to 50 mEq and for infants is about 1 to 3 mEq/kg of body weight daily.

Hyperkalemia

Hyperkalemia, or potassium excess, can be caused by acute or chronic renal failure; the release of large amounts of intracellular potassium in burns, crush injuries, or severe infections; overtreatment with potassium salts; or metabolic acidosis, including diabetic ketoacidosis, which causes a shift of potassium from the cells into the extracellular fluids.

Hyperkalemia causes interference with neuromuscular function, which may result in abdominal distention, diarrhea, weakness, and paralysis. Cardiac effects caused by hyperkalemia result from impaired conduction. The ECG shows widening and slurring of the QRS complexes, peaked T waves, depressed S-T segments, and possibly disappearance of P waves. Ventricular fibrillation and cardiac arrest may occur.

The treatment of hyperkalemia depends on the serum level of potassium and the electrocardiogram (ECG) patterns. Mild hyperkalemia is usually a serum level <6.5 mEq/L with ECG changes limited to peaking of the T waves, moderate hyperkalemia is a potassium serum level between 6.5 and 8 mEq/L, and severe hyperkalemia is serum levels >8 mEq/L with an ECG pattern of absent P waves, widened QRS complex, or ventricular dysrhythmias. For treatment of hyperkalemia, see the box on Management of Drug Overdose.

MANAGEMENT OF DRUG OVERDOSE

Treatment of Hyperkalemia

- For mild hyperkalemia, remove or treat the cause. For example, if the person is receiving potassium supplements or an ACE inhibitor, stop the medications. If metabolic acidosis is present, treat this condition.
- Moderate to severe hyperkalemia may require infusing hypertonic dextrose solutions with insulin to shift potassium into the cells. Sodium bicarbonate parenteral may be used to correct acidosis and also help shift serum potassium into cells. Calcium gluconate is administered intravenously under constant ECG monitoring for severe cardiac toxicity. Calcium counteracts the adverse effects of potassium on the neuromuscular membranes, so this is a temporary measure only. Lowering of the potassium levels is critical to reversing this situation.
- All the above methods do not remove potassium from the body. Sodium polystyrene sulfonate (Kayexalate), a cation exchange resin, can be given orally or rectally to remove potassium from the body.
- The oral adult dose of sodium polystyrene sulfonate is 15 g one to four times daily in water or preferably a 70% sorbitol solution to reduce the possibility of constipation. The rectal (retention enema) adult dose is 25 to 100 g of resin suspended in 100 to 200 ml of sorbitol or 10% dextrose in water. This dose may be administered every 6 hours.
- Laxatives must be used when the drug is given orally. Since its action is considered slow, the previously discussed treatments are indicated if ECG changes indicate severe potassium intoxication. Administration should be discontinued when the serum potassium level falls to 4 or 5 mEq/L.
- Side effects of sodium polystyrene sulfonate treatment include anorexia, nausea, vomiting, constipation, hypokalemia, and hypocalcemia. Fecal impaction has also been reported; it can be prevented with the use of laxatives (USP DI, 1998).

CALCIUM

Calcium (Ca^{++}) is essential for growth and bone ossification, neuromuscular transmission, cell membrane permeability, the maintenance of excitability in nerve fibers, hormone secretion and action, muscle contraction, maintenance of cardiac and vascular tone, many enzyme activities, and the normal coagulation of blood.

Almost all of the 1000 to 1200 g calcium in the normal adult is in the skeletal tissue, and only about 1% of the total body calcium is in solution in body fluids. About half the calcium in plasma is bound to complex organic anions (e.g., bicarbonate and phosphate). Nearly all unbound serum calcium is ionized. The normal serum calcium concentration is 4.5 to 5.5 mEq/L or 9 to 11 mg/100 ml.

The recommended dietary allowance of calcium for adults is 0.8 to 1.2 g daily. Pregnant or lactating women need 1.2 g; children 1 to 3 years of age need 0.4 to 0.8 g, and children 4 to 10 years of age need 0.8 g. The intake of calcium in a balanced diet is sufficient for normal body needs. Absorption of calcium depends on how well it is kept in solution in the digestive tract; an acid medium favors calcium solubility and absorption in the upper intestinal tract. Absorption is decreased by the presence of alkalis and large amounts of fatty acids. Adequate intake of vitamin D appears to promote calcium absorption. Calcium is excreted in the urine and feces as well as in perspiration. Estrogen deficiency promotes calcium loss.

The maintenance of a normal concentration of serum calcium depends on the interactions of three agents: parathyroid hormone, vitamin D, and calcitonin. Parathyroid hormone and vitamin D mobilize the removal of calcium from bone, the principal source of calcium for extracellular fluids. Parathyroid hormone also promotes renal tubular reabsorption of calcium and a slight increase in the intestinal absorption of calcium. Calcitonin synthesized in the thyroid gland moderates or decreases the rate of removal of calcium from the bone.

Hypocalcemia

Hypocalcemia, or a decrease in serum calcium, results from (1) hypoparathyroidism, (2) chronic renal insufficiency, (3) hypoalbuminemia, (4) malabsorption syndrome, and (5) deficiency of vitamin D. Hypoparathyroidism may follow thyroidectomy, since several parathyroid glands frequently are removed with this surgery. If the function of the remaining gland(s) is impaired, the result is depressed parathyroid activity.

Individuals who are bedridden tend to develop a negative calcium balance because the ion is lost from bones and excreted. This effect is likely to be serious when long immobilization of the patient is necessary.

Hypocalcemia increases excitability of the nerves and the neuromuscular junction, which leads to muscle cramps, muscle twitching, and tetany. Numbness and tingling of the fingers, toes, and lips occurs. Hypertonicity of muscle may cause tonic contractions of the hands and feet (carpopedal spasm) while increased neural excitability may cause convulsions, abnormal behavior, and personality changes. In children, prolonged hypocalcemia has resulted in mental retardation. The ECG shows a prolonged Q-T interval and an inverted T wave. In prolonged hypocalcemia, defects can occur in the nails, skin, and teeth; cataracts may appear; and calcification of the basal ganglia may occur.

Regardless of the underlying cause, severe hypocalcemia is treated initially with intravenous administration of rapidly available calcium ions. For latent tetany, mild symptoms of hypocalcemia, and maintenance therapy, an oral calcium salt is given. Vitamin D may also be prescribed. Overdosage of calcium may cause hypercalcemia, which results in anorexia, nausea, vomiting, weakness, depression, polyuria, and polydipsia.

Calcium must be administered cautiously to patients undergoing digitalis therapy, since calcium potentiates the effect of digitalis and may precipitate dysrhythmias. ECG monitoring of the patient is recommended when parenteral calcium is administered.

Calcium salts are used as a nutritional supplement, particularly during pregnancy and lactation. They are specific for the treatment of hypocalcemic tetany. They have also been used for their antispasmodic effects in cases of abdominal pain, tenesmus, and colic resulting from disease of the gallbladder or painful contractions of the ureters. The basic salts of calcium are also used as antacids. Approximately 1 to 1.5 g calcium per day has been recommended to prevent postmenopausal bone loss or osteoporosis.

The most widely used calcium salt is calcium carbonate, which requires an acid medium to form soluble calcium salts, since it is nearly insoluble in water. Absorption of or dissolution of calcium phosphate and calcium sulfate is also pH dependent, whereas calcium lactate, calcium citrate, and calcium gluconate are considered pH independent. In elderly persons and postmenopausal women, impaired stomach acid production is common. Therefore the high stomach pH or achlorhydric state results in a decreased solubility of the pH-dependent calcium salts.

Since the different calcium salts have different amounts of calcium present, many healthcare professionals choose the calcium salt with the highest percentage of calcium per gram because a smaller quantity of drug may be administered. For example, if the recommended daily dose of calcium is 1000 mg/day, then it would be necessary to administer nearly 10 g of calcium gluconate to reach this amount, whereas only 2.5 g of calcium carbonate per day would be required. This then requires the consumption of smaller quantities of tablets to obtain the same amount of calcium, assuming that the calcium is soluble under the conditions present in the patient (Table 61-5).

To improve calcium carbonate tablet solubility, especially in achlorhydric conditions, it is recommended the tablets be taken with meals when acid secretion is highest. Avoid taking the tablets on an empty stomach or at night because these are times when acid secretions are minimal. Calcium phosphates and tricalcium phosphate have little usefulness in possible achlorhydric states and, perhaps, even in the normal person. Both products have a very poor dissolution rate or pattern, thus reducing the possibility of calcium absorption. Perhaps in patients with known achlorhydric states, the soluble calcium salts (lactate or citrate) might be the appropriate form to use even though it will be necessary to use more tablets to provide sufficient quantities of calcium. Selected food consumption is another source for calcium (Table 61-6).

Hypercalcemia

Hypercalcemia, or elevated serum calcium levels, may be caused by neoplasms with or without bone metastases. Carcinoma of the ovary, kidney, or lung can synthesize and secrete a parathyroid-like hormone, causing hypercalcemia. Other common causes are hyperparathyroidism, thiazide

TABLE 61-5 Calcium Content of Various Calcium Salts

	Percent Calcium	Amount Calcium per Tablet	Tablets Needed for 1 g of Calcium
calcium carbonate	40	260 mg/650 mg	4
calcium gluconate	9	45 mg/500 mg	22
calcium lactate	13	42 mg/325 mg	24
calcium phosphate tribasic	39	600 mg/1565 mg	1.66

TABLE 61-6 Foods with High Calcium Content

Food	Calcium Content (mg)
Yogurt, lowfat (1 cup)	275-400
Skim milk (1 cup)	300
Cheese, Swiss (1 oz)	272
Cheese, cottage (1 cup)	215
Cheese, cheddar (1 oz)	200
Ice milk (3/4 cup)	132
Broccoli, raw (1 cup)	100
Ice cream (1/2 cup)	100

diuretic therapy, multiple myeloma, sarcoidosis, and vitamin D intoxication.

Clinical manifestations of hypercalcemia are highly variable and involve many organ systems because calcium may be deposited in various body tissues. The symptoms may include the following:

- *Gastrointestinal.* Anorexia, nausea, vomiting, constipation, and abdominal pain may occur.
- *Neurologic.* Weakness, apathy, depression, amnesia, confusion, stupor, and coma may occur.
- *Renal.* Polyuria and nephrocalcinosis may occur, seriously impairing renal function and possibly leading to edema, uremia, and hypertension, which may be irreversible.
- *Cardiovascular.* Increased cardiac contractility, ventricular extrasystoles, and heart block may be seen. ECG changes include a short Q-T segment and characteristic signs of heart block.

Treatment is variable and aimed at controlling the underlying disease. In dehydrated persons, restore extracellular fluid volume with normal saline infusions, which also increases calcium excretion. Furosemide may be prescribed to enhance diuresis, but thiazide diuretics should be avoided because they block or lower calcium excretion. Chelating (binding) agents such as disodium edetate have been used in acute hypercalcemia in selected individuals. It increases renal excretion of calcium by forming soluble complexes with the calcium that are not reabsorbed by the renal tubules.

Bisphosphonates

Bisphosphonates are analogs of pyrophosphate (normal component of bone); therefore these drugs are incorporated into bone where they inhibit bone resorption by decreasing osteoclasts activity, resulting in a decrease in serum calcium. The currently available bisphosphonates include alendronate (Fosamax), etidronate (Didronel), pamidronate (Aredia), risedronate (Actonel), and tiludronate (Skelid).

These agents are used to treat Paget's disease and hypercalcemia of malignancy; for the latter, however, pamidronate is more potent and usually the preferred agent. Parenteral etidronate is also used as adjunct therapy to treat hypercalcemia that is associated with neoplasms while alendronate is also indicated for the prevention and treatment of osteoporosis in postmenopausal women. An antineoplastic drug, plicamycin (Mithracin), also reduces serum calcium levels (Olin, 1998; Tang, Lau, 1995; USP DI, 1998).

Pharmacokinetics

Alendronate PO has low bioavailability (0.7%), which can be negligible if it is given with meals or up to 2 hours after breakfast. Therefore it should be administered on an empty stomach with 8 oz of water, at least 30 minutes before any food, beverage, or other medications. Etidronate is available orally and parenterally; absorption of the PO dosage form is approximately 1% in 5 mg/kg dosages up to 2.5% to 6% in 10 to 20 mg/kg dosages taken on an empty stomach. Pamidronate is available parenterally, whereas risedronate and tiludronate are oral dosage forms that also require an empty stomach for absorption. See Table 61-7 for bisphosphonate pharmacokinetics and dosing.

Drug interactions

The following effects may occur when the biphosphonates are given with the drugs listed below:

Drug	Possible effect and management
Food, beverages, and oral medications (including antacids)	Avoid concurrent use with oral preparations because decreased bisphosphonate absorption results.
Mineral supplements or any calcium, iron, magnesium or aluminum-containing substances	Avoid concurrent use with oral preparations because decreased bisphosphonate absorption results. Space apart by at least 2 hours.

Salicylates	Concurrent use increases the risk for gastric distress with alendronate. The absorption of iludronate is decreased by 50% if consumed within 2 hours after administration of tiludronate.
vitamin D, including calcifediol and calcitriol	Concurrent use with pamidronate antagonizes the effects of pamidronate in the treatment of hypercalcemia. Avoid concurrent use.

Side effects and adverse reactions

With alendronate these include gastric distress, dysphagia, heartburn, headache, muscle pain, and, the most serious effect, esophagitis (which can cause pain and ulceration). The latter effect is caused by alendronate not completely clearing the esophagus for the following reasons: the patient takes the drug while in a supine position or takes it with insufficient amounts of water, the patient lies down immediately after consuming the medication, or the patient has a preexisting esophageal constriction or condition that may be conducive to this effect. Advise all patients to take the medication with 8 oz of water while seated or standing and not to lie down for at least 30 minutes afterward.

Etidronate may cause diarrhea, nausea, anorexia, altered taste sensation, and bone pain, especially in patients with Paget's disease and osteomalacia (bone fractures, especially of the femur, which usually occurs in patients taking dosages higher than 20 mg/kg or, if therapy is continued longer than 6 months).

Pamidronate effects include fever, nausea, pain, and edema at the injection site, muscle stiffness, hypocalcemia (stomach cramps, confusion, and muscle spasms), and leukopenia (chills, fever, or sore throat).

Risedronate effects include dizziness, headache, chest or stomach pain, diarrhea, constipation, nausea, arthralgia, bone pain, leg cramps, weakness, peripheral edema, flu-like syndrome, and rash.

Tiludronate effects include back and generalized, body pain, gastric distress, joint pain, conjunctivitis, cough, dizziness, flu-type syndrome, and pharyngitis. (This medication can cause effects similar to those described for alendronate above. The same recommendations apply.) Other effects include rhinitis, rash, vomiting, upper respiratory tract infection, chest pain, glaucoma, and cataract.

Warnings

Use alendronate and tiludronate with caution in patients with hypocalcemia or vitamin D deficiency. Use etidronate with caution in persons with hyperphosphatemia, hypocalcemia, and hypovitaminosis D.

Contraindications

Avoid use in persons with bisphosphonates hypersensitivity. Avoid alendronate and tiludronate use in persons with GI disease and kidney function impairment, etidronate in persons with long bone fractures, cardiac heart failure, enterocolitis, and kidney function impairment, and pamidronate in persons with heart failure and kidney function impairment.

MAGNESIUM

Magnesium (Mg^{++}) is an important ion for the function of many enzyme systems.

Hypomagnesemia

Hypomagnesemia, a deficit of magnesium, may be encountered in chronic alcoholism, severe malabsorption, starvation, diarrhea, prolonged GI suction, vigorous diuresis,

TABLE 61-7 Bisphosphonate Pharmacokinetics and Dosing

Name	Pharmacokinetics	Adult Dose
alendronate (Fosamax)	D of A: 6 wk after single dose of 5 mg for osteoporosis; 6 mo in PD Excretion: primary in urine	PO: PD, 40 mg daily in morning (empty stomach); PMO, 10 mg daily in morning (empty stomach)
etidronate (Didronel)	O of A: PD, 1 mo; hypercalcemia, 24 hr. Peak effect: hypercalcemia, decrease in serum calcium peaks after third infusion. D of A: PD, up to 1 yr after drug was stopped Hypercalcemia: about 11 days Excretion: primarily in urine	PO: PD, 5 mg/kg/day for 6 mo; hypercalcemia, 20 mg/kg/day for 1-3 mo IV infusion: hypercalcemia 7.5mg/day for 3 days
pamidronate (Aredia)	Half-life: 1.6 hr (alpha), 27.2 hr (beta) Excretion: primarily in urine	IV infusion: 60 mg given over 4-24 hr for hypercalcemia or 90-180 mg total dose for PD
risedronate (Actonel)	Absorption: rapid Half-life: initial 1.5 hr, terminal 220 hr Excretion: primarily in urine	PO: PD, 30 mg daily for 2 mo, taken in morning (empty stomach); supplements or calcium and vitamin D necessary if dietary intake insufficient
tiludronate (Skelid)	Half-life: elimination 50 hr in healthy persons; 150 hr in PD patients Excretion: primarily in urine	PO: PD, 400 mg daily on empty stomach

From Olin, 1998; USP DI, 1998.
D of A, duration of action; O of A, onset of action; PD, Paget's disease; PMO, postmenopausal osteoporosis.

acute pancreatitis, and primary aldosteronism. Magnesium, the second most abundant intracellular cation, plays an important role in regulating the sodium-potassium adenosine triphosphaase (ATPase) pump function, neuromuscular transmission, cardiovascular function, and mitochondrial and other cellular functions in the body.

Magnesium deficiency may result in additional electrolyte problems (hypokalemia and hypocalcemia), cardiac dysrhythmias, and neurotoxicity. It may also cause an increase in neuromuscular irritability and contractility, coarse tremor, muscle spasm, delirium, athetoid movements, nystagmus, and tetany. It also causes tachycardia, hypertension, and vasomotor changes and increases the risk of digitalis toxicity in persons taking cardiac glycosides.

Hypomagnesemia may be treated with intravenous fluids containing magnesium, 10 to 40 mEq/day for severe deficit, followed by 10 mEq/day for maintenance. The use of intravenous fluids containing from 3 to 5 mEq magnesium per L may avert magnesium deficiency that arises from prolonged administration of intravenous solutions that do not contain magnesium.

Hypermagnesemia

Hypermagnesemia occurs primarily in individuals with chronic renal insufficiency. Adverse effects include flushing, sweating, hypothermia, areflexia, paralysis, and depression of cardiac, central nervous system (CNS), andrespiratory functions. Decreased muscle cell excitability is caused by blockade of the myoneural junction (inhibition of acetylcholine release). Cardiac depression effects result in an increase in conduction time with the ECG evidencing a lengthened P-R segment and a prolonged QRS complex. If the Mg^{++} concentration continues to increase, third-degree atrioventricular block and cardiac arrest may occur.

An excess of Mg^{++} may require dialysis. Because calcium acts as an antagonist to Mg^{++}, calcium salts may be given parenterally. The normal serum concentration is 1.5 to 2.5 mEq/L, with one third bound to protein and two thirds free. A toxic blood level is >4 mEq/L of magnesium. Magnesium has physiologic effects on the nervous system similar to those of calcium.

ADDITIONAL SINGLE-SALT SOLUTIONS

In addition to the previously discussed salt preparations, ammonium chloride injection and sodium lactate injection are also available for use.

Ammonium chloride injection is indicated to treat hypochloremia and metabolic alkalosis (not associated with severe liver disease) to prevent tetany or renal damage. Most patients respond to sodium chloride solution, but for the rare, nonresponsive situation, ammonium chloride is available. Ammonium chloride has been used as a urinary acidifier to promote excretion of alkaline substances. This product is available in 20-ml vials (100 mEq), and the dose selected depends on the individual (usually one to two vials) in normal saline infused slowly.

Sodium lactate injection available as a ⅙ molar solution contains 167 mEq/L each of sodium and lactate ions. It is used to treat metabolic acidosis when no evidence of an elevated lactic acid level exists. Sodium lactate is converted to sodium bicarbonate in the liver. In persons with lactic acidosis or impaired liver function, sodium bicarbonate is preferred.

MONITORING ELECTROLYTES

Laboratory tests are used to monitor the individual's electrolyte levels and to help determine replacement therapies when necessary for electrolyte deficiency. The normal plasma values are noted in the footnotes to Table 61-2. The healthcare professional should be aware of the difference between milligrams (mg) which reflects weight and **milliequivalents** (mEq) which measures the number of chemically active ions in solution. (A milliequivalent is the number of grams of the solute or electrolyte that is dissolved in 1 ml of a normal solution.) The latter is a more precise measure of the relative potency of an electrolyte solution and is the method the prescriber uses to order the electolytes.

SUMMARY

Fluids and electrolytes are administered intravenously to replace losses, correct acid-base imbalance, serve as a vehicle for other medications, measure renal function and changes in venous pressure, and administer essential nutrients. The bisphosphonates, analogs of pyrophosphate, are drugs that inhibit bone resorption and decrease serum calcium. This chapter reviews the type solutions, electrolytes, and various bisphosphonates available, and their proper usage in medical practice.

REVIEW QUESTIONS

1. Name the parenteral solutions that are used to treat intracellular dehydration and describe their effect in the body.
2. What are the causes and treatments for hypotonic, isotonic, and hypertonic dehydration?
3. Describe the mechanism of action, indications, significant drug indications, and major adverse effects of the bisphosphonates.
4. Explain the cause, effect, and treatment of hypomagnesemia and hypermagnesemia.

REFERENCES

American Hospital Formulary Service: *AHFS drug information '98*, Bethesda, Md, 1998, American Society of Hospital Pharmacists.

Johnson JA, Lalonde RL: Congestive heart failure. In DiPiro JT, Talber R et al, editors: *Pharmacotherapy, a pathophysiologic approach*, ed 2, Norwalk, Conn, 1993, Appleton & Lange.

Olin BR: *Facts and comparisons.* Philadelphia, 1998, JB Lippincott.

Tang I, Lau AH: Fluid and electrolyte disorders. In Young LY, Koda-Kimble MA, editors: *Applied therapeutics: the clinical use of drugs*, ed 6, Vancouver, Wash, 1995, Applied Therapeutics, Inc.

United States Pharmacopeial Convention: *USP DI: drug information for the health care professional,* ed 18, Rockville, Md, 1998, The Convention.

ADDITIONAL REFERENCES

Anderson KN et al, editors: *Mosby's medical, nursing, and allied health dictionary,* ed 5, St Louis, 1998, Mosby.

Brown RG: Disorders of water and sodium balance, *Postgrad Med* 93(4):227-228, 231, 234, 239-240, 244, 246, 1993.

Brown RO: Hypomagnesemia in critically ill patients: issues in pharmacotherapy, *ACCP Rep* 13(3):6, 1993.

CHAPTER 62

Enteral and Parenteral Nutrition

CHAPTER FOCUS

Malnutrition has been identified as a problem in selected hospitalized patients and institutional residents, especially those individuals who cannot consume sufficient nutrients from a balanced intake of food. Enteral and parenteral feedings were formulated to assist such patients and reduce or eliminate the complications of malnutrition, including muscle atrophy, reduced wound healing, impaired immune system, and infection. This chapter reviews these agents.

OBJECTIVES

After reading and studying this chapter, the student should be able to do the following:

1. *Define and describe the key terms.*
2. *Name and describe the four types of enteral formulations.*
3. *Identify and describe the three major drug-food interactions.*
4. *Distinguish between parenteral protein-sparing nutrition, peripheral vein parenteral nutrition, and central hyperalimentation. Also, name indications for their use.*
5. *Name the ingredients, functions, and their usual concentrations in total parenteral nutrition solutions.*
6. *Describe the potentially life-threatening drug interaction with total parenteral nutrition admixtures.*

KEY TERMS

amino acids, (p. 793)
enteral nutrition, (p. 790)
essential amino acids, (p. 793)
hyperalimentation, (p. 793)
negative nitrogen balance, (p. 793)
nonessential amino acids, (p. 793)
protein-sparing nutrition, (p. 794)
semiessential amino acids, (p. 794)
total parenteral nutrition (TPN), (p. 793)

To achieve and maintain good health requires a regular intake of sufficient amounts of protein (amino acids), carbohydrates, fats, vitamins, and minerals. Under normal conditions adequate nutrition can be achieved by the ingestion of a balanced diet, but there are situations when the nutritional needs of the body will not be met. Such conditions include malnutrition, severe inflammatory bowel disease and other gastrointestinal (GI) diseases, coma, postsurgical complications, major burns, and others. For such persons, nutritional support is necessary. Over the past 30 to 40 years, many advances have been recorded in the fields of both enteral and parenteral nutrition. Clinical nutrition is now a recognized and active entity for improving healthcare in all settings, including the individual's home, long-term care facilities, and hospitals. Today nutritional programs or specific products have been developed for individuals with specific disease states or illnesses. This chapter reviews enteral and parenteral nutrition, along with selected disease states and criteria for use of the specific nutritional products.

ENTERAL NUTRITION

Malnutrition among hospitalized persons and nursing home residents is associated with complications such as muscle atrophy, slow wound healing, impaired immunocompetence, infection, and death. Other complications include peripheral edema caused by reduced plasma proteins and its resultant decreased oncotic pressure, dry and flaky skin, and hair loss.

Malnutrition is also reflected in reduced total lymphocyte count, serum albumin, and transferrin levels (or iron-binding capacity). An increase in 24-hour urine urea nitrogen concentration reflects the protein catabolism that occurs with malnutrition.

Stress in relation to hospitalization may alter a patient's usual eating habits. Unfamiliar foods and general malaise resulting from illness also may cause patients to lose their appetites. An inadequate oral intake may result from oropharyngeal surgery, trauma, neoplasm, paralysis, or esophageal fistula. Fasting before surgery or for a diagnostic workup may also be nutritionally depleting. When sepsis, trauma, major surgery, inflammation, infection, or severe burns supervene, energy needs may be doubled. If the GI tract is functional, however, enteral or tube feedings may effectively supply essential nutrition. **Enteral nutrition** is the oral or tube feeding of an individual, usually via a nasogastric, nasoduodenal, nasojejunal, gastrostomy, or jejunostomy tube (Fig. 62-1). The cost per person for tube feedings is about equal to a regular hospital diet and provides more complete control and assessment of intake. Tube feedings also may be used to supplement inadequate oral intake and parenteral nutrition as it is being tapered.

Enteral feedings may be administered by bolus doses, typically 250 to 400 ml of formula every 4 to 6 hours; by intermittent feedings using a 20-to 30-minute drip; or by continuous gravity or enteral pumps. The continuous method over 16 to 24 hours is more successful because it helps prevent complications such as dumping syndrome and avoids the need for frequent tube irrigations. Dumping syndrome is the result of a sudden influx of feeding and the creation of a high osmotic gradient within the small intestine, which cause a sudden shift of fluid from the vascular compartment to the intestinal lumen. Plasma volume decreases, causing vasomotor responses such as increased pulse rate, hypotension, weakness, pallor, sweating, and dizziness. Rapid distention of the intestine produces a feeling of fullness, cramping, nausea, vomiting, and diarrhea.

Enteral feedings can be administered by the following routes: nasogastric, nasoduodenal, esophagostomy, gastrostomy, and jejunostomy. The last three are more invasive, requiring surgically created stomas, and thus are less preferred routes for short-term enteral feeding. Nasogastric, esophagostomy, and gastrostomy feedings allow for more natural digestion in the stomach. Aspiration is a risk with nasogastric tubes because the incomplete closure of the esophageal sphincter may result in gastric reflux.

Although feedings administered directly into the small intestine reduce the risk of aspiration, gastrointestinal distress and diarrhea may develop because of the sudden influx. Skin excoriation and infection are potential risks in gastrostomies and jejunostomies because the surgical opening penetrates the peritoneum. These complications are avoided in the cervical esophagostomy, a surgically created, skin-lined canal tunneled from the lower neck border and extending to below the cervical esophagus.

The selection of tube feeding formula depends on the individual's nutritional needs, concomitant disease states, lactose intolerance, and gastrointestinal competence, as well as on convenience, feasibility, and cost. Nutritional assessment may be based on anthropometric parameters, biochemical data, and physical findings, as well as on medical, diet, drug, and socioeconomic histories. Ideal body weight (IBW) can be used instead of actual weight because if an individual is obese, the adipose tissue would require less energy for maintenance. If the actual weight were used in the calculations, the patient would receive excessive calories. IBW is calculated as follows:

- *Men:* 106 lb (48 kg) for the first 5 ft (150 cm) plus 6 lb (2.7 kg) per inch (2.5 cm) over 5 ft (plus or minus 10%)
- *Women:* 100 lb (45 kg) for the first 5 ft plus 5 lb (2.2 kg) per inch over 5 ft (plus or minus 10%)

ENTERAL FORMULATIONS

Although many different enteral formulations are available, they can be broadly divided into oligomeric, polymeric, modular, and specialized formulations (Rollins, 1996).

1. Oligomeric formulations are chemically defined preparations that require minimum digestion and produce minimal residue in the colon. The two oligomeric subgroups include true elemental formulations that contain free amino acids and peptide-based formulations that

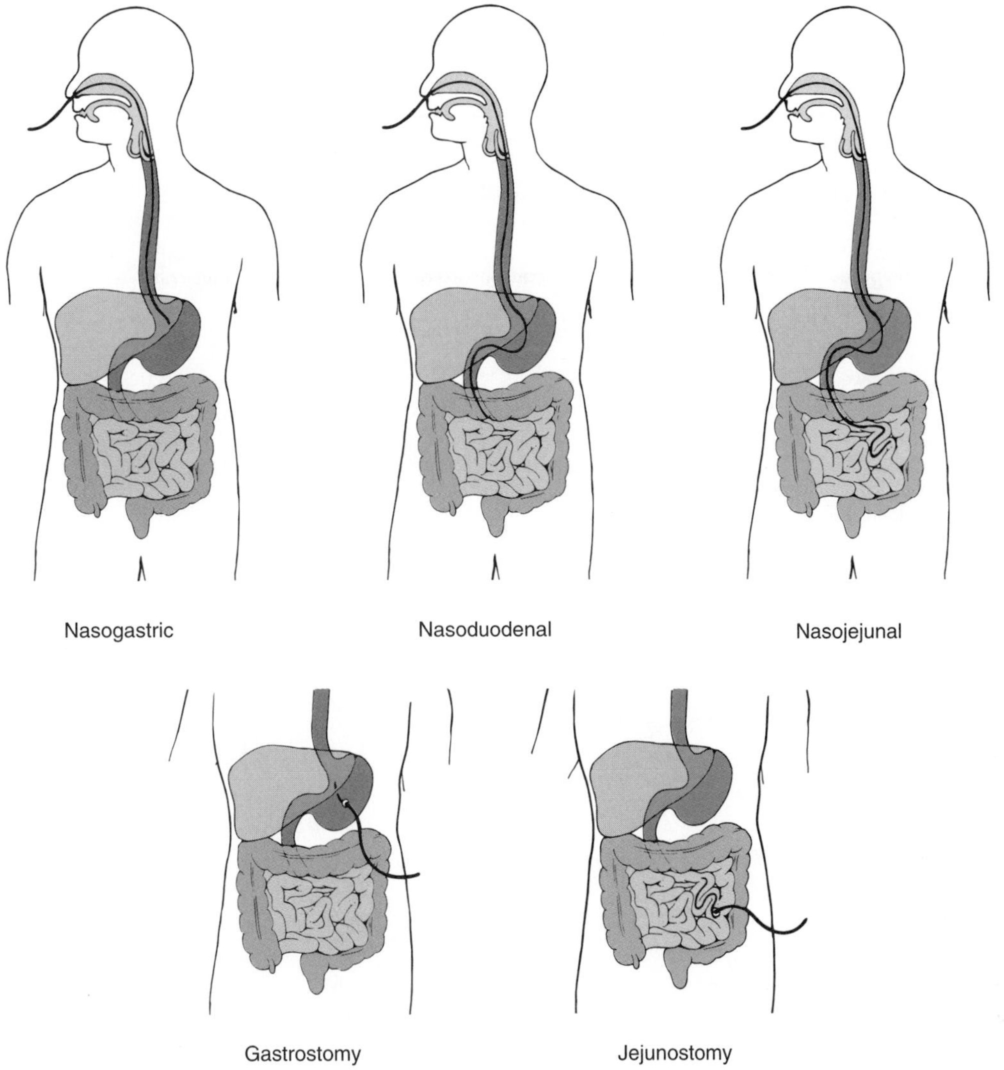

FIGURE 62-1
Tube feeding routes. *(Modified from Beare, Myers, 1998.)*

contain dipeptides and tripeptides and/or crystalline amino acids. These formulations are indicated for persons with partial bowel obstruction, inflammatory bowel disease, radiation enteritis, bowel fistulas, and short bowel syndrome.

2. Polymeric formulations are the most commonly prescribed complete enteral preparations. Such formulas contain complex nutrients: protein (e.g., casein and soy protein); carbohydrate (e.g., corn syrup solid and maltodextrins); and fat (vegetable oil or milk fat) and are preferred for persons who have a fully functional gastrointestinal tract and few or no specialized nutrient requirements. They should not be used in patients with a malabsorption problem. These formulas are preferred because the hyperosmolarity of the oligomeric preparations causes more gastrointestinal problems than the polymeric formulations.
3. Modular formulations are single-nutrient formulas, i.e., protein, carbohydrate, or fat. Such a formula can be added to a monomeric or polymeric formulation to provide a more individual specialized nutrient formulation.
4. Specialized formulations are indicated for individuals with specific disease states, such as genetic errors of metabolism (e.g., phenylketonuria, homocystinuria, or maple syrup urine disease) or acquired disorders of nitrogen accumulation (e.g., cirrhosis or chronic renal failure) and in persons who are catabolic because of injuries or infection (Table 62-1).

DRUG-FOOD INTERACTIONS

A number of drug-enteral nutrient interactions have been identified, but this possibility is often overlooked when enteral nutrient formulations are being administered. Because the interactions can be clinically significant, the major drug interactions with enteral or tube feedings are listed in Table 62-2.

TABLE 62-1 Examples of Commercial Enteral Formulations

Formulations	Comments
Oligomeric	
Elemental	
Vivonex TEN	Contains free amino acids, linoleic acid, vitamins, and minerals
Peptide-based	
Peptamen Liquid	Composed of hydrolyzed whey proteins, carbohydrates, fat, vitamins, and minerals
Polymeric	
Nutrient Source	
Blenderized	
Compleat Regular	Has beef, fruits, vegetables, nonfat milk, vitamins, and minerals; tube feeding preparation
Milk-based	
Sustacal powder	Composed of nonfat and whole milk, sugars, butter, vitamins, and minerals; contains high protein content and lactose
Lactose-free	
Ensure-Plus	Higher caloric formulation of protein, carbohydrates, fat, vitamins, and minerals that is lactose-free
Modular Components	
Carbohydrate	
Polycose	Glucose polymers derived from cornstarch; high source of calories from carbohydrate
Protein	
Amin-Aid	Contains essential amino acids, carbohydrates, and fat; has high caloric formula indicated for acute or chronic renal failure
Fats	
MCT Oil	Medium chain triglycerides that need less bile acid for digestion; does not provide any essential fatty acids
Specialized Formulations	
Renal Failure	
Amin-Aid	See above
Hepatic Failure	
Hepatic-Aid II	Contains amino acids (about 50% protein as branched-chain amino acids [BCAA]), carbohydrates, and fat; hepatic encephalopathy reportedly improved by increased serum levels of BCAA (Rollins, 1996); used for chronic liver disease
Pulmonary Disease	
Pulmocare	Composed of calcium and sodium caseinate, amino acids, carbohydrates, fats, vitamins, and minerals; has high caloric content; fat in this preparation is primarily from canola oil and corn oil (60%) plus 40% from MCT; persons with respiratory disease who received high-fat, low-carbohydrate diets demonstrated improvement in respiratory monitoring parameters (Rollins, 1996)

TABLE 62-2 Drug Interactions with Enteral and Tube Feedings

Drug	Comments
carbamazepine (Tegretol)	Bioavailability of carbamazepine suspension is affected if given through a polyvinyl nasogastric feeding tube. Serum levels also decreased when administered during enteral feedings. Recommended that suspension be diluted and given as described in phenytoin below.
phenytoin (Dilantin)	Lower serum phenytoin levels reported. Recommended approach is to stop enteral feeding for 2 hours before and after phenytoin administration. Flushing the tubing with 2 oz of water before giving phenytoin suspension is recommended.
warfarin (Coumadin)	Warfarin resistance reported when drug was administered with an enteral preparation. Interaction may be due to vitamin K in the feeding or to warfarin binding to protein ingredients in the formulation.

Closely monitor persons receiving the above and any other drugs in combination with enteral formulations. Laboratory tests such as serum drug levels or prothrombin time, when appropriate, may be ordered (Estoup, 1994). For additional information, see Miyagawa, 1993.

PARENTERAL NUTRITION

Parenteral nutrition is the treatment of choice for selected patients who are unable to tolerate and maintain adequate enteral intake. Often called **hyperalimentation** or **total parenteral nutrition** (**TPN**), it is the intravenous approach to complete nutrition. TPN can supply all the calories, dextrose, amino acids, fats, trace elements, and other essential nutrients needed for growth, weight gain, wound healing, convalescence, immunocompetence, and other health-sustaining functions. TPN provides these components in the ratio of a regular diet. It promotes anabolism by supplying all necessary nutrients in excess of those needed for energy expenditure, and it may be infused through a central vein, a peripheral vein, or both simultaneously.

Although related nomenclature has not yet been standardized, partial parenteral nutrition has come to denote parenteral nutrition therapy with intravenous solutions that are lacking some essential elements, notably fats. Although insulin and heparin (and several other medications) have been added to parenteral nutrition preparations for specific individuals, in general, the addition of medications to TPN solutions should be avoided because of the potential incompatibilities of the medication with the nutrients in the solution (Holcombe, 1996). The major parenteral systems for nutritional support are the following: (1) peripheral vein total parenteral nutrition and (2) central line venous hyperalimentation

PERIPHERAL VEIN TOTAL PARENTERAL NUTRITION

Peripheral vein total parenteral nutrition (PTPN) is prescribed for persons needing nutritional support for whom insertion of a central venous line for total parenteral nutrition may not be possible or necessary. The individual may be nutritionally healthy or have slight to moderate nutritional deficits without being in a hypermetabolic state. The individual's current health status indicates that a nutritional deficit will probably occur if nutritional therapy is not instituted.

PTPN is considered a temporary measure to provide an appropriate nitrogen balance in patients with mild deficits or who are receiving nothing by mouth (NPO) and have a slightly elevated metabolic rate. It may be prescribed to precede a procedure that imposes restrictions on oral feedings, for GI illnesses that prevent oral food ingestion, for anorexia caused by radiation or chemotherapy in cancer treatment programs, or after surgery, if the individual's nutritional deficits are minimal, but oral food consumption will not be instituted for 5 or more days. It is not indicated for nutritionally depleted patients with a hypermetabolic state. If used in such persons, it should be a temporary measure until central vein hyperalimentation can be initiated.

The solution is composed of 3% to 5% isotonic amino acids, mixed with a carbohydrate solution (usually dextrose 5% to 7%), vitamins, minerals, and electrolytes for administration through a peripheral vein. The solution will provide between 500 and 700 calories/day. The major advancement in this therapy is the use of a lipid as a nonprotein source of calories. Dextrose, when administered peripherally, must be limited to a 10% solution to avoid sclerosing of the veins. Some institutions also limit the concentration of electrolytes to be infused for the same reason.

Peripherally administered lipid preparations or intravenous fat emulsions (Liposyn, Intralipid, and others) are a source of additional calories for the individual.

CENTRAL HYPERALIMENTATION

In central hyperalimentation, a catheter is placed in a central vein, the subclavian vein most commonly, to administer solutions that contain hypertonic glucose and amino acids. Because of its blood flow, the central vein can accept the high osmolar concentrated solutions. Central hyperalimentation or total parenteral nutrition (TPN) is usually composed of the three major nutrients—dextrose, crystalline amino acids, and lipid emulsions—plus vitamins, minerals, trace elements, electrolytes, and water. The solutions may vary according to the individual's requirements and, in general, according to the supplier of the basic amino acid solution. Special preparations of amino acids are also available for the patient with a specific disease state.

Central hyperalimentation is used primarily for persons with nonfunctioning gastrointestinal tracts, for those who should not use the oral route for more than 5 to 7 days, or for persons who have either a limited peripheral access or whose needs cannot be met by peripheral formulations (Holcombe, 1996). For example, individuals with short bowel syndrome, acute pancreatitis, enteric or enterocutaneous fistulas, active inflammatory processes, gastrointestinal tract obstruction, major trauma, or burns for whom enteral feedings are not possible may need central hyperalimentation for survival.

SOLUTION FORMULATIONS

The basic total parenteral solution contains amino acids, carbohydrates (dextrose), lipids, and micronutrients (trace elements, vitamins, and others).

See Box 62-1 for a potentially life-threatening drug interaction.

Amino Acids

Amino acids are necessary to promote the production of proteins (anabolism), reduce protein breakdown (catabolism), and help promote wound healing. A **negative nitrogen balance** is a situation in which more nitrogen is excreted than taken in, leading to wasting of body tissue. Protein is composed of amino acids, which are identified as essential and nonessential. **Essential amino acids** cannot be synthesized by the body while **nonessential amino acids** can be synthesized from a nitrogen source (amino acids, ammonium salts, or urea). All natural amino acids are needed for growth and development and must be present concurrently

BOX 62-1 Potentially Life-Threatening Drug Interaction

The amount of calcium and phosphorus (or phosphates) in a TPN admixture must be closely monitored because of life-threatening events and deaths have been reported from calcium phosphate precipitation. The Food and Drug Administration (FDA) issued warnings concerning this drug interaction that include the following:

- Use an in-line filter whenever infusing TPN solutions centrally or peripherally.
- Start TPN admixtures within 24 hours after mixing or keep at room temperature. If refrigerated, start with 24 hours of rewarming.
- If acute respiratory distress symptoms occur, *stop infusion immediately.*

Special compounding instructions were issued to pharmacists on this safety alert.

From Mirtallo, 1994; FDA, 1994.

in the proper amounts for protein synthesis to occur. The adult can synthesize all but eight of these amino acids; these eight therefore are considered essential in adults. To the extent that oral intake of amino acids is limited, protein synthesis depends on an exogenous source. The **semiessential amino acids** (histidine, arginine) are not synthesized in adequate amounts during growth periods; thus 10 amino acids are considered essential in infants.

A healthy adult usually minimally requires approximately 0.9 g of protein per kg, whereas an infant or child needs from 1.4 to 2.2 g/kg. In undernourished or traumatized persons, this requirement can increase substantially, such as up to 6-fold in a traumatized or seriously ill individual, since this person's daily need is approximately 3 g/kg of body weight. A nonprotein source of calories must be provided with the amino acids to offset their use as an energy source.

Amino acid solutions contain crystalline amino acid (Aminosyn and many others); solutions are also available with electrolytes. Amino acid crystalline solutions contain synthetic amino acids but not peptides. This is the preferred form of amino acid because most persons are able to tolerate this formulation.

Dextrose usually is administered with these solutions because of the protein-sparing action of carbohydrates. If the protein is administered without adequate calories in the form of carbohydrate, the protein will be used for the body's caloric need rather than for repair and regeneration of tissue.

Protein-sparing nutrition is usually reserved for the patient who has minimal protein deficiencies and sufficient fat stores. A 3% to 5% isotonic amino acid is mixed with carbohydrate-free fluids, vitamins, minerals, and electrolytes that are administered by peripheral vein. The solution will provide approximately 400 to 600 calories/day. The individual will meet many energy requirements by using the free fatty acids and ketones derived from their endogenous adipose tissue, thereby preserving their protein compartment in the body. This type usually is used for short-term periods for patients who are not nutritionally compromised and are not in a hypermetabolic state.

Carbohydrates

Carbohydrates and lipids are used as the primary source of calories for the individual. One gram of d-glucose provides 3.4 calories, whereas fat supplies 9 calories/g and protein supplies 4 calories/g. Concentrations of dextrose solutions >10% are hyperosmolar and are too irritating to be given continuously peripherally; thus they should be administered through central venous catheters. Centrally, the concentration of dextrose solutions infused is usually between 25% and 35%.

When dextrose is administered without lipids as the primary source of calories, hyperglycemia usually occurs. Since dextrose requires insulin for utilization, using a combination of caloric sources, dextrose and lipids, will help decrease the potential for hyperglycemia and extra need for insulin in some individuals. Dextrose alone also increases the rate of metabolism and production of carbon dioxide, which may increase the patient's respiratory demands. Administering a combination caloric preparation of dextrose and lipids will reduce the increase in respiratory demands.

Other sources of calories available, although not as prevalent in usage, include alcohol in dextrose solution and invert sugar and electrolytes solution (Olin, 1998).

The dextrose used in formulations is derived from corn sugar; however, a very small portion of the population may be sensitive to corn derivatives. For such persons, invert sugar derived from cane or beet sugar is an alternative.

Alcohol is another substrate providing 7 kcal/g, and it does not require insulin for peripheral utilization. Providing enough calories would necessitate a quantity of alcohol that would produce a potential for intoxication and hepatotoxicity. Because dextrose is inexpensive and readily available, it is almost always the preferred product for administration.

Fats

lipid emulsions (Intralipid, Liposyn)

Fat constitutes 40% to 50% of the total calories supplied in the average North American diet. Fat emulsions are derived from either soybean or safflower oil, which provides a mixture of neutral triglycerides and unsaturated fatty acids. The two functions of intravenous fat emulsions in parenteral nutrition are to supply essential fatty acids and to be a source of energy or calories (9 calories/g).

Linoleic, linolenic, and arachidonic acids are essential in humans. Linoleic acid cannot be synthesized in the body, and it is the precursor to both linolenic and arachidonic acid. If linoleic acid is either unavailable or deficient, the enzyme system will act on oleic acid to synthesize eicosatrienoic acid, which is incapable of functioning like arachidonic acid. Essential fatty acid deficiency is noted with clinical signs of hair loss, scaly dermatitis, growth retardation, reduced wound healing, decreased platelets, and fatty liver. This necessitates the intravenous administration of a fat emulsion to correct the biochemical alteration.

The fat emulsions currently available are either safflower oil (Liposyn) or soybean oil (Intralipid) or a combination of both (Liposyn II). Fat emulsion particles are thought to be metabolized from the bloodstream in a manner similar to that of the chylomicrons, which appear in the blood postprandially. Fat emulsions may minimize hyperglycemia, hyperinsulinemia, and hyperosmolar syndrome, which often occurs in patients given dextrose as the only source of parenteral caloric nutrition. Fat emulsions pose some dangers for persons with severe liver disease, pulmonary disease, anemia, or blood coagulation disorders and for acutely ill patients with elevated serum concentrations of C-reactive protein. Fat emboli and accumulation of intravascular fat may occur in lungs of premature, preterm, or low-birth-weight infants (infusion rate not to exceed 1 g/kg in 4 hours). A normal diet should be 40% fat, 40% protein, and 20% carbohydrate.

Trace Elements and Electrolytes

Although some of the commercial parenteral nutrition solutions contain trace elements, or minerals, persons receiving long-term administration should be evaluated for trace element deficiencies. Trace element solutions are available individually (zinc, copper, manganese, chromium, and selenium) and in combination formulations (M.T.E. formulations and others). Several trace metal formulations are also available in combination with electrolytes (Tracelyte and others).

Examples of the signs and symptoms of trace element deficiency, normal serum levels, and primary excretion sites are noted in Table 62-3. It is also critical to monitor serum electrolyte levels, especially for the cations sodium, potassium, calcium, and magnesium and the anions chloride, phosphate, bicarbonate, and acetate. Generally, serum levels of trace elements are not routinely monitored.

If iron replacement is necessary, oral replacement is the preferred route of administration. If iron cannot be administered orally, then it can be given by intramuscular Z-track injection or by intravenous injection or infusion. Do not mix iron with other drugs or add it to parenteral nutrition solutions. For additional information on iron (iron dextran), refer to a current package insert or a current drug reference book.

Vitamins

The patient receiving parenteral feedings will also need additional vitamins. Usually a combination of multivitamin infusion and, perhaps, additional vitamins will be given on alternate days to meet the patient's needs for fat-soluble vitamins A and D and water-soluble vitamins B and C. Such preparations, if prescribed, can be added to the parenteral nutrition solution. Vitamin K is usually administered weekly by IM or SC injection. The specific dosage and frequency for vitamin regimens depend primarily on the individual patient's needs and the usual protocols of the prescriber.

SPECIAL FORMULATIONS OR ADMINISTRATION

Specially formulated amino acid preparations are available for patients with special disease conditions; such as renal failure, high metabolic stress, encephalopathy, and liver failure. For example, formulas such as HepatAmine are used for hepatic failure and Nephramine and others for renal failure.

Parenteral nutrition is often administered in a home setting, usually in one single container per day. Whenever possible, all the necessary nutrients are combined and administered on a cycling basis, depending on the individual. Cyclic therapy is the infusion of the feeding over less than 24 hours, to free the individual from constant therapy. Often such preparations are administered during the evening and night hours (Holcombe, 1996)

SUMMARY

Enteral and parenteral nutrition are important for the treatment of patients who cannot consume sufficient nutrients through the regular processes of ingestion. With enteral nutrition, the upper GI tract is bypassed in persons who have an adequate GI tract but cannot consume sufficient food by mouth. Parenteral nutrition is used to precede procedures that impose restrictions on oral feedings, such as GI illnesses that prevent oral food ingestion, anorexia caused by radiation or chemotherapy used to treat cancer, and after surgery

TABLE 62-3 Trace Elements

Elements	*Dose**	*Deficiency Symptoms*
Copper	0.5-1.5 mg	Decrease in red and white blood cells; hair and skeletal abnormalities; defective tissue growth
Chromium	10-15 μg	Neuropathy, confusion, impaired glucose tolerance, ataxia
Manganese	150-800 μg	Defective growth, nausea, vomiting, weight loss, skin rash, central nervous system alterations (ataxia, seizures)
Selenium	40-80 μg	Muscle aches, pain or tenderness, cardiomyopathy, kwashiorkor
Zinc	2.5-4 mg	Nausea, vomiting, diarrhea, weakness, anorexia, growth retardation, anemia, hypogeusia, rash, depression, eye lesions, defective wound healing, and hepatosplenomegaly

*Recommended daily adult dose.

if the individual will not be able to resume food consumption for 5 or more days. This chapter reviews the composition of the nutritional solutions, indications, and complications associated with these formulations.

REVIEW QUESTIONS

1. What precautions were issued by the FDA to help prevent the serious calcium and phosphorus drug interaction?
2. What is protein-sparing nutrition and in what situations is it indicated?
3. What is the purpose of fat emulsions in nutritional therapy? Name the available fat emulsions and describe their actions in the body.
4. Name the major five trace elements and the usual signs and symptoms of a deficiency.

REFERENCES

Beare PG, Myers JL: *Adult health nursing,* ed 3, St Louis, 1998, Mosby.

Estoup M: Approaches and limitations of medication delivery in patients with enteral feeding tubes, *Crit Care Nurse* 14(2):68, 1994.

Food and Drug Administration: Safety alert: hazards of precipitation associated with parenteral nutrition, *Am J Hosp Pharm* 51(6):1427-1428, 1994.

Holcombe BJ: Adult parenteral nutrition. In Young LY, Koda-Kimble MA, editors: *Applied therapeutics: the clinical use of drugs,* ed 6, Vancouver, Wash, 1995, Applied Therapeutics, Inc.

Mirtallo JM: The complexity of mixing calcium and phosphate, *Am J Hosp Pharm* 51(6):1535-1536, 1994.

Miyagawa CI: Drug-nutrient interactions in critically ill patients, *Crit Care Nurse* 13(5):69, 1993.

Olin BR: *Facts and comparisons.* Philadelphia, 1998, JB Lippincott.

Rollins CJ: Adult enteral nutrition. In Young LY, Koda-Kimble MA, editors: *Applied therapeutics: the clinical use of drugs,* ed 6, Vancouver, Wash, 1995, Applied Therapeutics, Inc.

ADDITIONAL REFERENCES

American Hospital Formulary Service: *AHFS drug information '98,* Bethesda, Md, 1998, American Society of Hospital Pharmacists.

Anderson KN et al, editors: *Mosby's medical, nursing, and allied health dictionary,* ed 5, St Louis, 1998, Mosby.

Beizer J: Enteral feeding in the LTC setting, *Long Term Care Forum* 2(2):8, 1992.

Lipman TO: Total parenteral nutrition: indications for hospitalized adults, *Drug Ther,* Jan, pp. 67-73, 1993.

Metheney N: Minimizing respiratory complications of nasoenteric tube feedings: state of the science, *Heart Lung* 22(3):213-222, 1993.

Mosby: *Mosby's GenRx,* St Louis, 1998, Mosby.

United States Pharmacopeial Convention: *USP DI: drug information for the health care professional,* ed 18, Rockville, Md, 1998, The Convention.

UNIT XVIII

Miscellaneous Agents

CHAPTER 63

Antiseptics, Disinfectants, and Sterilant Agents

CHAPTER FOCUS

The transmission of infections may occur by (1) airborne transmission (inhalation of the infectious materials), (2) transmission of the microorganism by an intermediate carrier, such as a mosquito, (3) contact transmission (direct or indirect contact with the infected source), and (4) enteric transmission (fecal to oral transmission by direct or indirect contact with feces or objects contaminated with feces). Healthcare professionals must practice and teach aseptic and sterile techniques to reduce the transmission of infection. In the latter two transmission methods (contact and enteric), antiseptics, disinfectants, and sterilant agents are used to decontaminate surfaces and equipment to prevent the spread of infection.

OBJECTIVES

After reading and studying this chapter, the student should be able to do the following:

1. *Define and describe the key terms.*
2. *Contrast the differences between a nosocomial infection and a community or home-acquired infection.*
3. *Define medical asepsis and surgical asepsis.*
4. *Differentiate between sterilization, antiseptics, and disinfectants.*
5. *Discuss the action and toxicity associated with hexachlorophene.*
6. *Present the indications for and limitations of silver nitrate.*
7. *Describe the indications for and effectiveness of iodine compounds and the iodophors.*

KEY TERMS

antiseptics, (p. 800)
bactericidal, (p. 800)
bacteriostatic, (p. 800)
disinfectants, (p. 800)
medical asepsis, (p. 800)
nosocomial infections, (p. 800)
sterilization, (p. 800)
surgical asepsis, (p. 800)

Infections and infectious diseases, although differing in type and character, occur in people in all settings—hospitals, institutions, the community at large, and the home.

Community-acquired infections in usually healthy individuals are often benign and are relatively responsive to treatment. *Streptococcus pneumoniae* or *Mycoplasma pneumoniae* infections are common in this population. **Nosocomial infections** are those that are acquired in a hospital and most frequently are due to gram-negative (*Pseudomonas, Proteus, Serratia, Providencia,* and others) infections (Bailey, Powderly, 1992). Nosocomial infections have been called one of the most significant current ecologic problems in North America. They are occasionally caused by virulent microorganisms resistant to antibiotics.

Urinary tract infections and postoperative wound infections account for the majority (approximately 70% or more) of the nosocomial infections detected in a hospital setting. The high-risk areas such as critical care, burn, and dialysis units usually have the highest incidence of infection outbreaks and of antibiotic resistance in the hospital.

MEDICAL AND SURGICAL ASEPSIS

Medical asepsis (absence of pathogenic organisms) and **surgical asepsis** (absence of all microorganisms) are used in healthcare to reduce the number and spread of organisms. These approaches presume the presence of pathogens (organisms capable of inducing disease or infection in human beings) or potential pathogens in the immediate environment and seek to limit their transmission.

Methods in surgical asepsis destroy all microorganisms, including spores; in medical asepsis, only pathogens are destroyed or inhibited. The focus in surgical asepsis is to keep all organisms out of a designated area (e.g., fresh wound), but in medical asepsis it is to remove or destroy the pathogens in the area and to contain the remaining nonpathogens there by conscious efforts. The former uses "sterile technique" (use of sterile equipment or sterile fields) and the latter uses "clean technique" (such as hygienic measures, cleaning agents, antiseptics, disinfectants, and barrier fields). Which is applied in any given situation depends largely on the susceptibility of the host, the organism's virulence, and other factors in the infectious cycle.

Sterilization

An object is sterile if it is free of all forms and types of life. **Sterilization** is a process that destroys all forms of life on an instrument or utensil, in a liquid, or within a substance. Living tissue (of patients, nurses, or surgeons) cannot be sterilized by any known means without damage to that tissue; therefore the process known as sterilization is applied only to objects. It is also important to grasp the concept put forth by the Council on Pharmacy and Chemistry that the terms "sterile," "sterilizer," and "sterilization" can be used only in the absolute sense; there is no acceptable concept of relative sterility. However, just because a piece of equipment is labeled "sterilizer" does not mean that it is totally and permanently effective for sterilizing. Nor does the term "sterilized" testify to an object's current condition of purity.

Several acceptable and practicable sterilization methods now exist. Steam under pressure (autoclaving) is preferred as the most effective. Ethylene oxide is a gas sterilant used for heat-labile materials, for sharp-edged instruments that could be dulled by steam, for electrical and anesthesia equipment, and for bedding. Hot-air ovens are used to sterilize glassware. Chemical sterilants are also used when necessary.

ANTISEPTICS AND DISINFECTANTS

Antiseptics and disinfectants are often chemical agents used to kill many of the pathogens within a given population of microorganisms. Their mechanisms of action are generally not very effective against spores of bacteria and fungi, many viruses, and some very resistant bacterial strains. As a group, the effects of disinfectants and antiseptics differ from sterilization largely in the degree and type of organisms destroyed. Disinfectants and antiseptics kill only pathogens, but sterilizing kills all types of organisms.

Although some literature uses the terms "disinfectant" and "antiseptic" interchangeably, this is erroneous and confusing. Disinfectants differ from antiseptics in the matter in which they are used and in their ability to destroy organisms. **Disinfectants** are used only on nonliving objects; they are toxic to living tissue. **Antiseptics** are chemicals typically applied only to living tissue, so they must be less potent or made more dilute to prevent cell damage. Such lessening of potency, although crucial to viable tissue, decreases effectiveness accordingly. Some definitions of antiseptics emphasize their inhibiting rather than destructive effects. The narrow range of tolerance by tissues to antiinfective topical preparations tends to limit the variety and number of acceptable antiseptic agents available. Therefore antiseptics may differ markedly from disinfectants in chemical composition or may simply be a dilute version of a disinfectant for use on intact tissue. Thus some chemical substances may be used either as an antiseptic or as a disinfectant, depending on concentration.

Antiseptics and disinfectants are further categorized as **bacteriostatic** or **bactericidal** in character. Antiseptics are most often bacteriostatic; they retard the growth and replication of bacteria but do not kill off the entire bacteria population. Disinfectants, as bactericides, actually kill bacteria but perhaps not all types (depending on the disinfectant, its specificity, and so on) and often not fungi, viruses, or spores. Other disinfectants—fungicides, virucides, and sporicides—act specifically on these organisms. Germicide is an all-encompassing term for agents that work against many types of "germs"—bacteria, fungi, viruses, and spores.

Organisms vary in sensitivity to disinfectants and antiseptics in general (Box 63-1). However, factors such as the dormant and impervious spore forms of some bacteria, the

BOX 63-1 Sensitivity of Organisms to Disinfectants and Antiseptics*

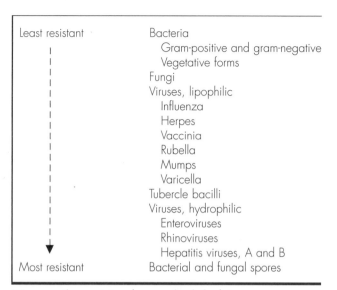

Least resistant	Bacteria
↓	Gram-positive and gram-negative
	Vegetative forms
	Fungi
	Viruses, lipophilic
	Influenza
	Herpes
	Vaccinia
	Rubella
	Mumps
	Varicella
	Tubercle bacilli
	Viruses, hydrophilic
	Enteroviruses
	Rhinoviruses
	Hepatitis viruses, A and B
Most resistant	Bacterial and fungal spores

*May vary with concentration of compound and other factors.

waxy envelopes of the tubercle bacilli, certain properties of some types of gram-positive bacteria (staphylococci and enterococci), some gram-negative bacteria (*Salmonella* and *Pseudomonas* species), and hepatitis viruses make them highly refractory to many forms of disinfectants or antiseptics.

The ideal all-around antiseptic/disinfectant does not yet exist. Such an ideal agent would have to do the following:

- Be destructive to all forms of microorganisms without being toxic to human cells.
- Have a low incidence of hypersensitivity.
- Be active in the presence of organic matter and soaps.
- Be stable, noncorrosive, nonstaining, and inexpensive.

The current criteria for an effective disinfectant, however, include the ability to destroy within 10 minutes all vegetative bacteria (not spores) and fungi, tubercle bacilli, animal parasites, and viruses (not hepatitis viruses). Many variables affect the relative efficiency of a product. These include the ingredients' ability to dissolve, mix, and work in the presence of organic matter such as blood or other exudate and also to penetrate into recesses. Other properties include chemical composition, concentration, pH, ionization, surface tension, temperature, and length of time required for action. Thus in actual clinical use, there may be extreme variability in the effectiveness of any given product, depending on the specific application and the situation. Although several standard tests for efficacy of these products are available, the results are subject to the same variables and may also be difficult to administer.

Currently there are few established guidelines for the specific approved use of any particular disinfectant: a disinfectant is considered a disinfectant whether it is to be used on corridor floors or on surgical instruments. This method of classifying permits widespread practices such as the common use of iodophor solutions as disinfectants when they have earned Food and Drug Administration (FDA) approval as antiseptics. Antiseptics are not required to be as potent as disinfectants. The relative usefulness of various antiseptics can be compared based on their therapeutic index. This index is the relationship between the specific antiseptic concentration proved to be effective against microorganisms without irritating tissues or interfering with healing. Other decisive factors are the potential for causing hypersensitivity reactions or systemic absorption. Thorough hand washing still predominates as the most effective measure for controlling the spread of infection.

To place the concepts of sterilization, disinfection, and antisepsis in perspective, it should be clear that these processes differ in the degree to which they destroy organisms. Thus anything that is sterile can also be considered both disinfected and antiseptic. (The converse is, of course, not true.) All of these processes correctly begin with hand washing, even when gloves are worn. It has been repeatedly demonstrated that clean, washed hands are crucial deterrents to microorganism growth, reproduction, and transmission in any environment.

Antiseptics and disinfectants may act in three ways:

1. They may bring about a change in the structure of the protein of the microbial cell (denaturation), which often proceeds to coagulation of protein with increased concentration of the chemical agent.
2. They may lower the surface tension of the aqueous medium of the parasitic cell, which increases plasma membrane permeability. This results in lysis or destruction of cellular constituents (the surface-active agents are thought to act this way).
3. They may alter a metabolic process in the microbial cells, which interferes with the cell's ability to survive and multiply.

PHENOLS

Phenol was used for more than 100 years as an antiseptic and disinfectant, but today it may be used in some facilities only as a disinfectant. All phenols are deadly poisons if taken internally or applied topically to abraded skin. They are also corrosive to equipment. Phenol and phenolic compounds should not come in contact with skin, especially if concentrations are greater than 2%.

hexachlorophene [heks' a klo roe feen] (pHisoHex, Septisol)

Hexachlorophene is a bacteriostatic agent that was incorporated into detergent creams, soaps, lotions, shampoos, and other topical products to reduce the incidence of pathogenic bacteria on the skin. Because of its toxicity, especially in infants, it is currently available only by prescription for surgical scrub purposes and as a bacteriostatic skin cleanser against staphylococci and other gram-positive bacteria. It is still used as a surgical scrub and bacteriostatic skin-cleansing agent, although other antiseptics such as chlorhexidine are more effective and safer agents.

Although single skin washing with hexachlorophene is no more effective than using soap in reducing the number of bacteria, this product has a cumulative antibacterial property and with repeated use will steadily decrease bacterial flora. However, cleansing with alcohol and repeated washing with soap removes its antibacterial residue.

Hexachlorophene is a toxic agent that can be absorbed through the skin causing gastric symptoms and central nervous system toxicity. Daily topical use on newborns or application several times daily to the skin or vagina in adults has resulted in confusion, diplopia, lethargy, convulsions, respiratory arrest, and death. Hexachlorophene is usually not routinely used or recommended for bathing infants. It also should not be used on mucous membranes or burned or denuded skin or for any prolonged skin contact without rinsing. Dermatitis and photosensitivity are also reported.

hexylresorcinol [hex ill re sore' sin ole]

Hexylresorcinol is a stainless and odorless antiseptic. Although quite irritating to body tissues, diluted solutions of hexylresorcinol are used to cleanse skin wounds and are also used in mouthwashes or pharyngeal antiseptic preparations. Occasionally a marked hypersensitivity reaction may occur.

DYES

Rosaniline dyes are a group of basic dyes used only occasionally today as antibacterial and antifungal agents. Most of these dyes (gentian violet, methyl violet, and others) have been removed from the market or have been replaced by other topical products.

Mercury Compounds

The FDA has banned all first-aid antiseptic mercury products which includes thimerosal, mercurochrome, and merthiolate because the products lack safety and effectiveness (FDA, 1998).

Silver Compounds

silver nitrate; silver protein, mild; silver sulfadiazine (Silvadene)

Locally applied, many inorganic silver compounds have antiseptic qualities. Those silver salts that are highly ionizable and soluble produce astringent or caustic actions. Free silver ions precipitate bacterial cellular proteins, resulting in bactericidal effects. The effectiveness of these agents is directly proportional to their concentration and duration of contact time. An immediate bactericidal effect occurs when silver solutions are applied to tissue. The silver proteinate that is formed slowly liberates small amounts of ionic silver, which provides continued bacteriostatic action. An unexplained strongly bactericidal quality resides in distilled water when it is in contact with metallic silver. Silver nitrate reacts with soluble chloride, iodides, and bromides to form insoluble salts, stopping the action of silver nitrate. Thus its action can be halted if necessary by irrigation of the area with sodium chloride solutions. This chemical characteristic explains why solutions of silver salts penetrate tissues slowly; apparently chlorides precipitate the silver ions and inactivate them.

Silver nitrate 1% solution is used to prevent gonorrheal ophthalmia neonatorum. Silver protein, mild (Argyrol S.S. 10%) is used to treat local mild inflammation in the eye, nose, and throat. Finally, silver sulfadiazine (Silvadene) is bactericidal for many gram-positive and gram-negative organisms and yeast, and it also inhibits bacteria resistant to other agents. It is used to prevent and treat infections in second and third degree burns.

Side effects and adverse reactions

With silver nitrate 1% solution, eye redness or irritation is the primary adverse reaction; with other silver nitrate preparations, it is skin irritation. With long-term use, it can cause permanent discoloration of the skin because of the deposit of reduced silver (argyria). Prolonged use of mild silver protein can result in permanent skin discoloration and conjunctival argyria. With silver sulfadiazine (Silvadene), allergic skin reactions may occur. Other adverse effects are difficult to attribute directly to silver sulfadiazine, since other therapeutic drugs are usually being administered concurrently. Leukopenia and perhaps systemic sulfonamide adverse reactions may occur.

Dosage and administration

With silver nitrate 1% solution, 2 drops of this solution are instilled and allowed to remain in the eyes for no longer than 30 seconds. The American Academy of Pediatrics endorsed a recommendation to eliminate eye irrigation after instillation of silver nitrate (Olin, 1996). In many hospitals, topical erythromycin or tetracycline ophthalmic ointments have replaced silver nitrate because they are effective against chlamydia and gonococcus eye infections (DiPiro, 1993).

For infections, instill 1 to 3 drops of silver protein, mild (Argyrol S.S.) in eye(s) every 3 to 4 hours for several days; for preoperative use, place 2 or 3 drops in eye(s), then rinse with a sterile irrigating solution.

Silver sulfadiazine (Silvadene) is applied with a sterile gloved hand once or twice daily to a 1/16-in thickness. Keep burn areas covered with this product at all times.

HALOGENS

Chlorine Compounds

Although chlorine can be bactericidal (it is ineffective against acid-fast bacteria), sporicidal, viricidal, and amebicidal, the elemental form of chlorine itself has limited usefulness as a disinfectant because the gas is difficult to handle. The antibacterial action of chlorine is said to be caused by the formation of hypochlorous acids, which results when chlorine reacts with water. Therefore chlorine-containing products that can release hypochlorous acid are in use today and include the following:

1. Sodium hypochlorite solution 1% is used to sterilize equipment while the 0.5% solution is used as an antiseptic for wound irrigation. This solution is of limited usefulness for wound irrigations, except for debridement purposes, because it is irritating to the skin and delays the clotting process. Common household bleaches are usually 5% solutions of sodium hypochlorite. Therapeutic solutions are unstable and must be freshly prepared before use.
2. Oxychlorosene (Clorpactin) is a combination product that contains hypochlorous acid, which when released is effective (bactericidal) against both gram-negative and gram-positive organisms, fungi, yeast, viruses, molds, and spores. It is indicated for the treatment of localized infections, especially if caused by resistant organisms; to cleanse and irrigate necrotic debris, wounds, sinus tract, and empyemas. Dilutions of this product are also used in urology and ophthalmology.

Iodine and Iodophors

iodine tincture; povidone-iodine solution

(Betadine)

Iodine is slightly soluble in water but is soluble in alcohol and in aqueous solutions of sodium and potassium iodide. Iodine is volatile, and solutions should not be exposed to air except during use. In its elemental or free form, iodine is very rapidly bactericidal, viricidal, fungicidal, and lethal to protozoa; it is less effective against spores. It is one of the most efficient chemical disinfectants and antiseptics currently in use.

Some iodine compounds are believed to be superior to other antiseptics because all types of bacteria may be destroyed with a single concentration of iodine, effective over a wide pH range. Organic matter interferes with the potency of iodine only when it is first applied; later, effectiveness increases because of diffusion as the iodine complexes dissociate. This initial delayed effect in the presence of organic material may also be offset by the increased strengths of the solution concentrations now on the market.

Iodine solution is used for the treatment of minor wounds, abrasions, and infected wounds whereas iodine tincture is preferred for intact skin procedures such as skin preparation before invasive procedures, Hickman catheter and parenteral nutrition dressing changes, and intravenous needle insertions. Aqueous solutions are thought to be as effective as tincture of iodine for similar therapeutic purposes, but because they are less irritating, they are used for abraded skin areas.

An aqueous solution of 5% iodine and 10% potassium iodide (Lugol's solution) can also be given orally for the treatment of goiter (see Chapter 40). The various iodine compounds marketed for antisepsis and disinfection include iodine topical and iodine tincture (the most commonly used iodine antiseptic). Although they both contain 2% iodine and 2.4% sodium iodide, the solution is in water while the tincture has 47% alcohol.

iodophor: povidone-iodine

(Betadine, Operand)

Iodophors have become widely used as antiseptics. This is the only purpose for which they have been approved by the FDA, although in practice they continue to be used for disinfection of certain equipment. Iodophors are a group of iodine compounds combined with povidone (carrier), which increases the water solubility of iodine and provides a slow release of iodine. It has the same germicidal action of iodine without producing irritation to skin and mucous membranes. Povidone-iodines are available in many formulations, such as solution, 2% scrub, spray, foam, vaginal gel and suppositories, ointment, mouthwash, or perineal wash.

Side effects and adverse reactions

Iodine is toxic if taken internally. It is locally corrosive to gastrointestinal tissues but is inactivated by gastrointestinal contents. Iodine tincture may be transiently quite painful when applied to open skin areas, but the aqueous solution form stings only slightly. These agents may be absorbed through the skin and with chronic use may affect thyroid function. Neonates have developed hypothyroidism after topical application of povidone-iodine. Marked hypersensitivity reactions do occur occasionally even with topical application. These are manifested by severe systemic reactions of fever and generalized skin eruptions.

OXIDIZING AGENTS

hydrogen peroxide

Hydrogen peroxide is a weak antiseptic that when in contact with a tissue enzyme (catalase) is converted to effervescent oxygen to produce an antibacterial action and cleansing effect on the wound. The presence of blood and pus, though, will decrease the efficacy of hydrogen peroxide (AHFS, 1996). The antiseptic action of hydrogen peroxide is fairly fast acting and short-lived; it acts as an antibacterial only as long as the bubbling action continues.

Oxygen that is released is particularly suited for destroying aerobic microorganisms in wounds, but as an antibacterial it is weak and slow. Its effervescence action, though, provides a mechanical effect to aid in removing foreign tissue debris. Several products containing hydrogen peroxide are marketed.

Hydrogen peroxide topical solution is available in a 3% solution in water and used to irrigate suppurating wounds and some extensive traumatic wounds. It should be used in areas where the oxygen can escape; therefore it should not be instilled into closed body spaces or abscesses (AHFS, 1996). It is not recommended for use for pressure ulcers because it and many other antiseptic agents are considered to be cytotoxic to normal tissues (Bergstrom et al, 1994).

The official hydrogen peroxide solution has been further diluted with water into a ½ or ¼ strength for most applications. The mouthrinse or mouthwash (Peroxyl) is a 1.5% solution.

Side effects and adverse reactions

If small amounts of diluted hydrogen peroxide solutions are swallowed, it rapidly decomposes in the stomach into relatively harmless molecular oxygen and water. Repeated use as a mouthwash may cause hypertrophied papillae of the tongue ("hairy tongue"), a reversible condition. The concentrated solutions used for hair bleaching may cause skin irritation and contact dermatitis.

BIGUANIDES

chlorhexidine [klor hex' i deen] (Hibiclens)

Chlorhexidine is a biguanide with antiseptic action against both gram-positive and gram-negative bacteria, such as *Pseudomonas aeruginosa.* Chlorhexidine acts by disrupting the bacterial cell's plasma membrane (particularly gram-positive organisms).

A bactericidal skin-cleansing solution containing chlorhexidine (Hibiclens) is useful as a surgical scrub, a hand-washing agent for personnel, and a skin wound cleanser. Chlorhexidine oral rinse (Peridex, PerioGard) is also used as an antibacterial dental product to treat gingivitis between dental visits.

For hand washing, Hibiclens is applied, water is added, and friction is applied for 15 seconds. Skin wounds should be washed gently with Hibiclens and rinsed. For surgical scrubs hands and forearms are scrubbed with approximately 5 ml of Hibiclens for 3 minutes without water, while using a brush or sponge. After hands and forearms are rinsed, washing is repeated for 3 more minutes.

Side effects and adverse reactions

Chlorhexidine is a relatively safe antiseptic. There have been reports of deafness occurring when these products came into contact with the middle ear through a perforated eardrum. Rare secondary effects include dermatitis, photosensitivity, and irritation of mucosal tissue. Physiochemical properties of these agents suggest that absorption through the skin is minimal.

SURFACE-ACTIVE AGENTS

benzalkonium chloride (Zephiran Chloride)

As wetting agents, emulsifiers, or detergents, surface-acting agents are considered superior to soaps because they can be used in hard water, are stable in acid or alkaline solutions, decrease surface tension more effectively, and are less irritating to the skin.

Benzalkonium chloride is a cationic (has a positive electric charge on the active portion of the agent) quaternary ammonium compound used in solution as a topical antiseptic or as a disinfectant. It is generally believed that benzalkonium chloride is not very reliable in either role. As an antiseptic it has a limited antibacterial spectrum; it lacks fast action and has a potential for inducing toxicity. As a disinfectant, the solution has to be changed regularly to maintain concentration and effectiveness. It is also inactivated by anionic substances, such as soap and organic materials.

The mechanism of action is not known for certain, but it may be due to bacteria enzyme inactivation.

This agent is slow acting in comparison to iodine. Therapeutic effects are thought to be in direct relation to the concentration of the solution used. Depending on the purpose and tissues or equipment to be treated, recommended dilutions range from 1:750 (tincture or aqueous solutions) on intact skin, minor wounds, and abrasions to 1:5000 or 1:10,000 (aqueous solution) for mucous membranes and broken or diseased skin. A variety of gram-positive and gram-negative organisms and many fungi and viruses (not hepatitis) are said to be susceptible. Tap water that contains metallic ions, organic matter, or resin-deionized water may reduce its effectiveness.

Side effects and adverse reactions

Chemical burns may occur if benzalkonium chloride is allowed to stay in contact with tissues, as in wet packs or occlusive dressings. Delicate tissues may be injured if specified dilution recommendations are not used. Ingestion only rarely causes toxicity. Hypersensitivity reactions can occur. The tincture and the spray formulations are flammable.

MISCELLANEOUS AGENTS

nitrofurazone (Furacin)

Nitrofurazone is a broad antibacterial topical agent active against many bacteria that cause local infections, including *Staphylococcus aureus, Streptococcus, Escherichia coli,* and others. It is indicated as adjunct therapy to patients with second- and third-degree burns when bacterial resistance to other agents is a problem and is also used during skin grafting when bacterial contamination may result in graft rejection or a donor site infection.

The 0.2% cream, ointment or solution may be applied directly on the area or to a gauze dressing for application. Efficacy is reduced in the presence of heavy microbial contamination, plasma, or blood. Resistance seldom develops.

Side effects and adverse reactions

Rash, itching, local edema (dermatitis), and allergic reactions have been reported. Hypersensitivity occurs early in the treatment of a few individuals. Bacterial and fungal superinfections may occur. Furacin is not absorbed significantly through mucosal or burned tissues, and systemic toxicity is rare. However, its propylethylene glycol base may be absorbed and challenge the patient with renal dysfunction.

ALCOHOLS

ethanol [eth' a nole] (ethyl alcohol)

isopropanol [eye soe proe' pa nole] (isopropyl alcohol)

A 70% alcohol solution is antiseptic. The 70% aqueous solution is more effective in reducing the surface tension of bacterial cells than absolute alcohol, which precipitates protoplasm at the periphery of the cell and thus tends to inhibit penetration of the agent. Alcohol also inhibits growth of bacteria, so it is often used as a preservative of biologic specimens and in some prepackaged injectables and medications. Alcohols may precipitate cellular proteins. They are potent viricidal agents.

Alcohol is used topically as a bactericidal, to prepare skin for minor invasive procedures (using commercially packaged skin wipes), and for disinfection of heat-labile instruments, polyethylene tubing, catheters, implants, prostheses, smooth hard-surfaced objects, hinged instruments, and inhalation and anesthesia equipment. Because of their rapid evaporation rate, dilute solutions of alcohols are still occasionally used as sponge baths to reduce fever, although systemic absorption may be especially harmful to neonates and children. Alcohols are also used as preservatives in solutions, as diluents, or to dissolve other drugs and in combination with many other drugs for over-the-counter purchase (often without rationale). Ethyl alcohol is also ingested purposefully as an intoxicating beverage.

Ethyl alcohol is slightly less effective as an antiseptic than isopropyl alcohol. Efficacy may depend on the concentration used and the amount of mechanical friction applied. The most effective solutions of ethyl alcohol are concentrations of 50% to 70%; stronger solutions are less effective. At concentrations of 70%, almost 90% of the bacteria on skin are killed within 2 minutes if the wet surface is allowed to dry naturally.

Toxicity

Essentially, all of the alcohols are poisonous drugs when taken internally, depending on the dose. Isopropyl alcohol is inherently highly poisonous; ethyl alcohol, pure alcohol made from vegetables, fruits, canes, and grains, is used in alcoholic beverages. The degree to which fractional distillation is carried out determines the resultant concentration.

Side effects and adverse reactions

When continuously inhaled or absorbed through the skin, alcohols can cause intoxication. Ethyl alcohol is irritating if left in contact with skin for prolonged periods. If ethyl alcohol is applied to open skin, a film that can harbor microorganisms develops. Isopropyl alcohol causes subcutaneous vasodilation, which can cause needle sites and incisions to bleed somewhat more freely.

ACIDS

acetic acid (vinegar); benzoic acid; lactic acid; boric acid

Various acids have been used as antiseptics or cauterizing agents, and of these vinegar is the most commonly used, especially in community health nursing, because of its practicality, availability, and low cost. Other acids that are used as antiseptics include benzoic acid (0.1%), which prevents bacterial and fungous growth; lactic acid, which is used primarily as a component of spermatocides in the United States and boric acid, which is so mild that it is used in eye and ear preparations. Of these other acids, most have lost credibility as effective antiseptics, for example, the implication of boric acid in cases of serious systemic intoxication by absorption.

Acetic acid provides an acid medium that inhibits the growth of organisms dependent on a neutral or alkaline medium. In a 5% concentration, acetic acid is germicidal to many organisms while it is bacteriostatic at lower concentrations. A mild vinegar solution is often recommended as a vaginal douche for antisepsis in the prevention or suppression of vaginal infections. Acetic acid may also be used as a mild antiseptic-deodorant for many other applications, such as bladder irrigation (0.25% concentration), and diaper soaks.

STERILANTS

ALDEHYDES

formaldehyde solution

Formaldehyde solution is a 37% concentration of formalin (by weight). It is a clear, colorless disinfectant liquid that on exposure to air liberates a pungent, irritating gas. In a concentration of 1% to 10%, it kills microorganisms and spores in 1 to 6 hours. It is effective against bacteria, fungi, and viruses and acts by combining with them to precipitate protein. It has been widely used as a disinfectant for instruments.

glutaraldehyde (Cidex)

Glutaraldehyde (Cidex), 2% alkaline solution, is a liquid disinfectant used as a germicidal agent to disinfect and sterilize some rigid optical instruments and prosthetic equipment. It kills some microorganisms in 10 minutes and spores in 10 hours. However, the solution is unstable and contact with skin should be avoided.

SUMMARY

Controlling the transmission of infection, especially in healthcare settings, is crucial to patient care. Frequent hand washing, medical asepsis, surgical asepsis, and the use of appropriate chemicals (antiseptics, disinfectants, and sterilants) are necessary to achieve this goal. Antiseptics are applied to living tissue whereas disinfectants are used on instruments or nonliving items; both are used to decrease the number of microorganisms present. Proper use of these agents is necessary to reduce the transmission of infection.

REVIEW QUESTIONS

1. What are the criteria for an ideal antiseptic/disinfectant? Compare the ideal to what is currently available.
2. Describe the action of hydrogen peroxide as an antiseptic. What substances interfere with its effectiveness?
3. What is the mechanism of action, indications, toxicity, and side effects and adverse reactions associated with the use of alcohol? Which alcohol is the more effective antiseptic: ethyl alcohol, or isopropyl alcohol? What concentrations are most effective?

REFERENCES

American Hospital Formulary Service: *AHFS drug information '98,* Bethesda, Md, 1998, American Society of Hospital Pharmacists.

Bailey TC, Powderly WG: Treatment of infectious disease. In Woodley M, Whelan A: *The Washington manual: manual of medical therapeutics,* ed 27, Boston, 1992, Little, Brown.

Bergstrom N, Bennett MA, Carlson CE et al: *Treatment of pressure sores: clinical practice guideline no 15,* AHCPR Pub No 95-0652, Rockville, Md, 1994, Agency for Health Care Policy and Research, US Department of Health and Human Services, Public Health Service.

ADDITIONAL REFERENCES

Anderson KN et al, editors: *Mosby's medical, nursing, and allied health dictionary,* ed 5, St Louis, 1998, Mosby.

DiPiro JT, Talber R et al, editors: *Pharmacotherapy, a pathophysiologic approach,* ed 2, Norwalk, Conn, 1993, Appleton & Lange.

Food and Drug Administration: Status of certain additional over-the-counter drug category II and III active ingredients, *Fed Register* 63(77):19799-19802, 1998.

Katzung BG: *Basic and clinical pharmacology,* ed 5, Norwalk, Conn, 1992, Appleton & Lange.

Mosby: *Mosby's GenRx,* St Louis, 1998, Mosby.

Olin BR: *Facts and comparisons.* Philadelphia, 1998, JB Lippincott.

United States Pharmacopeial Convention: *USP DI: drug information for the health care professional,* ed 18, Rockville, Md, 1998, The Convention.

CHAPTER 64

Diagnostic Agents

CHAPTER FOCUS

Diagnostic and laboratory tests are sources of information for the healthcare professional in the assessment, diagnosis, and ongoing monitoring of patients. The healthcare professional is also responsible for the preparation of the patient for diagnostic studies and for coordination of the completion of these tests. Many of these examinations require diagnostic agents with which the healthcare professional needs to be knowledgeable to appropriately instruct and care for patients undergoing diagnostic testing. The following objectives and key terms are important for a good understanding of this chapter.

OBJECTIVES

After reading and studying this chapter, the student should be able to do the following:

1. *Define and describe the key terms.*
2. *Describe the mechanism of action of radiopaque contrast medium.*
3. *State the method of absorption, metabolism, and excretion of barium sulfate and iodinated contrast media.*
4. *Explain the pharmacokinetics of diagnostic agents used as radioactive tracers and imaging agents.*
5. *State the indications, secondary effects, and management of common nonradioactive agents used for evaluating organ function and challenging glandular response.*
6. *Discuss common tests used for screening for selected health conditions.*

KEY TERMS

computed tomography (CT), (p. 811)
diagnostic agents, (p. 808)
nuclear magnetic resonance imaging (MRI), (p. 811)
radionuclide, (p. 810)
radiopharmaceutical, (p. 810)
ultrasonography, (p. 811)

Diagnostic agents are chemical substances used to diagnose or monitor a patient's condition or disease. As diagnostic agents, certain secondary chemical characteristics are used to confirm a diagnosis or prognosis or to guide therapy. For example, one type of diagnostic agent may interact with a bodily fluid specimen as a reagent to produce a color as an indicator, or it may induce an inflammatory response or an enhancement of a particular gland's functioning.

Other agents may act by contrasting and enhancing visibility on x-ray film of the lumens or cavities of internal body structures. Some, because of a special affinity and uptake by certain organs, permit critical assessment of organ function. Diagnostic agents may also have side effects and adverse reactions, just like any drug. Thus it is necessary that the healthcare professional know the agent used, its mechanism of action, and indications for use. Secondary effects are equally important as many agents have a somewhat narrow range of safety. Specialized training and professional education are necessary to administer some kinds of agents; others are packaged in simple kit form for over-the-counter sale. Because the field of diagnostics and its products are burgeoning, manufacturers' instructions should always be consulted to be assured of current information.

RADIOPAQUE AGENTS FOR VISUALIZING ORGAN STRUCTURE

When injected or instilled, radiopaque contrast agents make the body cavity or compartment more radiographically dense or opaque than neighboring anatomic structures. They are used when the structural integrity of a soft tissue organ system is under study. Ordinary x-ray examinations are useful only for studies of dense materials such as bone. Radiopaque contrast media may also permit visualization of organs' functional dynamics as part of associated diagnostic tests.

Many of these agents contain molecular iodine in the radiopaque contrast medium to provide the opacity necessary for outlining internal organ cavities, lumens, or ducts that would otherwise be invisible by x-ray examination or fluoroscopy.

Barium contrast media consist of barium sulfate powder and a vehicle such as hydrosol gum for mixing with a prescribed volume of water to provide a suspension for oral or rectal administration. Iodinated radiopaque agents consist of substituted, triiodinated, benzoic acid derivatives or water-soluble, triiodinated, benzoic acid salts. Check the manufacturers' instructions for ingredients.

The prescriber should be consulted when a patient reports a history of idiosyncratic response or hypersensitivity to iodine, shellfish, or contrast media or a history of multiple radiographic or radionuclide studies. The most common radiopaque contrast agents are barium sulfate suspensions and iodinated contrast materials. Table 64-1 lists medications, iodine content, and indications.

Indications

Barium-containing preparations are typically used to opacify the gastrointestinal (GI) tract, which is generally performed when ulcers, inflammatory bowel disease, or cancer is suspected. One of the most common uses of barium contrast media is in "double-contrast" studies for GI tract evaluation. Double contrast is a method of making an x-ray image by using two contrast agents, usually a gaseous medium and a water-soluble radiopaque agent.

The most frequent clinical uses of iodinated contrast media include intravenous urography and angiography. Iodinated contrast media are often used during computed to-

TABLE 64-1 Medications, Iodine Content, and Indications

Medication	*Indications*	*Iodine Content*
Contrast Media		
diatrizoate sodium injection (Hypaque Sodium)	Cerebral angiography Aortography Cholangiography	150 mg/ml (25% solution) 300 mg/ml (50% solution)
iocetamic acid (Cholebrine)	Oral cholecystography	465 mg/750 mg tablet
iopanoic acid (Telepaque)	Oral cholecystography	333 mg/500 mg tablet
ipodate (Oragrafin)	Oral cholecystography	3 g contains 61.7% iodine
tyropanoate (Bilopaque)	Oral cholecystography	430 mg/750 mg capsule
Other Agents		
amiodarone (Cordarone)	Antiarrhythmic	74 mg/200 mg tablet
iodoquinol (Yodoxin)	Antiprotozoal	134-416 mg/tablet
echothiophate iodide ophthalmic (Phospholine Iodide)	Antiglaucoma Cyclostimulant Diagnostic aid	5-41 μg/drop
idoxuridine ophthalmic (Herplex, Stoxil)	Antiviral	18 μg/drop

Modified from Farwell, Braverman, 1996; USP DI, 1998.

mography of the head and body to visualize vascular structures and to detect tumors.

Pharmacokinetics

Radiopaque agents may be administered by the oral, vaginal, rectal, intravenous, or intraarterial routes, or they may be instilled into other body cavities. Orally administered iodinated agents for visualization of the gallbladder are absorbed across the GI mucosa and enter the systemic circulation through the portal venous system. Orally or rectally administered iodinated media for delineation of the GI tract are absorbed only minimally, but enough so that the renal tract may also be visualized. Barium sulfate preparations are not absorbed. They are metabolized by the liver and gallbladder and excreted by the kidneys.

Drug interactions

The following effects may occur when the oral cholecystographic agents are given with the drugs listed below:

Drug	Possible effect and management
cholestyramine (Questran)	The cholestyramine will absorb the cholecystographic agents, thus interfering with the test. Avoid concurrent administration for at least 8 hours or more when tests involving these agents are scheduled.
iodipamide meglumine IV	Prior administration of the oral agents may block liver metabolism and excretion of this drug. Administration of both drugs within 24 hours is not recommended.
Urographic agents	Renal toxicity has been reported in patients with abnormal liver function when tests involving these agents were done after the oral urographic agents. Avoid concurrent administration.

Color type indicates an unsafe drug combination

The following interactions may occur when the radiopaque parenteral agents are given with the drugs listed below:

Drug	Possible effect and management
aspirin, nonsteroidal antiinflammatory drugs (NSAIDs), and other antiplatelet agents	May enhance the antiplatelet effect, since high levels of iodipamide meglumine, diatrizoate sodium, and diatrizoate meglumine all inhibit platelet aggregation. Monitor the patient for bleeding and also monitor platelet count.
Inotropic agents	May result in a paradoxic cardiac depressant effect, which is dangerous if patient has an ischemic myocardium. Monitor closely if agents must be administered concurrently.

Side effects and adverse reactions

Radiopaque agents are not without risk. Effects are diverse, mild to moderate in severity, and usually occur within 1 to 3 minutes. However, delayed reactions may occur up to 1 hour after injection. Anaphylaxis and hypersensitivity reactions are also reported.

Intravenous cholangiography has caused the highest number of reactions and has therefore been largely replaced by radionuclide diagnostics and retrograde duodenal examination. Excretory urography is performed frequently with only rare serious reactions. Milder reactions result from administration of oral cholecystographic agents. Certain agents are more likely to cause secondary effects than others; manufacturers' information should be consulted.

A history of allergy puts the person at twice the risk of reaction to contrast media, although, paradoxically, these are not true hypersensitivity reactions. Patients with a previous anaphylactoid reaction to contrast media may have an increased risk of 10-fold or more (Olin, 1998).

Barium sulfate preparations, since they are not absorbed internally, are only potentially hazardous when administered to persons with bowel perforations or fistulas. If allowed to remain in the colon, barium sulfate may cause constipation. Hospitalization and close observation during the procedures are recommended for persons who have a high potential for reactions or complications.

The most common side effects reported are nausea or flushing, with feelings of warmth over the abdomen and chest. Severely dehydrated patients, the elderly, infants, and the seriously ill tolerate these hemodynamic and hyperosmolar changes less well than do others. Rare adverse reactions include cerebral hematomas, hemodynamic alterations, sinus bradycardia, transient electrocardiogram (ECG) changes, ventricular fibrillation, and petechiae.

Rarely, diazoate salts inhibit blood coagulation, which may result in a severe thromboembolic event (AHFS, 1996). Platelet aggregation is inhibited by several of the agents. Exacerbations of sickle cell disease may result from intravascular injections of contrast media.

Renal system involvement may be manifested by nephrosis of proximal tubular cells in excretory urography, which may proceed to renal failure. Altered respiratory status may include rhinitis, cough, dyspnea, bronchospasm, asthma, laryngeal or pulmonary edema, and subclinical pulmonary emboli.

The senses may be impaired, for example distorted taste sensations or irritated, itching, tearing eyes, or conjunctivitis may be seen. Hypersensitivity reactions and anaphylaxis may occur. A history of allergy predisposes a person to reactions to contrast media.

AGENTS FOR EVALUATING ORGAN FUNCTION

Some diagnostic agents can be used to track and visualize the functional processes of organ systems. Inferences can be made about organ function by measurement of the degree or rate at which the agent is distributed, taken up, sequestered, secreted, or excreted from the target organ system or by measurement of the volume or flow rates. Some of these diagnostic agents are radionuclides (a species of radioactive atom characterized by higher atomic number than bodily tissues) whose gamma-ray emissions can be tracked or whose residues can be sampled. Other nonradioactive agents are dyes, polysaccharides, or other substances whose dissemination may be traced by color changes or chemical analysis.

RADIOACTIVE AGENTS

A **radionuclide** is an unstable form of a chemical element. **Radiopharmaceutical** agents are those in which one of the nonradioactive atoms has been replaced by a radioactive atom. They are either of natural origin or are produced by particle accelerators or generators. The process of neutron activation used in nuclear medicine to produce radionuclides describes the capture of a slow neutron into a stable nucleus with the subsequent emission of a gamma ray. Transmutation is a similar operation, using instead a fast neutron. After injection or ingestion of the resultant nuclide, its pharmacokinesis can be followed by a gamma-ray detector combined with either a rectilinear scanner, scintillation camera, Bender-Blau camera, or other radiation-display device. Some substances such as glucose, ^{14}C, air, blood, lymph, spinal fluids, urine, or biopsy specimens may be collected and the residual radioactivity analyzed or counted as it is excreted. These data are used to make inferences about organ disorders and the body's ability to absorb, metabolize, or excrete substances.

Ionizing Radiation

Much can be learned through the use of radiation that could not otherwise be discovered or diagnosed. Like any other diagnostic technique, a risk to benefit ratio must be determined. Ionizing radiation has the ability to knock electrons out of atoms, creating electrically charged ions. This radiation may be defined as electromagnetic radiation (x-rays and gamma rays) or particulate radiation (electrons, occasionally beta particles, protons, neutrons, or atomic nuclei with kinetic energy).

The impact by emitted radiation energy may disrupt bonds between atoms in crucial biologic molecules such as deoxyribonucleic acid (DNA). Disruption can lead to cell death, mutations, or defective mitosis. Energy that is absorbed by tissues can lead to acute effects (as in radiotherapy or radiation accidents) or chronic effects (as from multiple low radiation doses). Effects (such as cataracts) may appear only after long periods or in subsequent generations.

The amount of radiation absorbed by tissues during radiologic tests is determined by the dose administered, the half-life of the radionuclide, the energy, the mode of decay, and the length of time the agent dwells within the body. There is no known safe dosage of ionizing radiation despite limits set by the Nuclear Regulatory Commission and the National Council on Radiation, Protection and Measurements.

Estimations of the amount of radiation emitted, the effect, and the dose absorbed may be denoted by the following terms. A roentgen is the amount of gamma or x radiation that creates 1 electrostatic unit of ions in 1 ml of air at 0° C. A rem is the predicted effect on the human body of a 1-roentgen dose. A rad is a unit of measurement of absorbed ionizing radiation energy. One rad = 100 ergs of radiation energy per gram of matter.

Although arbitrary, annual limits for radiation for the general population and for any single gestational period have been set at 0.5 rem (for x-rays, 1 rem is equal to 1 rad) and for closely monitored occupational workers at about 3 rem/year. Most physicians, nurses, and other healthcare personnel are not routinely monitored for radiation exposure unless assigned to an area with high potential for exposure. Their risk for cumulative exposure is nonetheless higher than that of the general population.

Very little is known about the full effects of radiation. Certain increased risks are associated, however, as follows: infertility, birth defects, potential for certain malignant neoplasms, and manifestations of aging. Exposure to low-level ionizing radiation, such as that from radiographic examinations, and agents containing radionuclides add to the individual's total radiation history. Effects may be insidious, perhaps manifesting themselves in crucial enzyme defects many years after exposure. There is some evidence of the body's ability to repair chromosomal damage, but the scope of this ability is unknown.

"Excessive radiation exposure" is any unnecessary exposure above natural background levels. Although natural background radiation adds to the cumulative risk, medical and dental therapies account for the largest proportion of artificially generated exposure.

Indications

Most radionuclides in use today in radiology are for imaging of organs, evaluating organ function, or detecting or treating cancer. The role of nuclear imaging is gradually diminishing because of increased reliance on computed tomography, ultrasound, and magnetic resonance imaging.

Radionuclides are used as tracers to evaluate physiologic and biochemical functioning of organ systems. By imaging methods, extremely sensitive radioactivity sensing devices make it possible to detect, count, visualize, and analyze minute amounts of radionuclides. Uniquely useful applications of nuclear imagery include the following:

1. Thyroid enlargement or disease. Agents currently used include ^{131}I and ^{123}I. These are iodine isotopes that emit a type of radiation which can be mapped externally. Usually a 24-hour uptake study is used to determine the extent and areas of thyroid activity. A scan is then performed to evaluate any thyroid mass or enlargement. "Cold" tumors have a 20% to 25% probability of representing a thyroid cancer. Tumors that localize the radionuclide well are usually benign.
2. Screening individuals with diagnosed malignancies for metastases. Many patients treated for breast cancer, colon cancer, malignant melanoma, lymphoma, prostate cancer, and lung cancer, among others, are often successfully evaluated periodically by scintigrams of the liver, spleen, and skeletal system. A scintigraph is a photographic recording showing the distribution and intensity of radioactivity in various tissues and organs after the administration of a radiopharmaceutical. The risk to benefit ratio is very high, and information about new or recurrent disease can help the oncologist and the patient make crucial decisions about goals, management, prognosis, and so forth.
3. Evaluation of heart disease. This is a primary application of nuclear imagery. Computers are used to analyze data from the images to detect the extent of myocardial damage and wall motion abnormalities and to estimate the ejection fraction of the ventricles. Underlying coronary artery disease can also be estimated by the use of radionuclides before catheterization or other invasive procedures.
4. Tracking physiologic substances and assessment of the status of an organ (e.g., renal function, biliary excretion, and others). In addition to diagnostic uses, some radiopharmaceuticals may be administered therapeutically to deliver radiation to internal body tissues (e.g., ^{131}I for destruction of thyroid tissue in hyperthyroidism). Radioactive tracer substances may also be incorporated into a nonradioactive drug to track the second drug's pharmacokinetics for research purposes.

Computed tomography (**CT**) scans body parts in a series of contiguous slices with pencil-thin x-ray beams, which, after passing through the body, produce data from detectors positioned diametrically across from the beam source. Huge amounts of data are integrated and displayed by computer as a video image. CT presents a series of two-dimensional images representing a reconstructed "slice" in the axial plane. By viewing a series of these images, one can perceive the anatomy in a three-dimensional sense. CT therefore often conveys more information than other modalities about lesion density, location, and size.

CT has largely replaced older techniques such as pneumoencephalography and angiography in the diagnosis of intracranial disease, although angiography is still used for this application. CT may eliminate the need for other x-ray examinations, but it is not considered a first-line, or screening, technique. Radionuclide scans continue to be used for initial diagnostic screening and for specific tests for which their results are more fruitful. Radiation exposure from CT varies depending on the equipment used and the frequency of testing, but it is said to be equal to or sometimes considerably higher than ordinary x-ray techniques or radionuclides. Although CT is considered to be a noninvasive procedure, intravenous contrast material is frequently injected to enhance structures for differential diagnosis. This is referred to as CT with infusion.

Ultrasonography is a nonradioactive diagnostic modality with cardiovascular, abdominal, obstetric, and other applications. It is used with anatomic and physiologic information obtained by other nuclear medicine techniques. Ultrasound examinations yield data about organ contours and tissue consistency or, in the case of Doppler scanning, blood flow patterns. Results can be distorted in the presence of bone or gases in the body. The secondary effects of high-frequency sound waves on cellular structures and functions are not fully known, although such tests are considered to be noninvasive and innocuous by many in the field.

Nuclear magnetic resonance imaging (**MRI**) is a diagnostic modality that uses radio waves and a magnet, not radiation, drugs, biopsy specimens, or body fluids. Like CT, MRI provides sectioned imagery but gives more than the gross anatomic information gained by CT scanning. MRI supplies extremely detailed images of internal heart and brain structures, for example, and is capable of imaging areas of the spine, abdomen, and extremities. It can differentiate between lesions and normal tissue. Persons ineligible for diagnostics by MRI include those with metal prostheses or pacemakers, because the strong magnetic field surrounding the patient may move some metallic devices, or a metallic object may result in a distorted test image.

Pharmacokinetics

Each type of radionuclide emits alpha or beta particles or gamma rays or a combination of these. This spontaneous emission of charged particles is termed "radioactive decay" and eventually results in disintegration of the nucleus. The time it takes for the original radioactivity to decay to one half its original value is known as the physical or radioactive half-life of the particular radionuclide. Like a drug, the rate at which a tracer substance is excreted from the body also influences its effects, both valuable and undesirable.

Dosage and administration

Manufacturers' current directions should be reviewed. Dosages are not detailed here because they vary with individual needs.

The major considerations in radionuclide dosing are the amount of radioactivity that is administered to produce ef-

BOX 64-1 Selected Multiple Urine Tests

Measures	*Chemstrip GP*	*Combistix*	*HemaCombistix*	*Uristix-4*	*Keto-Diastix*	*Chemstrip 6*	*Labstix*	*BiliLabstix*	*Multistix SG**	*Multistix 7*	*Multistix 10 SG**	*Chemstrip 9*	*Multistix 9*	*Chemstrip 2LN*	*Multistix 2*
Glucose	X	X	X	X	X	X	X	X	X	X	X	X	X		
Protein	X	X	X	X		X	X	X	X	X	X	X	X		
pH		X	X			X	X	X	X	X	X	X	X		
Blood		X	X			X	X	X	X	X	X	X	X		
Ketones					X	X	X	X	X	X	X	X	X		
Bilirubin								X	X		X	X	X		
Urobilinogen									X		X	X	X		
Nitrite				X						X	X	X	X	X	X
Leukocytes				X		X				X	X	X	X	X	X

Modified and adapted from Olin, 1998.
*Also measures specific gravity.

fective readings and the secondary radionuclide effects. While the radioactive material is in the body, it is irradiating even after the study has been completed, whereas x-rays irradiate from an external source and do so only while the body is exposed during the examination. The radionuclide dosage unit for imaging or nonimaging doses of radionuclide is a microcurie (one millionth of a curie). A curie is a specified measure of radioactivity associated with a specific amount of a radioactive substance, e.g., a radionuclide. Recommended dosages are spelled out in manufacturers' literature. The patient's absorbed dose of each radionuclide has been predicted for each procedure with the following three factors being considered: (1) the biologic parameters that describe the uptake, distribution, retention, and release of the radiopharmaceutical in the body; (2) the energy released by the radionuclide and whether it is penetrating or nonpenetrating; and (3) the fraction of the emitted energy that is absorbed by the target.

The ultimate radiation dose to both the target organ and the whole body is somewhat less in radionuclide nonimaging procedures than in imaging procedures. It is considerably more in radiation therapy (not discussed here).

Shielding is a practical method to prevent or reduce excess radiation exposure of staff or patients during certain diagnostic examinations. Shielding reduces radiation intensity to acceptable limits in body areas not intended for exposure during the radiologic examination. Alpha and beta radiation require very little shielding. An alpha particle can be blocked by the thickness of a sheet of paper, a beta particle by an inch of wood, but several feet of concrete or several inches of lead are necessary to stop gamma or x radiation. "Half-value layer" is the term describing the thickness of any material required to reduce the intensity of an x-ray or gamma-ray beam to half its original value. Because of its characteristic density, lead is the material typically used in radiation shielding equipment and coverings such as aprons and gloves.

NONRADIOACTIVE AGENTS

Nonradioactive Agents for Evaluating Organ Function via Volumes and Flows

These relatively biologically inert and nonradioactive substances are commonly used to measure flow rates, fluid volumes, diffusion, concentration ability, and organ function. These compounds are mostly dyes, polysaccharides, or other substances that can be assayed chemically or detected by characteristic colors after administration. Many of the dye tests determine the rate of plasma clearance of the dye by the organ under study. The ability to measure certain parameters against known normal values at defined points in the procedure makes these compounds useful as diagnostic aids. They are used variously for evaluation of cardiac output, liver or kidney function or blood flows, circulation time, intestinal absorption, and so forth (Box 64-1).

These compounds are administered primarily by the intravenous or intramuscular routes. They are rapidly absorbed by the organ system under examination and are usually excreted by that system. These drugs are relatively pharmacologically inert and are used to measure specific physiologic functions without themselves significantly altering those functions (Table 64-2).

Nonradioactive Agents for Challenging Glandular Response

Certain compounds are used diagnostically to challenge a particular system, often glandular, to produce measurable responses. Secretory responses indicate whether there is functional integrity within the secreting gland or system.

TABLE 64-2 Selected Nonradioactive Agents for Evaluation of Organ Function

Agent	*Indication(s)*	*Secondary Effects*
aminohippurate sodium	Measure renal plasma flow and tubular secretory mechanism	Nausea, vomiting, cramping, flushing, and tingling
D-xylose (Xylo-Pfan)	evaluate intestinal absorption	Infrequent: nausea, vomiting, cramps, and diarrhea
indocyanine green (Cardio-Green)	Measure cardiac output, hepatic function, and used for ophthalmic angiography	Low incidence of side effects
inulin	Diagnostic for renal function	Minimal side effects
mannitol (Osmitrol)	Diuretic, antiglaucoma, antihemolytic	Dry mouth, thirst, headache, acidosis, dehydration; contraindicated in anuria, intracranial bleeding, severe dehydration, and pulmonary edema

Modified from AHFS, 1998; Olin, 1998.

Many of these testing agents are protein substances that mimic the action of naturally occurring bodily chemicals such as secretagogues for exocrine gland response and stimulants for endocrine secretion. Because most of theseagents are administered IM or IV, they move rapidly to the site of action. Degradation of these agents is equally rapid.

Nonradioactive agents are used to evaluate or enhance capabilities such as thyroid secretion, gallbladder contraction, insulin response, and gastric acid secretory function. These testing agents act on the targeted gland or site as releasing factors. Thus secondary effects may be as widespread and disruptive to bodily chemical balance as a large dose of the secretion or hormone itself (Table 64-3).

Epinephrine, antihistamines, corticoids, and a tourniquet should be readily available for all tests in case of severe reactions. Analgesics, nasogastric suction equipment, vasodilators (for histamine agents), intravenous glucose solutions (for tolbutamide), and atropine (for edrophonium) should also be kept available. Manufacturers' instructions should be followed very closely because nearly all these compounds are administered parenterally and in very small doses.

AGENTS FOR SCREENING AND MONITORING DISORDERS AND IMMUNE STATUS

Screening and monitoring agents may be extracts of common allergens (ragweed, grasses, trees, molds, animal dander, and foods) or purified derivatives or concentrates of microbial antigens, hormones, or animal cellular antigens, or they may be chemical reagents. Many chemical reagents for common diagnostic purposes are packaged in simple kit form for over-the-counter or prescribed purchase; they may also be used routinely in institutions and primary health-care settings.

Mechanism of action and pharmacokinetics

Antigens applied topically or intradermally cause antigen-antibody reactions, which may be manifested by a local inflammatory response at the test site. The test site is assessed after a prescribed time interval. A positive response is indicated by the presence of erythema and induration (a firm lump under the skin). In the case of microbial antigen challenge, this positive response may merely indicate a previous exposure to the microbe or its products, but not necessarily the presence of an active disease process. False-negative results may also occur, and further investigation may be necessary. The size of the erythematous area or induration may be measured to estimate the degree of the person's sensitivity or immune response. These responses may be short lived or of lifelong duration (see also Chapter 55).

Persons who are immunosuppressed because of cancer chemotherapy or radiation treatments, malnutrition, debilitation, or congenital or acquired immunodeficiency syndrome (AIDS) may demonstrate no response (anergy) when tested with a prescribed battery of antigen challenges. These persons are extremely vulnerable to infection and may need metabolic support and precautions to avoid infection. Test results may not be reliable in those who have viral infections, are febrile or uremic, or have recently received live viral vaccinations.

Indications

Some diagnostic agents measure a person's physiologic response or hypersensitivity to the agent as a specific chemical challenge. These agents are typically used in simple baseline screening procedures as part of an initial diagnostic workup. Some are used in skin tests by patch, prick, scratch, or intradermal injection to assess hypersensitivity (allergy), anergy (congenital or acquired inability to develop a cell-mediated reaction), cellular immunity, or antibody response (Table 64-4). Others are used as reagents in specimens of blood, urine, and bodily discharges for detection of the levels of certain components to facilitate diagnosis or to monitor known conditions (Table 64-5 and Box 64-1).

Side effects and adverse reactions

Local reactions to skin tests do not usually cause discomfort. Occasionally a highly positive reaction will result in ve-

TABLE 64-3 Common Nonradioactive Agents for Evaluating Body Response

Agent	Indications/Secondary Effects	Management
edrophonium (Tensilon)	Diagnostic: myasthenia gravis Secondary effects: severe cholinergic reaction; bradycardia or cardiac standstill; dysrhythmias	Have IV atropine 1 mg, available to relieve the adverse muscarinic effects of edrophonium. Monitor vital signs carefully. Have facilities available for CPR, cardiac monitoring, and respiratory assistance. A placebo may be administered first as if it were the test dose to evaluate baseline muscular capabilities. A number of drugs may be withheld for at least 8 hr; check with prescriber.
histamine	Diagnostic: gastric function Secondary effects: flushing, dizziness, headache, dyspnea, asthma, urticaria, hypotension or hypertension, tachycardia, GI distress, convulsions	Withhold food for 12 hr and fluids and smoking for 8 hr before test. Withhold medications: antacids, anticholinergics, alcohol, histamine, histamine receptor antagonists, insulin, parasympathomimetics, adrenergic blockers, corticosteroids. Keep epinephrine available for severe hypotension.
pentagastrin (Peptavlon)	Diagnostic: gastric function in pernicious anemia, Zollinger-Ellison and other GI conditions Secondary effects: hypersensitivity, stimulates pancreatic secretion, GI distress or bleeding.	Drug of choice for gastric secretion testing. Withhold food, liquids, and smoking after midnight before test. Inform patient a nasogastric tube will be passed. Withhold medications as above with histamine. After test, observe for GI distress. Resume usual diet and medications.
protirelin (Thypinone)	Diagnostic: thyroid function Secondary effects: blood pressure alterations, breast enlargement, nausea, increased urination, dizziness, dry mouth, headache	Have patient urinate and assume a supine position. Drug is administered as a bolus over 15-30 sec. Take blood pressure (BP) frequently over the first 15 min. Increases in BP (<30 mm Hg) are more common than decreases. Use caution in patients with whom rapid changes in BP would be dangerous.
sincalide (Kinevac)	Diagnostic: gallbladder and pancreatic function. Secondary effects: hypersensitivity, nausea, cramps, dizziness, flushing	Administered IV. Adverse effects usually occur immediately after the injection and last for a few minutes.
tolbutamide (Orinase Diagnostic)	Diagnostic: pancreatic islet cell function Secondary effects: severe hypoglycemia	Instruct patient to adhere to a 150-300 g/day carbohydrate diet for 3 days before test and to fast overnight. Avoid smoking during fast and the test. Tolbutamide not administered to patients with known sensitivities to the drug or other sulfonylurea drugs. Withhold medications: salicylates and other drugs known to potentiate the hypoglycemic action of tolbutamide for 3 days before the test (see Chapter 42). If severe hypoglycemia occurs during the test, administer 12.5-25 g of glucose in a 25%-50% IV solution.

siculation and necrosis of overlying skin; corticosteroids may be ordered. Transient tachycardia, malaise, or low-grade fever may occur separately from a local reaction. Occasionally, a person may report systemic allergic reactions of urticaria, sneezing, or dyspnea. Rarely an overwhelming antigen-antibody response may occur—an anaphylactic response—calling for emergency measures such as the administration of epinephrine and respiratory and circulatory support. All of these secondary effects are more likely to occur if hyposensitization therapy is begun, because this includes a well-controlled program of increasing dosages of the allergen in question.

Dosage and administration

For certain standardized tests such as that for coccidioidomycosis, the dosage is fixed (0.1 ml of a 1:100 dilution). Dosages for allergy testing are also very small (0.02 to 0.05 ml) but may be individualized. Manufacturers' instructions for all these diagnostic agents should be followed carefully.

TABLE 64-4 Biologic Agents for Diagnostic Tests

Biologic Product	***Indication/Adult Dose***
Tuberculin (purified protein derivative, [PPD], Mantoux Test) (Aplitest, Tuberculin Tine Test)	Diagnostic: tuberculosis Adult dose: 5 U.S. units, intradermal. Special instructions for application of Tine test should be followed.
Tuberculin (PPD) (Aplisol, Tubersol)	Diagnostic: tuberculosis Adult dose: 5 U.S. units, intradermal after specific instructions as noted by manufacturer or USP DI.
Allergenic extracts	Several hundred individual purified fluid allergens available for diagnosis and hyposensitization of allergies: pollens, poison ivy, foods, dusts, yeast and other allergens. Treatment: periodic subcutaneous injection of gradually increasing potent dilutions of specific allergen.

TABLE 64-5 Common Tests for Screening Selected Conditions

Identifies/Detects	***Test(s)***	***Available***
Ketones in blood or urine	Acetone tests: Acetest, Ketostix	Tablets, strips
Protein in urine	Albumin tests: Albustix	Strips
Nitrate, uropathogens, bacteria	Microstix-3, Uricult	Culture paddle, strips
Bilirubin in urine	Ictotest	Tablets
Urea nitrogen in blood	Azostix	Strips
Candida albicans, vaginal	Isocult for Candida, CandidaSure	Culture paddle Reagent slides
Chlamydia trachomatis	Chlamydiazyme, Sure Cell Chlamydia	Kits
Cholesterol	Advanced Care Cholesterol Test-for home use	Kit
Cryptococcal neoformans in cerebrospinal fluid and serum	Crypto-LA	Slide tests
Gastrointestinal duodenal fluid	Entero-Test	String capsules
stomach acid	Gastro-Test	String capsules
Glucose in blood	Chemstrip bG, Dextrostix, Diascan, Glucometer Encore, and others	Strips
Glucose in urine	Clinitest, Chemstrip bG, Clinistix, Tes-Tape	Tablets, strips
Gonorrhea	Biocult-GC, Gonozyme Diagnostic, others	Kits
Human immunodeficiency virus (HIV) tests	HIV-1 LA Recombigen, HIV-1 Latex Agglutination test, HIVAB HIV-1 EIA, others	Kits
Meningitis	Bactigen N Meningitidis	Slide tests
Mononucleosis	Mono-Diff, Mono-Latex, others	Kits
Occult blood screening	ColoCare, Colo-Screen, others	Kits
Ovulation tests	Answer Ovulation, Clearplan Easy, Ovu-Quick Self-Test, others	Kits
Human chorionic gonadotropin pregnancy tests	Advance, Answer Plus, Answer Quick & Simple, Fact Plus, others	Kits
Rheumatoid factor	Rheumatex, Rheumaton	Slide tests
Hemoglobin S sickle cell test	Sickledex	Kit
Staphylococcus aureus	Isocult for Staphylococcus	Culture paddles
Streptococci tests	Sure Cell Streptococci, Bactigen Strep B, others	Kits
virus tests, miscellaneous	Human T-Lymphotropic Virus Type, Sure Cell Herpes, Rubazyme for Rubella, others	Kits

SUMMARY

Diagnostic agents are chemical substances used to diagnose or monitor a condition or disease. Just like other drugs, they may also have side effects and adverse reactions. Radiopaque agents are used for visualizing organ structure. Examinations used for evaluating organ function involve radioactive agents, computed tomography, ultrasonography, and nuclear magnetic resonance imaging. Nonradioactive agents may be used for evaluating organ function via volumes and flows and challenging glandular response. Other agents are available for screening and monitoring the immune status and disorders. It is essential then that the healthcare professional knows the agent used, mechanism of action, and indications and how to prevent or minimize any adverse effects.

REVIEW QUESTIONS

1. Name and describe the risks associated with the use of radiopaque agents. Which test has the highest number of reactions reported?
2. Describe the action and potential adverse effects associated with the use of ionizing radiation.
3. What is a curie? What factors are used to describe the predicted dose of a radionuclide in patient care?
4. What is the difference between alpha, beta, and gamma radiation?

REFERENCES

American Hospital Formulary Service: *AHFS drug information '98,* Bethesda, Md, 1998, American Society of Hospital Pharmacists.

Farwell AP, Braverman LE: Thyroid and antithyroid drugs. In Hardman JG, Limbird LE, editors: *Goodman & Gilman's the pharmacological basis of therapeutics,* ed 9, New York, 1996, McGraw-Hill.

Olin BR: *Facts and comparisons.* Philadelphia, 1998, JB Lippincott.

United States Pharmacopeial Convention: *USP DI: drug information for the health care professional,* ed 18, Rockville, Md, 1998, The Convention.

ADDITIONAL REFERENCES

Anderson KN et al, editors: *Mosby's medical, nursing, and allied health dictionary,* ed 5, St Louis, 1998, Mosby.

DiPiro JT, Talber R et al, editors: *Pharmacotherapy, a pathophysiologic approach,* ed 2, Norwalk, Conn, 1993, Appleton & Lange.

Early PJ, Sodee DB: *Principles and practice of nuclear medicine,* ed 2, St Louis, 1991, Mosby.

Haaga JR, Alfidi RJ: *Computed tomography of the whole body,* ed 2, St Louis,1988, Mosby.

Jankowski CB: Radiation protection for nurses: regulations and guidelines, *J Nurs Admin* 17(2):30-34, 1992.

Mosby: *Mosby's GenRx,* St Louis, 1998, Mosby.

Pagana KD, Pagana TJ: *Mosby's diagnostic and laboratory test reference,* ed 3, St Louis, 1997, Mosby.

Singer CM et al: Exposure of emergency medicine personnel to ionizing radiation during cervical spine radiography, *Ann Emerg Med* 18(8):822, 1989.

Watson J, Jaffee MS: *Nurse's manual of laboratory and diagnostic tests,* ed 2, Philadelphia, 1995, FA Davis.

CHAPTER 65

Poisons and Antidotes

CHAPTER FOCUS

Accidental poisoning or intentional (or unintentional) drug overdose may result in a toxic or life-threatening situation. Assessing the situation and instituting the appropriate interventions is a requirement for healthcare professionals working in emergency departments and poison control centers. This chapter reviews the techniques of assessment, removal of the poison, and antidotes available for use in specific overdose situations.

OBJECTIVES

After reading and studying this chapter, the student should be able to do the following:

1. *Define and describe the key terms.*
2. *Name five clues or assessment techniques to determine a potential drug/chemical toxicity.*
3. *Describe the four grades of coma that are caused by a drug overdose.*
4. *Name at least six frequently ingested items that are considered to be nontoxic in small amounts.*
5. *List two drugs from each of the categories of drugs or chemicals that cause ataxia, coma, seizures, paralysis, constricted pupils, dilated pupils, and red flush.*

KEY TERMS

acute poisoning, (p. 818)
chronic poisoning, (p. 818)
gastric lavage, (p. 823)
poison, (p. 818)
toxicology, (p. 818)
toxidromes, (p. 819)

Regional poison control centers reported 1.8 million calls concerning drug or chemical exposures in the United States during 1991. Approximately 25% of this number required professional treatment, with 764 deaths reported (Watson, 1996). Although the incidence of poisoning in children is high, the mortality rate in this population is usually low. The majority of ingestions in children are accidental, whereas most adult drug overdoses are intentional, the result of a suicide attempt or drug abuse. Drug overdoses are reviewed in Chapter 6.

An unusual type of poisoning has resulted from the proliferation of battery-operated games, cameras, hearing aids, calculators, and watches. An estimated 500 to 600 miniature button or disk batteries are swallowed each year by persons of all ages. Their major component is aqueous potassium hydroxide, which also is used to unclog pipes. Children can mistake small batteries for candy; adults may mistake them for medication tablets. Batteries that lodge in the esophagus, cecum, or other areas of the gastrointestinal tract present two problems: (1) they are locally corrosive to mucosa, causing ulceration or perforation in 1 to 2 hours; and (2) they may cause mercury poisoning when certain battery contents leak. Endoscopic or surgical removal is necessary if the battery remains in the stomach for more than 24 hours, if gastric or peritoneal irritation develops, if radiologic evidence shows the battery lodging or leaking in the gastrointestinal tract, or if the particular type of battery is prone to leakage.

DETECTION OF POISONS

Toxicology is the study of poisons—their action and effects and methods of detection—and the diagnosis and treatment of poisoning. A **poison** can be defined as any substance that in relatively small amounts can cause death or serious bodily harm. All drugs are potential poisons when used improperly or in excess dosage. Poisoning may be acute or chronic. In **acute poisoning** the effects are immediate, whereas in **chronic poisoning** the effects are insidious because of cumulative effects of small amounts of poison absorbed over a prolonged period. Chronic poisoning causes chronic illness, which may or may not be reversible.

Cues that typically point to poisoning include sudden, violent symptoms of severe nausea, vomiting, diarrhea, collapse, or convulsions. If possible, it is important to find out what poison has been taken and how much. Additional information that might prove helpful to the physician in making a diagnosis includes answers to questions or reports of observed phenomena such as the following:

- Any reports of poison contact by the victim
- Poisoning in the "at-risk" age group of children 1 to 5 years of age
- Report of a history of previous poisonings or ingestion of foreign substances
- Diverse symptoms or signs referable to multiple organ system involvement that defy diagnosis
- A history of suicidal intent or thought
- Symptoms appearing suddenly in an otherwise healthy individual or a number of persons becoming ill about the same time, as might occur in food poisoning
- Anything unusual about the person, the clothing, or the surroundings; evidence of burns about the lips and mouth; discolored gums; needle (hypodermic) pricks, pustules, or scars on the exposed and accessible surface of the body or dilated or constricted pupils, as may be seen in drug addicts; any skin rash or discoloration
- The odor of the breath, the rate of respiration, any difficulty in respiration, and cyanosis
- The quality and rate of the pulse
- Appearance and odor of vomitus, if any, as well as accompanying diarrhea or abdominal pain
- Any abnormalities of stool and urine, any change in color or the presence of blood
- For signs of involvement of the nervous system, the presence of excitement, muscular twitching, delirium, difficulty in speech, stupor, coma, constriction or dilation of the pupils, and elevated or subnormal temperature

Coma caused by drug overdose is characterized by the following categories:

- *Grade I.* The individual is asleep but easily aroused, reacts to painful stimuli; deep tendon reflexes are present, pupils are normal and reactive, ocular movements are present, and vital signs are stable.
- *Grade II.* The pain response is absent, deep tendon reflexes are depressed, pupils are slightly dilated but reactive, and vital signs are stable.
- *Grade III.* Deep tendon and pupillary reflexes are absent and vital signs are stable.
- *Grade IV.* Respiration and circulation are depressed.

The healthcare professional should refrigerate in a covered container all specimens of vomitus, urine, or stool for examination and possible submission to the proper authority for analysis. This is of particular importance not only in making or confirming a diagnosis, but also in the event that the case has medicolegal significance.

Any of the signs listed earlier should be noted carefully for report to the poison control center or physician in charge. However, full reliance on signs and symptoms for clear-cut diagnosis and poison identification is fraught with danger. This is because these incidents may occur concurrently with an episode of acute disease, especially in children (e.g., aspirin intoxication), and symptoms may be similar or otherwise confusing. Also, more than one substance may be responsible for the signs of poisoning observed.

Not all substances commonly ingested accidentally are toxic if small amounts are taken only once. Poison control centers define a small amount as the quantity of a substance contained in "a taste," "one bite," or "a small piece," as opposed to "a mouthful." Although subjective, this is typical of data received when taking a poisoning history. A list of some frequently ingested products that are usually systematically nontoxic if taken in small amounts follows:

- Abrasives, bleaches (sodium hypochlorite, less than 5%)
- Chalk

BOX 65-1 Toxidromes*

atropine, scopolamine, anticholinergics: dry skin, tachycardia, beet-red skin color, agitation, dilated pupils, delirium, hyperthermia, hallucinations, coma

barbiturates, sedative-hypnotics, tranquilizers: ataxia, drowsiness, slurred speech (without an alcohol breath odor), respiratory depression, hypotension

cholinergics (such as organophosphates), **mushrooms** (*Amanita* or *Galerina*): salivation, lacrimation, involuntary urination and defecation, miosis, pulmonary congestion, seizures

opiods: miosis, respiratory depression, hypotension, slow respiratory, coma

salicylates: fever, vomiting hyperglycemia, mixed respiratory alkalosis and metabolic acidosis, hyperpnea

tricyclic antidepressants: anticholinergic signs and symptoms, plus dysrhythmias (prolonged QRS duration on electrocardiogram [ECG] report), convulsions, coma

*The drugs or drug types in bold are followed by clusters of signs of poisonings.

- Cigarettes, cigarette ash, cigars
- Cosmetics, perfume, cologne, deodorants
- Crayons (if labeled C.P., A.P., or C.S., 2 130-46)
- Glues, rubber cement
- Hydrogen peroxide (medicinal, 3%)
- Indelible pen or magic markers
- Ink in full cartridge of a ballpoint pen
- Paint (latex)
- Pencil (graphite or coloring)
- Saccharin and cyclamates
- Safety matches (ingestion of less than 20 books of matches)
- Soaps, liquid shampoos, household detergents (except dishwasher detergents)
- Toothpaste (unless heavy ingestion of fluorides)
- Vitamins (in amounts usually available for a single overdose, unless containing iron)

Ingestion of small amounts of these nonedible substances may produce mild gastric irritation but not systemic poisoning. However, contact with a poison control center or physician is important (essential, if symptoms exist), as no product or drug is entirely safe for ingestion and hypersensitivity reactions can occur.

In assisting with poisoning diagnosis and toxic substance identification, healthcare professionals, especially those working in emergency rooms, should familiarize themselves with certain clusters of signs associated with common drug poisonings or overdoses. These have been called **toxidromes** and are listed in the Box 65-1. Other common single signs and their associated causative toxins are listed in Table 65-1.

POISON CONTROL CENTERS

There are approximately 600 poison control centers in the United States; the majority are located near hospitals or in emergency rooms of large community hospitals. Their telephone numbers are listed in the local telephone book or may be obtained from a pharmacist. *Mosby's GenRx* and the *Physician's Desk Reference* (PDR) include a list of certified poison control centers that are open 24 hours/day and are staffed to answer specific questions from the public or from professionals about identification of ingredients in trade-named products, estimate their toxicity, and suggest specific treatment for poisonings.

CLASSIFICATION OF ACTION OF POISONS

The classification of poisons is as broad as the classification of drugs, since any drug is a potential poison when used in excess. Poisons may be classified in various ways such as: grouped according to chemical classifications as organic and inorganic poisons; as alkaloids, glycosides, and resins; or as acids, alkalis, heavy metals, oxidizing agents, halogenated hydrocarbons, and so on. Poisons also may be classified according to the organ or tissue of the body in which the most damaging effects are produced. Some poisons injure all cells they contact; they are sometimes called protoplasmic poisons or cytotoxins. Others have more effect on the kidney (nephrotoxins), the liver (hepatotoxins), or the blood-forming organs.

Poisons that affect the nervous system chiefly are called neurotoxin poisons. They must be studied separately because different symptoms characterize each one. Symptoms of toxicity are mentioned with each of these drugs in previous chapters. Although symptoms of this group of poisons are to some extent specific, certain symptoms are encountered repeatedly and are associated with many poisons. Drowsiness, dizziness, headache, delirium, coma, and convulsive seizures always indicate central nervous system (CNS) involvement. On the other hand, dry mouth, dilated pupils, and difficulty swallowing are associated with overdosage of atropine or one of the atropine-like drugs; ringing in the ears, excessive perspiration, and gastric upset may be associated with salicylate overdosage.

Many times the precise mechanism of action is not known; death may be caused by respiratory failure, but exactly what happens to cause depression of the respiratory center may not be known. The human body depends on a constant supply of oxygen if various physiologic functions are to proceed satisfactorily. Anything that interferes with the use of oxygen by the cells or with the transportation of

TABLE 65-1 Single Signs that Suggest Presence of Certain Toxins

Sign	*Inference*
Abdominal colic	Black widow spider bite Heavy metals Withdrawal from narcotic depressant
Ataxia	Alcohol Barbiturates Bromides Carbon monoxide Hallucinogens Heavy metals Organic solvents Phenytoin (Dilantin) Tranquilizers
Coma and drowsiness	Alcohol (ethyl) Antihistamines Barbiturates, other hypnotics Carbon monoxide Opiates Salicylates Tranquilizers
Convulsions or muscle twitching	Alcohol Amphetamines Antihistamines Boric acid Camphor Chlorinated hydrocarbon insecticides (DDT) Cyanide Lead Organophosphate insecticides Plants (azalea, iris, lily-of-the-valley, water hemlock) Salicylates Strychnine
Convulsions or muscle twitching—cont'd	Withdrawal from drugs: barbiturates, benzodiazepines (Valium, Librium), meprobamate
Paralysis	Botulism Heavy metals Plants (poison hemlock, etc.) Triorthocresyl phosphate (plasticizer)
Oliguria/anuria	Carbon tetrachloride Ethylene glycol (antifreeze) Heavy metals Hemolysis caused by naphthalene, plants, and so on Methanol Mushrooms Oxylates Petroleum distillates Solvents
Oral signs	
Breath odors	
Acetone	Acetone Alcohol (methyl or isopropyl) Phenol Salicylates
Alcohol	Ethyl alcohol
Bitter almonds	Cyanide
Coal gas	Carbon monoxide
Garlic	Arsenic Dimethyl sulfoxide (DMSO) Phosphorus Organophosphate insecticides Thallium

oxygen will produce damaging effects faster in some cells than in others. Carbon monoxide from automobile engines and unvented gas heaters is one of the most widely distributed toxic agents. It poisons by producing hypoxia and finally asphyxia. Carbon monoxide has a great affinity for hemoglobin and forms carboxyhemoglobin. Thus the production of oxyhemoglobin and the free transport of oxygen is interfered with; oxygen deficiency soon develops in the cells. Unless exposure to the carbon monoxide is terminated before 40% of hemoglobin has been changed to carboxyhemoglobin, anoxia may produce serious brain damage. Death occurs when 60% of the hemoglobin has been changed to carboxyhemoglobin.

The cyanides act somewhat similarly in that they bring about cellular anoxia, but they do so differently. They inactivate certain tissue enzymes so that cells are unable to use oxygen. Death may occur very rapidly. Curare and the curariform drugs in toxic amounts bring about paralysis of the diaphragm, and again the victim dies from lack of oxygen.

Certain drugs have a direct effect on muscle tissue from the body, such as that of the myocardium, or the smooth muscle of the blood vessels. Death results from the failure of circulation or cardiac arrest. The nitrites, potassium salts, and digitalis drugs may exert such toxic effects. Strong acids and alkalis denature and destroy cellular proteins. Examples of corrosive acids are hydrochloric, nitric, and sulfuric acids. Sodium, potassium, and ammonium hydroxides are examples of strong and caustic alkalis. Locally, these substances cause destruction of tissue, and death may result from hemorrhage, perforation, or shock. Corrosive poisons may also cause death by altering the pH of the blood or other body fluids, or they may produce marked degenerative changes on vital organs such as the liver or kidney.

TABLE 65-1 Single Signs that Suggest Presence of Certain Toxins—cont'd

Sign	*Inference*
Salivation	Arsenic Corrosive substances Mercury Mushrooms Organophosphate insecticides Thallium
Pupillary changes	
Dilated	Amphetamines Antihistamines Atropine Barbiturates (when combined with coma) Cocaine Ephedrine Lysergic acid diethylamide (LSD) (occasionally) Methanol Withdrawal from narcotic depressants (occasionally)
Constricted, pinpoint pupils	Mushrooms (Muscarinic) opiates Organophosphate insecticides
Nystagmus on lateral gaze	Barbiturates Minor tranquilizers (meprobamate, benzodiazepines), phenytoin (Dilantin)
Respiratory alterations	
Increased	Amphetamines Barbiturates (early sign) Carbon monoxide Methanol Petroleum distillates Salicylates
Paralysis	Botulism Organophosphate insecticides
Slowed or depressed	Alcohol (late sign) Barbiturates (late sign) Opiates Tranquilizers
Wheezing/pulmonary edema	Mushrooms (muscarinic) Opiates Organophosphate insecticides Petroleum distillates
Skin color changes	
Jaundice	Aniline dyes/coal tar colors Arsenic Carbon tetrachloride Castor bean Fava bean Mushroom Naphthalene (moth repellent/insecticide) Yellow phosphorus
Red flush	Alcohol Antihistamines Atropine Boric acid Carbon monoxide Nitrites Tricyclic antidepressants
Cyanosis	Aniline dyes Carbon monoxide Cyanide Nitrites Strychnine
Violent emesis (with or without hematemesis)	Aminophylline Bacterial food poisoning Boric acid Corrosives Fluoride Heavy metals Phenol Salicylates

SPECIFIC POISONS, SYMPTOMS, AND SUGGESTED EMERGENCY TREATMENT

Since the emphasis is on prompt treatment, healthcare may be best served by quick action by informed bystanders at the scene who apply first-aid measures while help is sought from the poison control center and while transportation to a hospital or other healthcare setting is arranged. A first-aid chart that offers instruction for various poisoning emergencies is included in Box 65-2.

The caller to the poison control center should have the following information, if available:

1. Physical appearance of the substance
2. Odor, color, and texture; distinguishing characteristics of the substance
3. Trade name or chemical name, if known
4. Purpose or how the substance was meant to be used
5. Label statements relating to "poison" content or flammability

After the events of the suspected poisoning have been assessed, prompt medical interventions must be instituted. Medical management will therefore be guided by the four major goals.

1. Vital functions (respirations, circulation, and others) will be maintained, supported, or restored.
2. The toxic substance will be removed or eliminated from the system as soon as possible.
3. The action of certain specific poisons may be counteracted, reversed, or antagonized by specific antidotes.
4. Recurrences will be reduced or prevented.

SUPPORT OF VITAL FUNCTIONS

Basic to the treatment of poisoning is intensive supportive therapy, good nursing care, and minimal dangerous invasive

BOX 65-2 First Aid for Possible Poisoning

Remember: any nonfood substance may be poisonous.

1. Keep all potential poisons—household products and medicines—out of children's reach.
2. Use "safety caps" (child-resistant containers) to avoid accidents.
3. Have 1 oz of ipecac syrup in your home and in your first-aid kit for camping, travel, and so on.
4. Keep your poison center's and your physician's phone number handy.

If you think an accidental ingestion has occurred:

1. Keep calm. Do not wait for symptoms—call for help promptly.
2. Find out if the substance is toxic; your poison control center or your physician can tell you if a risk exists and what you should do.
3. Have the product's container or label with you at the phone.
   a. If a poison is on the skin:
      Immediately remove affected clothing.
      Flood involved parts of body with water, wash with soap or detergent, and rinse thoroughly.
   b. If a poison is in the eye:
      Immediately flush the eye with water for up to 20 minutes.
   c. If a poison is inhaled:
      Immediately get the victim to fresh air. Give mouth-to-mouth resuscitation if necessary.
   d. If vomiting has been recommended:
      Give appropriate dose of ipecac syrup as instructed, followed by at least one glass (8 oz) of clear liquid. If the patient does not vomit within 15 to 20 minutes, give 1 more tablespoon of ipecac and more water. Do *not* use salt water.

Never induce vomiting if:

1. The victim is in a *coma* (unconscious).
2. The victim is *convulsing* (having a seizure).
3. The victim has swallowed a caustic or corrosive (e.g., lye).

For reemphasis:

1. Always call to be certain of possible toxicity before undertaking treatment.
2. Never induce vomiting until you are instructed to do so.
3. Do not rely on the label's antidote information, since it may be out of date. Call instead.
4. If you have to go to an emergency room, take the tablets, capsules, container, and/or label with you.
5. Do not hesitate to call your poison center or your physician a second time if the victim seems to be getting worse.

From Covington, 1996; Schauben, Spillane, 1990.

interventions. The medical care of the poisoned patient should focus on restoration, support, and maintenance of such vital functions as ventilation, circulation, and acid-base and fluid-electrolyte balance. Emotional support for the individual and others involved in this crisis is crucial.

A general assessment and history should be performed quickly and competently to determine the extent of any impairments of body systems or particular susceptibilities. Expert medical and/or nursing care is essential to observe the following for information indicating impending complications: (1) level of consciousness and (2) vital signs. Temperature may be elevated with certain CNS stimulants and salicylates and depressed with others. Transient cardiac dysrhythmias may occur; anticipate obtaining an electrocardiogram. Pulmonary congestion, airway obstruction, or apnea is common; aspiration of vomitus can occur.

Implemented plans may include: (1) turning, deep breathing, coughing, and suctioning; and (2) auscultation to demonstrate a need for chest x-ray examination, suctioning, tracheostomy, endotracheal intubation, blood gas determinations, supplemental oxygen, and a respirator/ventilator.

It is also essential that the victim be positioned to prevent aspiration of vomitus and that mouth care be attended to promptly after emesis. Moderate amounts of plain water by mouth (if a gag or swallow reflex is present) may be all that is needed to dilute or effectively inactivate many ingested poisons. Close attention to developing problems and responsive intervention can often fend off the need for more aggressive medical therapies that tax the already tenuous condition of the poisoned individual.

REMOVAL OR ELIMINATION OF POISON

Careful evaluation of the individual who has been affected by a toxic substance is essential to determine which of the foregoing steps take priority and by which route the poison should be removed or eliminated, if necessary. The route is largely determined by the manner of the poisoning. Removal of ingested substances can be attempted in several ways: (1) by directly removing it from the stomach, if the poisoning is discovered early; (2) by increasing the rate of transit of the poison through the colon, even though little or no absorption occurs there and thus may not be effective; or (3) if the substance has probably already been assimilated into the system or was injected, by attempting to remove or filter it from the bloodstream. Contact poisons may be flushed from the skin, eyes, and other external areas by copious volumes of plain, flowing water from a pitcher or other container. Inhaled toxins are treated by removing the patient to fresh air and administering artificial respiration or oxygen and other supportive measures as necessary.

Various methods exist for the removal or elimination of

poisons from the gastrointestinal tract or systemic circulation: emesis, gastric lavage, cathartics, diuretics, dialysis, or occasionally blood exchange transfusions or hemoperfusion through charcoal or exchange resins.

Emesis

Generally, if more than 4 hours have elapsed since a poison ingestion, emptying the stomach will be ineffective. Exceptions are poisonings by anticholinergic drugs, which slow gastric motility, and by salicylates, which promote pyloric spasm. Some drugs, such as ethanol, are absorbed too rapidly to be recovered after 1 hour. However, when situations have warranted emptying the stomach, whole tablets have occasionally been recovered even a day later. Because of this, some recommend emptying the stomach even after a delay.

The most effective method for removing ingested toxins is usually the most natural one: emesis, done as soon as possible. In some instances, however, emesis is contraindicated (Box 65-3). If vomiting does not or cannot occur naturally, ipecac syrup is usually administered. Apomorphine is no longer recommended for emesis because ipecac syrup is safer and a more convenient product to use (USP DI, 1998). However, neither emetic may be effective if the ingested substance is a sedative-hypnotic, a phenothiazine, or a tricyclic antidepressant, all of which have antiemetic properties.

ipecac syrup [ip' e kak]

The most commonly used emetic is ipecac syrup, which acts both centrally and locally by stimulating the vomiting center and by irritating the gastric mucosa. The usual dose for adults is 15 to 30 ml, followed immediately by 240 ml of water. Four to 8 oz of water are given with the following dosages: children 6 months to 1 year of age, a 5- to 10-ml dose (under special circumstances only); children 1 to 12 years of age, a 15-ml dose. Vomiting usually occurs in 15 to 30 minutes. The dose may be repeated once after 20 minutes if the first dose is not effective.

If vomiting does not occur within 30 minutes, gastric lavage should be performed. Ipecac is cardiotoxic if absorbed and may cause conduction disturbances, atrial fibrillation, or myocarditis. Ipecac syrup is available without a prescription in 1-oz (30-ml) bottles bearing the following instructions:

1. For emergency use to cause vomiting in poisoning. Before using, call physician, poison control center, or hospital emergency room immediately for advice.
2. Warning—Keep out of reach of children. Do not use if strychnine, corrosives such as alkalis (lye) and strong acids, or petroleum distillates such as kerosene, gasoline, fuel oil, coal oil, paint thinner, or cleaning fluid have been ingested.

Gastric Lavage

If the person is conscious, drug-induced vomiting is usually preferable to gastric lavage, particularly in children, since aspiration of vomitus is less likely to occur. Occasionally, induction of vomiting may be facilitated by stimulating the pharynx, but time should not be wasted in repeated futile attempts.

BOX 65-3 Contraindications for Induced Emesis in Poisonings

Infants up to 1 year of age
Comatose or convulsing patient
Absent gag and cough reflexes
Ingestion of
- Convulsion-inducing substances
- Sharp objects (e.g., glass, nails) along with toxic substance
- CNS poisons (e.g., camphor, strychnine), which must be removed more quickly by lavage

Acids, alkalis, or petroleum distillates, such as kerosene, gasoline, or paint thinner, etc.
Presence of hematemesis

From Schauben, Spillane, 1990; Wuest, Gossel, 1992.

If emesis cannot be induced, gastric lavage should be begun except under most of the same contraindicating conditions (e.g., untreated convulsions, absent reflexes, or ingestion of corrosives). **Gastric lavage** is the washing out of the stomach with sterile water or a saline solution. Lavage may be preferred treatment for pregnant women and for individuals who have ingested more than 2 ml/kg of body weight of a petroleum distillate and who should have endotracheal intubation to protect the airway. Lavage may be contraindicated in the presence of cardiac dysrhythmias.

An Ewald orogastric tube, no. 16 to 30 French, may be used for lavage in children; tube sizes for adult lavage range from no. 34 to 42. The newer, clear-plastic Levacuator tube also may be used. A standard nasogastric tube is too narrow for extraction of particulate matter such as intact tablets (Fig. 65-1). Stomach contents should be aspirated first and saved for toxicologic analysis if necessary.

Several liters of half-strength saline solution may be used in increments of 50 to 100 ml for children and 150 to 200 ml for adults during repeated lavages until return flows are clear. (Remember that dead space in the tube itself accounts for 20 to 25 ml of the fluid instilled.) Neither emesis nor lavage is guaranteed to empty the stomach completely.

Activated Charcoal

After emesis or lavage, activated charcoal prepared as a aqueous slurry may be administered to act as an absorbent. Activated charcoal should be given as soon after poison ingestion as feasible, but not after ipecac and emesis, since it will adsorb the ipecac. Activated charcoal adsorbs many substances, thus it is used as an adjunct in the treatment of oral poisonings with heavy metals, mercuric chloride, strychnine, phenol, atropine, phenolphthalein, oxalic acid,

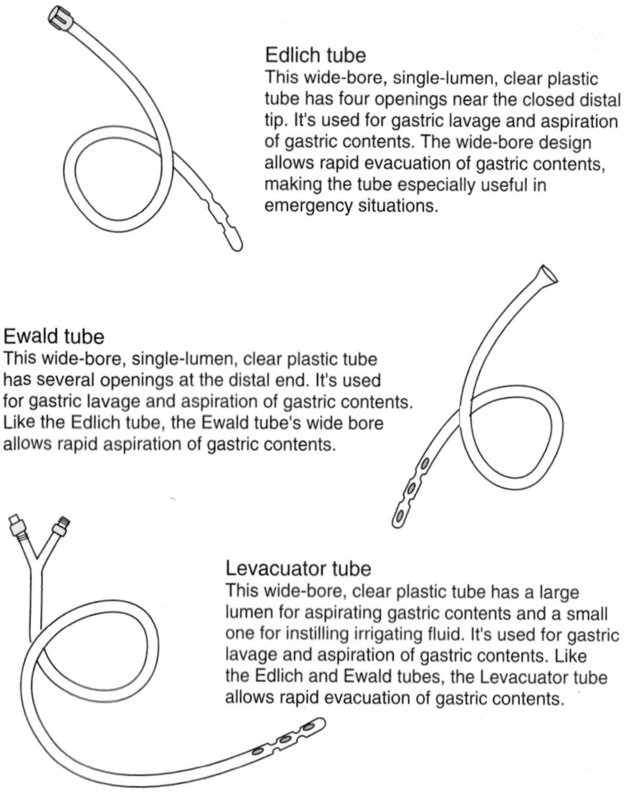
Edlich tube
This wide-bore, single-lumen, clear plastic tube has four openings near the closed distal tip. It's used for gastric lavage and aspiration of gastric contents. The wide-bore design allows rapid evacuation of gastric contents, making the tube especially useful in emergency situations.
Ewald tube
This wide-bore, single-lumen, clear plastic tube has several openings at the distal end. It's used for gastric lavage and aspiration of gastric contents. Like the Edlich tube, the Ewald tube's wide bore allows rapid aspiration of gastric contents.
Levacuator tube
This wide-bore, clear plastic tube has a large lumen for aspirating gastric contents and a small one for instilling irrigating fluid. It's used for gastric lavage and aspiration of gastric contents. Like the Edlich and Ewald tubes, the Levacuator tube allows rapid evacuation of gastric contents.

FIGURE 65-1
Various tubes used for lavage techniques.

poisonous mushrooms, aspirin, and most drugs. It is not effective for poisoning with ethanol, methanol, caustic alkalis, ferrous sulfate, boric acid, gas, kerosene, lithium, and mineral acids. The charcoal mixture need not be removed from the stomach afterward because no known adverse effects exist. Activated charcoal can also serve as a stool marker to indicate when further gastrointestinal absorption of the ingested poison has ended. Tablets or capsules of charcoal should not be used for treatment of poisoning, since they are less effective than the powder.

Other Treatments

Other ways used to block or eliminate toxins from the system include forced diuresis, cathartics and enemas, dialysis, hemoperfusion, and exchange transfusions. These methods should be reserved as treatment under certain conditions and for specific poisons because they are not universally effective and are much less commonly used than emesis or lavage.

Changing the pH of the urine by alkalinization (sodium bicarbonate) may enhance excretion of certain drugs such as salicylates and, possibly, tricyclic antidepressants. Forced acid diuresis is probably more potentially hazardous but is often recommended for poisoning with amphetamines and fenfluramine (Pondimin).

Clearance of poisons directly from the bloodstream by peritoneal dialysis or hemodialysis, hemoperfusion, or transfusion is occasionally done to augment other measures previously discussed. Peritoneal dialysis is less effective than hemodialysis or hemoperfusion. The degree to which they may be useful depends in part on the properties of the substance (i.e., whether it freely circulates or whether it is bound to plasma proteins or to tissues). Various lists of substances amenable to dialysis exist; some substances for which hemodialysis has not proved useful are as follows (USP DI, 1998; Aweeka, 1996): cefixime (Suprax), clindamycin (Cleocin), diazepam (Valium), cyclosporine, digoxin (Lanoxin), phenytoin (Dilantin), propranolol (Inderal), and zidovudine (Retrovir).

PREVENTION OF POISONING

Various creative graphic symbols appear on labels of poisonous substances to alert the adult and nonreading child to the potential hazard contained therein. "Mr Yuk," an ugly, green-faced, scowling image, is one of these. Tricky-to-open caps appear to delay if not totally prevent children's indiscriminate use of medicines. Others who have no need for these caps can request medication in the familiar easy-to-open caps.

Prevention has always been emphasized by healthcare professionals. Combined efforts with drug information centers and creative approaches have already had an impact on the frequency of certain categories of drug poisoning, notably aspirin poisoning.

There is much to learn about toxins in our environment, both apparent and potential, and therefore much to do in the way of poison prevention, but concerted, thoughtful efforts have already had a positive effect on statistics.

ANTIDOTES

The number of antidotes for specific toxins is minimal; no widely accepted "universal antidote" exists. Nevertheless, some general statements can be made about antidotes. Antidotes are more effective after the stomach is empty. The correct dose to reverse toxicity depends on the specific drug involved, its half-life, and the severity of toxicity shown. Antidotes work by any of the following mechanisms: (1) antagonizing or stimulating receptor sites that have been rendered hyperfunctional or dysfunctional by the poison; (2) interfering with enzyme inhibition; (3) administering the product of metabolism that has been interfered with; (4) inhibiting the biotransformation of a substance to a poisonous metabolite; (5) giving an agent that inactivates the toxic product; (6) chelation (forming highly stable complexes, tying up the substance—usually a heavy metal such as iron); and (7) producing immunotherapy—the use of antidrug antibodies to bind and inactivate drugs (e.g., there is a report of severe digoxin poisoning reversed with sheep digoxin-specific antibodies).

COMMON POISONS

Alcohols (ethanol, isopropyl, and methyl) are reviewed in Chapter 6 and acetaminophen is covered in Chapters 3 and

8. Carbon monoxide, iron, and organophosphate insecticides are reviewed here.

Carbon Monoxide

Carbon monoxide (CO) is an odorless gas produced by the incomplete combustion of carbon or carbonaceous materials. Sources of the gas include improperly maintained heating systems, improperly ventilated charcoal cookers or fireplaces, and industrial furnaces such as those in steel mills. Automobile exhaust contains 3% to 7% CO. No other poison causes as many deaths in the United States and Canada as does CO. Inhalation of automobile exhaust is a common method of suicide, while accidental home and industrial exposure to CO is much more common than generally appreciated.

Poisoning by CO results from pulmonary absorption of the gas, which readily combines with hemoglobin to form carboxyhemoglobin. The oxygen in hemoglobin is replaced, thus lowering available oxygen carried by the blood to the body tissues. With the addition of each CO molecule the oxygen molecules remaining on the hemoglobin become so tightly bound that they are not readily released to the oxygen-starved tissues. CO is measured in blood as the percent carboxyhemoglobin (% HbCO). Additionally, CO gas dissolved in blood but not bound to hemoglobin diffuses into the body tissues and poisons cytochrome enzymes necessary for cellular usage of oxygen.

The symptoms of CO poisoning are generally related to % HbCO. Clinically, only mild if any symptoms occur at 10% HbCO and cigarette smokers may have CO up to this level. The initial signs of poisoning usually occur at 10% to 30% HbCO; these signs include throbbing headache, nausea, vomiting, dizziness, weakness, and visual disturbances. These early symptoms of intoxication are nonspecific and may be attributed to a number of other causes unless a history of CO is available or laboratory tests demonstrate elevated % HbCO. At 40% to 50% HbCO, syncope, tachycardia, tightness in the chest, and tachypnea occur. HbCO has a cherry pink color rather than the red color of oxyhemoglobin; therefore the patient may have a cherry pink coloration of the skin. Percent HbCO in excess of 50% causes life-threatening convulsions, coma, dangerously compromised cardiopulmonary function, and possible death. Those who die from suicide or victims of fires often have % HbCO of 60% to 80%.

Treatment for CO poisoning is based on the patient's symptoms and % HbCO. Hyperbaric oxygen is the antidote of choice because oxygen under pressure is capable of replacing CO from hemoglobin and the iron-containing respiratory cytochrome enzymes in the tissues.

Ninety-five percent of absorbed CO is excreted by the lungs; however, once removed from the source of exposure, the half-life of CO in normal ambient air is 4 hours. If 100% oxygen is administered, the half-life ($t^{1/2}$) decreases to 40 minutes. Hyperbaric oxygen at 3 atm decreases the $t^{1/2}$ of CO to only 23 minutes. In severe poisoning, cardiopulmonary support is maintained throughout therapy. Additional drug therapy to control dysrhythmias, cerebral edema, and convulsions may be indicated.

Iron

Iron supplements are a leading cause of pediatric poisoning deaths in the United States; since 1986, over 110,000 accidental ingestions of iron preparations were reported that resulted in 33 deaths (FDA Consumer Update, 1994). Iron overdoses have also been noted to result in profound mental retardation; thus such products should be dispensed in child-resistant containers and stored in an area that is not readily accessible to small children.

Iron deficiency is a primary cause of anemia in both infants and adults. Thus iron is often added to infant formulas and foods and is available in more than 100 commercial products for adults, including multiple and prenatal vitamins. Available products use a number of forms of iron, various salts and chelates. The toxic effects of iron are caused by its elemental form; therefore the relative toxicity of iron salts is related to the percentage of elemental iron. For example, ferrous fumarate (33% iron) is more toxic on a weight basis than ferrous gluconate (12% iron).

On ingestion, large amounts of iron cause local corrosive actions on the gastric and duodenal mucosa and upper gastrointestinal tract. Initial symptoms of iron poisoning include nausea, vomiting, upper abdominal pain, and bloody diarrhea. The corrosive action destroys the normal mucosal barrier to iron absorption, allowing rapid absorption of large amounts of iron into the general circulation. These overdose concentrations of iron exceed the binding capacity of transferrin, the iron-carrying protein of the blood. The excess free iron readily diffuses into various tissues and binds to the sulfhydryl (SH) radicals of numerous enzymes and structural proteins. This binding of iron to compounds necessary for normal cellular function poisons the tissue cells.

Six to 24 hours after ingestion, symptoms of systemic intoxication—cyanosis, pulmonary edema, and possible cardiovascular collapse—start to occur. Within a few days, coagulation defects, hepatic necrosis, and renal failure may develop. As with adults, the initial symptoms of pediatric iron poisoning are characterized by repeated vomiting, abdominal pain, and diarrhea. However, frequently a latent phase occurs when the initial symptoms abate and the child appears well for a 6- to 12-hour period, which is followed by rapid illness and the development of shock. The determination of serum iron will indicate the severity of the intoxication and prevent the possible dangerous misinterpretation of this latency period.

Additionally, serum iron values indicate the necessity for the initiation of antidotal therapy. Serum iron concentrations of 350 μg/dl or less are rarely associated with clinical illness. Concentrations between 350 and 500 μg/dl call for observation of the patient for the development of clinical signs of intoxication. For concentrations >500 μg/dl, deferoxamine (an iron chelating agent) therapy is recommended.

The treatment for iron poisoning includes general supportive measures, and a specific antidote to bind the ingested iron. Emesis may be induced to expel unabsorbed iron tablets in the stomach; in addition, sodium bicarbonate lavage is indicated, since bicarbonate converts ferrous iron to ferrous carbonate, which is poorly absorbed. After lavage, 200 to 300 ml of the bicarbonate solution should be left in the stomach. When indicated by toxic serum iron concentrations (+500 mg/dl), deferoxamine, a chelating agent, should be administered.

Deferoxamine is a specific chelator that binds free serum iron and iron associated with hepatic and splenic stores. Deferoxamine does not bind with zinc, copper, or other trace metals. The deferoxamine-iron complex is nontoxic and freely excreted by the kidneys.

Organophosphate Insecticides

Organophosphate compounds are highly effective insecticides. Their chemical structure is unstable, resulting in their disintegration into nontoxic radicals within days after their application. Therefore they do not persist or accumulate in the environment or animal tissues as do the chlorinated insecticides such as DDT. This accounts for their addition to numerous commercial products from flea collars, bug bombs, and flypapers to most home and commercial insect sprays. This popularity accounts for the high potential for accidental poisoning by organophosphates.

Organophosphate compounds are powerful inhibitors of the enzyme acetylcholinesterase (AChE), which breaks down the neurotransmitter acetylcholine (ACh) (see Chapter 15). Organophosphates are generally rapidly absorbed in the body by all routes, although individual organophosphates display a wide variation in their ability to penetrate the skin, in oral absorption, and thus in their toxicity. For example, malathion does not penetrate the skin well and its oral toxicity is low, making it a popular insecticide for use in home products.

The signs and symptoms of organophosphate insecticide poisoning are related to inhibition of AChE, which results in an accumulation of ACh in the parasympathetic nervous system. Hence, all organs affected by ACh are overstimulated. The expected results of organophosphate poisoning are as follows: bradycardia, hypotension, dyspnea, wheezing, miosis, blurred vision, convulsions, muscular fasciculations, and profuse sweating. A common mnemonic for symptoms of organophosphate intoxication is SLUDGE: salivation, lacrimation, urination, defecation, gastrointestinal distress, and emesis. The usual mode of death is respiratory arrest caused by bronchospasm, decreased pulmonary muscle strength, and finally depression of central nervous system control of respiration. The sequence in which specific symptoms develop is related to the route of exposure. Respiratory tract effects appear first after inhalation, whereas gastrointestinal effects appear initially after ingestion. Skin absorption results in immediate profuse sweating and muscle weakness.

Therapy for organophosphate poisoning involves the support of cardiopulmonary function, clearance of respiratory tract secretions to maintain a clear airway, and the use of appropriate antidotes, atropine, and pralidoxamine (2-PAM, Protopam). Atropine competitively antagonizes the action of ACh at muscarinic receptors on organs innervated by postganglionic parasympathetic nerves and cholinergic sympathetic nerves (Chapter 15).

Atropine is effective in blocking muscarinic symptoms of bradycardia, bronchoconstriction, and excess secretions; however, muscular fasciculations are refractory to this antidote. These involuntary contractions and twitchings and respiratory paralysis are best treated with 2-PAM, a cholinesterase reactivator that removes organophosphates bound to AChE. This then frees AChE to break down the accumulated ACh, thereby resuming normal activity at the neuromuscular junction. 2-PAM also directly detoxifies certain organophosphates. Side effects of 2-PAM include dizziness, nausea, headache, and tachycardia.

SUMMARY

Poisoning, whether accidental or intentional, is a common problem in the United States. The majority of accidental poisonings usually involve children, while intentional drug overdoses are more likely to be secondary to a suicide attempt or an abused drug substance overdose. All poisonings require prompt drug or chemical identification, and appropriate interventions as necessary to save the life of the individual.

REVIEW QUESTIONS

1. What information (5 points) should the healthcare professional have available when they call a poison control center?
2. Name the four major goals for medical management of the person with a suspected poisoning.
3. Discuss the three methods for removal of ingested poisons.
4. What is a toxidrome? Describe two toxidromes.
5. Describe carbon monoxide toxicity, including its cause, symptoms, and treatment.

REFERENCES

Aweeka FT: Dosing of drugs in renal failure. In Young LY, Koda-Kimble MA, editors: *Applied therapeutics: the clinical use of drugs,* ed 6, Vancouver, Wash, 1995, Applied Therapeutics, Inc.

Covington TR, editor: *Handbook of nonprescription drugs,* ed 11, Washington, DC, 1996, American Pharmaceutical Association.

FDA Consumer Update: Preventive measures proposed for childhood iron poisoning, http://vm.cfsan.fda.gov/~dms (October 8, 1998)

Schauben JL, Spillane J: Poisoning: an overview for pharmacists, *Fla Pharm Today* 54(3):6, 1990.

United States Pharmacopeial Convention: *USP DI: drug information for the health care professional,* ed 18, Rockville, Md, 1998, The Convention.

Watson WA: Clinical toxicology. In Young LY, Koda-Kimble MA, editors: *Applied therapeutics: the clinical use of drugs,* ed 6, Vancouver, Wash, 1995, Applied Therapeutics, Inc.

Wuest JR, Gossel TA: A primer for pharmacists on treatment of poisoning, *Fla Pharm Today* 56(3):22, 1992.

ADDITIONAL REFERENCES

Anderson KN et al, editors: *Mosby's medical, nursing, and allied health dictionary,* ed 5, St Louis, 1998, Mosby.

Kwan T et al: Digitalis toxicity caused by toad venom, *Chest* 102(3):949-950, 1992.

Lammon CA, Adams MH: Organophosphate overdose: nursing strategies, *Dimens Crit Care Nurs* 11(6):310-317, 1992.

Melmon KL et al: *Clinical pharmacology,* ed 3, New York, 1992, McGraw-Hill.

Mosby: *Mosby's GenRx,* St Louis, 1998, Mosby.

Oderda GA, Jennings JC: Emetic and antiemetic products. In Covington TR, editor: *Handbook of nonprescription drugs,* ed 11, Washington, DC, 1996, American Pharmaceutical Association.

Olin BR: *Facts and comparisons.* Philadelphia, 1998, JB Lippincott.

Physicians' desk reference, ed 52, Montvale, NJ, 1998, Medical Economics Co.

Public Health Service, US Department of Health and Human Services: Jin bu huan toxicity in children—Colorado, *MMWR* 42(33):633-636, 1993.

Public Health Service, US Department of Health and Human Services: Lead poisoning associated with use of traditional ethnic remedies—California, 1991-1992, *MMWR* 42(27):521-524, 1993.

Wong DL et al: *Whaley and Wong's nursing care of infants and children,* ed 6, St Louis, 1999, Mosby.

Sugar-Free Products*

The following is a selection of sugar-free products by therapeutic categories. Check labels, though, because some of these medications may contain sorbitol, alcohol, or other sources of carbohydrate.

ANTACIDS

Alka-Seltzer Original
Alka-Seltzer, Lemon-Lime
Aluminum Hydroxide Gel
Gasicon Liquid
Gelusil Liquid
Maalox
Maalox HRF
Riopan
Riopan Plus
Titralac
Titralac Plus

ANALGESICS

Acetaminophen Oral solution, USP, Cherry
Arthritis Pain Formula
Aspirin, Delayed-Release
Bayer Aspirin
Bufferin Arthritis Strength
Bufferin Extra Strength
Excedrin Aspirin Free
Feverall Sprinkle Caps
Motrin IB
Nuprin
Panadol
Tempra Tylenol

COUGH, COLD, AND ANTIHISTAMINES

Benadryl Dye-Free
Benylin Adult Cough Formula
Benylin Expectorant Cough Formula
Cheracol Sore Throat
Diabetic Tussin Allergy Relief
Diabetic Tussin DM
Guaifenesin CF
Guaifenesin DM
Naldecon DX, Adult
Naldecon DX, Children's
Naldecon EX, Children's
Naldecon EX, Pediatric
Naldecon Senior DX
Naldecon Senior EX
Robitussin Pediatric Cough
Tussar-SF

FOOD SUPPLEMENTS

Criticare HN
Fibersource
Fibersource HN
Impact
Impact with Fiber
Isocal
MCT Oil
Vivonex T.E.N.

LAXATIVES

Doxidan
Dulcolax
Fiberall, Natural
Haley's M-O
Konsyl
Metamucil Sugar Free
Milk of Magnesia
Surfak

*Check label ingredients because manufacturers may alter or reformulate their products.

APPENDIX B

*Alcohol-Free Products**

ANALGESICS

Acetaminophen Oral Solution USP
Liquiprin, Infants'
Panadol, Children's
Panadol, Infants'
Tempra 1
Tempra 2
Tylenol, Children's Cherry Flavor
Tylenol, Children's Liquid
Tylenol, Infants'

ANTIASTHMATIC PRODUCTS

Alupent Syrup
Dilor G Liquid
Metaprel Syrup
Slo-Phyllin GG Syrup
Theolair Liquid

COUGH, COLD, AND ANTIHISTAMINES

Actifed
Benadryl
Benadryl Decongestant
Benylin Adult Cough Formula
Benylin Expectorant Cough Formula
Chlor-Trimeton Allergy
Demazin
Diabetic Tussin Allergy Relief
Diabetic Tussin DM
Diabetic Tussin EX
Dimetapp
Dimetapp Decongestant, DM
Dimetapp Decongestant, Pediatric
Drixoral Cough Liquid Caps
Guaifenesin DM
Naldecon DX, Adult
Naldecon DX, Children's
Naldecon DX Pediatric
Naldecon EX
Naldecon Senior DX
NyQuil Children's Cold/Cough
PediaCare Cough-Cold
Robitussin
Robitussin Night Relief
Robitussin PE
Sudafed Plus
Sudafed, Children's
Triaminic AM Cough & Decongestant Formula
Triaminic AM Decongestant Formula
Triaminic Expectorant
Tussar-DM
Tylenol Children's Cold Multi-Symptom
Vicks 44d Pediatric
Vicks DayQuil

GARGLE/MOUTHWASHES

Chloraseptic Gly-Oxide Liquid
Orabase-O
Orabase Plain
Oral-B Anti-Cavity Rinse

PSYCHOTROPICS

Haldol Concentrate
Stelazine Concentrate
Thorazine Syrup

*Check label ingredients because manufacturers may alter or reformulate their products.

APPENDIX C

Food-Drug Interactions

Drug Category/ Medication	***Foods to Avoid***	***Rationale***
Antacids		
calcium carbonate (Tums)	Avoid large amounts of dairy products If used as a calcium supplement, avoid concurrent administration of bran and whole grain breads or cereals.	Milk or cream may increase acid secretion. Reduces absorption of calcium
Antibiotics		
erythromycin, penicillins*	Meals, acidic fruit juices, citrus fruits, or acidic beverages, such as cola drinks	The antibiotics are acid labile (reduced absorption). Take medication 1 hour before meals or apart form acidic foods or 2 hours after meals.
tetracyclines	Calcium-containing foods: milk, ice cream, yogurt, cheeses, and others	Calcium may complex with tetracycline, resulting in reduced absorption of the antibiotic. Most tetracyclines, with the exception of doxycycline and minocycline, should be administered 1 hour before or 2 hours after meals.
Anticoagulants		
warfarin (Coumadin), dicumarol, heparin	Beef liver and green leafy vegetables contain vitamin K (spinach, cabbage, brussels sprouts)	Vitamin K can counteract therapeutic action of anticoagulants. A normal, balanced diet will not interfere with this medication. Fad or extreme diets with foods high in vitamin K can affect anticoagulant activity.
Laxative		
mineral oil (Agoral plain, Mineral Oil)	Take 2 hours apart from food. Do not administer at bedtime.	May decrease absorption of vitamins A, D, E, and K. Also reduces absorption of calcium. Aspiration of mineral oil may induce lipid pneumonitis.
MAO Inhibitors		
phenelzine (Nardil), tranylcypromine (Parnate)	Foods with high tyramine content, such as aged cheese (brie, cheddar, processed American, camembert, and others), aged meat, sour cream, yogurt, pickled herring, chicken liver, canned figs, raisins, bananas, avocados, soy sauce, yeast extract, meat tenderizers, alcoholic beverages such as beer and wine (chianti, sherry, or hearty red wines), sausages, chocolate, anchovies	Concurrent use may result in severe headache, nosebleed, chest pain, eyes sensitive to light, or severe hypertension, which may result in a hypertensive crisis.

*Erythromycin base (E-Mycin, Ery-Tab, E-Mycin Eryc) or stearates (Erypar, Erythrocin Stearate, Ethril, Wyamycin S) are best absorbed in the fasting state. Erythromycin ethylsuccinate (E.E.S.), estolate (Ilosone), and enteric-coated erythromycin may be given before or with meals. Penicillin, such as penicillin G, ampicillin, cloxacillin, cyclacillin, dicloxacillin, nafcillin, and oxacillin may have decreased absorption if given with food or acidic-type products.

Drugs That Change Urine or Stool Color

Medications That May Alter Urine Color

Drug	Possible Color Changes
amitriptyline (Elavil)	Blue-green
anticoagulants (coumarin and others	Pink, red, or dark brown (indicative of systemic bleeding)
cascara sagrada	In acid urine, brown; basic urine, yellow to pink; on standing, black
iron salts, dextran, and others	Brown to black
laxatives (danthron, senna)	Pink to red or brown
laxatives (phenolphthalein)	Pink to red
levodopa (Laradopa, Dopar)	May cause dark urine and sweat
methyldopa (Aldomet, Dopamet 🍁)	Pink, amber to dark urine
metronidazole (Flagyl)	Dark urine
nitrofurantoins (Furadantin, Macrodantin)	Yellow to rusty brown urine
phenazopyridine (Pyridium, Phenazo 🍁)	Orange red urine; may stain clothing
phenytoin (Dilantin)	Red-brown or darkening of urine
phenothiazines (chlorpromazine, or Thorazine, and others)	Pink, red, or orange urine
rifampin (Rifadin, Rofact 🍁)	Red, orange, or brown urine, stool, saliva, sweat, and tears

Medications That May Alter Stool Color

Drug	Possible Color Changes
antacids with aluminum salts (Maalox, Mylanta, and others)	White specks or discoloration of stools
anticoagulants (coumarin and others)	Red, orange, to black because of internal bleeding
bismuth or iron salts	Black
laxative (phenolphthalein)	Red
laxative (senna)	Yellow, orange to brown
phenazopyridine (Pyridium and others)	Orange, red

APPENDIX E

Time to Draw Blood for Specific Medications

Serum drug levels are used to aid the prescriber in (1) determining dosage adjustments for drugs with a narrow range between therapeutic effect and toxicity and (2) providing information to evaluate a suspected toxicity or noncompliance.

Blood samples are usually drawn according to the pharmacokinetics of the individual drug. For example, to obtain a steady state serum level, the blood sample should be drawn at approximately 5 drug half-lives after therapy was instituted.

Gentamicin (Garamycin) has a short half-life; therefore peak and trough levels are usually ordered to ensure adequate therapy. The peak serum level (P) is usually obtained 15 to 30 minutes after an intravenous dose or 1 hour after an intramuscular dose. The trough (Tr) serum level should be drawn just before the next scheduled dose. Trough serum levels are used to predict the risk of adverse reactions; a rising trough level or levels above 2 μg/ml have been associated with increased toxicity.

Therapeutic Ranges of Serum Drug Concentrations

	Serum Concentration		
Drug	***Ther (μg/ml)***	***Tr (μg/ml)***	***Time for Blood Sampling (Hours after Last Dose)****
Antibiotics			
amikacin (Amikin)	15-25	5	See previous discussion on gentamicin.
gentamicin (Garamycin)	4-10	2	See previous discussion on gentamicin.
netilmicin (Netromycin)	6-10	2	See previous discussion on gentamicin.
tobramycin (Nebcin)	4-10	2	See previous discussion on gentamicin.
Anticonvulsants			
carbamazepine (Tegretol)	4-12		SS 1-2 wk. Before morning dose (Tr).
phenobarbital	10-40		SS 10-30 days. Before morning dose (Tr).
phenytoin (Dilantin)	10-20		SS 1-4 wk. Oral (Tr), before next dose; IV, 2-4 hr after loading dose.
primidone (Mysoline)	5-12		SS 2-3 days for primidone; phenobarbital as above. Before next dose (Tr).
valproic acid (Depakene, Depakote)	50-100		SS 2-3 days. Before next dose (Tr).
Cardiovascular Drugs			
digoxin (Lanoxin)	0.8-2 ng/ml		SS 1 wk. Before next dose (Tr). At least 6 hr after last dose to allow for drug distribution in the body.
lidocaine (Xylocaine)	1.5-5		SS 7-12 hr. Anytime during IV infusion.
procainamide (Pronestyl)	4-10 mg/ml		SS 12-24 hr. Before next dose (Tr).
quinidine (various drugs)	3-6		SS 30 hr. Before next dose (Tr).
Respiratory Drugs			
theophylline (various drugs)	Asthma 10-20		SS 1-2 days in adults, up to 1 week in neonates. IV infusion, anytime; oral, before next dose (Tr).

**SS*, Time to reach drug steady state. The SS time is noted first, then the suggested appropriate time of blood sampling for the specific drug. *Tr*, Trough.

Appendix F

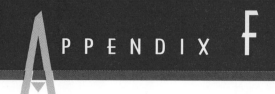

Additional Drug Product Information

Generic (Brand Name)	Drug Category	Indication	Usual Adult Dose	Comments
basiliximab (Simulect)	Immunosuppressant	Prophylaxis for organ rejection	20 mg IV before and after transplant	Used in combination with cyclosporine and corticosteroids.
becaplermin (Regranex Gel)	Topical	Diabetic foot ulcers	Apply daily.	See literature for dosage formula for application. This is a recombinant human platelet derived growth factor that enhances the formation of granulation tissue.
capecitabine (Xeloda)	Antineoplastic	Breast cancer, metastatic	2500 mg/m^2/day po in 2 divided doses for 2 weeks. Given on 3-week cycles	This is a prodrug that is converted to 5-fluorouracil (5-FU) in the body. SE/AR include nausea, vomiting, diarrhea, hand-foot syndrome, stomatitis, and cardiotoxicity.
cefdinir (Omnicef)	cephalosporin	Antibiotic	300 mg po bid	Used for acute bronchitis, sinusitis, tonsillitis, otitis media, pharyngitis, and uncomplicated skin infections.
citalopram (Celexa)	SSRI	Antidepressant	20-40 mg daily	Weak inhibitor of liver enzymes. SE/AR include nausea, dry mouth, sedation, insomnia, sweating, tremors, and diarrhea.
clopidogrel (Plavix)	Anti-platelet agent	Prevent MI and stroke in persons with atherosclerosis	75 mg daily	Drug is chemically similar to ticlopidine. Use with caution in patients at risk for bleeding.
dolasetron (Anzemet)	5-HT_3 antagonist	Antiemetic	100 mg po before chemotherapy (see insert for children's dose and postoperative dosing)	Use with caution in patients with cardiac conduction problems, hypokalemia, hypomagnesema, and patients taking diuretics.
eptifibatide (Integrilin)	Specific platelet inhibitor*	Acute coronary syndrome	N/A	Used to prevent complications of cardiac ischemia.
fenofibrate (Tricor)	Antihyperlipidemic	High triglycerides	67 mg/day	Used in conjunction with diet. DI: increases coumadin and cyclosporin serum levels: monitor closely
fenoldopam (Corlopam)	Vasodilator	Antihypertensive	IV infusion	Used for hypertensive emergency.
finasteride (Propecia)	Androgen inhibitor	Male pattern hair loss	1 mg daily	Finasteride is both Propecia (low dose) and Proscar (5 mg), which is used to treat benign prostatic hyperplasia. To assess effect in alopecia requires ≥3 months of therapy.
fomepizole (Antizol)	Antidote	Ethylene glycol poisoning	See current literature	Treatment blocks formation of toxic metabolites. Hemodialysis may also be necessary.

DI, Drug interactions; *SE/AR*, side effects/adverse reactions; *SSRI*, selective serotonin reuptake inhibitor; *po*, by mouth; *IV*, intravenously; *bid*, twice a day; *5-HT_3*, 5-hydroxytryptamine receptor antagonist; *N/A*, not available; *COMT*, catechol-O-methyl-transferase.
*platelet receptor (integrin), glycoprotein (GP) IIb-IIIa.

Generic (Brand Name)	***Drug Category***	***Indication***	***Usual Adult Dose***	***Comments***
interferon alfacon 1 (Infergon)	Recombinant interferon	Treatment of chronic hepatitis C virus	9 ug SC three times weekly	SE/AR: flu-like symptoms most common, depression also reported. Monitor triglyceride, thyroid, and blood.
ivermectin (Stromectol)	Anthelmintic	Treat of *Strongyloidiasis* and *Onchocerciasis* parasites	Dosed by body weight	Take with water. SE/AR: pruritus, rash, fatigue, tremors, anorexia.
lepirudin (Refludan)	Anticoagulant	Heparin-induced thrombocytopenia	Dosed by body weight	Directly inhibits thrombin. Monitor closely as there is no antidote if overdose or severe bleeding occurs. Follow guidelines as noted in insert.
montelukast (Singulair)	Leukotriene Antagonist	Asthma, prophylaxis	5-10 mg daily	This is not for acute asthma. May be used with bronchodilator inhaler.
Naratriptan (Amerge)	5-HT_1 agonist	Migraine	1-2.5 mg dose	Caution patients about possibility of photosensitivity (i.e., use sunscreen or protective clothing if exposed to ultraviolet or sunlight).
oprelvekin (Neumega)	Human interleukin 11	Prophylaxis for thrombocytopenia	SC: 50 ug/kg/daily	SE/AR: edema, headache, fever, rash, nausea, vomiting, dyspnea, rhinitis, tachycardia, dizziness, and insomnia.
raloxifene (Evista)	Selective estrogen receptor modifier	Prevent osteoporosis	60 mg daily	This drug does not reduce hot flashes. Advise patient to take calcium and vitamin D supplements if dietary intake is not sufficient.
rifapentine (Priftin)	Bactericidal	Pulmonary tuberculosis	600 mg po twice weekly	Advise patient that drug may cause red urine, sweat, sputum, and tears and may discolor contact lenses permanently. May affect oral contraceptives: use alternative methods.
rizatriptan (Maxalt)	Serotonin (5-HT_1) agonist	Migraine	5-10 mg dose	May be taken without water. Separate repeat doses by 2 hours; no more than 30. 30 mg in a 24 hour time period.
sodium hyaluronate (Hyalagan)	Hyaluronic acid derivative	Osteoarthritis of the knee	2 ml intraarticular in affected knee weekly	Product made from chicken/rooster, do not give to patients allergic to avian proteins and egg. Transient pain and swelling may occur. Avoid strenuous activity for 2 days after treatment.
thalidomide (Thalomid)	Immunomodulator	Leprosy	100-300 mg/day	Restricted drug to professionals in S.T.E.P.S. program. Before use, woman must have negative results on pregnancy tests. Has many warnings, side effects, etc., (see current literature).
tirofiban (Aggrastat)	Antiplatelet	Acute coronary syndrome	0.4 ug/kg IV for 30 minutes, then 0.1 mg/kg/min	SE/AR: bleeding, episodes. Monitor closely.
tizanidine (Zanaflex)	α_2-adrenergic Agonist	Central-acting skeletal muscle relaxant	8 mg po q 6-8 hours, max 3 doses in 24 hours	May lower blood pressure, monitor. SE/AR: sedation, weakness and dizziness.
tolcapone (Tasmar)	COMT Inhibitor	Antiparkinsonian	100-200 mg tid	Maximum daily dose is 600 mg per day. Warn patients about nausea and possibly an increase in dyskinesia or dystonia.
tolterodine (Detrol)	Antimuscarinic	Urinary frequency	1-2 mg bid	Highly protein bound with active metabolites. Use with caution in patients with liver impairment, GI obstruction, and narrow angle glaucoma.
trovafloxacin/ alatrofloxacin (Trovan I.V.)	Fluoroquinolone	Antibacterial	100-300 mg IV/po daily	po: contains Trovafloxacin, IV: contains alatrofloxacin DI: Dose at least 2 hours apart from antacids and sucralfate. Administer morphine IV at least 2 hours after oral dosage form and at least 4 hours later if oral is taken with food.
zolmitripatan (Zomig)	Serotonin 5-Ht_1 agonist	Migraine	$\leq$2.5mg-5mg	Use caution in patients with liver disease. Increase blood pressure reported in some patients.

Disorder Index

*See General Index for cross-reference.

D

E

Index

A

H

J

K

M

Q

T